Clinical Monitoring for *Anesthesia & Critical Care*

Clinical Monitoring for *Anesthesia & Critical Care*

Second Edition

CAROL L. LAKE, M.D.

Professor and Chair
Department of Anesthesiology
University of California, Davis
Sacramento, California

W.B. SAUNDERS COMPANY
A Division of Harcourt Brace & Company
Philadelphia London Toronto Montreal Sydney Tokyo

W.B. SAUNDERS COMPANY
A Division of
Harcourt Brace & Company

The Curtis Center
Independence Square West
Philadelphia, Pennsylvania 19106

Library of Congress Cataloging-in-Publication Data

Clinical monitoring for anesthesia and critical care / [edited by]
Carol L. Lake.—2nd ed.

p. cm.

Rev. ed. of: Clinical monitoring 1990.

Includes bibliographical references.

ISBN 0–7216–5269–7

1. Anesthesia. 2. Critical care medicine. 3. Patient monitoring.
I. Lake, Carol L. II. Clinical monitoring.

[DNLM: 1. Monitoring, Physiologic—methods. WB 142 C6415 1994]

RD82.C55 1994

616.07′5—dc20
DNLM/DLC 93–41600

CLINICAL MONITORING FOR ANESTHESIA AND CRITICAL CARE,
SECOND EDITION ISBN 0–7216–5269–7

Printed in the United States of America

Last digit is the print number: 9 8 7 6 5 4 3 2 1

Contributors

JEROME H. ABRAMS, M.D., F.A.C.S.
Associate Professor, Department of Surgery, University of Minnesota Medical School—Minneapolis; Staff Surgeon, University of Minnesota Hospital and Clinic and Veterans Affairs Medical Center; Associate Director, Surgical Critical Care, University of Minnesota Hospital and Clinic, Minneapolis, Minnesota.
Patient Data Management Systems

WILLIAM P. ARNOLD III, M.D.
Associate Professor of Anesthesiology, University of Virginia, School of Medicine; Anesthesiologist, University of Virginia Hospital and Virginia Ambulatory Surgery Center, Charlottesville, Virginia.
Perioperative Biochemical Monitors

JOHN L. ATLEE, III, M.D.
Professor of Anesthesiology, Medical College of Wisconsin; John L. Doyne Hospital, Department of Anesthesiology, Milwaukee, Wisconsin.
Electrocardiography: Monitoring for Arrhythmias

STEVEN J. BARKER, Ph.D., M.D.
Professor and Chair, Department of Anesthesiology, University of California, Irvine, College of Medicine, Irvine; Chairman, Department of Anesthesiology, University of California, Irvine, Medical Center (Orange), Orange, California.
Monitoring of Oxygen

FRANK E. BLOCK, JR., M.D.
Associate Professor of Anesthesiology, University of Arkansas for Medical Sciences, Little Rock, Arkansas.
Human Factors and Alarms

HOWARD R. BROMLEY, M.D.
Associate Professor of Anesthesiology, Critical Care and Pain Management; Consulting Staff, Medical University of South Carolina College of Medicine; Chief, Anesthesiology Service, Veterans Affairs Medical Center; Consulting Staff, Charleston Memorial Hospital, Charleston, South Carolina.
Metabolic Monitoring

F. CLEMENTS, M.D.
Associate Professor of Anesthesiology and Assistant Professor of Internal Medicine, Department of Anesthesiology, Division of Cardiac Anesthesia, Duke University Medical Center, Durham, North Carolina.
Electrocardiography: Monitoring for Ischemia

D. RYAN COOK, M.D.
Professor of Anesthesiology, University of Pittsburgh School of Medicine; Director of Anesthesiology, Children's Hospital of Pittsburgh, Pittsburgh, Pennsylvania.
Monitoring Peripheral Nervous System Function

ROBERT W. COOK, B.A., R.R.T., R.C.P.
Technical Director, Respiratory Therapy Department, Medical University of South Carolina College of Medicine, Charleston, South Carolina.
Metabolic Monitoring

N. DEBRUIJN, M.D.
Associate Professor of Anesthesiology and Assistant Professor of Surgery and of Internal Medicine, Department of Cardiac Anesthesia, Duke University Medical Center, Durham, North Carolina.
Electrocardiography: Monitoring for Ischemia

VEDRAN DELETIS, M.D., Ph.D.
Research Assistant Professor, Department of Anesthesiology, New York University School of Medicine, New York, New York.
Evoked Potentials

CHARLES G. DURBIN, JR., M.D., FCCM
Professor of Anesthesiology and Surgery, University of Virginia School of Medicine; Director, Surgical Intensive Care Unit and

Department of Respiratory Care, University of Virginia Health Science Center, Charlottesville, Virginia.
Arterial Blood Gas Analysis

JAN EHRENWERTH, M.D.
Professor, Department of Anesthesiology, Yale University School of Medicine; Attending Anesthesiologist, Yale-New Haven Hospital, New Haven, Connecticut.
Electrical Safety

THOMAS J. GAL, M.D.
Professor of Anesthesiology, University of Virginia School of Medicine; Attending Anesthesiologist, University of Virginia Health Sciences Center, Charlottesville, Virginia.
Monitoring the Respiratory System

PATRICIA M. GRAMLING-BABB, M.D.
Assistant Professor of Anesthesiology, Medical University of South Carolina College of Medicine; Co-Director, Pain Clinic, Veterans Administration Medical Center, Charleston, South Carolina.
Metabolic Monitoring

STEVEN C. HALL, M.D.
Associate Professor, Department of Anesthesia, Northwestern University Medical School; Arthur C. King Professor of Pediatric Anesthesia and Anesthesiologist-in-Chief, Children's Memorial Hospital, Chicago, Illinois.
Monitoring in Radiology

BERNICE R. HECKER, M.D.
Attending Anesthesiologist, Virginia Mason Medical Center; Clinical Assistant Professor of Anesthesiology, University of Washington School of Medicine, Seattle, Washington.
Monitoring Anesthetic Gases

ZAK HILLEL, M.D., Ph.D.
Associate Professor, Department of Anesthesiology, Columbia University College of Physicians and Surgeons; Director of Cardiothoracic Anesthesia, St. Luke's-Roosevelt Hospital Center, New York, New York.
Perioperative Echocardiography

JOHN W. HOYT, M.D., FCCM
Clinical Professor of Anesthesiology/Critical Care Medicine, University of Pittsburgh School of Medicine; Chairman, Department of Critical Care Medicine, St. Francis Medical Center, Pittsburgh, Pennsylvania.
Patient Data Management Systems

GAVIN N. C. KENNY, B.Sc. (Hons.), M.B., Ch.B., M.D., FRCA
Department of Anaesthesia, Glasgow Royal Infirmary, Glasgow, Scotland.
Computers in Monitoring

KEITH D. KNOPES, M.D.
Department of Anesthesiology, Virginia Mason Hospital, Seattle, Washington.
Monitoring Anesthetic Gases

STEVEN KONSTADT, M.D.
Associate Professor of Anesthesiology, Department of Anesthesiology, Mount Sinai School of Medicine of the City University of New York; Co-Director, Division of Cardiothoracic Anesthesiology, The Mount Sinai Hospital, New York, New York.
Perioperative Echocardiography

STUART C. LAW, M.D.
Chief of Cardiac Anesthesia, Western Pennsylvania Hospital, Pittsburgh, Pennsylvania.
Monitoring Peripheral Nervous System Function

WARREN J. LEVY, M.D.
Associate Professor of Anesthesia, University of Pennsylvania School of Medicine; Philadelphia, Pennsylvania.
Electroencephalography

ROBERT G. LOEB, M.D.
Assistant Professor of Anesthesiology, University of California, Davis; Attending Physician and Director of Ambulatory Surgery, University of California, Davis, Medical Center (Sacramento), Sacramento, California.
Intravascular Pressure Monitoring Systems

WAYNE K. MARSHALL, M.D.
Associate Professor, Department of Anesthesia, Pennsylvania State University College of Medicine, Hershey; Milton S. Hershey Medical Center, Hershey, Pennsylvania.
Monitoring of Intracranial Pressure

ROGER A. MOORE, M.D.
Associate Professor, University of Pennsylvania School of Medicine, Philadelphia, Pennsylvania; Chairman, Anesthesiology, Deborah Heart and Lung Center, Browns Mills, New Jersey.
Monitoring Hemostasis

ALAN W. MURRAY, M.B., Ch.B., FRCA
Department of Anaesthesia, Glasgow Royal Infirmary, Glasgow, Scotland.
Computers in Monitoring

ERIC PERSILY, M.D.
Instructor in Anesthesia, West Virginia University School of Medicine; Charleston Area Medical Center, Morgantown, West Virginia.
Specialized Neurophysiologic Monitoring

THERESA PIURKOWSKY, M.Ed., R.R.T., C.P.F.T., R.C.P.
Department Head, Allied Health/Rehabilitative Services at Trident Technical College; Clinical Faculty, Respiratory Therapy, HCA Trident Regional Medical Center, Veterans Affairs Medical Center, Medical University Hospital, Roper Hospital, Charleston Memorial Hospital, and St. Francis Xavier Hospital, Charleston, South Carolina.
Metabolic Monitoring

WILLIAM T. ROSS, JR., M.D.
Professor of Anesthesiology, University of Virginia School of Medicine; Professor of Anesthesiology and Medical Director, Ambulatory Surgery Center, University of Virginia Health Sciences Center, Charlottesville, Virginia.
Monitoring the Anesthesia Machine

JEFFREY J. SCHWARTZ, M.D.
Assistant Professor, Department of Anesthesiology, Yale University School of Medicine; Attending Anesthesiologist, Yale-New Haven Hospital, New Haven, Connecticut.
Electrical Safety

KAREN J. SCHWENZER, M.D.
Assistant Professor of Anesthesiology, University of Virginia School of Medicine; Associate Director, Surgical Intensive Care Unit, University of Virginia Health Sciences Center, Charlottesville, Virginia.
Venous and Pulmonary Pressures

DAVID S. SMITH, M.D., Ph.D.
Associate Professor, Department of Anesthesia, University of Pennsylvania School of Medicine; Director, Division of Neuroanesthesia, Hospital of the University of Pennsylvania, Philadelphia, Pennsylvania
Specialized Neurophysiologic Monitoring

M. STAFFORD SMITH, M.D., C.M, F.R.C.P.(C)
Fellow in Cardiac Anesthesia, Department of Anesthesiology, Division of Cardiac Anesthesia, Duke University Medical Center, Durham, North Carolina.
Electrocardiography: Monitoring for Ischemia

DANIEL M. THYS, M.D.
Professor, Department of Anesthesiology, Columbia University College of Physicians and Surgeons; Director, Department of Anesthesiology, St. Luke's-Roosevelt Hospital Center, New York, New York.
Perioperative Echocardiography

KEVIN K. TREMPER, Ph.D., M.D.
Professor and Chair, Department of Anesthesiology, University of Michigan Medical School; Chairman, Department of Anesthesiology, The University of Michigan Hospitals, Ann Arbor, Michigan.
Monitoring of Oxygen

ANDREW M. WOODS, M.D.
Associate Professor of Anesthesiology, University of Virginia Health Sciences Center; Medical Director, Postanesthesia Care Unit and Surgical Admissions, University of Virginia Health Sciences Center, Charlottesville, Virginia.
Maternal and Fetal Monitoring

Preface

Monitoring, defined as continuous or repeated observation and vigilance, is an essential component of anesthesia and critical care practice. More than 50% of critical incidents occurring during anesthesia result from inadequate or incomplete monitoring of the patient, the anesthesia machine, or the patient-machine interface. Two major causes of anesthesia-related injuries are equipment failure and human error.

The first reason for monitoring is patient safety—by reducing preventable patient injury through positive identification of all physiologic parameters during cardiac procedures, neurosurgical procedures, and other complicated procedures, including postoperative critical care.

The second reason for monitoring is objective evaluation of the individual anesthesiologist or intensive care specialist's performance. Nevertheless, no electronic device can replace the totally aware physician or nurse who is looking, listening, and sensing significant changes in the anesthetized or critically ill patient.

The second edition of *Clinical Monitoring for Anesthesia and Critical Care* describes both invasive and noninvasive devices as well as automated and nonautomated monitoring methods for all types of anesthetized and critically ill patients. The approach to monitoring in this book is through the role of monitoring as a subspecialty of anesthesiology.

This book is intended for attending anesthesiologists with broad and general interests in clinical practice or with specific interests in monitoring of patients' receiving cardiac anesthesia, neuroanesthesia, obstetric anesthesia, and intensive care. It is also intended for residents and fellows in anesthesiology as well as for nurse anesthetists.

As with the first edition, the intended goal of the second edition is to provide complete, authoritative information without the bias or the inclusion of the monitoring methods as utilized in or applicable to research-oriented institutions only.

Acknowledgments

The inspiration and support for writing and editing this text have come from many people. The editor extends sincere thanks to the many contributors who gave of their time, experience, and expertise in the writing of the individual chapters in this text. A special debt of gratitude is owed to the families, friends, and colleagues of these contributors for their share in the hard work that made this text a reality.

Special thanks are due to Avé McCracken, Senior Medical Editor at W.B. Saunders Company, whose diligence resulted in the timely publication of this second edition. Finally, I am most grateful to my former colleagues at the University of Virginia for their encouragement, guidance, and assistance in the preparation of the manuscript.

Contents

SECTION ONE

Principles of Monitoring

CHAPTER 1

Monitoring: History and Philosophy

CAROL L. LAKE, M.D.

In perioperative patient care, monitoring can be defined as continuous or repeated observation and vigilance.[1] The best monitor is the totally aware anesthesiologist who is looking, listening, and sensing significant changes in the patient. No electronic device can (or should, given the number of false alarms) replace this function. Most of the anesthesiologist's time (59.1%) is spent in direct (44.8%) or indirect (via monitors—14.3%) monitoring; record-keeping is a distant second at 10.9%.[2] A high level of vigilance among anesthesiologists has been documented[3] but varies inversely with workload.[4]

The goal of monitoring is to identify trends and to prevent untoward events. Repeated observations must be performed frequently, intermittently, semi-continuously, or continuously to record trends. Machines make repetitive measurements at frequencies impossible for humans. The value of any specific monitor in the achievement of this goal is how likely a change in a particular monitored variable predicts poor outcome or contributes directly to it. Adequate warning time to change conditions and alter outcome is implicit in the definition of monitoring. For these reasons, use of a variable to establish a diagnosis is not monitoring. An example is the placement of an intra-arterial catheter in a critically ill patient. The direct measurement of arterial pressure allows identification of hypotension while there is time to reverse it rather than making the diagnosis of hypertension as blood pressure determination does in a outpatient. Another example is the oxygen analyzer which detects a condition of reduced oxygen delivery but fails to pinpoint the source of the problem. Although this monitor functions well to prevent injury, correct action (increased oxygen delivery) must be taken to assure a good outcome.[5]

The importance of perioperative monitoring in the past decade has been increasingly promulgated by the founding of the Society for Technology in Anesthesia, the emphasis on patient safety by the Anesthesia Patient Safety Foundation, the publication of the *Journal of Clinical Monitoring,* societal pressure for Continuous Quality Improvement, and the demonstration of reduced mortality with oximetry and capnometry in the Anesthesia Closed Claims Study.[6] Resident training and anesthesiologist performance evaluation are likely to rely heavily on the use of anesthesia simulators.[7] The developing practice guidelines in many aspects of anesthesia and critical care practice rely heavily on monitoring technologies.[8] Thus, the efficacy, risk, and benefit of a monitored variable must be carefully assessed as practice guidelines are formulated.

HISTORY OF MONITORING

The monitoring technology of the twentieth century is best appreciated in the light of history. Most of the early historical observations centered on the physiology of the circulatory, respiratory, and central nervous systems. The need to monitor equipment functions (e.g., analysis of inspired/expired gas content and volume) is a more recent development.

PULSE

Herophilus, around 300 B.C., used a water clock for counting the pulse, on which he placed considerable importance as an index of health or disease.[9] Galen also detailed the role of the pulse as a predictive variable.[9] Changes in the pulse volume such as pulsus paradoxus and pulsus alternans were described in 1873 and 1892, respectively.[10]

STETHOSCOPY

Clinical observations were restricted to external observations, palpation, percussion, or postmortem examination until Laënnec's development of the stethoscope in 1816.[10] It permitted judgment on the patient's internal conditions, specifically position of organs, presence of fluid, and location of lesions. Laënnec's original stethoscope was a wooden tube, 9 inches long and 1.5 inches in diameter. Piorry improved the monaural stethoscope, introduced the trumpet chestpiece, and improved the earpieces. The binaural stethoscope was developed by Cammann in 1852. Microphonic amplification stethoscopy was used in 1878.[11] In 1909, Sprague invented the combined stethoscope with both bell and diaphragm chestpieces. Use of the precordial stethoscope in the operating room is attributed to Cushing.[12]

BLOOD PRESSURE

The first person to measure or monitor a physiologic function was Stephen Hale, who directly measured the blood pressure of a horse in 1733. Hale inserted a brass pipe into the crural artery; attached to the pipe was a 9-foot length of glass tubing. Release of an arterial ligature allowed blood to rise in the tube to a distance of 8 feet 3 inches above the heart. Hale also noted that the blood in the tube rose and fell different amounts with each pulse; greater excursions of 12–14 inches alternated with lesser changes. During hemorrhage of the animal, Hale noted that the amount of blood loss failed to correlate with the decrease in pressure. However, it was more than 150 years later before the importance of measuring blood pressure was appreciated.

Sphygmomanometry

Over the years, attempts were made to measure blood pressure either by direct cannulation or with a sphygmograph. One of the links between direct arterial measurement and noninvasive methods was made by Poiseuille in 1828 when he used a U-shaped tube containing mercury (which counterbalanced the pressure of the blood) to replace the long glass tube into which blood flowed from a cannulated artery. Herisson invented an instrument that showed the pulse in a column of mercury, thus obviating the need for intra-arterial measurement of blood pressure. This instrument was later combined with a kymographion (a pen-and-drum recorder), creating the sphygmograph. The sphygmograph consisted of a series of levers that could be loaded until arterial pulsations were abolished. The levers also recorded the movements that the pulse imparted and measured the force necessary to impede the arterial pulse completely.

Basch in 1881 modified the sphygmograph by using a rubber ball, which communicated with a mercury manometer, to compress the artery. However, Basch's instrument was inaccurate. Riva Rocci stressed the importance of monitoring blood pressure and its variation. In his sphygmomanometer, blood pressure equalled the pressure in the inflated cuff, compressing the arm at the point where the pulse was felt during cuff deflation. Riva Rocci described the stress produced by the pressure on the arterial wall in 1896 in *A New Sphygmomanometer.* His sphygmomanometer was intended for rapidly repeatable measurement of radial artery pressure. However, in 1905 Korotkoff, using the stethoscope to monitor the pulse, discovered that the pulse sounds disappeared as cuff pressure declined, at the point roughly corresponding to ventricular diastole, the diastolic pressure.[13]

Intraoperative Blood Pressure Measurement

Intraoperative recording of blood pressure was introduced by Cushing, who recognized its value to indicate physiologic condition.[14] Crile also advocated blood pressure monitoring with the Gärtner tonometer, but neither his nor Cushing's recommendation for routine use of blood pressure measurement during surgery was widely accepted in the first decade of the twentieth century. However, by the time of publication of Gwathmey's book, *Anesthesia,* in 1914, a section on the intraoperative monitoring of blood pressure by McKeson was included.[15] Rovenstine in 1934 promoted systematic data collection for statistical purposes in anesthesia.[16] Collected observations of blood pressure, pulse, and respiration became the first anesthesia records.[17]

INTRAVASCULAR PRESSURES

Intracardiac pressures were measured in 1928 by Wiggers using a glass, fluid-filled cannula that could be directly introduced into the heart. One end of the cannula was covered by a distensible rubber membrane with a mirror attached to it.[18] The oscillations of the mirror were recorded by a reflected beam of light on a photographic plate. A thistle-shaped glass vessel, called a cardiometer, placed over the ventricle and connected to a piston recorder, was used to determine volume changes in animal hearts.

Both direct and indirect methods were employed to measure venous pressure. The indirect method was the amount of external pressure required to collapse a small superficial vein or the pressure that prevented its refill. Venous pressure was measured directly by insertion of a needle connected by a rubber tube to a manometer into the median basilic vein. Pressure changes in the central venous system were measured in the jugular vein by placing a small metal cup over the vein and connecting it to a Marey tambour. Refinements in the measurement of pressure and flow in the heart were made by Cournand and Richards in the early 1940s.[13] In addition to percutaneous intra-arterial cannulation introduced in the 1960s, the right-heart flotation catheter of Swan and Ganz, developed in 1970, was a twentieth-century milestone in circulatory monitors.

ELECTROCARDIOGRAPHY

The electrocardiogram (ECG) was first described by Einthoven.[19] In the Einthoven galvanometer, a fine silvered glass fiber was suspended in an electromagnet. Minute oscillations occurred when current passed through the fiber.

The shadow of the oscillating fiber was magnified and projected on a photographic plate. Adjustment of the tension of the fiber allowed a potential difference of 1V between the two ends of the fiber to cause a 1-cm deflection. Intracavitary electrograms using saline-filled catheters were described in 1949.[20] The development of closed chest cardiac resuscitation and defibrillation in the 1960s increased the need for continuous monitoring of the ECG in the operating room or critical care unit.

CARDIAC OUTPUT

The Fick principle to measure cardiac output was theorized in 1870 but was not in common use until the 1930s.[21] Collection of mixed venous blood from humans was difficult. The Fick principle forms the basis for dye dilution and thermodilution cardiac output determinations in modern times.

ECHOCARDIOGRAPHY

The Doppler principle, that transmitted sound will reflect from a moving object and return to the point of transmission at a frequency shift relative to the velocity and direction of the moving object, was described in 1842. Devices based on the Doppler principle were initially used in monitoring arterial pulse and blood pressure in the early 1970s. Its application in transesophageal echocardiography, however, did not occur until 1976, when Frazin first introduced M-mode technology.[22]

THERMOMETRY

Although the importance of body temperature was recognized by Hippocrates, the first thermometer was probably constructed by Galileo in 1592. However, his thermometer had no measurement scale, was influenced by atmospheric pressure, and gave only gross indications of temperature alteration.[13] Essential steps toward clinical measurements came with the development of fixed temperature scales by Christian Huygens (Centigrade scale) and Gabriel Fahrenheit (Fahrenheit scale).[11] Boerhaave introduced the thermometer to clinical practice in the seventeenth and eighteenth centuries, but it did not become an integral part of medical monitoring until the nineteenth century with the publication of Carl Wunderlich's *The Temperature in Diseases* in 1868.[11, 13] Early thermometry was complex and cumbersome, which precluded its acceptance even though its significance was apparent. The present-day clinical thermometer was designed in 1870 by Albutt.[13]

RESPIRATORY MONITORS

Hutchinson, in his monograph *On the Capacity of the Lungs, and on the Respiratory Functions, with a View of Establishing a Precise and Easy Method of Detecting Disease by the Spirometer,* defined five variables for measurement of respiratory performance. These were vital capacity (quantity expelled during greatest exhalation after deepest inspiration), residual air (amount of air remaining in lungs after deepest breathing), reserve air (amount of air left after gentle expiration), complemental air (amount beyond normal inspiration by deep breathing), and breathing air (normal inspiration and expiration).[11] Hutchinson's spirometer did not require skilled interpretation, and he verified the association between pulmonary disease and alterations in spirometric variables.[9]

The principle of pulse oximetry was recognized in the 1930s, and infrared absorbance detection of carbon dioxide was described in 1952.[23] Mass spectrometry became available in the 1970s, but its expense and susceptibility to malfunction precluded its widespread acceptance until smaller, more reliable, multiplexed devices became available in the 1980s.

LABORATORY MEDICINE

Evaluation of the appearance and chemical properties of the blood and urine initially was done in the late eighteenth century to diagnose chronic conditions such as diabetes and renal disease. Electrodes for the measurement of partial pressures of oxygen and carbon dioxide in the blood were developed by Clark and Severinghaus in the 1950s.[24, 25] Frequent, intraoperative measurements of blood glucose, hematocrit, electrolytes, and arterial gases are a development of the past two decades. The importance of laboratory evaluation was demonstrated by the development of "ward labs," a precursor of the present-day "stat lab."

PHILOSOPHY OF MONITORING

More than 50% of the critical incidents occurring during anesthesia result from inadequate or incomplete monitoring of the patient, the anesthesia machine, or the patient-machine interface. Equipment failure is one of the recurring causes of anesthesia-related injuries.[26] Problems with ECG, blood pressure monitors, or other monitoring devices; disconnections or incorrect connections in breathing circuits; and incorrect types or flows of gases or vapors are frequent causes of critical perioperative incidents. Although the monitoring device itself may be the source of the incident, failure to use an adequate array of monitors, inadequate recognition of the changes displayed, and failure to respond to a undesirable monitored event constitute most anesthetic management problems.

Human error continues to play a major role in anesthetic mishaps.[27] In this regard, inexperience and exchange of personnel are critical factors. Either the relief of one person by another or the return of the primary caretaker may permit detection and control of untoward events.[27] (See Chapter 2.)

However, the proliferation of new monitors and safety features often has occurred without regard to the ability of humans to assimilate the additional information. There is a need to limit the complexity of control and information displays (i.e., to increase their manageability or make them more "user friendly") so that adverse outcomes are prevented, not caused.[28]

The vast array of monitors currently available for use in the perioperative period allows the anesthesiologist or critical care physician greater access to variables measured by machines but may actually reduce the amount of direct personal observation of the patient. The British anesthetist Pask suggested in 1965 "that the best patient-monitoring device would be a tube of contact adhesive: Place a small dab of it over the patient's temporal artery, another small dab on one of the anaesthetist's fingers and bring these two into contact so that they could not be readily separated."[29] Although times have changed, there is still much truth in these words.

REASONS FOR MONITORING

Two of the major reasons promulgated for perioperative monitoring are physiologic monitoring and patient safety. Physiologic monitoring includes the ECG and devices that monitor intravascular pressures, intracranial pressure, neuromuscular function, cardiac output or ventricular function, and biochemical variables. Patient safety monitors include breathing circuit oxygen analyzers and breathing circuit disconnect alarms. Other such monitors of the anesthesia delivery system are included as well as devices such as capnographs or pulse oximeters, which monitor the patient-anesthesia machine interface. Whitcher and colleagues suggest that a minimally acceptable monitoring configuration should permit positive identification of all major pathways of patient injury.[30] They further suggest that the expected savings in the prevention of injuries outweighs the costs of sophisticated monitors.[30] The emphasis is on *preventable* injuries such as disconnection of the anesthetic circuit, esophageal intubation, hyperthermia, and the like.

ESSENTIAL MONITORING

Establishment of minimal monitoring standards has been difficult, although the goals of such standards are clear. Monitors may be essential for the conduct of the anesthetic (e.g., respirometers, oxygen analyzers, breathing circuit alarms, volatile anesthetic vapor analysis), for the conduct of perioperative care for a specific procedure (pulmonary artery and intra-arterial catheters, intracranial cannulas), or for general perioperative management (blood pressure, pulse, ECG, temperature measurement, pulse oximetry, capnography).[31]

Eichhorn and associates suggest that standards for monitoring codify accepted practices, provide the means for objective evaluation of individual practice, reduce patient injury from anesthesia accidents, and apply collective experience to rare events (occurring one or two times in the career of an individual anesthesia practitioner).[32] The essential monitors proposed by Whitcher and coworkers in 1988 were automatic sphygmomanometer, pulse oximeter, capnograph, spirometer, halometer, breathing circuit oxygen analyzer, stethoscope, electrocardiograph, and thermometer.[30] Most essential monitors provide continuous, as opposed to intermittent, information. The value of these devices to prevent or limit mishaps is detailed in Figure 1–1. However, the use of monitors must be realistic and easily attainable for the average practitioner. Cost-benefit ratios must be considered in detailing standards. However, the cost of maintenance and disposable components, which is not always considered in the cost-benefit ratio, must also be included.

Others have suggested different values for the monitors proposed by Whitcher and colleagues for the detection of various critical events and have recommended different essential arrays (Fig. 1–2).[28, 30, 33] Block suggests that the essential monitors are pulse oximeter, capnograph with waveform display, autosphygmomanometer, electrocardiogram, thermometer, electroencephalogram, transcutaneous oxygen and carbon dioxide tension, and neuromuscular function monitor.[33]

Philip and Raemer noted other factors—such as predictability (freedom from aberrant output or malfunction), specificity (few false-positive results), sensitivity (few false-negative results), simplicity of use, distraction of caregiver, cost, and availability—that must be considered when recommendations for equipment or guidelines for monitoring are regarded as standards. The optimal monitoring array must be effective, noninvasive, manageable, and economical.[28]

An automated anesthesia record also has been suggested as an essential "monitor."[31] This suggestion results from the diagnostic information derived from trend plots, which form patterns of great clinical importance (see Chapter 21).

Monitoring Standards

Standards for the monitoring of patients during anesthesia have been developed worldwide, including those of the Association of Anaesthetists of Great Britain, the French Society of Anesthesia, the Faculty of Anaesthetists Royal Australasian College of Surgeons, the Belgian Society of Anesthesia and Reanimation, and the Scandinavian Society of Anaesthesiologists, among others.[34–36] Standards of practice for minimal monitoring accepted by the Harvard Department of Anesthesia in 1985 are presented in Table 1–1. The House of Delegates of the American Society of Anesthesiologists accepted on October 21, 1986 a set of standards for basic intraoperative monitoring, which are similar in content to the Harvard standards. These standards were amended in 1992 to strongly encourage the use of capnometry (Table 1–2). These documents affirm the need to monitor oxygenation, respiration, circulation, and temperature in either a continual ("repeated regularly and frequently in steady succession") or continuous ("prolonged without interruption at any time") manner. However, the

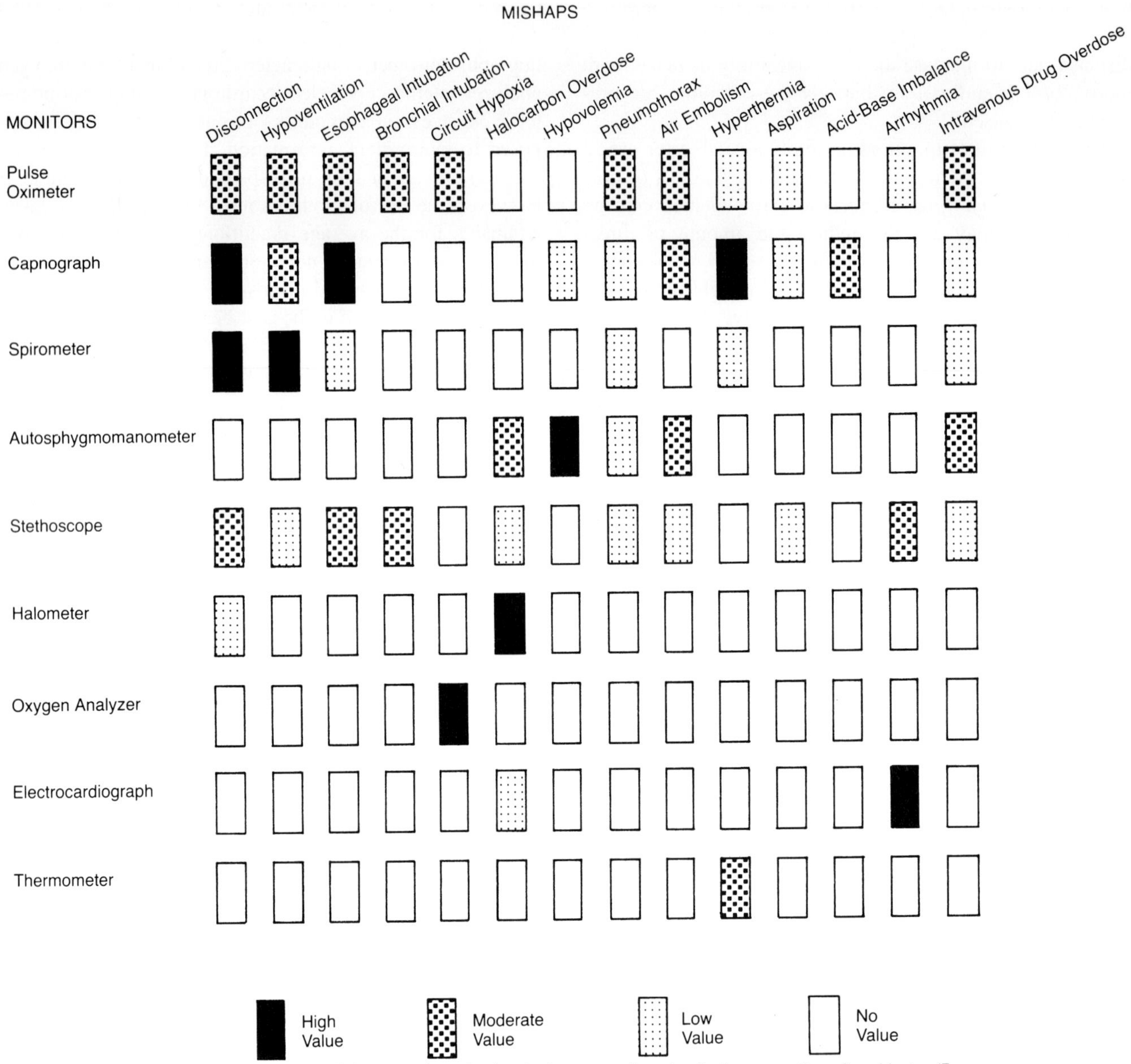

Figure 1–1. A matrix of the type of monitoring device versus its value in the prevention of accidents. (From Whitcher C, et al: Anesthetic mishaps and the cost of monitoring: A proposed standard for monitoring equipment. J Clin Monit 1988; 4:11. With permission.)

inability to utilize such monitoring at all times and in all patients is recognized. In fact, the "essential nature" of any given monitor may be confirmed by the unwillingness of the anesthetic caregiver to proceed in its absence. Finally, no matter how valuable, the acceptance of any particular monitor as a standard of care in the legal sense is always controversial.

ESSENTIAL NONINVASIVE MONITORING FUNCTIONS

Monitoring devices also can be classified as invasive, minimally invasive, or noninvasive, with some overlap of functions such as the use of an invasive pulmonary artery catheter to measure thermodilution cardiac output.

INSPECTION

Very little monitoring in perioperative patient care is by inspection only. However, the color of the skin, blood, mucous membranes, and conjunctiva can be noted easily and provide important information about perfusion, oxygenation, and hematocrit. Pupillary reflexes, pupil size, eye movement, and presence or absence of tearing provide information about depth of anesthesia. Inspection of the nose is necessary if nasal tubes of any type are present. The chest is routinely and frequently inspected to assure ade-

	Mishap																								
Monitor	Disconnection	Hypoventilation	Esophageal Intubation	Bronchial Intubation	Circuit Hypoxia	Halocarbon Overdose	Hypovolemia	Pneumothorax	Air Embolism	Hyperthermia	Aspiration	Acid Base Imbalance	Arrhythmia	Intravenous Drug Overdose	Hypotension	Hypoxia	Cerebral Ischemia	Airway Obstruction	Circuit Valve Malfunction	Anesthetic Agent Error	Pulmonary Edema	Inadequate Cardiac Output	Inadequate Peripheral Perfusion	Residual Neuromuscular Blockade	Hypothermia
Pulse Oximeter	1	2	1	1	1	1	1	1	1	1	1	0	2	1	2	3	0	1	1	0	2	3	3	0	0
Capnograph	3	3	3	2	0	0	2	2	2	3	1	2	0	1	2	1	0	3	3	0	1	2	1	2	2
Spirometer	3	3	1	0	0	0	0	1	0	1	0	0	0	1	0	0	0	3	2	0	1	0	0	1	0
Autosphygmomanometer	0	0	0	0	0	2	2	1	1	0	0	0	0	2	3	0	0	0	0	0	1	2	2	0	0
Stethoscope	2	1	2	2	0	1	0	1	1	0	1	0	1	0	1	0	0	2	0	0	2	1	0	0	0
Halometer	1	0	0	0	0	3	0	0	0	0	0	0	0	0	0	0	0	1	0	1	0	0	0	0	0
Oxygen Analyzer	1	0	0	0	3	0	0	0	0	1	0	0	0	0	0	0	0	0	0	0	0	0	0	0	0
Electrocardiograph	0	0	0	0	0	1	0	0	0	2	0	0	3	0	0	1	0	0	0	0	1	0	0	0	0
Thermometer	0	0	0	0	0	0	0	0	0	1	0	0	0	0	0	0	0	0	0	0	0	0	0	0	3
Electroencephalograph	0	1	0	0	1	3	1	0	2	0	0	2	0	3	2	3	3	0	0	1	0	3	3	0	1
Evoked Potentials	0	0	0	0	0	2	1	0	1	0	0	1	0	0	2	2	2	0	0	1	0	2	1	0	1
Airway Pressure	3	1	1	2	0	0	0	2	1	0	1	0	0	0	0	0	0	3	1	0	2	0	0	0	0
Agent-specific Halometer	1	0	0	0	0	3	0	0	0	0	0	0	0	0	0	0	0	1	0	3	0	0	0	0	0
Nitrogen Analyzer	1	0	0	0	1	0	0	0	3	0	0	0	0	0	0	0	0	0	0	0	0	0	0	0	0
Cardiac Output	0	0	0	0	0	2	2	1	2	0	0	0	1	2	2	1	0	0	0	1	2	3	2	0	1
Two-Dimensional Echocardiograph	0	0	0	0	0	2	3	0	3	0	0	0	2	2	1	0	0	0	0	1	1	2	1	0	0
Continuous Blood Pressure	0	0	0	0	0	2	3	1	2	0	0	0	0	2	3	0	0	0	0	0	1	2	2	0	1
Pulse Plethysmograph	0	0	0	0	0	2	3	2	2	0	0	0	2	2	2	0	0	0	0	0	2	3	3	0	2
Transcutaneous Po_2	1	1	1	3	2	1	2	3	2	1	3	1	0	1	2	3	0	1	1	0	3	3	3	0	1
Transcutaneous Pco_2	1	3	1	1	1	1	2	1	2	3	1	2	0	0	2	2	0	1	1	0	2	1	1	0	0
Neuromuscular Twitch	0	0	0	0	0	0	0	0	0	0	0	0	0	0	0	0	0	0	0	0	0	0	0	3	0

Figure 1–2. Capability of different monitors to detect critical events during administration of anesthesia. 3 = high value, 2 = moderate value, 1 = low value, and 0 = no value. (From Block FE: A proposed standard for monitoring equipment: What equipment should be included? J Clin Monit 1988; 4:1–4. With permission.)

quate, symmetric motion without retraction. Abdominal contraction should be absent if respiration is unobstructed and depth of anesthesia is adequate.

However, monitoring of equipment requires considerable inspection. The gas supply, flowmeters, pressure gauges, inspiratory and expiratory valves, cables to pressure transducers, ECG, electroencephalograph (EEG), oximeter, and automated blood pressure cuff all must be inspected to ensure continuity and function.

Positioning of the patient during surgery also requires careful inspection to avoid pressure on superficial nerves, venous congestion, or arterial occlusion.[37] Airways and endotracheal tubes should be taped to avoid compression of the lip or tongue between teeth, endotracheal tube, or oropharyngeal airway. The ears should be flat against the head, without kinking or compression.[37] Neither excessive flexion nor extension of the neck should be permitted. Excessive flexion may cause the endotracheal tube to compress the recurrent laryngeal nerve, resulting in vocal cord paralysis. Neck extension or rotation can limit cerebral arterial blood flow, particularly in elderly patients with extracranial occlusive disease. Postoperative neck pain occurs after excessive extension in patients with cervical arthritis. The extremities should be inspected to prevent dependent edema, neural compression, arterial insufficiency, or malfunction of intravascular catheters (infiltration, extravasation, or arterial occlusion).

PALPATION

Palpation of the arterial pulse for heart rate, volume, cardiac rhythm, and determination of blood pressure are simple, readily learned monitoring tasks. The position of the endotracheal tube cuff frequently can be verified by laryngeal palpation. Laryngeal motion, also detected by palpation, occurs in the anesthetized patient with incomplete neuromuscular blockade. Symmetry of respiratory excursion can be documented by palpation. Palpation easily reveals gastric or bladder distention, allowing drainage to be performed before gastric aspiration or the hemodynamic sequelae of a distended bladder occur. Palpation of the

TABLE 1–1. HARVARD MEDICAL SCHOOL STANDARDS FOR ANESTHESIA MONITORING PRACTICE

These standards apply for any administration of anesthesia involving department of anesthesia personnel and are specifically referable to preplanned anesthetics administered in designated anesthetizing locations (specific exclusion: administration of epidural analgesia for labor or pain management). In emergency circumstances in any location, immediate life support measures of whatever appropriate nature come first with attention turning to the measures described in these standards as soon as possible and practical. These are minimal standards that may be exceeded at any time based on the judgment of the involved anesthesia personnel. These standards encourage high-quality patient care, but observing them cannot guarantee any specific patient outcome. These standards are subject to revision from time to time, as warranted by the evolution of technology and practice.

Anesthesiologist's or Nurse Anesthetist's Presence in Operating Room

For all anesthetics initiated by or involving a member of the department of anesthesia, an attending or resident anesthesiologist or nurse anesthetist shall be present in the room throughout the conduct of all general anesthetics, regional anesthetics, and monitored intravenous anesthetics. An exception is made when there is a direct known hazard, e.g, radiation, to the anesthesiologist or nurse anesthetist, in which case some provision for monitoring the patient must be made.

Blood Pressure and Heart Rate

Every patient receiving general anesthesia, regional anesthesia, or managed intravenous anesthesia shall have arterial blood pressure and heart rate measured at least every 5 minutes, where not clinically impractical.*

Electrocardiogram

Every patient shall have the electrocardiogram continuously displayed from the induction or institution of anesthesia until preparing to leave the anesthetizing location, where not clinically impractical.*

Continuous Monitoring

During every administration of general anesthesia, the anesthetist shall employ methods of continuously monitoring the patient's ventilation and circulation. The methods shall include, for ventilation and circulation each, at least one of the following or the equivalent:†

—*For Ventilation.* Palpation or observation of the reservoir breathing bag, auscultation of breath sounds, monitoring of respiratory gases such as end-tidal carbon dioxide, or monitoring of expiratory gas flow. Monitoring end-tidal carbon dioxide is an emerging standard and is strongly preferred.

—*For Circulation.* Palpation of a pulse, auscultation of heart sounds, monitoring of a tracing of intra-arterial pressure, pulse plethysmography/oximetry, or ultrasound peripheral pulse monitoring. It is recognized that brief interruptions of the continuous monitoring may be unavoidable.

Breathing System Disconnection Monitoring

When ventilation is controlled by an automatic mechanical ventilator, there shall be in continuous use a device that is capable of detecting disconnection of any component of the breathing system. The device must give an audible signal when its alarm threshold is exceeded. (It is recognized that there are certain rare or unusual circumstances in which such a device may fail to detect a disconnection.)

Oxygen Analyzer

During every administration of general anesthesia using an anesthesia machine, the concentration of oxygen in the patient breathing system will be measured by a functioning oxygen analyzer with a low concentration limit alarm in use. This device must conform to the American National Standards Institute No. Z.79.10 standard.*

Ability to Measure Temperature

During every administration of general anesthesia, there shall be readily available a means to measure the patient's temperature.

—*Rationale.* A means of temperature measurement must be available as a potential aid in the diagnosis and treatment of suspected or actual intraoperative hypothermia and malignant hyperthermia. The measurement/monitoring of temperature during *every* general anesthetic is not specifically mandated because of the potential risks of such monitoring and because of the likelihood of other physical signs giving earlier indication of the development of malignant hyperthermia.

From Eichhorn JH, Cooper JB, Cullen DJ, et al: Standards for patient monitoring during anesthesia at Harvard Medical School. JAMA 1986; 256:1017–1020. Copyright 1986, American Medical Association.

*Under extenuating circumstances, the attending anesthesiologist may waive this requirement after so stating (including the reasons) in a note in the patient's chart.

†Equivalence is to be defined by the chief of the individual hospital department after submission to and review by the department heads. Department of Anaesthesia, Harvard Medical School, Boston.

peripheral pulse provides an index of both blood pressure and cardiac output.

AUSCULTATION

The heart sounds can be assessed repeatedly through a stethoscope applied over the sternal notch or precordium. Likewise, depth, rate, equality, and quality (presence of wheezing, rhonchi, rales) of breathing are noted similarly. Blood pressure can be determined using the traditional Riva Rocci method of auscultation for the onset and loss of Korotkoff sounds.

NONINVASIVE OR MINIMALLY INVASIVE METHODS

Most essential monitoring is either noninvasive or minimally invasive. In addition to inspection, palpation of pulses, and blood pressure determinations, it includes such devices as oximeters, temperature, ECG, and neuromuscular transmission. Among the minimally invasive devices are temperature probes inserted in the esophagus, nasopharynx, rectum, or tympanic membrane; esophageal stethoscopy; and insertion of needle electrodes for electroencephalographic or neuromuscular function monitoring. Insertion of a bladder catheter is usually minimally invasive, although it always carries the risk of urinary tract infection. External monitoring of fetal heart rate or uterine tone is minimally invasive. Highly invasive devices such as intravascular, intracranial, and intracardiac catheters or probes, which pose the greatest risks, are not usually considered as minimally essential monitors.

Even when invasive monitors are present, noninvasive or minimally invasive methods to monitor the same functions should be present in the event of failure of the invasive device (e.g., placement of an automated sphygmomanometer with an arterial catheter). Such duplication also permits easy calibration of the monitor. The choice of monitoring equipment must be made by the responsible anesthesiolo-

TABLE 1–2. STANDARDS FOR INTRAOPERATIVE MONITORING ACCEPTED BY THE AMERICAN SOCIETY OF ANESTHESIOLOGISTS

These standards apply to all anesthesia care although, in emergency circumstances, appropriate life support measures take precedence. These standards may be exceeded at any time based on the judgment of the responsible anesthesiologist. They are intended to encourage quality patient care, but observing them cannot guarantee any specific patient outcome. They are subject to revision from time to time, as warranted by the evolution of technology and practice. This set of standards addresses only the issue of basic intra-operative monitoring, which is one component of anesthesia care. In certain rare or unusual circumstances, (1) some of these methods of monitoring may be clinically impractical, and (2) appropriate use of the described monitoring methods may fail to detect untoward clinical developments. Brief interruptions of continual† monitoring may be unavoidable. *Under extenuating circumstances, the responsible anesthesiologist may waive the requirements marked with an asterisk (*); it is recommended that when this is done, it should be so stated (including the reasons) in a note in the patient's medical record.* These standards are not intended for application to the care of the obstetrical patient in labor or in the conduct of pain management.

Standard I

Qualified anesthesia personnel shall be present in the room throughout the conduct of all general anesthetics, regional anesthetics and monitored anesthesia care.

—Objective

Because of the rapid changes in patient status during anesthesia, qualified anesthesia personnel shall be continuously present to monitor the patient and provide anesthesia care. In the event there is a direct known hazard, e.g., radiation, to the anesthesia personnel which might require intermittent remote observation of the patient, some provision for monitoring the patient must be made. In the event that an emergency requires the temporary absence of the person primarily responsible for the anesthetic, the best judgment of the anesthesiologist will be exercised in comparing the emergency with the anesthetized patient's condition and in the selection of the person left responsible for the anesthetic during the temporary absence.

Standard II

During all anesthetics, the patient's oxygenation, ventilation, circulation and temperature shall be continually evaluated.

Oxygenation

—Objective

To ensure adequate oxygen concentration in the inspired gas and the blood during all anesthetics.

—Methods

1. Inspired gas: During every administration of general anesthesia using an anesthesia machine, the concentration of oxygen in the patient breathing system shall be measured by an oxygen analyzer with a low oxygen concentration limit alarm in use.*
2. Blood oxygenation: During all anesthetics, a quantitative method of assessing oxygenation such as pulse oximetry shall be employed.* Adequate illumination and exposure of the patient is necessary to assess color.*

Ventilation

—Objective

To ensure adequate ventilation of the patient during all anesthetics.

—Methods

1. Every patient receiving general anesthesia shall have the adequacy of ventilation continually evaluated. While qualitative clinical signs such as chest excursion, observation of the reservoir breathing bag and auscultation of breath sounds may be adequate, quantitative monitoring of the CO_2 content and/or volume of expired gas is encouraged.
2. When an endotracheal tube is inserted, its correct positioning in the trachea must be verified by clinical assessment and by identification of carbon dioxide in the expired gas.* End-tidal CO_2 analysis, in use from the time of endotracheal tube placement, is strongly encouraged.
3. When ventilation is controlled by a mechanical ventilator, there shall be in continuous use a device that is capable of detecting disconnection of components of the breathing system. The device must give an audible signal when its alarm threshold is exceeded.
4. During regional anesthesia and monitored anesthesia care, the adequacy of ventilation shall be evaluated, at least, by continual observation of qualitative clinical signs.

Circulation

—Objective

To ensure the adequacy of the patient's circulatory function during all anesthetics.

—Methods

1. Every patient receiving anesthesia shall have the electrocardiogram continuously displayed from the beginning of anesthesia until preparing to leave the anesthetizing location.*
2. Every patient receiving anesthesia shall have arterial blood pressure and heart rate determined and evaluated at least every 5 minutes.*
3. Every patient receiving general anesthesia shall have, in addition to the above, circulatory function continually evaluated by at least one of the following: palpation of a pulse, auscultation of heart sounds, monitoring of a tracing of intra-arterial pressure, ultrasound peripheral pulse monitoring, or pulse plethysmography or oximetry.

Body Temperature

—Objective

To aid in the maintenance of appropriate body temperature during all anesthetics.

—Methods

There shall be readily available a means to continuously measure the patient's temperature. When changes in body temperature are intended, anticipated or suspected, the temperature shall be measured.

Standards for Basic Intraoperative Monitoring. House of Delegates, Oct. 21, 1986—amended Oct. 21, 1992. Reprinted with permission of the American Society of Anesthesiologists, 520 N. Northwest Highway, Park Ridge, Illinois 60068-2573. (See page 709 of ASA Directory.)

†Note that "continual" is defined as "repeated regularly and frequently in steady succession," whereas "continuous" means "prolonged without any interruption at any time."

gist, critical care physician, surgeon, or other medical personnel after careful consideration of patient disease process and anticipated perioperative changes.

ACQUISITION OF NEW EQUIPMENT

Patient monitoring is a rapidly changing field. Therefore, the need to purchase new devices is inevitable. Specifications for purchase of new monitoring systems should be prepared jointly by physicians, nurses, and biomedical engineers. The user groups should determine needed devices; available technology; equipment reliability; requirements for space, service, or attendant personnel; and cost. First and foremost, the specifications must translate specific clinical monitoring needs into technical details recognized by industry and regulatory groups (National Fire Protection Association, Association for the Advancement of Medical Instrumentation, American National Standards Institute, and others—see Chapter 23). The specifications also should include requests for schematic wiring diagrams and computer programs for all equipment supplied by the manufacturer to permit troubleshooting by qualified, in-house personnel, detailed safety instructions, human factor engineering details, and environmental requirements such as susceptibility to temperature variations, power failure, or electrical interference. Evaluation of proposed equipment by these same groups is essential to avoid acquisition of unsuitable devices. Most hospitals and universities have rigorous procedures to ensure that equipment acquisition is performed in a fair and equal manner for all vendors while providing carefully negotiated, cost-effective contracts for the buyer.

Commonality of monitoring equipment throughout the operating suite, critical care units, emergency room, and other areas of a hospital should be encouraged. Interchangeability of monitors permits rapid, easy transfer of patients between hospital locations without loss of monitored data, ready replacement of equipment during calibration or repair, and speedy training of new personnel. Multivariable, integrated monitoring equipment offers a space-saving, cost-effective alternative to the individual devices of past decades. Whenever possible, the same monitoring capability should exist during patient transport as exists at any other time.

TECHNICAL SUPPORT PERSONNEL

Another essential feature of any monitoring operation is the presence of adequate support personnel who are expert in the care, application, troubleshooting, and maintenance of the sophisticated monitors.[38] Educational requirements are a bachelor's degree at least. The duties of such personnel vary from institution to institution, as does their training. In some hospitals, these technicians may also be responsible for autotransfusion systems and intra-aortic balloon counterpulsation. They may also care for the anesthesia machine, its ventilator, anesthetic gas tanks, and anesthesia hoses and connectors. Such personnel maintain logs of scheduled preventive maintenance, calibration, and emergency service calls. They are also responsible for the important, but often overlooked, responsibility of keeping equipment in a clean and undamaged condition. Abuse resulting from soilage by fluid, thermal damage from undissipated heat, and direct physical injury from collisions are common in the hospital environment. Although there have been no controlled studies of the impact of technical support personnel on the efficiency of anesthesia and critical care services, the unique contributions of such workers are unquestioned.[38]

REFERENCES

1. Nobel JJ, Kostinsky H: Selection of monitoring equipment. *In* Saidman LJ, Smith NT (eds): Monitoring in Anesthesia. New York: John Wiley & Sons, 1978; 261.
2. McDonald JS, Dzwonczyk R, Gupta B, Dahl M: A second time-study of the anaesthetist's intraoperative period. Br J Anaesth 1990; 64:582–585.
3. Morris R, Montano S: Monitoring the monitors: How quickly do anaesthetists react to an alarm? Anaesth Intens Care 1993; 21:241–242.
4. Loeb RG: A measure of intraoperative attention to monitor displays. Anesth Analg 1993; 76:337–341.
5. Durbin CG. Personal communication. March 1, 1988.
6. Tinker JH, Dull DK, Caplan RA, Ward RJ, Cheney FW: Role of monitoring devices in prevention of anesthetic mishaps: A closed claims analysis. Anesthesiology 1989; 71:541–546.
7. Gaba DM: Improving anesthesiologists' performance by simulating reality. Anesthesiology 1992; 76:491–494.
8. American Society of Anesthesiologists Task Force: Practice guidelines for pulmonary artery catheterization: A report. Anesthesiology 1993; 78:380–394.
9. Hamburger WW: Development of knowledge concerning the measurement and rhythm of the pulse. J Mt Sinai Hosp 1941; 8:585–591.
10. White PD: The evolution of our knowledge about the heart and its diseases since 1628. Circulation 1957; 15:915–923.
11. McGrew RE: Encyclopedia of Medical History. New York: McGraw Hill, 1985; 64–66, 71–77, 126–127, 317–318.
12. Cushing H: Some principles of cerebral surgery. JAMA 1909; 52:184.
13. Lyons AS, Petrucelli RJ: Medicine. An Illustrated History. New York: Abradale Press, 1987; 432–436, 592.
14. Cushing H: On the avoidance of shock in major amputations by cocainization of large nerve trunks preliminary to their division. With observations on blood pressure in surgical cases. Ann Surg 1902; 36;321–345.
15. McKeson EI: The interpretation of pulse, respiration, and blood pressure with special reference to surgical shock. *In* Gwathmey JT (ed): Anesthesia. New York: Appleton and Company, 1914; 410–413.
16. Rovenstine EA: A method of combining anesthetic and surgical records for statistical purposes. Anesth Analg 1934; 13:122–128.
17. Beecher HK: The first anesthesia records (Codman, Cushing). Surg Gynecol Obstet 1940; 71:689–693.
18. Wiggers CJ: The Pressure Pulse in the Cardiovascular System. New York: Longmans, Green and Company, 1928; 15.
19. Einthoven W: Die galvanometrische registrirung des menschlichen capillar-elektrometers in der physiologie. Arch Ges Physiol 1903; 99:472–480.
20. Hellerstein HK, Pritchard WH, Lewis RL: Recording of intracavitary potentials through single lumen, saline filled cardiac catheters. Proc Soc Exp Biol Med 1949; 71:58–60.
21. Fick A: Uber den Messung der blut quantum inden Herzentrikeln. Ver Phys Med Ges Wurzburg 1870; 16:1872.
22. Frazin L, Talano JV, Stephanides L, et al: Esophageal echocardiography. Circulation 1976; 54:102–108.
23. Smith BE: Universities and the clinical monitoring industry: Feckless independents or fruitful partners? Int J Clin Monit Comput 1990; 7:249–258.
24. Clark LC: Monitor and control of tissue O_2 tensions. Trans Am Soc Artif Intern Organs 1956; 2:41–48.
25. Severinghaus JW, Bradley AF: Electrodes for blood PCO_2 and PCO_2 determination. J Appl Physiol 1958; 13:515–520.
26. Harrison GG: Anesthetic accidents. Clin Anesth 1983; 1:415–429.
27. Cooper JB, Newbower RS, Long CD, McPeek B: Preventable anesthesia mishaps: A study of human factors. Anesthesiology 1978; 49:399–406.
28. Philip JH, Raemer DB: Selecting the optimal anesthesia monitoring array. Med Instrum 1985; 19:122–126.
29. Pask EA: Hunt and signal. Proc R Soc Med 1965; 58:757–766.
30. Whitcher C, Ream AK, Parsons D, et al: Anesthetic mishaps and the cost of monitoring. A proposed standard for monitoring equipment. J Clin Monit 1988; 4:5–15.
31. Gravenstein JS: Essential monitoring examined through different lenses. J Clin Monit 1986; 2:22–28.
32. Eichhorn JH: Standards for monitoring. JAMA 1986; 256:1017–1020.
33. Block FE: A proposed standard for monitoring equipment: What equipment should be included? J Clin Monit 1988; 4:1–4.
34. Belgian Anesthesia Patient Safety Steering-Committee: Belgian standards for patient safety in anesthesia. Acta Anaesth Belg 1989; 40:231–238.
35. Rosenberg P, Gisvold SE, Flaaten H, et al: Guidelines for anaesthesia care in the Nordic countries. Acta Anaesthesiol Scand 1992; 36:741–744.
36. Sage D: Monitoring during anaesthesia. N Z Med J, 1989; 102:313.
37. Gravenstein JS, Paulus DA: Clinical Monitoring Practice. Philadelphia: JB Lippincott, 1987; 415–425.
38. Frazier WT, Kelly PM, Lewis JE: The anesthesia instrumentation and monitoring specialist. Med Instrum 1985; 19:113–118.

CHAPTER 2

Human Factors and Alarms

FRANK E. BLOCK, JR., M.D.

Good-nature and good sense must ever join; To err is human, to forgive, divine.

ALEXANDER POPE [1688–1744]

An Essay on Criticism (1709), Part II, lines 524–525 [1]

DEFINITIONS AND BACKGROUND

"Human factors" is a body of scientific knowledge about human characteristics.[2] It includes human requirements, talents, and deficiencies as well as the way people interact with their environments. Human factors engineering refers to the design of devices so that they can be used by people. Thus, psychologic principles are applied to engineering designs. In Europe, the term "ergonomics" is used in the same way. Most of the literature employs the two terms interchangeably.

Human factors engineering includes the performance of the human-machine (or in our case, the human-monitor) system as a whole. Instead of focusing merely on the technical characteristics of a monitoring device, engineers and designers are now beginning to view the human-monitor system as a single unit. The failures and successes of all sorts of modern devices have been noted by ordinary people and described in the lay press by Donald Norman in *The Psychology of Everyday Things.*[3]

Norman cites several basic principles of good human factors design. In a sense these factors should be obvious, but, as Norman points out, we live in a world of poorly designed devices of all sorts. A key element of success is that of user-centered design. Devices should make our lives simpler, not more complicated. Equipment should be designed to make use of common knowledge. Logical mappings should be used whenever possible. The possibility—indeed the probability—of error should be considered in the design. Forced constraints should be employed when appropriate, but only when appropriate. And if processes are unavoidably complex or potentially confusing, they should be standardized.[3]

Examples of reasonable human factors design can be found in aviation cockpits and in nuclear power stations. The typical anesthesia workplace today, however, is a terrible example of design. Equipment and monitors are commonly in disarray. Monitor displays cover a wide range of arc, including positions behind the anesthesia care team. Incompatible components operate separately instead of as a unified whole. Multiple separate devices and their associated alarms compete for the anesthesiologist's attention.

Today's multiparameter monitors—the ones that measure the electrocardiogram, invasive and noninvasive pressure, pulse oxygen saturation, temperature, and often cardiac output and anesthetic gases—generally have the same technical capabilities. They differ sharply, however, in the intuitiveness of their design, their ease of being understood, and their ease of operation. The more successful devices make good use of human factors engineering. They have been specifically designed to be utilized in operating room and/or intensive care environments by physicians and nurses not by engineers and programmers.

To design a monitor so that it can be used is a complex task. Computer programmers have long realized that the input and output of a program are far more complex than the algorithms that will crunch the data. A major subspecialty of computer science now deals with the human-machine interface.[4] Only now are medical equipment companies beginning to utilize the expertise of consultants in human factors. The result will be a new generation of monitors that will be easier to understand and easier to operate, especially in a crisis situation.

The Association for the Advancement of Medical Instrumentation (AAMI) has developed a set of guidelines for human factors engineering,[5] which is now undergoing revision.[6] Preferred locations for consoles, displays, and controls, with regard to the range of height, hand size, and strength of men and women, are presented in detail. Keyboards, knobs, displays, illumination, and other ergonomic issues are also described. The guidelines, of course, are no substitute for knowledge of and experience with human factors. Adherence to the guidelines does not guarantee successful design of a medical device.[7] Checklists for designers have been developed,[8] but these, too, have their limitations. User testing is essential in the actual operating environment at all stages of the design process. Testing and retesting are the most important features of good human factors engineering.

Some functions of devices are impossible to design in a simple and straightforward fashion. In these instances, standardization is a key factor. User training and familiarity can overcome design deficiencies and design impossibilities.

TASKS OF THE ANESTHESIOLOGIST

Most of the key human factors have not been studied specifically during the practice of anesthesiology. Thus, it is necessary to draw upon the human factors experience in other fields. Several investigators have used time-motion studies to identify the specific tasks performed by an anesthesiologist.[9–13] Much time is spent in direct patient monitoring (over 30%) and in writing the anesthetic record (about 10–15%). Always there is some amount of "idle time." Studies have attempted to ascertain whether the automated anesthesia record requires more or less time than the manual record. One study showed no significant difference in recordkeeping time.[14]

Anesthesiologists must be vigilant. Few studies have attempted to assess vigilance. One study suggested that automated noninvasive blood pressure devices impaired residents' abilities to detect the loss of breath and heart sounds from a stethoscope.[15] A similar study found that loss of breath and heart sounds from a stethoscope was detected in 34 seconds ± 59 (mean ± SD), with 13% delayed beyond 1 minute and 2% beyond 4 minutes.[16] One question about the studies is whether anesthesiologists do, or should, rely as heavily on heart and breath sounds in the era of pulse oximetry and capnography as they did in previous times. Another study required residents to press a button when an abnormal vital sign was artificially displayed on a monitor. The majority of abnormal readings were detected within 1 minute; only 16% were undetected within 5 minutes.[17]

In addition, beginning residents have multiple duties, not the least of which is to learn the basic operation of the monitors and the anesthesia machine, and the general procedures for the conduct of anesthesia. These new residents are perhaps subject to different workloads. In particular, when they are busy with manual tasks (e.g., airway management, cannula placement), vigilance is decreased.[18]

HUMAN ERROR IN ANESTHESIA

There are two major kinds of errors: slips and mistakes. Slips are behaviors that are nearly automatic but that are based on errors in classification, intention, timing, or spatial location, or on wrong data. Mistakes are intended actions, but are based on faulty or incomplete knowledge or training.[3]

In an ideal world, every anesthesiologist would have perfect medical knowledge, perfect diagnostic skills, and perfect technical skills, and would apply these perfect talents 100% of the time. In the real world, people have traditionally avoided talking about the errors of health care personnel. Errors of commission and omission are often misstated, denied, or excused. In an anonymous mail survey, however, over 18% of anesthesiologists who replied admitted having made a lethal error.[19]

In his classic work, Cooper et al have shown that 82% of preventable accidents involved human error.[20] Lack of experience, lack of familiarity with a device, carelessness, fatigue, and distraction were among the many reasons cited for these errors. A later study confirmed these findings and documented that true equipment failure contributed to only 4% of the incidents.[21] Thus, humans are far more often the problem than the equipment! Such knowledge seems especially important when we hear that pulse oximetry saves lives or that increased monitoring saves lives. Both Whitcher et al and Eichhorn suggested that an improved array of monitors (pulse oximetry and capnography in particular) would allow detection of many anesthesia mishaps, would reduce the incidence of serious patient complications, and would save enough money from anesthesia malpractice judgments to pay for the additional monitors.[22, 23] In an editorial, I suggested applying the savings to a fantastic array of monitors, including electroencephalography.[24] Critical statistical evaluation points out, however, the difficulty or impossibility of proving such claims.[25] "Increased" monitoring does not necessarily mean "improved" monitoring.

HOW DOES HUMAN ERROR CAUSE INJURY?

In most instances, human errors are promptly detected and promptly corrected, long before any injury can occur. As time passes before the problem is detected, however, the probability of permanent damage becomes greater. For example, an anesthesiologist might place an endotracheal tube into the patient's esophagus. In the great majority of instances, the absence of breath sounds, the gastric distention, and particularly the absence of expired carbon dioxide on the capnogram would permit a prompt diagnosis.

Under other circumstances, additional errors might occur. A fatigued anesthesiologist might hear sounds of air entry over the chest and conclude that breath sounds were present but abnormal. Abdominal distention might be attributed to the patient's disease process. The absent capnogram could be blamed on a faulty monitor. Furthermore, time might be wasted in obtaining a new monitor, a chest radiograph, or a consultant to help diagnose the problem.

In many instances, anesthesiologists make fixation errors—they become "locked in a frame." In a problem situation, the anesthesiologist makes a tentative diagnosis. As more data become available (laboratory data, radiographic reports), the anesthesiologist attempts to fit the new data into his or her tentative diagnosis. Even as more and more data arrive to suggest that an alternative diagnosis is more likely, the anesthesiologist continues to believe his or her initial diagnosis. Often in such cases, an outside consultant who is presented the data *de novo* can more easily reach the correct conclusion. Such a pattern is seen in anesthesiology and in industrial areas such as nuclear power.[26–29]

In anesthesiology, of course, time is of the essence. A combination of monitors and other devices, with alarms where appropriate, plus a skillful anesthesiologist, should minimize the time required to make a definitive diagnosis and begin essential therapy. During the time required, the patient passes through a sequence of states: normal (safe) → abnormal (still safe but with potential for temporary derangement or permanent injury) → abnormal (temporary derangement but no permanent injury) → abnormal (permanent injury or death). In most instances, problems are detected during the second or third levels. An example is a sedated patient under monitored anesthesia care. If the patient hypoventilates, the oxygen saturation will start to decrease. A brief period of hypoxia hardly ever causes problems; if the hypoxia is unrecognized and uncorrected, however, a permanent injury could occur. Again, effective medical devices, engineered for human factors, and a competent, vigilant anesthesiologist offer the best defense against these temporary derangements and permanent injuries. Simulators and good crisis management skills also are helpful.[30]

ENVIRONMENTAL FACTORS AND LIMITATIONS OF ANESTHESIOLOGISTS

Members of the anesthesia care team suffer from the same weaknesses, foibles, and aging processes as the rest of society. Approximately 8% of the United States male population have deficient red-green color vision. Medical devices should be designed to take this limitation into account, and color should never be the sole visual clue. Instead, size, shape, or text should be varied to prevent confusion in color-deficient users. In the fifth decade of life, many anesthesiologists will require bifocal lenses for presbyopia. A number of anesthesiologists have complained of difficulty in seeing monitors and gauges located both high and low on the anesthesia machine, because of their difficulty in accommodation.

Both young and old anesthesiologists may have hearing deficits. Most of today's alarm sounds are not designed to accommodate even the normal decrease of hearing with the aging process.[31] The noisy environment of the operating room may even compromise the ability of those with normal hearing to accurately detect changes in breath sounds and to monitor signal sounds and alarms. Some persons with normal hearing are "tone-deaf" and unable to hear the pitch change as intended on a pulse oximeter.[32] Additional engineering considerations apply to the design of monitors to be used by elderly and physically challenged clinicians.[33]

Noise, lighting, temperature, and humidity all affect performance. An older study suggested that the operating room approximates the noise level of a garbage disposal or a food blender, and it is frequently louder than a freeway.[34] A later study suggests that the operating room may be even noisier than was previously believed. A stainless steel bowl that falls 2 m onto the floor produces a sound level of 108 decibels.[35] At a minimum, noise impairs communication among team members and affects short-term memory and vigilance. Although noise causes a beneficial increase in arousal when it first begins, it also causes distractions.[36] High-level noise commonly increases stress through sympathetic activation.[37]

Operating room lighting may vary from near darkness for endoscopic procedures to flood lighting for videotaping. Monitors and other medical devices must be designed for use under all lighting conditions. Under bright lights, glare from display screens can be a major problem. Contrast and size of type fonts must be carefully chosen to ensure legibility under varying lighting conditions.

Speed is increased in moderate heat and decreased at normal temperatures or severe heat. Errors are more common in both moderate and severe heat.[38] Increased environmental temperature increases body temperature and heart rate, and leads to dehydration. Low humidity can also result in dehydration, which impairs performance.[37]

SLEEP DEPRIVATION AND FATIGUE

Physicians have traditionally been expected to work long hours without breaks or to remain on call all night and work through the following day. Most anesthesiology departments, however, have opted for limited call schedules that normally include the day off after call. It is difficult to separate the effects of fatigue and sleep deprivation, since the two phenomena often go together. In addition, humans function on a circadian cycle, with performance usually best between 10 A.M. and 3 P.M. and poorest between about 2 A.M. and 6 A.M.

The few studies that have addressed these issues in physicians often have been flawed. For example, a study by Deaconson et al showed that surgical residents who were on call every other night had similar performances on the days of call and on the days after call.[39] As several letters to the editor pointed out,[40] however, this study was flawed because the residents were chronically fatigued! One study confirmed that interns were less able to detect arrhythmias on the electrocardiogram after sleep loss.[41] A study by Jacques et al found that third-year family practice residents who had lost one night's sleep scored about the same on the residency in-training examination as fully rested first-year residents.[42] Another study showed that anesthesia residents scored more poorly on a vigilance test after 24 hours of in-house call than when they were rested.[43]

Anecdotal medical stories suggest that fatigued residents may provide dangerous medical care.[44] Thus, there are many arguments in favor of limiting the hours of residents but such limitations will have substantial costs.[45]

Studies in other fields suggest that fatigued subjects experience physical symptoms and psychologic aversion to further work. Fatigued subjects demonstrate decreased arousal, exhibit variable responses and timing, pay less attention to peripheral instruments, and take short-cuts that may be dangerous. Morale is commonly decreased. Often subjects do not recognize that they are fatigued and that their performance is impaired. On the other hand, sufficiently motivated fatigued subjects may exhibit near-normal performance on a short task.

Vigilance decreases after only 25–30 minutes on a task and decreases rapidly after 2 hours on a task. Performance decreases after 4 hours and again after 18 hours of a task. Other environmental factors may affect this decrement. Tasks that require vigilance should be done for periods of less than 4 hours, but such limitations hardly seem possible in medical situations.

Rest breaks usually are perceived as beneficial, though the benefit may result more from relief of boredom than from anything else. Rest breaks have been shown not to reduce work output and indeed may result in increased productivity. Cooper et al have suggested that, although the process of relieving anesthesia personnel may contribute to an error, the more common phenomenon is for the relieving person to discover an error.[46] The use of a checklist for the process of anesthesia relief is recommended (Table 2–1).

Sleep cannot be stored. After one or more nights of complete or near-complete sleep loss, decrements in performance may be as high as 70%. Sleep loss impairs reaction time, vigilance, and perception, and it causes changes in affect. Physical tasks may be less affected than cognitive tasks. Chronic sleep loss (sleeping less than 6 hours), night after night, has a cumulative effect on performance—a fact ignored in some of the studies on physicians.[39]

A surprising finding is the effect of naps. In military studies, a 2-hour nap was useless, a 3-hour nap was helpful, and a 4-hour nap was required for baseline performance. But a common side effect of napping is ''sleep inertia.'' Immediately after a nap, a subject may show a decreased level of arousal and decreased vigilance for as long as 3 hours. For this reason, naps shorter than 2 hours cannot be recommended. It is better to stay awake than to nap for less than 2 hours!

Shift work, especially rotating shift work, disturbs circadian rhythms. Rotating shifts cause sleep loss and disturbance because of the redistribution of sleep. Cognitive performance often is impaired. The traditional practice of rotating shifts has been a counterclockwise rotation (days to nights to evenings). The natural circadian rhythm suggests that clockwise rotation (days to evenings to nights) would be preferable. It may take two weeks to adjust to a new circadian rhythm, and persons over age 50 may have more trouble in adjusting to a new shift. It is best to immediately establish a new sleep cycle on the new shift. Nightshift workers may have a 10% decrease in efficiency and an increased incidence of ulcers. Premium overtime pay does not make workers less tired, and does not increase their alertness![47] An exhaustive discussion of the effects of sleep deprivation and related issues is beyond the scope of this chapter. The reader is referred to reviews by Weinger and Englund,[37] Krueger,[48] and Comperatore and Krueger.[49]

TABLE 2–1. RELIEF EXCHANGE PROTOCOL

When one anesthetist relieves another, the reliever should determine the following *before* the original anesthetist exits:

A. Situation
1. Patient's diagnosis, procedure, notable past history, allergies, abnormal lab values, chest film, electrocardiograph
2. Anesthetic technique and logic

B. Status
1. Anesthetic course
2. Progress of surgical procedure
3. Fluids and blood products given; blood loss
4. IV and arterial catheters, ports
5. Present level of anesthesia (going up or down)
6. Labeling of drugs and concentrations on administration apparatus and syringes
7. Current gas flows, anesthetic concentration, and reading of oxygen analyzer; cylinder and pipeline supply pressures
8. Clinical signs and vital signs

C. Future
1. Need for anesthetics, fluids, and drugs
2. Availability of blood products
3. Plan for postoperative respiratory and drug support
4. Time when the relieved anesthetist will return

From Cooper JB: Do short breaks increase or decrease anesthetic risk? J Clin Anesth 1989; 1:228–231.

Note: Record time of relief exchange and reliever's name on anesthetic record.

MUSIC AND READING

Few topics elicit more emotions than playing music in the operating room and whether it is permissible for anesthesia care team members to read (and if reading is permitted, what sorts of materials may be read). Music is commonly played because those in the operating room enjoy hearing it, although disputes may arise over the kind of music and the listening volume. Music may serve as a source of noise and may interfere with communication and the hearing of breath sounds, monitoring signals, and alarms. It can produce relaxation or tension.

Music composers, both classical and modern, use musical techniques specifically to build and release the tension of the music. Some workers have caustically denounced the playing of music in the operating room.[50, 51] Others have pointed out its value, although one author suggested that jazz and rock music would be ''totally unacceptable.''[52]

When music is played, one must remember that an awake patient will hear the music also. Patients have become upset when they have heard various sorts of music, ranging from hymns such as ''Nearer My God to Thee''[53] to Don McLean's *American Pie* (with the lyrics ''This will be the day that I die''). However, patients may benefit from background music played over headphones.[54, 55]

Reading remains controversial. Some department chairs forbid reading altogether, whereas others restrict reading to necessary material (such as equipment instruction manuals or a drug package insert) or to medical materials. Some anesthesiologists use reading or puzzle-solving as a "secondary task" to help maintain alertness when they are fatigued. The nuclear power plant in Loviisa, Finland specifically permits the power plant operators to listen to music and to read newspapers while they are on duty.[56]

INTERACTIONS AMONG PERSONNEL

Members of the anesthesia care team must work with each other and with surgeons, operating room nurses, perfusionists, and technicians of all sorts. These interactions often play a role in permitting safe and efficient care of the patient—or in preventing it! Little work has been done in this field of "ethnography in the operating room." The operating room itself is a culture, with expected and "normal" patterns of behavior. Here, cultural behaviors, religions, social relationships, personal and family relationships, various roles in the operating room and perceived authority of those roles, and the possibility of arguments make up the framework for personal interactions. There are times in the operating room when it is not clear who is in charge of what aspects of medical care.[57]

STRESS

Stress in the workplace can arise from three factors. The first is the work environment, including its social and physical properties. The second is the tasks involved and the workload required. The third is the individual's health and personality.[58]

The internship and residency process itself is stressful. One study compared mood factors of medical interns at the beginning of their internship year and throughout the year. Anger-hostility scores increased by December and remained elevated through the rest of the year. Vigor activity scores were higher at orientation than at the end of the year.[59] The practice of anesthesiology also can be stressful. One study documented heart rate increases among anesthesia personnel during induction and intubation.[60] Additional stresses may arise during crisis situations. Even in the midst of a crisis, an anesthesiologist may be fearful of legal and quality assurance ramifications! Such fears and tensions may impair the smooth delivery of medical care needed during the crisis.

Stress from mental tasks may result in deleterious physiologic effects, such as silent myocardial ischemia in persons with coronary artery disease.[61]

THE IMPAIRED PHYSICIAN

A major concern is the chemically dependent physician. Such persons often deny the problem and, in the early stages of addiction, may be able to conceal all traces of their substance abuse. The American Medical Association suggests that 1–2% of practicing physicians are addicted to drugs and that 7–8% are now or will become alcoholics.[62] Anesthesiologists may be even more likely to be substance abusers.[63]

Aircraft pilot simulations show that even blood alcohol levels well below the "legally drunk" level can significantly impair performance.[64] Even the next morning, a "hangover" may affect a person's ability to function.[65] The Federal Aviation Administration prohibits pilots from flying within 8 hours of alcohol consumption, although 14 hours may be a safer duration.[37]

In one survey of anesthesiologists, slightly less than 10% of respondents admitted to giving anesthesia while hung over, but 40% admitted to having occasionally given anesthesia within 12 hours of alcohol consumption.[66] Sedating antihistamine drugs, marijuana, and perhaps cigarettes also can impair performance. Small doses of caffeine, however, can increase performance without elevating mood.[67]

TRAINING AND SIMULATION

Thorough training on a device can compensate for limitations in the design of the device. In other words, anesthesia personnel can learn to adapt to peculiarities in the operation of a device and improvise solutions to encountered problems. Although nurses have long recognized the importance of in-training sessions and certification in the operation of specific devices, physicians have long resisted such efforts. The Joint Commission on the Accreditation of Healthcare Organizations (JCAHO) now requires documentation of adequate training of all personnel on medical devices that they are expected to operate.

In strict terms, a training device recreates some aspect of the environment. A simulator, on the other hand, attempts to duplicate the entire environment. Despite the technical distinction, these terms are often used interchangeably. The first anesthesia simulator, Sim One, was developed in 1967 at the University of Southern California. This simulator was far ahead of its time. It included a lifelike manikin that could change skin color, a realistic pharynx and larynx, and computer-controlled responses to injection of drugs.[68–70] Computer simulations of anesthetic uptake and distribution were developed in the 1980s. ANSIM,[71] GUS,[72] and GAS MAN[73] simulate anesthetic uptake and distribution.

Howard Schwid has developed several computer programs that run on IBM PC–compatible computers; the Anesthesia Simulator-Recorder simulates the effects of many anesthetic drugs. It also teaches and evaluates management of critical incidents.[74] Another of Schwid's programs teaches management of cardiac arrest according to the Advanced Cardiac Life Support (ACLS) guidelines.[75]

More complete simulators have now been developed to simulate the entire anesthesia environment. A simulator developed at the University of Florida[76] allows the application of most brands of physiologic monitors to a manikin to measure the noninvasive blood pressure, temperature, and inspired and expired gases, as well as to perform electrocardiography and pulse oximetry. The manikin can even ''breathe'' spontaneously, and appropriate gas concentrations can be measured at the airway! Problem scenarios, stored on computer, are displayed in the workings and malfunctions of various monitors and anesthesia machines. This simulator has been used in anesthetic training and has been particularly helpful in training inexperienced residents.[77]

A different simulator was designed at Stanford University. In this version, a complete operating room, with surgeons and nurses, is provided. The manikin and the outputs on the monitors are controlled by a computer under direct human control. An instructor directs the computer operator as to what to simulate. The control operator can then simulate any scenario in real time, based on the responses of those undergoing the simulation.[78, 79]

Simulators are very expensive. An airline simulator may cost millions of dollars. A full anesthesia simulator may cost $200,000. There is also an ongoing cost to pay people to run the simulator and to remove people from clinical duties to use it. The simulator can also be used by surgeons, cardiologists, traumatologists, and other personnel.

One idea to lower cost is that multiple anesthesia training programs in a single city might share the simulator. There is also the problem of duplicating the simulation in another medical center, because the approaches to a problem may vary among institutions. Videotapes of anesthesia personnel who are dealing with a crisis situation on a simulator may be almost as effective in teaching crisis management as the simulator itself. Several computer simulations related to anesthesiology are now commercially available (ASC Anesthesia Simulator Consultant, AneSoft Corp., Bellevue, WA; Emergencies in Anesthesiology: Interactive Simulations, Roche Laboratories, Nutley, NJ; Virtual Anesthesiology, CAE-Link Corp., Binghamton, NY; Cardiac Arrest!, Alpha Media, Santa Monica, CA; and others).

As in airline simulators, the advantage of the anesthesia simulators is that one may try different approaches to a problem without endangering people's lives. A favorite stunt in the airline simulator is to take off from an airport, turn off the engines, and (without power) turn around 180° and land on the takeoff runway! (Personal communication, Denny Reynolds, United Airlines, March, 1992.)

Unfortunately, anesthesia simulators do not simulate the entire patient. Although it is relatively straightforward to simulate anesthetic uptake and distribution and cardiovascular responses to drugs and infusions, it is much more difficult to incorporate the interactions between various organ systems. Therefore, most anesthesia simulators are relatively incomplete, and unexpected modalities of treatment and unexpected incidents may not be understood by the simulators.[80]

THE HUMAN-MACHINE INTERFACE AND AUTOMATION

A machine may be designed so that it will perform nearly flawlessly once it is set up and operating. But that machine may be so complicated that it is nearly impossible to understand, to set up, or to get operating! The usability of devices is critical. Most devices—medical, industrial, and consumer—undergo a series of five phases, shown in Table 2–2.

Automation has both benefits and pitfalls. Certainly, automation is already in the operating room in the form of infusion and syringe pumps, but it is appearing in new forms such as automatic controllers for blood pressure; neuromuscular blockade; end-tidal carbon dioxide; anesthetic agent; and, perhaps someday, depth of anesthesia. A major problem of automation is that although it may make the work load easier when situations are calm and ordinary, it often makes tasks more difficult in crises or in busy times such as anesthetic induction and emergence. This is what Wiener calls ''clumsy automation.''[81]

Human-centered automation, rather than machine-centered automation, should be the goal. Human-centered automation assumes cooperative problem-solving between people and machines. This same issue applies to such fields as aviation. As aircraft become controlled more and more by computers, what happens to the roles of the pilot and the computer?[82] Weiner suggests that we should avoid the common position of seeing our automated devices and wondering, ''What is it doing? Why is it doing that? What will it do next?''[81] Instead, the human should be clearly in charge.[83]

INPUT DEVICES

Any monitor or medical device requires some sort of control. These controls may take a variety of forms, most of which are commonly found on commercial equipment and home appliances.

VOICE RECOGNITION

Voice recognition would seem a natural data entry form for medical devices. Earlier voice recognition software had several limitations. For instance, in the voice recognition module that was previously included in the Diatek Arkive Anesthesia Information Management System (Diatek Corp., San Diego, CA), the user had to train the device to his or her own voice. For a vocabulary of 400 words, this training process often required an hour. Data entry via voice required a stylized syntax—for instance, ''Thiopental, 2, 5, 0, Enter.'' The computer would speak back (in its own voice) through an earphone, ''Thiopental, 2, 5, 0, milligrams, Correct?'' and the user would say ''Yes'' or ''No'' (or press the ''Enter'' key). One curious problem was that

TABLE 2–2. FIVE PHASES OF THE DESIGN OF A PRODUCT

Phase	Functionality	Features	Operation
1	Limited	Few, simple	Complex, manual
2	Limited	Few, simple	Simple, automatic
3	Full	Many, complex	Complex, manual; user must make selection of desired features and displays
4	Full	Many, complex	Simple, automatic; complex internal operations are hidden from user; device tells only what the user needs to know
5	Device replaced by new technology		

the system had a high recognition rate for about 3 or 4 weeks and then the recognition rate fell sharply. The problem was that users began to speak the way the computer spoke, instead of the way that they had trained the system! Retraining usually solved the problem. Although recognition rates over 90% could be attained, the recognition was lower in the noisy operating room environment than in the laboratory environment.[84] Unfortunately, although a recognition rate of 90% would seem to be excellent, for the five-word example cited, the total recognition rate would be only 0.90^5 (0.90 raised to the fifth power) or 59%! Some users became quite proficient in voice entry, but most users became frustrated.[85]

Voice recognition hardware and software are improving constantly. It is likely that a future voice recognition scheme will have more success in the operating room than did the Arkive system. Another future possibility is that of data entry through brain waves, with electrodes attached to the head of the patient. Such a system will require considerably more research, however.[86]

BAR CODES

Bar codes are familiar to most as the Universal Product Code (UPC) in grocery stores. Bar codes have the advantage that the error rate in reading them is less than 1 in 1 million. Dr. Howard Apple was the first to propose bar codes for drug identification. The Duke Automatic Monitoring Equipment (DAME) system utilized pages of bar codes for controlling the monitoring system.[87] The bar code readers on the DAME system were an early design, and the bar codes could not be read well in that application. A computerized patient documentation system has made successful use of bar codes for standardized text entries that describe all aspects of the patient's condition (VITALNET Patient Manager System, Critikon, Tampa, FL). The contents of four computer screens of menus can be contained in two pages of bar codes. Data entry is extremely user-friendly and fast. The American Association of Blood Banks (AABB) employs a system of bar coding on most blood products. Greater use of bar coding in medical applications is likely in the future.

SWITCHES, BUTTONS, AND KEYS

This category includes on-off switches, buttons to cycle through a series of modes, and fixed (or "hard") keys. Normally, each key will be labeled with its function. Keys can be arranged for engineers (as in a line or a grid), but a better arrangement is by function. Grouping common functions together and indicating the hierarchy of functions improves understanding and usage.

At one time, it would have been almost unthinkable to put a standard typewriter or computer keyboard into an operating room. Now automated anesthesia recordkeepers and hospital information system terminals are found in many operating rooms. Most of today's anesthesia care team members have been exposed to computers in high school and college. In contrast to the older generation of practitioners who did not know how to type,[87] most anesthesiologists today can reasonably be expected to be able to type on a standard keyboard. Unfortunately, the QWERTY keyboard (named for the letters at the left-hand end of the top row) is the standard and will remain the standard, despite the fact that the arrangement of letters was specifically chosen to *slow down* the typing of operators who would jam the machines by typing too fast![3]

Keypads are especially convenient for entry of digital data. Although most people are more familiar with a telephone-style keypad, with 1-2-3 at the top, computer keyboards generally follow the accounting keyboard practice of having 7-8-9 at the top. Studies indicate no difference in speed of data entry with the two styles of keyboard. Either style of keypad may be used.[88]

Equipment that will be used in foreign countries also can cause problems, because of additional letters and accents not found in English. The ASCII code, which is the standard for computer storage of characters, does not include any foreign characters!

KNOBS, WHEELS, AND SLIDERS

A knob is an obvious interface, similar to a volume control knob or a radio tuning knob. Such knobs are an easy way to adjust the height of an electrocardiogram waveform or the loudness of a pulse oximeter beep.

Convention dictates that turning a knob clockwise will mean "on," or will increase a variable, or will move a cursor or highlight clockwise, upwards, or to the right. An opposite convention prevails for mechanical flow valves, such as the flowmeters on an anesthesia machine. For these valves, counter-clockwise means opening the valve and increasing the flow. Confusion may arise in future anesthesia gas machines that may have electronic flowmeters, and it will be necessary to determine which way to turn the knob!

Knobs also can be coded by shape and thus by feel. For instance, the oxygen flow knob on an anesthesia machine has a fluted shape, whereas the other flow knobs are round.[89]

Some medical monitors allow selection of menu items via a ''push and turn'' knob. Such knobs have been found on industrial electronic equipment and evoked potential monitors. The knob is rotated to highlight a desired menu selection, then pressed in to confirm the selection.

Sliders are mechanical devices that function as a knob. They are used for coarse setting of alarm limits on medical monitors.

INPUT DEVICES FROM COMPUTERS

Mouses, trackballs, joysticks, touch screens, light pens, and pen-based interfaces have been transferred from computers to medical monitors. The transfer has not been entirely successful, however, in part because of problems of space and of blood and fluid contamination. Trackballs may be preferable to mouses because of space limitations.

Some designs of touch screens may pose problems to personnel who are wearing gloves. One disadvantage of a touch screen is that the needed information is hidden below the finger at the time of pressing, thus preventing instant confirmation of the desired function. Occasionally an accidental press occurs. Frequent touching results in oil and grease on the screen and the need for cleaning.

Many prefer the touch screen over all other interfaces. Some touch screen entry systems are nearly effortless to operate. For instance, on some Fukuda-Denshi monitors, three trends may be displayed by touching the name of the desired trend and the slot in which one wishes the trend to appear (Fig. 2–1).

A new version of the touch screen is called the ''touch mouse'' and is achieving some popularity in medical as well as other systems. In this system, pressing one's finger onto the screen activates no function but causes a small arrow or cursor to appear on the screen just above the tip of the finger. In this way the finger does not hide needed information on the screen. In case of an error in placing the finger, the user drags the finger to the proper location, and release of the finger from the screen activates the function. Thus, a touch mouse is able to solve most of the problems associated with a standard touch screen.

PEN COMPUTERS

One advance allows the use of a grid over the screen and a stylus to enter data into the computer. The stylus can be utilized like a mouse, in that touching the stylus to the screen is the equivalent of moving the mouse cursor to that location. It is easy to check off items on a list with the stylus. In addition, character recognition software allows the computer to identify numbers that are handwritten onto the grid. Letters are more difficult, but these often can be recognized as well.

Although at least two companies are experimenting with pen computer interfaces for automated anesthesia recordkeepers, the technology of the pen computer itself is probably not yet advanced enough to work smoothly.

MENU SELECTION

Most computers and medical monitors perform functions through menus. A panel of fixed function keys or, more often, soft keys or an on-screen menu will be used. One common formation from the Apple computer[90] or from Microsoft Windows is the ''pull-down'' menu. In this system, a menu of choices appears across the top of the screen. By selecting one choice in the top row, a submenu appears, this time running vertically down the screen. In some IBM-compatible systems, one ''clicks'' the mouse by pressing the mouse button on the desired option. In other systems, one ''drags'' the mouse (by sliding the mouse while holding down the mouse button) until the desired menu option is reached and then one ''drops'' the mouse by releasing the button. Different people have different preferences for these two kinds of systems. Once a menu item is selected, often a submenu or subwindow will be opened to allow adjustment or some other operation of the item.

Menu design is important for ease of use. Menus are often an excellent design choice for novices, but they may frustrate experts. Experts know exactly the function they want but that function may be 10 steps away from the top-level menu! Thus, expert users often wish for a short-cut or advanced mode of operation.

Traditional wisdom suggests that menus should be not more than ''seven wide and three deep.'' In other words, each visible menu should have a maximum of seven possible selections, and the whole menu structure should not go deeper than a top-level menu, a set of submenus, and a set of sub-submenus. Research into human factors has shown, however, that although a long, unordered list of options is terrible, a single-level menu with the options in a logical order is an excellent entry system.

Most medical functions do not fit neatly into seven-wide and three-deep menus. Nevertheless, it is important to design the menu levels in a clear and organized fashion. Perhaps the most common problem that users experience in the operation of a menu-driven monitor is knowing the desired function but not knowing where to find it. For example, is the high heart rate alarm set on the electrocardiogram menu or on the alarm menu? Where is the volume adjustment for the beep on each QRS complex? Is the setup for the pressure waveforms found under each pressure variable or under the ''monitor setup'' selection? Often a better design will involve making options available through two or more menus.

Perhaps the best design approach is to offer excellent

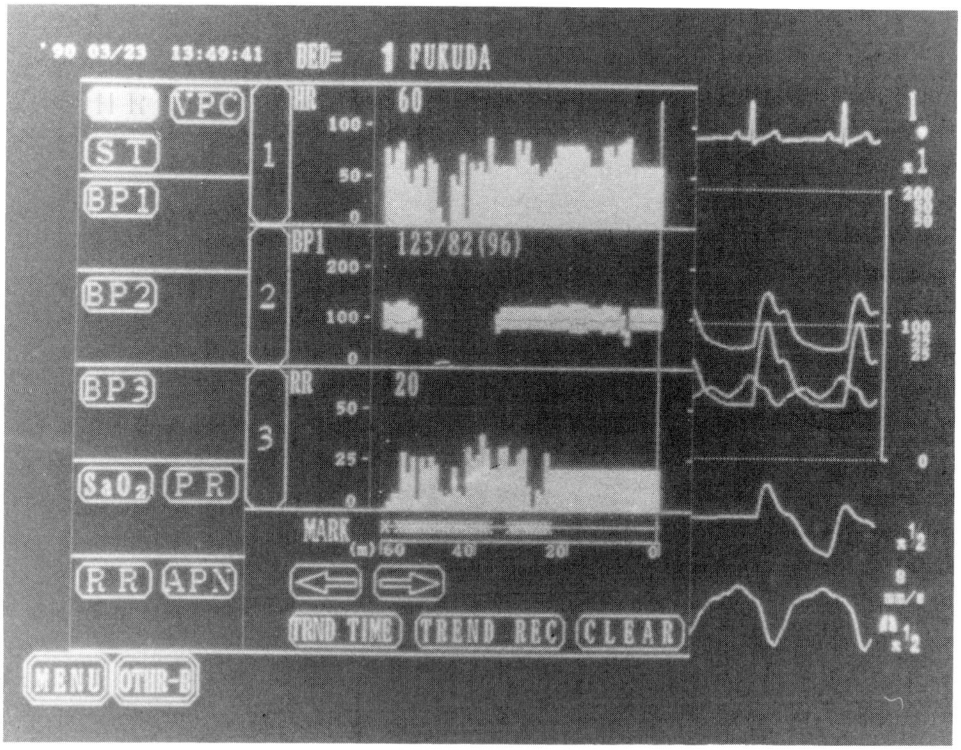

Figure 2–1. The trend page of the Fukuda-Denshi monitor. The user touches the name of the desired trend and then the desired location. (Courtesy of Fukuda-Denshi America.)

''on-line help.'' On-line help refers to information available through the monitor itself, such as through a ''help'' key. Unfortunately, such help often consists of a handful of standard pages of information that come up in the same order every time. It is still necessary to sift through the pages in search of the needed information. More modern approaches include context-sensitive help and alphabetical help. In context-sensitive help, the displayed help page is determined by the user's location in a menu or submenu. In this way, a page of information on cardiac output setup can appear instead of general information about how to use the monitor. In alphabetical help, an index is provided so that users can look up a specific desired function. Cross-referencing can be provided, so that the process for zeroing an arterial pressure can be found in alphabetical order under ''Arterial pressure, zeroing'' and under ''Calibration, pressure'' and under ''Pressure, zeroing'' and under ''Zeroing, pressure.'' In this way the user can use alternative terms and still find the answer!

In any menu system, it is common to ''select'' an item from a menu, and then to ''adjust'' it. An example is adjustment of the high heart rate alarm limit. First the high limit must be selected, and then it must be adjusted. With many monitors, often it is unclear whether one is ''selecting'' or ''adjusting'' the limit. Confusion can result in accidentally changing a limit—and then forgetting what the original setting was! These problems may occur particularly with push-and-turn knob systems. Another problem in choosing menu items is that the knob can be turned continuously, well beyond the top of the menu, or, for instance, beyond the highest possible alarm setting.

VIDEO SHUTTLE KNOB

Block proposed a ''video shuttle knob'' as a monitor interface.[91] The video shuttle knob is found on commercial videotape machines and is now beginning to appear on the more expensive home video recorders. This is a large knob, about 2 inches (5 cm) in diameter (Fig. 2–2). The internal mechanics of the knob contain a brake and a clutch, which are controlled by software. The brake stops rotation of the knob in one direction and could well be used at the top or bottom of a menu. The clutch determines if the knob is free-wheeling or if it has ''clicks'' (detents) as it is turned. One solution to the select versus adjust problem is to use the clicking mode for menu selection, and then, after the knob is pressed, to use the free-wheeling mode to adjust. In this way, the mode can be determined from the feel of the knob.

NOUN-VERB MENU SYSTEM

Another proposed system recognizes that most functions in a multiparameter monitor are really the same. Only a limited number of things can be done to a variable or a waveform, whether it is an electrocardiogram or a capnogram.

Thus the noun buttons would include the electrocardiogram, noninvasive blood pressure, various invasive pressures, cardiac output, temperature, oxygen saturation, various gases, alarms, trends, and monitor setup. The verb buttons would include help, setup, zero/calibrate, select/label/lead, size/scale, speed, on/start/unfreeze, off/stop/

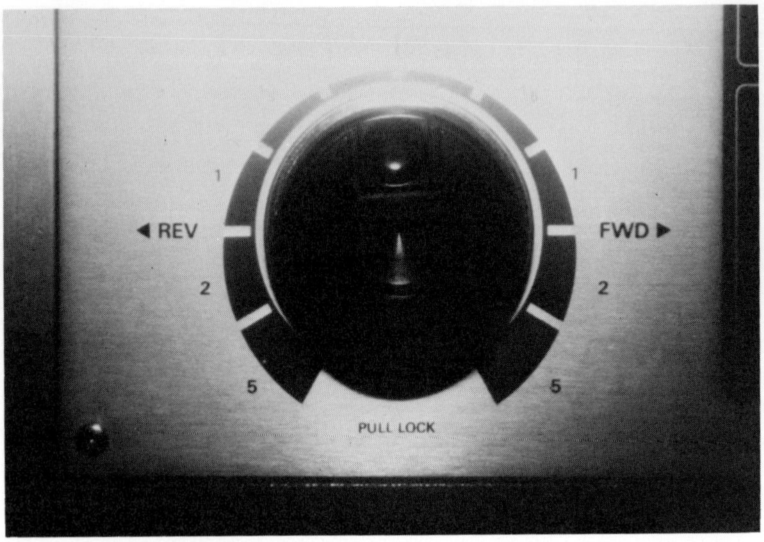

Figure 2–2. One design of video shuttle knob. (Courtesy of Jimmy Pilbeam.)

freeze, display, trend, record, set high alarm, and set low alarm. In this way, nearly all functions could be mapped onto a reasonable number of fixed keys, with two key presses sufficient for each function. Such a system would be easy to implement and easy to use for both novices and experts.

OUTPUT DEVICES

Monitors must communicate data and information to the user. Most communication will be via vision or hearing. Proper design and use of monitors requires an appreciation of the issues involved in the design of output devices.

MECHANICAL AND METER DISPLAYS

Mechanical displays remain in common use. Aneroid gauges display pipeline and cylinder pressure, and flowmeter bobbins display gas flows on anesthesia machines. Mechanical thumbwheels may be used to set and display a respiratory rate and an alarm limit.

Electrical meter displays also may be utilized. An example of a meter display is a needle that pointed to the voltage on older voltmeters, or the display gauge that indicated the instantaneous carbon dioxide reading on older capnographs.

DIGITAL DISPLAYS

More common today are digital displays. These are often liquid crystal displays (LCDs), which require ambient lighting or a separate internal light source for visibility. Such displays may be hard to read in a darkened operating room. In addition, most LCDs can be seen only from a limited viewing angle. Users at angles far from a perpendicular to the display panel may find it difficult or impossible to read the display. Some monitors incorporate a contrast knob that can make the display legible from different viewing angles in the vertical plane. Unfortunately, it is often difficult to adjust the knob while standing in the position from which viewing will take place!

Light-emitting diode (LED) displays also can be used. Because these displays supply their own light power in the display itself, they can be seen in darkness and from a wider range of viewing angles than LCDs can. The commonly used red LED displays may be invisible when red goggles are worn during Nd:YAG laser use.[6]

INTEGRATED DISPLAY SCREENS

Most multiparameter patient monitors incorporate an integrated display screen. Often a cathode ray tube (CRT) display, similar to a standard television screen, will be used, although LED and LCD screens also can be used. Key issues include resolution, flicker, and monochrome versus color.

The older electrocardiogram monitors for the operating room had an ''analog'' display instead of the more modern digital display. In an analog display, a continuous voltage allows a smooth waveform to be displayed on the screen, because every point on the screen can be scanned. In the more modern digital display screens, only discrete points (dots or ''pixels'') on the screen can be scanned.

Resolution refers to the number of pixels that make up the display. As an example, the IBM-compatible video graphics array (VGA) uses an array of dots that are as follows: 640 × 480 i.e., 640 horizontal by 480 vertical. Displays with even higher resolution are available; 1024 × 768 displays are common. Most medical monitors have higher than VGA resolution.

As resolution increases, waveform detail increases, and the characters appear smoother on the screen. In general, resolution will be better with a monochrome screen than with a color screen, because the color screen requires three dots per location (red, green, and blue) instead of only one.

Closely related to resolution is the issue of vectoring for

waveforms. Vectoring refers to the drawing of lines between discrete points on the screen. The vectoring problem is most often found on lower-resolution screens and is identified by a stair-stepping appearance of QRS complexes on the electrocardiogram, often with each QRS complex slightly different in appearance. The same phenomenon can occur with higher-resolution screens, however.

Flicker is a subjective phenomenon and is not perceived in the same way by all subjects. Flicker is related to the problem of persistence of vision, and it is akin to the operation of motion pictures and television. Images from motion pictures and television are not presented to the eye continuously but as separate discrete pictures. These images appear at such a rapid rate that the human brain fills in the gaps between pictures. In the United States, television screens are transmitted at 30 Hz, which is 30 frames per second. These pictures are ''interlaced,'' however, so that the odd-numbered horizontal lines are transmitted first, followed by the even-numbered lines. The effective rate is thus 60 Hz. In Europe, television screens are scanned at an effective rate of only 50 Hz, which may cause noticeable flicker.

Flicker is most noticeable in brightly illuminated areas of the screen, such as large areas of white. Flicker may be seen more easily in one's peripheral vision. Users who observe flicker in a monitor screen will commonly experience fatigue when watching the monitor for long periods. Scan rates of 70–72 Hz or higher generally will eliminate flicker. Often an engineering trade-off between resolution and flicker is required.

Color in anesthesia monitors is problematic for two reasons. One is that many monitors have been designed with pure, bright colors, perhaps to attract customers into a sales booth. The properties of the lens of the human eye (or of any lens) are such that it is impossible to focus on red and blue at the same time. The different wavelengths of light refract to a different distance. The result is that a pure red adjoining a pure blue produces a shimmering image as the eye attempts to accommodate to two focal lengths. Such images produce observer fatigue.

Better use of color involves avoidance of pure colors. Blended colors are easier to look at. Pleasing images may be generated with shades of the same color, for instance, yellows and browns. Colors with slighter contrasts are more harmonious than dramatic contrasts. Blue is commonly used as a background color and may be well used for background material, such as dots or lines of a grid or scale. Brown, gray, and black are often excellent choices for background colors, despite the fact that many potential customers note the ''waste'' of a color monitor to use blacks and grays!

The second problem with color on most of today's monitors is that most are available in both a monochrome version and in a higher-priced color version. The monitor is designed for full functionality in the monochrome version, and thus the color display adds little or nothing in terms of the information content of the display!

It is possible, of course, to use color in an effective way. Color coding of waveforms has become commonplace, with the electrocardiogram and pulmonary artery waveform usually yellow or green, the arterial waveform red, and the central venous waveform blue. Displays of the concentrations of inspired/expired gases also can be color coded—oxygen is green in the United States but white in Europe; nitrous oxide is blue in the United States and in most countries; carbon dioxide is gray; halothane is red; enflurane is orange; isoflurane is purple; desflurane is blue; and sevoflurane is yellow. Such color coding of the various gases is a logical mapping from the colors of the cylinders and agent bottles. For all these, however, blended colors are preferable to pure colors for these waveforms. Commonly, the numeric digits are color coded to the waveforms, although it is better to align the numbers with the waveforms than to rely on color coding alone.

NOVEL DISPLAY FORMATS

A monitoring screen with a series of waveforms running from left to right and associated numbers in one or two columns on the left or right side of the screen is the most familiar. Some investigators have wished for an integrated display, in which monitored variables and their relationships can be seen at a glance.

Over many centuries, scientists and authors have worked to present data in as clear and concise a fashion as possible.[92, 93] One classic example is that of Napoleon's march to Moscow (Fig. 2–3). In this drawing by Charles Joseph Minard (1781–1870), the size of the army is shown by the width of the band. From 422,000 men at the start, only 10,000 returned. The lower graph shows the temperature, as many froze to death on the march back.

One improved display is the bar graph display. Early versions of bar graphs offered no distinct advantage, since it was still necessary to scan each bar for a value within the proper range. A newer idea for medical monitors is the center-normal bar graph, found on the Narkomed 4 anesthesia machine ''Datascan'' display (North American Dräger, Telford, PA) (Fig. 2–4). This display system includes a reset button, which sets monitored variables to the center of the bar. Changes above and below the setpoint are readily identified by bars lengthening above or below the setpoint.

Another display is the polygon display, which has been employed for some years in industrial applications. Such a display is found on the Ohmeda Modulus CD anesthesia machine (Fig. 2–5). Half a dozen monitored variables are displayed as the spokes of a six-pointed wheel. Establishing the setpoint fixes the lengths of the spokes to a single length. The data points of the spokes are connected to form a normal polygon. Changes in the current variables up and down may be identified as lengthening or shortening of the spokes.

Other display formats, including icons of the human body, lungs, blood pressure cuffs, and the like, also have been proposed.[94]

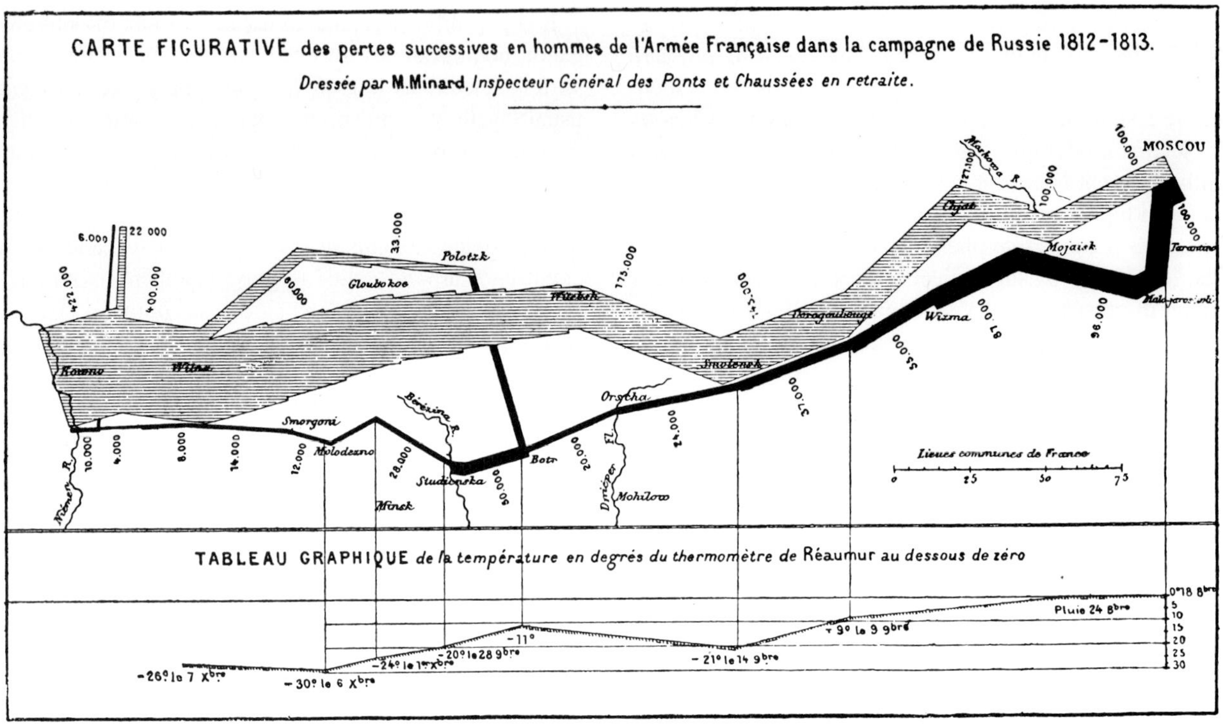

Xbre = December 9bre = November 8bre = October

Figure 2–3. Napoleon's march to Moscow, by Charles Joseph Minard (1781–1870). (From Tufte ER: The Visual Display of Quantitative Information. Cheshire, CT: Graphics Press, 1983, with permission.)

CLUTTERED DISPLAYS

The effort to present all data on a single screen often results in clutter. The list of monitored variables in anesthesia is extensive on a simple case and nearly unending on a complex case! Yet some manufacturers seem determined to place all the data on a single screen.

Multiple screens may be preferable. Screens should be separated by function and not by engineering module. For instance, anesthesia machine ventilator and gas delivery data belong with monitored respiratory volume, pressure, and gas analysis data. It seems appropriate to have one screen for cardiovascular variables, one for ventilator and gas delivery variables, and one for trending and record keeping. A case could be made to add a separate screen for setup and control, another screen for alarms, and still another screen for communication with the outside world (for laboratory data and other reports). Thus the number of screens could be easily expanded to six! Although this might seem to be too many screens, an anesthesiologist could easily process the data if all information was always in a predictable location. For example, if the end-tidal carbon dioxide reading and waveform appear in a consistent place, the user will always be able to find it.

Putting the data on a screen is hardly sufficient. The purpose of the screen is to transfer *information* more than data. In the Apollo 13 moon mission, poor data presentation delayed the diagnosis of the oxygen tank explosion. The three Screens A, B, and C in Figure 2–6 show the reconstructed displays on one of several monitors. In *A,* the pressure in oxygen tank 2 (at the bottom center, below the label 02-2) is 906—slightly high but not dangerously high. One minute later, in *B,* the pressure has risen to 1008.3, a dangerous level. Six seconds after that, in *C,* the tank has exploded and the pressure is only 19. No one noticed what had happened to the pressure in the few seconds before the low reading. Confusion in realizing that the pressure had first risen and that the tank had exploded caused a delay of nearly an hour in diagnosing the cause of the emergency. An alternative display format for the two oxygen tanks would have made the situation obvious, as in Figure 2–6*D.*[95]

"HEAD-UP" DISPLAYS

Head-up displays (often erroneously called "Heads-up" displays) refer to displays that are positioned directly in front of the user's field of vision, on a visor or other mount. Such devices offer the advantage of being always visible, regardless of the user's location. Such industries as aviation already are utilizing this technology,[96] and it has been proposed for automobiles.[97]

A lower-cost device, the "Private Eye" (Reflection Technology, Cambridge, MA), has become available and may be applied to medical settings as well as to industry.[98] This device is worn on a headband and can be located in a "reading bifocal" position (Fig. 2–7). The apparent focal depth can be adjusted from 22.9 cm (9 inches) to infinity.

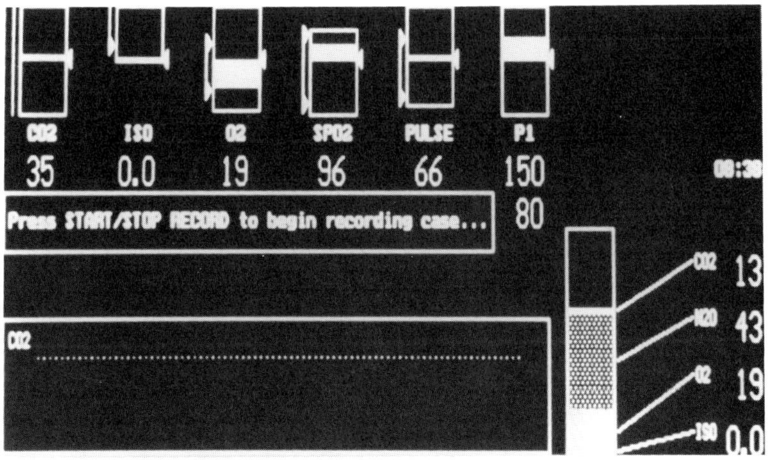

Figure 2–4. The North American Dräger "Datascan" display. (Courtesy of North American Dräger.)

If the device is placed directly in front of the eye, some users with good binocular vision will be able to learn to focus on both the work area and the screen display (similar to numbers superimposed on a television screen). This device has been tested in an operating room environment. Most users would be willing to test the device further if it could duplicate the waveforms and digital display of a standard monitor screen.[99]

AUDIO DISPLAYS

At first it seems illogical to refer to a sound as a "display," but hearing is one of the primary means of human learning. Audio displays include monitoring signals, alarm sounds, and spoken alarms.

MONITORING SIGNALS

The most familiar monitoring signal is the beep that occurs on each QRS complex. Of course, in pulse oximetry, the pitch of the beep on each heartbeat commonly varies with pulse oxygen saturation. The ability to detect the change in pitch as the manufacturers intended has been questioned: approximately 10% of naive listeners are unable to detect the change in pitch.[32] Even so, the pitch change remains a sought-after feature. Many listeners view the falling pitch of the pulse oximeter as an "alarm"!

Additional monitoring signals include the "ready beep" available on some noninvasive blood pressure devices. This tone signals the completion of a blood pressure determination and indicates that new data are available. A final example is a tone to indicate detected breaths, as via impedance respiratory monitoring (SpaceLabs, Redmond, WA) or as proposed for capnography.[100]

ALARMS

The word "monitor" comes from the Latin *monere,* "to warn." In today's practice, that warning is often in the form of alarms. A formal definition of an alarm on a medical device might be as follows: An alarm on a medical device is a sound or other signal intended to attract the operator's attention to a problem or a change in the condition of either the patient or the device. As such, alarms should decrease the time required to locate and correct a

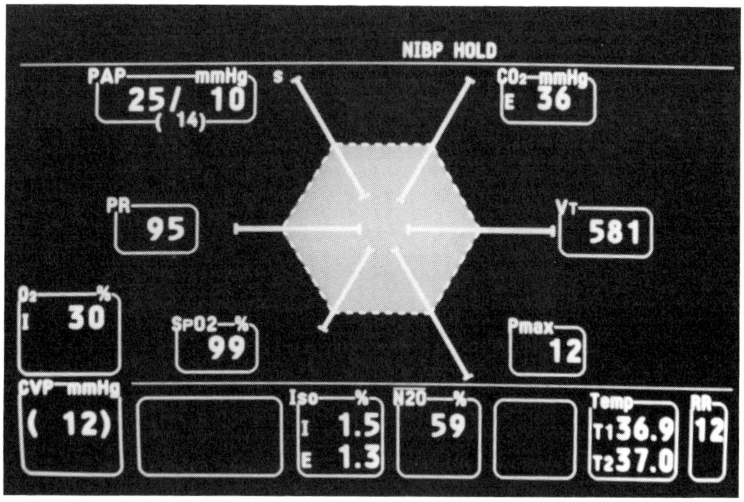

Figure 2–5. The Ohmeda Modulus CD "polygon" display. (Reprinted with permission of Ohmeda. Copyright 1993, BOC Health Care Inc.)

```
LM12839                          CSM ECS-CRYO TAB                                      0613

CTE 055:46:51     (          )     GET 055:53:47        (          )          SITE
-------LIFE SUPPORT--------                         -----PRIMARY COOLANT-----
GF3571  LM CABIN P        PSIA|                     CF0019  ACCUM QTY PCT           34.4
CF0001  CABIN   P         PSIA|   5.1               CF0016  PUMP P     PSID         45.0
CF0012  SUIT    P         PSIA|   4.3               SF0260  RAD IN T       F        73.8
CF0003  SUIT   ΔP       IN H20   -1.68
CF0015  COMP   ΔP       P PSID|   0.30
CF0006  SURGE   P       P PSIA|  891                CF0020  RAD OUT T      F        35
        SURGE QTY           LB|   3.67              CF0181  EVAP IN T      F        45.7
   02  TK  1  CAP     ΔP PSID|  21                  CF0017  STEAM T        F   |    64.9
   02  TK  1  CAP     ΔP PSID|  17                  CF0034  STEAM P    PSIA    |     .161
                                                    CF0018  EVAP OUT T     F        44.2
CF0036  02 MAN P          PSIA   105
CF0035  02 FLOW          LB/HR     0.181
                                                    SF0266  RAD VLV 1/2             ONE
CF0008  SUIT T               F|   50.5              CF0157  GLY FLO LB/HR          215
CF0002  CABIN                F|   65                ----SECONDARY COOLANT----
CF0005  CO2 PP            MMHG     1.5              CF0072  ACCUM QTY PCT      |    36.8
------------H20------------                         CF0070  PUMP P     PSID    |     9.3
CF0009  WASTE              PCT|   24.4              SF0262  RAD IN T       F   |    76.5
        WASTE               LB|   13.7              SF0263  RAD OUT T      F   |    44.6
CF0010  POTABLE            PCT|  104.5              CF0073  STEAM P    PSIA          .2460
        POTABLE             LB|   37.6              CF0071  EVAP OUT T  F           66.1
CF0460  URINE NOZ T          F|   70                CF0120  H20-RES    PSIA         25.8
CF0461  H20 NOZ T            F|   72                TOTAL FC CUR       AMPS
--------CRYO SUPPLY-------------------02-1------02-2-------H2-1-----------H2-2---
SC0037-38-39-40 P            PSIA     876.5     906        225.7(03-1)    235.1
SC0032-33-30-31 QTY          PCT       77.63    O/S         73.24          74.03
SC0041-42-43-44-T             F      -189      -192        -417           -416
A            QTY             LBS      251.1     260.0       20.61          20.83
```

```
LM12839                          CSM ECS-CRYO TAB                                      0613

CTE 055:54:45     (          )     GET 055:54:47        (          )          SITE
-------LIFE SUPPORT--------                         -----PRIMARY COOLANT-----
GF3571  LM CABIN P        PSIA|                     CF0019  ACCUM QTY PCT           34.4
CF0001  CABIN   P         PSIA|   5.1               CF0016  PUMP P     PSID         45.0
CF0012  SUIT    P         PSIA|   4.1               SF0260  RAD IN T       F        73.8
CF0003  SUIT   ΔP       IN H20   -1.68
CF0015  COMP   ΔP       P PSID|   0.32
CF0006  SURGE   P       P PSIA|  892                CF0020  RAD OUT T      F        35
        SURGE QTY           LB|   3.68              CF0181  EVAP IN T      F        45.7
   02  TK  1  CAP     ΔP PSID|  20                  CF0017  STEAM T        F   |    64.9
   02  TK  1  CAP     ΔP PSID|  15                  CF0034  STEAM P    PSIA    |     .161
                                                    CF0018  EVAP OUT T     F        44.2
CF0036  02 MAN P          PSIA   105
CF0035  02 FLOW          LB/HR     0.163
                                                    SF0266  RAD VLV 1/2             ONE
CF0008  SUIT T               F|   50.2              CF0157  GLY FLO LB/HR          215
CF0002  CABIN                F|   66                ----SECONDARY COOLANT----
CF0005  CO2 PP            MMHG     1.5              CF0072  ACCUM QTY PCT      |    36.8
------------H20------------                         CF0070  PUMP P     PSID    |     9.3
CF0009  WASTE              PCT|   24.2              SF0262  RAD IN T       F   |    76.5
        WASTE               LB|   14.2              SF0263  RAD OUT T      F   |    44.6
CF0010  POTABLE            PCT|  104.5              CF0073  STEAM P    PSIA          .2460
        POTABLE             LB|   37.6              CF0071  EVAP OUT T  F           66.1
CF0460  URINE NOZ T          F|   71                CF0120  H20-RES    PSIA         25.8
CF0461  H20 NOZ T            F|   72.1              TOTAL FC CUR       AMPS
--------CRYO SUPPLY-------------------02-1------02-2-------H2-1-----------H2-2---
SC0037-38-39-40 P            PSIA     874.9    1008.3      225.7(03-1)    235.1
SC0032-33-30-31 QTY          PCT       75.45    60          73.24          74.03
SC0041-42-43-44-T             F      -190      -160        -417           -416
B            QTY             LBS      251.1     O/S         20.61          20.83
```

Figure 2–6. *See legend on opposite page.*

problem. In this way, one hopes that the problem would be identified and corrected before the patient is harmed.

An alarm is designed specifically to attract attention. The valid assumption is that, at least some of the time, the operator's attention will not be focused on the device! A clinician is unable to stare at the monitor screen and at nothing else for a period of several minutes, much less for several hours. Alarms are necessary precisely because a clinician has many other duties in the operating room or indeed in any patient care area. Everyone has a limited

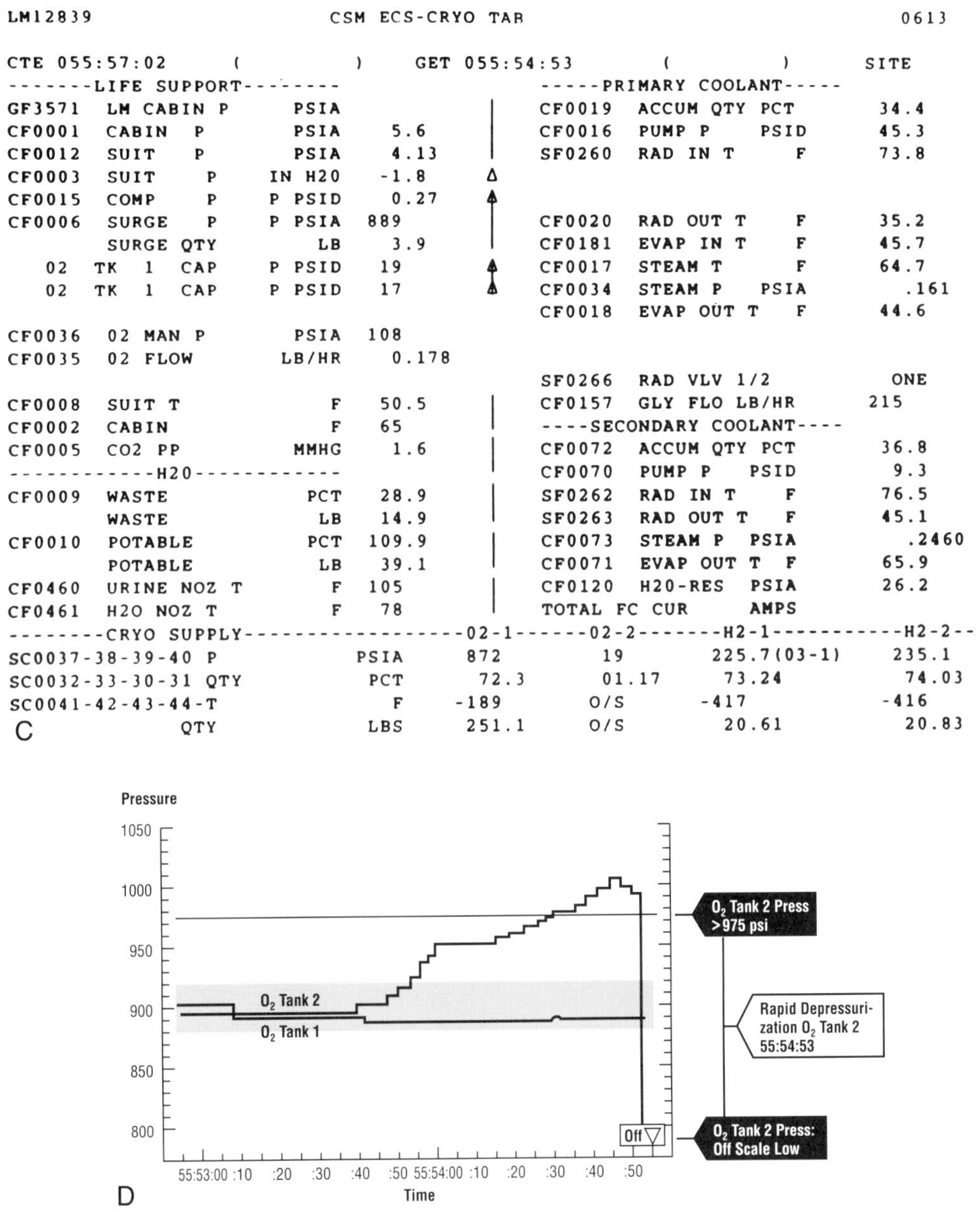

Figure 2–6. Reconstructed display screens from the Apollo 13 moon mission *(A–C)* and an alternative data representation *(D)*. See text for full explanation. (From Woods DD: Towards a theoretical base for representation design in the computer medium: Ecological perception and aiding human cognition. In Flach J, Hancock P, Caird J, Vicente K (eds): The Ecology of Human-Machine Systems. Hillsdale, NJ: Erlbaum, in press. Figures copyright 1992 by Woods and Holloway, used by permission.)

ability to perceive different signals simultaneously from more than one sensory source. Indeed, even within a single visual display screen, it is usually necessary to draw attention to an offending variable. The purpose of the alarm, then, is to call attention to the device and thus to the patient when something is amiss. In particular, it should alert patient care personnel to a problem, without startling them or annoying them. It should be easy to determine the reason for the alarm.

Few topics generate as much discussion as alarms. In general, anesthesiologists are frustrated by the large number of alarms, by false alarms, and by the inability to identify which of several medical devices is in an alarm condition. The result is that many, if not most, anesthesiologists frequently turn off the alarms.[101] If the alarms are not turned off, the first response to a sounding alarm is to try to silence it.

Indeed, there are too many false alarms. A study by Kestin et al reported a mean of 10 alarms per case with a mean frequency of one alarm every 4.5 minutes. The alarms were classified as patient risk (3%), change outside the alarm limits but not a risk to the patient (22%), and false alarms (75%).[102] Some of Kestin's false alarms resulted from the use of older equipment, such as pulse oximeters that were extremely sensitive to interference from electrocautery.[103] Some false alarms are really the fault of the user.

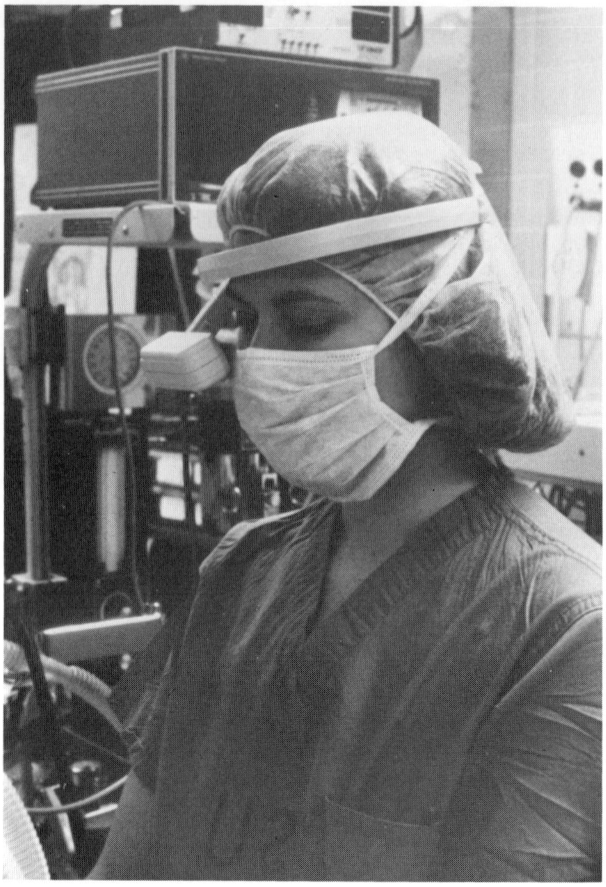

Figure 2–7. The "Private Eye" head-up display.

For instance, if the pulse oximeter is placed on the same arm as a noninvasive blood pressure cuff, many monitors will generate false alarms on the loss of pulse. Placing the blood pressure cuff on the ankle eliminates this problem.[104] A short delay in the sounding of the alarm also will eliminate many false alarms.[105]

Manufacturers seem compelled, however, to include a raucous alarm on every possible monitored variable. The implied intention is be able to claim someday in a courtroom, ''We had an alarm!''

Numerous issues arise in the rational design of an alarm system. One is the issue of enabling alarms. If an alarm sounds constantly whenever the electrocardiogram leads are disconnected, it will be necessary to turn off the monitor between patients. A better design would be to have the alarm remain silent until, for instance, five valid QRS complexes have been detected within a minute. At that point the alarm would be enabled in case of asystole. Such an approach is not without hazards. If a gas monitor required several breaths to enable the apnea alarm, disconnection for suctioning the endotracheal tube, reconnection, and ventilator failure early after reconnection might be missed.

Another issue is the concept that ''loss of the signal equals loss of the patient.'' This guiding principle began in industry and should be applied to medical devices. Unfortunately, it can become a nuisance, particularly for those who do not understand the principle. If a patient is monitored only with a pulse oximeter, and if the oximeter probe falls off, a high-priority alarm should sound, just as if the patient were in asystole. (Priority levels of alarms will be discussed later.) The usual response from users is, ''But it was only the probe falling off.'' The point is, though, that if the probe is off, the monitor does not know whether the patient is in asystole or not!

In the previous example, however, it is proper to make use of a ''staged alarm.'' In a staged alarm, the alarm begins more quietly, and becomes louder and more urgent if it is unattended. This sort of system would allow a nonirritating alarm for the few seconds it might take to replace the oximeter probe.

Still, there is a desire for multiparameter devices to make use of redundant alarms. If the electrocardiogram is being monitored and a lead falls off, but an integral pulse oximeter documents the presence of a pulse, the patient is not in asystole! In this instance, the asystole alarm need not sound.

Nearly all of today's monitors include the ability to set alarm limits. A typical monitored variable may have both a high limit and a low limit, and if that threshold is equaled or exceeded, the alarm will sound. Of course, narrow alarm limits allow a high sensitivity at the cost of poor specificity—that is, an inordinate number of false alarms. Wider alarm limits cause a lower sensitivity but higher specificity. The danger, of course, is that an alarm with wide limits might not sound until it is too late to prevent harm to the patient (Fig. 2–8).

Another issue is the ability to store alarm configurations. Almost all monitors are shipped with a set of ''factory default'' alarm settings. Typically these limits are set fairly wide, to numbers that would not be dangerous in the average or typical patient. These limits are thus safety limits rather than clinical care limits. Often, however, users wish to store their own alarm settings. Some monitors allow the user to store one set, or sometimes more than one set, of user alarm limits.

A problem can arise, however, when two monitors have an identical outward appearance yet different software functions for alarms and other features. Perhaps the best solution to this problem is as follows: In general, at power-up, a device should revert to the factory default alarm settings. If the device stores a single set of user defaults, then alternatively these may be activated at power-up, provided that the monitor displays a message that user alarm limits are in use. If the device stores more than one set of user alarm limits, the factory limits should be the default at power-up and the user limits should require deliberate activation by the user. It should always be possible to choose ''factory default'' alarm limits as an option. In any case, persons responsible for monitor installations should consider how alarm and setup features are handled across the various monitors in their facilities.

Another often-debated issue is that of latching versus nonlatching alarms. A latching alarm, once sounded, con-

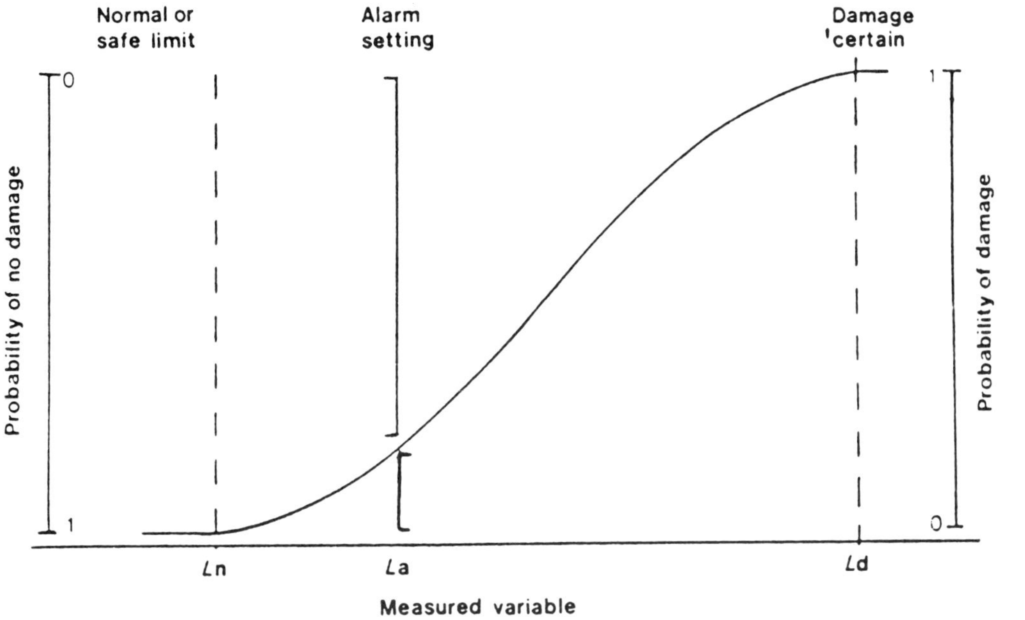

Figure 2–8. The relationship between a safe value for a measured variable (Ln) and a value that will harm the patient (Ld). Where should the alarm setting (La) be? (From Kerr JH: Warning devices. Br J Anaesth 1985; 57:696–708.)

tinues to sound until the user silences it, even if the condition that caused the alarm has cleared itself. A nonlatching alarm is reset automatically once the condition has cleared. There are strong advocates on both sides of this issue. In either case, it should be possible to identify the cause of the alarm once it has been silenced. It is very frustrating to approach a monitor that was in an alarm condition and be unable to determine why the alarm had been activated. An alarm log that can be viewed or printed on request, or retention of the alarm message for several seconds after silencing, can help avoid this problem.

An additional concern is that many users wish to silence the alarms. Some standards, and some individuals, specifically forbid the permanent silencing of certain alarms. In a perfect world, it should never be necessary to silence alarms. Unfortunately, particularly in multiparameter monitors, a module or a section of the monitor can break, and then the alarm sounds constantly. Sometimes the only available alternative is to turn off the entire monitor.

A better alternative would be to permit permanent silencing of alarms, subject to several strict criteria: (1) Silencing should require deliberate action; for instance, two or more steps. (2) During the sequence of steps for silencing a life-critical alarm, the user should be warned that he or she is about to permanently silence a life-critical alarm. (3) There must always be a visible indication that the alarm is silenced, such as a prominent "bell-with-a-slash-through-it." (4) A silenced life-critical alarm usually should be annunciated at intervals of several minutes with a periodic audible reminder or "reminder tone." A reminder tone could be, for instance, a short beep or "ding-dong" sound to remind the user every 2–5 minutes that the alarm is silenced. (5) The audible alarm should be automatically re-enabled at the next power-up of the device.

Another issue is that of displaying the alarm limits and the alarm status. The Emergency Care Research Institute (ECRI) has advocated that all alarm limits should be continuously displayed or at least readily available for display.[106] For an integrated monitoring device that already has a cluttered screen, the addition of high and low alarm limits for each variable may be impossible. A better approach is a separate alarms screen that can be viewed on request. An excellent example is the Datex AS/3 integrated anesthesia monitor (Datex Instrumentarium Oy, Helsinki, Finland) (Fig. 2–9). Here the high and low alarm settings are shown as the top and bottom lines of center-normal bar graphs. If an alarm is turned off, the limit still appears as a number but with a slash through it. Ten-minute trends of each variable are shown within each bar. In this way, it is possible to readily identify which variable is or was in an alarm condition, as well as those variables that may be close to their alarm limits. The top or bottom portions of the bars change color when an alarm sounds, as will be explained later.

AUTOMATIC ALARM LIMITS

Some monitors allow automatic setting of alarm limits, to a certain interval and/or percentage above and below the current values. The idea is that fairly narrow alarm limits can be set around stable variables in a stable patient, such as a patient during the maintenance phase of anesthesia. In some monitors, the interval and/or percentage may be adjusted by the user; in others, the formula for the automatic

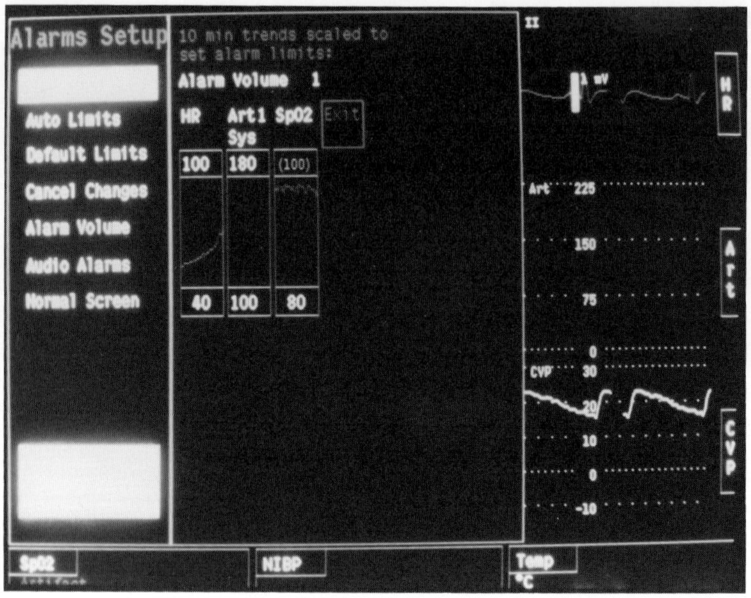

Figure 2–9. The Alarms Setup screen of the Datex AS/3 integrated anesthesia monitor. Each bar graph shows high and low alarm limits, with a 10-minute trend scaled to the alarm limits. (Courtesy of Datex Instrumentarium Oy.)

limits is fixed by the manufacturer. In many instances, these automatic alarm limits are so narrow as to cause frequent alarms. Another problem is that most monitors do not provide an easy exit from the automatic limits, for instance, when the patient is to be awakened from anesthesia. (This is another reason to allow users to select factory default alarm limits!) Setting the automatic alarm limits against the range of values that have occurred in the last 2–5 minutes, rather than against the current value; allows for electronic noise, the precision of the transducer and the monitor, and the patient noise or variability.

SMART ALARMS AND ARTIFICIAL INTELLIGENCE

''Smart alarms'' could replace the limit alarms of today. On present monitors, nearly every alarm is a univariate alarm—that is, it is linked to a single variable. When that variable meets or exceeds a certain limit threshold, the alarm sounds. Redundant sources of information might prevent excessive alarms; for instance, from multiple sources of heart rate information. Work has begun toward developing sophisticated integrated alarm schemes.[107]

A ''smart alarm'' system would have some sort of ''intelligence'' in deciding about an alarm condition. Perhaps the monitor would be able to pinpoint the source of the alarm, rather than merely announcing that a certain limit has been violated. Smart alarms normally make use of one of two artificial intelligence techniques.

The older technique of artificial intelligence is the rule-based expert system. In these systems, a human expert or a panel of experts composes a series of rules that are then implemented via computer. For example, if the heart rate is low and the blood pressure is low, a rule-based cardiac expert might announce, ''Consider increased vagal tone.'' If the heart rate is low but the blood pressure is high, the expert might announce, ''Consider hypertension with reflex bradycardia.'' Of course, in many instances there would be a long list of differential diagnoses, and it is often difficult to achieve a consensus about what condition the expert system should report! A rule-based expert system has generated an algorithm to provide alarms on a ventilator for the proposed Space Station.[108]

One advance has been the development of expert-system ''shell'' programs. These programs allow a relatively naive user to enter specific examples: a set of conditions and the associated result. The shell program then builds the rules required for the expert system to run. The rules also can be edited manually. Such an expert system shell program has produced a troubleshooting program for an automated anesthesia recordkeeper.[109]

One approach to artificial intelligence involves neural networks. A neural network is a computer-based representation with a layer of input nodes, hidden layers of nodes, and a layer of output nodes. Figure 2–10, for example, shows how a mouse or a computer might decide if another animal is or is not a cat. The neural network is first ''trained'' by presenting example data, much like the artificial intelligence shell program described. In the case of an artificial neural network, however, thousands of input values and output results may be presented to the network in a program that may require a night to run. Since real data are used, the input data may be conflicting, erroneous, or incomplete. Through computer trial and error, appropriate weighting factors are assigned to the various paths that connect the nodes. When unknown cases are then presented to the trained neural network, the network often can determine the correct answer anyway. Of course, in our example, the mouse or the computer might misidentify a Manx cat with no tail![110] A favorite neural network example is that of backing a tractor-trailer truck up to a loading dock.

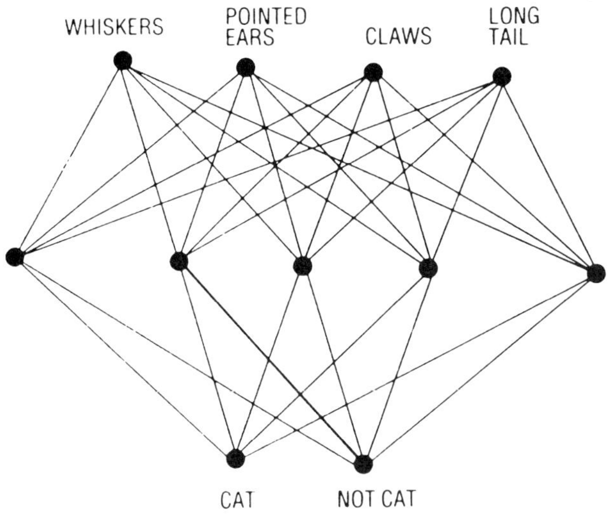

Figure 2–10. An example of a neural network: How a mouse can determine if an animal is or is not a cat. Each node in the input layer acquires data about one feature of the animal. In the training phase, the correct answer is given to the output layer, namely, "cat" or "not cat." The computer then assigns weights to each path. When an unknown animal is then presented to the network, the network has a high probability of determining if it is a cat or not. (From "Artificial Neural Networks." No. 11 of "Anesthesia Advances." Nutley, NJ: Roche Pharmaceutical, 1992.)

Through trial and error, the correct angle of the truck's wheels can be determined as a function of the truck's position.[111]

The number of hidden layers must be chosen carefully. Often, human trial and error are necessary to find the number of layers required for the neural network to function properly. Once the neural network is trained, new data can be presented to the neural network in real time, and the neural network supplies output data in accordance with the way it has been trained.

Neural networks have been created to analyze pulse oximeter and cardiac output waveforms to distinguish between valid and invalid waveforms.[112, 113] One neural network may improve the accuracy of noninvasive blood pressure monitoring.[114] A neural network can categorize the sound spectrum of an air embolus detected through precordial Doppler monitoring.[115] Another neural network can use airway pressure and flow measurements, plus the capnogram, to pinpoint faults in an anesthesia breathing circuit. Such a system has been shown to provide faster response times than conventional alarms.[116]

Although neural networks often can achieve a high percentage of correct diagnoses, they always will make some errors. One disadvantage of a neural network system is that there is no way to determine why it reached the conclusion that it did! In contrast, an erroneous answer from a rule-based system can be traced back and the rule can be revised to yield the correct answer.

Both rule-based expert systems and neural networks hold great promise for the future of alarms. These techniques will bring us closer to the goal of 100% sensitivity and 100% specificity for alarm systems.

PRIORITY OF ALARMS

Nearly all devices and all standards recognize that there are different levels of alarm urgency. Traditionally, these were called warning, caution, and advisory, but the current terminology refers to them as high priority, medium priority, and low priority. A high-priority alarm means that immediate operator action is required; a medium-priority alarm means that prompt operator action is required; a low-priority alarm means that operator awareness is required. These terms are used consistently in the standards literature.[117] This system coordinates well with the staged alarms described earlier, because an unattended problem may progress from low to medium to high priority.

A flashing red light is the visible signal of a high-priority alarm. This requirement poses a problem for manufacturers with monochrome display screens, so an exception was made to omit the red light if the user could determine the priority of the alarm from a distance. A flashing yellow light is the visible signal of a medium-priority alarm. A steady yellow light is the visible signal of a low-priority alarm. These colors illustrate an occasional problem of standards. As noted, red lights may not be visible through the red goggles used with Nd:YAG lasers. In addition, it is now known that a flashing blue light is more attention-getting than a flashing red light. Nonetheless, the color convention for alarms is unlikely to change.

ATTENDED VERSUS UNATTENDED DEVICES

Different devices have different requirements for alarms, depending on the person who is operating the device. An anesthesia machine has different requirements than an intensive care monitor—which is in turn different from a patient-controlled anesthesia device on a hospital ward, which is different from an intravenous pump designed for home use. In every case, it is important to consider whether a qualified person is near the device. In the operating room, for instance, it is reasonable to assume that a qualified member of the anesthesia care team is present at all times! Loud, constant alarms are not required. On a patient ward, however, a device may need to alarm loudly so that nursing personnel can hear the device in the hallway. Again, a successful design will often include a staged alarm, so that the alarm sounds persist and become louder only if the alarm condition remains uncorrected.

VISUAL ALARM DISPLAYS

Except for life-threatening conditions, most alarms should be announced visually. Common techniques include (1) color changes (to yellow or red); (2) flashing the variable that is out of range; (3) "reverse video" in which the background and foreground colors are interchanged; (4) highlighting a variable with a box, an underline, an arrow, or an asterisk; and (5) separate alarm messages that appear in a designated alarm area.

Flashing numerals require careful design consideration. If the flashing numeral has an On:Off period of 1:1, half the time the numeral appears to have disappeared! It is better to flash reverse video and the normal numeral, so that the numeral is always visible.

AUDIO ALARMS

An audio alarm is, of course, a form of audio display. Much debate has surrounded the effort to standardize alarms. There are major problems with audio alarms. First, because of variations among manufacturers, the same alarming variable may have different sounds, or the same sound may indicate any of several different variables. Second, alarm sounds commonly bear no relation to their urgency.[118] Third, because of poor choice of frequency components, it is often impossible to localize the source of an alarm. Often monitoring alarms compete with other devices in the room. For example, during an ophthalmology procedure, I endured a high-pitched alarm that could not be located despite 30 minutes of searching by all in the room. The alarm was finally identified as the low-battery alarm on a pocket pager! Fourth, many manufacturers appear to have attempted to design the loudest possible alarm, to ensure that it will be heard above all others. And fifth, the notion arose that all alarms must be either a constant, steady tone or an unending beep-beep-beep sound.

As a result of these factors, most anesthesiologists are unable to identify the alarm sounds in their operating rooms. Human factors studies in other industries suggest that one can reliably identify no more than five to eight different alarm sounds. Loeb et al found similar results among anesthesiologists: clinicians were able to identify the alarm source only 34% of the time.[119]

These same problems with alarms are found in other fields, such as aviation. Dr. Roy Patterson, of the Applied Psychology Unit, Medical Research Council, Cambridge, England, is an acoustician who is one of the world's experts on alarms. He has extensive experience with the design of alarms for aviation, railroads, and the like.[120] His research has led him to the concept of an alarm composed initially of pulses, then bursts, and finally the entire warning sound (Fig. 2–11). Each pulse is an individual note, tapered at the beginning and end, to avoid a "startle" reaction that would occur from a sudden loud noise. The pulse contains various audio components (harmonics) to give it a distinguishing sound spectrum (such as that of a specific musical instrument) and to aid in localization of the alarm. Each burst is a melody or sequence of pulses, with a distinctive rhythm. The entire warning sound includes several bursts, with several seconds of silence between each burst. For example, the burst might be played twice at a moderate level, then twice more at a higher level if the alarm remains unattended. Then it would drop to a softer level, only to return as a loud sound if the alarm condition persists.

Some years ago, Patterson developed a scheme of prototype alarm sounds for the operating room. His scheme included a longer and more urgent form, plus a shorter cautionary form, for six organ system sounds (cardiovascular, ventilation, oxygenation, temperature, drug infusion, and artificial circulation). There was also a warning and a cautionary form for a general alarm sound. These tones are similar to a set of tones in aviation,[121] and they have been described in the anesthesia literature in an article on warning devices.[122] To an individual who does not understand the design rationale for the Patterson alarm sounds, they sound like a meaningless series of electronic noises. These sounds were discussed quite seriously by several standard-setting organizations, yet they generally evoked sentiments of amusement or terror when discussed by anesthesiologists.[123] In fact, I proposed an alternative scheme of alarm sounds, based on the melodies of familiar songs. For instance, the cardiovascular alarm might be to the tune of "I Left My Heart in San Francisco."[124]

Several key points of Patterson's proposed sounds were misinterpreted. First, he never planned that all the different sounds would coexist in a single environment. His intention was that most alarms would be mapped onto the general warning sound, with an integrated visual display to indicate the source of the alarm. In some settings, perhaps one other organ-specific sound would be permitted as well. For instance, in a coronary care unit, one might find the general sound plus the cardiovascular sound. The six systems were provided to allow for the occurrence of a nonintegrated piece of monitoring equipment, some sort of "stand-alone" device that would not be connected to the central monitoring system. Through the six sounds, every device—and indeed every variable on every device—would have the option of being mapped to the general sound or to its organ-specific sound.

Second, Patterson intended that only truly life-threatening conditions would be announced by audio alarms. Non–life-threatening conditions would be indicated visually. Third, the Patterson alarm bursts could be mapped to a logical mnemonic for the alarms they represent. Thus the cardiovascular alarm sounds like the word "cardiovascular." Such mnemonics can be made to work in French and German as well as in English.

Fourth, work with similar alarm sounds and naive subjects suggests that the alarm sounds could be learned almost as rapidly as they could be played for the subjects. Finally, Dr. Patterson never intended that his would be the final alarm sounds. They were intended solely for demonstration purposes.

Acoustic techniques allow the creation of alarm sounds with different levels of urgency. For example, a faster rhythm is more urgent than a slower rhythm.[125] Thus while retaining the basic identifiable pattern, a more urgent form of the sound can be used for a high-priority alarm, and a less urgent form can be used for a medium-priority alarm. A low-priority alarm might sound only once, perhaps as a "ding-dong" somewhat like a door chime. Alternatively, a low-priority alarm may have no sound at all but only a visual message. A major need is to abandon today's contin-

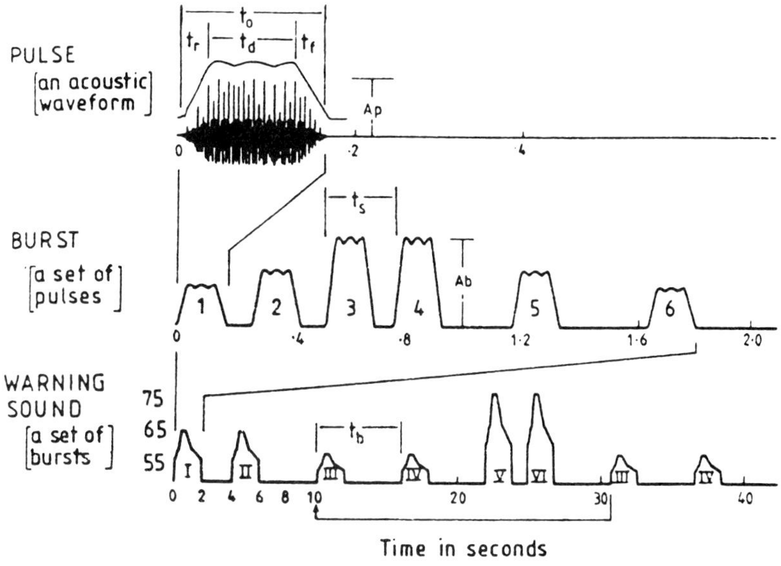

Figure 2–11. The components of a prototype warning sound. The pulse is an acoustic waveform with tapered onsets and offsets. Each pulse is an individual note. The burst is a sequence of pulses with a characteristic melody and rhythm. The warning sound consists of several bursts at different volumes. (Courtesy of Dr. Roy Patterson.)

uous and repeated pulsating (beep-beep-beep) alarms and to replace them with intermittent patterns such as the Patterson sounds.

At the 1993 meeting of the Society for Technology in Anesthesia, Dr. Patterson lamented the fact that the world of medical monitoring has labored with unsatisfactory alarm sounds for a decade since he proposed his alarm sounds. Surprisingly, the majority of that audience indicated a preference for all the organ system sounds over a single sound! Perhaps the Patterson sounds are an idea whose time has finally come.

In the intensive care unit, postanesthesia care unit, or ward area, there is often an additional problem with alarm sounds. In these areas, it may be difficult to tell which of several patients is generating an alarm. A central station might identify the patient on a display screen. But a nurse at a bedside might hear the alarm sound of a nearby patient and be unable to ascertain which patient it is. There are at least four possible solutions. One is that flashing lights, preferably something like a strobe light, could attract attention to the patient who was the source of the alarm. Second, alarm sounds with a better choice of frequency components would be easier to localize. Third, some companies' monitors allow the fundamental frequency of the alarm pitch to be changed by the user. In this way, different frequencies might identify different patients. Finally, I have proposed standardized alarm pitches, but altering the timbre of the sounds to resemble different instruments such as a piano, violin, flute, guitar, and xylophone. If these instrument sounds could be easily distinguished, a specific patient could be keyed to a specific instrument. (An organ or a harp would probably be inappropriate.)[124]

TALKING ALARMS

Along with progress in computer voice recognition have come advances in computerized speech and in digital speech recording. Many have advocated talking alarms, also known as verbal or spoken alarms. One suggestion is to present these alarms to the anesthesiologist's earpiece—assuming that the anesthesiologist is, in fact, wearing the earpiece!

Talking alarms have proved successful in aviation, but only under carefully controlled circumstances. First, they are used only in situations not often susceptible to false alarms. Second, they are limited to a handful of truly critical conditions. Third, they provide specific instructions on what to do, such as "Pull up! Pull up!"

Limitations on verbal alarms in a clinical setting include the concerns listed in Table 2–3. Only if these concerns can be adequately addressed should talking alarms be considered for use in clinical environments.

Acknowledgment

The speakers at the 1993 Annual Meeting of the Society for Technology in Anesthesia in New Orleans, Louisiana, provided considerable input and ideas that have been included in this chapter.

TABLE 2–3. LIMITATIONS OF VERBAL ALARMS

1. In an intensive care or ward setting, patients might hear other patients' alarm messages and become upset because they think that the messages apply to themselves.
2. Talking alarms should be presented in the native language of the user. In a device used all over the world, or in a country with many people who immigrated from other countries, a complex device capable of many languages would be required.
3. Talking alarms may compete with, and not be heard over, other conversations with care team members. Alternatively, talking alarms may distract personnel from necessary communication.
4. In many situations, when one alarm sounds, several others will soon follow. In this case, there would be multiple messages presented sequentially or simultaneously.
5. Depending on the gender of the voice of the talking alarm, and the gender of the user, there may be an emotional response counterproductive to the intended message.

REFERENCES

1. Elwin W: The Works of Alexander Pope, Vol 2. New York: Gordian Press, 1967; 66.
2. Military Standard: Definitions of Human Factors Terms. MIL-STD-1908, 24 December, 1992.
3. Norman DA: The Psychology of Everyday Things. New York: Basic Books, 1988.
4. Shneiderman B: Designing the User Interface: Strategies for Effective Human-Computer Interaction, 2nd Ed. Reading, MA: Addison-Wesley, 1992.
5. AAMI HE-1988: Human factors engineering guidelines and preferred practices for the design of medical devices. Arlington, VA: Association for the Advancement of Medical Instrumentation, 1988.
6. AAMI HE48-R-92 (December 1992 revision of AAMI HE-1988, proposed): Human factors engineering guidelines and preferred practices for the design of medical devices. Arlington, VA: Association for the Advancement of Medical Instrumentation, 1992.
7. Cook RI, Woods DD, McDonald JS, Potter S: Human factors standards for operating room equipment: Do they work? Does it matter? Anesthesiology 1989; 71:A335.
8. Ravden SJ, Johnson GI: Evaluating usability of human-computer interfaces: A practical method. Chichester, West Sussex, England: Ellis Horwood Ltd., 1989.
9. Drui AB, Behm RJ, Martin WE: Predesign investigation of the anesthesia operational environment. Anesth Analg 1973; 52:584–591.
10. Kennedy PJ, Feingold A, Wiener EL, Hoesk RS: Analysis of tasks and human factors in anesthesia for coronary artery bypass. Anesth Analg 1976; 55:374–377.
11. Boquet G, Bushman JA, Davenport HT: The anaesthetic machine—A study of function and design. Br J Anaesth 1980; 52:61–67.
12. McDonald JS, Dzwonczyk RR: A time and motion study of the anaesthetist's intraoperative time. Br J Anaesth 1988; 61:738–742.
13. McDonald JS, Dzwonczyk R, Gupta B, Dahl M: A second time-study of the anaesthetist's intraoperative period. Br J Anaesth 1990; 64:582–585.
14. Dzwonczyk R, Allard J, McDonald JS, Block F, Yablok D: The effect of automatic record keeping on vigilance and record keeping time. Anesth Analg 1992; 74:S79.
15. Kay J, Neal M: Effect of automatic blood pressure devices on vigilance of anesthesia residents. J Clin Monit 1986; 2:148–150.
16. Cooper JO, Cullen BF: Observer reliability in detecting surreptitious random occlusions of the monaural esophageal stethoscope. J Clin Monit 1990; 6:271–275.
17. Loeb RG: Intraoperative vigilance toward a physiologic monitor. Anesth Analg 1992; 74:S190.
18. Gaba DM, Herndon O, Zornow M, Weinger M, Dallen L: Task analysis, vigilance, and workload in novice residents. Anesthesiology 1991; 75:A1060.
19. McDonald JS, Peterson S: Lethal errors in anesthesiology. Anesthesiology 1985; 63:A497.
20. Cooper JB, Newbower RS, Clong CD, McPeek B: Preventable anesthesia mishaps: A study of human factors. Anesthesiology 1978; 49:399–406.
21. Cooper JB, Newbower RS, Kitz RJ: An analysis of major errors and equipment failures in anesthesia management: Considerations for prevention and detection. Anesthesiology 1984; 60:34–42.
22. Whitcher C, Ream AK, Parsons D, et al: Anesthetic mishaps and the cost of monitoring: A proposed standard for monitoring equipment. J Clin Monit 1988; 4:5–15.
23. Eichhorn JH: Prevention of intraoperative anesthesia accidents and related severe injury through safety monitoring. Anesthesiology 1989; 70:572–577.
24. Block FE Jr: A proposed standard for monitoring equipment: What equipment should be included? [Editorial]. J Clin Monit 1988; 4:1–4.
25. From RP, Pearson K, Tinker JH: Did monitoring standards influence outcome? Anesthesiology 1989; 71:808–809.
26. Perrow C: Normal accidents: Living with high-risk technologies. New York: Basic Books, 1984.
27. Gaba DM, Maxwell M, DeAnda A: Anesthetic mishaps: Breaking the chain of accident evolution. Anesthesiology 1987; 66:670–676.
28. Cook RI, McDonald JS: Cognitive tunnel vision in the operating room: Analysis of cases using a frame model. Anesthesiology 1988; 69:A497.
29. Gaba DM: Improving anesthesiologists' performance by simulating reality [Editorial]. Anesthesiology 1992; 76:491–494.
30. Howard SK, Gaba DM, Fish KJ, Yang G, Sarnquist FH: Anesthesia crisis resource management training: Teaching anesthesiologists to handle critical incidents. Aviat Space Environ Med 1992; 63:763–770.
31. Wallace MS, Ashman MN: Volume and frequency of anesthetic alarms: Are the current alarm systems appropriate for normal human ear aging? J Clin Monit 1991; 7:134.
32. Schulte GT, Block FE Jr: Can people hear the pitch change on a variable-pitch pulse oximeter? J Clin Monit 1992; 8:198–200.
33. Honeywell Inc: Human factors design guidelines for the elderly and people with disabilities, Revision 3 draft, May 1992. Minneapolis: Honeywell Inc., 1992.
34. Shapiro RA, Berland T: Noise in the operating room. N Engl J Med 1972; 287:1236–1238.
35. Hodge B, Thompson JF: Noise pollution in the operating theatre. Lancet 1990; 335:891–894.
36. Poulton EC: A new look at the effects of noise: A rejoinder. Psychol Bull 1978; 85:1068–1079.
37. Weinger MB, Englund CE: Ergonomic and human factors affecting anesthetic vigilance and monitoring performance in the operating room environment. Anesthesiology 1990; 73:995–1021.
38. Epstein Y, Keren G, Moisseiev J, Gasko O, Yachin S: Psychomotor deterioration during exposure to heat. Aviat Space Environ Med 1980; 51:607–610.
39. Deaconson TF, O'Hair DP, Levy MF, Lee MB, Schueneman AL, Condon RE: Sleep deprivation and resident performance. JAMA 1988; 260:1721–1727.
40. Letters to the editor. JAMA 1989; 261:859–863.
41. Friedman RC, Bigger JT, Kornfeld DS: The intern and sleep loss. N Engl J Med 1971; 285:201–203.
42. Jacques CHM, Lynch JC, Samkoff JS: The effects of sleep loss on cognitive performance of resident physicians. J Fam Pract 1990; 30:223–229.
43. Denisco RA, Drummond JN, Gravenstein JS: The effect of fatigue on the performance of a simulated anesthetic monitoring task. J Clin Monit 1987; 3:22–24.
44. Asch DA, Parker RM: Sounding board: The Libby Zion case: One step forward or two steps backward? N Engl J Med 1988; 318:771–775.
45. Thorpe KE: House staff supervision and working hours: Implications of regulatory change in New York State. JAMA 1990; 263:3177–3181.
46. Cooper JB, Long CD, Newbower RS, Philip JH: Critical incidents associated with intraoperative exchanges of anesthesia personnel. Anesthesiology 1982; 56:456–461.
47. Krueger GP: Presentation at Society for Technology in Anesthesia Annual Meeting, New Orleans, 1993.
48. Krueger GP: Sustained work, fatigue, sleep loss and performance: A review of the issues. Work Stress 1989; 3:129–141.
49. Comperatore CA, Krueger GP: Circadian rhythm desynchronosis, jet lag, shift lag, and coping strategies. Occup Med 1990; 5:323–341.
50. Daly WM: A dangerous fad [Letter]. JAMA 1974; 228:1370.
51. Schneider AJ, Biebuyck JF: Music in the operating-room. Lancet 1990; 335:1407.
52. MacClelland DC: Music in the operating room. AORN J 1979; 29:252–260.
53. Ayre P: Editorial. Anaesthesia 1980; 35:233–234.
54. Gulledge SL, Kline OR Jr: Use of stereo headphones for patient relaxation during cataract surgery under local anesthesia. Ophthalmic Surg 1981; 12:289–290.
55. Naidu KRC: Music sedation for local analgesia. Anaesthesia 1982; 37:354.
56. Imatran Voima Oy: Loviisa Power Plant. Helsinki. No date.
57. Gild WM: Ethnography in the operating room. *In* Abstracts of the Society for Technology in Anesthesia Annual Meeting, New Orleans, 1993.
58. Weinger MB: Performance shaping factors in anesthesiology. Presentation at Society for Technology in Anesthesia Annual Meeting, New Orleans, 1993.
59. Gordon GH, Hubbell FA, Wyle FA, Charter RA: Stress during internship: A prospective study of mood states. J Gen Intern Med 1986; 1:228–231.
60. Toung TJK, Donham RT, Rogers MC. The stress of giving anesthe-

sia on the electrocardiogram (ECG) of anesthesiologists. Anesthesiology 1984; 61:A465.
61. Rozanski A, Bairey CN, Krantz DS, et al: Mental stress and the induction of silent myocardial ischemia in patients with coronary artery disease. N Engl J Med 1988; 318:1005–1012.
62. Steindler EM: The Impaired Physician. Chicago: American Medical Association, 1975.
63. Spiegelman WG, Saunders L, Mazze RI: Addiction and anesthesiology. Anesthesiology 1984; 60:335–341.
64. Henry PH, Davis TQ, Engleken EJ, Triebwasser JH, Lancaster MC: Alcohol-induced performance decrements assessed by two Link trainer tasks using experienced pilots. Aerospace Med 1974; 45:1180–1189.
65. Franck DH: "If you drink don't drive" motto now applies to hangovers as well. JAMA 1983; 250:1657–1658.
66. Herndon OW, Weinger MB, Englund C: Indices of substance abuse and psychological disturbances in a population of anesthesia providers. Anesthesiology 1992; 77:A1047.
67. Lieberman HR, Wurtman RJ, Emde GG, Roberts C, Coviella ILG: The effects of low-dose caffeine on human performance and mood. Psychopharmacology 1987; 92:308–312.
68. Denson JS, Abrahamson S: A computer-controlled patient simulator. JAMA 1969; 208:504–508.
69. Abrahamson S, Denson J, Wolf R: Effectiveness of a simulator in training anesthesiology residents. J Med Educ 1969; 44:515–519.
70. Hoffman KI, Abrahamson S: The "cost-effectiveness" of Sim One. J Med Educ 1975; 50:1127–1128.
71. Tanner GE, Angers DG, Van Ess DM, Ward CA: ANSIM: An anesthesia simulator for the IBM PC. Comput Methods Programs Biomed 1986; 23:237–242.
72. Philip JH: Gas Man—An example of goal oriented computer-assisted teaching which results in learning. Int J Clin Monit Comput 1986; 3:165–173.
73. Block FE Jr: A controlled, randomized evaluation of the Puritan-Bennett Gas Uptake Simulation (GUS) Computer-Assisted Learning Program. Anesthesiology 1989; 71:A953.
74. Schwid HA, O'Donnell D: The Anesthesia Simulator-Recorder: A device to train and evaluate anesthesiologists' responses to critical incidents. Anesthesiology 1990; 72:191–197.
75. Schwid HA, O'Donnell D: Anesthesiologists' management of simulated critical incidents. Anesthesiology 1992; 76:495–501.
76. Good ML, Gravenstein JS: Anesthesia simulators and training devices. Int Anesthesiol Clin 1989; 27:161–168.
77. Good ML, Gravenstein JS, Mahla ME, et al: Can simulation accelerate the learning of basic anesthesia skills by beginning anesthesia residents? Anesthesiology 1992; 77:A1133.
78. Gaba DM, DeAnda A: A comprehensive anesthesia simulation environment: Re-creating the operating room for research and training. Anesthesiology 1988; 69:387–394.
79. Gaba DM, DeAnda A: The response of anesthesia trainees to simulated critical incidents. Anesth Analg 1989; 68:444–451.
80. DeAnda A, Gaba DM: Unplanned incidents during comprehensive anesthesia simulation. Anesth Analg 1990; 71:77–82.
81. Wiener EL: Human Factors of Advanced Technology ("Glass Cockpit") Transport Aircraft. Washington, DC: NASA Ames Research Center, Technical Report 117528, 1989.
82. Chambers AB, Nagel DC: Pilots of the future? Human or computer? Communications ACM 1985; 28:1187–1199.
83. Mitchell CM: Machine centered vs. human centered automation. *In* Abstracts of the Society for Technology in Anesthesia Annual Meeting, New Orleans, 1993.
84. Smith NT, Brien RA, Pettus DC, Jones BR, Quinn ML, Sarnat A: Recognition accuracy with a voice-recognition system designed for anesthesia record keeping. J Clin Monit 1990; 6:299–306.
85. Block FE Jr: The Diatek Arkive Patient Information Management System. Balliere's Clin Anaesth 1990; 4:159–170.
86. McDonald CJ: Input technology. MD Comput 1990; 7:201–204.
87. Block FE Jr, Burton LW, Rafal MD, et al: Two computer-based anesthetic monitors: The Duke automatic monitoring equipment (DAME) system and the MicroDAME. J Clin Monit 1985; 1:30–51.
88. ANSI/HFS 100-1988: American national standard for human factors engineering of visual display terminal workstations. Santa Monica, CA: The Human Factors Society, Inc., 1988.
89. ASTM F 1161-88: Standard specification for minimum performance and safety requirements of components and systems of anesthesia gas machines. Philadelphia: American Society for Testing and Materials, 1988.
90. Apple Computer: Human Interface Guidelines: The Apple Desktop Interface. Reading, MA: Addison-Wesley, 1987.
91. Block FE Jr: Quality control of data input and output. Int J Clin Monit Comput, in press.
92. Tufte, ER: The Visual Display of Quantitative Information. Cheshire, CT: Graphics Press, 1983.
93. Tufte, ER: Envisioning Information. Cheshire, CT: Graphics Press, 1990.
94. van der Aa JJ, Beneken JEW, van Oostrom JH, Gravenstein JS: Integrated information transfer: A summary display of patient status. J Clin Monit 1992; 8:153–154.
95. Woods DD: Towards a theoretical base for representation design in the computer medium: Ecological perception and aiding human cognition. *In* Flach J, Hancock P, Caird J, Vicente K (eds): The Ecology of Human-Machine Systems. Hillsdale, NJ: Erlbaum, in press.
96. Stokes A, Wickens C, Kite K: Head-Up (HUD) displays. *In* Display Technology: Human Factors Concepts. Warrendale, PA: Society of Automotive Engineers, 1990; Chap 8.
97. Sojourner RJ, Antin JF: The effects of a simulated head-up display speedometer on perceptual task performance. Hum Factors 1990; 32:329–339.
98. McDonald CJ: Private eye and continuous-use clinical computers. MD Comput 1990; 7:352–353.
99. Block FE Jr, Swan JF, Yablok DO, McDonald JS: Clinical evaluation of the "Private Eye": A "heads-up" display of anesthesia data. Anesthesiology 1990; 73:A534.
100. Omogui S, Glass P, Martel DLJ, et al: Blind nasal intubation with audio-capnometry. Anesth Analg 1991; 72:392–393.
101. McIntyre JWR: Ergonomics: Anaesthetists' use of auditory alarms in the operating room. Int J Clin Monit Comput 1985; 2:47–55.
102. Kestin IG, Miller BR, Lockhart CH: Auditory alarms during anesthesia monitoring. Anesthesiology 1988; 69:106–109.
103. Block FE Jr, Detko GJ Jr: Minimizing interference and false alarms from electrocautery in the Nellcor N-100 pulse oximeter. J Clin Monit 1986; 2:203–205.
104. Schulte GT, Block FE, Jr: Comparison of non-invasive blood pressure measurements on the arm and the ankle. Anesthesiology 1989; 71:A408.
105. Pan PH: False alarm distribution in intra-operative pulse oximetry. Anesthesiology 1992; 77:A494.
106. ECRI. Multiple medical gas monitors. Health Devices 1990; 19:207–240.
107. Navabi MJ, Watt RC, Hameroff SR, Mylrea KC: Integrated monitoring can detect critical events and improve alarm accuracy. J Clin Eng 1991; 16:295–306.
108. Brunner JX, Westenskow DR, Zelenov P: Prototype ventilator and alarm recognition algorithm for the NASA space station. J Clin Monit 1989; 5:90–99.
109. Block FE Jr, McDonald JS: An expert system to teach how to troubleshoot common problems of an automated anesthesia record-keeper. Anesthesiology 1990; 73:A1087.
110. Artificial Neural Networks. No. 11 of "Anesthesia Advances." Nutley, NJ: Roche Laboratories, 1992.
111. Westenskow DW: Artificial intelligence. Presentation at Society for Technology in Anesthesia Annual Meeting, New Orleans, 1993.
112. Egbert TP, Westenskow DR: Detection of artifact in pulse oximetry signals using a neural network. Anesthesiology 1992; 77:A521.
113. Baker PD, Küch K, Orr JA, Westenskow DR: Improved thermodilution cardiac output using neural networks. Anesthesiology 1992; 77:A476.
114. Narus SP, Egbert TP, Lee TK, Lu J, Westenskow DR: An artificial neural network oscillometric algorithm for the temporal artery. Anesthesiology 1992; 77:A549.
115. Strong KM, Fine PG, Orr JA, Westenskow DR: Neural network quantification of air embolism using Doppler ultrasound. Anesthesiology 1992; 77:A516.
116. Westenskow DR, Orr JA, Simon FH, Bender H, Frankenberger H: Intelligent alarms reduce anesthesiologist's response time to critical faults. Anesthesiology 1992; 77:1074–1079.
117. ISO 9703-1:1992(E). Anaesthesia and respiratory care alarm signals—Part 1: Visual alarm signals. Geneva: International Organization for Standardization, 1992.
118. Finley GA, Cohen AJ: Perceived urgency and the anaesthetist: Re-

sponses to common operating room monitor alarms. Can J Anaesth 1991; 38:958–964.
119. Loeb RG, Jones BR, Leonard RA, Behrman K: Recognition accuracy of current operating room alarms. Anesth Analg 1992; 75:499–505.
120. Patterson RD: Guidelines for the design of auditory warning sounds. Proc Inst Acoust 1989; 11(5):17–24.
121. Patterson RD: Guidelines for auditory warning systems on civil aircraft. London: Civil Aviation Authority Report 82017, 1982.
122. Kerr JH: Warning devices. Br J Anaesth 1985; 57:696–708.
123. Weinger MB: Proposed new alarm standards may make a bad situation worse [Letter]. Anesthesiology 1991; 74:791–792.
124. Block FE Jr: Evaluation of users' abilities to recognize musical alarm tones. J Clin Monit 1992; 8:285–290.
125. Edworthy J, Loxley S, Dennis I: Improving auditory warning design: Relationship between warning sound parameters and perceived urgency. Hum Factors 1991; 33:205–231.

CHAPTER 3

Electrical Safety*

JEFFREY J. SCHWARTZ, M.D.
and JAN EHRENWERTH, M.D.

Although the importance of a finger on the pulse and an eye on the patient cannot be diminished, monitoring of the anesthetized patient in the 1990s requires a multitude of electronic devices. This equipment is often intentionally connected to the patient and used in an environment in which saline solutions spill and catheters enter the heart. Certainly, no one would feel perfectly comfortable adjusting a radio while standing in a bathtub; the operating room presents similar hazards. In hospitals, 40% of electrical accidents occur in the operating room (OR).[1] Fortunately, electrocution is a rare event in the OR. This is due, in part, to various safeguards incorporated into both the electrical supply and the monitoring equipment. It is the responsibility of anesthesiologists to be familiar with electrical safety matters so that they may protect the patient and the operating room personnel.

PRINCIPLES OF ELECTRICITY

It is impossible to understand the principles of electrical safety without a basic understanding of electricity and its biologic effects. Electrical current (I), the flow of electrons through a resistance (R) in a complete circuit, is measured in amperes. The drive that moves the electrons is the voltage or the electromotive force (E), measured in volts. The relationship between the applied voltage and the resulting current is given by Ohm's law:

$$E = I \times R$$

Practitioners may find that the relationship between the driving force of the circulation and the flow of blood, MAP = CO × SVR, where MAP is mean arterial pressure, CO is cardiac output, and SVR is systemic vascular resistance, makes Ohm's law more intuitive. Electric power is measured in watts and can be calculated by the formula W = E × I, where W is the power dissipated. The energy or work performed by electricity is equal to the power multiplied by the duration of the current flow. Some numeric examples may clarify these relationships.

Consider a 1200-W hair dryer that is powered by a conventional 120-V household outlet. The current flow through the dryer is 1200 W / 120 V = 10 A (W = E × I). The resistance of the hair dryer is 120 V / 10 A = 12 Ω (E = I × R). If the dryer is used for 6 minutes, one tenth of an hour, the energy dissipated is 1200 W × 1/10 hour = 120 watt-hours or, more conventionally, 0.12 kilowatt-hours.

Dry intact skin has a resistance of approximately 100,000 Ω. If a person with this skin resistance accidentally becomes part of a 120-V electrical circuit, a current of 120/100,000 = 1.2 mA would flow through that person. As discussed below, this current is not dangerous and is, in fact, barely perceptible. However, wet skin may have a resistance as low as 1000 Ω. If a person then contacts the same 120 V, a current of 120/1000 = 120 mA will flow, which would likely be fatal.

ALTERNATING CURRENT

When electron flow is always in one direction it is termed "direct current" (DC). Batteries generate DC. When the flow of current periodically reverses itself, it is referred to as "alternating current" (AC).[2] Commercial utility companies in the United States generate electricity as AC to allow for easier distribution. The physics of AC is somewhat more complicated than that of DC. Surprisingly, a coiled piece of wire that would offer virtually no resistance to direct current will impede alternating current.[3] Conversely, a circuit that contains a gap or no physical connection may allow alternating current to pass. The sum of the forces that oppose current flow in an AC circuit is termed "impedance" and is designated by the letter Z.

A capacitor is defined as any two conductors separated by an insulator. A capacitor can store a charge on its con-

*Adapted in part from Ehrenwerth J: Electrical safety. *In* Barash PG, Cullen BF, Stoelting RK (eds): Clinical Anesthesia, 2nd Ed. Philadelphia: JB Lippincott, 1992.

ductors when a voltage is applied; the quantity of that charge, in proportion to the voltage, is the capacitance (C). When a DC voltage is initially applied to a capacitor, current flows briefly through the wires, but not across the capacitor, and charges accumulate on the conductors.[4] If an AC voltage is applied, the capacitor will alternately charge and discharge, and there will be a constant AC current in the wires. The opposition to electron flow in a capacitor is called the "capacitive impedance" and is inversely proportional to the frequency of the applied voltage. Direct current is blocked by a capacitor; high-frequency alternating currents pass easily.

A capacitor need not be a fixed, constructed device. Any two conductors separated by an insulator will have some capacitance, known as "stray capacitance."[5] The patient or the anesthesiologist may be one of the conductors. This situation implies that despite being apparently physically disconnected and apart from electrical sources, small and possibly dangerous currents still may flow.

Any wire with a current flowing through it is associated with a magnetic field. The ability to store energy in the magnetic field is the wire's inductance (L). If the current is changing, as in AC, the magnetic field will be changing; this changing magnetic field actually opposes electron flow. This opposition is inductive impedance and is directly proportional to frequency. Inductance is less relevant than capacitance to electrical safety.

PHYSIOLOGY OF ELECTRIC SHOCK

What exactly is the risk from electrical shock and how does it come about? Electrical shocks occur when a person becomes part of or completes an electrical circuit. Thus, to receive a shock, one must contact the electrical circuit at two different points at different voltages. By Ohm's law, a current will then flow that is proportional to the voltage difference and inversely proportional to the impedance. Birds can sit happily on high voltage wires because they are contacting only one part of a circuit.

The physiologic effects of electric shock depend on the current (which, by Ohm's law, is determined by the voltage and impedance), the duration of contact, the frequency at which the current changes direction, and the area through which the current flows. Electrical shock may be divided into two categories, essentially depending on the path of current flow. Macroshock refers to large amounts of current flowing through intact skin, which can cause injury. Microshock refers to very small amounts of current that are dangerous because they are applied directly to the myocardium.[6, 7]

This can occur in the electrically susceptible patient (i.e., one who has an external conductor in direct contact with the heart). This may be a pacemaker wire or a saline-filled central venous catheter. Currents as low as 80 μA, when delivered through such a catheter, may cause ventricular fibrillation, because all the current is concentrated over a small area.[8] This is 1/1000th the current that could cause fibrillation if applied externally.

Table 3–1 lists the effects of progressively increasing currents applied to the skin. Note that, as discussed in the numeric examples above, widely different currents may flow, depending on the skin resistance. The longer the duration of contact, the more energy that will be dissipated in the victim. Significant thermal burns are uncommon with household current but are a feature of lightning injuries and high-tension accidents. Ventricular fibrillation is more likely to develop with prolonged contact because of stimulation during the relative refractory period of the heart.

Electrical shock does most of its damage by interfering with electrically excitable tissue: brain, nerve, heart, and skeletal muscle. Nerve stimulation leads to pain, whereas muscle stimulation leads to sustained contraction. Indeed, a current of 10–20 mA leads to sustained contractions and to the inability of a conscious victim to release an energized wire. This is the "let-go" current, more properly termed the "can't-let-go" current.[9, 10] Stimulation of the heart can lead to ventricular fibrillation and cardiac tetany. Of course, DC applied to the chest wall can also treat fibrillation. Current through the brain can lead to unconsciousness and respiratory paralysis.

The electrosurgical unit (ESU) illustrates the influence of frequency on the danger of electric current. Surgeons regularly "electrocute" their patients with high-amperage, high-frequency current. The only ill effect is a thermal burn at the tip of the ESU pencil, which occurs because the operating frequency of the ESU is so high that cardiac and neural tissues are not excited. Interestingly, the frequency of commercial electricity in the United States—60 Hz—is probably the most dangerous one in terms of electrical shock hazard.[11]

GROUNDED POWER

The electric company supplies electrical current via two wires. The voltage between these wires is well maintained at about 120 V. An uncommon mechanism of injury is simultaneous contact with both wires, thus completing a circuit. Pets and toddlers may lick or chew electric outlets or wires to produce such an injury.

The electric company, to increase safety in the distribution and delivery of electrical power, connects one of the two wires to earth ground, usually via a large conducting rod buried deep in the earth. This wire is the neutral wire; the other is called the hot wire. The electrical power is thus considered grounded.

This arrangement, unfortunately, makes electrocution easier (Fig. 3–1). To reiterate, in order for a person to sustain an electrical shock, he or she must become part of an electric circuit. If a person is in electrical contact with the earth, he or she has already made one of the contacts to complete a circuit. Only one additional contact point is necessary to complete the circuit and to receive an electrical shock. The reasoning behind the classic admonition not to

TABLE 3–1. EFFECTS OF 60-Hz AC ON THE AVERAGE HUMAN FOR A 1-SECOND DURATION OF CONTACT

Current	Effect
Macroshock	
1 mA (0.001 A)	Threshold of perception
5 mA (0.005 A)	Accepted as maximum harmless current intensity
10–20 mA (0.01–0.02 A)	"Let-go" current before sustained muscle contraction
50 mA (0.05 A)	Pain, possible fainting, mechanical injury; heart and respiratory functions continue
100–300 mA (0.1–0.3 A)	Ventricular fibrillation will start but respiratory centers remain intact
6000 mA (6 A)	Sustained myocardial contractions, followed by normal heart rhythm; temporary respiratory paralysis; burns if current density is high
Microshock	
10 μA (0.01 mA)	Recommended maximum allowable 60–Hz leakage current
100 μA (0.1 mA)	Ventricular fibrillation

A = ampere; mA = milliampere; μA = microampere.

touch a bathroom light switch while standing in a puddle of water is now apparent. In this situation, current could flow from a faulty switch through the person, out through the feet, and through the puddle, which might be in contact with a water pipe, which is connected to the earth, which is where the electric company has connected its neutral wire.

A similar situation could occur in the OR. There is a 120-V potential difference between the hot wire and the neutral wire as well as between the hot wire and earth ground. Over time, the insulation covering wires may deteriorate, and the bare hot wire may internally come into contact with the case of an electrical instrument and constitute a shock hazard. Touching the equipment while contacting earth ground will lead to an electrical shock, because the person is contacting the circuit at two points.

Modern electrical wiring and equipment provide a safety feature to decrease the risk when contacting an energized chassis. In addition to the hot and neutral wires, a third equipment ground wire is part of the electrical distribution system to all electrical outlets. This is the part of the electrical outlet that is round rather than flat. This wire is also connected to the earth ground. Most modern electrical equipment connects the chassis to the ground wire via the third prong. When the chassis is connected to the equipment ground wire, the equipment is said to be grounded. Normally, no current would be expected to flow through the ground wire. However, if the chassis were to become energized, the bulk of the electrical current would be shunted to earth ground via the equipment ground wire (Fig. 3–2). If the current were large enough, the circuit breaker would trip. (It should be noted that fuses or circuit breakers interrupt current to a circuit when the current flow exceeds a designated amount. They are intended to prevent electrical fires due to overheating of wires. They do little to protect against electrical shock because they generally do not trigger until the current is well above lethal levels.) If a person contacts an energized but grounded chassis, he or she might receive a shock, but it would unlikely be fatal. This safety feature requires the consistent use of grounded equipment and the utter avoidance of "cheater plugs" that allow a three-pronged piece of equipment to plug into a two pronged outlet without connection of the third prong to earth ground.

ISOLATED POWER

Because a large part of the potential risk for electrical shock appears to be due to the grounding of the electrical power supply and the ubiquitous connections of people to earth ground, it seems reasonable to utilize an ungrounded, or isolated, power supply to decrease this risk. In this case, neither of the two wires supplying current is connected to earth ground.

Grounded electrical power can be converted to isolated power by means of an isolation transformer. This device uses electromagnetic induction to induce current in the ungrounded secondary winding of the transformer from energy supplied to the grounded primary winding. There is no electrical connection between the electrical power supplied

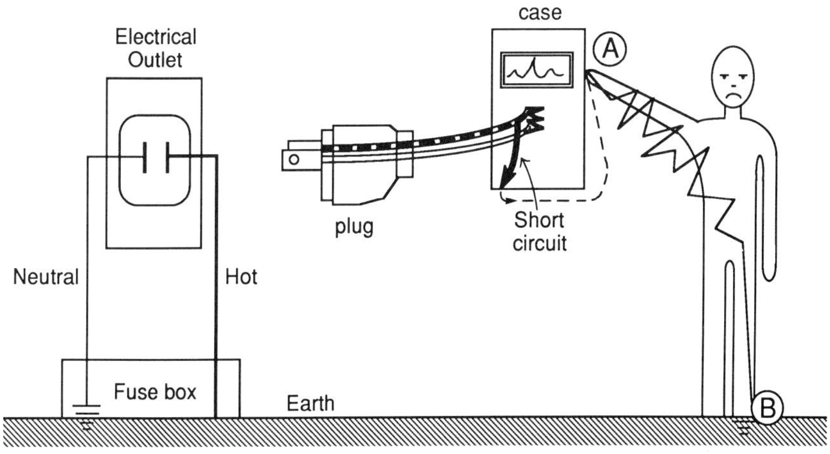

Figure 3–1. When a faulty piece of equipment without an equipment ground wire is plugged into an electric outlet that does not incorporate a ground wire, the case of the instrument will become hot. If an individual touches the hot case (point A), he or she will receive a shock, because standing on the earth (point B) completes the circuit. The current (dotted line) will flow from the instrument through the individual touching the hot case. (From Ehrenwerth J: Electrical safety. *In* Barash PG, Cullen BF, Stoelting RK (eds): Clinical Anesthesia, 2nd Ed. Philadelphia: JB Lippincott, 1992.)

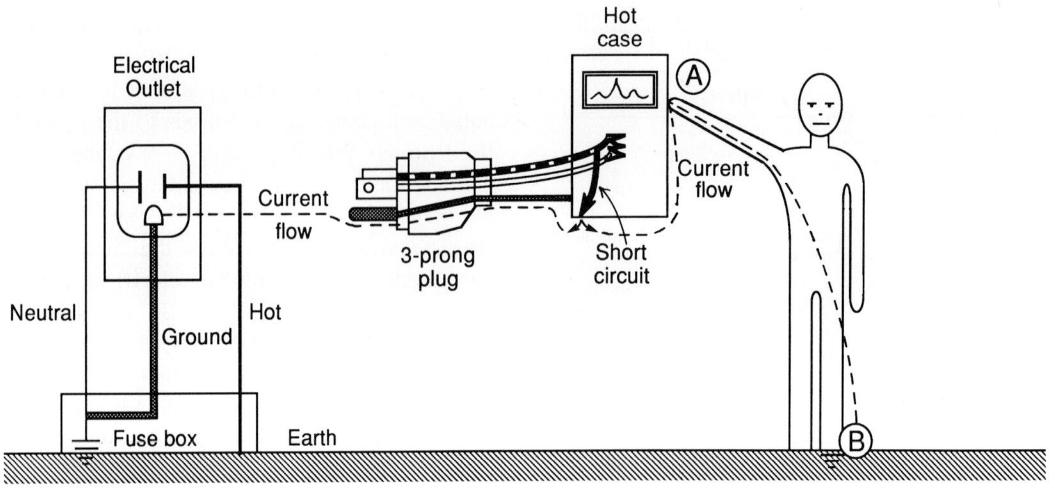

Figure 3–2. When a faulty piece of equipment that incorporates an equipment ground wire is properly connected to an electric outlet with a grounding connection, the current (dotted line) will preferentially flow through the low-resistance ground wire. A person touching the case (point A) and standing on the ground (point B) will still complete the circuit; however, only a small part of the current will flow through the person. (From Ehrenwerth J: Electrical safety. *In* Barash PG, Cullen BF, Stoelting RK (eds): Clinical Anesthesia, 2nd Ed. Philadelphia: JB Lippincott, 1992.)

by the utility company and the power delivered to the electrical outlets. Thus, for safety reasons, in the isolated power system the equipment ground wire is still connected to earth ground; however, the power supply to the electrical outlets has no earth ground connection. The two secondary wires have a 120-V potential difference between them and no relationship to ground. The terms ''hot'' and ''neutral'' no longer make sense, so the wires are designated ''line 1'' and ''line 2'' (Fig. 3–3).

In an isolated power system, if our potential victim is standing in a puddle of water, is connected to earth ground, and contacts one part of the isolated power circuit through a faulty chassis, he or she does *not* complete any circuit and will not receive a shock. That person has contacted one point of one circuit (isolated) and another point in an electrically distinct circuit (grounded). Because this person does not contact either the isolated or the grounded circuit at two points, there is no current flow (Fig. 3–4).

The use of an equipment ground wire and connection of the chassis of the instrument to earth ground is still important in the isolated power system. Should one of the wires fray and come into contact with the chassis, no current will flow to ground, and there is no shock hazard. The system will no longer be isolated from ground, however, and will, in fact, be identical to the original grounded power electrical system. It will require a second mishap (i.e., another piece of faulty equipment) to pose an electrical hazard. In that unlikely event, the ground wire will still shunt most of the current to earth ground. It is a distinct advantage of the isolated power system that the first faulty piece of equip-

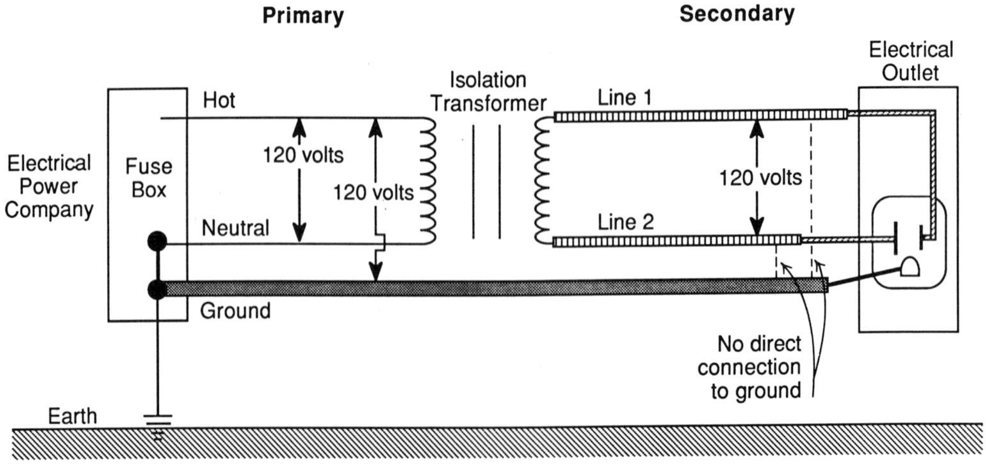

Figure 3–3. In the operating room, the isolation transformer converts the grounded power on the primary side to an ungrounded power system on the secondary side of the transformer. A 120-volt potential difference exists only between line 1 and line 2. There is no direct connection between the power on the secondary side and the ground. The equipment ground wire is still present, however. (From Ehrenwerth J: Electrical safety. *In* Barash PG, Cullen BF, Stoelting RK (eds): Clinical Anesthesia, 2nd Ed. Philadelphia: JB Lippincott, 1992.)

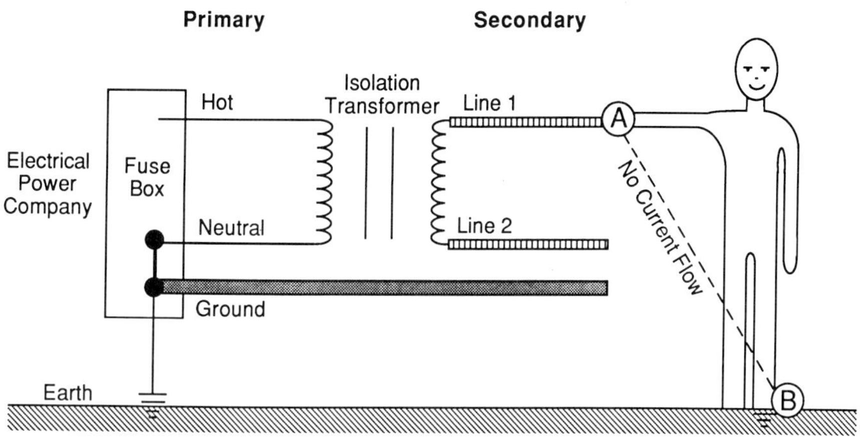

Figure 3–4. A safety feature of the isolated power system is illustrated. A person contacting one side of the isolated power system (point A) and standing on the ground (point B) will not receive a shock. In this instance, the person is not contacting the circuit at two points and thus is not completing the circuit. Point A *(cross-hatched lines)* is part of the isolated power system, and point B is part of the primary or grounded side of the circuit *(solid lines)*. (From Ehrenwerth J: Electrical safety. *In* Barash PG, Cullen BF, Stoelting RK (eds): Clinical Anesthesia, 2nd Ed. Philadelphia: JB Lippincott, 1992.)

ment will continue to function safely, because it may be life supporting equipment.

It was somewhat incorrect to state that there was no electrical connection between the earth ground and secondary circuit of the isolation transformer. As discussed earlier, stray capacitance exists between any two conductors and, when AC is involved, small leakage currents may flow from the isolated power lines to ground, thus degrading the isolation. These currents generally are small, 1–2 mA in total, and may be perceptible, but not dangerous.

The integrity of the isolation is key to its acting as a safety feature. Because a malfunctioning device will continue to work normally in an isolated power supply, there must be some means for detecting the problem before a second fault can occur. This detector is the line isolation monitor (LIM). The LIM continually checks the impedance between each of the isolated power lines and ground (Fig. 3–5). Rather than display the impedance, the LIM calculates how much current would flow to ground in the event of a first fault. Normally and ideally, the impedance would be infinite and the current would be zero. The inevitable stray capacitance and leakage currents reduce the impedance somewhat. Modern LIMs are set to trigger an audible and visual alarm when the current exceeds 5 mA.[12] By Ohm's law, this represents an impedance of 24,000 Ω (120 V/0.005 A). Older LIMs triggered at 2 mA (60,000 Ω).

The LIM will trigger an alarm when a faulty piece of equipment is connected to the isolated power circuit. This will be a true fault to ground with a small impedance from one line to ground. The system is now equivalent to a grounded power supply but is still perfectly safe. It would require another fault, in the same or in a different device,

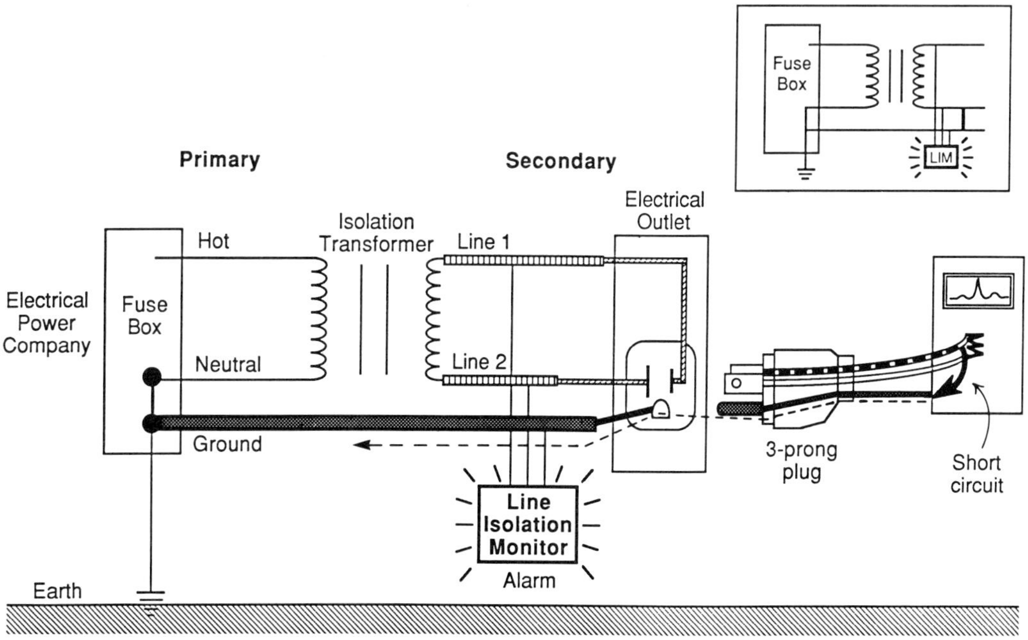

Figure 3–5. When a faulty piece of equipment is plugged into the isolated power system, it will decrease markedly the impedance from line 1 or line 2 to the ground. This change will be detected by the LIM, which will sound an alarm. (From Ehrenwerth J: Electrical safety. *In* Barash PG, Cullen BF, Stoelting RK (eds): Clinical Anesthesia, 2nd Ed. Philadelphia: JB Lippincott, 1992.)

to pose a true risk of shock. The device that triggered the LIM should be removed from operation and serviced as soon as possible but, because there is no immediate threat, the device may continue to be used if it is essential to the care of the patient.

The LIM also may trigger an alarm if many pieces of normally functioning equipment are all connected to the same isolated power supply. Although each piece may have a small leakage current, the sum may exceed the 5-mA threshold. For instance, if 30 devices, each with a 200-μA leakage current, are connected to the same power supply, the total leakage current would be 6 mA, and the LIM would trigger. The change in threshold from 2 mA to 5 mA was prompted by an attempt to prevent this false alarm.

When the LIM alarm sounds, the anesthesiologist should unplug each device in the room, one at a time (generally the most recently plugged items first), until the alarm disappears. This device should be removed for servicing unless it is essential at the time. If no faulty device is found, the possibility should be considered that too many functioning devices are causing the total leakage current to exceed threshold, thus triggering the LIM.

The equipment ground wire becomes more important in the isolated power system. If this wire is broken or defeated with a cheater plug, a faulty piece of equipment that is plugged into an outlet will operate normally, but the LIM will not alarm. The LIM can only sense the reduced impedance to ground and lack of isolation if the device's equipment ground wire is connected to ground.

GROUND FAULT CIRCUIT INTERRUPTERS

A ground fault circuit interrupter (GFCI) is an inexpensive, alternative method of decreasing the risk of shock when isolated power is not utilized. In a working electrical circuit, the current in the hot wire must be equal to the current in the neutral wire; what goes in must come out. If a person becomes part of the circuit, some of the current will pass through that person to ground. Therefore, there will be a difference in current between the two limbs of the circuit. The GFCI monitors both sides of the circuit for equality of current flow. If the difference between the currents exceeds a threshold, typically 5 mA, the GFCI will interrupt the power to the circuit. GFCIs are reliable devices. Modern building codes actually require them in ''wet locations'' such as bathroom, kitchen, and outdoor outlets. Curiously, ORs are not always considered wet locations in the building codes. The main disadvantage of the GFCI in the operating room is that the first warning that a piece of equipment is defective is that it turns off. A GFCI may be monitoring several devices, all of which will lose power if one of them is faulty. In addition, before the power can be restored, the faulty device must be identified and unplugged. This can be a serious problem if the equipment is life-supporting, such as a ventilator or cardiopulmonary bypass pump.

OPERATING ROOM CONSTRUCTION

The anesthesiologist is frequently called upon to help design new ORs. In 1984, the National Fire Protection Association (NFPA) revised its standards regarding isolated power systems in operating rooms. Currently, only ORs in which flammable agents are used are required to have isolated power systems. Operating rooms in which nonflammable agents are used may have isolated power systems, GFCIs or maybe even no protection at all. If the area is considered a wet location, isolated power systems or GFCIs are required.

Anesthesiologists need to be aware of these changes and to insist that some form of protection be installed for patients and operating room personnel. It is best to have isolated power because this system is safe *by design* and will limit fault current to less than 5 mA. GFCIs are acceptable, but they are an active system and require a fault current to be flowing before they interrupt the circuit. As noted above, if many outlets are protected by one GFCI, serious problems could result from patient monitors or life support equipment being shut off. If GFCIs are used, the best system is to have each electrical outlet in the room be its own branch circuit and be protected by an individual GFCI. It would be foolhardy to eliminate these important safety systems in order to obtain a small reduction in the cost of constructing the operating room.[13, 14]

MICROSHOCK

Neither isolated power nor GFCIs can protect an electrically susceptible patient from the minuscule currents that represent a microshock hazard. When applied directly to the myocardium, currents as low as 80 μA may cause ventricular fibrillation.[15, 16] This is well below the threshold of perception (1000 μA) and well below the 5000-μA current that would trigger an LIM or a GFCI.

The stray capacitance that is part of any AC-powered circuit can cause a significant charge to build up on the chassis of a piece of equipment. The anesthesiologist who touches this chassis and then contacts the electrically susceptible patient may cause a lethal, though imperceptible current to flow directly into the heart. The principal protection against microshock is the presence of an intact, functional equipment ground wire in all OR devices. Just as it provides a low resistance path to ground for large currents that may flow in the event of a fault, the ground wire also provides a low-resistance path for pervasive leakage currents. Figure 3–6 illustrates a situation involving a patient who has a saline-filled catheter in the heart, with a resistance of approximately 500 Ω. The equipment ground wire has a resistance of 1 Ω. A leakage current of 100 μA due to stray capacitance will only cause 0.2 μA to flow into the patient while 99.8 μA take the lower-resistance path to ground. If the ground wire were broken, all 100 μA would flow into the patient. Extra care must be taken when man-

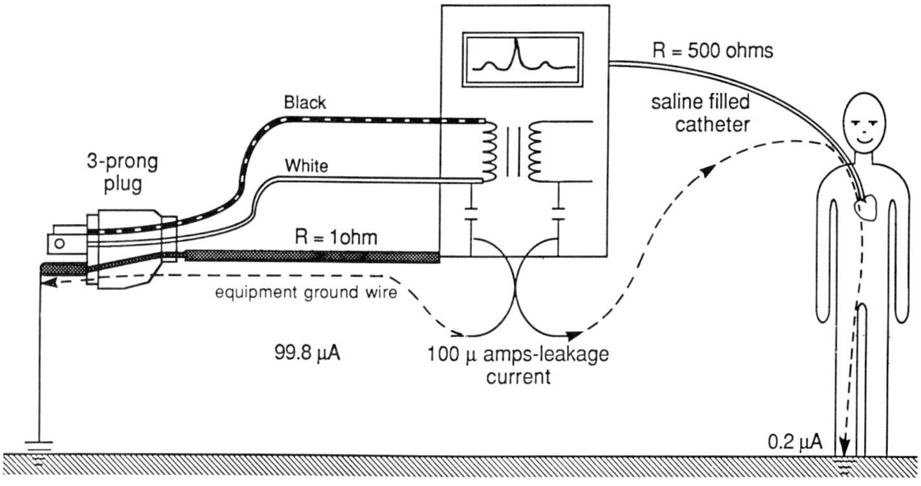

Figure 3–6. The electrically susceptible patient is protected from microshock by an intact equipment ground wire. The equipment ground wire provides a low-impedance path along which most of the leakage current *(dotted lines)* can flow. (From Ehrenwerth J: Electrical safety. *In* Barash PG, Cullen BF, Stoelting RK (eds): Clinical Anesthesia, 2nd Ed. Philadelphia: JB Lippincott, 1992).

aging the electrically susceptible patient. Gloves should be worn when touching intracardiac catheters or pacemaker wires. Medical personnel should not simultaneously touch these catheters and other electrical devices.

Additional protection against microshock is obtained by attempting to isolate any electrical connection to the patient, such as electrocardiogram leads, from the power supply of the monitor. The original OR electrocardiogram actually intentionally connected the patient to the power supply to reduce the noise in the signal.[17] This is now recognized as foolhardy. Optical isolators, transformers, and high-impedance amplifiers assure that leakage current is minimal between the monitor and the patient while allowing easy passage of the physiologic signal.

ELECTROSURGERY

The electrosurgical unit (ESU) operates by generating very-high-frequency currents (500,000 to 5,000,000 Hz). Heat is produced whenever a current flows through a resistance. The amount of heat produced is the product of the resistance and the square of the current and is inversely proportional to the area through which the current passes.[18] By concentrating the current at the tip of the ESU pencil, very localized cutting and coagulation can be achieved. As discussed, these high-frequency currents are not an electrical shock hazard. The risk is of thermal burns at unintended sites.[19–24] The ESU current must return to the ESU generally through a dispersive or return electrode (often mistakenly given the misnomer "ground plate") of large surface area. The large surface assures that the area of contact is large and that the current density is small when it exits. If the plate is improperly applied or becomes dislodged so that it covers only a small area, the patient may sustain a burn where the current exits as well as a burn where it enters. The plate usually is the path of least resistance for the return current. If it is improperly applied or the cord connecting it to the unit is malfunctioning, the current will seek a lower-resistance alternative return pathway. If the return pathway is of a small area, such as an ECG electrode, a similar burn can result. Although modern ESUs use a power supply isolated from ground, not unlike the isolated power to the OR, it is impossible to totally isolate the energy. Capacitive impedance decreases as frequency increases; therefore, high-frequency current may travel easily through stray capacitance.

All OR personnel must be vigilant for proper application of the dispersive plate. The plate should be removed as far as possible from ECG leads, pacemaker units, and metal implants. If a surgeon requests a higher power because a proper cut is not being made, this should arouse suspicion that the plate is poorly applied.

REFERENCES

1. Bruner JMR, Aronow S, Cavicchi RV: Electrical incidents in a large hospital: A 42 month register. J Assoc Adv Med Instrum 1972; 6:222–230.
2. Bruner JMR: Hazards of electrical apparatus. Anesthesiology 1967; 28:396–425.
3. Miller F: College Physics, 2nd Ed. New York: Harcourt Brace and World, 1967;457–459.
4. Leonard PF, Gould AB: Dynamics of electrical hazards of particular concern to operating-room personnel. Surg Clin North Am 1965; 45:817–828.
5. Leonard PF: Characteristics of electrical hazards. Anesth Analg 1972; 51:797–809.
6. Weinberg DI, Artley JL, Whalen RE, McIntosh HD: Electric shock hazards in cardiac catheterization. Circ Res 1962; 11:1004–1009.
7. Starmer CF, Whalen RE: Current density and electrically induced ventricular fibrillation. Med Instrum 1973; 7:158–161.
8. Raftery EB, Green HL, Yacoub MH: Disturbances of heart rhythm produced by 50-Hz leakage currents in human subjects. Cardiovasc Res 1975; 9:263–265.
9. Harpell TR: Electrical shock hazards in the hospital environment: Their causes and cures. Can Hosp 1970; 47:48–53.
10. Wald A: Electrical safety in medicine. *In* Skalak R, Chien S (eds): Handbook of Bioengineering. New York: McGraw-Hill, 1987;341.
11. Buczko GB, McKay WPS: Electrical safety in the operating room. Can J Anaesth 1987; 34:315–322.
12. Bernstein MS: Isolated power and line isolation monitors. BioMed Instrum Technol 1990; 24:221–223.
13. Pashayan AG, Ehrenwerth J: Lasers and electrical safety in the operating room. *In* Ehrenwerth J, Eisenkraft JB (eds): Anesthesia Equipment: Principles and Applications. St. Louis: Mosby-Yearbook, 1993;436–469.

14. Matjasko MJ, Ashman MN: All you need to know about electrical safety in the operating room. *In* Barash PG, Deutsch S, Tinker J (eds): ASA Refresher Courses in Anesthesiology, Vol 18. Philadelphia: JB Lippincott, 1990;251.
15. Hull CJ: Electrocution hazards in the operating theatre. Br J Anaesth 1978; 50:647–657.
16. Watson AB, Wright JS, Loughman J: Electrical thresholds for ventricular fibrillation in man. Med J Aust 1973; 1:1179–1182.
17. Bruner JMR, Leonard PF: Electricity, Safety and the Patient. Chicago: Year Book, 1989;43.
18. Dornette WHL: An electrically safe surgical environment. Arch Surg 1973; 107:567–573.
19. Meathe EA: Electrical safety for patients and anesthetists. *In* Saidman LJ, Smith NT (eds): Monitoring in Anesthesia, 2nd Ed. Boston: Butterworth, 1984;497.
20. Rolly G: Two cases of burns caused by misuse of coagulation unit and monitoring. Acta Anaesthesiol Belg 1978; 29:313–316.
21. Parker EO: Electrosurgical burn at the site of an esophageal temperature probe. Anesthesiology 1984; 61:93–95.
22. Schneider AJL, Apple HP, Braun RT: Electrosurgical burns at skin temperature probes. Anesthesiology 1977; 47:72–74.
23. Bloch EC, Burton LW: Electrosurgical burn while using a battery-operated doppler monitor. Anesth Analg 1979; 58:339–342.
24. Becker CM, Malhotra IV, Hedley-Whyte J: The distribution of radiofrequency current and burns. Anesthesiology 1973; 38:106–122.

SECTION

TWO

Monitors of Cardiovascular Function

CHAPTER 4

Electrocardiography: Monitoring for Ischemia

M. STAFFORD SMITH, M.D., C.M., F.R.C.P.(C), F. CLEMENTS, M.D., and N. DEBRUIJN, M.D.

Since the discovery that ischemic myocardium produced alterations in the electrocardiogram (ECG), various ways of displaying these changes have been introduced. Advances in electronics have made ECG diagnosis more accurate and have allowed for its automated analysis. This technology has resulted in the emergence of a vast amount of new information about both symptomatic and silent ischemia over the past few years. Automated on-line ECG analysis facilitates the recognition of abnormalities and trends that previously went unnoticed even in critically ill patients monitored in the operating room or intensive care unit. The significance of ST segment changes occurring in the absence of pain or hemodynamic changes is the subject of many ongoing investigations. It is the intent of this chapter to bring the reader up to date with current theory and technology pertaining to ECG monitoring for ischemia.

ECG MONITORING

The ECG is a graphic recording of the electrical potentials produced by the beating heart. Impulse formation and conduction create small electrical currents that may be detected over the entire body surface. From the infinite number of possible electrode locations, standardized lead systems have been defined for ECG monitoring. Careful application of electrodes is required if maximum information is to be gained from the ECG.

ECG LEAD APPLICATION AND PROBLEMS

Poor signal fidelity is often the primary factor in decreasing the usefulness of an ECG tracing or computer-generated ECG waveform analysis. Attention to electrode placement frequently improves signal quality.[1] An ideal electrode adheres firmly to skin and is easy to remove, while producing minimal electrical noise, electrode-skin impedance, or polarization. Electrodes should not be placed over broken skin or bony prominences. Skin preparation involves hair removal, followed by alcohol cleansing to dislodge oils that may contribute to increased impedance and poor electrode adhesion. Mild superficial abrasion can reduce impedance still further by thinning the keratinized skin layer. Measured impedance of an ECG lead can be reduced from greater than 100,000 Ω in unprepared skin to below 5000 Ω (and often below 3500 Ω) with proper skin preparation.

ECG monitoring is generally a safe noninvasive procedure associated with very few risks. Electrical shock and burns rarely result from ECG monitoring. Failure of operating room electrical safety mechanisms may permit current to pass through the ECG leads that is dense enough at the heart to initiate dysrhythmias, most notably ventricular fibrillation. Use of isolation transformers, line isolation monitors, and ground fault interrupters are designed to reduce the shock hazard. Guidelines demand that leakage current from ECG monitor chassis be below 100 μA, and below 50 μA from ECG leads.[2] When using electrocautery, a large grounding pad with a wide area of contact is essential to disperse current, which when concentrated at the tip of an electrocautery probe is sufficient to vaporize tissue. If the grounding pad has poor or no contact with the patient, the ECG electrodes in some circumstances may offer an alternative route for current passage. Because the electrodes have a relatively small surface area, current is concentrated and may cause burns at the site of electrode application. See Chapter 3.

ECG LEAD SYSTEMS

Twelve standardized leads have been defined for the standard ECG. These fall into three groups: bipolar leads I, II, and III, described by Einthoven and associates[3]; augmented unipolar leads aVR, aVL, and aVF, described by Goldberger[4]; and the unipolar precordial leads defined by Wilson.[5]

Electrodes for the bipolar leads are placed on the right and left arms and on the left leg. The classic approach has been to postulate geometric uniformity around the recording lead system and to construct a reference frame accordingly. Einthoven used a triangle to represent the "axis" of the bipolar limb leads I, II, and III.[3] Einthoven's triangle is an equilateral triangle, positioned in the frontal plane, with its corners representing the two arms and the left leg (Fig. 4–1). This is obviously an oversimplification because several factors are not taken into consideration: the heterogeneous conducting characteristics of the body, the size and shape of the body, and the eccentric position of the heart within the chest. Nevertheless, the three bipolar leads are extremely useful for the detection of rate and rhythm disturbances and of myocardial ischemia.

In 1932, Wilson introduced a new method to measure body surface potentials by referencing them to a "central terminal."[5] Technically this is accomplished by connecting the three bipolar electrodes by 5-KΩ resistors in series to an indifferent central terminal. The potential difference between this common electrode and one of the other active electrodes, designated the "exploring" electrode, then becomes the actual measured potential. This lead system is known as a unipolar lead system. A slightly different technique allows for an approximately 50% augmentation in amplitude of the potentials derived from the unipolar leads; this modification is now routinely employed, accounting for the leads aVR, aVL, and aVF.

The precordial leads (Fig. 4–2) also constitute a unipolar lead system, in which the standard leads form a neutral electrode. The exploring electrode is positioned in one of six locations on the chest wall:

V_1—fourth intercostal space at the right sternal border
V_2—fourth intercostal space at the left sternal border
V_3—equidistant between V_2 and V_4
V_4—fifth intercostal space in the left midclavicular line
V_5—same horizontal plane as V_4, at anterior axillary line
V_6—same horizontal plane as V_4, at midaxillary line

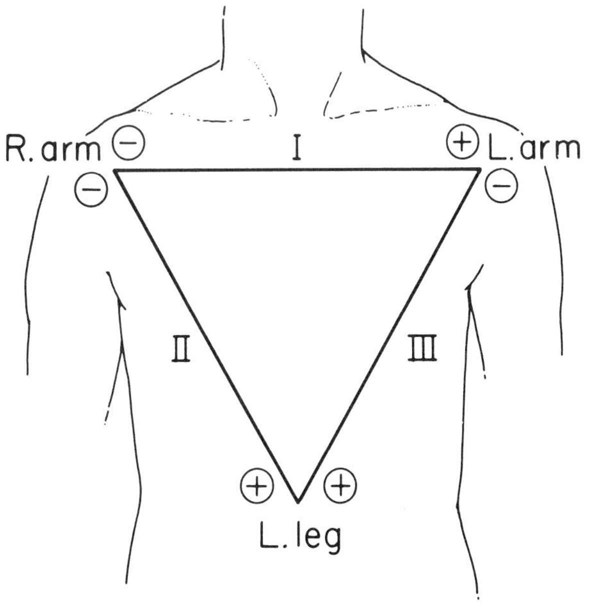

Figure 4–1. Einthoven's triangle: an equilateral triangle in the frontal plane with its corners representing the two arms and the left leg. (From Thys DM: The normal ECG. *In* Thys DM, Kaplan JA. [eds]: The ECG in Critical Care. New York: Churchill Livingstone, 1987; 3.)

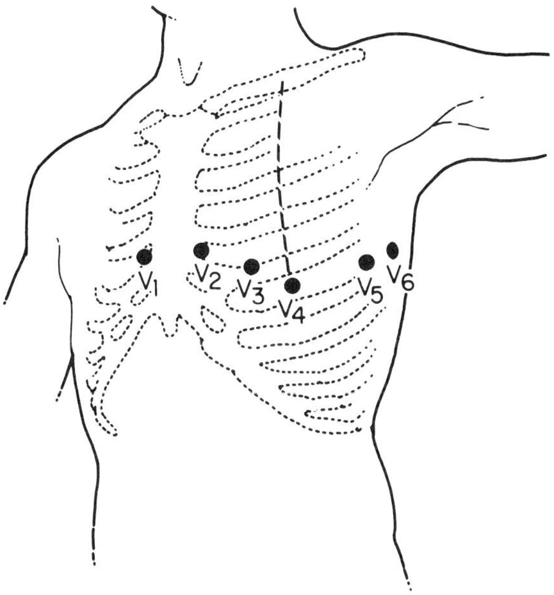

Figure 4–2. Electrode positions for the precordial unipolar leads. The dashed line indicates the midclavicular line. (From Thys DM: The normal ECG. *In* Thys DM, Kaplan JA [eds]: The ECG in Critical Care. New York: Churchill Livingstone, 1987; 6.)

LEAD SELECTION

Precordial leads are more sensitive than the standard leads in the detection of ischemia and are valuable in the diagnosis of left ventricular hypertrophy and bundle-branch block. Information derived from treadmill testing in the 1960s and 1970s showed that over 90% of all exercise-related ischemic episodes detectable from 12-lead ECG are observable in leads II and V_5, with V_5 being the most sensitive single lead for ischemia.[6] Hence, most anesthesiologists chose to monitor leads II and V_5 intraoperatively. The increases in heart rate and cardiac output seen with exercise are not prominent features of most general anesthetics, making exercise a poor model for the cardiovascular changes that precipitate ischemia under anesthesia. London et al in 1988 used 12-lead ECG to monitor 51 intraoperative ischemic episodes in 105 patients with known or suspected coronary artery disease (Fig. 4–3).[7] They noted lead V_5 to be the best single lead for detecting ischemia (74% of episodes), but could only increase the sensitivity to 80% with the addition of lead II. In contrast, lead V_4 alone was the second best lead, demonstrating 61% of ischemic episodes, and the combination of leads V_4 and

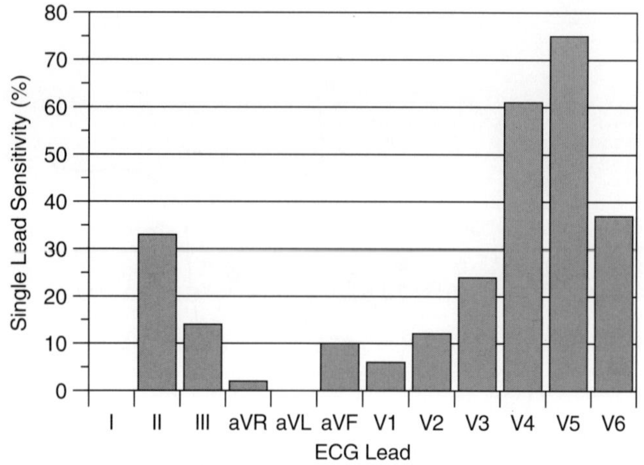

Figure 4–3. Single-lead sensitivity for detection of myocardial ischemia during noncardiac surgery. (From London MJ, Hollenberg M, Wong MG, et al: Intraoperative myocardial ischemia: Localization by continuous 12-lead electrocardiography. Anesthesiology 1988; 69:232–241.)

V_5 increased sensitivity to 90%. The authors concluded that leads II, V_4, and V_5 were the best monitoring combination because they provided 96% sensitivity for ischemic episodes and allowed superior detection of arrhythmias because of the inclusion of lead II.

In certain specialized facilities such as the intensive care unit and the operating room, simultaneous monitoring of several leads is impractical. Therefore, for continuous monitoring, a number of modified bipolar chest leads have been suggested. Some of these are more suited to the detection of arrhythmias than of ischemia. For example, MCL_1 is commonly employed in the intensive care unit because it provides a good P wave; however, CS_5, CM_5, CB_5, and CC_5 have been found more useful for the detection of ischemia.[8, 9] It can be seen from Figure 4–4 and from the subscript ''5'' on each of these named leads that the positive, exploring electrode is placed in the V_5 position on the chest wall. The negative, ''central'' electrode is what varies, as shown. Of these leads, the CS_5 is most often used intraoperatively. Either the CS_5 or the CM_5 lead is a good alternative to a true V_5 lead.

The localization of ischemia with the ECG has been clearly demonstrated.[10] Leads II, III, and aVF reveal disease in the right coronary artery, which supplies the basal part of the left ventricular posterior wall, the posterior third of the interventricular septum, and a large part of the right ventricle. The V leads correspond to anterior, anteroseptal, lateral, and apical ischemia within the distribution of the left anterior descending (LAD) and circumflex coronary arteries. The LAD artery supplies the anterior wall of the left ventricle, the anterior two thirds of the interventricular septum, and part of the right ventricle. In a 12-lead system, V_1, V_2, and V_3 reflect anteroseptal ischemia; V_3, V_4, and V_5 suggest anteroapical ischemia; and V_4, V_5 and V_6 indicate anterolateral ischemia. True posterior wall ischemia produces changes in leads aVL and V_1.

ECG MANIFESTATIONS OF ISCHEMIA

The ECG has long been recognized to change in a predictable fashion with the onset of myocardial ischemia and infarction. However, its limitations as a diagnostic tool must be recognized, because the typical ECG changes of ischemia and infarction may be mimicked or obscured in certain circumstances. As technologies have developed, allowing monitoring of other changes in the cascade of events that herald myocardial ischemia, the ECG has been challenged for its position as the primary perioperative monitor for cardiac ischemic events.

ECG CHANGES WITH ISCHEMIA AND INFARCTION

Electrocardiographic manifestations of ischemia are the result of alterations in repolarization of ischemic myocardium. Depolarization is not primarily affected. Repolarization is delayed in an area of ischemic myocardium. Decreased oxygen supply results in a delayed and abnormal electrical charging of the myocardial cells manifested as changes in the ST segment and the T wave. The sequence of repolarization, proceeding from epicardium to endocardium, is exactly opposite to that of depolarization, giving

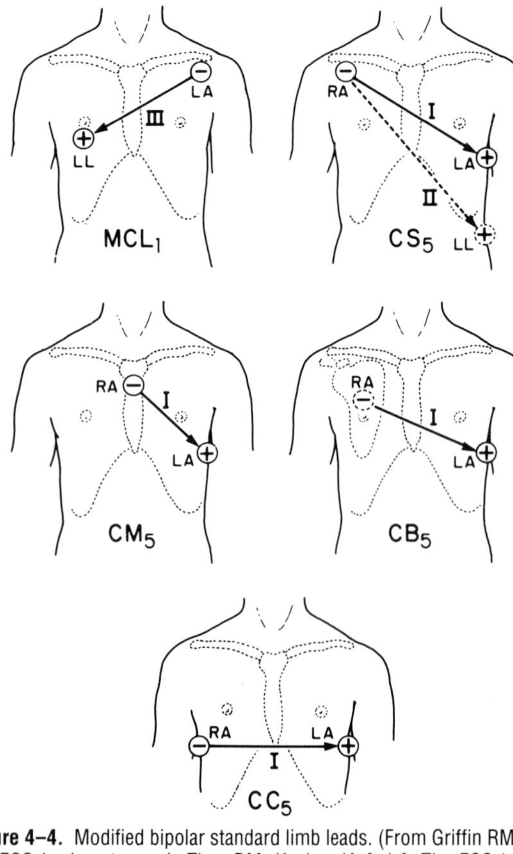

Figure 4–4. Modified bipolar standard limb leads. (From Griffin RM, Kaplan JA: ECG lead systems. *In* Thys DM, Kaplan JA [eds]: The ECG in Critical Care. New York: Churchill Livingstone, 1987; 19.)

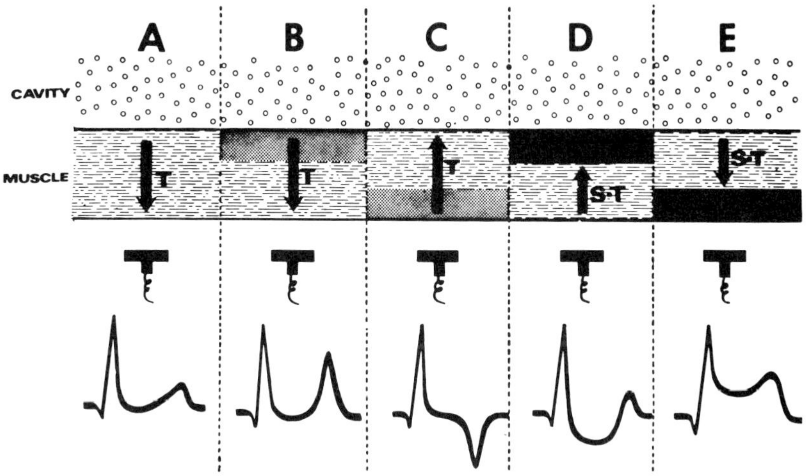

Figure 4–5. *A*, The normal endocardial to epicardial T wave vector. *B*, The T wave vector of subendocardial ischemia. *C*, The T wave vector of subepicardial ischemia. *D*, The ST segment vector of subendocardial injury. *E*, The T wave vector of subepicardial injury. (From Schamroth L: The Electrocardiography of Coronary Artery Disease. Oxford: Blackwell, 1984; 7.)

rise to an upright T wave following an upright QRS complex (Fig. 4–5*A*).

Symmetric T wave changes are manifestations of ischemia, abnormal ST segment changes represent an injury pattern, and abnormal Q waves show myocardial necrosis. Ischemia tends to begin in the subendocardium, which is the last region to receive blood flow from the epicardially situated coronary arteries. When ischemia is confined to the subendocardium, the forces of repolarization are increased, resulting in tall, peaked T waves (Figs. 4–5*B* and 4–6). However, when ischemia is transmural, implying subepicardial involvement, the direction of repolarization is reversed and travels from endocardium to epicardium. The T wave then becomes inverted (Fig. 4–5*C*). Note that in leads aVR, V_1, and V_2, where the QRS complex and T wave are normally negative, the polarity of the T wave is reversed and becomes upright.

Ischemic changes may be seen only in leads that "face" the affected myocardium. Thus, anterior wall ischemia may be evident only in a V lead and not in any limb leads. However, reciprocal changes may appear in leads on the opposite side of the heart such that posterior wall ischemia, for example, may produce an upright T wave in V_1. Other factors that affect ST segment and T waves, such as digoxin, quinidine, electrolyte imbalances, or left ventricular hypertrophy, tend to affect all leads, unlike ischemia, which is almost always a localized process.

With persistent or more severe ischemia, the ECG may develop a pattern that is characteristic of a reversible myocardial injury, and this may precede the development of a true infarction. Two currents of injury are recognized: diastolic and systolic. The diastolic current occurs in resting cells because of the electrical gradient that exists between tissue with a normal resting potential and ischemic tissue, which has an altered, more positive, resting potential.[11] The systolic current of injury occurs during myocardial activation when the wavefront is distorted by the altered properties of the ischemic tissue. As the stimulus passes through the ischemic region, the partially depolarized cells either do not depolarize further or generate a modified action potential with an early repolarization.

Current flows from regions of relative positivity to regions of relative negativity. In the resting state, the diastolic injury current flows from ischemic to normal tissue. An ECG recording from an electrode overlying the ischemic area exhibits depression of the TP segment (Fig. 4–7) with a subepicardial injury. As electrical activation proceeds from normal into ischemic tissue, the action potentials become distorted and shortened with early repolarization. Injured tissue becomes relatively more negative than the nor-

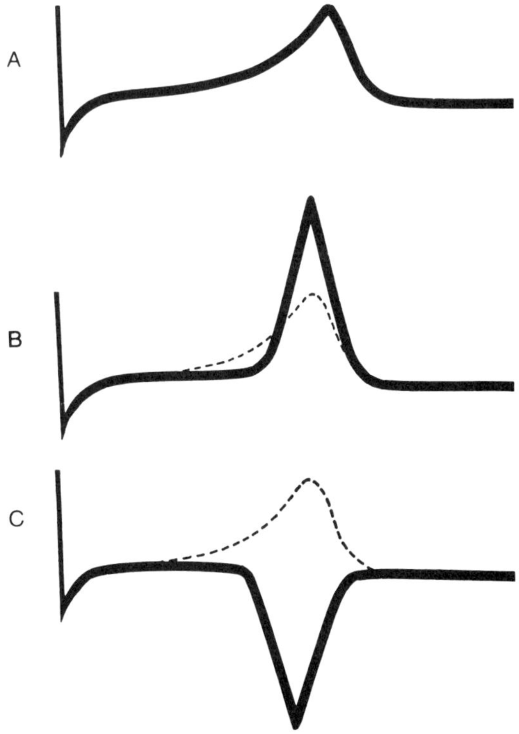

Figure 4–6. *A*, Normal ST segment and T wave. *B*, *C*, The T wave of myocardial ischemia. (From Schamroth L: The Electrocardiography of Coronary Artery Disease. Oxford: Blackwell, 1984; 5.)

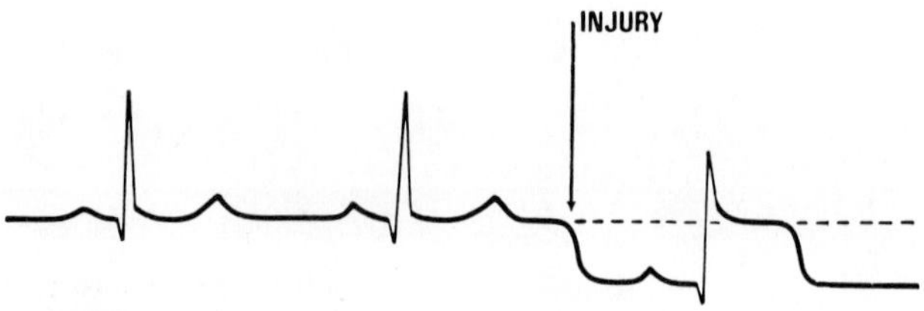

Figure 4–7. Depression of the TP segment at the onset of myocardial injury. (From Schamroth L: The Electrocardiography of Coronary Artery Disease. Oxford: Blackwell, 1984; 22.)

mal tissue, and the current of injury is reversed. Thus, true ST segment elevation occurs (systolic current of injury). The ST segment elevation apparent on the surface ECG with subepicardial ischemia (see Fig. 4–5*E*) can therefore be simulated by TP or ''baseline'' depression, or it may involve true elevation of the ST segment. This differs from the appearance of subendocardial ischemia (see Fig. 4–5*D*), in which the recording electrode records a positive resting diastolic current (TP elevation) and a negative systolic current (ST depression). Once again, the resultant ST deviation (now depression) appears because of both of these factors. Thus, the ST-segment is depressed with subendocardial ischemia and is elevated with subepicardial or transmural ischemia.

Ellestad and colleagues have defined myocardial ischemia as greater than 1 mm of horizontal or downsloping ST segment depression at a point 0.06 seconds from the J point.[12] Much debate has centered around the importance of defining ischemic ST segment depression at a point 0.06–0.08 seconds after the J point, because it is recognized that J point depression and upsloping ST segments are common occurrences, unassociated with ischemia. However, Stuart and Ellestad noted that subjects with an upsloping ST segment, but with 2 mm of ST segment depression, measured at 0.08 seconds after the J point, had the same incidence of two- and three-vessel coronary disease as did subjects with horizontal ST depression.[13] Downsloping ST segments have been correlated with an increased mortality and with an increased number of diseased coronary vessels, when compared with horizontal ST segments.[14, 15] In addition, the degree of ST segment depression has been correlated with the amount of myocardium involved and the severity of the ischemia.[12] Similarly, the degree of ST segment depression occurring perioperatively has been related to the development of myocardial infarction in patients undergoing coronary artery bypass surgery (Fig. 4–8).[16]

In summary, depressed ST segments occur with subendocardial ischemia. As the ischemia becomes more profound, the ST segments progress from upsloping to horizontal to downsloping, at which time the ischemia may be transmural. ST elevation is also indicative of transmural ischemia, and it may occur in association with evolution of a myocardial infarction.

Progression of ischemia is associated with binding of calcium to the membranes along the intercalated disks, which limits potassium flux. Thus, injury current is ultimately prevented from flowing between cells, and ST segment changes disappear. After the disappearance of the acute ST and T wave changes, myocardial infarction is represented on the ECG only by the Q wave. A Q wave longer than 0.03 seconds correlates well with the presence of a myocardial infarction, except in the presence of bundle-branch block. Fortunately, when there is normal conduction, Q waves of myocardial infarction are localized to a few leads, indicating the site of the infarction. In this circumstance, the presence of Q waves are false-positive findings for infarction only 4% of the time.[17]

ST-SEGMENT DEPRESSION AS A MARKER FOR ISCHEMIA: CONFOUNDING FACTORS

If computer-assisted ST segment trend analysis is to be useful as a reliable indicator of myocardial ischemia, it must be both sensitive and specific. Some of the design features of ECG monitors may reduce the detection of real ischemic ST segment changes. Many factors besides ischemia depress the ST segments, including exercise, left ventricular hypertrophy, bundle-branch blocks, digoxin therapy, hypokalemia, and even postural changes.

Artifacts Due to Electronic Filtering Mechanisms

Electronic-related artifacts are more often encountered with bedside monitoring than during performance of the 12-lead standard ECG, during which the patient does not move or speak. A bedside monitor filters out extraneous signals derived from movement of the patient and preserves the general pattern of the ECG. The potential difference generated by the heart between two surface electrodes is approximately 1 mV, whereas there may be 20 mV across the skin. The latter, however, is a much lower-frequency signal that can be excluded by a filter with a low-frequency cut-off of 0.5 Hz. This frequency cut-off unfortunately may interfere with reproduction of the ST segment, which is a relatively low-frequency portion of the ECG complex—as low as 0.14 Hz.[18] Thus, for closer examination of the ST segment, it is desirable to have a frequency cut-off below this level. Many ECG monitors allow for the manual selection of one of two levels: a monitor mode with a frequency

	Perioperative ST Segment Depression		
	None	0.10–0.19 mV	≥0.2 mV
Number of patients	646	291	86
Incidence of PMI (%)*	2.5	6.2	9.3

* $P < 0.005$ by multiple chi-square.

Figure 4–8. The relationship between the degree of ST segment depression and the incidence of perioperative myocardial infarction (PMI). (From Slogoff S, Keats AS: Does perioperative myocardial ischemia lead to postoperative myocardial infarction? Anesthesiology 1985; 62:107–114.)

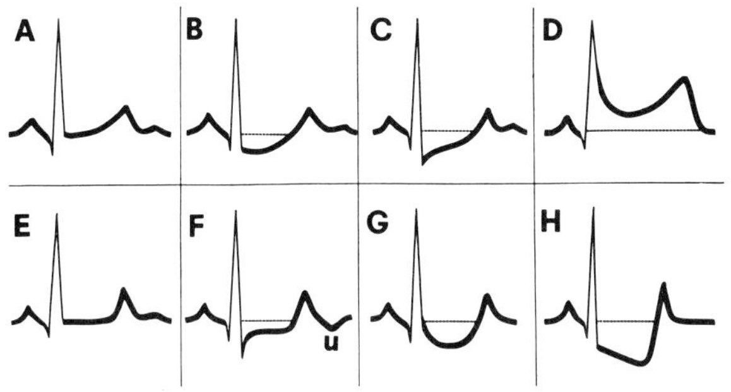

Figure 4–9. *A*, Normal P-QRS-T complex. *B*, Junctional ST segment depression. *C*, Upward sloping ST segment depression. *D*, ST segment elevation and T wave amplitude increase caused by variant angina pectoris. *E*, Horizontality of the ST segment with a sharply angled ST-T junction. *F*, Plane ST segment depression with U wave inversion. *G*, Sagging ST segment depression. *H*, Downward sloping ST segment depression. (From Schamroth L: The Electrocardiography of Coronary Artery Disease. Oxford: Blackwell, 1984; 140.)

cut-off of 0.5 Hz and a diagnostic mode with a cut-off of 0.05 Hz. The diagnostic mode is automatically used by most computer-assisted ST segment analysis programs because it allows for a more faithful display of the ST segment, but it may also introduce more baseline wandering owing to other low-frequency signals.

In addition to filtering artifacts, other interference may appear on the ECG. Intraoperatively, electrocautery is the most frequent problem, but one that is generally intermittent and short-lived. More sustained artifacts are created by other machinery in the operating room such as the roller pumps of an extracorporeal oxygenator and suction devices.

Exercise

Much interest has been shown in the ST segment changes induced by exercise, which causes J point depression and an upsloping ST segment (Fig. 4–9*C*). Unfortunately, this pattern is indistinguishable from that seen with the onset of ischemia; only continuation of exercise can separate the two. Normal subjects maintain the upsloping ST segment, whereas ischemic subjects show progressive flattening and then downsloping of the ST segment (Fig. 4–9*F*, *H*). The slope of the ST segment, therefore, has received a good deal of attention. A slope of more than 40% at a paper speed of 25 mm/second is "probably normal."[11] However, evidence shows that the slope is less important than the presence of continued ST segment depression at a point 0.06–0.08 seconds after the J point. In patients undergoing exercise stress testing, where significance was 2 mm of ST segment depression 0.08 seconds after the J point, Stuart and Ellestad found the same incidence of coronary disease in patients with upsloping ST segment depression as in those with horizontal ST segment depression.[13] The prognosis for patients with downsloping ST segments was worse than that for patients with either horizontal or upsloping ST segments.[13]

Left Ventricular Hypertrophy

Left ventricular hypertrophy changes many ECG features. The increased mass of the left ventricle increases the voltage of the QRS complex and alters the time course and direction of ventricular activation. A widening of the QRS-T angle can result in a shift of the ST-segment opposite in direction to that of the QRS. In Estes' criteria for the diagnosis of left ventricular hypertrophy, this carries as much weight as voltage criteria, and even more if the ST segment shift is part of a "strain" pattern.[19] Strain develops in longstanding hypertrophy, especially with the onset of left ventricular dilatation and failure. However, its mechanism and significance are not well understood. Classic "strain" is characterized by ST segments that slope downward, with an upward convexity, into an inverted T wave (Fig. 4–10*B*). Such strain is seen in the lateral precordial leads V_5 and V_6, and in limb leads having a qS pattern.[19]

Conduction Defects

Abnormal ventricular activation sequences, such as occur with the bundle-branch blocks, alter repolarization, making the interpretation of ST segments more difficult. In addition, sudden changes in the conduction pattern in patients with Wolff-Parkinson-White syndrome simulate the onset of ischemia. On the other hand, ischemia may precipitate a right bundle-branch block. Indeed, the most common cause of bundle-branch block is coronary artery disease. Because Q waves may disappear in left bundle-branch blocks, the diagnosis of myocardial infarction is obscured. Bundle-branch blocks are characterized by widened QRS complexes and wide S waves. However, it appears that acute changes in the ST segments, monitored carefully, still reflect ischemia. Notably, these may not always be frank ST depression; ischemia developing in the presence of right bundle-branch block may appear as a flattening of the ST segment, restoring it closer to the baseline, whereas the T waves appear more symmetric and taller.

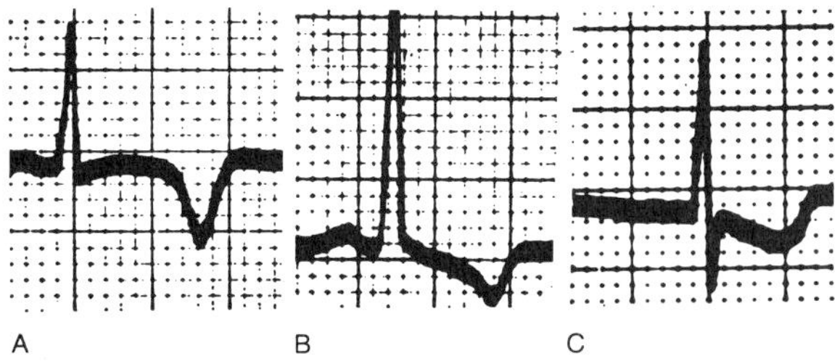

Figure 4–10. Electrocardiograms showing ST segment and T wave in: *A*, Coronary artery disease with a sharply pointed, symmetric, deep T wave and an ST segment that hugs the isoelectric line for a relatively long period. *B*, Left ventricular hypertrophy and strain with a depressed, minimally upward concave ST segment that is not isoelectric for any period; the T wave is blunt, shallow, and asymmetric. *C*, Digitalis effect with which the ST segment is not isoelectric for any period and shows a downward slope with a sharp terminal rise ending in a blunt T wave. (From Schamroth L: The Electrocardiography of Coronary Artery Disease. Oxford: Blackwell, 1984; 313.)

Digoxin

The response of the ECG to digoxin is variable. The resulting ECG may or may not reveal ST segment depression and may differ from the ECG taken during exercise. The amount of ST segment depression has not been closely correlated with the serum digoxin concentration, although in general, there appears to be more ST segment depression at higher serum levels, indicating some dose-dependence.[20]

Because of the effects of digoxin on the ST segment, it is often discontinued 1–2 weeks before exercise testing. During exercise, more ST segment depression may be seen, but it does not inexorably progress with time as is typical for the ST segment depression of ischemia (Fig. 4–10*C*). However, exercise studies done in the presence of digoxin yield conflicting results.

Hypokalemia

Hypokalemia produces significant flattening and depression of the ST segment. In addition, however, the T wave is usually diminished in amplitude, the Q-T interval becomes prolonged, and a U wave may appear (Fig. 4–11).

Posture

Postural changes affect the ECG. Shifting of the heart within the chest alters the axis of the ECG. Older literature suggests that a number of leads may show ST-T wave changes during movement from supine to sitting positions.[21] With improvements in electrodes, electronic amplification, and filtering techniques, the relative importance of this problem has diminished.

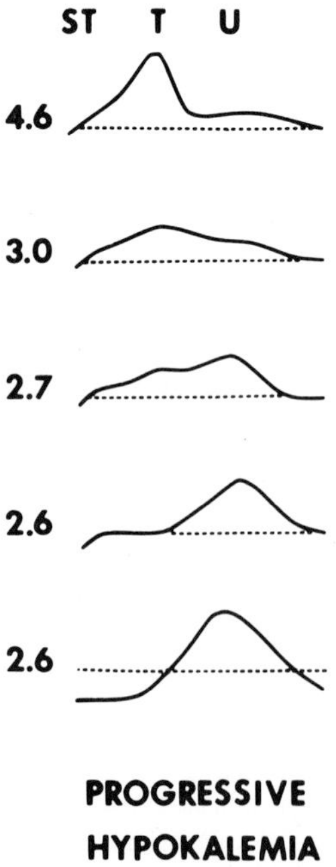

Figure 4–11. The ECG effects of hypokalemia. There is progressive development of the U component of the ST-T-U wave as the serum potassium levels decrease. The T wave itself becomes progressively flatter. (From Braunwald E: Heart Disease: A Textbook of Cardiovascular Medicine. Philadelphia: WB Saunders, 1980; 247.)

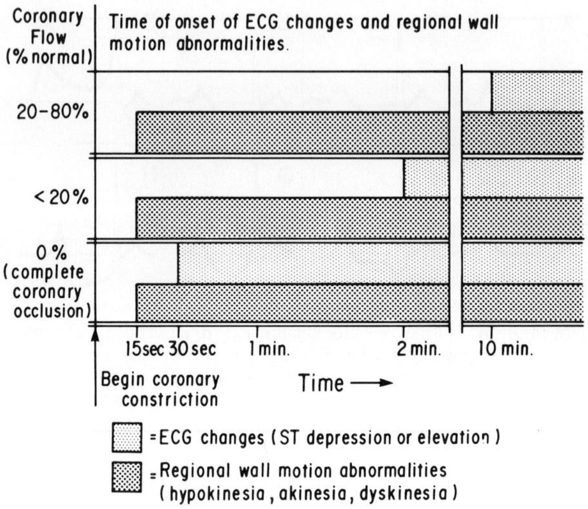

Figure 4–12. Temporal relationship between acute coronary constriction and onset of ECG and regional wall motion abnormalities. The figure summarizes data from several animal and human studies. (From Clements FM, deBruijn NP. Anesth Analg 66:249–261, 1987.)

ST SEGMENT CHANGES COMPARED WITH OTHER MYOCARDIAL ISCHEMIA INDEXES

The cascade of metabolic and physiologic events that occur with the onset of myocardial ischemia continues to be a focus of research. The goal is to determine a parameter that could be monitored to reliably alert the physician to myocardial ischemia. An ideal monitor not only would allow early intervention, but would give information on the response to therapy and have a proven resulting benefit on final outcome. In clinical practice, the onset of ischemia is more frequent and of more interest than a completed myocardial infarction.

Ventricular wall motion and wall thickening abnormalities occur earlier during the development of myocardial ischemia than do ST segment changes (Fig. 4–12) and are more sensitive indicators of ischemia.[22–24] Several clinical studies have compared intraoperative monitoring of ventricular wall motion using transesophageal echocardiography (TEE) with ECG monitoring. Despite the compelling logic that intraoperative regional wall motion abnormalities (RWMAs) should be a more sensitive predictor of postoperative adverse cardiac events, this has only been confirmed in a few high-risk patient groups. Smith et al showed that in a group of 50 patients with coronary disease undergoing major vascular or cardiac surgery, 24 developed new wall motion abnormalities.[25] There were three perioperative myocardial infarctions; only one of these patients had intraoperative ST segment changes recorded on 12-lead ECG, but all of them exhibited new regional wall motion abnormalities. Leung et al, using perioperative CC_5 and CM_5 ECG and TEE monitoring, demonstrated immediate postbypass RWMAs to be a predictor of adverse cardiac outcome in a group of 50 patients undergoing coronary artery bypass graft (CABG) surgery.[26] No patients had adverse cardiac outcomes without RWMA. Of the 18 patients with RWMAs after bypass, 6 went on to have significant cardiac events (cardiac death, perioperative myocardial infarction, or ventricular failure). ST segment changes had no predictive value at any point during surgery. In contrast, London et al[27] and Eisenberg et al[28] used intraoperative 12-lead ECG and TEE to monitor 156 and 332 patients respectively with known or suspected ischemic heart disease undergoing noncardiac surgery. They were unable to find any association between RWMAs or ECG changes and any perioperative ischemic cardiac outcome.

The pulmonary capillary wedge pressure waveform has also been studied as an early indicator of ischemia. In a group of 40 patients undergoing CABG surgery, ischemia was defined as 1 mm of ST depression or the development of an abnormal wedge tracing with an A and C wave greater than 15 mm Hg, or a V wave greater than 20 mm Hg. Ten patients met wedge tracing criteria only, three met ECG criteria only, and five met both. The authors concluded that a wedge pressure tracing could be more sensitive than the ECG for the detection of ischemia.[29] Several studies, however, have been unable to confirm the usefulness of pulmonary artery wedge pressure or pulmonary artery diastolic pressure as a reliable predictor of myocardial ischemia.[30, 31]

Properly applied, the ECG remains both an economical and convenient way to monitor patients for ischemia and a standard of care unlikely to be replaced. It is clear, however, that it is not the most sensitive tool available and that certain patients may benefit from additional monitoring.

PERIOPERATIVE USE OF ECG FOR ISCHEMIA DETECTION

Because most perioperative ischemia is not perceived by the patient, monitoring takes on an important role in documenting myocardial ischemic episodes during an operation. Routine ECG monitor observation fails to detect many episodes of ischemia.[32, 33] Transient small changes in ST depression are difficult to detect unless hard-copy waveforms are painstakingly compared over time. As newer ECG monitors have gained credibility for their accuracy, interest has developed in automated on-line ST segment analysis and trend recordings. Perioperative ST segment analysis not only enhances detection of ischemia but has significant prognostic value and provides continuous feedback following therapeutic interventions.

INCIDENCE OF PERIOPERATIVE ISCHEMIA

Several studies have shown that in patients with coronary artery disease, most episodes of myocardial ischemia causing ST segment depression are painless.[34, 35] With the availability of monitors for ST segment analysis, the concept of silent ischemia has emerged as a prominent feature of coronary artery disease. However, silent ischemia appears to carry the same prognosis as painful ischemia.[36, 37] Thus, symptoms of coronary artery disease are recognized to be only "the tip of the iceberg"; the concept of the "total ischemic burden" has evolved as a more accurate indicator of myocardial oxygen balance in the long term. McCann et al[38] showed a 38% incidence of ischemia in a group of 50 patients undergoing peripheral vascular reconstructions monitored with a modified bipolar V_5 lead pre-, intra-, and post-operatively.[38] All ischemic events were unaccompanied by angina except for some episodes in one patient. The occurrence of ischemia was significantly correlated with unfavorable outcomes ($p < 0.02$). To reduce perioperative cardiac morbidity and mortality, the goal of medical therapy may therefore be a significant reduction in the total ischemic burden, or the total duration of ischemic time, rather than merely the amelioration of symptoms. As more attention is directed toward silent ischemia in the perioperative period, it is useful to examine the data pertaining to silent ST segment depression in subjects with and without coronary disease and in those with and without anginal symptoms.

Preoperative Ischemia

In the absence of confounding factors, typical ST segment changes of ischemia are extremely rare in asymptomatic patients without cardiovascular disease.[39, 40] However, in some populations of asymptomatic patients (e.g., middle-aged men), the prevalence of silent ischemia indicating underlying coronary disease may be as high as 2.5–10%.[34, 41–43] The incidence of silent myocardial ischemia in asymptomatic patient populations is a derived estimate from studies using coronary angiography to validate positive results in treadmill and ambulatory ECG studies.

In contrast, 60–80% of patients with symptomatic, stable angina have daily episodes of ischemia or 5–10 episodes of ischemia per week, with a median duration of 17 minutes (range 1–90).[44] From 70% to 85% of these ischemic episodes are silent, or painless.[36, 37] Painful episodes of ischemia tend to last longer than painless episodes (e.g., 21 ± 7 minutes versus 16 ± 5 minutes), but there has been no correlation between the degree of ST depression and the occurrence of pain.[45] Also, 70% of ischemic episodes occur with only minimal physical activity and may be more related to levels of mental activity. Interestingly, the heart rate at onset of ischemia during ambulatory monitoring is significantly lower than the heart rate at onset of ischemia during exercise testing. Thus, factors other than increased myocardial oxygen demand alone must play a significant role. Patients with early positive stress tests experience more silent ischemia during ambulatory monitoring. Episodes occur most frequently between the hours of 6:00 A.M. and 10:00 A.M., which mirrors the peak time of occurrence of myocardial infarction and sudden death.[46]

Finally, patients with unstable angina receiving maximum medical therapy in a coronary care unit have a demonstrated 50% incidence of silent ischemia.[47] Moreover, silent ischemia is a better predictor of poor outcome than is the presence of continued chest pain.[47] In the group of patients exhibiting ischemia, duration of ischemia was significant in that patients with more than 60 minutes of ischemia per 24 hours were more likely to have unfavorable outcomes than were patients with less ischemia.

INTRAOPERATIVE AND POSTOPERATIVE ISCHEMIA

For patients with proven coronary artery disease, the incidence of intraoperative myocardial ischemia detected by ECG during noncardiac surgery has been reported to range from 18% to 74%.[31, 48] This parallels the 26–78% incidence reported during CABG surgery. Kotter and coworkers reported ischemic ECG changes before cardiopulmonary bypass in 11.9% of patients.[49] In their study, the incidence was lower in patients undergoing initial CABG surgery (8.1%) than in patients having repeat CABG surgery (23.5%). The highest incidence was observed in patients with combined CABG-valve operations (35.3%). Knight et al demonstrated that the intraoperative and postoperative frequency of ischemia in 50 CABG surgery patients was not significantly different from that observed preoperatively, as determined by two-lead ambulatory ECG recording for 48 hours before surgery.[50] They suggested that the preoperative ischemia pattern may be useful in predicting the likelihood of perioperative ischemia. Dodds et al confirmed this observation in a group of 39 patients undergoing noncardiac surgery.[51]

SIGNIFICANCE OF PREOPERATIVE ISCHEMIA

Preoperative Ischemia

Preoperative evidence of ischemia has been shown to have predictive value for postoperative cardiac morbidity in selected patient groups.[52–55] Pasternack and coworkers identified silent ischemia and angina at rest as the only preoperative patient characteristics predictive of perioperative myocardial infarction in 200 patients undergoing major vascular surgery.[52] Raby et al used ambulatory ECG (AECG) to monitor inferior and lateral bipolar leads for 48 hours preoperatively in 176 elective peripheral vascular surgery patients.[53] Twelve of the thirty-two patients demonstrating preoperative ischemic episodes suffered a major postoperative ischemic cardiac complication, compared with only 1 of the 144 patients without recorded ischemic episodes. A second study by the same group on 115 patients produced similar results.[54] Fleischer et al confirmed these findings using modified V_1 and V_5 AECG to monitor 79 general, gynecologic, and orthopedic surgical patients for a minimum of 12 hours preoperatively.[55] Three of eight patients with preoperative ischemic episodes by AECG suffered major postoperative ischemic complications, compared with only 1 of 70 patients in the group without ischemic episodes. Mangano et al were unable to confirm this association using CC_5 and CM_5 Holter AECG monitoring in a group of 474 patients with or at risk for coronary artery disease undergoing noncardiac surgery.[56]

Intraoperative Ischemia

In a well-known study by Slogoff and Keats examining 1023 patients, ischemia occurred in 36.9% of all patients undergoing CABG surgery, and perioperative myocardial infarction was three times as frequent in patients with ischemia—6.9% versus 2.5%.[16] Some have questioned the validity of this study because the 18% incidence of myocardial ischemia present at the time of arrival in the operating room is much greater than usually seen in this patient population (e.g., 0.3%, Kotter et al[49]). Raby et al used AECG to monitor lateral and inferior bipolar leads in 115 peripheral vascular surgical patients throughout the perioperative period.[54] Six of twenty-one patients with intraoperative ischemia went on to have major postoperative cardiac complications, compared with 10 of 94 patients without evidence of intraoperative ischemia. Though associated, intraoperative ischemia was not felt by this group to be as strongly predictive of postoperative cardiac morbidity as preoperative or postoperative ischemia. Mangano and coworkers were unable to show an association between intraoperative ischemia (documented by CC_5 and CM_5 AECG) and adverse cardiac events in 474 patients with or at risk for coronary artery disease undergoing noncardiac surgery.[56]

The use of intraoperative prophylactic nitroglycerin to prevent myocardial ischemia is controversial. Three groups have reported that 0.9–1 μg/kg/minute of nitroglycerin was effective in decreasing intraoperative ischemia.[33, 57, 58] However, other investigators have noted that similar doses of nitroglycerin were ineffective.[51, 59, 60]

A single preoperative dose of beta-adrenergic blocking agent has been shown to protect against intraoperative myocardial ischemia in two studies.[61, 62] In Kotter and coworkers' study of 50 CABG surgery patients, preoperative nitrates, calcium channel blockers, or beta blockers did not affect the occurrence of ischemia.[49]

Postoperative Ischemia

The study by Raby et al cited above found postoperative evidence of ischemia to be strongly associated with cardiac complications in peripheral vascular surgical patients.[54] Fourteen of thirty-five patients with postoperative ischemia went on to have major ischemic cardiac events, compared with only 2 of 80 patients without postoperative ischemia. Mangano et al found postoperative ischemia, as documented by CC_5 and CM_5 AECG, to be associated with a 9.2-fold increase in the incidence of postoperative ischemic cardiac events in 474 patients with or at risk for coronary artery disease undergoing noncardiac surgery.[56]

In summary, ECG evidence of myocardial ischemia at any time during the perioperative period has been associated with increased risk for major postoperative ischemic complications in some high-risk patient groups. The association appears to be strongest in the postoperative period. The role of pharmacologic interventions to prevent myocardial ischemia remains unclear, but interventions to control myocardial oxygen supply and demand via manipulation of hemodynamic parameters are probably effective.

In spite of its limitations, ECG remains one of the most important tools to detect perioperative ischemic episodes. Recent technologic improvements and the development of automated ST segment analysis have significantly enhanced the value of ECG and have facilitated early diagnosis of perioperative myocardial ischemic events.

ST SEGMENT MONITORING SYSTEMS

Ambulatory ECG Monitors

Ambulatory ECG (AECG) monitors were first introduced by N.J. Holter in 1961.[63] Soon after their introduction, it was noted that patients with documented coronary artery disease manifested frequent episodes of ST segment deviation, only 25% of which were accompanied by angina.[64, 65] Because 80% of these episodes could be reduced by administration of nitroglycerin, it was felt that these ST deviations truly represented ischemia.[45] However, the ability of amplitude-modulated (AM) recording systems to record frequencies below 10 Hz was found to be limited. Indeed, narrow bandwidths used to eliminate baseline wandering and other artifacts tended to specifically distort the frequency spectrum that includes the ST segment.[66] Thus, ambulatory monitors were somewhat discredited for the purpose of ST segment monitoring. Further doubt of their usefulness was engendered by studies that did not distinguish between J point depression and horizontal or downsloping ST segment depression persisting for 60 or 80 msec.

In the past several years, however, ambulatory monitoring has regained favor by virtue of improvements in technology and validation studies of various systems. For example, studies comparing the detection of ST segment depression by simultaneous two-channel Holter monitoring and 12-lead ECG during exercise testing have shown a concordance of 96%.[67] The sensitivities of the two methods were similar—81% and 84%, respectively—and the specificity for both was 85%.

A standard ambulatory ECG study involves gathering data, usually from one or two bipolar ECG leads, for 24–48 hours. The first units available for this task were frequency-modulated (FM) or AM analog tape and playback recorders. Despite the concerns regarding distortion at the lower frequencies, both of these methods have been shown to be sufficiently accurate for clinical use[68], and hence have endured. Processing of recorded tapes requires analog-to-digital conversion and computer scanning by a programmable playback instrument system, involving significant operator interaction to interpret and tabulate results. The advent of solid-state microcomputer systems capable of real-time analysis offered the advantage of rapidly available processed information that required much less operator interaction. Critics of these systems, however, pointed out that despite the greater accuracy inherent in digitally recording ECG complexes, the real-time ST segment detection algorithms used to analyze them were unproven.[69] This concern was especially real because the first digital systems lacked enough memory to record more than selected samples of ECG abnormalities for verification. Since 1986, solid-state Holter monitors have been available that utilize data compression techniques and improved technology to allow storage of all ECG complexes.[70] The establishment of a standardized database for evaluating systems for the analysis of ST segments has further validated this monitoring technique.[71, 72] Studies comparing analog and digital Holter recordings to standard ECG monitoring of the same leads confirmed both the ability of the two techniques to identify significant ST segment changes and the greater accuracy of digital AECG.[73]

Useful additions to all Holter monitors have included time and event markers, which allow correlation of symptoms with ECG observations. Some real-time analysis Holter monitors also offer ECG surveillance, making selected information immediately available to the patient (e.g., ST segment depression) and early therapeutic intervention possible. Several perioperative AECG studies have been performed using QMed Holter monitors.[38, 52, 61] The operating algorithms and features of these monitors are described as an example of present real-time analysis monitor technology.[72]

The QMed System

Monitors marketed by QMed, Inc., are real-time analysis microcomputer systems with the ability to identify and trend (1) heart rate, (2) arrhythmias and conduction disturbances, and (3) ST segment deviations. Units such as the MONITOR ONE system (QMed Inc., Laurence Harbor, NJ) (Fig. 4–13) are programmable and possess both an event marker and the ability to communicate ECG occurrences to the patient in real time. Models vary in their memory capacity for full disclosure of all ECG complexes. Downloading of formatted trend reports, along with event histograms and ECG samples, is achieved via an infrared optical interface to a dot-matrix printer.

A 65C02 microprocessor interrogates incoming ECG signals 256 times each second. The computer identifies a QRS complex when the three inflection points representing the Q, R, and S waves are found within a span of 120 msec. The Q is noted when the slope of the line increases beyond a threshold value; similarly, the J point is defined when the slope falls to zero following the QRS complex. A point 60 msec after the J point is then taken for comparison with the isoelectric segment of the PR interval (Fig. 4–14). The amount (0.1–0.3 mV) and duration (40–60 seconds) of ST segment depression considered significant can be pro-

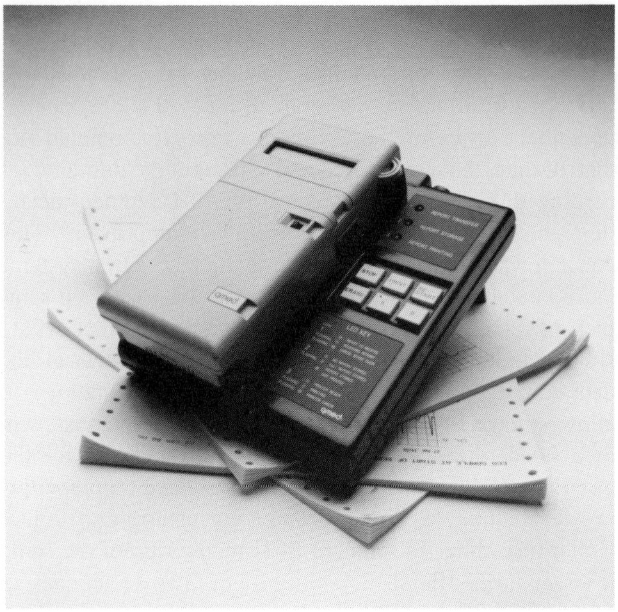

Figure 4–13. The QMed MONITOR ONE system. (Courtesy of QMed Inc., Laurence Harbor, NJ.)

grammed. If an abnormal ST segment is identified, the algorithm accepts it only after confirming that the slope between the J point and the J + 60 point is less than 2.5×10^{-3} mV/msec and that the signal is free of noise. Tracings rejected by the algorithm as QRS complexes and those for which an ST segment cannot be analyzed are shown in Figure 4–15. When significant ST segment depression occurs, an ischemic event is recorded and a 5-second sample of the most severe ECG changes is stored (Fig. 4–16).[72, 74] The end of an ischemic event is marked when no ST segment depression has occurred for 40–60 seconds.

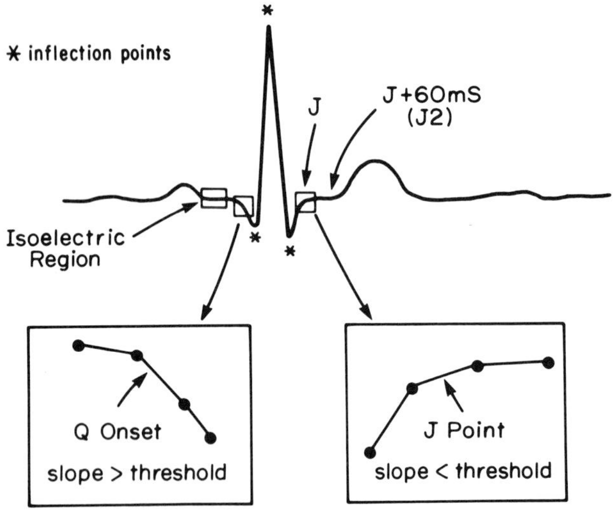

Figure 4–14. QRS analysis by computer algorithm in the Qmed system marks the inflection points (∗) of the complex. The Q and J points are identified by the changing slope of the analog signal (see text). (From Levin RL, Cohen D, Frisbie W, et al: Potential for real-time processing of the continuously monitored electrocardiogram in the detection, quantitation, and intervention of silent myocardial ischemia. Cardiol Clin 1986; 4:735–745.)

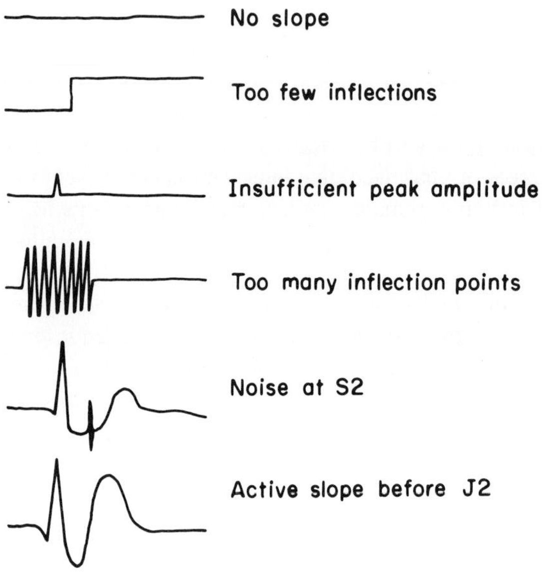

Figure 4–15. Examples of "beats" rejected for QRS-1 analysis by the computer algorithm (Qmed system). The first four traces would be rejected as QRS complexes; the last two would be recognized as QRS complexes but rejected for ST analysis. (From Levin RI, Cohen D, Frisbie W, et al: Potential for real-time processing of the continuously monitored electrocardiogram in the detection, quantitation, and intervention of silent myocardial ischemia. Cardiol Clin 1986; 4:735–745.)

Automated ST-Segment Monitors

A recent addition to several ECG monitoring systems designed for use in operating rooms and intensive care units has been computerized ST segment analysis and trending. The concept of automated ST segment analysis is appealing because simple observation of the ECG signal by anesthesiologists and cardiologists has been shown to be a poor way of identifying ischemic ECG changes. Roy et al showed that using observation alone, anesthesiologists identified only 2 of 11 episodes of significant ST segment depression recorded by Holter monitor in a group of 29 patients undergoing noncardiac surgery.[32] Cardiologists asked to review ECG tracings on an oscilloscope from patients admitted to a coronary intensive care unit were able to identify only 42% of significant episodes of ST segment depression.[75] Although automated ST segment analysis and trending technology has received far less scrutiny than ambulatory ECG, American Heart Association standards have been established[1], and ambulatory ECG has been widely accepted in both operating rooms and the intensive care units.

The first intraoperative ST segment monitors were no more than modified exercise/arrhythmia ECG monitors.[76] These modified monitors were used to provide real-time information during cardiac surgery. The use of ST segment monitoring has since spread widely, and subsequent generations of ST segment monitors have been tailored to provide the practitioner with multiple graphic displays and programming capability.

To understand the way these monitors assess the ST segment, one must review several basic features that are

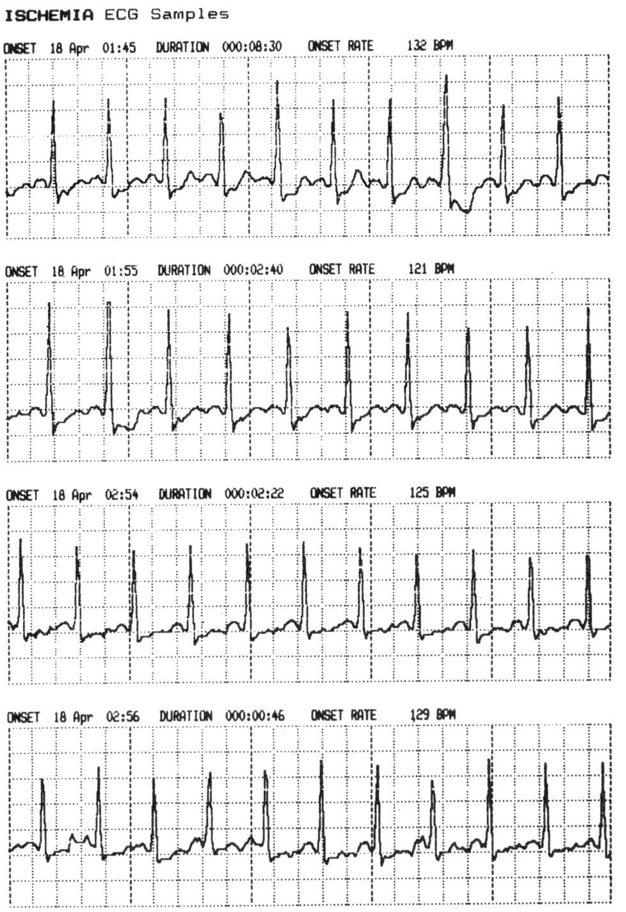

Figure 4–16. Five-second ECG traces recorded by a Qmed ambulatory monitor during ischemic episodes (1-mm ST segment depression) occurring shortly before an extensive anterior wall myocardial infarction. (From Clements FM, McCann RL, Levin RI: Continuous ST-segment analysis for the detection of perioperative myocardial ischemia. Crit Care Med 16(7); 710–711, © Williams & Wilkins, 1988.)

common to all presently available ST segment monitors. When an ST segment monitor is activated, it automatically switches the ECG to a mode with a frequency response of approximately 0.05–100 Hz; this is usually the diagnostic (unfiltered) mode. Some monitors (e.g., Siemens) claim an advantage from remaining in the monitoring (low-frequency filtered) mode, which they achieve by using a ''corrective filter'' to retrieve low-frequency signals. Several complexes are then sampled, compared, and averaged to form baseline (''dominant'') templates for each ECG lead being monitored (usually two or three leads). A dominant QRS template is only generated if a minimum number of similar complexes occur during the sampling period (usually 15–20 seconds).

''Incremental averaging'' is used by some systems (e.g., Marquette, Siemens) to form the dominant template—a method that prevents a single beat containing artifact (noise) from excessively influencing the averaged complex. The computer then uses the templates to identify and reject subsequent abnormal complexes and pacemaker beats. Markers of (1) the isoelectric reference point (usually between the P and Q waves) and (2) the ST analysis point (measured from the J point, or the peak of the R wave) are automatically set for each template; these are often open to inspection and can be adjusted by the clinician (Fig. 4–17). In some monitors, the J point is also displayed and may be modified (e.g., SpaceLabs). ST segment deviation is calculated from the isoelectric point and not the J point in most ST segment monitors. After template formation, complex sampling occurs in 15 to 20-second epochs. For each epoch, confirmed dominant complexes are averaged (or incrementally averaged) to form a current template from which ST segment deviation for that epoch is determined.

Some monitors display each current template for direct comparison with the dominant and other recorded templates (e.g., SpaceLabs), whereas others simply superimpose the current complex on the dominant template. ST segment measurements are also displayed numerically and trended over time for each lead. The Marquette monitors create an ''ST segment index'' by summing the absolute amount of ST segment deviation in leads I, II, and V_5 for each epoch; this index is displayed as a trend over the preceding 28 minutes (Fig. 4–18). An upward trend indicates more ST segment deviation, and a downward trend indicates a return to baseline. The goal of this index is to amplify any ST segment changes, making them more obvious to the observer than those seen in any single lead. The division of ST segment information between the primary monitoring screen and secondary screens is highly variable between manufacturers. Strip-chart recorders allow hard-copy versions of ST segment information to be produced. Adjustable alarms alert the clinician to the onset of ST segment changes. All monitors have algorithms that cause monitoring to cease with events such as lead disconnection or persisting grossly abnormal QRS complexes (e.g., during cardiopulmonary bypass with cardioplegic arrest).

Very few studies have attempted to validate ST segment

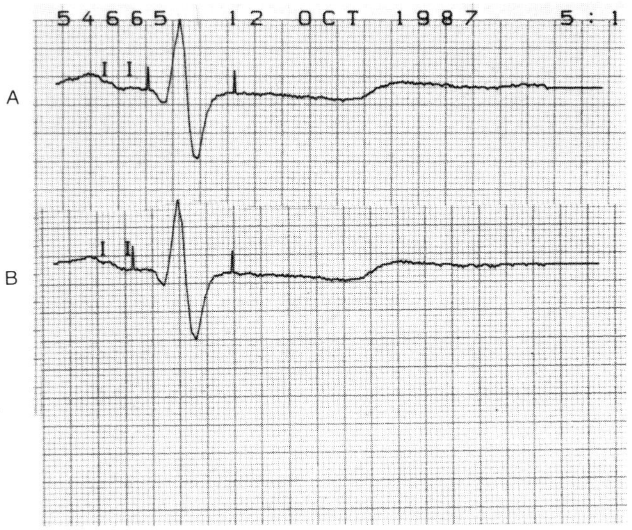

Figure 4–17. Automated ST segment analysis and display on the Marquette monitor (Marquette Electronics, Milwaukee, WI). *A*, The default isoelectric and ST segment points are shown. *B*, The isoelectric point has been manually shifted to select an earlier point prior to the QRS complex.

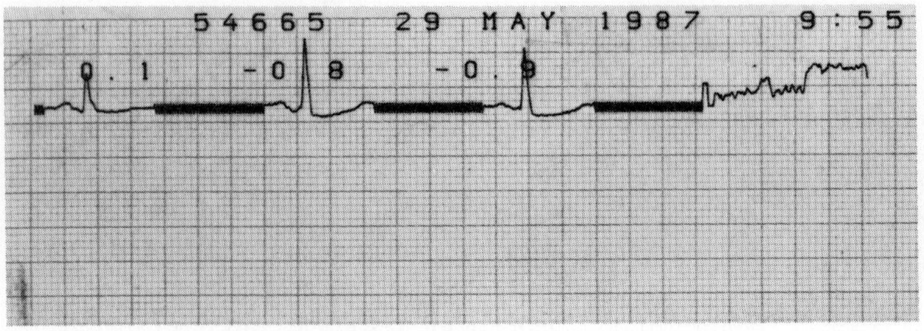

Figure 4–18. ST segment index display on the Marquette monitor (Marquette Electronics, Milwaukee, WI). ST deviation for the previous 28 minutes is shown. The rising line on the right indicates recent development of ischemia, with ST depression in leads II and V. (See text.)

monitors. London tested the response of a PC2 bedside monitor (SpaceLabs, Inc., Redmond, WA) to digitally simulated horizontal ST segment elevation and depression, and to downsloping ST segment depression.[77] Seventy-nine percent of horizontal ST segment elevation and 95% of downsloping ST segment depression were measured within an accuracy of ±0.5 mm, although some samples of horizontal ST elevation were consistently misread. In contrast, only 10% of horizontal ST segment depression examples were accurate to within ±0.5 mm.

Burns and coworkers compared ST segment values generated by a SpaceLabs, Inc. (Redmond, WA) bedside ST segment monitor against reference digitally recorded and computer analyzed ST segment values in 14 coronary care unit patients over a total period of 66.2 hours.[78] Of the 3970 samples taken at 1-minute intervals, 92.6% of the ST segment monitor values were reported to be within ±0.5 mm, and 98% within ±0.75 mm of the reference value. However, all results from 3 patients, representing 489 data points, were excluded from analysis because of systematic errors in the bedside monitor ST segment determination. One patient had ST elevation that exceeded the trending limits of the device. A second had ectopic complexes that resembled the dominant complex and therefore were not rejected from analysis by the monitor (Fig. 4–19). The third patient had an intermittently widened QRS complex caused by a subtle conduction defect, which was accepted by the monitor. This moved the ST segment analysis point to a rapidly rising ST segment, causing significant error (Fig. 4–20).

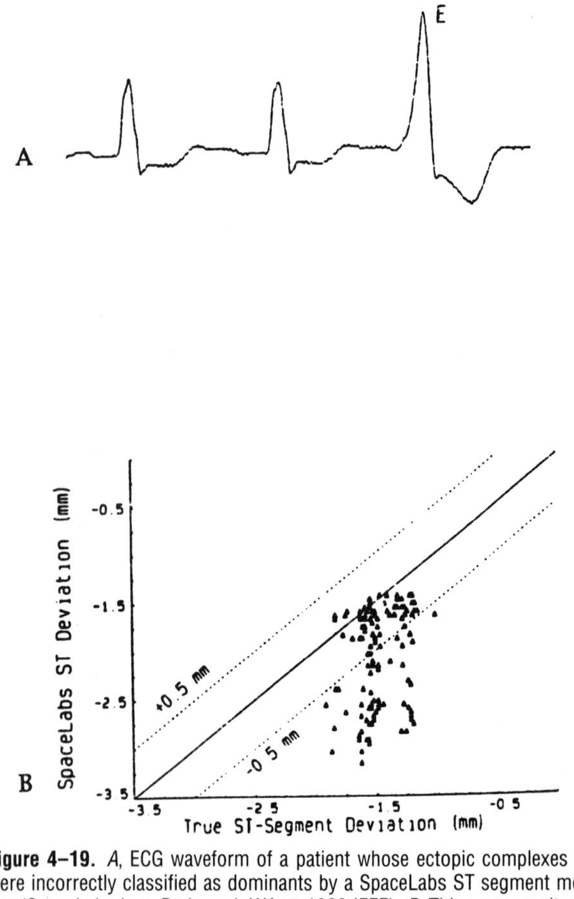

Figure 4–19. *A*, ECG waveform of a patient whose ectopic complexes (E) were incorrectly classified as dominants by a SpaceLabs ST segment monitor (SpaceLabs Inc., Redmond, WA © 1988 IEEE). *B*, This error resulted in inaccurate ST segment measurements when graphed against reference values. (From Burns PM, Downs WG: Clinical evaluation of a bedside ST segment monitor. Proc Comput Cardiol 1988; 97–100.)

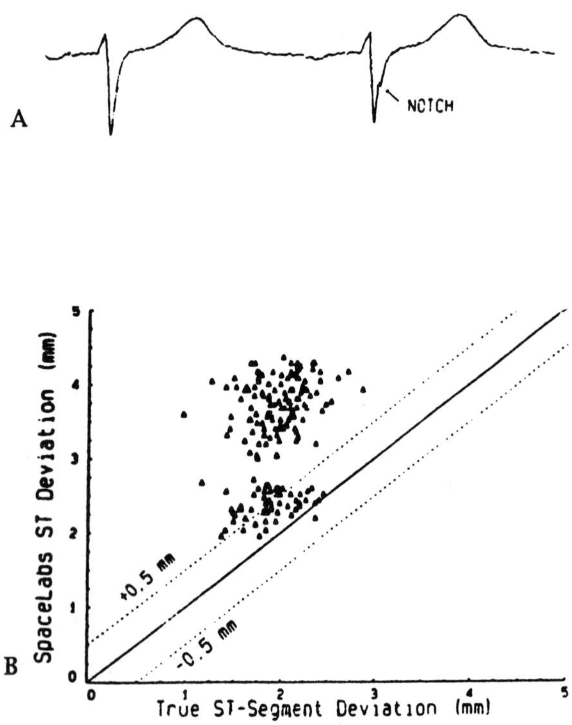

Figure 4–20. *A*, Two ECG waveforms of a patient with a variable ventricular conduction defect and a steeply sloped ST segment. Note the notch and longer QRS duration in the right waveform. Abnormally conducted QRS complexes were incorrectly classified as dominants by a SpaceLabs ST segment monitor (SpaceLabs Inc., Redmond, WA © 1988 IEEE). *B*, This error resulted in inaccurate ST segment measurements when graphed against reference values. (From Burns PM, Downs WG: Clinical evaluation of a bedside ST-segment monitor. Proc Comput Cardiol 1988; 97–100.)

Ellis et al studied 44 patients at several times during noncardiac surgery using printed 8-lead ECG (assessed by a blinded cardiologist), and two types of ST segment monitors.[79] The Hewlett Packard 78534C monitor (Hewlett Packard, Waltham, MA) was used in all patients, and showed a 75% sensitivity (6 of 8 episodes) for ischemic events diagnosed by 8-lead ECG. The Marquette 7000 ST segment trend monitor (Marquette, Milwaukee, WI) was used concurrently in only 23 patients, for whom it displayed a 100% sensitivity (5 of 5 espisodes). In the group in which both types of ST segment monitors were used, there was no significant difference in ability to detect ischemia.

A small number of studies document differences in management and outcome that are attributable to ST segment monitors. Two case reports[76, 80] describe ischemic episodes during cardiac surgery, one related to silent graft occlusion, which were first identified by ST segment monitoring and prompted therapeutic interventions. Kotter and coworkers monitored ST segments prior to cardiopulmonary bypass in 312 cardiac surgical patients using a modified stress/arrhythmia ECG monitor.[49] Over the 30 months of the study, they noted a decrease in the incidence of ischemia from 17% (8 episodes in 47 patients) in the first 6 months to 6% (12 episodes in 200 patients) in the subsequent 24 months ($p < 0.01$). They attributed this difference in part to the heightened awareness to subtle ST segment changes, and to prompt remedial action possible with information from the ST segment monitoring.

In summary, although ST segment monitors appear to be a significant improvement on real-time visual inspection for identifying ischemic episodes, they are by no means an infallible tool. The sparse validation data available for ST segment monitoring endorses no particular system. Studies to further validate these technologies, including their role in patient management and outcome, are required.

REFERENCES

1. Mirvis DM, Berson AS, Goldberger AL, et al: Instrumentation and practice standards for electrocardiographic monitoring in special care units. Circulation 1989; 79: 464–471.
2. American National Standard for Safe Current Limits for Electromedical Apparatus (ES-1/95): Arlington, VA: Association for the Advancement of Medical Instrumentation ANSI/AAMI,1985.
3. Einthoven W, Fahr G, de Waart A: On the direction and manifest size of the variations of potential in the human heart and on the influence of the position of the heart on the form of the electrocardiogram. Am Heart J 1950; 40:163–178.
4. Goldberger E: Unipolar Lead Electrocardiography and Vector Cardiography. Philadelphia: Lea & Febiger, 1953.
5. Johnson FD, Lepeschkin E (ed): Selected Papers of Dr. Frank N. Wilson. Ann Arbor: JW Edwards, 1955.
6. Blackburn H, Katigbak R: What electrocardiographic leads to take after exercise? Am Heart J 1964; 67:184–185.
7. London MJ, Hollenberg M, Wong MG, et al: Intraoperative myocardial ischemia: Localization by continuous 12-lead electrocardiography. Anesthesiology 1988; 69:232–241.
8. Griffin RM, Kaplan JA: Comparison of ECG leads V_5, CS_5, CB_5 and II by computerized ST segment analysis. Anesth Analg 1986; 65:S65.
9. Bazaral MG, Norfleet EA: Comparison of CB_5 and V_5 leads for intraoperative electrocardiographic monitoring. Anesth Analg 1981; 60:849–853.
10. Robertson D, Kostok WJ, Ahuja SP: The localization of coronary artery stenosis by 12-lead ECG response to graded exercise test. Am Heart J 1976; 91:437–444.
11. Braunwald E: Heart Disease: A Textbook of Cardiovascular Medicine. Philadelphia: WB Saunders, 1980.
12. Ellestad MH, Cooke DMJ, Greenberg PS: Stress Testing: Principles and Practice. Philadelphia: FA Davis, 1980.
13. Stuart RJ, Ellestad MH: Upsloping ST-segments in exercise stress testing. Am J Cardiol 1976; 37:19–22.
14. Robb GP, Marks H: Post-exercise electrocardiogram in arteriosclerotic heart disease. JAMA 1967; 200:918–926.
15. Goldschlager N, Selzer A, Cohn K: Treadmill stress tests as indicators of presence and severity of coronary artery disease. Ann Intern Med 1976; 85:277–286.
16. Slogoff S, Keats AS: Does perioperative myocardial ischemia lead to postoperative myocardial infarction? Anesthesiology 1985; 62:107–114.
17. Horan LG, Flowers NC, Johnson JC: Significance of the diagnostic Q wave of myocardial infarction. Circulation 1971; 43:428–436.
18. Berson A, Pipberger HV: The low-frequency response of electrocardiographs, a frequent source of recording errors. Am Heart J 1966; 71:779–789.
19. Marriott HJ: Practical Electrocardiography. Baltimore: Williams & Wilkins, 1983.
20. Sundqvist K, Atterhog JH, Jogestrand T: Effect of digoxin on the electrocardiogram at rest and during exercise in healthy subjects. Am J Cardiol 1986; 57:661–665.
21. Lachman AB, Semler HJ, Gustafson RH: Postural ST-T wave changes in the radioelectrocardiogram simulating myocardial ischemia. Circulation 1965; 31:557–563.
22. Waters DD, da Luz P, Wyatt HL, et al: Early changes in regional and global left ventricular function induced by graded reductions in regional coronary perfusion. Am J Cardiol 1977; 39:537–543.
23. Tomoiki H, Franklin D, Ross JJ: Detection of myocardial ischemia by regional dysfunction during and after rapid pacing in conscious dogs. Circulation 1978; 58:48–56.
24. Tomoiki H, Franklin H, McKown D, et al: Regional myocardial dysfunction and hemodynamic abnormalities during strenuous exercise in dogs with limited coronary flow. Circ Res 1978; 42:478–496.
25. Smith JS, Cahalan MK, Benefiel DJ, et al: Intraoperative detection of myocardial ischemia in high risk patients: Electrocardiography vs. two-dimensional transesophageal echocardiography. Circulation 1985; 75:1015–1021.
26. Leung J, O'Kelly B, Browner W, et al: Prognostic importance of postbypass regional wall-motion abnormalities in patients undergoing coronary artery bypass graft surgery. Anesthesiology 1989; 71:16–25.
27. London MJ, Tubau JF, Wong MG, et al: The ''natural history'' of segmental wall motion abnormalities in patients undergoing noncardiac surgery. Anesthesiology 1990; 73:644–655.
28. Eisenberg MJ, London MJ, Leung JM: Monitoring for myocardial ischemia during noncardiac surgery. A technology assessment of transesophageal echocardiography and 12-lead electrocardiography. JAMA 1992; 268(2):210–216.
29. Kaplan JA, Wells PH: Early diagnosis of myocardial ischemia using the pulmonary artery catheter. Anesth Analg 1981; 60:789–793.
30. Haggmark S, Hohner P, Ostman M, et al: Comparison of hemodynamic, electrocardiographic, mechanical, and metabolic indicators of intraoperative myocardial ischemia in vascular surgical patients with coronary artery disease. Anesthesiology 1989; 70:19–25.
31. Mangano DT: Perioperative cardiac morbidity. Anesthesiology 1990; 72:153–184.
32. Roy WL, Edelist G, Gilbert B: Myocardial ischemia during noncardiac surgical procedures in patients with coronary artery disease. Anesthesiology 1979; 51:393–397.
33. Coriat P, Daloz M, Bousseau D, et al: Prevention of intraoperative myocardial ischemia during non-cardiac surgery with intravenous nitroglycerin. Anesthesiology 1984; 61:193–196.
34. Cohn PF: Silent myocardial ischemia in patients with a defective anginal warning system. Am J Cardiol 1980; 45:697–702.
35. Deedwania PC, Carbajal EV: Silent myocardial ischemia: The cardiologist's perspective on mechanisms, prevalence, and treatment. Anesthesiol Clin North Am 1991; 9:493–519.
36. Deanfield JE, Kensett M, Wilson RA, et al: Silent myocardial ischemia due to mental stress. Lancet 1984; 2:1001–1005.
37. Shea MJ, Deanfield JE, Wilson R, et al: Transient ischemia in angina pectoris: Frequent silent events with everyday activities. Am J Cardiol 1985; 56:34E–38E.

38. McCann RL, Clements FM: Silent myocardial ischemia in patients undergoing peripheral vascular surgery: Incidence and association with perioperative cardiac morbidity and mortality. Vasc Surg 1989; 9:583–587.
39. Stern S, Tzivoni D: Dynamic changes in the ST-T segment during sleep in ischemic heart disease. Am J Cardiol 1973; 32:17–20.
40. Deanfield JE, Ribeiro P, Oakley K, et al: Analysis of ST-segment changes in normal subjects: Implications for ambulatory monitoring in angina pectoris. Am J Cardiol 1984; 54:1321–1325.
41. Langou RA, Huang EK, Kelley MJ, et al: Predictive accuracy of coronary artery calcification and abnormal exercise test for coronary artery disease in asymptomatic men. Circulation 1980; 62:1196–1203.
42. Eriksson J, Thoulaw E: Follow-up of patients with asymptomatic myocardial ischemia. *In* Rutisauser W (ed): Silent Myocardial Ischemia. Berlin: Springer-Verlag, 1980;154–164.
43. Froelicher V, Yanowitz F, Thompson A, et al: The correlation of coronary angiography and the electrocardiographic response to maximal treadmill testing in 76 asymptomatic men. Circulation 1973; 48:597–604.
44. Deanfield JE, Selwyn AP, Chierchia S, et al: Myocardial ischemia during daily life in patients with stable angina: Its relation to symptoms and heart rate changes. Lancet 1983; 2:753–758.
45. Schang SJJ, Pepine CJ: Transient asymptomatic ST depression during daily activity. Am J Cardiol 1977; 39:396–402.
46. Mullen JE, Stone PH, Turi ZG, et al: Circadian variations in the frequency of the onset of acute myocardial infarction. N Engl J Med 1985; 313:1315–1322.
47. Gottlieb SO, Weisfeldt LM, Ouyant P, et al: Silent ischemia as a marker for early unfavorable outcomes in patients with unstable angina. N Engl J Med 1986; 314:1214–1219.
48. Coriat P, Harari A, Daloz M, Viars P: Clinical predictors of intraoperative myocardial ischemia in patients with coronary artery disease undergoing non-cardiac surgery. Acta Anaesth Scand 1982; 26:287–290.
49. Kotter GS, Kotrly KJ, Kalbfleisch JH, et al: Myocardial ischemia during cardiovascular surgery as detected by an ST-segment trend monitoring system. Cardiothorac Anesth 1987; 1:190–199.
50. Knight AA, Hollenberg M, London MJ, et al: Perioperative myocardial ischemia: Importance of the preoperative ischemic pattern. Anesthesiology 1988; 68:681–688.
51. Dodds TM, Stone JG, Coromilas J, et al: Prophylactic nitroglycerin infusion during non-cardiac surgery does not reduce perioperative ischemia. Anesth Analg 1993; 76:705–713.
52. Pasternack PF, Grossi EA, Baumann FG, et al: The value of silent myocardial ischemia monitoring in the prediction of perioperative myocardial infarction in patients undergoing peripheral vascular surgery. J Vas Surg 1989; 10:617–625.
53. Raby KE, Goldman L, Creagher M, et al: Correlation between preoperative ischemia and major cardiac events after peripheral vascular surgery. N Engl J Med 1989; 321:1296–1300.
54. Raby KE, Barry J, Creager MA, et al: Detection and significance of intraoperative and postoperative myocardial ischemia in peripheral vascular surgery. JAMA 1992; 268:222–227.
55. Fleisher LA, Rosenbaum SH, Nelson AH, et al: The predictive value of preoperative silent ischemia for postoperative ischemic cardiac events in vascular and nonvascular surgery patients. Am Heart J 1991; 122:980–986.
56. Mangano DT, Browner W, Hollenberg M, et al: Prediction of cardiac morbidity and mortality in patients undergoing noncardiac surgery. N Engl J Med 1990; 323:1787–1788.
57. Lell WA, Johnson P, Plagenhoef J, et al: Effect of prophylactic nitroglycerin infusions on the incidence of wall motion and ST abnormalities in CABG patients [Abstract]. Presented at the Society of Cardiovascular Anesthesiologists 15th Annual Meeting, San Diego, 1993:238.
58. Fusciardi J, Godet G, Bernard JM, et al: Roles of fentanyl in prevention of myocardial ischemia associated with laryngoscopy and tracheal intubation in patients undergoing operations of short duration. Anesth Analg 1986; 65:617–624.
59. Gallagher JD, Moore RA, Jose AB: Prophylactic nitroglycerin infusions during coronary artery bypass surgery. Anesthesiology 1986; 64:785–789.
60. Thompson IR, Mutch WAC, Culligan JD: Failure of intravenous nitroglycerin to prevent intraoperative myocardial ischemia during fentanyl-pancuronium anesthesia. Anesthesiology 1984; 61:385–393.
61. Pasternack PF, Grossi EA, Baumann FG, et al: Beta blockade to decrease silent myocardial ischemia during peripheral vascular surgery. Am J Surg 1989; 158:113–116.
62. Stone JG, Foex P, Sear JW, et al: Myocardial ischemia in untreated hypertensive patients: Effect of a single small oral dose of a beta-adrenergic blocking agent. Anesthesiology 1988; 68:495–500.
63. Holter NJ: New methods for heart studies. Science 1961; 134:1214.
64. Bellet S, Roman L, Kostis J, et al: Continuous electrocardiographic monitoring during automobile driving. Am J Cardiol 1968; 22:856–862.
65. Cohn PF: Severe asymptomatic coronary artery disease: A diagnostic, prognostic and therapeutic puzzle. Am J Med 1977; 62:565–568.
66. Balasubramanian V, Lahiri A, Green HL, et al: Ambulatory ST-segment monitoring. Problems, pitfalls, solutions, and clinical applications. Br Heart 1980; 44:419–425.
67. Tzivoni D, Benhorin J, Gavish A, Stern S: Holter recording during treadmill testing in assessing myocardial ischemic changes. Am J Cardiol 1985; 55:1200–1203.
68. Shook TL, Balke W, Kotilainen PW, et al: Comparison of amplitude-modulated (direct) and frequency-modulated ambulatory techniques for recording ischemic electrocardiographic changes. Am J Cardiol 1987; 60:895–900.
69. Kennedy HL, Wiens RD: Ambulatory (Holter) electrocardiography using real-time analysis. Am J Cardiol 1987; 59:1190–1195.
70. Kennedy HL: Ambulatory (Holter) Electrocardiography technology. Cardiol Clin 1992; 10(3):341–359.
71. Taddei A, Edmin M, Pisani P, et al: The European ST-T database: Standard for evaluating systems for the analysis of ST-T changes in ambulatory electrocardiography. Eur Heart J 1992; 13:1164–1172.
72. Levin RI: Quantitation of transient myocardial ischemia by digital, ambulatory electrocardiography. Am J Cardiol 1988; 61:13B–17B.
73. Silber S, Bajaj RK, Kirk KA, et al: Accuracy of digital Holter monitoring of extent and duration of ischemic episodes compared to analog recording. Am J Cardiol 1990; 65:383–388.
74. Levin RI, Cohen D, Frisbie W, et al: Potential for real-time processing of the continuously monitored electrocardiogram in the detection, quantitation, and intervention of silent myocardial ischemia. Cardiol Clin 1986; 4:735–745.
75. Biagini A, Labbate A, Testa R, et al: Unreliability of conventional visual electrocardiographic monitoring for detection of transient segment changes in a coronary care unit. Eur Heart J 1984; 5:784–791.
76. Kotrly KJ, Kotter GS, Mortara D, et al: Intraoperative detection of myocardial ischemia with an ST-segment trend monitoring system. Anesth Analg 1984; 63:343–345.
77. London MJ: Validation testing of commercially available ST-segment analysis software using a digital ST-segment simulator [Abstract]. Presented at the Society of Cardiovascular Anesthesiologists 15th Annual Meeting, San Diego, 1993:273.
78. Burns PM, Downs WG: Clinical evaluation of a bedside ST-segment monitor. Proc Comput Cardiol 1988; 97–100.
79. Ellis JE, Shah MN, Briller JE, et al: A comparison of methods for the detection of myocardial ischemia during non-cardiac surgery: Automated ST-segment analysis systems, electrocardiography, and transesophageal echocardiography. Anesth Analg 1992; 75:764–772.
80. Kotter GS, Bernstein JS, Kotrly KJ: ECG changes detect coronary artery bypass graft occlusion without hemodynamic instability. Anesth Analg 1984; 63:1133–1135.

CHAPTER 5

Electrocardiography: Monitoring for Arrhythmias

JOHN L. ATLEE, III, M.D.

Perioperative arrhythmias are quite common, with incidences as high as 84% reported in anesthetized surgical patients.[1] Fortunately, most cardiac arrhythmias do not produce immediate, life-threatening hemodynamic compromise requiring urgent therapeutic intervention. However, new or altered forms of arrhythmias often signify some imposed physiologic imbalance which, uncorrected, could harm the patient. Consequently, prompt detection and proper diagnosis of cardiac arrhythmias by anesthesiologists or critical care physicians is important. This chapter discusses incidence, surveillance, and significance of cardiac arrhythmias; mechanisms for arrhythmias; electrocardiographic (ECG) monitoring; ECG diagnosis of arrhythmias; ECG manifestations of altered physiologic states; and ECG diagnosis of artificial pacemaker function.

INCIDENCE AND SURVEILLANCE OF ARRHYTHMIAS

The reported incidence of perioperative cardiac arrhythmias depends on the ECG methods used for surveillance. Incidence of all types of arrhythmias during anesthesia and surgery, excluding sinus bradycardia and noncompensatory sinus tachycardia, often exceeds 60% when continuous ECG methods (e.g., Holter monitoring) compared with visual inspection are used.[1–7] However, it should be noted that studies with continuous monitoring are usually quite limited in size (<200 patients), and often concern selected anesthetic agents and surgical procedures.[1–8] Large, multicenter, prospective studies of arrhythmia incidence and associations with continuous ECG monitoring are needed. Such studies could identify important risk factors and causes for arrhythmias, and determine patient outcomes with specific management. In the absence of such studies, available evidence suggests that (1) arrhythmias are more likely in patients with underlying cardiovascular or major systemic disease, (2) arrhythmias are most commonly associated with thoracic, cardiovascular, and intracranial surgery, (3) arrhythmias most commonly occur during anesthetic induction, tracheal intubation, and periods of maximal surgical stimulation, and (4) aside from underlying cardiac or major systemic disease, imbalance produced by drugs and altered physiologic states is the most common cause for arrhythmias.[8–10]

SIGNIFICANCE OF ARRHYTHMIAS

Although new or altered forms of cardiac arrhythmias in perioperative or intensive care settings usually signify some imposed physiologic imbalance, which may or may not be easily corrected, they may also adversely affect circulatory dynamics or myocardial O_2 balance or lead to lethal forms of arrhythmias.

CIRCULATORY IMPACT

Cardiac arrhythmias can adversely affect the patient's hemodynamic status because of bradycardia, tachycardia, mechanically ineffective contractions, or loss of atrial transport function.

Bradycardia

Cardiac output is the product of heart rate and stroke volume. Therefore, if stroke volume remains constant, cardiac output must decrease with reduced heart rate, and vice versa. What constitutes hemodynamically significant bradycardia for a given patient, however, will depend on the origin of the bradycardia and the status of myocardial function. For example, sinus bradycardia of 40 beats/minute might be tolerated by resting or anesthetized healthy adults. However, the inability to adequately increase heart rate during major stress could compromise vital organ perfusion even in healthy patients. Sinus bradycardia of less than 40 beats/minute, or atrioventricular (AV) junctional or idioventricular rhythm of less than 50 beats/minute is unlikely to be tolerated by any patient, regardless of underlying myocardial function. Finally, bradycardia is poorly tolerated in patients with dilated cardiomyopathy.[11]

Tachycardia

With excessive heart rate, hemodynamics are compromised by reduced diastolic filling time. Because ventricular systole requires about 200 msec and most filling (except that due to atrial contraction) occurs over 150–200 msec,[12] cardiac output is expected to decrease at rates much over 150 beats/minute (cycle length = 400 msec), even in patients with normal hearts. Tolerance of tachycardia (>120 beats/minute in adults) varies considerably among patients, but is least tolerated by patients with coronary artery disease and hypertrophic cardiomyopathy (e.g., patients with aortic stenosis, hypertension).[13]

Mechanical Effect

Disorganized and ineffective contractions of the atria or ventricles occur with fibrillation. With atrial fibrillation, flow from the atria to ventricles is only passive (i.e., loss of "atrial kick"), with the effect on cardiac output most dependent on ventricular compliance. With ventricular fibrillation, insufficient pressure is generated by the ventricles to maintain vital organ perfusion.

Atrial Transport Function

Contractions of the atria and ventricles are dissociated with AV heart block, atrial fibrillation, and AV junctional or ventricular rhythm disturbances. With AV dissociation, circulation is adversely affected by lost atrial transport function, and possibly also because of the effects of regurgitant blood flow. The importance of the atrial contribution to ventricular filling was appreciated by William Harvey, who wrote ". . . that the auricles beat, contract and push blood into the ventricles."[14] The hemodynamic importance of atrial contraction was demonstrated by Gesell, who showed that properly timed atrial contractions could augment ventricular stroke volume by as much as 50%, and that randomly associated atrial and ventricular systoles produced large beat-to-beat fluctuations in systolic blood pressure.[15–17] Application of these physiologic principles to management of patients with heart disease, however, required understanding of the implications of impaired ventricular diastolic function and development of "physiologic" artificial cardiac pacemakers.[11, 18–22] In essence, it can be deduced from this work that arrhythmias with AV dissociation are expected to have the greatest negative hemodynamic impact on patients with ventricular diastolic dysfunction (impaired relaxation, increased stiffness). Left ventricular diastolic function is altered by most cardiac disease processes[11, 18–20] and by volatile inhalation anesthetics.[23]

MYOCARDIAL OXYGEN BALANCE

Myocardial O_2 supply must equal or exceed supply in order to avoid ischemia. Myocardial ischemia and hypoxia are important causes for cardiac arrhythmias.[24] Aside from arterial O_2 content, major factors affecting myocardial supply and demand are listed in Table 5–1. Except for coronary artery diameter and contractility, arrhythmias might adversely affect any of these factors and further promote arrhythmogenesis. Most important, however, is the effective cardiac rate with arrhythmias. Tachycardia, which increases myocardial O_2 demand, is particularly dangerous in patients with reduced O_2 supply (e.g., patients with coronary artery disease, anemia, hypovolemia, myocardial hypertrophy). Thus, arrhythmias not normally considered life-threatening (e.g., supraventricular tachycardia) can become so if sustained and associated with ischemia. Ischemia, in turn, promotes deterioration to lethal ventricular tachyarrhythmias.

PREDISPOSITION TO LETHAL ARRHYTHMIAS

Do certain lesser atrial or ventricular arrhythmias (e.g., frequent, complex, or closely coupled extrasystoles) predispose to or trigger potentially lethal tachyarrhythmias and thus require antiarrhythmic drug treatment? For example, it has been widely assumed by anesthesiologists that lesser ventricular arrhythmias will trigger ventricular tachycardia (VT) or ventricular fibrillation (VF). Although such predisposition has been repeatedly confirmed for lesser ventricular arrhythmias in the setting of acute myocardial infarction, there is no compelling evidence for it in other circumstances, including during anesthesia or with catecholamines.[9, 10, 26, 27] Results of the Cardiac Arrhythmia Suppression Trials—CAST I and II—support this contention.[28, 29] In both CAST I and CAST II, class 1c antiarrhythmic drugs were administered to post–myocardial infarction patients with lesser ventricular arrhythmias to reduce the risk of sudden death from arrhythmias. Instead of reducing the incidence of sudden death, drugs actually increased morbidity and mortality from arrhythmias, a phenomena termed "proarrhythmia." Although the proarrhythmic potential of antiarrhythmic drugs in surgical or critical care settings must be established because of their depressant circulatory and other systemic effects, as well as their potential for adverse interactions with other drugs,[9, 10] I think that antiarrhythmic drugs should not be used indiscriminately to treat lesser arrhythmias in perioperative settings or critical care units.

TABLE 5–1. MAJOR FACTORS AFFECTING MYOCARDIAL O_2 SUPPLY AND DEMAND

O_2 Supply	O_2 Demand
Aortic diastolic pressure	Heart rate
LV end-diastolic pressure	Contractility
Coronary artery diameter	Myocardial wall tension

MECHANISMS FOR ARRHYTHMIAS

Only a brief overview of cellular mechanisms for cardiac arrhythmias is given here. A more detailed discussion can be found elsewhere.[9, 23, 24, 30] Arrhythmias are disturbances of cardiac impulse generation, propagation, or both. Disturbances of impulse generation include altered normal and abnormal forms of automaticity, as well as triggered activity and automaticity. Disturbances of impulse propagation include reentrant excitation and sinoatrial (SA) or AV conduction block. Parasystole, whereby a discreet and separate automatic focus is ''protected'' by a region of conduction block, is a disturbance of both impulse initiation and propagation.

NORMAL CARDIAC ELECTROPHYSIOLOGY

Cardiac Action Potential (AP)

Most cardiac fibers are electrically quiescent, with the level of cell transmembrane potential (TMP) during quiescence termed the ''resting membrane potential'' (RMP). The cardiac AP describes the changes in TMP that occur with excitation. The AP of a quiescent Purkinje fiber, including major ionic fluxes responsible for it, is depicted in Figure 5–1, *top*. Only very small amounts of ions, in proportion to their intra- or extra-cellular concentrations, move across the cardiac cell membrane during depolarization and repolarization. The AP has five distinct phases, created by ionic fluxes due to the passive movement of ions across the cell membrane through specific ion channels and to active ion exchange pumps within the cell membrane.[9, 23, 30] Ion pumps derive their energy from the hydrolysis of adenosine triphosphate. Phase 0 depolarization and overshoot (phase 1) are due to the rapid inward movement of sodium ions. The AP plateau (phase 2) is maintained by the slower inward movement of calcium ions. Final rapid repolarization (phase 3) is due mainly to the net outward movement of potassium ions. Finally, the sodium-potassium exchange pump and other ion exchange pumps restore normal intra- and extra-cellular ion concentrations during phase 4.

Refractory Periods

During the AP plateau, fibers are absolutely refractory; that is, they cannot be reexcited regardless of stimulus strength (Fig. 5–1, *bottom*). The primary reason for this is inactivation of the inward sodium current during the plateau phase; full repolarization is required before reopening can occur. In Purkinje and other fast-response fibers, restoration of the normal resting membrane potential is usually sufficient for full recovery of excitability. There is a period between the end of absolute refractoriness and full recovery of excitability when the fibers may respond partially to excitation—the so-called ''relative refractory period'' (Fig. 5–1, *bottom*).

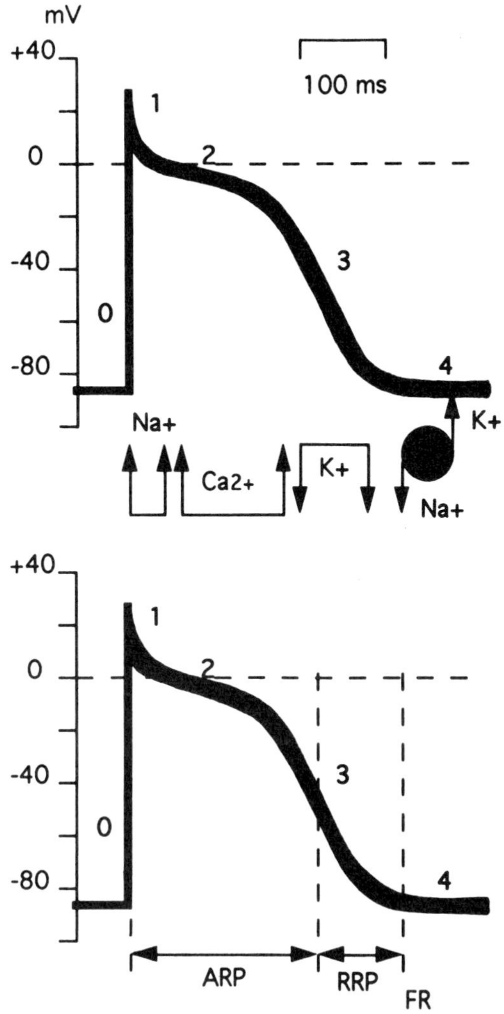

Figure 5–1. Schematic representation of Purkinje fiber action potentials (APs). *Top*, Phases of AP and major ionic fluxes ($\uparrow$ = influx; $\downarrow$ = efflux) across cell membrane during the cardiac cycle. Phase 0—rapid depolarization and overshoot; phase 1—initial rapid repolarization; phase 2—plateau; phase 3—final rapid repolarization; phase 4—electrical diastole. The sodium-potassium exchange pump is indicated by the black circle. *Bottom*, Responsiveness of fiber to electrical stimulation during the cardiac cycle. ARP—absolute refractory period; RRP—relative refractory period; FR—full recovery. See text for further discussion.

Action Potentials of Different Cardiac Fibers

Cardiac APs vary throughout the heart (Fig. 5–2). There is a progressive increase in the duration of the AP from fibers of the atria to those of the ventricles. APs of the SA and AV nodes have distinctly rounded contours, and AP upstrokes depend more on the slow-inward movement of calcium (i.e., ''slow-response fibers''). In contrast, AP upstrokes in atrial and ventricular muscle fibers, as well as those of fast-conducting fibers of the specialized AV conducting system—Purkinje fibers—depend more on the fast inward movement of sodium (i.e., ''fast-response fibers'').

Impulse Generation (Automaticity)

Some cells of the heart do not remain electrically quiescent during diastole (phase 4); rather, they depolarize

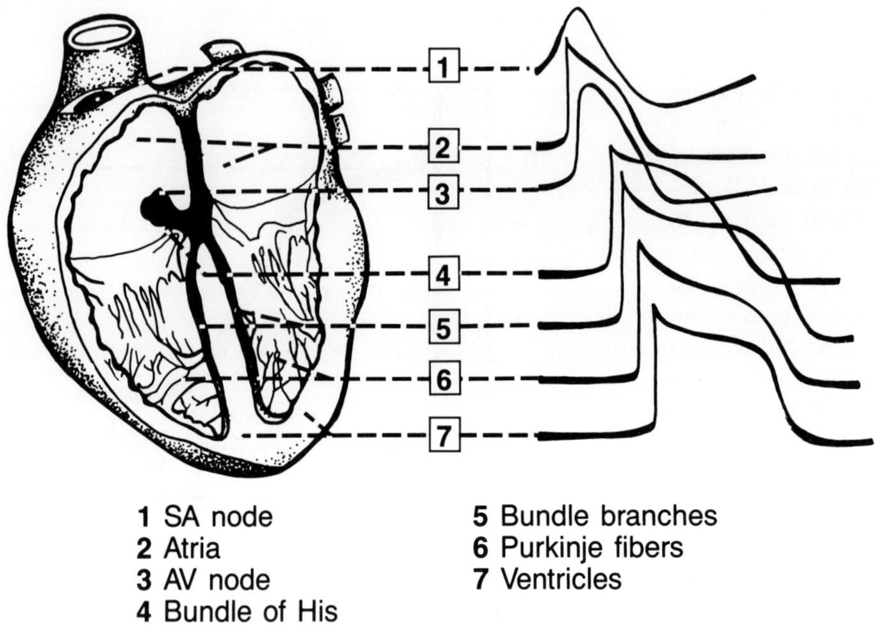

Figure 5–2. Schematic representation of heart and APs from various cardiac fiber types. Note that APs increase in duration from the atria to ventricles. Note also that APs of the SA and AV nodes have rounded contours ("slow response" APs), whereas those of the other fibers ("fast response" APs) have distinct overshoots at end of phase 0 and plateau phases. See text for further discussion.

slowly until they reach threshold for rapid phase 0 depolarization. This process, termed "phase 4 depolarization" or "automaticity," is a property of primary pacemaker cells found in the SA node (Fig. 5–2). It is also characteristic of secondary (latent, subsidiary) pacemakers found in the atria, AV junction, and His-Purkinje system. However, secondary pacemakers are usually overdriven by faster discharging cells of the SA node (overdrive suppression of automaticity). Secondary pacemakers may escape to become the heart's pacemaker for one or more beats if the SA node defaults or automaticity is enhanced relative to that of the SA node. Automaticity in cardiac fibers results from a net reduction in the outward movement of positive charges. This is due to a progressive reduction in an outward current, an increase in inward current, or both.[9, 23, 30] Ionic currents responsible for automaticity are different in SA node and in Purkinje fibers.[9, 23, 30]

Impulse Propagation (Conduction)

The rate of conduction of cardiac APs depends on properties of the current source and of the sink.[9, 23, 30] The former includes AP rate of rise, overshoot, amplitude, and duration. The latter is primarily longitudinal cellular resistance. The relation between the current source and sink determines whether conduction will be successful or if only local, nonpropagated (electrotonic) effects will result following excitation of adjacent cells. For example, excitation of adjacent fast-response fibers with high resting membrane potentials, AP amplitudes, etc., is likely to result in successful impulse propagation. In contrast, excitation of adjacent slow-response or depressed fast-response fibers is more likely to result in electrotonic effects. Finally, during impulse conduction, the excess of activation current over the amount just required to produce successful impulse propagation is termed the "safety factor of conduction." Fast-response fibers have a high safety factor, whereas slow-response or depressed fast-response fibers have a low safety factor of conduction.

ABNORMAL CARDIAC ELECTROPHYSIOLOGIC PROPERTIES

Abnormal cardiac electrophysiologic properties include conduction of the depressed fast response DFR, abnormal automaticity, triggered activity and automaticity, and reentry of excitation. These result when normal electrophysiologic processes are disrupted by pathophysiologic processes. A common mechanism underlying some abnormal electrophysiologic properties (notably, abnormal automaticity and re-entry) is loss of membrane potential (LMP) in fast-response fibers.[9, 24] LMP frequently occurs as the result of myocardial hypoxia or ischemia. With LMP, fast-response cells have lower resting membrane potentials and reduced sodium channel availability. Because of this, conduction is slower in depressed fast-response fibers, refractoriness is prolonged, and cells that do not normally exhibit automaticity may become automatic (abnormal automaticity).

Depressed Fast-Response Conduction

Because loss of membrane potential is not a uniform process, slowed conduction and prolonged refractoriness due to the DFR tend to be uneven. This is conducive to reentry of excitation. DFR conduction velocities may be only slightly slower than those normally observed in nondepressed fast-response fibers (up to several meters per second), or similar to those in slow-response fibers of the SA and AV nodes (<0.1 m/second). Severely depressed conduction can cause heart block.

Abnormal Automaticity

Abnormal automaticity is distinguished from altered normal automaticity.[9, 24] With altered normal automaticity, the ionic mechanism for automaticity is normal, except that the kinetics or magnitude of the ionic currents responsible for depolarization are altered. The net result is acceleration or deceleration of automaticity. With abnormal automaticity, the ionic mechanism for automaticity is substantially different from that for normal automaticity in the same fiber type (e.g., a Purkinje fiber), or it may be observed in fibers that do not normally exhibit automaticity (e.g., atrial or ventricular muscle). Depolarization of Purkinje, atrial, or ventricular muscle fibers by disease or other interventions can accelerate existing spontaneous activity or induce abnormal automaticity in previously quiescent fibers. Abnormal automaticity is believed to be responsible for AV junctional and idioventricular rhythms early (in the first 48–72 hours) after myocardial infarction, and with myocardial ischemia and reperfusion.[9, 23, 24]

Triggered Activity and Automaticity

This is abnormal rhythmic activity of the heart that critically depends on prior impulses for its initiation.[9, 24] These prior impulses are early or delayed afterdepolarizations. Triggered automaticity is sustained rhythmic activity following early afterdepolarizations (EADs—depolarizations before full AP repolarization). Triggered activity is sustained rhythmic activity following delayed afterdepolarizations (DADs—depolarizations after full AP repolarization). Extensive evidence exists both in animal models and in human studies to suggest DAD-triggered activity as the probable mechanism for atrial and ventricular tachyarrhythmias with digitalis toxicity, and EAD-triggered automaticity as the mechanism for torsades de pointes or polymorphic ventricular tachycardia with congenital long QT interval syndrome.[9, 24]

Re-Entry of Excitation

Re-entry of excitation occurs when the propagating cardiac impulse does not die out following excitation.[9, 24] Instead, it returns to re-excite tissue before the arrival of the next normal impulse from above. There are a number of possible mechanisms for re-entry, including circus movement around an anatomic obstacle, linear re-entry, reflection, and leading circle re-entry. Depressed conduction and/or altered refractoriness may create the substrate for re-entrant tachycardia, whether of atrial or of ventricular origin. Re-entry has not been conclusively demonstrated as the mechanism for any clinical tachyarrhythmia, except for AV nodal re-entrant tachycardia, atrial flutter, and AV reciprocating tachycardia in patients with the Wolff-Parkinson-White syndrome. Nevertheless, there is strong circumstantial evidence (e.g., electrophysiologic mapping, initiation of arrhythmias by premature stimulation) for re-entry in many clinical tachyarrhythmias.

MECHANISTIC APPROACH TO PREVENTION AND TREATMENT

The described cellular arrhythmia mechanisms are relatively easy to demonstrate in animal models of arrhythmias but more difficult in patients. Nevertheless, there is at least strong presumptive evidence that all the identified cellular mechanisms are responsible for specific clinical arrhythmias. For this reason, a mechanistic approach to the prevention and treatment of cardiac arrhythmias has become the standard for successful management. Based on accepted clinical cardiac electrophysiologic criteria, cellular electrophysiologic mechanisms are correlated with specific clinical arrhythmias, diagnostic features, and suggested therapeutic strategies, as listed in Table 5–2.

ELECTROCARDIOGRAPHIC MONITORING TECHNIQUE

As with ECG monitoring for myocardial ischemia (see Chapter 4), leads are selected that maximize the opportunity for detection and diagnosis. For detection and diagnosis of arrhythmias, the leads selected are ones that maximize P waves such as esophageal and intracavitary leads.

MAXIMIZING P WAVES

Critical to diagnosis of arrhythmias is establishing the relation between atrial (P wave) and ventricular depolarization (QRS complex). If P waves always result in QRS complexes (i.e., if they are "associated"), the arrhythmia must be of supraventricular origin—regardless of QRS appearance. If P waves are dissociated or result from the QRS, the disturbance must be of AV junctional or ventricular origin. Although the QRS complex is easily recognized in most conventional surface ECG leads, P waves are best seen in the inferior (standard) limb leads (II, III), unipolar (augmented) extremity lead aVF, or unipolar precordial (chest) lead V_1. Today, most operating rooms and critical care units employ 5-electrode ECG monitoring systems. In some, however, three-electrode systems (i.e., modified bipolar leads) may be used. With modified bipolar leads, a subscript number indicates the position of the exploring (positive) electrode on the chest, according to the usual chest lead position.[31] Also, the negative electrode is designated as central (C) followed by its position (e.g., CL—central lead, left arm). The letter M before C designates a modified position for the central lead (e.g., MCL—a central lead moved from the left arm to beneath the left clavicle). The letter B after C designates that the negative electrode is over the center of the right scapula. Of the modified bipolar leads, MCL_1 and CB_5 appear to be the best for P wave detection.[31]

ESOPHAGEAL AND INTRACAVITARY LEADS

Detection of P waves for arrhythmia diagnosis is greatly enhanced by positioning electrodes close behind the left

TABLE 5–2. MECHANISTIC APPROACH TO DIAGNOSIS AND TREATMENT OF CARDIAC ARRHYTHMIAS: CORRELATION OF CELLULAR MECHANISMS WITH CLINICAL ARRHYTHMIAS, DIAGNOSTIC FEATURES, AND THERAPEUTIC STRATEGY

Cellular Mechanism	Clinical Arrhythmias	Diagnostic Features	Therapeutic Strategy
Altered normal automaticity	Sinus bradycardia/tachycardia; sinus arrhythmia/wandering pacemaker; AV junctional/ventricular escape rhythms	Gradual decrease/increase in rate or shifting pacemaker	Correct imbalance; temporary pacing/ chronotropes; prevent tachycardia with α_2 agonist
Abnormal automaticity	AV junctional/ventricular rhythms with ischemia/reperfusion; some automatic atrial tachycardia	Gradual warm-up in rate vs. sudden (paroxysmal) increase; uniform QRS appearance	Treat hypoxia/ischemia; BB, CCB, or $MgSO_4$; physiologic* temporary pacing; mechanical support; avoid catecholamines
Triggered activity/ automaticity	DAD: VT 2° reperfusion/ischemia; catecholamine-mediated VT; digitalis toxicity EAD: torsades de pointes VT with QT interval prolongation	More abrupt onset DAD: First beat of tachycardia occurs late in electrical diastole vs. early with re-entry EAD: Facilitated by slow heart rates	DAD: Treat cause (digitalis, catecholamines); CCB, BB, or $MgSO_4$ (if low $Mg_2{}^+$); pacing EAD: $MgSO_4$, BB; stellate ganglion block
Re-entry of excitation	AV reciprocating tachycardia (WPW); PSVT; most VT late following MI; atrial flutter; atrial or ventricular fibrillation	Abrupt (paroxysmal) onset or termination after spontaneous or stimulated premature beats	PSVT: adenosine, BB, CCB; pacing/ cardioversion VT: cardioversion/defibrillation; lidocaine, bretylium, BB

*Physiologic pacing—Select pacing mode/rate that preserves atrial transport function and that optimizes hemodynamic profile.

AV, atrioventricular; BB, β-blocker; CCB, calcium channel blocker; DAD, delayed afterdepolarization; VT, ventricular tachycardia; CAD, coronary artery disease; WPW, Wolff-Parkinson-White syndrome; PSVT, paroxysmal supraventricular tachycardia; MI, myocardial infarction.

atrium within the esophagus or by recording from catheter electrodes within the atria or atrial epicardial leads during cardiac surgery.[31] Enhanced P waves recorded from a prototype transesophageal ECG recording and pacing stethoscope[32] are shown in Figure 5–3. Either unipolar or bipolar electrograms can be recorded from esophageal or intracavitary locations. With unipolar esophageal or intracavitary ECG, one lead from the electrode pair is substituted for the V position in a 5-lead, pin adapter assembly. Unipolar ECG can also be recorded from within the esophagus[31, 33] or right atrium[34, 35] using intravascular wires and alligator clip leads or special adapters (e.g., RAECG adapter, Arrow International, Reading, PA). With bipolar ECG, each lead from a pair of electrodes is substituted for the right and left arm positions of the electrode pin adapter, and lead I is selected. One advantage of bipolar over unipolar esophageal or intracavitary ECG is decreased baseline drift with respiration.

REGULARITY OF RHYTHM DISTURBANCE

Concerning the regularity of the rhythm disturbance, ''irregularly irregular'' rhythms (no constancy or recurring variation in R-R intervals), regardless of QRS appearance (supraventricular vs. ventricular), suggest underlying atrial fibrillation. A ''regularly irregular'' disturbance (recurring variation in R-R intervals) is compatible with sinus arrhythmia, wandering atrial pacemaker, or the presence of SA or AV heart block. Sinus arrhythmia is cyclical variation in heart rate, usually (phasic form) but not always (nonphasic form) linked to respiration. If the P wave appearance also varies cyclically, the arrhythmia is termed ''wandering atrial pacemaker.''

CAUSE OF VENTRICULAR ABERRATION

A widened and bizarre QRS does not necessarily signify a ventricular origin for the beat. Impulses of supraventricular origin may be conducted abnormally (i.e., with ventricular aberration) because of changes in heart rate, anomalous AV conducting pathways, altered electrophysiologic properties, metabolic disorders, electrolyte imbalance, drug toxicity, and other conditions.[31] As currently used, ventricular aberration does not include fixed organic conduction defects. Aberration most commonly occurs with a right bundle-branch block pattern, sometimes also with a left anterior fascicular block pattern.[36] Left bundle-branch block pattern

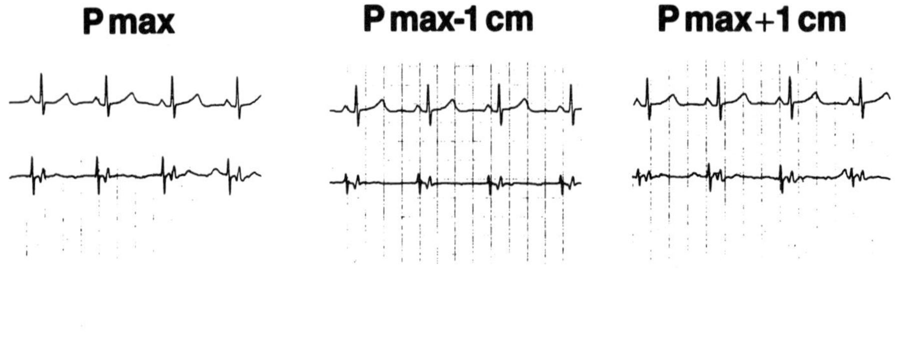

Figure 5–3. Transesophageal, bipolar, left atrial electrogram recorded with a prototype ECG recording and pacing esophageal stethoscope (Arzco Medical Systems, Inc., Vernon Hills, IL). The top tracing in each panel is surface ECG lead II, and the bottom tracing is esophageal ECG. Recordings from left to right are at the position of a maximal amplitude esophageal P wave (Pmax), 1 cm proximal to Pmax (Pmax − 1), and 1 cm distal to Pmax (Pmax + 1).

aberration is much less common and nearly always due to heart disease, although the disease may not be clinically evident.[37] To distinguish supraventricular beats with ventricular aberration from ventricular-origin beats, it is necessary to establish the relation between P waves and ventricular activity.

DIAGNOSTIC MONITORING MODES

Older ECG monitoring oscilloscopes (i.e., the "bouncing ball" type) had a toggle switch to choose between monitoring and diagnostic modes. In the *monitoring mode*, all signals below 0.5 Hz and above 45 Hz were eliminated to reduce artifacts and baseline drift. Although this effectively "cleaned up" the ECG for improved arrhythmia diagnosis, it also reduced the amplitude of P and T waves. The *diagnostic mode* filtered frequencies below 0.05 Hz and above 100 Hz, and provided the detail necessary for accurate interpretation of the T wave and ST segment for diagnosis of myocardial infarction or ischemia. However, the diagnostic mode transferred more artifact to the waveform (sometimes making P wave recognition difficult), including significant baseline drift with respiration. The phosphor screens used in contemporary ECG monitors have lower resolution than the older cathode ray tubes (i.e., they cut off frequencies above 30–35 Hz). Therefore, contemporary operating room monitors do not feature selection specifically of the former diagnostic and monitoring modes. With the monitors of one manufacturer (Marquette Electronics), the low-pass filter roll-off is set at 25 Hz by the manufacturer, and this is adjustable by software (not by the user). In some units of this manufacturer, aggressive linear filtering is used to minimize baseline wandering (drift). In other units, there may be selectable low-frequency break points (e.g., 0.005, 0.5, and 5 Hz) to minimize baseline drift, because the lower the low-frequency response is, the more likely baseline drift is.

MICROSHOCK HAZARD AND ELECTROCAUTERY INTERFERENCE

There is the danger of fibrillation when a sufficient amount of electrical current passes across a sufficient mass of atrial or ventricular myocardium. According to Ohm's law, the amount of current (in amperes) transferred depends on the potential difference (in volts) between two points divided by the resistance (in ohms). For example, if 100 V is applied across each arm and dry skin resistance is 200,000 Ω the current flow through the body would be 0.5 mA. This amount of current would be barely perceived, and falls into the category of *macroshock*.

Approximately 100 mA is required with macroshock to cause ventricular fibrillation, although there could be increased susceptibility to fibrillation with myocardial imbalance (e.g., hypothermia, electrolyte imbalance, ischemia). Line isolation monitors formerly used in anesthetizing locations approved for flammable anesthetics typically caused alarms at leakage currents of 2–10 mA.

For transvenous catheter or epicardial electrodes in direct contact with the myocardium, much smaller amounts of current are required to cause fibrillation. This amount of current (about 100 μA) is termed the *microshock* level. The level of current from esophageal electrodes to cause fibrillation has not been determined, but in all probability is minimally greater because the esophageal lumen is from 0.5 to 3.0 cm behind the left atrium and ventricle.[38] All ECG monitoring devices are electrically isolated to prevent leakage current $\geq$ 100 μA. To reduce microshock danger to the patient, it is recommended that rubber gloves be worn when handling intracavitary or transesophageal leads.

TABLE 5–3. STEP-WISE APPROACH TO ECG INTERPRETATION

1. Use leads with maximal information (II, III, aVF, V_1, intracavitary, esophageal)
2. Are P waves present? If so, AV association, VA association, or AV dissociation?
3. Regularity of the disturbance? Regular, regularly irregular, irregularly irregular?
4. Widened, bizarre QRS? Ventricular origin vs. QRS aberration?

ECG DIAGNOSIS OF ARRHYTHMIAS

The anesthesiologist or intensivist does not need to be an expert in ECG diagnosis to make initial management decisions. A step-wise approach to ECG interpretation is suggested (Table 5–3), and a strip-chart recording capability should be available. The reasons for obtaining a permanent record of cardiac rhythm disturbances are listed in Table 5–4. Although contemporary operating room monitors do feature software for automated arrhythmia detection and diagnosis, I caution against relying too much on these, particularly in electrically contaminated environments. Arrhythmia detection and diagnosis programs should provide artifact messages, and the algorithm of at least one manufacturer (Marquette Electronics) will suspend itself in the presence of strong electromagnetic interference. Nevertheless, it is possible that some electrical or mechanical artifact will be misdiagnosed by software. Thus, the prudent physician will base his or her management decisions on visual inspection of the ECG monitor screen or strip-chart record, using the automated arrhythmia detection and diagnosis software more for prompting.

TABLE 5–4. REASONS FOR MAKING ECG STRIP-CHART RECORDINGS

1. Ability to carefully examine disturbance facilitates diagnosis
2. Permanent record of disturbance in chart for later comparisons
3. Permanent record of response(s) to therapeutic intervention(s)

SUPRAVENTRICULAR ARRHYTHMIAS

Disturbances of Sinus Rhythm

Sinus bradycardia (Fig. 5–4*B*) exists when normal P waves (lead II—upright, rounded contour, uniform appearance) occur at a rate < 50 beats/minute in adults, with a P-R interval ≥ 0.12 seconds. Faster rates (<100 beats/minute) are considered bradycardia in neonates. *Sinus arrhythmia* (Fig. 5–4*B*) is sinus rhythm with a cyclical variation in sinus rate (cycle length variation > 120 msec). With *respiratory (phasic) sinus arrhythmia*, the P-P interval varies with respiration, with shorter cycle lengths (faster rate) during inspiration and longer ones (slower rate) during expiration. Phasic sinus arrhythmia is common in healthy young adults and athletes. With *nonphasic sinus arrhythmia*, the cyclical variation in sinus rate is not linked to respiration and is usually a manifestation of underlying sinus node disease. *Wandering atrial pacemaker* (Fig. 5–4*C*) also termed ''multiform supraventricular rhythm,'' is a variant of sinus arrhythmia. In addition to cycle length variation, there is variation in P wave morphology and P-R intervals as well. Although the variation in P wave morphology might be explained by variation in atrial dimensions with changes in atrial filling, it might also be explained by pacemaker shifts from the sinus node to locations of subsidiary atrial pacemakers along the sulcus terminalis[39–41] or more remote atrial sites.

Sinus pause or *arrest* results from impaired SA node automaticity. The P-P interval with sinus pause or arrest is not some multiple of the basic P-P interval (Fig. 5–5*A*). With *sinoatrial (SA) block*, the P-P interval between conducted beats (i.e., due to SA conduction) is some multiple of the basic P-P interval (Fig. 5–5*B*). First-degree SA block cannot be recognized in the surface ECG, and third-degree SA block is seen as complete absence of any P waves of sinus origin. With type I, 2° (Wenckebach) SA block, the P-P intervals progressively shorten prior to the pause, and the duration of the pause is less than two preceding P-P cycles.

Sick sinus syndrome is not a rhythm disturbance. Rather, the term encompasses a number of possible rhythm disturbances resulting from sinus node dysfunction, usually due to underlying heart disease: (1) persistent sinus bradycardia, with or without ectopic atrial beats, not due to extrinsic causes; (2) apparent sinus arrest with subsidiary pacemaker escape beats and rhythm; (3) established SA block; (4) combined SA and AV conduction defects; (5) alteration of paroxysms of atrial tachycardia with periods of slow atrial or ectopic escape rhythms (i.e., the bradycardia-tachycardia syndrome).[42]

Sinus tachycardia. Sinus tachycardia is the most common intraoperative ''arrhythmia.'' The diagnosis is made when there are morphologically normal P waves at a rate >100 beats/minute in adults. Fast sinus tachycardia (>150 beats/minute) is difficult to distinguish from paroxysmal supraventricular tachycardia due to SA node re-entry, ex-

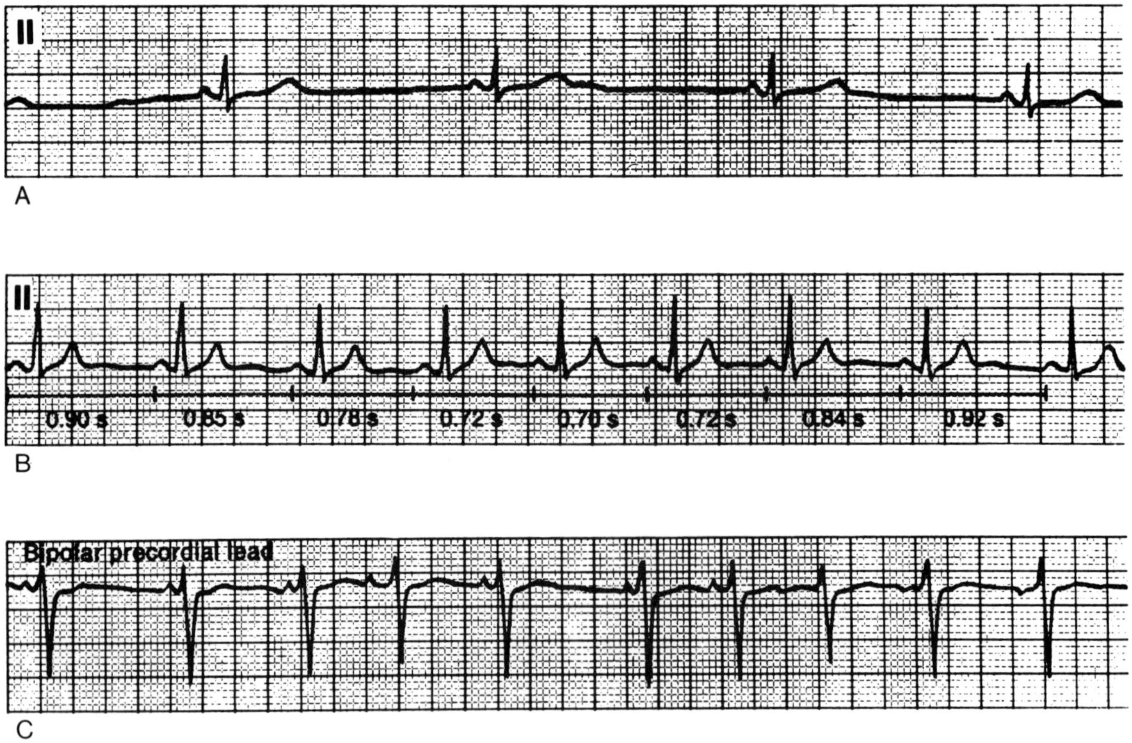

Figure 5–4. Supraventricular rhythms. *A*, Sinus bradycardia at 36 beats/minute. *B*, Sinus arrhythmia with cyclical rates from 65 to 86 beats/minute. Note the slight variation in P wave morphology, which could be due to varying atrial filling or to shifts in atrial pacemaker location (see text). *C*, Wandering atrial pacemaker; also termed ''multiform supraventricular rhythm.''

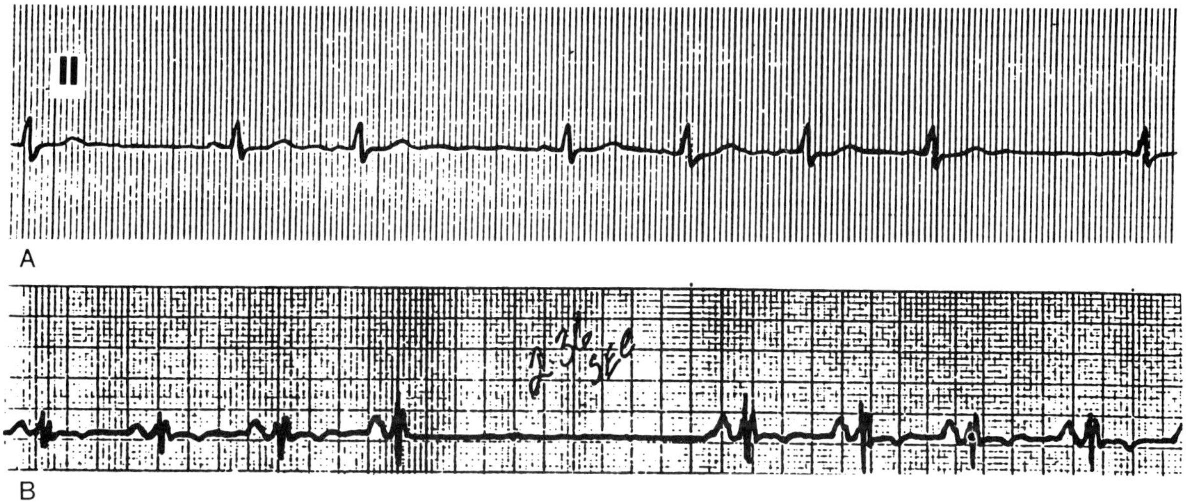

Figure 5–5. Disorders of sinus rhythm. *A*, Sinus pause or arrest. Note that prolonged P-P intervals are not exact multiples of the preceding P-P intervals, as they would be with SA block. *B*, Sinus rhythm with 3:1 SA exit block. The pause is exactly three times the preceding P-P interval.

cept that the latter is characterized by a more abrupt onset and termination. Sinus tachycardia may be compensatory or noncompensatory. The former could be in response to hypovolemia, hypoxia, anemia, fever, or hemorrhage. The latter may be due to pain, increased catecholamines, light anesthesia, drug side effects, or nonapparent causes.

AV Junctional Rhythm Disturbances

AV junctional escape beats occur when the rate of supraventicular pacemakers slows enough to release the AV junctional pacemakers from overdrive suppression of automaticity. The ECG diagnosis of junctional escape beats is made when a prolonged R-R interval is followed by a normal QRS complex not preceded by a P wave. Junctional escape beats may or may not be followed by a retrograde P wave. *AV junctional premature beats* have a similar appearance to AV junctional escape beats, except that the R-R interval is shorter than that of the underlying, dominant rhythm.

AV Junctional Rhythm. When the AV junctional pacemakers take over control of the ventricles, either by default of supraventricular pacemakers or enhanced automaticity of the junctional pacemakers, *AV junctional rhythm* exists (Fig. 5–6*A*). The rate of AV junctional rhythm is usually between 50 and 70 beats/minute. AV junctional rhythm is commonly associated with *isorhythmic dissociation* (Fig. 5–6*B*).[43] With the latter, the supraventricular and AV junc-

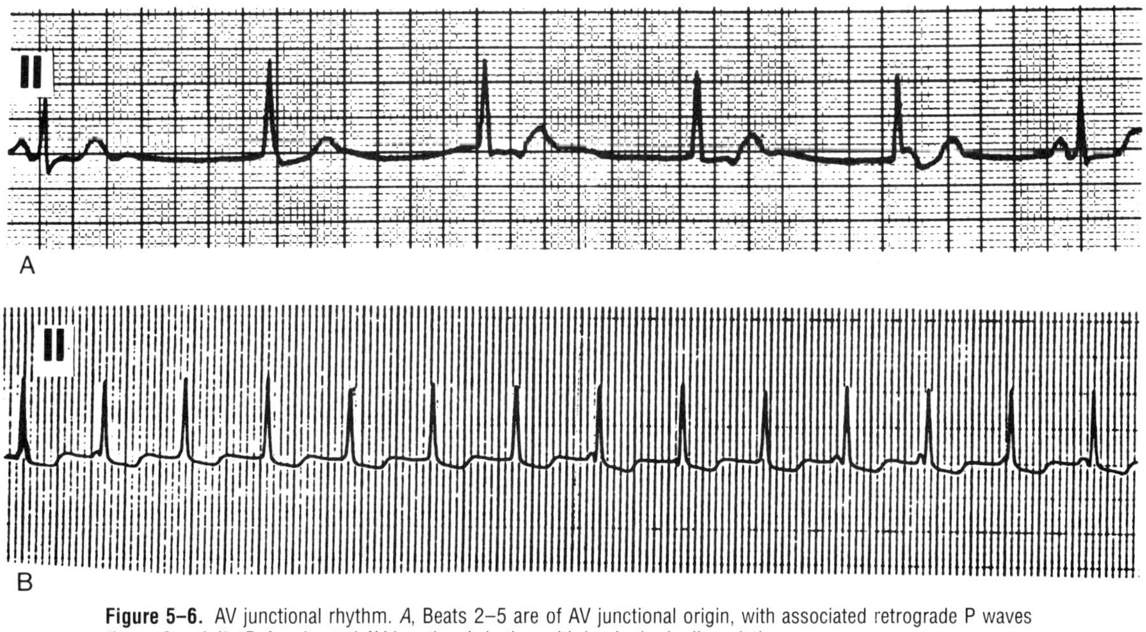

Figure 5–6. AV junctional rhythm. *A*, Beats 2–5 are of AV junctional origin, with associated retrograde P waves (beats 3 and 4). *B*, Accelerated AV junctional rhythm with isorhythmic dissociation.

tional rates are nearly the same, so that the two pacemakers become synchronized. When synchronization has occurred, junctional pacemaker discharge causes the AV node to be refractory, thereby interfering with conduction of impulses from above. On the ECG, such AV dissociation by interference is recognized by upright P waves that appear to march in or out of the QRS complex (Fig. 5–6*B*).

AV Junctional Tachycardia. Any AV junctional rhythm faster than 70 beats/minute is considered *AV junctional tachycardia* or *accelerated AV junctional rhythm* (Fig. 5–6*B*). Normally, AV junctional tachycardia is not faster than 110–120 beats/minute, and the disturbance is not uncommon with digitalis intoxication or myocardial ischemia, or following reperfusion of ischemic myocardium.

Supraventricular Tachycardia

Supraventricular tachycardia (SVT) is a generic term, encompassing a variety of tachycardic, supraventricular rhythm disturbances (including sinus tachycardia). Any SVT with an abrupt onset and termination is termed "paroxysmal." In contrast, nonparoxysmal tachycardia has a more gradual onset ("warm-up") and termination. Paroxysmal SVT is ascribed to re-entry whereas nonparoxysmal SVT is due to disturbed normal automaticity, abnormal automaticity, or triggering.

Paroxysmal (Re-Entrant) SVT. Paroxysmal SVT (PSVT) is often initiated by a premature atrial beat (Fig. 5–7*A*) and terminates suddenly followed by a variable period of sinus pause or arrest due to overdrive suppression of SA node automaticity (Fig. 5–7*B*). AV node re-entry accounts for 40–45% of PSVT, and SA node or atrial re-entry accounts for 10–20%.[44] The rate of PSVT varies from 150 to 250 beats/minute, but is commonly 180–200 beats/minute in adults. Vagal maneuvers may terminate or slightly slow the rate of PSVT. With PSVT due to AV node re-entry, inverted P waves are occasionally seen following the QRS complex (best seen in the inferior leads). P waves during PSVT due to SA node re-entry may be difficult to distinguish from those of sinus tachycardia.

AV Reciprocating Tachycardia. PSVT due to AV reciprocation includes both the atrium and ventricle in the re-entry circuit, as well as the AV node and a *manifest* or *concealed accessory AV pathway*. A "manifest" accessory pathway (AP) is capable of conducting in the anterograde direction during sinus rhythm to cause ventricular pre-excitation, the delta wave in patients with the Wolff-Parkinson-White (WPW) syndrome. However, an AP may conduct only in the retrograde direction, in which case it cannot produce ventricular pre-excitation, and is said to be "concealed." AV reciprocation with re-entry over a manifest or concealed AP accounts for 40–45% of PSVT.[44] Further, in patients with the WPW syndrome, 80% of all tachycardias are due to AV reciprocation.[44] AV reciprocating tachycardia is usually between 150 and 240 beats/minute (typically > 200 beats/minute).[45] There are two types of AV reciprocating tachycardia: orthodromic and antidromic AV reciprocating tachycardia (Fig. 5–8). The orthodromic variety is said to be 10–15 times more common.[45]

Nonparoxysmal (Automatic, Ectopic) Atrial Tachycardia. Automatic, or ectopic, atrial tachycardia (Fig. 5–9*A* and *B*) is distinguished from re-entrant SVT because of its more gradual onset and termination, certain associations, and its ECG appearance. In patients receiving digitalis, with hypokalemia, or with significant heart disease, automatic atrial tachycardia may be accompanied by second-degree AV heart block (Fig. 5–9*B*). This occurrence has been (incorrectly) termed "paroxysmal atrial tachycardia (PAT) with block."[44] The P waves during automatic atrial tachycardia differ from those of sinus origin, and there may be slight irregularity in the P-P intervals. The P-R intervals are influenced by the rate of tachycardia (140–200 beats/minute) and by cardiovascular drugs. Vagal maneuvers do not terminate automatic atrial tachycardia, but may produce transient AV block. Finally, in contrast to paroxysmal SVT in which P waves of the initial and subsequent beats of tachycardia differ, P waves for the initial and subsequent beats of automatic atrial tachycardia are the same.

Multiform (Chaotic) Atrial Rhythm. Multiform atrial tachycardia is characterized by atrial rates between 100 and

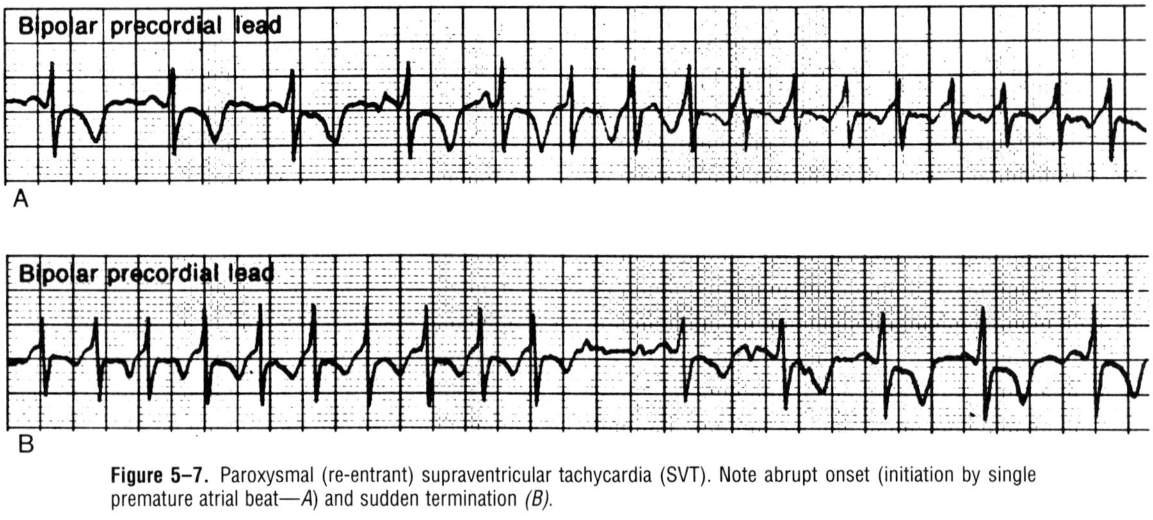

Figure 5–7. Paroxysmal (re-entrant) supraventricular tachycardia (SVT). Note abrupt onset (initiation by single premature atrial beat—*A*) and sudden termination *(B)*.

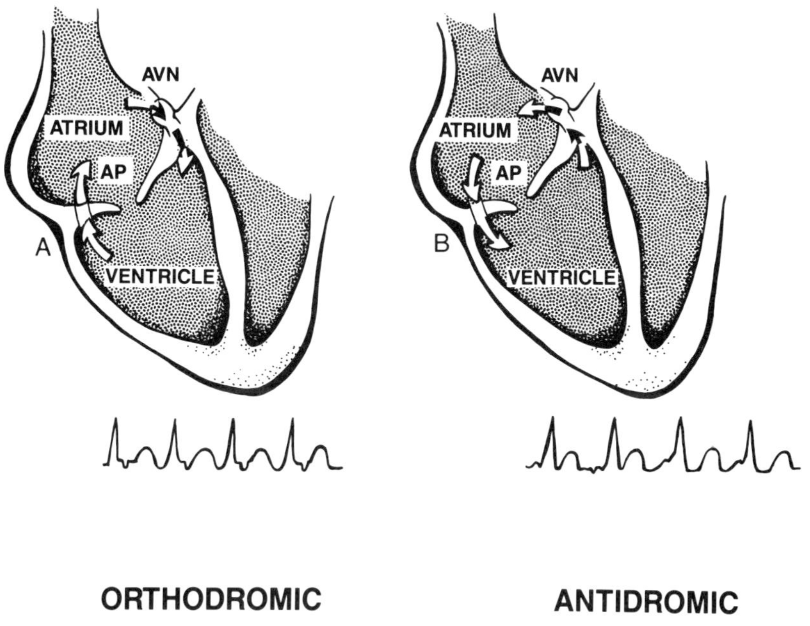

Figure 5–8. AV reciprocating tachycardia. Schematic representations of re-entry circuits and ECG appearance of tachycardia. *Left,* Orthodromic AV reciprocating tachycardia. During tachycardia, conduction proceeds from the atrium to ventricle (i.e., in an anterograde direction) via the AV node (AVN), and back to the atrium (i.e., in a retrograde direction) via the accessory AV pathway (AP). Note that an inverted P wave occurs in the left half of the R-R interval (i.e., "short R-P, long P-R"). This finding during narrow QRS tachycardia suggests orthodromic AV reciprocating tachycardia. *Right,* Antidromic AV reciprocating tachycardia. During tachycardia, anterograde conduction proceeds over the AP, and retrograde conduction occurs via the AVN. Because ventricular activation during tachycardia occurs solely via the AP, the QRS complexes during tachycardia have a maximally pre-excited pattern. Also, because retrograde conduction via the AVN is slow compared to anterograde conduction over the AP, the P-R interval is shorter during antidromic AV reciprocating tachycardia (i.e., "long R-P, short P-R"). However, this latter feature is rarely of diagnostic value, because the rapid rate of tachycardia and maximally pre-excited QRS complexes usually result in nondiscernible P waves.

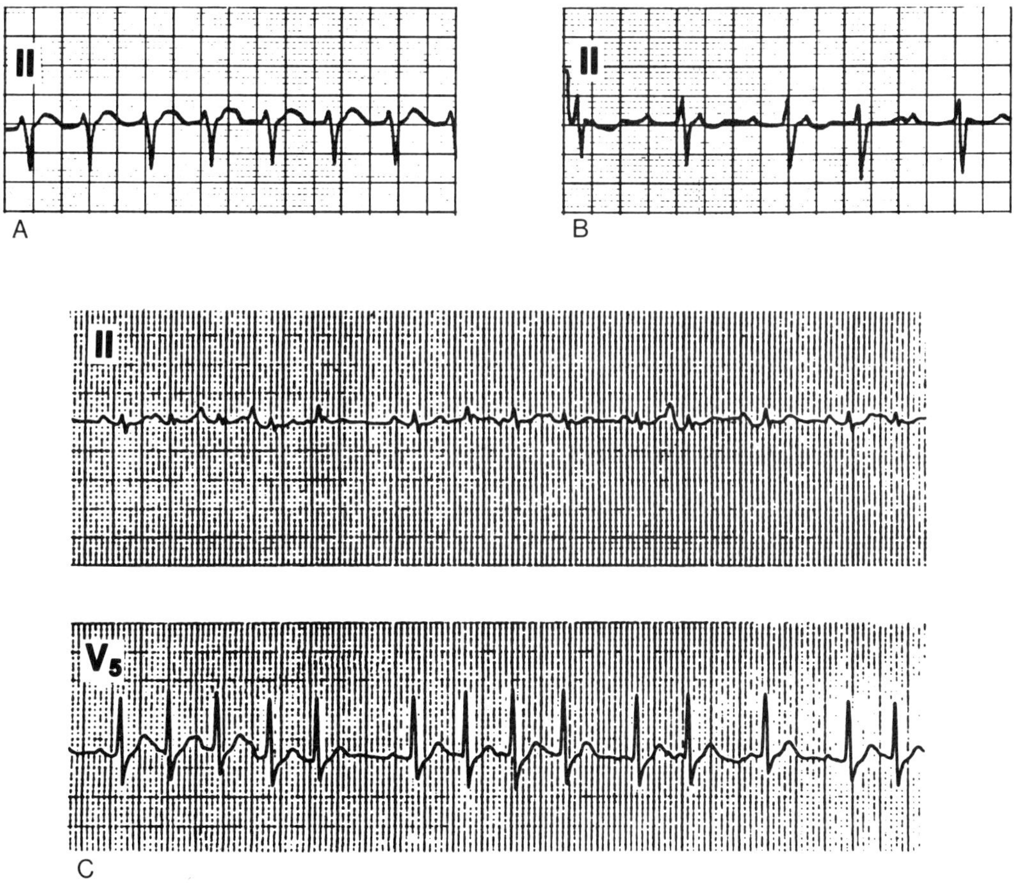

Figure 5–9. Automatic (ectopic) atrial tachycardias. *A,* Automatic atrial tachycardia with block. *B,* Nonparoxysmal (automatic) atrial tachycardia. Note that the P waves of the initial and subsequent beats of tachycardia are the same. *C,* Multiform (chaotic) atrial tachycardia.

150 beats/minute with marked variation in P wave morphology and totally irregular P-P intervals (Fig. 5–9*C*). In general, at least three different P wave contours are noted in a single lead, and most P waves are conducted to the ventricles.

Atrial Flutter and Fibrillation

Atrial Flutter. With type I atrial flutter, there are identical, recurring flutter waves with sawtooth appearance and no isoelectric interval between them (rate 240–340 beats/minute). Usually, the ventricular rate is one half the atrial rate (Fig. 5–10*A*). If the AV conduction ratio remains constant, the ventricular rhythm will be regular. If not, the ventricular rhythm will be ''regularly irregular'' because of some recurring pattern of AV conduction block. Type I atrial flutter is usually affected and often terminated by rapid atrial pacing. In contrast, with type II atrial flutter, the atrial rate is between 340 and 440 beats/minute and rapid atrial pacing has no effect on the disturbance.

Atrial Fibrillation. Atrial fibrillation is characterized by totally fragmented and disorganized atrial electrical activity. With atrial fibrillation, atrial activity may not be recognized in all leads. In the absence of apparent atrial activity, atrial fibrillation is recognized by the totally irregular R-R intervals (i.e., ''irregularly irregular''). With atrial fibrillation, the QRS complexes may appear normal or may be conducted aberrantly (Fig. 5–10*B*). It is important to appreciate the frequency of ventricular aberration in patients with atrial fibrillation, because aberrantly conducted beats may be misdiagnosed (and incorrectly treated) as ventricular ectopic beats. Ventricular aberration is especially likely when, during atrial fibrillation, lengthening of the R-R interval is immediately followed by a short R-R interval. This is termed the ''Ashman phenomenon'' (Fig. 5–10*B*).

VENTRICULAR ARRHYTHMIAS

Ventricular Ectopic Beats

Ectopic beats arising below the bifurcation of the common (His) bundle can be grouped as *premature* or *escape beats.* Premature ventricular beats include extrasystolic, parasystolic, and unclassified beats, all of which end cycles that are shorter than that of the dominant rhythm. Ventricular escape beats are postmature and end a cycle that is longer than that of the dominant rhythm. The typical *ventricular extrasystole* bears a constant relation to the preceding beat of the dominant rhythm (Fig. 5–11*A*). *Parasystolic beats* bear a definite mathematical relation to each other, but not the dominant rhythm (Fig. 5–11*B*). Therefore, with parasystolic beats, intervals between successive ventricular

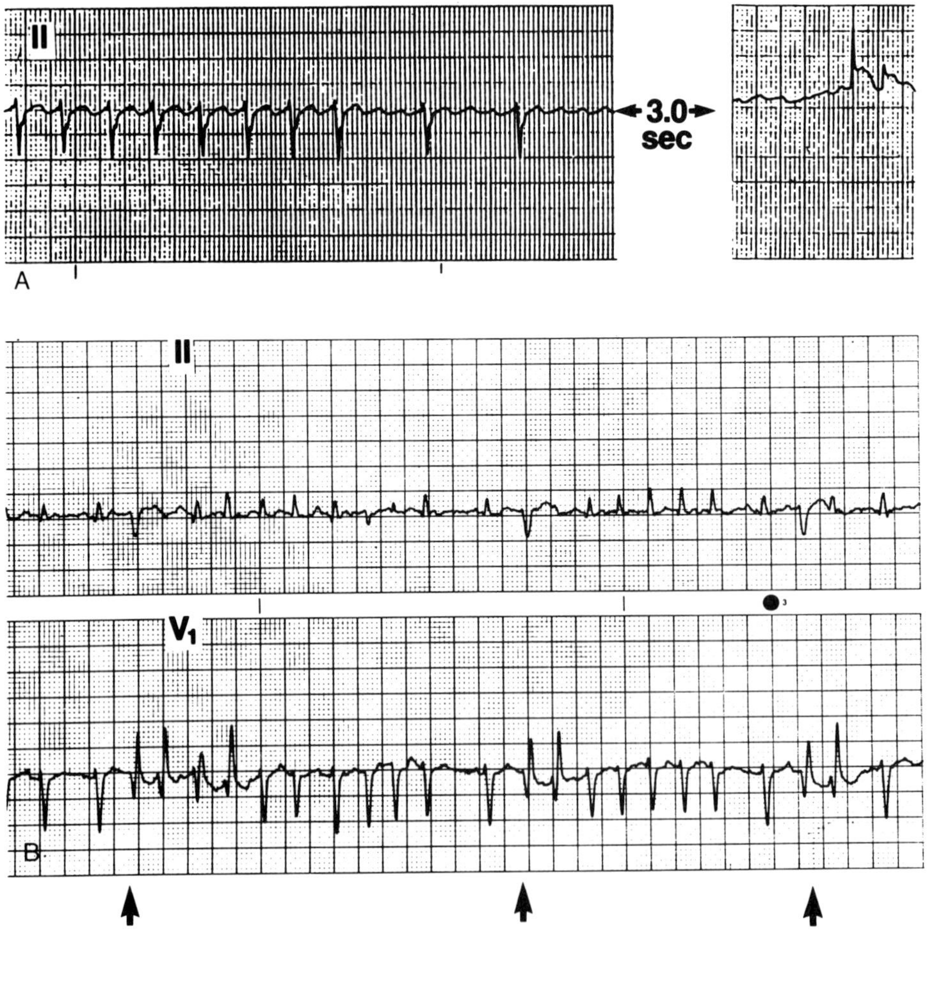

Figure 5–10. *A*, Atrial flutter (type 1) with 2:1 AV block. Application of carotid sinus massage increases the block to 4.1, followed by an approximate 5-second period of complete heart block before a ventricular escape beat. During advanced or complete heart block, the atrial mechanism for tachycardia is revealed. *B*, Atrial fibrillation. Note that three beats indicated with arrows (lead II) are conducted with ventricular aberration. Since the beats with aberration occur with a short R-R interval following a relatively prolonged R-R interval, aberration is likely due to the Ashman phenomenon.

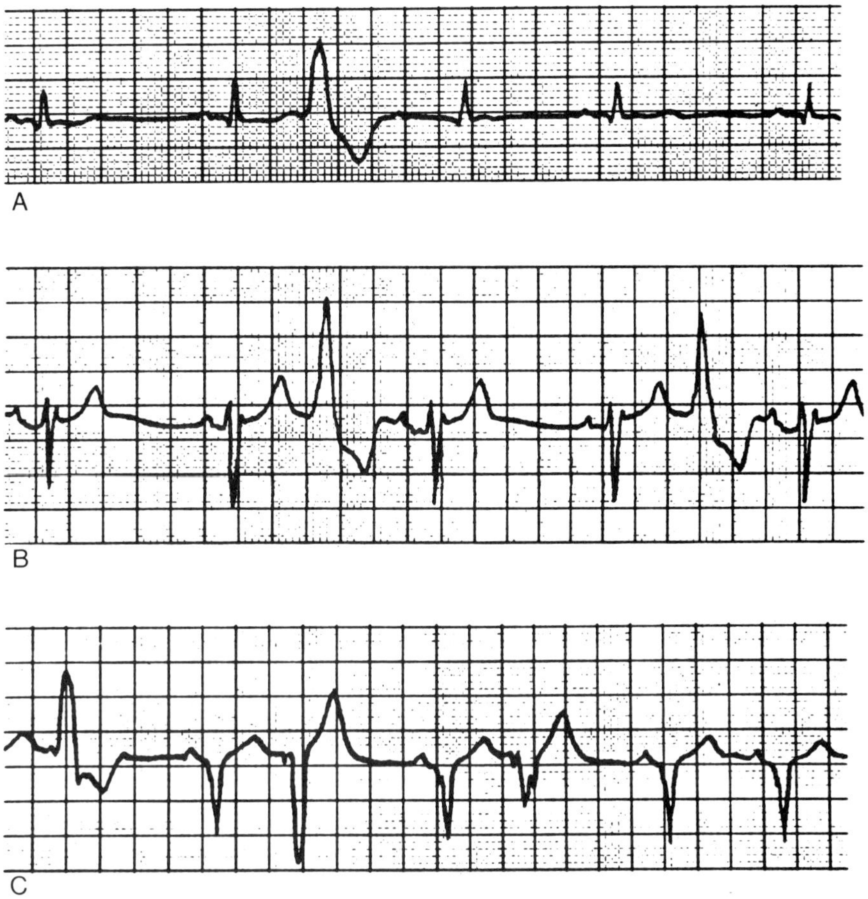

Figure 5–11. Ventricular premature beats. *A*, Single ventricular extrasystole. Note that retrograde penetration of the AV node by the ventricular premature beat causes delay in the conduction of the next sinus-origin beat (prolonged P-R interval). *B*, Possible parasystolic ventricular beats. These beats do not appear to affect, nor are they affected by, the dominant rhythm. To prove parasystole would require a much longer rhythm strip. *C*, Unclassified, multiform ventricular extrasystoles. These ventricular extrasystoles bear no relation to each other or to the dominant rhythm.

extrasystoles will be some multiple of each other, but not of the underlying rhythm. *Unclassified beats* occur randomly, that is, they bear no relation to each other or to the preceding beat (Fig. 5–11*C*). A premature beat is characterized by the premature occurrence of a bizarre QRS complex that is typically wider than 0.12 seconds, but that may vary some among leads. However, more important than the width of the QRS is its different morphologic features from those of surrounding, normally conducted beats. In fact, the premature beat may appear remarkably similar to normally conducted beats in some leads, so that multiple leads may have to be examined when there is doubt. If a premature beat conducts retrogradely to the atria (may cause a retrograde P wave), it could reset automaticity of the SA node to cause a compensatory pause. However, the compensatory pause is not a hallmark of ventricular premature beats. Ectopic atrial or AV junctional beats (conducted with ventricular aberration) can also reset automaticity of the SA node. If the ventricular premature beat is interpolated, it does not affect the cycle length of the dominant rhythm, or it does so only minimally (incomplete interpolation). Premature ventricular beats may have different morphologic features in the same ECG lead, in which case they are said to be "multiform" or "polymorphic." The term "multifocal" is not used because it is not known whether multiple foci are discharging, or whether conduction of impulses from one focus is changing. If premature beats follow each beat of the dominant rhythm, the term "bigeminy" is used. If they follow two or three normal beats, the terms "trigeminy" and "quadrigeminy" are used, respectively. Finally, two or three successive ventricular premature beats are termed a "couplet" or a "triplet," respectively. Arbitrarily, more than three beats in succession constitute ventricular tachycardia.

Idioventricular and Accelerated Idioventricular Rhythm

Idioventricular rhythm occurs when an ectopic ventricular pacemaker controls the ventricles for successive beats, usually at 30–45 beats/minute. With accelerated idioventricular rhythm (AIR), the rate exceeds 45 beats/minute, but rarely 110 beats/minute. The ectopic ventricular rate is usually close to the sinus rate, so that control of the ventricles may pass back and forth between the SA node and ventricular ectopic focus, indicated by the presence of capture and fusion beats (Fig. 5–12). AIR is commonly associated with inferior wall myocardial infarction,[46] digitalis excess,[44] and reperfusion of ischemic myocardium.

Ventricular Tachyarrhythmias

Useful Diagnostic Criteria. Any wide QRS tachycardia should be presumed to be of ventricular origin until proved

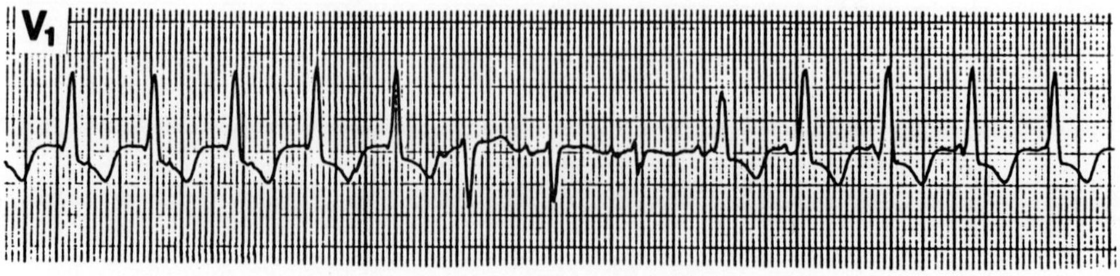

Figure 5–12. Accelerated idioventricular rhythm with V-A association (beats 1–3), A-V dissociation (beats 4, 5, 10–13), and A-V association with capture beats (beats 6 and 7) or fusion beats (beats 8 and 9).

otherwise. There may not be time or sufficient ECG leads to differentiate the two causes for wide QRS tachycardia (ventricular ectopy vs. aberration). The presence of *fusion* or *capture beats* during the course of a wide QRS tachycardia (Fig. 5–13) provides maximum support for the diagnosis of ventricular tachycardia, except that fusion or capture beats are rarely seen, and then only at rates below 160 beats/minute. A *fusion beat* has an appearance somewhere between one of supraventricular or ventricular origin, since it is the result of simultaneous activation from both sites. A *capture beat* is ventricular activation by an atrial impulse during AV dissociation with ventricular tachycardia. The timing of the atrial impulse must be such that it reaches the AV junction and ventricles when they are not refractory. Finally, the presence of AV dissociation during a wide QRS tachycardia is strong presumptive evidence for ventricular tachycardia. However, discerning P waves during a rapid wide QRS tachycardia can be difficult. Esophageal or intravascular atrial leads may be required.

Rate and Appearance. Three or more successive ventricular beats at rates from 100 to 250 beats/minute is ventricular tachycardia (VT). QRS complexes with VT may have a uniform (monomorphic) or multiform (polymorphic) appearance, and the R-R intervals during VT may be regular or may vary somewhat. As with SVT, the onset of VT may be sudden (paroxysmal) or more gradual (nonparoxysmal). Arbitrarily, VT is sustained if tachycardia lasts longer than 30 seconds.

Specific Patterns or Types of VT. *Accelerated idioventricular rhythm* is considered by some to be a slow form of monomorphic VT. *Torsades de pointes VT* is characterized by QRS complexes that constantly change in amplitude, appear to twist around the ECG isoelectric line, and occur at rates from 200 to 250 beats/minute (Fig. 5–14*A*). It occurs only in association with acquired or congenital long QT syndrome.[47] When VT morphologically similar to torsades occurs without QT interval prolongation, it is classified as *polymorphous VT*. With *bidirectional VT* (Fig. 5–14*B*), the QRS complexes alternate in polarity, and the rhythm is regular. *Repetitive monomorphic VT* (RMVT) is the repetitive occurrence of three or more ventricular beats of uniform appearance with only brief intervening periods of normal sinus beats.

Ventricular Flutter and Fibrillation. The ECG distinction between ventricular flutter and fibrillation is moot, because either disturbance is lethal if not promptly terminated. Ventricular flutter gives the ECG appearance of sine wave oscillations around the isoelectric line at a rate of 150–300

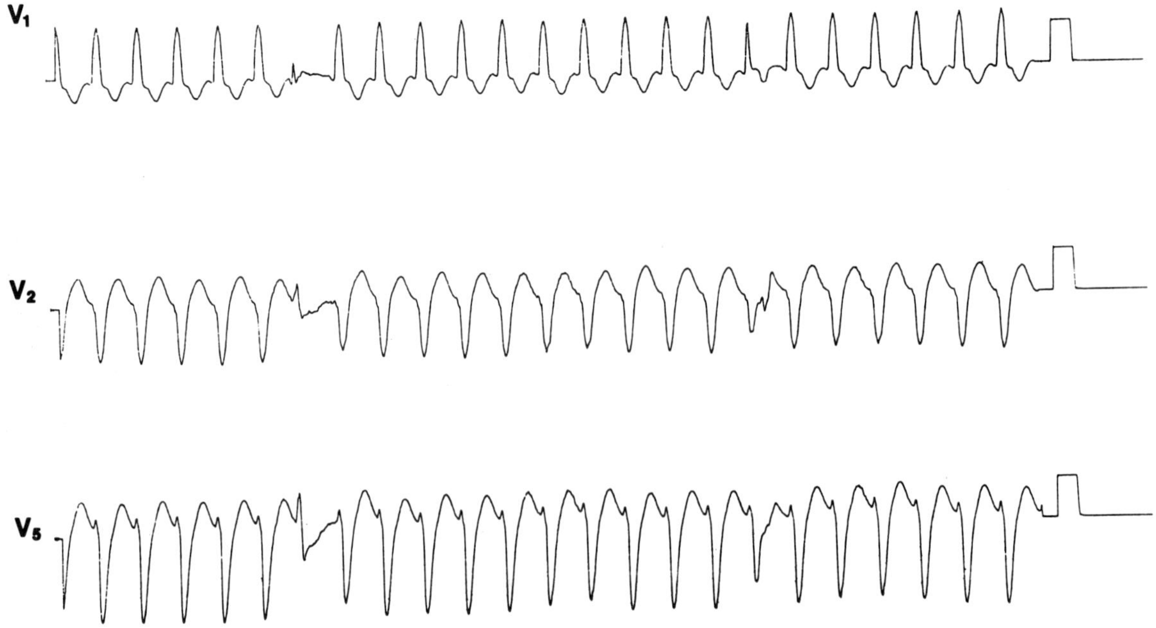

Figure 5–13. Monomorphic ventricular tachycardia with capture (beat 7) and fusion beats (beat 18). The presence of capture and fusion beats is maximum evidence that this tachycardia is ventricular.

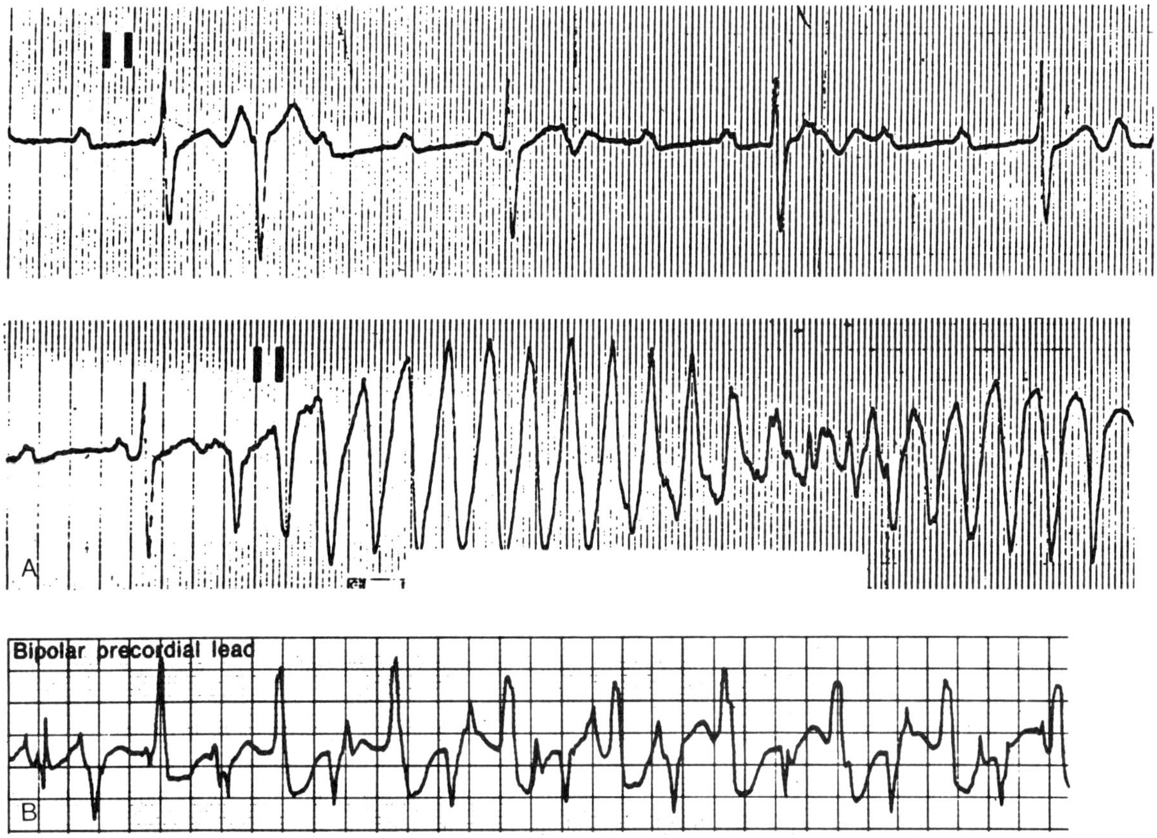

Figure 5–14. Specific patterns of ventricular tachycardia (VT). *A*, Torsades de pointes VT in patient with complete heart block. *B*, Bidirectional VT in patient with severe digitalis intoxication.

beats/minute. Ventricular fibrillation is recognized by irregular undulations in the ECG baseline, with no distinct QRS complexes, ST segments, or T waves.

HEART BLOCK

Heart block is a temporary or permanent disturbance of impulse conduction due to anatomic or functional impairment of AV conduction. It is not the same as *interference*, whereby physiologic refractoriness induced by a preceding impulse affects transmission of the subsequent impulse. Heart block can occur anywhere in the heart where impulses are conducted. It is recognized on the ECG as occurring between the SA node and atria (*SA block*), in the atria (*intra-atrial block*), between the atria and ventricles (*AV block*), or in the ventricles (*intraventricular block*). AV heart block may occur within the AV node, the common (His) bundle, or the bundle branches.

First-, Second-, and Third-Degree AV Heart Block

With *first-degree AV heart block*, all supraventricular impulses are conducted to the ventricles, but with a P-R interval >0.21 seconds in adults (normal 0.12–0.21 seconds). P-R interval prolongation can result from conduction delay within the AV node, the His-Purkinje system, or both. If the QRS complex in multiple surface leads has a normal contour, the delay is almost always within the AV node.[44] If first-degree block occurs in the AV node, acceleration of heart rate or enhanced vagal tone may increase block.

Second-degree AV heart block is characterized by the failure of some, but not all, atrial impulses to cause ventricular depolarization. With *type I (Wenckebach) second-degree AV heart block* (Fig. 5–15*A*), there is progressive prolongation of the P-R interval prior to dropped beats. Type I second-degree AV block almost always occurs within the AV node, especially with normal QRS complexes. With *type II (Mobitz) second-degree AV heart block* (Fig. 5–15*B*), there is no progressive P-R interval prolongation prior to dropped beats. *Advanced second-degree AV heart block* exists when, in the absence of physiologic interference and at reasonable atrial rates (<140 beats/minute), two or more successive atrial beats fail to conduct to the ventricle. Type II or advanced second-degree AV block with abnormal QRS complexes usually signifies disease within the His-Purkinje system.

Third-degree (complete) AV heart block is present when no atrial beats are conducted to the ventricles (Fig. 5–15*C*). Consequently, the atria and ventricles are controlled by independent pacemakers and are completely dissociated. The ventricular rate is usually 40 beats/minute or less, but could be faster (60–65 beats/minute) with congenital third-degree AV heart block.

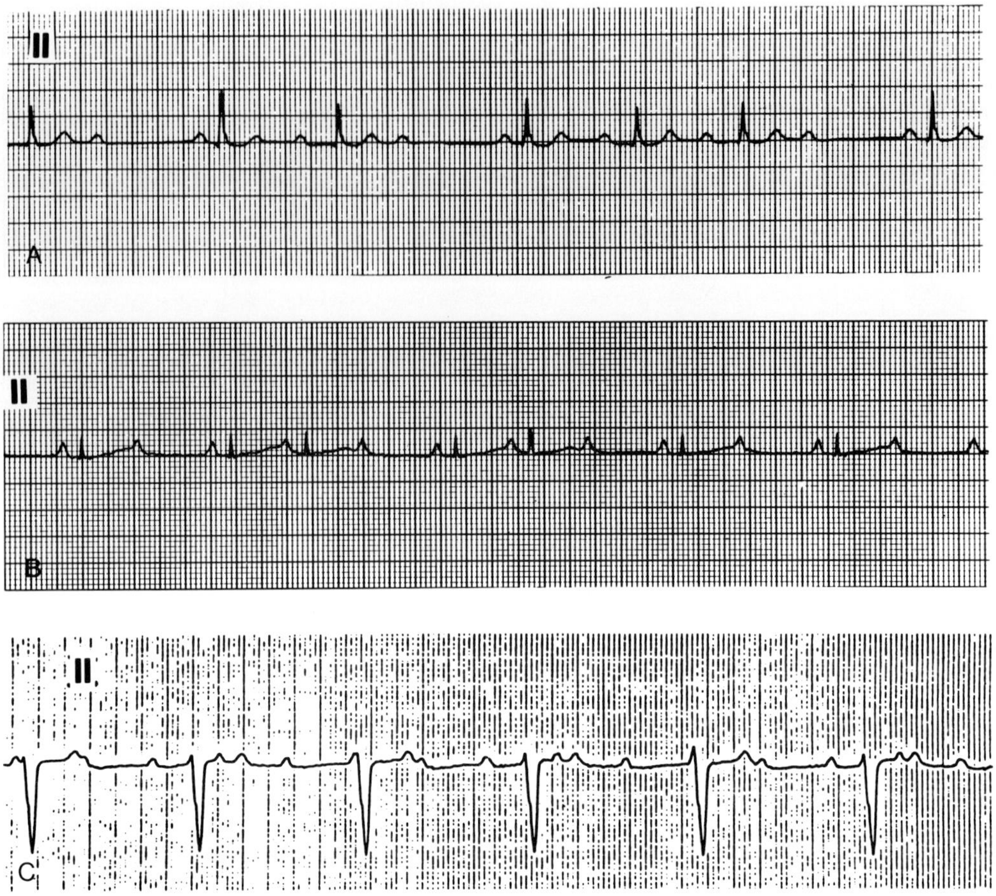

Figure 5–15. Second- and third-degree AV heart block. *A*, Type 1 (Wenckebach) second-degree AV heart block. *B*, Type 2 (Mobitz II) second-degree AV heart block. *C*, Third-degree (complete) AV heart block.

Bundle-Branch and Fascicular Heart Block

Bundle-branch and fascicular blocks are not really cardiac rhythm disturbances. Rather, they are ECG patterns associated with conduction block (organic or functional) in the right or left bundle branch, or in the major subdivisions of the left bundle branch. Recognition of these patterns is helpful for the diagnosis of many arrhythmias, because these patterns may be confused with more serious arrhythmias. Examples include SVT in a patient with left bundle-branch block that is mistaken for ventricular tachycardia and premature atrial beats conducted with functional right bundle-branch aberration that is mistaken for premature ventricular beats. The characteristic ECG feature of complete *right bundle-branch block* is the late and delayed electrical force of right ventricular depolarization oriented to the right and anteriorly. This produces a QRS of 0.12 seconds or greater, and a wide S wave in leads I and V_4 to V_6 (Fig. 5–16). The anterior component of the late force is responsible for the wide R′ waves in the right precordial leads (V_1 and V_2). The ST segment and T wave are opposite in direction to the late force of ventricular depolarization, resulting in ST segment and T wave inversion in V_1 and V_2. Finally, as result of normal septal activation (oriented to the right and anteriorly), a small initial r wave will be recorded in V_1 and V_2 (q in V_4 to V_6).

With complete *left bundle-branch block*, the ECG patterns in the standard and augmented leads vary with heart position,[48] whereas the precordial leads show less variation due to heart position. For the horizontal heart position (most common), the QRS is 0.12 seconds or longer with a frontal plane axis of 0 to −30 degrees. There are wide and slurred R waves with depressed ST segments and inverted T waves in leads I and II (Fig. 5–17). Lead aVL is similar, except possibly for small r and s waves preceding a wide and slurred R′. Lead aVF has a qrS, QS, or rS complex with an elevated or isoelectric ST segment and upright T wave. A more vertical heart position is illustrated in Figure 5–17 with an RR′ and depressed ST segment with inverted T wave. The right precordial leads (V_1 and V_2) may record an initial Q from left to right septal activation followed by a small R wave from normal right ventricular activation. Delayed left ventricular activation produces a deep, wide S wave. The left precordial leads (V_4 and V_6) record the typical left ventricular epicardial pattern of a wide, notched R wave or rsR′ complex, with depressed ST segments and inverted T waves. The left bundle branch has two major divisions or fascicles (anterior and posterior); block of either fascicle is termed *fascicular heart block.* Left anterior fascicular block is by far more common than posterior fascicular block, and frequently occurs in association with

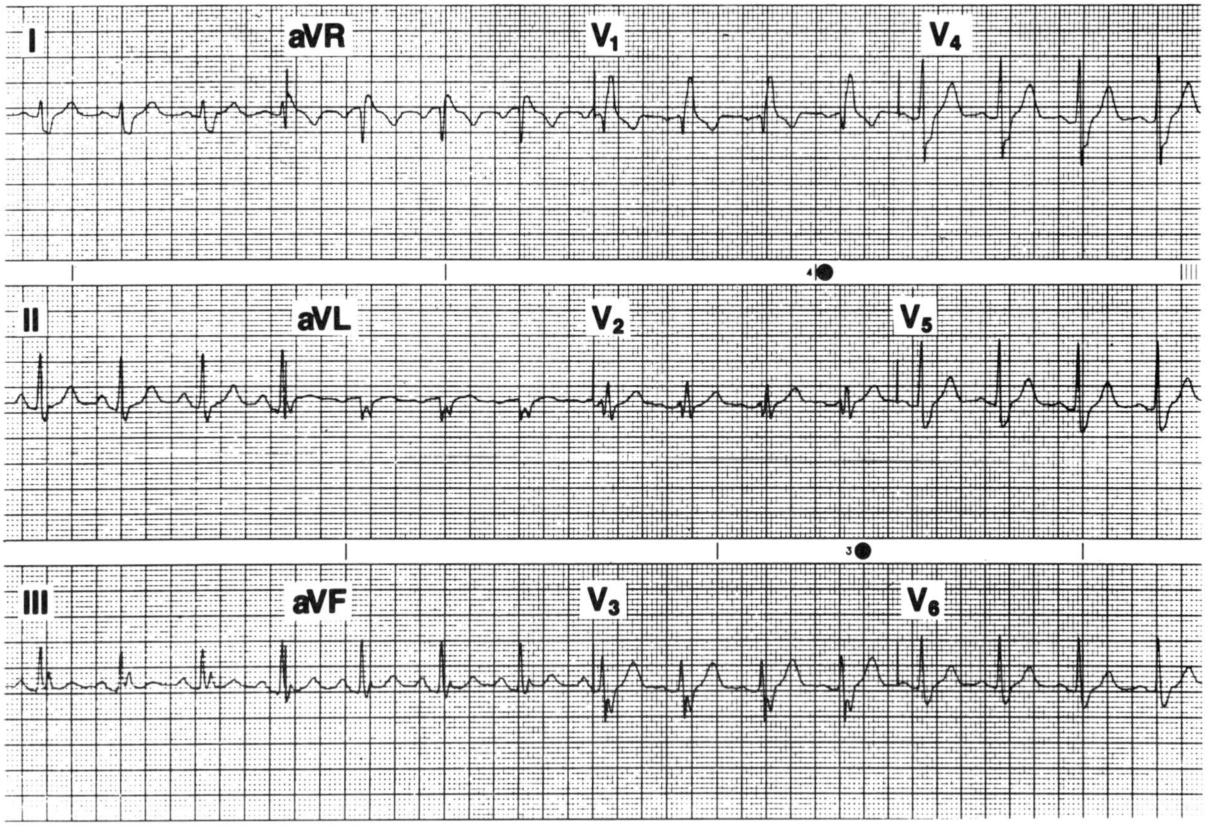

Figure 5–16. Typical 12-lead ECG changes of complete right bundle branch block.

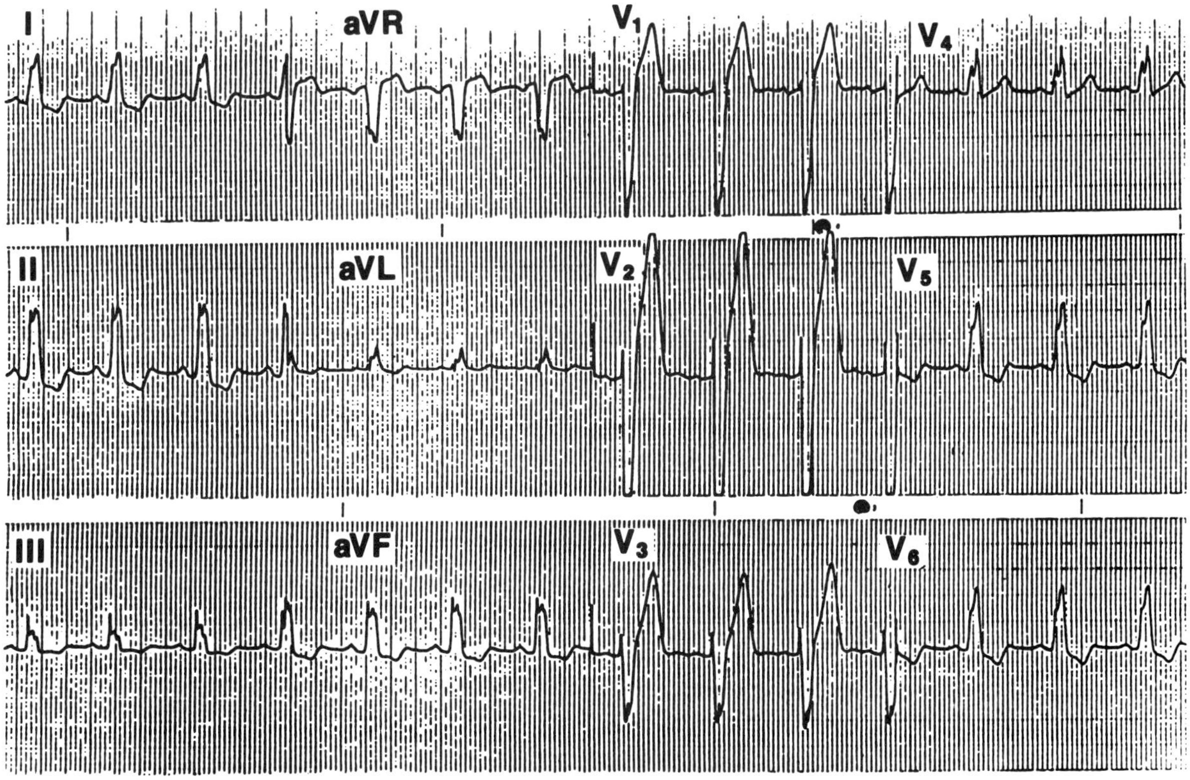

Figure 5–17. Typical 12-lead ECG changes of complete left bundle branch block.

right bundle-branch block (an association termed "bifascicular heart block"). Fascicular blocks are described in standard ECG references.

VENTRICULAR PRE-EXCITATION

Pathways

Ventricular pre-excitation exists if the ventricle or some part of the ventricle is activated earlier than it would when activation occurs solely by the normal pathways. There are several possible pathways by which the ventricles can be activated earlier than expected, including (1) *accessory AV pathways* (Kent's bundle), (2) *nodofascicular, nodoventricular,* or *fasciculoventricular fibers* (Mahaim fibers), and (3) *intranodal bypass tracts* (James fibers). By far the most common are accessory AV pathways. These are responsible for ventricular pre-excitation and AV reciprocating tachycardia in patients with the WPW syndrome. The other pathways are rare and are demonstrated by sophisticated electrophysiologic techniques.

ECG with Pre-excitation

When there is dual activation of the ventricles via normal and accessory AV pathways, a fusion QRS complex results—the so-called delta wave (Fig. 5–18). The configuration of the fusion complex depends on the location of the accessory pathway in relation to the SA node, the size of the atria, the relative contribution of accessory and normal pathways (AV node and His-Purkinje system) to ventricular activation, and the ECG lead selected.[44, 50] The extent of contribution of the accessory and normal pathway activation wave fronts to ventricular depolarization depends on their relative activation times. This can vary from beat to beat. Typically, however, with fast atrial rates or premature atrial beats, there will be increased AV nodal delay, so that ventricular depolarization will result at least in part from activation via the accessory pathway. In other words, fusion beats (or delta waves) are more likely at faster heart rates. In contrast, with slow heart rates or with accessory pathways located far from the SA node, more ventricular depolarization will result from activation via the normal pathway.

Tachyarrhythmias with Pre-excitation

The term "WPW syndrome" is used when (1) there is evidence of pre-excitation and (2) the patient has symptoms of tachyarrhythmia. Patients with WPW are prone to develop extremely rapid AV conduction (via an accessory AV pathway) during atrial flutter or fibrillation (Fig. 5–19). The maximal possible ventricular rate with atrial flutter or fibrillation in patients with the WPW syndrome is limited by the refractory period of the accessory pathway. Ventricular rates of ≥300 beats/minute are possible with short (≤200 msec) refractory periods.[49]

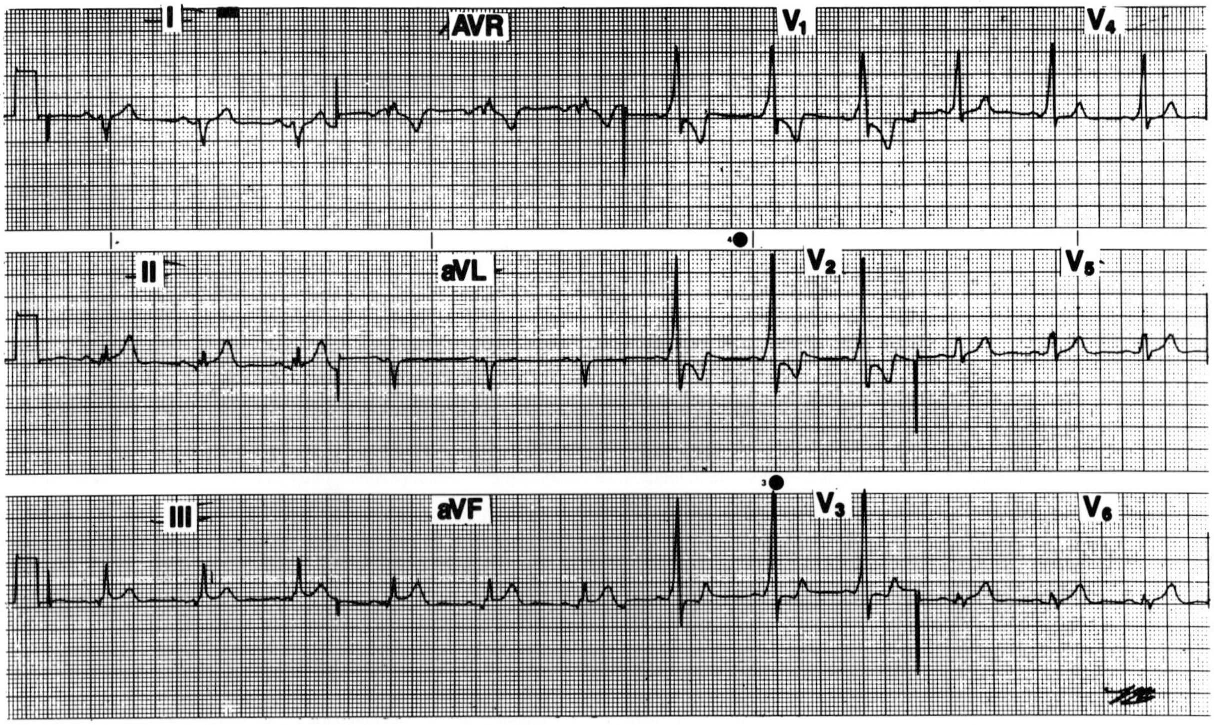

Figure 5–18. Twelve-lead ECG from patient with Wolff-Parkinson-White syndrome and evidence of ventricular preexcitation during sinus rhythm. The short P-R interval and slurring of the initial upstroke of the R wave (i.e., "delta wave") are most pronounced in leads V_1 to V_3.

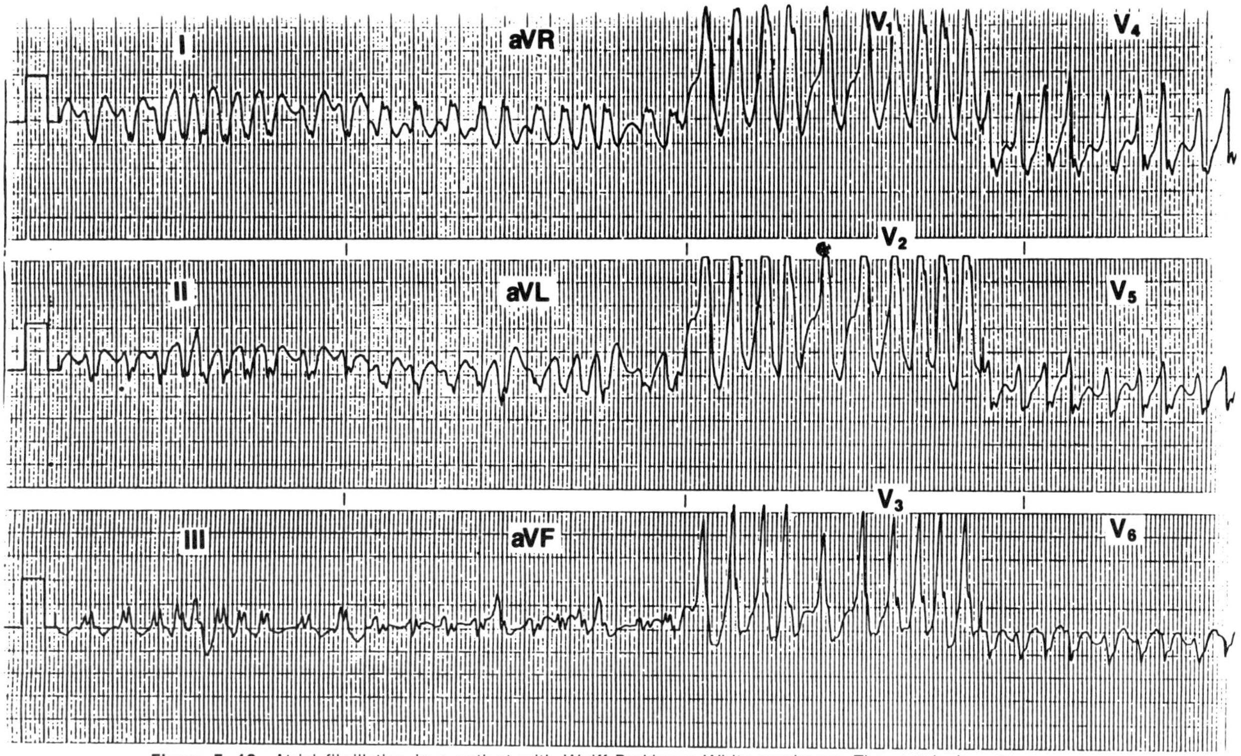

Figure 5–19. Atrial fibrillation in a patient with Wolff-Parkinson-White syndrome. The ventricular rate ranges from 180 to 285 beats/minute for the portion of rhythm shown.

ECG MANIFESTATIONS OF ALTERED STATES

Altered physiologic states can be the cause of life-threatening cardiac rhythm disturbances. Fortunately, they are also associated with fairly specific ECG patterns. The ability to recognize these ECG patterns, with prompt correction or removal of the imbalance, may be all that is required to prevent more troublesome occurrences.

EFFECTS OF ELECTROLYTE DISTURBANCES

Potassium

Hypokalemia. Hypokalemia is probably more likely than hyperkalemia to cause arrhythmias. Hypokalemia usually results from potassium-wasting diuretics, metabolic alkalosis, overventilation of patients (respiratory alkalosis), insulin administration, or use of β-adrenergic agonists. Hypokalemia facilitates or causes arrhythmias due to re-entry and disturbed or abnormal automaticity. Arrhythmias in patients with severe hypokalemia are similar to those in patients with digitalis toxicity, including ectopic beats, automatic atrial tachycardia (with AV block), ventricular tachycardia, and fibrillation. Hypokalemia, similar to digitalis, intensifies the effects of vagal stimulation. There is reasonable correlation between ECG changes and potassium levels below 2.5–3.0 mEq/L.[31, 51] Hypokalemia is characterized by an exaggerated U wave without significant prolongation of the QT interval (Fig. 5–20). ST segment depression and gradual fusion with the U wave, less commonly T wave inversion, and an increase in amplitude of the QRS complex may also be manifestations of hypokalemia. However, these same changes are not specific for hypokalemia, and may be associated with digitalis, other drugs, or even ventricular hypertrophy.

Hyperkalemia. In perioperative and critical care settings, hyperkalemia is usually associated with chronic renal disease, depolarizing neuromuscular blocking drugs in susceptible patients (e.g., patients with burns or neuromuscular disease),[47] or overly aggressive potassium replacement in hypokalemic patients. Patients with chronic, moderate hyperkalemia (<7.5 mEq/L) rarely have atrial or ventricular ectopy or AV conduction defects.[57] Possibly, this seeming "antiarrhythmic effect" of moderate hyperkalemia is explained by depression of automaticity in ectopic pacemakers, or by termination of re-entry with improved conduction.[52] The effect of acute potassium administration on cardiac rhythm and conduction depends on the integrity of the myocardium, the beginning extracellular potassium concentration, the amount of potassium administered, and the rate of change in extracellular potassium.[31] The dependence of fibers of the SA and AV node on the slow-inward (calcium) current is thought to explain their relative resistance to effects of increased potassium compared to atrial, His-Purkinje, or ventricular fibers.

The peaked (also termed "tented") T wave (Fig. 5–20) is the earliest ECG abnormality associated with hyperkalemia. Its pointed, symmetric appearance and narrow base help to differentiate the effect of hyperkalemia from other

Normal tracing (serum potassium 4-5.5 mEq/L): PR interval=0.16 sec; QRS interval=0.06 sec; QT interval=0.4 sec (normal for an assumed heart rate of 60).

Hypokalemia (serum potassium ± 3.5 mEq/L): PR interval=0.2 sec; QRS interval=0.06 sec; ST segment depression. A prominent U wave is present following the T wave. The QT interval remains 0.4 sec. If the U wave is erroneously considered a part of the T, a falsely prolonged QT interval of 0.6 sec will be measured.

Hypokalemia (serum potassium ± 2.5 mEq/L): The PR interval is lengthened to 0.32 sec; the ST segment is depresssed; the T wave is inverted; a prominent U wave is seen. The true QT interval remains normal.

Hyperkalemia (serum potassium ± 7 mEq/L): The PR and QRS intervals are within normal limits. Very tall, slender, peaked *"tented"* T waves are now present.

Hyperkalemia (serum potassium ± 8.5 mEq/L): There is no evidence of atrial activity; the QRS complex is broad and slurred, and the QRS interval has widened to 0.2 sec. The T waves remain tall and slender. Further elevation of the serum potassium will result in ventricular tachycardia and ventricular fibrillation.

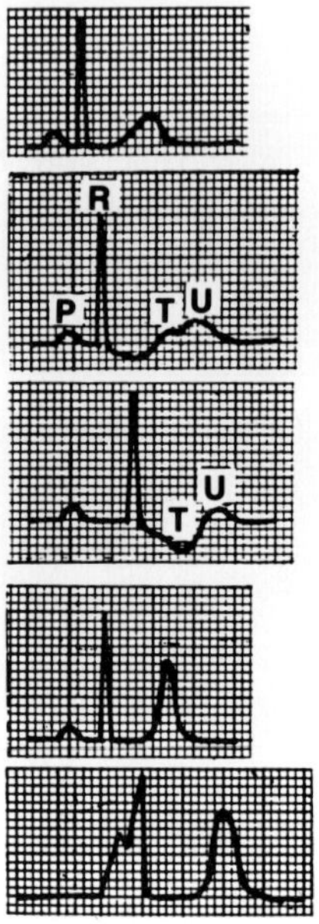

Figure 5–20. Correlation of serum potassium level and the ECG. It is assumed that the serum calcium remains normal. The diagrammed complexes are from left precordial leads. (From Goldman MJ: Principles of Clinical Electrocardiography, 12th Ed. Los Altos, CA: Lange Medical Publications, 1986.)

causes of tall T waves. However, T waves suggestive of hyperkalemia are seen in only about 20% of patients with hyperkalemia[53] and are best seen in the inferior and precordial leads. Decreased R wave amplitude, prominent S waves, widening of the QRS complex, and ST segment depression (or occasionally elevation) appear as the potassium concentration approaches 8–9 mEq/L.[53] Decreased amplitude and widening of the P wave with prolongation of the P-R interval may make diagnosis of arrhythmias with hyperkalemia extremely difficult. Finally, the depression of intraventricular conduction associated with hyperkalemia is characteristically diffuse and fairly uniform, and results in prolongation of the initial and terminal portions of the QRS complex (Fig. 5–20).

Calcium and Magnesium. Only extreme extracellular *hypercalcemia* is likely to produce electrophysiologic abnormalities of clinical importance.[52] The most striking change with hypercalcemia is shortening of the Q-T interval, particularly the distance from the beginning of the QRS to the apex of the T wave—QTa interval.[54] In some cases, the P-R interval is also prolonged, and there may be a widespread increase in the QRS amplitude and diphasic T waves. *Hypocalcemia* prolongs the plateau (phase 2) of the cardiac action potential, reflected in the surface ECG by prolongation of the Q-T interval and the ST segment. The QTa and QT intervals are prolonged, but the QTc interval (i.e., QT corrected for heart rate) rarely exceeds 140% of normal.[51] Administration of magnesium salts significantly shortens the Q-T interval. Abnormalities of the ST segment caused by chronic hypermagnesemia cannot be identified on the ECG because the changes are dominated by calcium.[51] Hypomagnesemia cannot be recognized on the ECG.

EFFECTS OF PHARMACOLOGIC AGENTS

None of the *inhalation* or *intravenous anesthetics, opiates, neuromuscular blockers,* or *anesthetic adjuvant drugs* have characteristic ECG effects of their own. Although the potent volatile anesthetics may produce small prolongation of specialized cardiac conduction (AV node, ventricular), this effect with clinical doses is small and nonapparent on the surface ECG.

Digitalis inhibits the sodium-potassium exchange pump, which increases intracellular sodium followed by accumulation of intracellular calcium. The latter contributes to arrhythmias with digitalis toxicity, and almost any type of cardiac rhythm disturbance can be observed. Except for automatic atrial tachycardia with block, no arrhythmia is really specific. Alterations of the ST segment and T wave are the earliest recognizable changes caused by digitalis and are therefore considered evidence of digitalis effect. The T wave amplitude is reduced, and the ST segment is depressed and shortened (''sagging'') with the occasional appearance of a prominent U wave. Expected ECG effects of digitalis are some prolongation of the P-R interval, slowing of the ventricular rate with atrial flutter or fibrillation and the appearance of isolated AV junctional escape beats with atrial fibrillation.

Class 1 antiarrhythmic drugs, including the class 1a drugs (quinidine, procainamide, disopyramide) and 1c drugs (encainide, flecainide, propafenone) all can produce Q-T interval prolongation and polymorphic ventricular tachycardia as a manifestation of toxicity.

Tricyclic antidepressants (e.g., amitriptyline, imipramine) are myocardial depressants that also impair AV conduction. In therapeutic doses, these drugs may prolong the P-R interval, QRS complex, and Q-T interval; alter the ST segment and T wave; and induce both atrial and ventricular arrhythmias.[31] Toxic doses of these drugs, in addition, may cause second-and third-degree AV block.

ECG changes caused by the *phenothiazines* include prolongation of the Q-T interval and widening and notching of the T wave. These changes are most common with thioridazine and less likely with other phenothiazines.[31] The amplitude of the U wave may be increased, but the ST segment is usually unaffected. At higher doses, the amplitude of the T wave decreases, and it may become inverted. The P wave and QRS complex are not altered. Large doses of the phenothiazines may induce ventricular arrhythmias and even cause sudden death. The most common ECG abnormalities associated with *lithium* are T wave changes.[31] SA node dysfunction (bradycardia, pause, arrest, SA block) and heart block are more characteristic of toxicity. Lithium has no recognizable effects on the QRS complex.

ACID-BASE IMBALANCE OR CENTRAL NERVOUS SYSTEM (CNS) LESIONS

Clinically observed derangements of *acid-base balance* do not produce characteristic ECG changes nor do they directly cause arrhythmias. However, associated autonomic imbalance, electrolyte disorders, and cellular hypoxia are causes for ECG changes and arrhythmias. The most common ECG abnormalities with *CNS lesions*, especially acute subarachnoid hemorrhage, are Q-T interval prolongation, ST segment elevation or depression, inverted or tall T waves, and occasionally Q waves that mimic those with acute myocardial infarction.[55] Bradycardia and hypertension occur with severely increased intracranial pressure (>50 mmHg).

ARTIFACTS

ECG artifacts are most commonly the result of poor electrode contact, patient movement, muscle contractions (e.g., tremors, fasciculations, shivering), electromagnetic or mechanical interference (e.g., electrocautery, bone saws and drills, infusion pumps), lead or electrode movement, and improper standardization. Some examples of artifacts are provided in Figure 5–21. It cannot be emphasized strongly enough how important good electrode contact is for correct ECG diagnosis. Disposable electrodes should be checked for adequate contact gel, and the skin surface should be

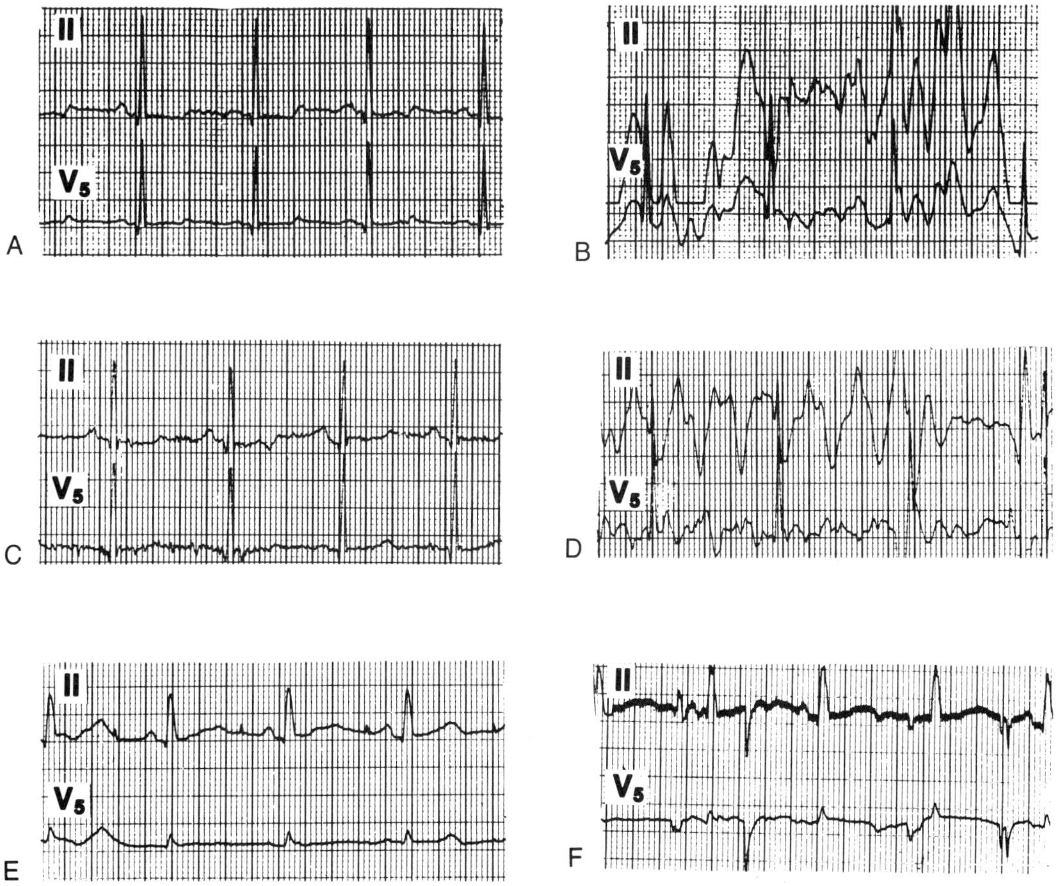

Figure 5–21. Examples of ECG artifacts on monitored leads. *A*, Improperly applied (poor skin contact) left leg electrode. Baseline in lead II simulates fine atrial fibrillation, except that R-R intervals are regular. *B*, Detached left leg lead. Note that no organized activity is present in lead II, but that QRS complexes are seen in V_5. *C*, Improperly applied ground (right leg lead). Baseline in all leads will simulate fine atrial fibrillation. *D*, Mechanical (motion) artifact due to manipulating or touching leads. Artifact simulates ventricular tachycardia (lead II) or fibrillation (lead V_5), except that regular QRS complexes are evident in both leads. *E*, Artifact produced by neuromuscular stimulator (1.0-second twitches). *F*, Artifact produced by neuromuscular stimulator (50 Hz tetanus).

properly prepared. Artifacts produced by improper electrode contact can lead to incorrect diagnosis and sometimes to overtreatment. Before making any ECG diagnosis, first exclude artifact.

ELECTRONIC (ARTIFICIAL) PACEMAKERS

TERMINOLOGY

Electronic cardiac pacemakers are temporary or permanent devices that electrically stimulate the heart to contract. Pacemakers are most commonly used for the treatment of bradycardic rhythm disturbances, but newer pacemakers may have programmable antitachycardia features, including an internal cardioversion-defibrillation capability.[56] Pacemakers consist of a *power source* (battery) that supplies energy for stimulation and other pacemaker functions, *circuitry* for sensing and regulating stimulus timing, and *leads* that connect the power source to *electrodes* used for cardiac sensing or stimulation. *Epicardial* or *endocardial* (transvenous) electrodes are used for most temporary and for all permanent pacing applications, although some temporary pacing utilizes the transcutaneous or transesophageal routes. All modern pacemakers, including most temporary devices, are considered *programmable.* This means that it is possible to reversibly alter such functions as stimulus timing, current and duration, sensing parameters, and refractory periods. Sensing and stimulation are performed with atrial and/or ventricular electrodes. Electrode pairs may be connected directly to the myocardium in close proximity to each other (*bipolar configuration*), or one electrode may be myocardial and the other remote (*unipolar configuration*).

PACEMAKER IDENTIFICATION CODE

The 5-position ICHD (Inter-Society Commission for Heart Disease Resources) code is widely used as short-hand notation to indicate modes of pacing (Table 5–5). The *first position* designates the chamber paced, the *second position* the chamber sensed, and the *third position* the response to sensed events. The *fourth* and *fifth positions* designate programmable and special antitachycardia features, and are little used except by pacemaker technologists or implanting physicians. However, the letter R may be seen after a hyphen following the third position (e.g., VVI-R, DDI-R) to indicate *sensor-modulated, rate-adaptive pacing.* This type of pacing is used in patients with sinus node chronotropic incompetence or atrial tachyarrhythmias to sense changing body metabolic requirements. Some physiologic markers that have been or are currently being used for sensor-modulated, rate-adaptive pacing include the Q-T interval, body temperature, pH, endocardial evoked potentials, preejection interval, O_2 saturation, and right atrial pressure.[57, 58]

DIAGNOSIS OF FUNCTION

With anticipation of anesthesia and surgery, or with stress occasioned by surgery or critical care circumstances, it is not uncommon for pacemaker patients to have adequate spontaneous rhythm. Thus, the functional status of the pacemaker will be unknown to the casual observer. For the surgical candidate, time-permitting, pacemaker function should be evaluated in a pacemaker clinic or by a consultant physician prior to surgery. The type of pacemaker and the indications for its implantation should be noted. Also, any special recommendations for perioperative management should be provided. Sometimes it is necessary to ascertain the functional status of a pacemaker that has been suppressed by spontaneous rhythm under more urgent circumstances. A Valsalva maneuver or carotid sinus massage can be performed to slow the rate of spontaneous rhythm. Alternatively, drugs such as esmolol or edrophonium might be given to temporarily slow the rate. Any of these should only be carried out with continuous ECG monitoring and emergency chronotropic drugs available. The ECG can also provide additional information concerning pacemaker function. If the device is functioning properly, unless inhibited, a stimulus artifact should precede each P wave or QRS complex, or both, depending on the chambers paced. If the unit is pacing the patient, a rate other than the programmed rate could indicate impending power source depletion. The programmed rate can be learned from a pacemaker identi-

TABLE 5–5. ICHD FIVE-POSITION PACEMAKER CODE

I Chamber Paced	II Chamber Sensed	III Response Mode	IV Programmability	V Antitachycardia
V—ventricle	V—ventricle	T—triggered	P—simple†	B—bursts
A—atrium	A—atrium	I—inhibited	M—multiple	N—normal rate competition‡
D—dual	D—dual	D—double	C—communicating	S—scanning§
	O—none	O—none	O—none	E—external¶
		R—reverse*		

*Pacemaker activated on sensing tachycardia as opposed to bradycardia.
†Rate and/or output only.
‡Paces at slow rate on sensing tachycardia (*i.e.,* underdrive pacing).
§Some scanning response, such as timed extrastimuli.
¶External control (activated by magnet, radiofrequency, or some other means).

fication card or notes in the patient's chart concerning programmed parameters or from the implanting physician or pacemaker follow-up clinc. Pacing modes used for the management of bradyarrhythmias are summarized in Table 5–6. ECG illustrations of single- and dual-chamber pacing modes are provided in Figures 5–22 and 5–23. For further discussion concerning pacemaker function (e.g., sensing and blanking refractory periods, rate hysteresis, AV intervals, interference modes), the interested reader is referred elsewhere.[31, 59, 60]

PACEMAKER MALFUNCTION

Because of built-in interference modes, operation of modern pacemakers is quite dependable, even with substantial potential for malfunction (e.g., ionizing radiation, lithotripters, electrocautery).[60] Nevertheless, the anesthesiologist should know the causes and signs of pacemaker malfunction.

Failure to Pace

The failure to produce paced (capture) beats is recognized on the ECG by absent pacing stimuli (when expected) or pacing stimuli that fail to result in P waves or QRS complexes. Failure to capture is also readily apparent in pulse oximetry or direct arterial pressure waveforms. The principal cause for this type of malfunction is a defective power source or defective leads. Other causes include lead fracture, dislodgement, or migration, or an increase in pacing thresholds. Failure to pace may be misdiagnosed if stimuli are delivered during the refractory period of myocardium.

TABLE 5–6. ICHD CODE, NOMENCLATURE, AND DESCRIPTION OF BRADYCARDIA PACING MODES

Code	Nomenclature
AOO	Atrial asynchronous (fixed-rate) pacing. No atrial sensing.
VOO	Ventricular asynchronous (fixed-rate) pacing. No ventricular sensing.
DOO	Dual-chamber asynchronous (fixed-rate) pacing. No atrial or ventricular sensing.
AAI(R)*	Atrial noncompetitive (demand) pacing. Sensed A inhibits A output.
VVI(R)*	Ventricular noncompetitive (demand) pacing. Sensed V inhibits V output.
VAT	Atrial synchronous (tracking) pacing. Sensed A triggers V output.
VDD	Atrial synchronous (tracking) pacing. Sensed A triggers V output if sensed V does not inhibit V output.
DVI	AV (dual) sequential pacing. Dual-chamber pacing with V output inhibited by sensed V.
DDD(R)*	AV universal pacing. Atrial sensing inhibits atrial output. Atrial sensing (or output) triggers V output, if sensed V does not inhibit V output.
DDI (R)*	No official nomenclature. Atrial sensing inhibits atrial output, but atrial sensing (or output) does not trigger ventricular output. Ventricular sensing (within a preset AV interval) inhibits ventricular output.

*Addition of (R) after an ICHD code designation indicates the addition of sensor-modulated, rate-adaptive pacing (see text).

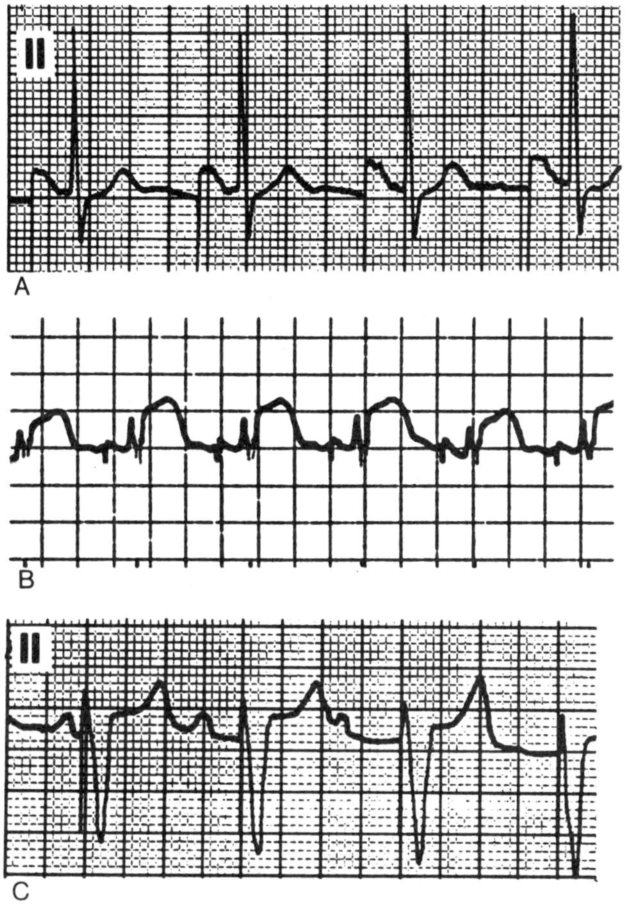

Figure 5–22. Single-chamber pacing modes. *A*, Atrial asynchronous (AOO) pacing. Note that a pacing spike is responsible for every P wave. This could also be a record from a patient with an atrial-inhibited pacemaker (AAI), except that there was no spontaneous atrial activity during this portion of the record to inhibit atrial output. *B*, Atrial-triggered (AAT) pacing. Note that pacing artifacts occur during inscription of each P wave. *C*, Ventricular asynchronous (VOO) pacing. Note that a pacing spike precedes every QRS complex. This could also be from a patient with a ventricular-inhibited pacemaker (VVI), except that there was no spontaneous ventricular activity during this portion of the record to inhibit ventricular output.

Oversensing

Oversensing occurs when the pacemaker detects signals other than the ones it is supposed to detect such as muscle movements (Fig. 5–24*A*), unusually large T waves with hyperkalemia, delayed T waves with hypokalemia, long Q-T interval, or hypocalcemia. Additionally, a dislodged ventricular electrode in the right ventricular outflow tract may sense atrial myopotentials in addition to or instead of the ones it is supposed to detect. A ventricular electrode may sense atrial pacing stimuli artifacts leading to inhibition of ventricular output (i.e., ''cross-talk''). Atrial sensing modes may sense ventricular myopotentials if the atrial signals are too small. Sensing of skeletal myopotentials, electromagnetic interference (EMI—e.g., from electrocautery, drills, saws, lithotripter, radiation fields), and mechanical interference leading to inappropriate pacemaker inhibition also are examples of oversensing. Oversensing caused by EMI or mechanical interference is corrected by reprogramming the pacemaker to an asynchronous mode of operation.

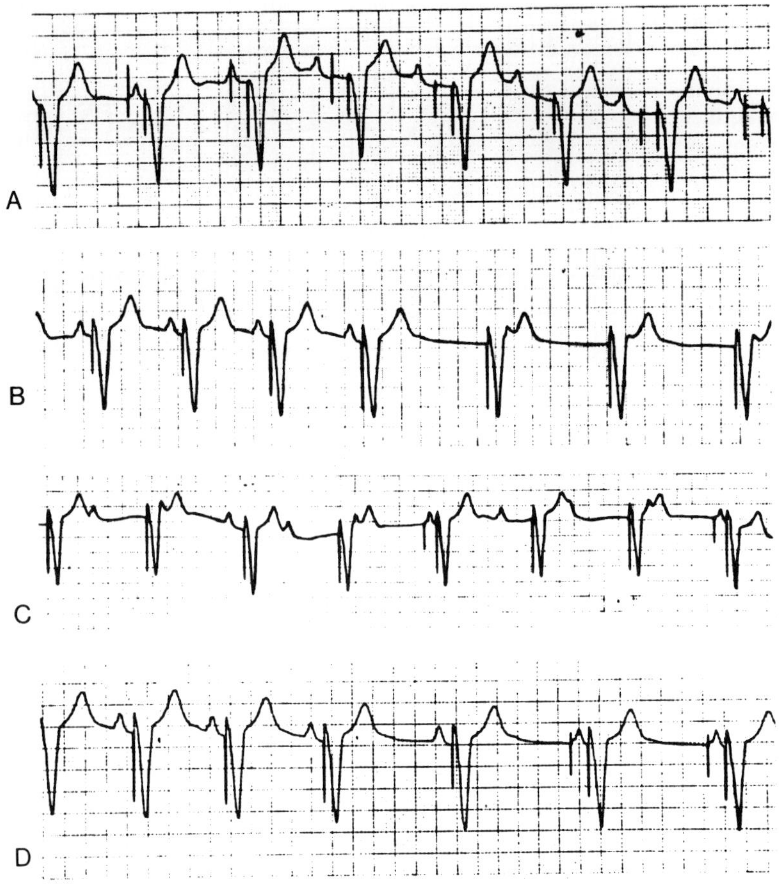

Figure 5–23. Dual-chamber pacing modes. *A*, Dual-chamber (AV sequential) asynchronous pacing (DOO). Note that atrial and ventricular pacing spikes precede all beats. The atrial spikes occur independent of spontaneous P waves and, except for the first beat, fail to depolarize the atria (which are refractory from previous spontaneous depolarization). Since all ventricular complexes are paced (i.e., there is no evidence of ventricular inhibition), this is a record of DOO as opposed to DVI A-V sequential pacing. *B*, Atrial synchronous (tracking) pacing (VDD). The first 4 paced ventricular beats are triggered by spontaneous atrial beats after a preset A-V interval. Atrial asystole after the fourth beat causes ventricular-asynchronous pacing at a slower rate. There are no spontaneous ventricular beats in this portion of the record to indicate that this pacemaker's ventricular output is inhibited by sensed ventricular myopotentials. *C*, Unofficially designated ICHD mode, intermediate between DVI and DDD ("DDI"—see Table 5–6). Sensed spontaneous atrial or ventricular activity inhibits atrial or ventricular output, although there is no ventricular inhibition evident in this portion of the record. Note the atrial pacing spikes with the fifth and eighth beats. The DDI mode prevents one-to-one ventricular tracking of fast atrial rates that is possible with the VAT, VDD, and DDD pacing modes. *D*, AV universal pacing (DDD). Atrial sensing triggers ventricular pacing for the first four beats. There is no evidence of ventricular inhibition with any ventricular beat; all are paced. There is slowing of the spontaneous atrial rate with the last two beats. When the atrial sensing amplifier determines that atrial rate is below the lower rate cut-off, the atria are paced, followed by the ventricles, at the preset A-V interval.

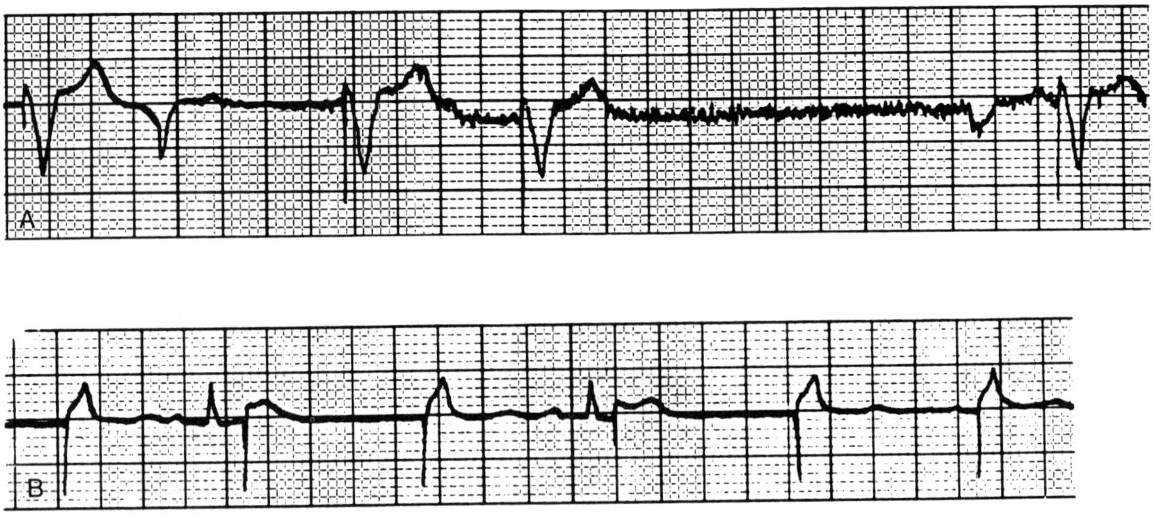

Figure 5–24. Pacemaker malfunction. *A*, Oversensing due to interference from skeletal muscle myopotentials during VVI pacing. The second beat is a ventricular premature beat that inhibits pacemaker output. Pacemaker output also is inhibited by pectoral muscle contractions occurring after the third beat—note the 2-second pause after the fourth beat. *B*, Undersensing due to reduced amplitude of spontaneous ventricular myopotentials during VVI pacing. Note that pacing spikes occur during the S-T segment of beats 2 and 4, when spontaneous ECG activity should have inhibited the pacemaker.

Failure to Sense

Sensing failure is commonly due to lead dislodgement, connector defects, or pulse generator component failure. Another cause could be changes in the shape or size of myopotentials produced by the effects of disease, drugs, or altered states (Fig. 5–24*B*). Improper programming of sensing parameters can cause sensing failure. Sensing failure may be misdiagnosed if spontaneous myopotentials coincide or fuse with pacing stimuli, or if the pacemaker has unknowingly been reprogrammed to an asynchronous mode.

Pacing at an Altered Rate

Unless one knows the programmed, intended operation of a particular pacemaker unit, diagnosis of this type of malfunction cannot be made. Causes include the following: (1) oversensing that leads to inappropriate inhibition or triggering of pacemaker stimuli, (2) rate drift or reduction due to component aging or power source depletion, and (3) accelerated rate (i.e., "runaway pacemaker") or no stimulus output consequent to component failure. *Endless-loop tachycardia* (an AV reciprocating tachycardia caused by sensing retrograde P waves) and *pacemaker-mediated tachycardia* (an atrial tracking pacemaker tracks SVT to cause a "paced" ventricular tachycardia) are not strictly examples of pacing at an altered rate, but might be misdiagnosed as such. Misdiagnosis of pacing at an altered rate can also be made if the pacemaker has been programmed with *rate hysteresis.* With rate hysteresis, the pacemaker *escape interval* (i.e., the time it waits to sense spontaneous events) is programmed to be longer than the *automatic interval* (i.e., the rate at which the pacemaker paces the heart once pacing has begun). Hysteresis is commonly programmed in VVI pacemakers to maximize the hemodynamic benefit of sinus rhythm in patients with sinus node dysfunction.

REFERENCES

1. Bertrand CA, Steiner NV, Jameson AG, et al: Disturbances of cardiac rhythm during anesthesia and surgery. JAMA 1971;216:1615–1617.
2. Kuner J, Enescu V, Utsu F, et al: Cardiac arrhythmias during anesthesia. Dis Chest 1967; 52:580–587.
3. Rodrigo MRC, Moles RM, Lee PK: Comparison of the incidence and nature of cardiac arrhythmias occurring during isoflurane or halothane anesthesia. Studies during dental surgery. Br J Anaesth 1986; 58:394–400.
4. Sorensen O, Waaben J, Andersen KB, et al: The incidence of cardiac arrhythmias and arterial hypotension subsequent to standardized surgical stimuli in patients undergoing thoracotomy. With reference to enflurane and halothane. Acta Anaesthiol Scand 1986; 30:630–632.
5. Damen J: Ventricular arrhythmias during insertion and removal of pulmonary artery catheters. Chest 1985; 88:190–193.
6. Dewar ML, Rosengarten MD, Blundell PE, et al: Perioperative Holter monitoring and computer analysis of dysrhythmias in cardiac surgery. Chest 1985; 87:593–597.
7. Casey WF, Wynands JE, Ramsay JG, et al: The incidence of prebypass dysrhythmias in patients undergoing coronary artery surgery. J Cardiothorac Anesth 1988; 2:123–129.
8. Atlee JL: Perioperative cardiac dysrhythmias in perspective. *In* Atlee JL: Perioperative Cardiac Dysrhythmias, 2nd Ed. Chicago: Year Book, 1990; 1–13.
9. Atlee JL, Bosnjak ZJ: Mechanisms for cardiac dysrhythmias during anesthesia. Anesthesiology 1990; 72:347–374.
10. Atlee JL: Causes for perioperative cardiac dysrhythmias. *In* Atlee JL: Perioperative Cardiac Dysrhythmias, 2nd Ed. Chicago: Year Book, 1990; 187–273.
11. Baig MW, Perrins EJ: The hemodynamics of cardiac pacing: Clinical and physiological aspects. Prog Cardiovasc Dis 1991; 33:283–298.
12. Smith JJ, Kampine JP: The heart: Structure and function. *In* Smith JJ, Kampine JP: Circulatory Physiology: The Essentials, 3rd Ed. Baltimore: Williams & Wilkins, 1990; 31–46.
13. Andriakos PG, Hughes CW, Thomas SJ: Anesthesia for cardiac surgery. *In* Barash PG, Cullen BF, Stoelting RK (eds): Clinical Anesthesia. Philadelphia: JB Lippincott, 1989; 979–1013.
14. Harvey W: Movement of the Heart and Blood in Animals. An Anatomical Essay (translated by Franklin). Oxford: Blackwell Scientific, 1957;34.
15. Gesell RA: Auricular systole and its relation to ventricular output. Am J Physiol 1911; 29:32–63.
16. Gesell RA: Initial length, initial tension and tone of auricular muscle in relation to myo- and cardiodynamics. Am J Physiol 1916; 39:239–267.
17. Gesell RA: Cardiodynamics in heart block as affected by auricular systole, auricular fibrillation and stimulation of the vagus nerve. Am J Physiol 1916; 40:267–313.
18. Stauffer J-C, Gaasch WH: Recognition and treatment of left ventricular diastolic dysfunction. Prog Cardiovasc Dis 1990; 32:319–332.
19. Dean JW, Poole-Wilson PA: Therapeutic implications of diastolic dysfunction in heart failure. Postgrad Med J 1990; 66:932–937.
20. Bonow RO: Regional left ventricular nonuniformity. Effects on left ventricular diastolic function in ischemic heart disease, hypertrophic myopathy, and the normal heart. Circulation 1990; 81(Suppl 3):54–65.
21. Packer M: Abnormalities of diastolic function as a potential cause of exercise intolerance in chronic heart failure. Circulation 1990; 81(Suppl 3):78–86.
22. Mahmarian JJ, Pratt CM: Silent myocardial ischemia in patients with coronary artery disease. Possible links with diastolic left ventricular dysfunction. Circulation 1990; 81(Suppl 3):33–40.
23. Bosnjak ZJ, Warltier DC: New aspects of cardiac electrophysiology and function: Effects of inhalational anaesthetics. *In* Conzen P, Peter K (eds): Inhalation Anaesthesia. London: Bailliere Tindall, 1993.
24. Atlee JL: Abnormal electrical activity of the heart. *In* Atlee JL: Perioperative Cardiac Dysrhythmias, 2nd Ed. Chicago: Year Book, 1990; 57–118.
25. Lown B, Wolf M: Approaches to sudden death from coronary heart disease. Circulation 1971; 44:130–144.
26. Myerburg RJ, Kessler KM, Luceri RM: Classification of ventricular arrhythmias based on parallel hierarchies of frequency and form. Am J Cardiol 1984; 54:1355–1358.
27. Bethge K-P: Classification of arrhythmias. J Cardiovasc Pharmacol 1991; 17(Suppl 6):13–19.
28. The Cardiac Arrhythmia Suppression Trial (CAST) Investigators: Preliminary Report: Effect of encainide and flecainide on mortality in a randomized trial of arrhythmia suppression after myocardial infarction. N Engl J Med 1989; 321:406–412.
29. The Cardiac Arrhythmia Suppression Trial II Investigators: Effect of the antiarrhythmic agent moricizine on survival after myocardial infarction. N Engl J Med 1992; 327:227–233.
30. Atlee JL: Normal electrical activity of the heart. *In* Atlee JL: Perioperative Cardiac Dysrhythmias, 2nd Ed. Chicago: Year Book, 1990; 14–56.
31. Atlee JL: Clinical electrocardiography and electrophysiology. *In* Atlee JL: Perioperative Cardiac Dysrhythmias, 2nd Ed. Chicago: Year Book, 1990; 119–186.
32. Atlee JL, Pattison CZ, Mathews EL, Bilof RM, Hedman AG: Evaluation of transesophageal atrial pacing stethoscope in adult surgical patients under general anesthesia. PACE 1992; 15:1515–1525.
33. Brown DL, Greenberg DJ: A simple device for monitoring the esophageal electrocardiogram. Anesthesiology 1983; 59:482–483.
34. Artru AA, Colley PS: The site of origin of the intravascular electrocardiogram recorded from multiorificed intravascular catheters. Anesthesiology 1988; 69:44–48.

35. Artru AA, Colley PS: Placement of multiorificed CVP catheters via antecubital veins using intravascular electrocardiography. Anesthesiology 1988; 65:132–135.
36. Marriott HJL, Myerburg RJ: Recognition of arrhythmias and conduction abnormalities. *In* Hurst JW (ed): The Heart, 5th Ed. New York: McGraw-Hill, 1982; 532.
37. Fisch C, Zipes DP, McHenry PL: Rate-dependent aberrancy. Circulation 1973; 48:714–724.
38. Benson DW Jr: Transesophageal electrocardiography and cardiac pacing: State of the art. Circulation 1987; 75(Suppl 3):86–90.
39. Jones SB, Euler DE, Fishman DL, Randall WC: Atrial ectopic foci in the canine heart: Hierarchy of pacemaker automaticity. Am J Physiol 1980; 238:H788–H793.
40. Randall WC, Rinkema LE, Jones SB, Moran JF, Brynjolfsson G: Functional characterization of atrial pacemaker activity. Am J Physiol 1982; 242:H98–H106.
41. Polic S, Atlee JL, Laszlo A, Kampine JP, Bosnjak ZJ: Anesthetics and automaticity in latent pacemaker fibers. II. Effects of halothane and epinephrine or norepinephrine on automaticity of dominant and subsidiary atrial pacemakers in the canine heart. Anesthesiology 1991; 75:298–304.
42. Pick A, Langendorf R: Interpretation of Complex Arrhythmias. Philadelphia: Lea & Febiger, 1979; 177–178.
43. Schubart AF, Marriott HJL, Gorten RJ: Isorhythmic dissociation: Atrioventricular dissociation with synchronization. Am J Med 1958; 24:209–214.
44. Zipes DP: Specific arrhythmias: Diagnosis and treatment. *In* Braunwald E (ed): Heart Disease, 3rd Ed. Philadelphia: WB Saunders, 1988; 658–715.
45. Morady F: The spectrum of tachyarrhythmias in preexcitation syndromes. *In* Benditt DG, Benson DW (eds): Cardiac Preexcitation Syndromes. Boston: Martinus Nijhoff, 1986; 119–139.
46. Marriott HJL, Myerburg RJ: Recognition of arrhythmias and conduction abnormalities. *In* Logue RB, Rackley CE, Schlant RC, et al (eds): The Heart, 6th Ed. New York: McGraw-Hill, 1986; 433–475.
47. Atlee JL: Causes for perioperative dysrhythmias. *In* Atlee JL: Perioperative Cardiac Dysrhythmias, 2nd Ed. Chicago: Year Book, 1990; 187–273.
48. Goldman MJ: Principles of Clinical Electrocardiography. Los Altos, CA: Lange Medical, 1986; 113–141.
49. Klein GJ, Sharma AD, Milstein S: Initial evaluation of patients with the Wolff-Parkinson-White syndrome. *In* Benditt DG, Benson DW (eds): Cardiac Preexcitation Syndromes. Boston: Martinus Nijhoff, 1986; 305–319.
50. Wellens HJJ, Brugada P, Penn OC: The management of preexcitation syndromes. JAMA 1987; 257:2325–2333.
51. Fisch C: Electrocardiography and vectorcardiography. *In* Braunwald E (ed): Heart Disease, 3rd Ed. Philadelphia: WB Saunders, 1988; 180–222.
52. Surawicz B: The interrelationship of electrolyte abnormalities and arrhythmias. *In* Mandel WJ (ed): Cardiac Arrhythmias, 2nd Ed. Philadelphia: JB Lippincott, 1987; 81–100.
53. Fisch C: Electrolytes and the heart. *In* Hurst JW (ed): The Heart, 5th Ed. New York: McGraw-Hill, 1982; 1599.
54. Marriott HJL: Practical Electrocardiography, 8th Ed. Baltimore: Williams & Wilkins, 1988; 511–534.
55. Taylor AL, Fozzard HA: Ventricular arrhythmias associated with CNS disease. Arch Intern Med 1982; 142:232–233.
56. DeBelder MA, Malik M, Ward DE, Camm AJ: Pacing modalities for tachycardia termination. PACE 1990; 13:231–248.
57. Furman S: Rate-modulated pacing. Circulation 1990; 82:1081–1094.
58. Tyers GFO: Current status of sensor-modulated rate-adaptive cardiac pacing. J Am Coll Cardiol 1990; 15:412–418.
59. Atlee JL: Cardiac pacing and electroversion. *In* Kaplan JA (ed): Cardiac Anesthesia, 3rd Ed. Philadelphia: WB Saunders, 1993; 877–904.
60. Atlee JL, Gombotz H, Tscheliessnigg KH (eds): Perioperative Management of Pacemaker Patients. Berlin: Springer-Verlag, 1992.

CHAPTER 6

Intravascular Pressure Monitoring Systems

ROBERT G. LOEB, M. D.

Arterial blood pressure monitoring, along with pulse rate, is historically and currently one of the most frequently monitored physiologic parameters during anesthesia. Invasive monitoring of arterial blood pressure in anesthesia and critical care is common. Invasive monitoring is more advantageous than noninvasive monitoring because continuous observation of the waveform is possible, arterial blood samples can be readily obtained, and it is the gold standard. Invasive blood pressure monitoring is deceptively simple, as exemplified by the misnomer ''direct pressure monitoring.'' As explained in this chapter, clinical monitoring of intravascular pressure is not direct but indirect through transducers, filters, amplifiers, and displays. Attention to detail and an understanding of the frailties of such systems are necessary to avoid inaccuracy and misinterpretation.

COMPONENTS OF A PRESSURE MEASUREMENT SYSTEM

Common clinical pressure measurement systems consist of four main subsystems (Fig. 6–1): the mechanical coupling system, the transducer, the electronic components, and the display. The mechanical coupling system transmits the pressure from the source to the transducer. The transducer converts the pressure into an electrical analog (usually voltage). The electronic components change the electrical analog into a form suitable for display and extract features of the waveform. The display converts the electrical signal and features into a visible form. The mechanical coupling system consists of an intravascular catheter, tubing, stopcocks, and sometimes a transducer dome. The electronic components include amplifiers, filters, and analog or digital circuits for peak detection and averaging.

CALIBRATION AND PERFORMANCE

STATIC CALIBRATION

The most important factor for ensuring the accuracy of a blood pressure measurement is the calibration of the system. Static calibration refers to the calibration of the system against a known static pressure. Clinical pressure monitoring systems are assumed to be linear; that is, the pressure input versus the system output is described by a straight line. Therefore, a two-point calibration is sufficient.

Two-Point Calibration

Static calibration is performed by first exposing the mechanical coupling system to atmospheric pressure (this is usually performed by opening a stopcock to air). The electrical ''zero'' control is then adjusted to bring the displayed pressure to zero. On digital systems, a ''zero'' button is pressed. Either way, this results in balancing of the preamplification circuitry to produce a zero voltage. Second, a known pressure is presented to the mechanical coupling system at the same site and level that the zero reading was taken. The known pressure is usually generated with a mercury manometer, but a water manometer (1.35 cm H_2O = 1 mmHg) or any calibrated manometer is acceptable. With the system exposed to a known pressure, the electrical ''gain'' control is adjusted to bring the displayed pressure to the calibrated value. This adjusts the gain of the preamplifier circuits to match the sensitivity of the transducer.

Two-point calibration should be performed prior to attaching a patient to the system. Because pressure transducers have a standard sensitivity of 5.0 μV/V/mmHg, it can be argued that one-point calibration is sufficient. However, reusable transducers are subject to abuse and, when

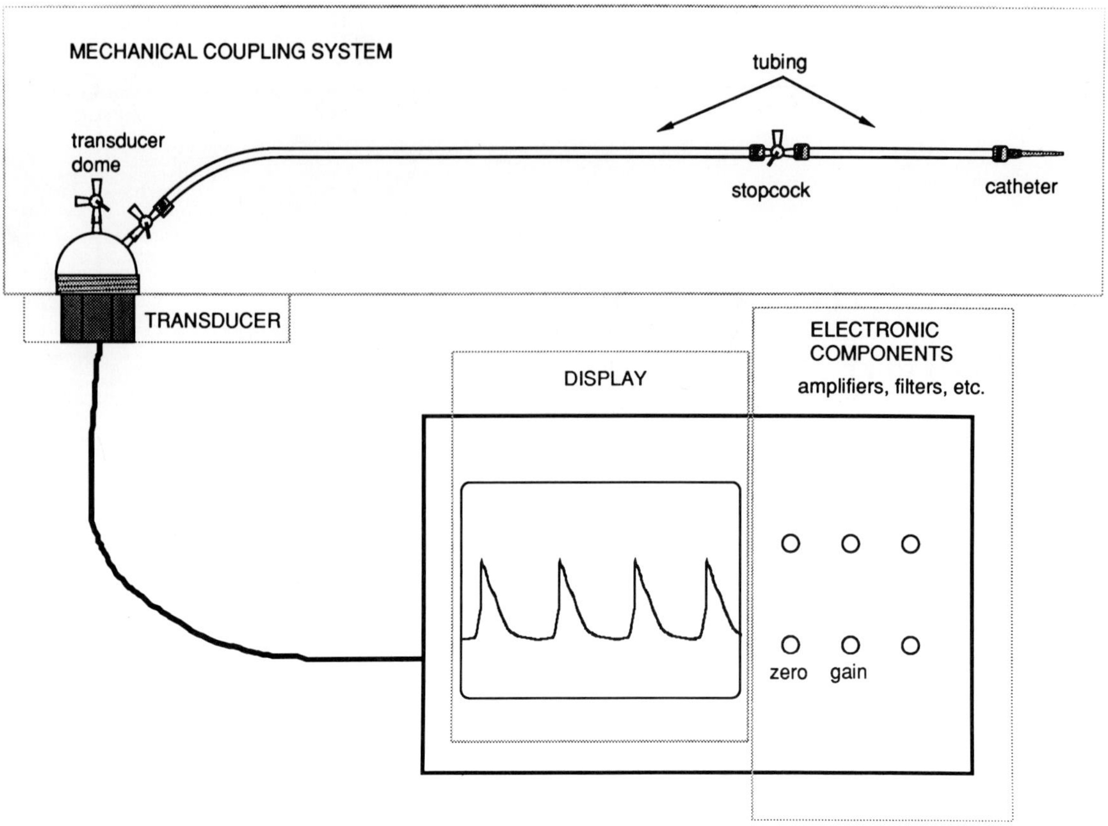

Figure 6–1. The four subsystems of a clinical pressure measurement system: mechanical coupling system, transducer, display, and electronic components.

used with transducer domes containing a diaphragm, the method of applying the dome affects the sensitivity.[1] The only way to verify accuracy is by two-point calibration of the entire system. Disposable transducers are calibrated at the factory but may be damaged during shipping. Although the quality control of these devices seems to be good, two-point calibration prior to use identifies the rare defective unit.[2] Transducer cable malfunction can also result in artifactual hypotension if two-point calibration is not performed prior to use.[3, 4] Two-point calibration should be repeated during use if it is suspected that the transducer has malfunctioned.[5]

Drift. The system should be rezeroed, without changing the gain, periodically during use. Transducer drift occurs over time. Usually, the zero drifts with little change in sensitivity.[2] Drift may lead to inaccuracy, especially when low pressures (e.g., venous or intracranial) are being measured. Two main causes of drift are thermal effects on the transducer[2] and the effect of transducer domes containing diaphragms. Temperature changes of 10°C usually change the measured pressure by less than 1 mmHg.[2]

Transducer domes with diaphragms create larger inaccuracies. Gradual drifts of the baseline of 15 mmHg over 3 hours have been reported.[6] Inadvertent loosening of the transducer dome during use has caused 80-mmHg negative offsets.[7] It is recommended, therefore, that the system be rezeroed and that transducer domes be tightened at frequent intervals during use. Transducer offset may also occur during electrocautery.[8] Therefore, pressure values obtained while electrosurgical units are active may not be accurate.

Reference Points. The pressure reference point varies with the pressure being measured and the position of the patient. Central venous pressure is measured at the level of the middle of the right atrium. Intracranial pressure is measured at the tragus of the ear. The pressure reference point for arterial blood pressure may be the middle of the right atrium when the patient is in the supine position or the level of the brain in neurosurgical procedures performed with the patient in a sitting position.

The column of fluid between the transducer and the pressure reference point represents a static pressure.[9] This static pressure can be zeroed mechanically or electrically. Mechanical zeroing is achieved by ensuring that the transducer is at the level of the pressure reference point. Electrical zeroing is achieved by rezeroing the system with a stopcock open at the pressure reference point, disregarding the level of the transducer. Either procedure needs to be repeated whenever the level of the transducer changes with respect to the pressure reference point. (Fig. 6–2).

DYNAMIC CALIBRATION

Measuring static pressure is relatively straightforward. Accurately measuring dynamic pressures is more difficult

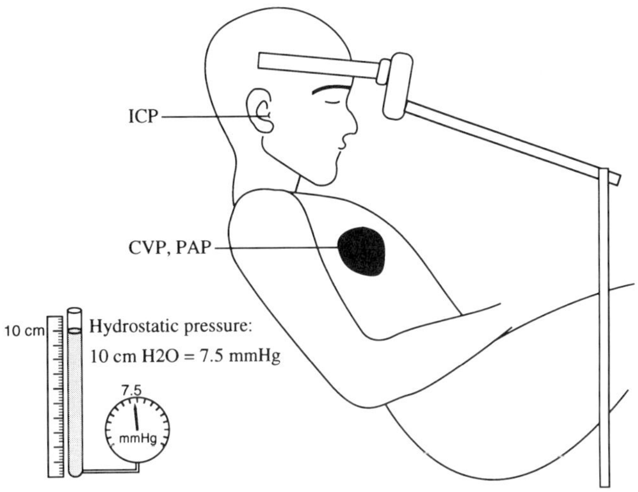

Figure 6–2. Zero reference points in the sitting position for intracranial pressure (ICP), central venous pressure (CVP), and pulmonary artery pressure (PAP). Arterial pressure is zeroed at the base of the skull to measure cerebral perfusion pressure (ICP = zero when the dura is open). To calculate cardiovascular indices, such as systemic vascular resistance, 7.5 mmHg must be added to the arterial pressure for each 10 cm that the base of the skull is above the heart.

by an order of magnitude. Fundamental to understanding the potential distortion is a conceptual knowledge of the behavior of oscillating systems. (For a mathematical description of the behavior of oscillating systems, see this chapter's appendix.)

There are many examples of oscillating systems: vibrating strings, pendulums, and waves on a pool of water. The vascular tree, the mechanical coupling subsystem, the pressure transducer, and electrical amplifier circuitry are also oscillating systems.

All oscillating systems have two energy storage compartments between which energy is transferred. In mechanical systems, the energy storage compartments are mass (which stores kinetic energy as inertia when in motion) and elasticity (which stores potential energy when distorted). Oscillations decrease with time, owing to friction, when no energy is added to the system (there are no perpetual motion machines). Damping or viscosity is a measure of the friction that counteracts the kinetic energy of the mass. To summarize, an oscillating system can be described by the coefficients of mass, stiffness (the inverse of elasticity), and damping.

Natural Frequency

All oscillating systems have a natural frequency. The natural frequency is the oscillating frequency of the undamped system. Oscillations at the natural frequency generate the largest displacement for a given input energy. The qualitative effects of changes in mass and stiffness on natural frequency can be observed with piano strings. The low notes (slow oscillations) are generated by long, heavy, thick strings that are loosely stretched to be less stiff; high notes are generated by short, thin, light strings that are tightly stretched to be more stiff. Natural frequency decreases with increased mass and decreased stiffness.

Damping

Damping can be understood qualitatively by imagining a vibrating string immersed in honey. Two things would be noticed when comparing oscillations in honey with those in air; the oscillations in honey extinguish more quickly and the string oscillates at a lower frequency. That the oscillating frequency increases as damping decreases can also be demonstrated by the increasing pitch of the voice after inhaling a low density gas such as helium. The resonant frequency is the oscillating frequency of a damped system. It is a function of the natural frequency and the damping coefficient (Fig. 6–3).

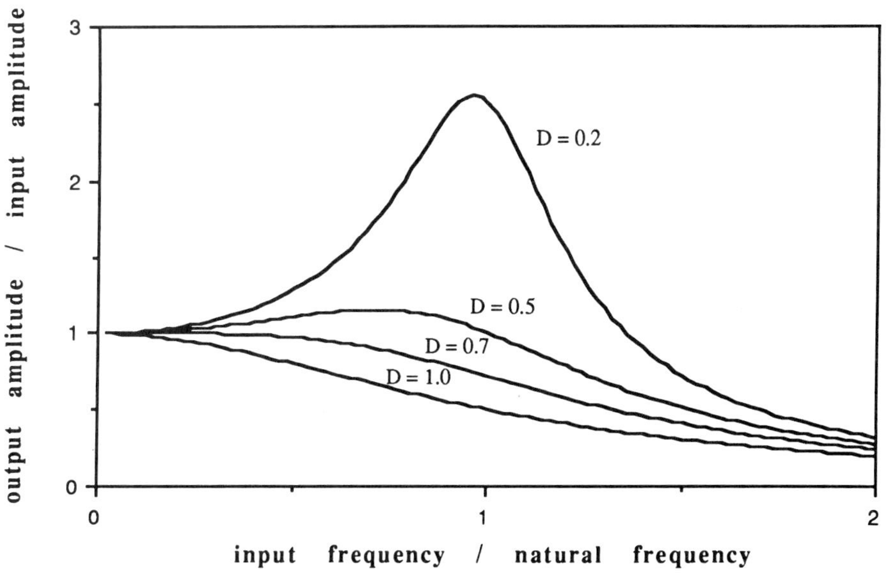

Figure 6–3. The effect of damping on the frequency response. Increasing the damping coefficient (D) results in less overshoot from oscillations near the natural frequency of the system. It also decreases the oscillating frequency. A damping coefficient around 0.7 is optimal because it yields an output-to-input amplitude ratio close to unity over the widest frequency range.

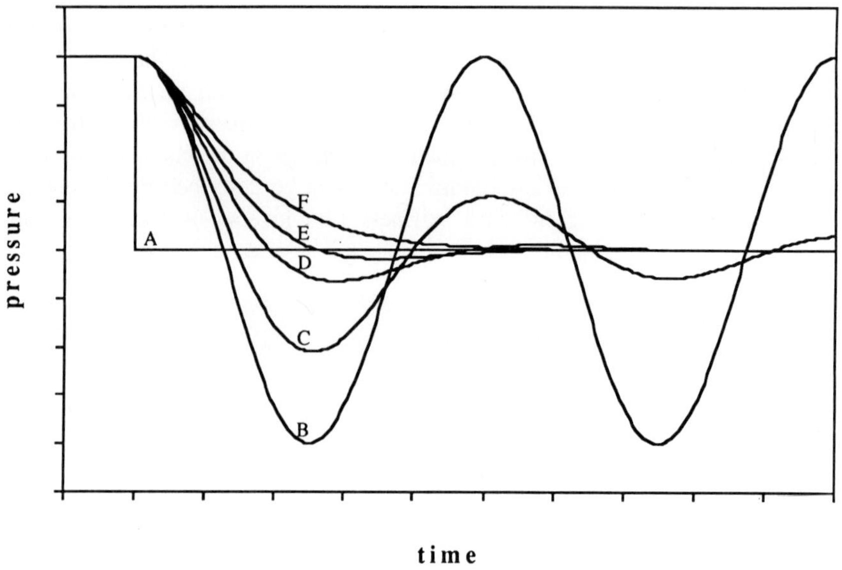

Figure 6–4. The effect of damping on the system response to a step change in pressure: *A*, The input signal. *B*, Response of a system with zero damping. *C*, Response of a system with a damping coefficient of 0.2. *D*, Response of a system with a damping coefficient of 0.5. *E*, Response of a system with an optimal damping coefficient of 0.7. *F*, Response of a system with a critical damping coefficient of 1.0. Note that a damping coefficient around 0.7 yields the best compromise between fast response time and small overshoot.

Figure 6–4 illustrates the effect of increasing the coefficient of damping on the response of an oscillating system to a sudden input of energy. Increasing the coefficient of damping decreases the overshoot but increases the response time of the system. (Response time is the time required to reach some fraction of the final value.)

MECHANICAL COUPLING SUBSYSTEM

The mechanical coupling subsystem (catheter, stopcock, tubing, dome) contains the elements of an oscillating system. The mass is represented by the mass of fluid within the system. The distensibility of the plastics from which the components are made gives the system its elasticity. Damping is a function of the frictional resistance to movement of the fluid and distortion of the plastics.

NATURAL FREQUENCY

Numerous studies have described the natural frequency and damping coefficient of commercial pressure monitoring systems. Bare transducers have resonant frequencies of 100–500 Hz.[1, 10] Transducer-tubing systems have much lower natural frequencies of 5–50 Hz.[11–14] The length of the tubing has a profound influence on the natural frequency.[13] Five feet of low-compliance tubing results in a natural frequency of 6.5 Hz, compared with 33 Hz for 6 inches of tubing. This may be especially important when using disposable systems with an option of patient- versus pole-mounted transducers. In one study, the natural frequencies of seven brands of pole-mounted disposable units ranged from 19 to 28 Hz; mounting the same transducers on the patient increased the natural frequencies to a range of 41–73 Hz.[15]

The presence of a diaphragm in a disposable transducer dome also causes a decrease in natural frequency. A study of five transducer models showed natural frequencies of 270–545 Hz when domes without diaphragms were used; the same transducers had natural frequencies of 54–423 Hz when used with domes containing diaphragms.[1] More important, the method of application of the transducer dome significantly affected the natural frequency. Consistently, the lowest natural frequencies resulted when the dome was applied without water between the diaphragm and the dome.[1]

The final factor influencing the natural frequency of the mechanical coupling system, and a factor that is too frequently ignored by clinicians, is the presence of air bubbles. Air bubbles are compressible and increase the elasticity of the system. Most clinicians only know that air bubbles increase the damping coefficient of the mechanical coupling system. However, air bubbles also cause a significant decrease in the natural frequency. The addition of 0.03 ml of air to pole-mounted disposable pressure transducer systems decreases the natural frequency from a range of 18–28 Hz to a range of 8–13 Hz.[15]

DAMPING COEFFICIENT

The length of tubing, the presence of diaphragms in transducer domes, and the presence of air bubbles also affect the damping coefficient. Five feet of low-compliance tubing results in a damping coefficient of 0.1 compared with 0.3 for 6 inches of tubing.[13] The damping coefficients for five transducers without diaphragms ranged from 0.023 to 0.1; the same transducers had damping coefficients from 0.035 to 0.125 when used with domes containing diaphragms.[1] The addition of 0.3 ml of air to pole-mounted disposable pressure transducer systems increases the damping coefficient from a range of 0.14–0.22 to a range of 0.16–0.28.[15]

FREQUENCY CONTENT

To predict the effect of any combination of resonant frequency and damping coefficient on the accuracy of reproduction of a pressure waveform, one first needs to know the frequency content of the pressure waveform. Fourier analysis is a mathematical method of extracting the simple sine and cosine waves that sum to form a complex wave. Fourier analysis of blood pressure waveforms is demonstrated in Figure 6–5. Multiple studies have concluded that the original blood pressure waveform can be accurately reproduced by summing the first 5 to 10 harmonics.[10, 16] Because heart rate normally is in the range of 60–180 beats/minute (1–3 Hz), the fifth to tenth harmonics encompass a range of 5–30 Hz. Re-examination of Figure 3–2 reveals that amplitude distortion occurs around the natural frequency of the system. Small damping factors allow amplitude overshoot, whereas large damping coefficients result in low relative amplitudes below the natural frequency.

Two methods to preserve an accurate amplitude response are to increase the natural frequency of the system and to optimize the damping coefficient. Gardner published a study that experimentally derived the adequate dynamic response range of invasive blood pressure measurement systems used for monitoring in intensive care units and operating rooms.[11] His results indicate the combinations of natural frequency and damping coefficient that accurately reproduce arterial blood pressure waveforms (Fig. 6–6). Two ranges are depicted. Systems with adequate response accurately reproduce pressures at slow heart rates. Systems with optimum response may be necessary to accurately reproduce blood pressure waveforms at fast heart rates or when fast upstrokes are present in the pressure waveform.[15]

The largest error introduced by inadequate dynamic response is an inaccurate systolic pressure. Because the systolic upstroke of the pressure waveform contains the highest frequency components, these components are the most difficult to reproduce accurately. Figure 6–6 demonstrates the effect of dynamic response on the measured systolic pressure. Systolic pressure is underestimated by an overdamped system and is overestimated by an underdamped system. Diastolic pressure is less sensitive to suboptimal dynamic response, but it is underestimated by underdamped systems and is overestimated by overdamped systems. Mean pressure is least affected by the dynamic response of the measuring system.

CLINICAL DETERMINATION OF DYNAMIC RESPONSE

There are two methods of determining the natural frequency and damping coefficient of a blood pressure measurement system. In the clinical laboratory, a pressure generator can be used to produce a constant amplitude sine wave pressure at progressively increasing frequency (sine wave method). Natural frequency and damping coefficient can be determined by comparing the pressure tracing recorded by the system under investigation with the pressure tracing recorded by a reference transducer (Fig. 6–7). In the operating room or intensive care unit, the natural frequency and damping coefficient of a pressure measurement system can be determined by the response of the system to a square wave pressure input. A square wave pressure can be generated by opening, then quickly closing the fast-flush valve of a continuous flush mechanism (square wave method). Figure 6–8 demonstrates this method of determining the dynamic response of the system from the measured pressure waveform. Figure 6–9 provides a graph and table for determining the damping coefficient from the amplitude ratio.[11] It is generally accepted that the sine wave and square wave methods of determining dynamic response yield identical results.[15] However, differences in results obtained with these two methods have been documented.[17, 18] Large differences in damping coefficients obtained with the two techniques have been attributed to damping effects of the catheter within the artery when the flush method is used *in vivo*.

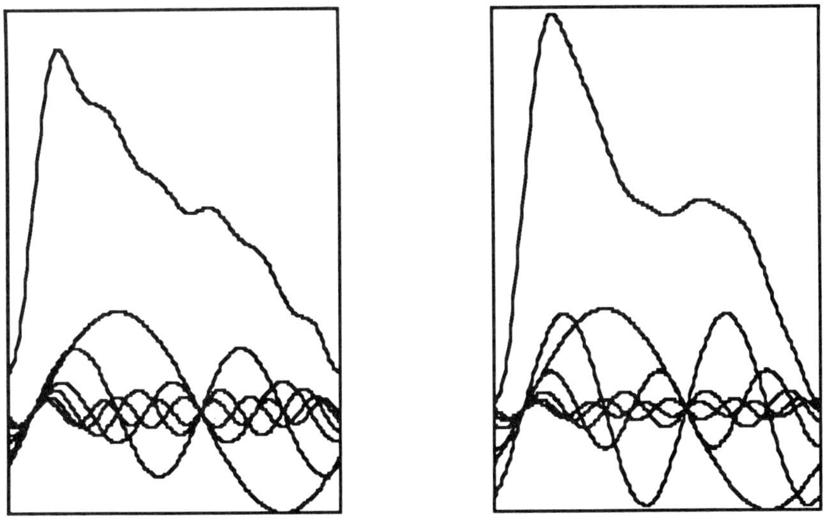

Figure 6–5. Two examples of Fourier analysis of a blood pressure waveform. The upper trace in each example is the original waveform. The lower traces in each example are the sine wave harmonics, which sum to yield the original waveform. The period of each sine wave is an integral multiple of the period of the original waveform. The only difference between the examples is the relative amplitude of each sine wave harmonic.

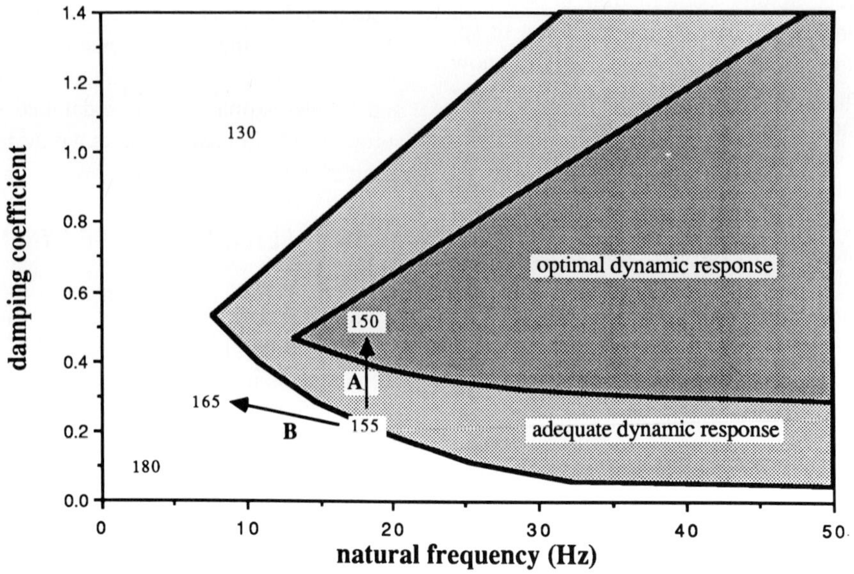

Figure 6–6. The adequate and optimal dynamic response ranges for invasive blood pressure measurement systems. The numbers are examples of output systolic pressures for a systolic input pressure of 150 mmHg. Increasing the damping coefficient decreases the systolic pressure. Systems with a high natural frequency have a wider range of acceptable damping coefficients. Systems with a natural frequency below 7.5 Hz are never adequate. *Arrow A* shows the effect of changing the damping coefficient of the mechanical coupling system with a commercial device for that purpose. *Arrow B* shows the effect of introducing an air bubble into the mechanical coupling system. (Modified from Gardner RM: Direct blood pressure measurement: Dynamic response requirements. Anesthesiology 1981; 54:227–236.)

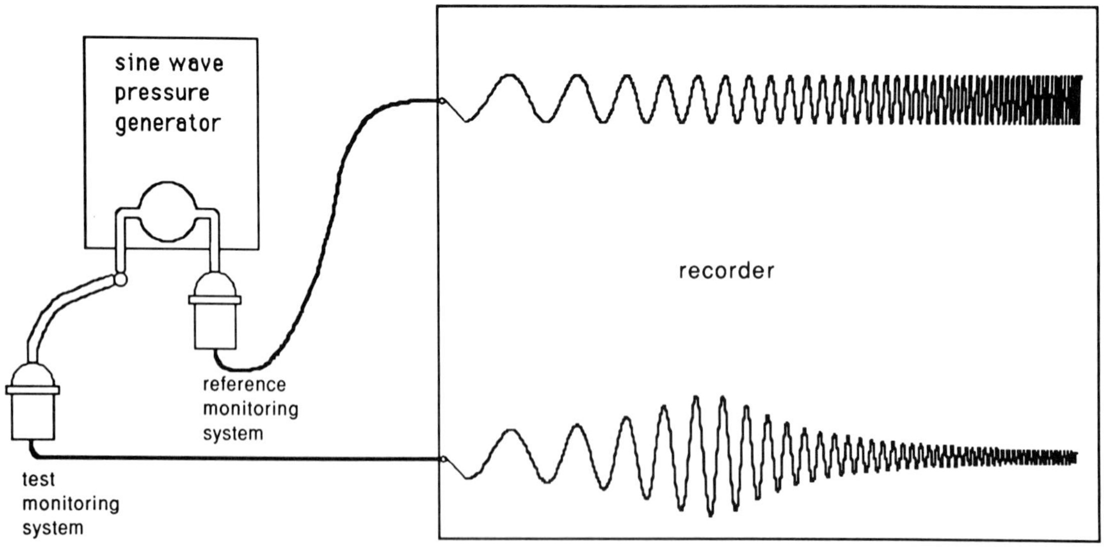

Figure 6–7. The sine wave method of determining dynamic response. A sine wave pressure of increasing frequency is simultaneously measured by a reference and a test system. The reference system should have a flat response; the test system should have an output defined by the natural frequency and damping coefficient. Two measurements are made: the frequency at which there is peak amplitude from the test system (oscillating frequency) and the ratio of test system amplitude to reference system amplitude at the oscillating frequency. The damping coefficient and natural frequency can be calculated from these numbers (see this chapter's appendix for formulas).

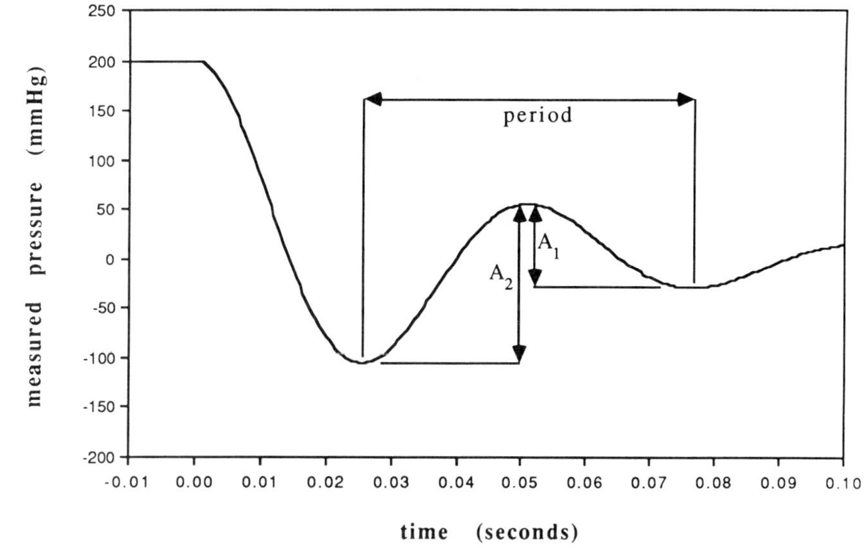

Figure 6–8. The square wave method of determining dynamic response. A square wave is generated by opening, then quickly closing, the fast flush valve of a continuous flush mechanism. Two measurements are then made from the recorded output: the oscillating frequency, which is the inverse of the period, and the amplitude ratio of two successive peaks, A_1/A_2. In this example, the oscillating frequency is 19 Hz (1/0.052 seconds) and the amplitude ratio is 0.51. The damping coefficient and natural frequency can be derived from these numbers (see this chapter's appendix and Fig. 6–9).

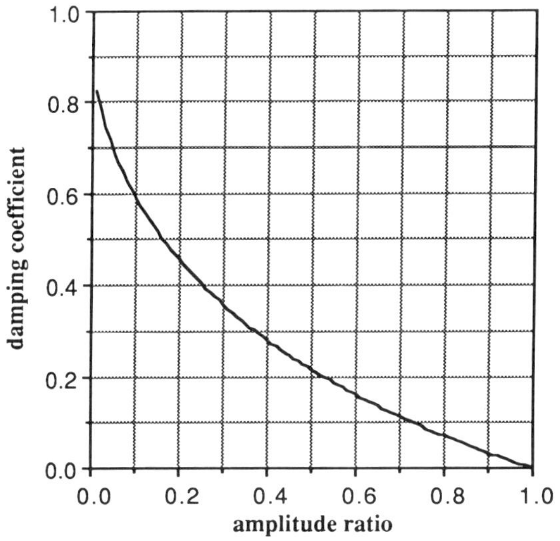

	0.00	0.01	0.02	0.03	0.04	0.05	0.06	0.07	0.08	0.09
.0	1.000	0.826	0.780	0.745	0.716	0.690	0.667	0.646	0.627	0.608
.1	0.591	0.575	0.559	0.545	0.531	0.517	0.504	0.491	0.479	0.467
.2	0.456	0.445	0.434	0.424	0.414	0.404	0.394	0.385	0.376	0.367
.3	0.358	0.349	0.341	0.333	0.325	0.317	0.309	0.302	0.294	0.287
.4	0.280	0.273	0.266	0.259	0.253	0.246	0.240	0.234	0.228	0.221
.5	0.215	0.210	0.204	0.198	0.192	0.187	0.181	0.176	0.171	0.166
.6	0.160	0.155	0.150	0.146	0.141	0.136	0.131	0.126	0.122	0.117
.7	0.113	0.108	0.104	0.100	0.095	0.091	0.087	0.083	0.079	0.075
.8	0.071	0.067	0.063	0.059	0.055	0.052	0.048	0.044	0.041	0.037
.9	0.034	0.030	0.027	0.023	0.020	0.016	0.013	0.010	0.006	0.003
1.0	0.000									

Figure 6–9. Two methods of determining the damping coefficient from the square wave method amplitude ratio. The conversion can be read from the graph or, if greater accuracy is desired, from the table. For example, an amplitude ratio of 0.51 yields a damping coefficient of 0.210.

Methods to Improve Dynamic Response

Most commercial blood pressure measurement systems are underdamped, with a borderline natural frequency for arterial blood pressure measurement.[14] What can the clinician do if the measured dynamic response of his or her system is outside the acceptable range? To optimize the dynamic response, the natural frequency should be as high as possible; a natural frequency below 7.5 Hz is never acceptable.[11] This is accomplished by using the shortest practical tubing (definitely less than 4 feet) and the fewest number of stopcocks (not more than one) between the transducer and the patient.[13] Tubing should be noncompliant; compliant devices such as T-connectors with injection ports should not be used.

Air bubbles should be meticulously removed from the mechanical coupling system.[19] Bubbles often hide in stopcocks and transducer domes. Air embolization through arterial and venous catheters is associated with significant patient morbidity, especially in children[20, 21]; air should be aspirated into a syringe when it is detected.[20] To reduce the incidence of invisible bubbles, air should be removed from the intravenous bag before it is pressurized, the intravenous solution may be warmed or exposed to ultrasonic waves prior to use, and a filter may be used to trap air distal to the fast-flush mechanism.[20, 22]

After all measures have been taken to increase the natural frequency of the system, the dynamic response may still be inadequate owing to suboptimal damping. Two hydraulic devices are commercially available to increase the damping coefficient of the system without decreasing the natural frequency.[18, 23] The ROSE (Resonance OverShoot Eliminator, Gould Instruments Inc., Cleveland, OH) is a nonadjustable device that increases the damping coefficient by adding a second resonating element in parallel with the pressure measurement system. The Accudynamic (Sorenson, Salt Lake City, UT) is an adjustable device that operates on the same principle. The effect of using either device is illustrated in Figure 6–6.[11, 12] Schwid has developed a semiautomatic electronic method for improving the dynamic response of a catheter-manometer system.[23] With that method, a computer automatically determines the natural frequency and damping coefficient of the monitoring system after the clinician performs a fast flush. The computer then adapts calculations to the specific system to remove resonance artifacts and display an undistorted pressure waveform.

TRANSDUCERS

A transducer is a device that converts one form of energy into another. All pressure transducers first convert pressure into movement. An elastic device, such as a Bourdon tube or a diaphragm, is exposed to the pressure, and its deflection is measured.

HISTORICAL DEVELOPMENT

Geddes has written a fascinating summary of the historical development of blood pressure transducers.[10] Early transducers measured the deflection of a Bourdon tube using mechanical linkages, a method still used today in blood pressure manometers. However, purely mechanical manometers have a very low frequency response owing to the need for a large sensing element with a large displacement volume. This is an inherent requirement, because the energy to move the mechanical parts must come from the event being measured. A significant advance was made in the fidelity of blood pressure measurement with the development of mechano-optical transducers. These devices, developed between 1903 and 1945, further transduced the movement of the sensing element to the deflection of a beam of light. Ultimately, high fidelity was achieved using miniature low-elasticity glass membrane sensing elements to deflect the light beam. These devices, although useful in the physiology laboratory, were never clinically used because pressure recordings required a darkened room and photographic techniques. However, new optical transducers that attach to standard monitors have been developed.[24] They may be especially useful for measuring pressure during magnetic resonance scanning.[25]

Given the advanced state of electrical technology, it is not surprising that modern blood pressure transducers convert movement of the sensing element into current or voltage. This conversion is usually accomplished by inducing a change in capacitance, inductance, or resistance. High-frequency response is achieved using small sensing elements with low fluid displacement.

TYPES

Capacitance Transducers

In a capacitance transducer, the sensing element is one plate of the capacitor (Fig. 6–10). As pressure is applied, the two plates of the capacitor move closer together and capacitance increases. An oscillating voltage is applied across the plates of the capacitor, which results in an alternating current that varies with the pressure on the sensing element results. This alternating current is then demodulated (converted to direct current) for further processing. Capacitance transducers have a number of practical problems.[10, 26, 27] They have poor temperature stability and require separate temperature-compensating circuitry. Electrical cables are themselves capacitors; therefore, the oscillator and demodulator must be built into the transducer housing to avoid interference. This increases the size of the unit. Further, in order to be used with biologic amplifiers, the current produced must first be converted to voltage.

Inductance Transducers

Inductance is an electrical property of coils produced by the forces of an induced magnetic field that causes the coil to resist changes in current flow. The inductance of a coil is affected by the position of an iron core within the coil. Inductance transducers have a core attached to the sensing element (Fig 6–10). As pressure is applied, the core is displaced into the coil and inductance increases. Like capacitance, inductance is measured with an oscillating current. Therefore, the transducer housing usually contains oscillators and demodulators. Inductance transducers have a number of advantages. They are stable over a useful temperature range and can be designed to have a large electrical output for a small mechanical displacement. The most sensitive transducers based on the property of inductance use a miniature linear variable differential transformer. These units use a core and four coils to produce a multivolt output for 0.001-inch deflection of the sensing element.

Resistance Transducers

Change in resistance is the most common way of measuring displacement of the sensing element. The principle of measurement is based on the fact that the resistance of a wire increases as it is stretched (Fig. 6–10). Nondisposable pressure transducers are usually bonded strain gauges. In these, a resistor or a group of resistors is bonded to the back of the diaphragm. As pressure is applied to the diaphragm, the resistors are distorted and their resistance changes. Resistive-type transducers have a major advantage over capacitance- and inductance-type transducers. Change in resistance is easily converted to change in voltage by a Wheatstone bridge. Therefore, bulky circuits for modulation-demodulation are not necessary. Strain gauges are temperature-sensitive, but the Wheatstone bridge can be designed with two or four active arms to be temperature-compensated. The popular disposable pressure transducers are resistive-type transducers. The diaphragm is a piece of silicon with the resistive elements etched onto it.

Intravascular Transducers

Most clinical pressure transducers are for external use, but intravascular transducers can be of the inductive, capacitance, or resistive type. The advantage of intravascular transducers is that there is no mechanical coupling system to distort the pressure waveform. The frequency response of an intravascular transducers system can be flat to over 100 Hz.

Unfortunately, intravascular transducers have a number of drawbacks. They are expensive and fragile, a bad combination for clinical devices. Although they are miniature compared with external transducers, they are too large to be passed through a catheter smaller than 18 gauge. Finally, they cannot be recalibrated during use. The result is that intravascular transducers are not widely used for clinical measurement of intravascular pressures.

STANDARDIZATION

Manufacturers have adopted a standard blood pressure transducer output of 5 microvolts per volt excitation per mmHg input pressure (5 μV/V/mmHg). This standardization means that transducers from different manufacturers are functionally interchangeable. The interface plug between the transducer and the preamplifier has not been standardized, so a conversion unit may still be required to connect any particular combination of transducer and monitor.

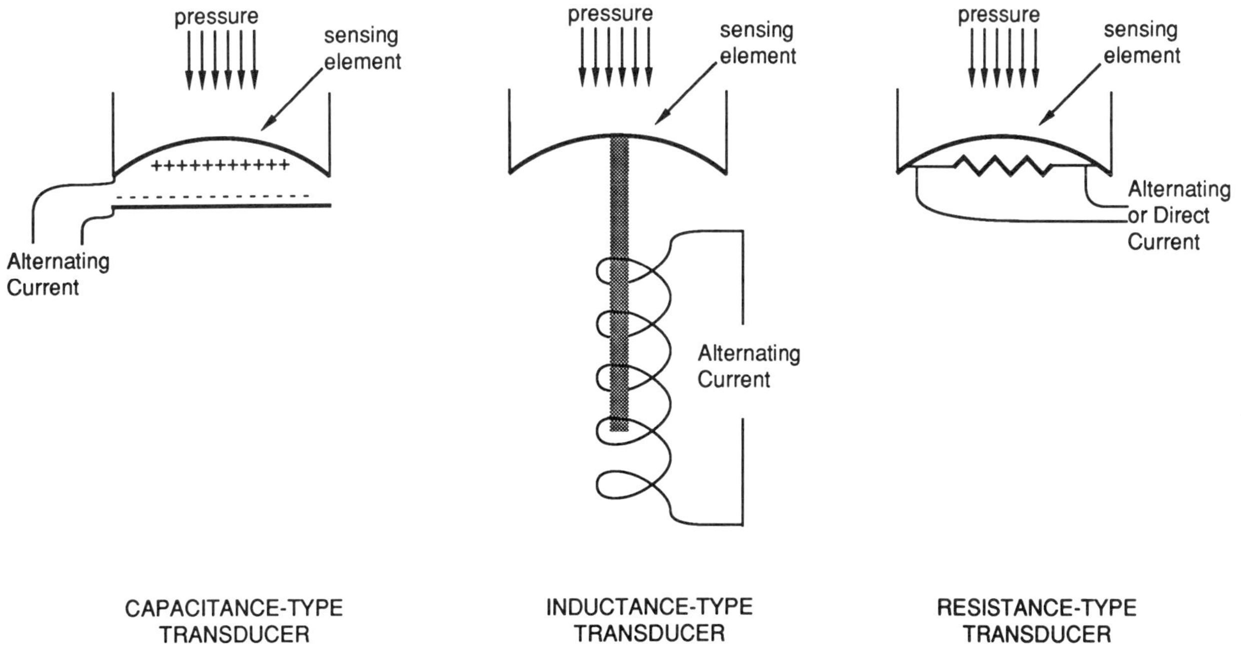

Figure 6–10. The three common types of electronic pressure transducers.

AMPLIFIERS AND FILTERS

Electrical amplification and filtering occurs between the generation of the electrical analog at the transducer and the display of the pressure waveform. Many modern monitors also perform analog-to-digital conversion of the signal at this point. The actual mechanism of this ''electronic massage'' for any given monitor is unimportant and proprietary, but the specifications of the amplifiers, filters, and analog-to-digital converters are important because they influence the waveform and derived values. Amplifiers are used to increase the voltage and power of the signal. They contain oscillating electronic circuits but have a frequency response 100 times better than that of the mechanical coupling system.

Low-pass filters are included for three reasons: to remove high-frequency noise due to electrocautery; to smooth the waveform, which is often reconstructed from discretely sampled points; and to give the waveform a more pleasant appearance. Removal of electrocautery noise is clinically necessary. However, filtering to yield a more rounded appearance of the waveform is unwarranted. Filtering is a serious problem because it is not standardized, and the filters affect the frequencies of interest. For example, Hewlett-Packard monitor models 78353/4 and 78833/4 (Hewlett-Packard Co., Waltham, MA) have a bandwidth of 0–12 Hz, whereas the Tektronix model 414 monitor (Tektronix, Inc., Beaverton, OR) has a bandwidth of 0–20 Hz. (Bandwidth is the frequency range over which the output has between 70% and 140% the power of the input.) Nonstandardization may cause discrepancies, especially in systolic values and derived cardiovascular parameters, whenever a patient is moved from one monitor to another.

There are two reasons that a waveform may be sampled as discrete points and then reconstructed. Some monitors electronically disconnect the transducer hundreds of times per second (chop the signal) and subtract any baseline voltage during that time to maintain baseline stability of the internal electronic components. More important, most modern monitors convert the analog voltage to a digital value. This process, known as analog-to-digital conversion, occurs 60 to a few hundred times per second. The advantages of having the information in a digital form are that it can be stored and manipulated. Stored values allow display of frozen waveforms and trends. Digital computer manipulation of the values allows feature detection, automatic calculation of derived variables, and other sophisticated algorithms that are discussed later.

ELECTRONIC SIGNAL ANALYSIS

The shape of the pressure waveform is important to detect artifact, to judge the effect of arrhythmias on blood pressure (see Chapter 5), and perhaps to estimate the inotropic and volume status of the cardiovascular system. In addition to displaying the waveform, clinical monitors extract and digitally display four features: rate, systolic pressure, diastolic pressure, and mean pressure. These values are used, either directly or in derived parameters, to guide diagnostic and therapeutic decisions. These values are affected by dynamic and static calibration and electronic filtering as well as by the method of signal analysis.

What information is important from a physiologic viewpoint? Heart rate is one description of cardiovascular status. Cardiac output is affected by heart rate, especially in children. Heart rate also affects the oxygen supply-to-demand ratio of the heart. Heart rate variability with respiration indicates active autonomic control, and variability with surgical stimulus helps one evaluate depth of anesthesia. Therefore, the absolute value of heart rate and some measure of heart rate variability are clinically useful parameters.

The systolic blood pressure—that is, the average aortic pressure during systole—estimates left ventricular afterload. The mean blood pressure indicates tissue perfusion pressure. Perfusion pressure of the coronary arteries is influenced by the diastolic pressure—that is, the average aortic pressure during diastole. Normally, these systemic pressures are relatively uniform, beat to beat, over the respiratory cycle. However, hypovolemia is associated with increased variability with respiration. For systemic pressures, the clinically useful values are the average systolic pressure, the average diastolic pressure, the average mean pressure, and some measure of blood pressure variability.

Central vascular pressures (central venous pressure, pulmonary artery pressure, and pulmonary capillary wedge pressure) are used as correlates of atrial filling pressure and end-diastolic volume. These pressures are dramatically affected by respiration, especially in critically ill patients. The physiologically important values occur at end-expiration when the intrathoracic pressure is closest to atmospheric pressure. Therefore, for central vascular pressure, the average end-expiratory mean pressure is the most desirable measurement.

In the past few decades, there has been a shift in technology in clinical monitors from analog to digital techniques of signal analysis. However, there are still many analog monitors in use. Analog averaging is usually accomplished by using a resistor-capacitor circuit. These circuits output a voltage that is the exponentially weighted average of the input voltage. The effect is that all previous values are averaged, the more recent values being weighted exponentially more than the older values. A step change in input results in an exponential approach to the change in output. The response time of the circuit can be adjusted by changing the relative values of the resistor and capacitor. The output of these circuits is not very different from a moving average for an oscillating signal, but their response to a step change is quite different. There are also analog circuits that detect and hold a peak or nadir voltage. These circuits are used to detect systolic and diastolic values, actually maximum systolic and minimum diastolic pressures. In the older equipment, the averaging and peak detection circuits were reset every few seconds; the output was then a mean, peak, or nadir pressure detected over a constant period. This tended to emphasize the highest systolic and lowest diastolic pressures during the respiratory cycle and was especially inaccurate at slow heart rates.

Later analog devices reset the averaging and peak detection circuits in synchrony with the heart rate. This allows calculation of beat-to-beat values of mean, peak, and nadir pressures that are averaged prior to display. Heart rate can be determined from the blood pressure waveform by taking the first derivative of the waveform and counting the rate of strongly positive values or by counting the number of times the pressure changes from a value below the mean pressure to a value above the mean pressure. Either event triggers an electronic pulse that is fed into an averaging circuit whose output voltage then correlates with the average heart rate. In summary, monitors using analog signal processing to extract waveform parameters display the exponentially weighted average of heart rate, maximum systolic pressure, minimum diastolic pressure, and exponentially weighted mean pressure. Maloy and Gardner have experimentally demonstrated that these values may not equal those determined by a clinician reading from a calibrated strip-chart recording.[28] The systolic pressure is the most inaccurate value displayed, especially in patients with hypertension, pulsus paradoxus, or arrhythmias.

DIGITAL PROCESSING ALGORITHMS

Digital signal processing is also employed in most of the new blood pressure monitors. It is performed by one or more internal microprocessors. Digital processing algorithms are proprietary, and manufacturers rarely reveal the details of their methods. In general, algorithms are used to determine the beginning and end of a cardiac cycle. The maximum and minimum pressures during that cycle are then selected as systolic and diastolic values. These values, averaged over a constant period, are displayed. Mean pressures are also calculated beat to beat. Digital algorithms do perform better than analog algorithms. Maloy and Gardner found that the numeric values displayed by monitors using digital technology agreed more closely with clinicians' readings than did monitors using analog technology.[28] Even using current digital algorithms, systolic values are less reliable than diastolic values, and machine-generated values are sensitive to artifacts in the waveform.

New algorithms are being devised to remove the effect of respiratory artifact on central vascular pressures. Currently, the recommendations are for the clinician to determine these pressures from a calibrated paper-strip recording at end-exhalation.[29, 30] Simultaneous measurement of airway pressure accurately identifies end-expiration.[31] Alternatively, stable digital values can be obtained during a prolonged expiratory pause in the paralyzed and anesthetized patient.[5] However, this procedure risks morbidity from failure to reinitiate mechanical ventilation. With current algorithms, the displayed mean value of central vascular pressures during mechanical ventilation is completely inaccurate and should not be used as either an absolute value or a trend.[30, 32]

A number of methods have been described in an attempt to automatically determine end-expiratory values of pulmonary artery pressures. The goal of each of these algorithms is to detect end-expiration. This is done most accurately by measuring the pressure, temperature, flow, or carbon dioxide concentration in the respiratory gas.[31, 33] Unfortunately, these techniques require additional measuring equipment.

An alternative method is described by Ellis.[34] He noted that the beat-to-beat mean pressure fluctuates least during end-expiration whenever expiratory time exceeds or equals inspiratory time. He used this observation to develop an algorithm that identifies end-expiration from information present in the pressure waveform itself.[34]

After end-expiration is identified, end-expiratory pressures can be estimated in a number of ways. One way is to average all values but to give greater weight to the values with less beat-to-beat variability.[34] This method is currently used in some monitors. Another way is to average only the end-expiratory values.[33] These methods are slightly more accurate than simple averaging techniques but become inaccurate at high respiratory rates. They also have the disadvantage of not displaying the pressure waveform with the respiratory artifact removed.

Mitchell and coworkers reported a microprocessor-based method of removing the respiratory artifact from the pressure waveform.[35] To separate the cardiac and respiratory components, they use an adaptive filter that changes its characteristics based on the measured heart rate. They then determine the mean intravascular pressure using Ellis's algorithm and add this offset to the cardiac component. The result is a continuous pulmonary artery pressure waveform with the respiratory artifact removed. The method is equally applicable to central venous pressure and pulmonary capillary wedge pressures.

Commercially available monitors utilize simple analog or digital methods, or both, to determine average systolic, mean, and diastolic pressures. Algorithms are being developed to remove or identify artifact in invasive pressure waveforms. It is hoped that future commercial monitors will use more sophisticated electronic signal analysis.

DISPLAYS

Most clinicians are familiar with the variety of displays available on commercial monitors. Early blood pressure monitors used a simple oscilloscope to display the waveform. Systolic, diastolic, and mean values were displayed on separate analog or digital meters. Today, monitor displays have increased in complexity and sophistication. Waveforms and numbers are displayed simultaneously on a cathode ray tube. Display format can be partially defined by the user and can automatically change as different combinations of transducers are connected to the monitor. Remote displays are available; these are classified as "smart" or "dumb." Dumb terminals simply echo the monitor's integrated display. They are usually large screens used in operating rooms so that all members of the surgical team can observe cardiovascular parameters. Smart terminals allow various levels of display control from a remote location. These are most frequently used in intensive care units to display information from multiple monitors in a central location.

Displays have undergone two major improvements: color and trend displays. Color displays help the user to find and focus her or his attention on a particular waveform or value. This is important because displays often contain multiple waveforms and values from a number of sources. Many commercial monitors now have the ability to store a few hours of information and display it on a compressed time scale. The immediate advantages are twofold: (1) A clinician who has not been in constant attendance has access to an accurate record of the patient's physiologic status during the clinician's absence. (2) The clinician can view physiologic parameters on a compressed time scale to detect trends that may not be apparent in real time. Trend displays are underutilized by clinicians. Most clinicians are used to the standard monitor display of real-time waveforms; this is the most frequently selected display for continual observation in the operating room and intensive care unit.

No studies have been done to determine whether physiologic stability can be better maintained with real-time waveforms or with trend displays as feedback, but trend displays may be the better choice under many circumstances. Humans are very effective in detecting patterns, but their memory limits their ability to detect patterns occurring over a span of time. By allowing the clinician to focus on the changes in relevant physiologic variables over a relevant period, trend displays aid in the detection and treatment of undesirable conditions.

EFFECTS OF CATHETERS

Superficial arteries are commonly cannulated for pressure measurement. Barr first reported the use of an over-the-needle catheter that is inserted percutaneously for indwelling use.[36] Central arteries and veins are commonly cannulated using the method first described by Seldinger (see Chapters 7 and 8).[37]

CATHETER SIZE AND TYPE

The size of the catheter influences the rate of complications and the dynamic response of the system. Bedford studied the incidence of temporary radial artery occlusion as a function of catheter size. He found a 34% incidence of occlusion 24 hours after insertion with 18-gauge catheters, compared with 8% with 20-gauge catheters.[38] The incidence of arterial occlusion is directly related to the percentage of the vessel lumen that is occupied by the catheter. Wrist circumference is a noninvasive measurement that is well correlated with the risk of radial arterial occlusion; a wrist circumference of less than 18 cm is associated with a greater than 25% incidence of occlusion using an 18-gauge catheter.[39] Although radial artery occlusion is usually temporary, persistent occlusion can result.[40] The lower incidence of thrombosis with smaller catheters is an advantage to the clinician. Distal occlusion of the radial artery causes overshoot of the measured systolic pressure owing to increased wave reflection, whereas proximal occlusion causes a reduction in measured pulse pressure owing to overdamping.[41] Small catheters have an additional effect of improving the dynamic accuracy of the system. Although small catheters have a slightly lower resonant frequency than do large catheters, they have a significantly larger damping coefficient.[42, 43] Because most blood pressure monitoring systems are underdamped, this results in increased accuracy of the system. The major clinical disadvantage of smaller catheters is that they kink more easily.

CATHETER COMPOSITION

The material from which the catheter is made also influences the rate of complications. Intravascular catheters are commonly manufactured from polyethylene, polypropylene, polyvinylchloride, or polytef (Teflon). Numerous studies have documented the increased thrombogenicity of polypropylene and polyethylene over Teflon.[41, 44–47] Polyvinylchloride is comparable to Teflon in its incidence of thrombus formation.[46, 48] Thrombogenicity is also affected by the smoothness of the catheter surface; roughened Teflon catheters are more thrombogenic than polyethylene catheters.[45] This may be clinically important, because pulmonary artery catheters have a higher incidence of thrombus formation when they are passed through introducers or protective sleeves.[49] Heparin impregnation of catheters decreases the incidence of thrombus formation initially, especially in larger vessels, but the effect is lost after 48 hours, probably because the heparin leeches out of the catheter.[46, 50] However, improved methods to attach heparin to surfaces are being developed.[50] In addition to initial thrombus formation, polyethylene catheters cause injuries to the vessel, which could serve as a nidus for atherosclerotic plaques.[51]

A notable exception to the findings presented here are the data from Slogoff and coworkers. In their study of 1699 patients after radial artery cannulation, they were unable to find any correlation between the risk of thrombus and catheter size (18 or 20 gauge) or catheter composition (Teflon or polypropylene).[52] They did report a statistically higher incidence of thrombosis in women (who tend to have a smaller wrist circumference).[52]

MAINTENANCE OF CATHETER PATENCY

Catheters for pressure monitoring are kept patent by one of three methods: intermittent bolus of heparin-containing solution, continuous flush of heparin-containing solution, or continuous flush of non–heparin-containing solution.

Intermittent Bolus Technique

Historically, the intermittent bolus of the heparin-containing solution was the only method available. There are two major problems with the intermittent bolus technique. First, it is not particularly effective in preventing catheter thrombosis, which leads to waveform damping.[46] Wesseling and Smith report that the duration of waveform loss owing to damping with the intermittent bolus technique is 2–10 times that with the continuous flush technique.[53] More important, significant patient morbidity can result from a manual bolus when thrombotic or air emboli are forced retrograde into the central or cerebral circulation.[21] The volume of the bolus necessary to reach the central circulation correlates with the height of the patient. Therefore, extreme care is necessary during bolus injection in pediatric patients.

Continuous Flush Technique

In 1970, Gardner and colleagues published a report of the first commercial continuous flush device for clinical use.[54] Such devices, which infuse fluid through the catheter at a nominal rate of 3–6 ml/hour, are now widely used. Advantages of continuous flush include effectiveness, ease of use, and the ability to maintain a closed sterile system. An additional advantage is that constantly wedged pulmonary artery catheters may be identified by a steady increase in the measured pulmonary artery pressure with loss of the waveform.[55]

There are, of course, some disadvantages with continuous flush. A static error is introduced in the pressure measurement. The magnitude of the error depends on the infusion rate and the resistance to flow through the catheter. Static errors between 0.1 and 2.5 mmHg have been reported.[22, 54] For arterial pressure monitoring, this error is clinically insignificant. A more important disadvantage is the potential for inadvertent excess fluid administration. This can occur if the flush mechanism is defective.[56] However, in neonates and children, even a flow of 3–6 ml/hour through multiple pressure monitoring lines may exceed the fluid requirements for a particular patient. In such cases, the standard system can be modified so that the fluid for the flush device is dispensed from a syringe pump or volumetric infusion pump.[57] A final potential problem of continuous flush is the introduction of air into the pressure monitoring system. If the fluid source for the flush device is a pressurized bag of fluid that contains air, an air embolism may occur when the bag empties. This may be avoided if all the air is removed from the bag prior to applying pressure. Smaller amounts of air can also be introduced during a fast flush. This occurs owing to the vortex created when a stream of fluid enters the drip chamber. The best solution is to inspect the system for air after a fast flush or to use an appropriate filter.

The final issue in maintaining catheter patency is whether to use heparin in a continuous flush solution. Most practitioners use 1 or 2 U of heparin/ml of flush solution.[58] However, heparin administration carries the risk of heparin-induced thrombocytopenia or accidental heparin overdose.[59] Two small studies have investigated whether heparin is necessary in a continuous flush solution to maintain arterial catheter patency. Heparin at a concentration of 2.5 U/ml did not maintain catheter patency better than lactated Ringer's solution in a nonrandomized unblinded study of 50 adult patients.[60] However, catheter occlusion *was* more frequent when heparin (4 U/ml) was omitted from the continuous saline flush in a blinded and randomized study of 30 medical intensive care patients.[61] Thus, the use of heparin in arterial line flush solutions is still controversial, and a multisite study is in progress to further investigate its need.[58]

PRESSURE ALTERATION IN VASCULATURE

The preceding discussions imply that systems with an optimal dynamic response accurately measure blood pressure. However, although the pressure at the site of measurement is accurately reproduced, the pressure may already be distorted where it is measured. The vascular tree is a complex oscillating system that acts to change the blood pressure at different areas of the body. Usually, the pressures in peripheral arteries contain more high-frequency components than do central arteries; the systolic pressure is usually higher in peripheral arteries.[62, 63] However, there are exceptions. Multiple studies have demonstrated that the systolic pressure is often lower in peripheral arteries than it is in central arteries immediately after cardiopulmonary bypass.[62, 64–66] Iatrogenic compression of an upstream artery can also cause a falsely low peripheral blood pressure—for example, during sternal retraction.[67, 68] In neonates, the peripheral pressure correlates well with the central umbilical artery pressure.[69]

Three major factors cause the vascular tree to change peripheral blood pressure: oscillations, wave reflections, and phase shift. The effects of oscillation on pressure measurements have been discussed previously. The vascular tree acts like many oscillating segments connected in series.[70] The damping coefficient and resonant frequency of each segment are functions of the vascular tone and blood volume. Computer modeling demonstrates how changes in vascular compliance and resistance alter the radial artery pressure independent of central aortic pressure. Not only are the systolic, diastolic, and mean pressures affected, the entire shape of the pressure waveform is changed.[70] The dicrotic notch of the radial artery pressure waveform is an artifact;[63, 70] there is no correlation between it and the dicrotic notch of the central aortic pressure waveform.

The influence of wave reflection and phase shift on the

resultant peripheral pressure is probably less than that of oscillations. Wave reflections occur when the pressure wave reaches the resistance arterioles.[71] At the arterioles, some of the energy of the pressure wave forces blood past the resistance, some of the energy is absorbed by the vessel, and the remainder is reflected. The tone of the arterioles influences the amount of energy reflected. Normal femoral vascular beds reflect 80% of the incident wave; reflections are decreased to almost zero after intra-arterial vasodilator injections.[71] The location of the pressure measurement site with respect to the wave reflection site and the elasticity of the arterial tree influence the effect of reflected waves on the measured pressure. Reflected waves coincident with the systolic part of the incident waveform cause an increased systolic pressure; those transmitted more slowly or detected a farther distance away contribute to a diastolic peak.[71]

Wave reflection is easily demonstrated. When pressure is applied with the finger over the intravascular portion of an arterial catheter, an increase in the systolic pressure is observed.[41] This is because a situation is created in which there is 100% energy reflection coincident with the systolic pressure. A similar situation occurs when there is thrombosis obstructing the artery distal to the site of measurement.[41]

Phase shift occurs because higher frequencies are transmitted at different rates than lower frequencies.[72] This distorts the peripheral pressure, causing the leading edge of the systolic pressure to be exaggerated.[16]

Because the pressure waveform in peripheral vessels is so different from that in the central aorta, care should be used in interpreting peripheral invasive blood pressures. The pressures in peripheral arteries differ from the aortic pressures to which the heart is exposed. Derived values that are meaningful when calculated from aortic pressures are meaningless when calculated from peripheral pressures. For example, the ratio of the area under the diastolic portion of the aortic pressure to the area under the systolic aortic pressure (DPTI/SPTI) has been used to predict the myocardial oxygen supply-to-demand ratio. This ratio is magnified by 25% when peripheral instead of aortic pressures are used.[73] Similarly, derivations of myocardial contractility and stroke volume from the peripheral blood pressure are inaccurate.[70]

Invasive blood pressure measurements are used clinically to judge the cardiovascular status of the patient. Extrapolations are made from arterial blood pressure to flow conditions in the brain, heart, kidney, and other organs; to the work of the heart; and even to cardiovascular volume status. The vascular tree and measurement devices modulate the pressure waveform in complex and dynamic ways. It is appropriate to use blood pressure trends to direct therapy; however, one should avoid placing too much confidence in the absolute value displayed on the blood pressure monitor.

REFERENCES

1. Fox F, Morrow DH, Kacher EJ, Gilleland TH: Laboratory evaluation of pressure transducer domes containing a diaphragm. Anesth Analg 1978; 57:67–76.
2. Disposable Pressure Transducers—Evaluation. Health Devices 1984; 13:268–290.
3. Navedo AT, Wald A: Erroneous measurement with invasive monitoring of blood pressure [Letter]. Anesth Analg 1991; 73:96–97.
4. Raines DE, Hogue CJ, Wickens C, *et al*: Artifactual hypertension due to transducer cable malfunction. Anesthesiology 1991; 74:1149–1151.
5. Barbieri LT, Kaplan JA: Artifactual hypotension secondary to intraoperative transducer failure. Anesth Analg 1983; 62:112–113.
6. Gordon VL, Welch JP, Carley D, *et al*: Zero stability of disposable and reusable pressure transducers. Med Instrum 1987; 21:87–91.
7. Sisko F, Hagerdal M, Neufeld GR: Artifactual hypotension without damping, a hazard of disposable diaphragm domes. Anesthesiology 1979; 51:263–264.
8. Milne B, Cervenko FW, Henderson MB, Westra PJ: Transducer offset by electrocautery resulting in erroneous blood pressure measurement. Can J Anaesth 1986; 33:234–236.
9. Fernandez-Cano F: A simple accurate technique for establishing zero reference levels for pressure measurements [Letter]. Anesthesiology 1984; 61:478.
10. Geddes LA: The Direct and Indirect Measurement of Blood Pressure. Chicago: Year Book, 1970; 1–69.
11. Gardner RM: Direct blood pressure measurement—Dynamic response requirements. Anesthesiology 1981; 54:227–236.
12. Abrams JH, Olson ML, Marino JA, Cerra FB: Use of a needle valve variable resistor to improve invasive blood pressure monitoring. Crit Care Med 1984; 12:978–982.
13. Boutros A, Albert S: Effect of the dynamic response of transducer-tubing system on accuracy of direct blood pressure measurement in patients. Crit Care Med 1983; 11:124–127.
14. Shinozaki T, Deane RS, Mazuzan JE: The dynamic responses of liquid-filled catheter systems for direct measurements of blood pressure. Anesthesiology 1980; 53:498–504.
15. Hunziker P: Accuracy and dynamic response of disposable pressure transducer-tubing systems. Can J Anaesth 1987; 34:409–414.
16. Geddes LA, Baker LE: Principles of Applied Biomedical Instrumentation. New York: John Wiley & Sons, 1968; 446–467.
17. Schwid HA: Frequency response evaluation of radial artery catheter-manometer systems: Sinusoidal frequency analysis versus flush method. J Clin Monit 1988; 4:181–185.
18. Hipkins SF, Rutten AJ, Runciman WB: Experimental analysis of catheter-manometer systems in vitro and in vivo. Anesthesiology 1989; 71:893–906.
19. Wade LD, Krejcie TC: The effect of air bubbles on the dynamic response of invasive pressure monitoring systems [Abstract]. Anesth Analg 1983; 62:S289.
20. Soule DT, Powner DJ: Air entrapment in pressure monitoring lines. Crit Care Med 1984; 12:520–522.
21. Lowenstein E, Little JW, Lo HH: Prevention of cerebral embolization from flushing radial-artery cannulas. N Engl J Med 1971; 285:1414–1415.
22. Gardner RM, Bond EL, Clark JS: Safety and efficacy of continuous flush systems for arterial and pulmonary artery catheters. Ann Thorac Surg 1977; 23:534–538.
23. Schwid HA: Semiautomatic algorithm to remove resonance artifacts from the direct radial artery pressure. Biomed Instrum Technol 1989; 23:40–43.
24. Roos CF, Carroll FE Jr: Fiber-optic pressure transducer for use near MR magnetic fields. Radiology 1985; 156:548.
25. Hackman CH, Tan PS, Chakrabarti MK, Whitwam JG: A new optical transducer for arterial pressure measurement. Br J Anaesth 1991; 67:346–352.
26. Rushmer RF: Cardiovascular Dynamics. Philadelphia: WB Saunders, 1976; 36–75.
27. Lee APB: Biotechnological principles of monitoring. Int Anesthesiol Clin 1981; 19:197–207.
28. Maloy L, Gardner RM: Monitoring systemic arterial blood pressure: Strip chart recording versus digital display. Heart Lung 1986; 15:627–635.
29. Schmitt EA, Brantigan CO: Common artifacts of pulmonary artery and pulmonary artery wedge pressures: Recognition and interpretation. J Clin Monit 1986; 2:44–52.
30. Maran AG: Variables in pulmonary capillary wedge pressure: Variation with intrathoracic pressure, graphic and digital recorders. Crit Care Med 1980; 8:102–105.
31. Berryhill RE, Benumof JL, Rauscher LA: Pulmonary vascular

pressure reading at the end of exhalation. Anesthesiology 1978; 49:365–368.
32. Riedinger MS, Shellock FG, Swan HJC: Reading pulmonary artery and pulmonary capillary wedge pressure waveforms with respiratory variations. Heart Lung 1981; 10:675–678.
33. Oden R, Mitchell MM, Benumof J: Detection of end-exhalation period by airway thermistor: An approach to automated pulmonary artery pressure measurement. Anesthesiology 1983; 58:467–471.
34. Ellis DM: Interpretation of beat-to-beat blood pressure values in the presence of ventilatory changes. J Clin Monit 1985; 1:65–70.
35. Mitchell MM, Meathe EA, Jones BR, *et al*: Accurate, automated, continuously displayed pulmonary artery pressure measurement. Anesthesiology 1987; 67:294–300.
36. Barr PO: Percutaneous puncture of the radial artery with a multipurpose Teflon catheter for indwelling use. Acta Physiol Scand 1961; 51:343–347.
37. Seldinger SI: Catheter replacement of the needle in percutaneous arteriography. Acta Radiol 1953; 39:368–376.
38. Bedford RF: Radial arterial function following percutaneous cannulation with 18- and 20-gauge catheters. Anesthesiology 1977; 47:37–39.
39. Bedford RF: Wrist circumference predicts the risk of arterial occlusion after cannulation. Anesthesiology 1978; 48:377–378.
40. Weiss BM, Gattiker RI: Complications during and following radial artery cannulation: A prospective study. Intensive Care Med 1986; 12:424–428.
41. Kim JM, Arakawa K, Bliss J: Arterial cannulation: Factors in the development of occlusion. Anesth Analg 1975; 54:836–841.
42. Browning DH, Graves SA, van der Aa J: Catheters for arterial pressure monitoring in pediatrics [Abstract]. Anesthesiology 1981; 55:A131.
43. Goodwin SR, Graves SA, van der Aa J: Umbilical catheters and arterial blood pressure monitoring. J Clin Monit 1985; 1:227–231.
44. Davis FM, Stewart JM: Radial artery cannulation. Br J Anaesth 1980; 52:41–47.
45. Mortensen JD, Schaap RN: Further experience with an acute intraarterial implantation screening test for thrombogenicity of intravascular catheters. Trans Am Soc Artif Intern Organs 1980; 26: 284–288.
46. Downs JB, Chapman RL Jr, Hawkins IF Jr: Prolonged radial-artery catheterization. Arch Surg 1974; 108:671–673.
47. Bedford RF: Percutaneous radial-artery cannulation—Increased safety using Teflon catheters. Anesthesiology 1975; 42:219–222.
48. Brown AE, Sweeney DB, Lumley J: Percutaneous radial artery cannulation. Anaesthesia 1969; 24:532–536.
49. Youngberg JA, Texidor M, Cantrell C, Theriot T, Wolf R: Introducers and protective sleeves increase thrombogenicity of pulmonary artery catheters [Abstract]. Anesthesiology 1985; 63:A181.
50. Eberhart RC, Clagett CP: Catheter coatings, blood flow, and biocompatibility. Semin Hematol 1991; 28:42–48.
51. Madsen JK, Garbarasch C, Nielsen PE: Endothelial injury of arteries following catheterization with polyethylene tubes: Experimental studies on rabbit aorta using the Seldinger technique. Cardiovasc Res 1979; 13:541–546.
52. Slogoff S, Keats AS, Arlund C: On the safety of radial artery cannulation. Anesthesiology 1983; 59:42–47.
53. Wesseling KH, Smith NT: Availability of intraarterial pressure waveforms from catheter-manometer systems during surgery. J Clin Monit 1985; 1:11–16.
54. Gardner RM, Warner HR, Toronto AF, Gaisford WD: Catheter-flush system for continuous monitoring of central arterial pulse waveform. J Appl Physiol 1970; 29:911–913.
55. Shin B, Ayella RJ, McAslan C: Pitfalls of Swan-Ganz catheterization. Crit Care Med 1977; 5:125–127.
56. Morray J, Todd S: A hazard of continuous flush systems for vascular pressure monitoring in infants. Anesthesiology 1983; 58:187–189.
57. Johnson DL: Invasive pressure monitoring: A modified system for pediatrics. Dimens Crit Care Nurs 1986; 5:93–96.
58. Ledbetter C, Ahrens T, Brown B, Gawlinski A, Quinn A, Walsh S: Comparison of normal saline and heparin solutions for maintenance of arterial catheter patency [Letter]. Heart Lung 1991; 20:316.
59. Silver D, Kapsch DN, Tsoi EKM: Heparin-induced thrombocytopenia, thrombosis, and hemorrhage. Ann Surg 1983; 198:301–305.
60. Hook ML, Reuling J, Luettgen ML, Norris SO, Elsesser CC, Leonard MK: Comparison of the patency of arterial lines maintained with heparinized and nonheparinized infusions. Heart Lung 1987; 16:693–699.
61. Clifton GD, Branson P, Kelly HJ, *et al*: Comparison of normal saline and heparin solutions for maintenance of arterial catheter patency. Heart Lung 1991; 20:115–118.
62. Gallagher JD, Moore RA, McNicholas KW, Jose AB: Comparison of radial and femoral arterial blood pressures in children after cardiopulmonary bypass. J Clin Monit 1985; 1:169–171.
63. Bruner JMR: Handbook of Blood Pressure Monitoring. Littleton, MA: PSG, 1978.
64. Mohr R, Lavee J, Goor DA: Inaccuracy of radial artery pressure measurement after cardiac operations. J Thorac Cardiovasc Surg 1987; 94:286–290.
65. Rulf EN, Mitchell MM, Prakash O, *et al*: Measurement of arterial pressure after cardiopulmonary bypass with long radial artery catheters. J Cardiothorac Anesth 1990; 4:19–24.
66. Stern DH, Gerson JI, Allen FB, Parker FB: Can we trust the direct radial artery pressure immediately following cardiopulmonary bypass? Anesthesiology 1985; 62:557–561.
67. Saka D, Lin TY, Oka Y: An unusual cause of false radial-artery blood-pressure readings during cardiopulmonary bypass. Anesthesiology 1975; 43:487–489.
68. Diamant M, Arkin DB: False radial-artery blood-pressure readings [Letter]. Anesthesiology 1976; 44:273.
69. Butt WW, Whyte H: Blood pressure monitoring in neonates: Comparison of umbilical and peripheral artery catheter measurements. J Pediatr 1984; 105:630–632.
70. Schwid HA, Taylor LA, Smith NT: Computer model analysis of the radial artery pressure waveform. J Clin Monit 1987; 3:220–228.
71. O'Rourke MF, Yaginuma T: Wave reflections and the arterial pulse. Arch Intern Med 1984; 144:366–371.
72. Remington JW: Contour changes of the aortic pulse during propagation. Am J Physiol 1960; 199:331–334.
73. Reitan JA, Martucci RW, Levine NA: A computer evaluation of the ratio of the diastolic pressure-time index to the time-tension index from three arterial sites in dogs. J Clin Monit 1986; 2:95–99.

Appendix

The oscillating behavior of the mechanical coupling system can be described by this differential equation

$$M \frac{d^2x}{dt^2} + R \frac{dx}{dt} + Ex = P(t) \qquad \textbf{6–1}$$

which describes the displacement of the fluid (x) for a given pressure waveform, P(t). M is the kinetic fluid mass of the system, R is the viscous damping, and E is the effective modulus of volume elasticity.

With zero damping, the system oscillates at the natural frequency (f_n) in response to a sudden input pressure:

$$f_n = \frac{1}{2\pi} \sqrt{\frac{E}{M}} \qquad \textbf{6–2}$$

E can be calculated from the physical characteristics of the transducer:

$$E = A^2 \frac{\Delta P}{\Delta V} \qquad \textbf{6–3}$$

where A is the exposed area of the transducer sensing element and $\Delta P/\Delta V$ is the change in pressure required to cause a volume of fluid to enter the transducer.

M can also be related to the physical characteristics of the system:

$$M = \frac{4}{3}\left(\frac{A}{a}\right)^2 la\rho + LA\rho \qquad \textbf{6–4}$$

where a is the cross-sectional area of the tubing, ρ is the density of the fluid, and L and l are the lengths of the columns of fluid in the transducer and tubing, respectively. Of course, the cross sectional area is related to the diameter of the tubing, d by

$$a = \frac{\pi d^2}{4} \qquad 6\text{–}5$$

Thus the natural frequency is increased by decreasing the elasticity and surface area of the transducer sensing element, by using short wide-bore tubing, and by using a fluid of low density.

The damping coefficient (D) is the viscous damping of the system expressed as a fraction of the critical damping. The damping coefficient can be calculated from the physical characteristics of the system:

$$D = \frac{16\eta}{d^3}\sqrt{\frac{3L}{\pi\rho E}} \qquad 6\text{–}6$$

where η is the fluid viscosity. Note that damping is inversely related to the cube of the diameter of the tubing.

The natural frequency and damping coefficient can be calculated by measuring the output of the system for a step pressure input or an increasing frequency sine wave input. In either case, the damped resonant frequency (f_d) of the system is measured. The damped resonant frequency is related to the natural frequency as follows:

$$f_d = f_n\sqrt{1 - D^2} \qquad 6\text{–}7$$

Using the step pressure method, the damping coefficient is calculated by measuring the amplitude ratio of two successive peaks (A_S) (see Fig. 6–8):

$$D = -\ln\left[\frac{A_S}{\sqrt{\pi^2 + (\ln A_S)^2}}\right] \qquad 6\text{–}8$$

Using the sine wave method, the damping coefficient is calculated by measuring the amplitude ratio of the test system to the reference system at the frequency of test system peak amplitude (Ar_{fd}):

$$D = \sqrt{\frac{1 - \sqrt{1 - \dfrac{1}{(Ar_{fd})^2}}}{2}} \qquad 6\text{–}9$$

Once the damping coefficient and natural frequency have been determined, the response of the system to a step pressure input and an increasing frequency sine input can be predicted. The output of the system over time to a step pressure input is

$$P(t) = P_0 - \frac{P_0}{\sqrt{1 - D^2}} e^{-D2\pi f_n t} \sin\left(2\pi f_n t\sqrt{1 - D^2} + \sin^{-1}\sqrt{1 - D^2}\right) \qquad 6\text{–}10$$

for $0 < D \leq 1$. The output-to-input ratio amplitude ratio (A_r) for any sine wave input frequency (f) (Fig. 6–3) is

$$A_r = \frac{1}{\sqrt{\left(\dfrac{f}{f_n}\right)^4 + 2\left(\dfrac{f}{f_n}\right)^2(2D^2 - 1) + 1}} \qquad 6\text{–}11$$

CHAPTER

7

Monitoring of Arterial Pressure

CAROL L. LAKE, M.D.

PHYSIOLOGY

ARTERIAL PULSE

The arterial pulse results from the wave of vascular distention initiated by the impact of the stroke volume on the closed vascular system. This wave begins at the base of the aorta and radiates throughout the arterial system. There is both a fast-moving (10 m/second) pressure wave and a slower (0.5 m/second) flow element in the pressure pulse.[1] The pulse waveform results from both the forward-propagating pressure wave and its reflectance back toward the heart from various portions of the circulation. The major source of wave reflection is the arteriole, which provides the majority of peripheral vascular resistance.[2] Peak aortic blood flow acceleration produces the initial rate of rise of the pressure pulse, whereas the ejection of ventricular volume fills out and sustains the pulse waveform.[1] The initial peak of the arterial waveform is the direct continuation of its initial upstroke. It is followed by a more or less well defined notch and subsequently by a second peak. The second peak falls away to the descending limb of the waveform, which often contains a dicrotic notch (Fig. 7–1).[1] The height of the dicrotic notch is unrelated to systemic vascular resistance.[3] The lowest point of the waveform is diastolic pressure.

As it moves peripherally, the arterial waveform changes dramatically (Fig. 7–1). The pulse waveform becomes more peaked and increases in amplitude because the initial slope of the upstroke continues for a longer time. Systolic pressure is higher and diastolic pressure is lower. The waveform has a greater amplitude, lower mean pressure, and more pronounced diastolic wave.[2] Mean pressure must decrease peripherally for flow to continue, although mean pressure changes less than either systolic or diastolic pressure. Karamanoglu et al described a transfer function that would permit determination of central aortic pressure from peripheral pressure.[4]

Pulse contour also varies with physiologic conditions. Compared with that of children, wave reflection in the elderly occurs earlier in the cardiac cycle, increasing systolic and decreasing diastolic pressure. Although pulse pressure increases as the pressure wave travels from the central aorta to the periphery in young subjects, there may be little change in elderly persons because the loss of elasticity with age reduces the degree of waveform amplification.

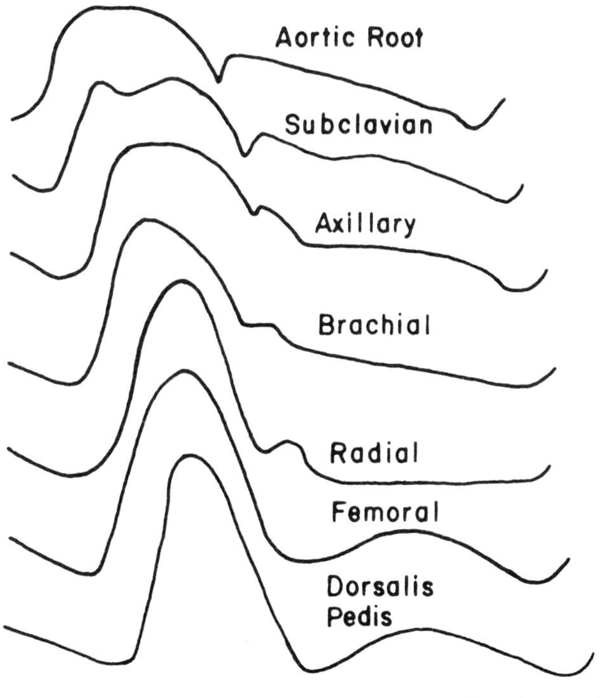

Figure 7–1. The pulse waveform changes as it moves from the central circulation to the periphery because of forward wave propagation and wave reflection. In the periphery, systolic pressure is higher, diastolic and mean pressures are lower, and the waveform displays greater amplitude. (From Bedford RF: Invasive blood pressure monitoring. In Blitt CD [ed]: Monitoring in Anesthesia and Critical Care Medicine. New York: Churchill Livingstone, 1985; 50).

Pulse wave velocity depends on vessel elasticity. In the least distensible arteries such as the aortic arch, the pulse wave travels about 3–5 m/second; in large distensible arteries such as the subclavian artery, about 7–10 m/second; and in small nondistensible peripheral arteries, 15–30 m/second. Thus, the aortic waveform precedes the brachial waveform by 0.05 seconds. Shock decreases pulse wave velocity because of hypotension, peripheral vasoconstriction, and increased heart rate (decreases duration of systole).

BLOOD PRESSURE

Blood pressure is the lateral pressure exerted on the walls of the vessels by blood in the vasculature. Mean arterial pressure is the product of systemic vascular resistance (in resistance units) and the cardiac output. If the arterial waveform is normal, mean pressure is approximately one third of the difference between systolic and diastolic pressure. Mean arterial pressure probably best estimates systemic perfusion. Systolic pressures are particularly useful in the assessment of myocardial oxygen demand, whereas diastolic pressures relate to supply. Pulse pressure, the difference between systolic and diastolic pressure, narrows with hypovolemia or hemorrhage. Increased pulse pressure opens collapsed capillary beds.

INDICATIONS FOR ARTERIAL PRESSURE MONITORING

Although arterial pressure was measured in an animal in 1731, indirect recordings in humans were not made until 1855; in 1904, a committee at the Massachusetts General Hospital recommended *against* the adoption of routine blood pressure monitoring during surgery. Today it is essential to use either noninvasive or invasive methods to measure systolic, diastolic, mean, and pulse pressures during all surgical procedures.

Invasive methods are usually reserved for the critically ill and when hemodynamic compromise is likely as a result of the surgical procedure or for when multiple blood specimens are required. Because of measurement errors, the greater energy required to generate a Korotkoff sound than a direct signal, changes in arterial compliance, and differences in equipment, pressures measured by different noninvasive methods often correlate poorly with direct measurements (Table 7–1).[1,5]

However, industry standards require that blood pressure measurement systems accurately measure static pressures to within 2% or 1 mmHg at pressures up to 250 mmHg.[6] Such systems must not deliver erroneous reading on abnormal waveforms. Other safety requirements include minimum and maximum pressures of 10 and 330 mmHg, respectively, and cuff inflation adjustments near previous values for subsequent inflations (usually 30–50 mmHg). Automatic cuff cycling at user-chosen intervals is available on most automated oscillometric blood pressure monitors. For further recommendations on specific blood pressure monitoring devices, the reader is referred to reference 6.

TABLE 7–1. CAUSES OF INACCURACY IN NONINVASIVE MEASUREMENT OF ARTERIAL PRESSURE

Improper cuff size (too small or large)
Observer error (hearing of sounds, visualization of meter needle oscillation)
Improper cuff application to limb (too tight or loose)
Too-rapid cuff deflation (difficulty assessing sound disappearance on auscultation)
Too-slow cuff deflation (venous congestion)
Uncalibrated gauges
Circulatory alterations (shock, vasoconstriction)

INDIRECT MEASUREMENT OF ARTERIAL PRESSURE

Methods to measure arterial pressure indirectly include (1) palpation, (2) detection of Korotkoff sounds with an occlusive cuff (Riva Rocci method), (3) Doppler, (4) oscillotonometry using either a standard oscillotonometer or an automated method, and (5) plethysmography. The American Heart Association recommends standard procedures and methods to minimize errors in noninvasive determination of blood pressure (Table 7–1).[7]

PALPATION METHOD

The simplest method of blood pressure determination is by palpation of the pulse as an occluding cuff is inflated to a pressure above expected arterial pressure and then gradually deflated until the first pulse is palpable. In infants, the "flush" method is a variation of the palpation method wherein the pressure at which limb color returns is noted. The flush method depends highly on speed of cuff deflation, peripheral perfusion, and operator skill. Oscillations of aneroid manometers during cuff deflation provide very subjective endpoints of the start and maximum of flicker oscillation that roughly estimate blood pressure.[1] More sophisticated modifications of the palpatory method are observation of return of the pulse by Doppler, direct arterial cannula, or oximeter when cuff deflation is performed.[8]

KOROTKOFF METHOD

Technique

The best-known method of noninvasive determination of arterial blood pressure is the auscultatory method employing Korotkoff sounds.[9] Stethoscopes and sphygmomanometers are relatively inexpensive, readily available, and reasonably reliable and accurate. Korotkoff sounds are produced with resumption of blood flow through a previously collapsed artery. Inflation of the cuff to a pressure above the expected systolic pressure and gradual deflation permits identification of the maximum audible (systolic) and minimum audible (diastolic) pressures. The inflation device is a simple rubber bulb with a one-way valve that is reliable and easily replaced. Attached to the inflation device is the deflation valve, allowing deflation at 2–4 mm Hg per heartbeat. Very rapid deflation decreases the resolution of the pressure determination.[10] Too-rapid deflation underestimates systolic pressure and either overestimates or underestimates diastolic pressure, depending on individual assessment of sound disappearance.[10] Too-slow deflation allows venous congestion to occur, which attenuates the Korotkoff sounds near the diastolic pressure.[10]

A transducer with a wide frequency response reveals the presence of three components to the pulse recorded during cuff deflation.[11] These components are K_1, K_2, and K_3, with K_2 a triphasic signal appearing at systolic pressure and disappearing at diastolic pressure, roughly corresponding the audible Korotkoff sounds. The K_2 signal is more accurate than standard auscultatory methods and is similar to intra-arterial measurements.[11]

Equipment

The pressure sensor in the sphygmomanometer is either a mercury manometer or an aneroid gauge. For accuracy, the mercury manometer must be vertical and have a clean, unbroken column of mercury resting at the zero point. The aneroid gauge is a simple device containing a diaphragm of hollow, corrugated metal disks that expands or contracts as pressure changes. Diaphragmatic motion is transmitted to a rod connected to a gear operating a pointer. Aneroid gauges must be calibrated against mercury to ensure accuracy because the diaphragm and transmitting parts will malfunction over time or after mechanical or thermal shocks. A stethoscope, microphone, or other sensor used to auscultate the pulse is the signal detector placed over the artery.

Appropriate cuff size is essential to sphygmomanometric pressure measurements. The artery is collapsed by an occlusive cuff that must be 20% larger than the diameter of the limb. If the cuff is too small, the systolic and diastolic pressures are artificially increased, and vice versa.[12] All air should be expelled from the cuff when it is applied. Snug application to the limb is essential because loosely fitting cuffs falsely increase pressure measurements.[10] Tight application of the cuff causes venous distention and patient discomfort.

Compared with intra-arterial pressures, auscultatory pressures differ by 1–7 mmHg systolic and 8–18 mmHg diastolic, with correlation coefficients of 0.73 (Fig. 7–2).[5, 13–16] Inaccuracies also result from the continuous nature of the task of blood pressure measurement in an operating room or intensive care unit. When the caregiver's attention is diverted to other tasks, recordings are not made, incorrect measurements are made, incorrect numbers are recorded, and the human ear is unattuned to the Korotkoff sounds.[5, 17] For all of these reasons, manual determinations of blood pressure have been largely replaced by automated indirect or direct measurements in operating rooms and critical care settings.

Changes in the circulation affect pressure measurement. Detection of the Korotkoff sounds is difficult when peripheral vasoconstriction or hypotension is present. In shock, Korotkoff sounds are gradually attenuated until they are inaudible.[10] Auscultation is also impossible in the absence of pulsatile flow, as during cardiopulmonary bypass. In a hyperdynamic circulatory state, auscultatory sounds are present before the systolic pressure is reached, overestimating systolic and underestimating diastolic pressure.[10]

DOPPLER METHODS

Technique

The Doppler effect is the principle by which frequency is changed when waveform energy is reflected from a moving surface. The pitch of the sound is proportional to the

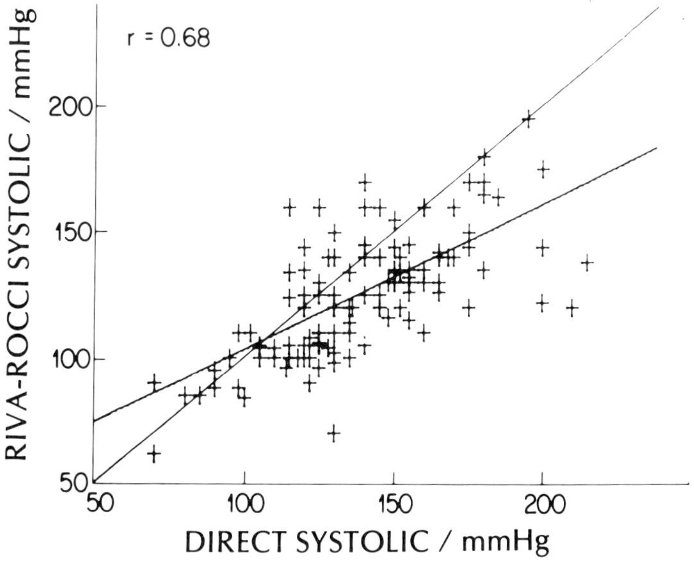

Figure 7–2. The comparison of direct intra-arterial systolic pressures with those measured by the Riva Rocci auscultatory method show considerable scatter (r = 0.68). (Modified from Bruner JMR, et al: Comparison of direct and indirect methods of measuring arterial blood pressure, part III. Med Instrum 1981; 15:184. Association for the Advancement of Medical Instrumentation. Arlington, Virginia.)

velocity of the reflective surface. The volume of the sound is proportional to the area of the moving reflective surface.[18] Blood pressure is measured with a 10-Hz ultrasound transducer and receiver assembly, which detects the difference in frequency between the transmitted and reflected ultrasound in response to occlusion and deflation of a proximally located cuff.[18, 19]

A Doppler-shift signal is detected when blood flow causes movement of the arterial wall at systolic pressure. No Doppler-shift signal is detected while the artery is closed. Diastole is a soft sloshing sound that is difficult to detect clinically.[20] Differences between Korotkoff sounds and Doppler-shift sounds are listed in Table 7–2.[20]

Doppler measurements of blood pressure are higher than those obtained with palpation or flush techniques but lower than those with direct arterial pressures.[21] Figure 7–3 demonstrates the close correlation of Doppler pressures to intra-arterial measurements. One of the major advantages of the Doppler technique is the ability to measure pressure during low flow states, such as the mean arterial pressure during cardiopulmonary bypass and cardiopulmonary resuscitation.[22]

TABLE 7–2. DIFFERENCES BETWEEN KOROTKOFF AND DOPPLER SOUNDS

1. Korotkoff sounds are heard only during opening of artery; Doppler sounds are heard during opening and closure.
2. Korotkoff sounds require vibratory motion in audible range; any arterial motion generates a Doppler signal.
3. Korotkoff sounds depend on the properties of the resonant biologic system in which it operates; Doppler signals are altered by changes in operating frequency.

Data from Stegall HF, et al: Indirect measurement of arterial blood pressure by Doppler ultrasonic sphygmomanometry. J Appl Physiol 1968; 25:793.

OSCILLOMETRIC METHOD

Standard Technique

The oscillotonometer, first described by Von Recklinghausen in 1931,[23] consists of a double-cuff system with the proximal cuff occluding the artery while the distal cuff senses the onset of arterial pulsation. Systolic and diastolic pressures are obtained by noting the oscillation of a mercury column or an aneroid manometer. Slow deflation of the cuff is essential to accurately measure systolic pressure because there is considerable observer variation in the detection of needle oscillation.[24] Fast rates of deflation produce a greater decrease in cuff pressure between heartbeats, making the change in oscillation of the needle more apparent.

Oscillometry is the only noninvasive method that directly estimates mean blood pressure. The minimum occlusive pressure at which maximum oscillation occurs is the mean arterial pressure. Diastolic measurements, regardless of deflation rate, are quite inaccurate.[24] The pressure waves do not change dramatically but only decrease in amplitude, which complicates recognition of a diastolic endpoint. Several cardiac cycles are required for oscillotonometric determination of arterial blood pressure because the measurement depends on the heart rate, blood pressure, initial cuff inflation pressure, and rate of cuff deflation.[18]

Automated Technique

Automated techniques have the advantages of independence from Korotkoff sounds, greater accuracy, and limited operator intervention. In automated oscillometric techniques using devices such as the Dinamap (*d*evice for *i*ndi-

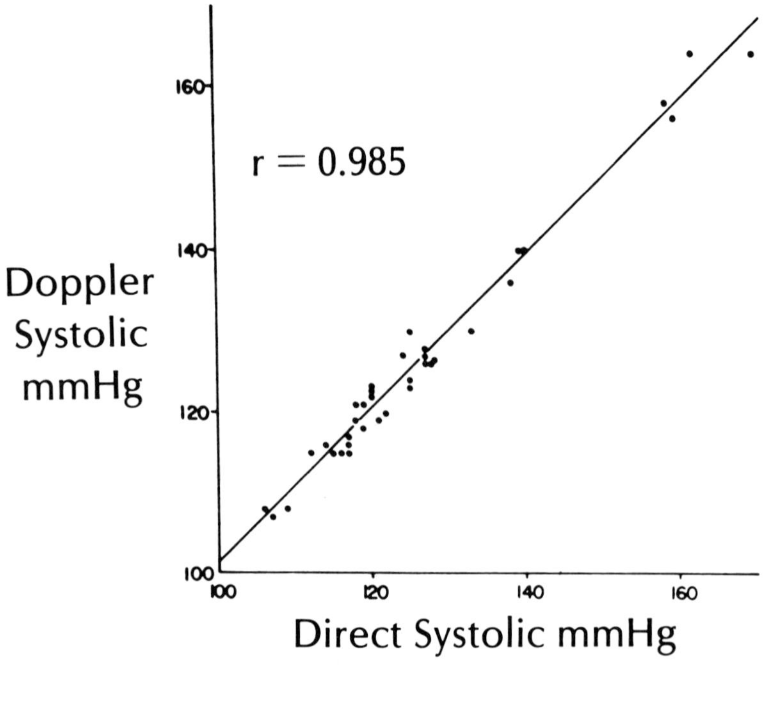

Figure 7–3. The relationship of systolic arterial pressures measured using a Doppler-shift signal is compared with direct intra-arterial measurements. Good correlation is seen (r = 0.985). (Modified from Stegal HF, et al: Indirect measurement of arterial blood pressure by Doppler ultrasonic sphygmomanometry. J Appl Physiol 1968; 25:796.)

rect *n*oninvasive *a*utomatic *m*ean *a*rterial *p*ressure—Critikon, Tampa, FL), the cuff is both actuator and transducer (Fig. 7–4). An electric pump generates pressure to inflate the single-bladder cuff, initially to a pressure above systolic pressure. A solenoid valve incrementally deflates the cuff. Pressure is sensed by a pressure transducer enclosed within the instrument case. The cuff has two tubes, one to inflate the cuff from a pump and the other for transmission of the sensed pressure to the pressure transducer within the instrument. A microprocessor controls the cuff inflation-deflation sequence. The cuff itself is the signal sensor, which responds to pressure oscillations in the limb. Specific placement of the cuff over an artery is unnecessary. However, an appropriately sized cuff for the extremity must be used as described previously.

Two cardiac cycles are compared at each increment if ''noise'' conditions are low. With increased noise (patient or cuff movement), inflation is held until successive comparative beats occur. Under these conditions, measurement becomes time-dependent, although normally the entire sequence from measurement to display is 20–45 seconds.[17] The averaged pairs of oscillations and the corresponding cuff pressures are stored and analyzed electronically to determine the systolic, diastolic, and mean pressures. Systolic pressures correspond to the rapid increase in the amplitude of oscillation and diastolic pressures to the rapid decrease in oscillation after maximum oscillation. The lowest cuff pressure at which maximum oscillation occurs is the mean arterial pressure.[25] The heart rate is the median of rates obtained by analysis of all pressure pulses in a given determination.

Problems with Measurement

The accuracy of the automated oscillometric measurements utilizing arm or leg cuffs compared with pressures measured directly in the aorta or a peripheral artery has been documented (Fig. 7–5).[25–28] Under ideal conditions, automated noninvasive methods are accurate to ±10 mmHg. Other investigators noted good correlations only for systolic pressures.[29] Oscillometric diastolic pressures are 8–13 mmHg higher as compared to direct arterial measurements.[28] They are also accurate in premature or term infants.[30, 31] However, finger oscillometric cuffs are not sufficiently accurate for routine use.[32] Noninvasive devices cannot replace direct arterial measurements when substantial beat-to-beat variability in the pressure is present.[26] Automated oscillometric measurements are difficult during patient movement because the instrument considers the movement as a large oscillation. Failure to evacuate air from the cuff prior to application to a vasoconstricted patient results in attenuation of oscillations by the residual air volume. Although mean arterial pressure is measured under these conditions, systolic and diastolic are usually not.[10] Overall, automated oscillometry is the most accurate noninvasive method.[5]

PLETHYSMOGRAPHY

Technique

Penaz used the principle of unloading of the arterial wall to measure a calibrated pressure waveform in the finger.[33] Further modification of the cuff and other components by Wesseling and associates led to the currently available device known as the Finapres (*fin*ger *a*rterial *pres*sure).[34, 35] The Finapres consists of a small finger cuff containing an infrared photoplethysmograph volume transducer and an inflatable bladder. The photoplethysmograph diode and the light detector are positioned on the medial and lateral aspects of the finger near the digital arteries to record finger volume. A servo control system regulates the pressure ap-

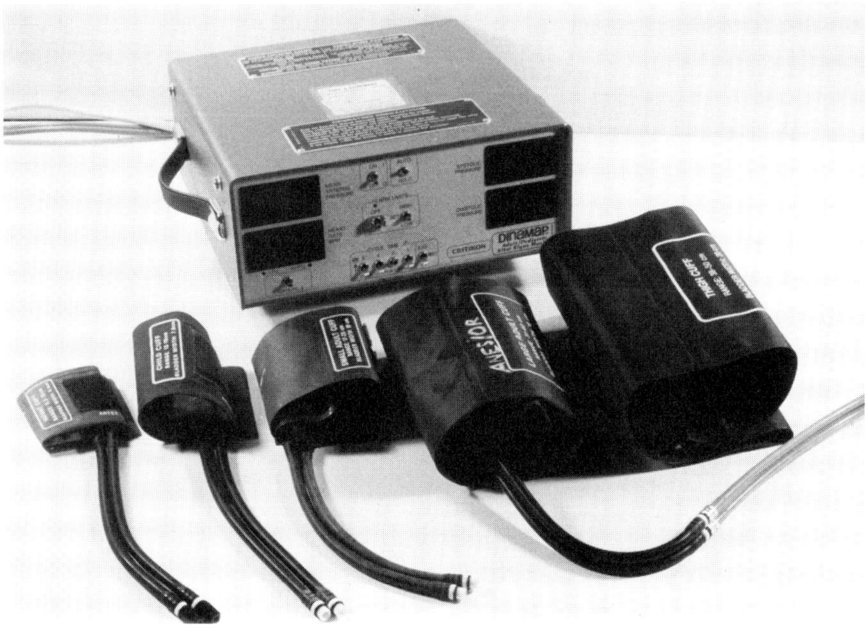

Figure 7–4. The Dinamap is an automated noninvasive device for measurement of arterial blood pressure by the oscillometric technique. Cuffs suitable for use in infants, children, and adults (arm or thigh) are shown. A switch alters the algorithm controlling cuff inflation pressures to ranges suitable for infants and adults.

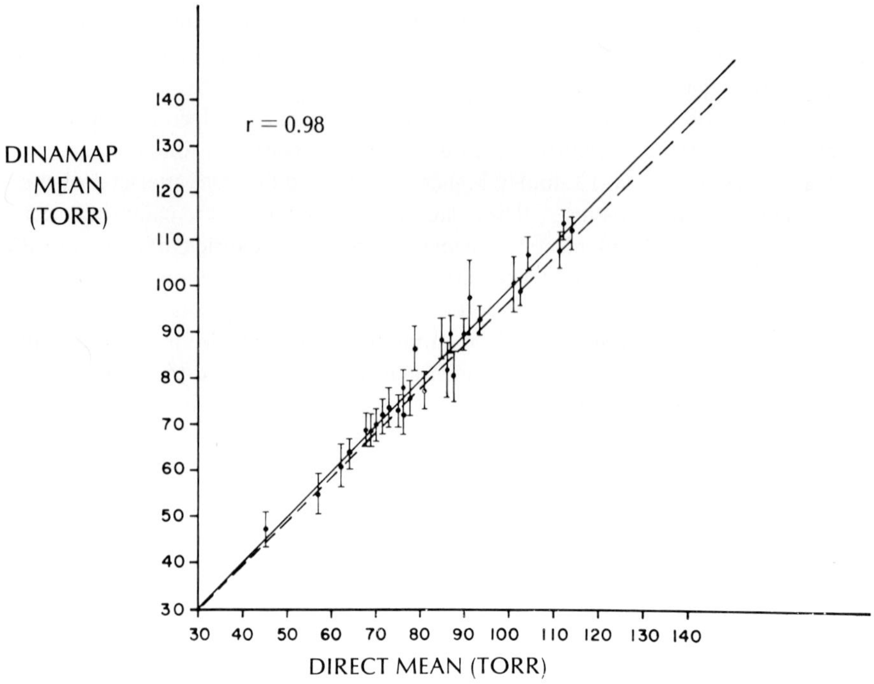

Figure 7–5. The correlation of direct intra-arterial measurement of mean arterial pressures with those measured by Dinamapp shows a correlation coefficient of 0.98. (Modified from Ramsey M: Noninvasive automatic determination of mean arterial pressure. Med Biol Eng Comput 1979; 17:11–18.)

plied by the cuff to the arterial wall. As the arterial wall expands with an increase in blood pressure, the volume differential is measured by the transducer. In response to the increasing volume, cuff pressure increases until original arterial blood volume and pressure are restored (servo mode of operation). The external pressure of the cuff closely matches the arterial pressure of the finger so that the external pressure is a function of arterial blood pressure. Both the arterial waveform and pressures are displayed. Such devices can be used for long-term portable noninvasive blood pressure measurement as in patients on antihypertensive therapy.[36]

Problems with Measurement

The accuracy of this device compared with conventional Riva Rocci technique,[35] automated indirect brachial,[37] or radial arterial pressure[38] has been documented. Pressures measured in the thumb correlate with intra-arterial pressure better than do pressures measured in other digits.[39] Changes in hemoglobin saturation affect the transmission of light to the device but not the pressure readings.[39]

Safety with long-term use has been confirmed, although the pressure in the cuff is at or near mean arterial pressure for prolonged periods.[40] Pressures are above venous levels, resulting in slight digital swelling.[41] Capillary oxygen tension decreases significantly within 2.5 minutes of cuff inflation, and oxygen saturation determined by oximetry demonstrates desaturation.[41] Numbness of the finger after 60 minutes of monitoring has been noted, but resolved within 1 minute of discontinuation.[41] The possibility of digital nerve injury must be considered. Whether the interposition of periods without monitoring alters neural ischemia is unclear, because capillary PO_2 is actually reduced by ''rest'' periods.[41]

Arterial spasm may preclude measurements in some patients, particularly those with cardiopulmonary bypass or other circulatory stresses (administration of phenylephrine, peripheral vasoconstriction).[39, 42] During peripheral vasoconstriction, systolic pressures measured with Finapres were 7 mmHg above, and diastolic and mean pressures were 9 mmHg below, those of the upper arm.[43] During induced hypotension, agreement with directly measured intra-arterial pressure was insufficient for clinical practice.[44]

CONTINUOUS NONINVASIVE BLOOD PRESSURE MONITORING

Two techniques, arterial tonometry and pulse wave delay detection, are currently being investigated as noninvasive methods to continuously assess arterial pressure. In the pulse wave delay method, photometric sensors are placed at different locations such as a digit and the forehead to detect the delay in pulse wave propagation.

ARTERIAL TONOMETRY

The arterial tonometry method partially compresses a systemic artery, usually the radial, to flatten the arterial wall but not totally occlude the artery. A microtransducer then determines the arterial pressure by detection of the pressure wave of arterial pulsation. The circumferential tension in the flattened arterial wall toward the transducer is negligible. In a comparison of arterial tonometry with direct arterial measurements, Kemmotsu et al found limits of agreement of 0 ± 10 (SD) mmHg for systolic, diastolic, and mean pressures during normotension and hypotension.[45, 46] Sato noted near equality of the tonometric waveform with a direct arterial waveform except during the early systolic phase in normotensive and hypertensive subjects.[47] Accurate measurements require absence of motion artifacts and specific positioning of the transducer over the artery.

RISKS OF NONINVASIVE MEASUREMENTS

Despite their noninvasive nature, cuff techniques for blood pressure measurement are not without risk. With electrically operated devices, the possibility of shock always exists. Failure of cuff deflation increases venous congestion and arterial hypoperfusion, causing tissue or neural ischemia. Ulnar nerve damage was reported when a cuff, applied too distally on the arm, caused direct compression of the ulnar artery in the ulnar groove.[48] Intravenous injection of irritating substances during cuff inflation may cause tissue damage due to a locally increased concentration. Accidental injection of succinylcholine into a vein distal to the inflated cuff of an automated device during a rapid sequence anesthetic induction may preclude timely intubation.

INVASIVE MEASUREMENT OF BLOOD PRESSURE

Although indirect measurements of blood pressure by palpation, oscillometry, and auscultation demonstrate close agreement, the values are always lower than directly measured pressures (underestimating systolic and overestimating diastolic pressure).[1, 5] Direct techniques measure arterial pressure, whereas indirect methods often depend on detection of blood flow beneath an occlusive cuff.[1]

With the exception of the plethysmographic technique, noninvasive methods of pressure determination usually do not display an arterial pressure waveform. Arterial pressure waveforms qualitatively approximate alterations in the circulation. The area beneath the curve is affected by myocardial performance, peripheral vascular resistance, and stroke volume.

Indwelling arterial cannulae are utilized in all procedures requiring cardiopulmonary bypass, in most major vascular surgery procedures and in intrathoracic procedures, and in critically ill patients (adult respiratory distress syndrome and those receiving vasoactive drugs or positive end-expiratory pressure). Single uncomplicated radial arterial punctures produce no changes in blood flow.[49] However, if more than three to four arterial blood specimens are required daily, a indwelling arterial catheter should be inserted.[50]

TECHNIQUE OF CANNULATION

A technique for percutaneous cannulation of an artery was first reported by Peterson and Dripps in 1949.[51] Cannulation techniques are similar in all sites (Fig. 7–6). The technique described below is specific to the radial artery, and pertinent details for other sites are discussed elsewhere in this chapter.

Adequate preparation is essential for successful arterial cannulation. The patient's arm should be comfortably supported on an armrest. Good lighting over the site is helpful and the operator should be seated. The patient's wrist should be dorsiflexed over a folded towel or other support. The course of the artery is traced on the skin. Povidone iodine skin preparation is performed distal to the tracing. Local anesthesia is infiltrated into the area over the artery, taking care not to puncture the artery or to obliterate its pulsation. A small nick with a 20-gauge needle is made in the skin over the anticipated puncture site to prevent catheter damage. Through the skin nick, a 20-gauge catheter is introduced at an angle of 30° to the skin.[52] Twenty-two gauge catheters are commonly used in children under the age of 5 years (Fig. 7–7).

Three techniques for arterial cannulation are commonly employed (1) direct cannulation, (2) the transfixion technique, and (3) the Seldinger technique. In the direct technique, the cannula is advanced until arterial pulsation is transmitted to the cannula. The artery is then pierced, the angle of the cannula to the skin is reduced to 10° and the cannula is advanced from the needle into the artery (Fig. 7–6). A pressure transducer is then connected to verify the arterial waveform. Blood should be aspirated to ensure free flow. The Seldinger technique requires passage of a guidewire through the cannula after arterial puncture, followed by advancement of the cannula over the guidewire (Fig. 7–7 [bottom]; see Chapter 8). Although catheters 2–3 cm in length are most commonly used, longer 18- or 20-gauge catheters may be threaded into brachial or axillary arteries from a radial insertion site.[53]

In the transfixion method, the posterior wall of the artery is punctured before the needle is withdrawn from the cannula. The cannula is slowly withdrawn until freely flowing blood is obtained. At that point, the cannula is advanced into the vessel lumen and connected to a pressure transducer. Success rates for cannulation at the initial radial artery site have been reported at 92%.[54]

Fixation of the catheter to the skin with tape or a suture to prevent accidental removal is essential. Iodophor ointment is applied to the puncture site after successful cannulation. The support used to dorsiflex the wrist is removed to prevent median nerve damage.

DIFFICULT ARTERIAL CANNULATION

If passage of the catheter-needle unit to a distance of 2 cm beneath the skin fails to obtain freely spurting blood flow, the stylet should be removed and the catheter slowly withdrawn. Inadvertent penetration of the posterior wall of the artery is common and often recognized only during withdrawal. Once free flow is obtained, an attempt to advance the catheter should be made.

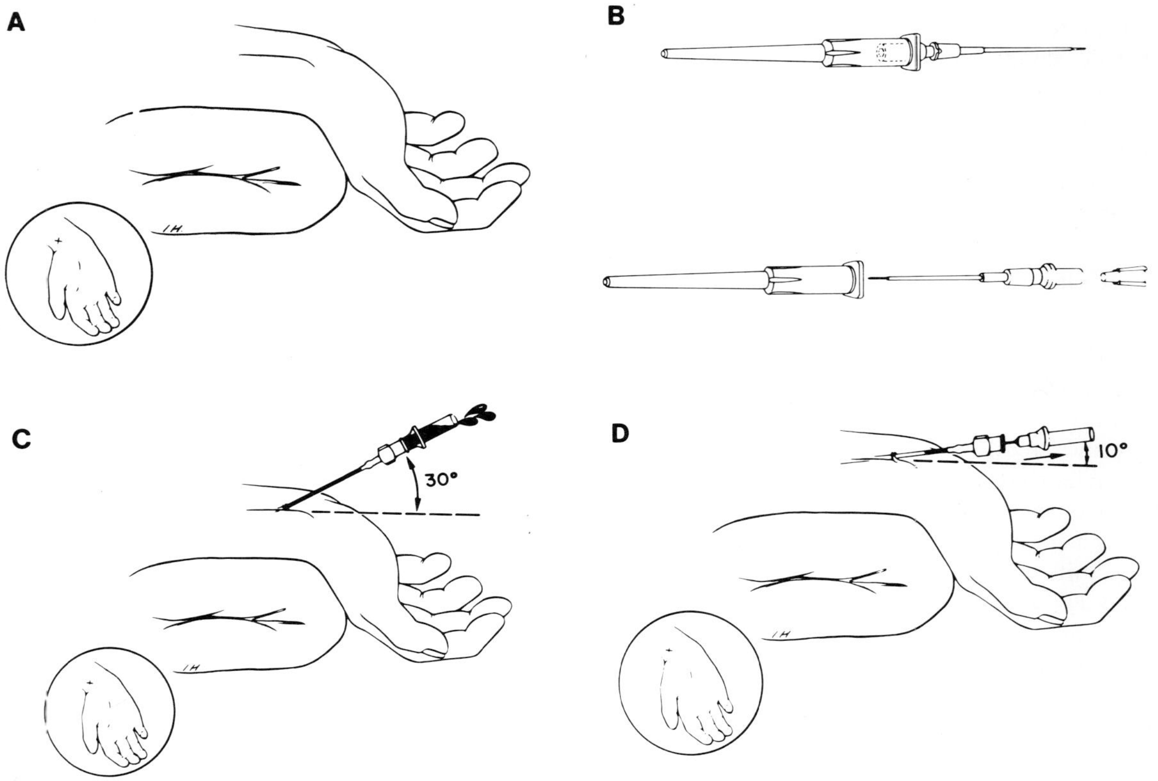

Figure 7–6. The technique of cannulation of a peripheral artery is similar for almost all arteries. The direct technique for the radial artery is demonstrated. *A*, Proper hand position with the hand dorsiflexed over a small roll. *B*, Technique of placing the catheter cover over the end of the catheter. This technique allows visualization of free flow of blood without environmental contamination. (Personal communication, KR Grosslight, MD.) *C*, The catheter is inserted at an angle of 30–40 degrees to the plane of the wrist until spurting blood flow is obtained. *D*, The angle of the catheter is reduced to 10 degrees while the plastic catheter is advanced into the artery. (From Lake CL: Cardiovascular Anesthesia. New York: Springer-Verlag, 1985; 54.)

If no blood flow is obtained on withdrawal, the catheter-needle unit should be reassembled, the needle should be flushed with heparinized saline, and another attempt should be made after confirming the palpable course of the artery. The number of attempts should be limited to reduce trauma to the artery. Catheters that cause a grating sensation on passage through tissue or artery should be removed because a damaged catheter tip may cause injury to the arterial intima.[55] Doppler transducers may facilitate cannulation of weakly palpable arteries or those in infants (Fig. 7–8).[56–58] Placement of a pulse oximeter distal to the proposed cannulation site and repeated palpation over the area determines the arterial course by observation of cessation of the distal pulse.[59] This technique is particularly useful in obese patients.

Flushing of an intra-arterial catheter causes one of two

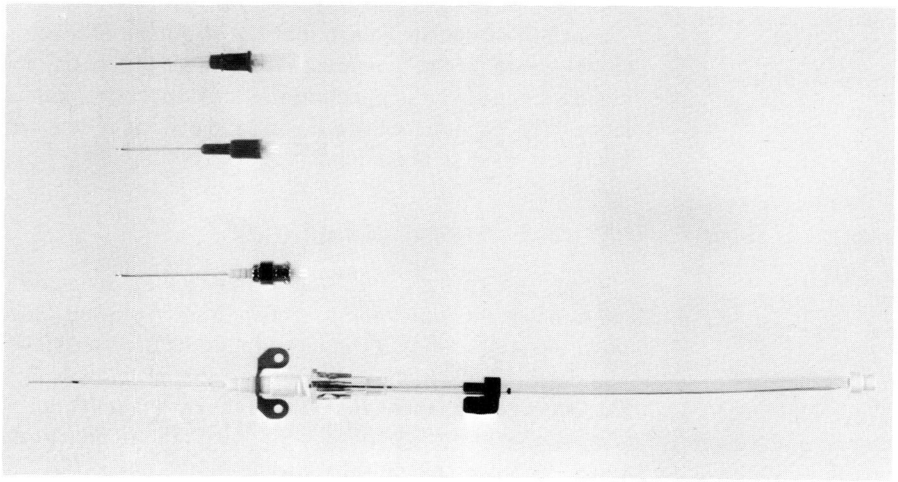

Figure 7–7. Various types of arterial catheters are commonly used. Twenty-two-gauge catheters (*top*), either tapered or straight, are used in infants and children under the age of 5 years. In adults, 20-gauge catheters are placed either directly or using a wire guide (*bottom*).

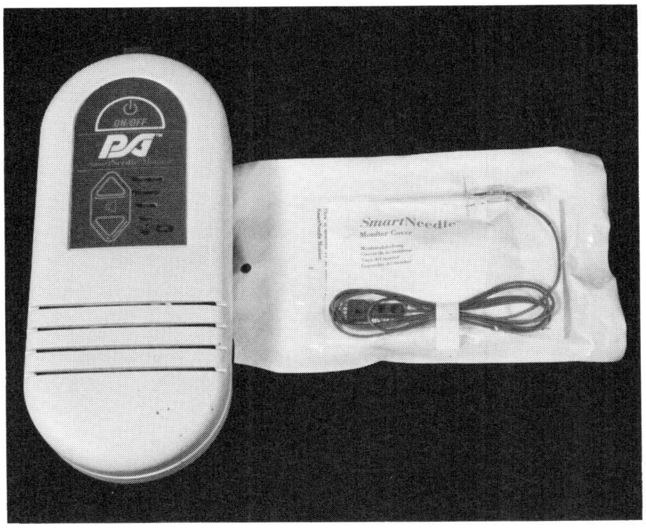

Figure 7–8. The Smart Needle Doppler device for cannulation of peripheral arteries and central veins with ultrasound localization. Both 18- and 20-gauge cannulas may be inserted using this technique.

responses: a localized area of a few square centimeters of intense blanching or a generalized transient area of slight pallor (the preferable response).[60] Careful adjustment of the position of the catheter tip usually converts a localized response to a generalized response, which indicates less interference with local cutaneous circulation by the flushing solution.

ARTERIAL CANNULATION SITES

Cannulation of the arterial circulation is performed most commonly in the radial artery. Other sites that have been safely used include the femoral, dorsalis pedis, posterior tibial, brachial, axillary, ulnar, dorsal radial, superficial temporal, and umbilical arteries (Fig. 7–9).[61–69]

Radial

Evaluation of Collateral Flow

Both radial arteries should be assessed to determine equality of pulsation prior to cannulation. In patients with generalized arteriosclerosis, determination of blood pressure in both arms prevents inadvertent cannulation of a radial artery distal to innominate or subclavian stenosis. Likewise, cannulation distal to a brachial or axillary cannulation site (as after angiography) should be avoided because pulse volume is often diminished. Raynaud's phenomenon is also a contraindication because ischemia requiring digital amputation has been reported.[70]

In almost 90% of humans, the ulnar artery provides most of the arterial perfusion to the hand.[71] However, the arterial

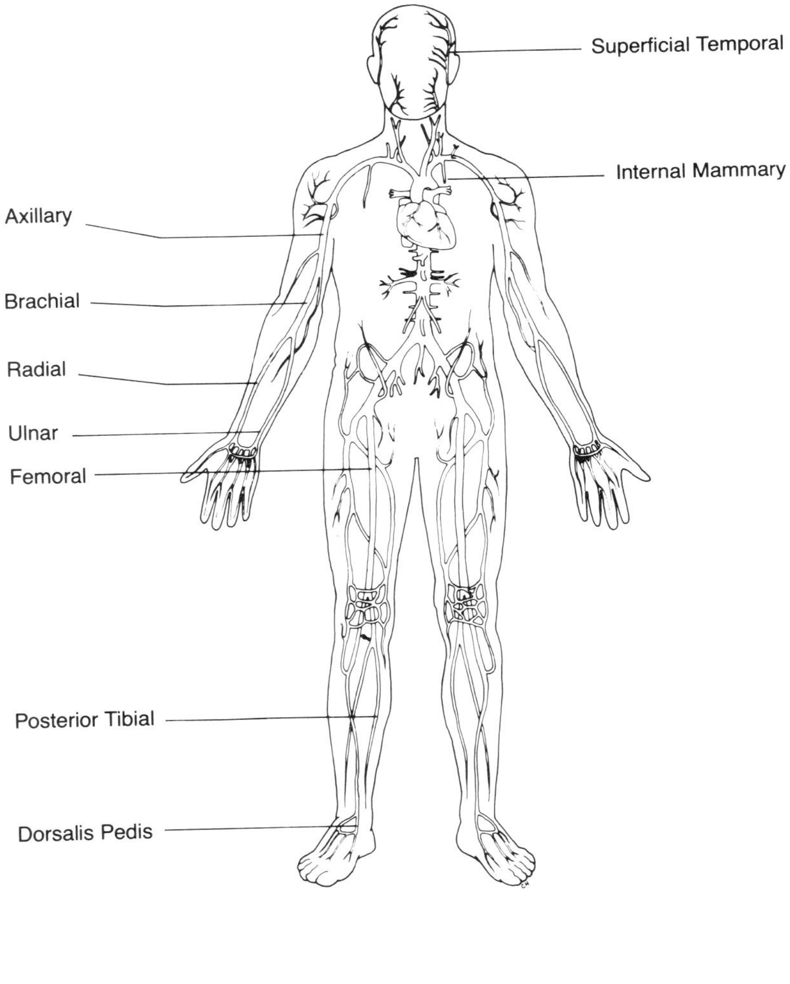

Figure 7–9. Sites for cannulation of the systemic arterial circulation. Although the most common location for catheterization is the radial artery, other sites (axillary, brachial, femoral, dorsalis pedis, superficial temporal) are used when radial collateral circulation is inadequate or radial pressures may be erroneous. Not demonstrated is the umbilical artery cannulation site.

anatomy of the hand is quite variable.[72] The adequacy of ulnar collateral flow is assessed using Allen's test. Allen's test determines the dominant vessel supplying the hand. Whenever possible, the nondominant vessel should be cannulated. To perform Allen's test, the examiner compresses both radial and ulnar arteries while the patient flexes and extends his fingers four or five times to blanch the hand. If the palmar arterial arch is intact, release of either artery permits rapid restoration of color to the hand (within 5–7 seconds).[72]

However, if the arterial circulation is compromised, release of the occluded artery prevents the normal reactive hyperemia. In addition to observation of reflow, Husum and colleagues suggest measurement of the blood pressure in the thumb, because the arterial pressure in the thumb can be inadequate in the presence of an Allen's test demonstrating adequate collateral flow.[73] Chronic occlusion of both radial and ulnar arteries with the only blood supply through numerous palmar collaterals has been reported.[74] Some investigators suggest that arterial occlusion be performed near the proposed location of the tip of the arterial cannula.[75] Such a technique avoids subsequent occlusion of aberrant arteries supplying the palmar arterial arch.[75] In one series, almost 22% of hands had an incomplete palmar arch.[76]

In anesthetized patients, Allen's test is modified by having an assistant passively clench the fist while radial and ulnar arteries are compressed. Alternatively, the pulse in a finger is checked using a Doppler or pulse oximeter during radial and ulnar compression to document patency of the transpalmar arch.[77, 78] The time for return of a pulse oximeter reading with release of ulnar compression should be less than 15 seconds.[79]

Wide separation or marked hyperextension of the fingers permits the palmar fascia to occlude the transpalmar arch so that flow appears inadequate.[80, 81] Another cause of apparently inadequate collateral flow is arterial spasm in the ulnar artery caused by compression of the radial artery.[74]

The necessity of Allen's test is often questioned. Slogoff and colleagues cannulated the radial arteries of 16 patients who required longer than 15 seconds for refill without subsequent ischemic damage.[82] Another large series in which Allen's test was routinely used to determine the cannulation site demonstrated a similar incidence of ischemic complications and flow abnormalities after decannulation, as seen in the series of Slogoff and colleagues.[83] Conversely, hand ischemia requiring amputation has been reported in the presence of adequate collateral circulation as demonstrated by Allen's test.[84] However, there has not been a large prospective study performing radial arterial cannulation in patients without ulnar pulses or flow except through the cannulated radial artery.

Ulnar

The technique and complications of ulnar cannulation are similar to those of the radial artery described previously. However, it should be noted that the ulnar artery is usually the primary source of blood flow in the hand.

Brachial

Cannulation of the brachial artery is performed with either an 18- or a 20-gauge catheter at the elbow where it lies medial to the biceps tendon. Although one of the major risks is median nerve damage because the nerve lies just medial to the artery at the elbow,[85] the safety of brachial cannulation in cardiac surgical patients has been documented.[61, 68, 86] Another risk is thrombosis, necessitating surgical exploration. Brachial arterial pressures are usually similar to femoral pressures.[87]

Axillary

Axillary arterial catheters are inserted at the junction of the pectoralis major with the deltoid muscle. The patient's arm is abducted.[61, 68] The Seldinger technique (see Chapter 8) is recommended to place an 18- or 20-gauge, 12- to 15-cm catheter.[69] The left axillary artery is preferentially used to minimize the possibility of cerebral air embolism during flushing of the catheter. Axillary arterial cannulation is a useful option in patients with severe peripheral vascular disease.[88] Concomitant sympathetic blockade of the upper extremity using continuous brachial plexus blockade further protects the arm by increasing its blood flow.[88]

Femoral

The femoral artery is cannulated directly in adults with an 18-gauge catheter, 5–15 cm in length. Alternatively, the Seldinger technique of passing a wire through a 20-gauge, 2- to 3-cm catheter is used to cannulate the vessel with a larger, longer catheter.

Minor complications such as local hemorrhage and ecchymoses are occasionally seen.[61] Disadvantages of the femoral approach are its position within the surgical field during cardiovascular surgery and its temporary discontinuation if an intra-aortic balloon must be placed in the same artery. Massive retroperitoneal hematoma has been reported after unsuccessful femoral cannulation.[89]

In children, 18- or 20-gauge, 5- to 10-cm catheters are often more easily placed in the femoral than in the radial arteries. However, cannulation of the femoral artery is often avoided in children because of its proximity to the peritoneum, the risk of hip capsule puncture, and the potential for decreased limb growth with thrombosis. In the series reported by Glenski and coworkers, femoral catheterization was performed in 151 children undergoing cardiac surgery with only a 3.6% failure rate.[90] Decreased limb perfusion occurred in 25% of neonates, but the overall rate was only 6 in 165 catheterizations.[90] No permanent complications were noted. Rosenthal and colleagues noted no reduction in leg growth after femoral cannulation.[91]

Dorsalis Pedis

Evaluation of Collateral Flow

The arterial supply to the foot is the anterior tibial, posterior tibial, and peroneal arteries. Anterior and posterior tibial arteries are terminal branches of the popliteal artery. The posterior tibial artery divides near the medial malleolus to form the lateral and medial plantar arteries. In the foot, the anterior tibial continues as the dorsalis pedis artery, which divides to form the deep plantar and first dorsal metatarsal arteries. An alternative site for cannulation is the anterior peroneal artery just medial to and above the anterior aspect of the lateral malleolus.[64] A plantar arterial arch is formed by anastomoses between the deep and lateral plantar arteries. However, the pedal circulatory pattern is quite variable.[92, 93]

Collateral circulation via the posterior tibial artery is evaluated by occlusion of the dorsalis pedis and compression of the great toenail. Flow via the lateral plantar artery is adequate if the toe flushes. An alternative method, suggested by Youngberg and Miller, is compression of both dorsalis pedis and posterior tibial arteries together with compression of great and second toes.[94] Adequate collateral is verified by both flushing of the toes and a Doppler probe on the dorsalis pedis when posterior tibial compression is released. Flow can also be evaluated by pulse plethysmography.[93]

Cannulation should not be performed unless circulation is restored within 10 seconds of posterior tibial release.[95] Palm and colleagues also recommend measurement of great toe pressure with compression of the dorsalis pedis. In 99 of 200 feet studied, blood pressure in the great toe decreased to 44% of control with dorsalis pedis compression.[95]

Technique of Cannulation

A 20-gauge catheter is used to cannulate the dorsalis pedis artery as it lies subcutaneously on the dorsum of the foot, parallel and lateral to the extensor hallucis longus tendon.[96]

Problems and Complications

Systolic and pulse pressure in the dorsalis pedis artery are higher than either the brachial or radial pressures (systolic and pulse). However, dorsalis pedis mean arterial and diastolic pressures are lower than in the radial artery. Severe peripheral vascular disease often causes the dorsalis pedis to be nonpalpable or to have inadequate collateral flow. The incidence of thrombosis ranges from 6.7% to 25%.[67, 94] Arterial recannulation occurs, but often fails to restore the vessel to its previous condition.[67]

Superficial Temporal

The temporal artery is a branch of the external carotid artery that passes anterior to the tragus of the ear. Temporal cannulation may be useful during thoracic aortic procedures. Cannulation of the superficial temporal artery is performed by first delineating the often variable arterial course with a Doppler probe.[65] Arterial puncture is performed at the superior edge of the helix of the ear,[66] either percutaneously or through a 3-mm to 2-cm incision (depending on patient size) with the catheter-needle device in a bevel-down position.[65] The bevel-down position prevents posterior arterial perforation. Proper positioning of the catheter tip is critical. An optimal location is in the external carotid at the junction with the external maxillary artery.[65, 66] The superficial temporal artery is often quite tortuous and difficult to cannulate. Other risks include thrombosis with scalp ischemia and catheter malposition that permits emboli to reach the cerebral circulation via the internal carotid artery. Because of the site, it is often difficult to secure the catheter so that it does not become dislodged.[66]

Umbilical

The umbilical arteries branch from the internal iliac arteries, crossing over the ureters and passing inferiorly on either side of the dome of the bladder to course in the anterior abdominal wall to the umbilicus. Either a percutaneous or a cutdown technique is used to cannulate the umbilical artery of infants soon after birth. With the percutaneous method, a 16-gauge short catheter is initially inserted; through this, a longer 3.5- or 5-F catheter is guided into the aorta. The cutdown method requires placement of a suture at the base of the umbilicus prior to cutting the umbilical cord several millimeters above the skin. An umbilical artery is identified and a probe is inserted to dilate the vessel prior to passage of the catheter (a 3.5- or 5-F catheter). Spasm at the junction of hypogastric and iliac arteries is the most common cause for failure to catheterize the umbilical artery.[97] After the catheter is successfully inserted, the suture at the umbilical base is tied around the catheter.

Optimal locations for the catheter tip are just above the aortic bifurcation,[98] below the inferior mesenteric artery, or at the middorsal aorta above the diaphragm. Undesirable locations include the celiac plexus, renal, or superior mesenteric arteries (Fig. 7–10).[63]

Complications of umbilical arterial cannulation include abdominal organ ischemia if the catheter becomes dislodged into specific intra-abdominal vessels, aortic thrombosis, embolism, lower extremity ischemia secondary to arterial vasospasm, and vascular perforation causing hemorrhage.[63, 99, 100] Factors contributing to complications include prolonged use and repeated manipulation. Methods to avoid complications include radiographic confirmation of catheter tip location, avoidance of catheter manipulation, nonthrombogenic catheters, and timely removal of catheters when no longer indicated.[101]

INDICATIONS FOR REMOVAL OF INTRA-ARTERIAL CATHETERS

Arterial cannulae can remain for 3 or more days in the absence of infection, arterial insufficiency, and hematoma.

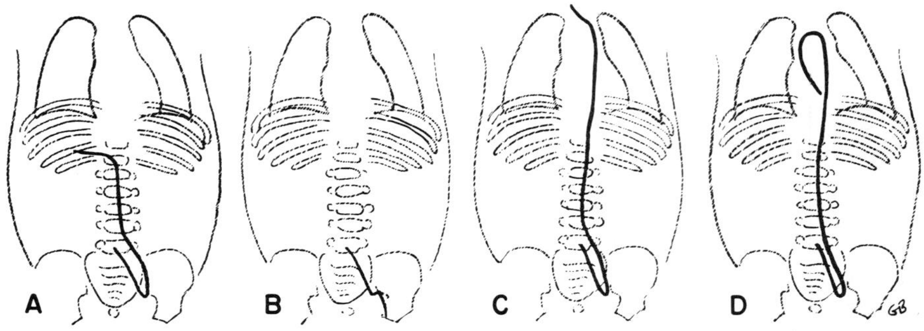

Figure 7–10. Abnormal locations of umbilical arterial catheters are demonstrated. *A*, The tip of the catheter has been displaced into one of the abdominal vessels (hepatic, superior mesenteric, or renal). *B*, The catheter coursed downward to lie in the external iliac artery. *C*, Excessive passage of the catheter, such that its tip is in carotid or innominate arteries. *D*, The excessive length of catheter inserted results in passage around the aortic arch, across the aortic valve, and into the left ventricle. (From Paster SB, Middleton P: Roentgenographic evaluation of umbilical artery and vein catheters. JAMA 1975; 231: 742–746. Copyright 1975, American Medical Association.)

However, after prolonged cannulation they become nonfunctional because of thrombus accumulation. Feeley described a technique for thrombectomy if continued arterial pressure monitoring is required.[101]

Technique

Bedford suggested that radial arterial cannulae be removed with continuous aspiration during proximal and distal arterial occlusion.[102] Thrombotic material, potentially contributing to arterial occlusion, might be removed from other cannulation sites in a similar manner. After decannulation, compression is applied for 10 minutes or longer to prevent hematoma formation (Fig. 7–11).

COMPLICATIONS

Although most of the studies of complications concern radial artery cannulation, complications such as hematomas, decreased peripheral circulation distal to the cannula site, infection, vasospasm, thrombosis, embolism, aneurysm formation, and infection are applicable to all sites. Embolism due to clots or air flushed into the cerebral circulation are most likely with radial, brachial, axillary, and temporal cannulation sites. From the radial artery, 3–12 ml of flushing solution in adults and 0.3–5 ml in children produce retrograde flow.[103–105] Chang and coworkers documented passage of air from a radial arterial cannula into the vertebral artery of an animal.[104] The volume of flush solution necessary to reach the central circulation correlates well with patient height.[103] Another source of emboli are bubbles in the constant infusion system, particularly with rapid flushing or the use of a microdrip chamber.[106, 107]

Hemorrhage resulting from inadvertent disconnection of an arterial catheter from the transducer tubing is potentially lethal because about 500 ml of blood per minute are lost if cardiac output is normal.[50] Ischemic complications may be more likely in patients with severe atherosclerosis, diabetes, low cardiac output, and peripheral vasoconstriction, particularly from vasoactive drugs.

Reported complications specific to the radial artery include pseudoaneurysm (caused or complicated by infection),[108] expanding aneurysm,[109] forearm amputation in two patients, one with complicated tetralogy and another with type V hyperlipoproteinemia,[110, 111] vasospasm,[112] ecchymoses and induration of the skin,[113, 114] arteriovenous fistula, and nerve injuries (median and radial from compression by hematomas). Neural compression is more common after multiple arterial punctures than with indwelling catheters.[115]

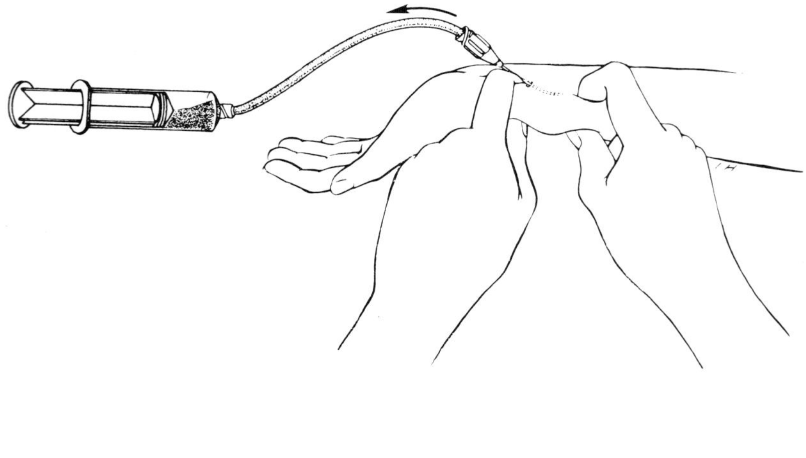

Figure 7–11. The technique recommended by Bedford[102] for removal of arterial cannulas includes compression of the artery proximal and distal to the catheter site while the catheter is removed during continuous aspiration. This method allows aspiration of thrombotic material surrounding the catheter.

Thrombosis

Thrombosis of the radial artery is a common complication, occurring in 34% of patients when 18-gauge catheters are used, decreasing to 8% when 20-gauge catheters are used. (Figs. 7–12 and 7–13).[114, 116] During ulnar compression, a decrease in the arterial pressure to 10 mmHg or less in the thumb is diagnostic of occlusion.[117] Other factors contributing to an increased incidence of thrombosis include use of polypropylene rather than polytef (Teflon) catheters,[118] tapered rather than straight catheters,[119] increased duration of cannulation,[109] increased proportion of vessel lumen occupied by catheter,[112] and smaller wrist circumference (47% incidence of occlusion with wrist circumferences of less than 18 cm versus 21% with larger wrists), (Figs. 7–14 and 7–15).[116] However, thrombosis is unaffected by the method of cannulation (perforation of the posterior arterial wall versus nonperforation).[121] Treatment with aspirin prior to cannulation decreases the incidence of thrombosis from 39% to 13%.[122] This effect is particularly prominent in women (smaller arteries), for whom the incidence of thrombosis decreased from 63% to 22%.[122] Thrombosis can be delayed for several days after decannulation (Table 7–3).[113] Recanalization eventually occurs after occlusion but requires an average of 13 days (Fig. 7–16).[60, 123]

The etiology of ischemia of the hand in the presence of a radial artery catheter can be difficult to determine.[124] Proximal pulses should be examined; if they are absent, an arteriogram should be performed to eliminate embolism. Vessel occlusion distal to an arterial cannula has been demonstrated by Kim and coworkers.[123] The presence or absence of a change in the arterial waveform during occlusion of the cannulated artery distal to the puncture site is noted. With a patent artery, obstruction of flow increases arterial pressure and changes the configuration of the waveform as the blocked flow is converted to increased pressure. However, if the artery is occluded, additional occlusion distal to the occluded segment fails to alter either pressure or arterial waveform.

TABLE 7–3. FACTORS CONTRIBUTING TO ARTERIAL THROMBOSIS*

Catheter size[120]
? Tapered catheters[52, 119]
Increased duration of cannulation[113]
Increased proportion of vessel lumen occupied by catheter[116]
Smaller size of wrist[120]
Polypropylene catheters[118, 119]

*Thrombosis is unaffected by method of cannulation, but is decreased by aspirin pretreatment.[121, 122]

Infection

Bacteremia and positive blood culture results have been reported after catheters remained in situ for more than 4 days.[125, 126] Other factors contributing to catheter-related infections are nondisposable transducer domes, use of dextrose instead of saline for the flushing solution, and location of the continuous flush device near the insertion site instead of just distal to the transducer.[125, 127, 128] However, another study in 68 children demonstrated no positive catheter or fluid cultures after 59 hours of cannulation.[129]

Special Problems with Radial Arterial Catheters

Problems with measurement of direct arterial pressure occur frequently enough to warrant the presence of a second measuring device such as a noninvasive automated oscillometer. Despite widespread use of radial catheters for more than two decades, occasional difficulties with accurate

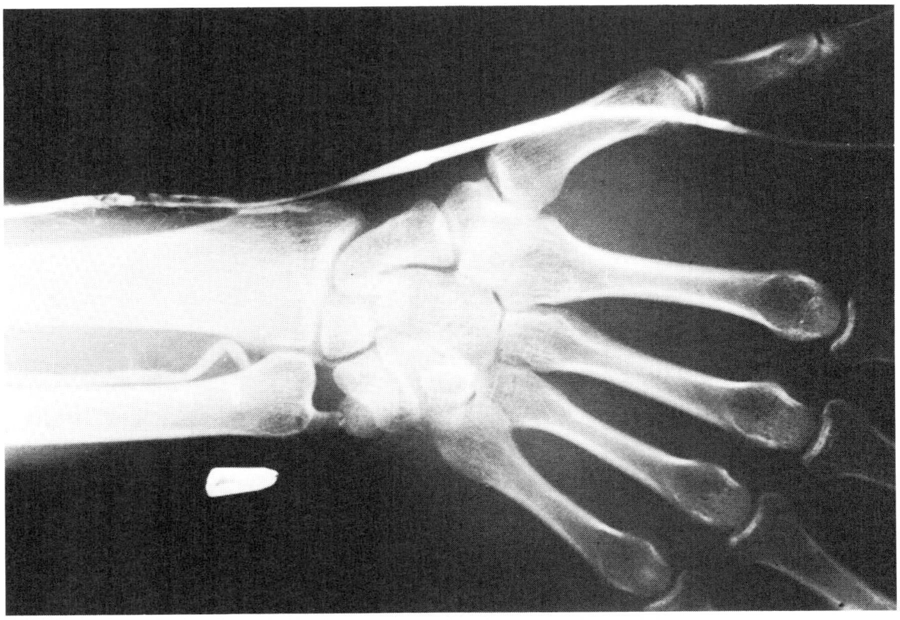

Figure 7–12. Radial artery occlusion after cannulation with a tapered polypropylene catheter is demonstrated in this arteriogram performed through the catheter. There is no antegrade flow around or beyond the catheter, only retrograde flow toward the brachial artery. (From Bedford RF: Percutaneous radial-artery cannulation. Increased safety using Teflon catheters. Anesthesiology 1975; 42:221.)

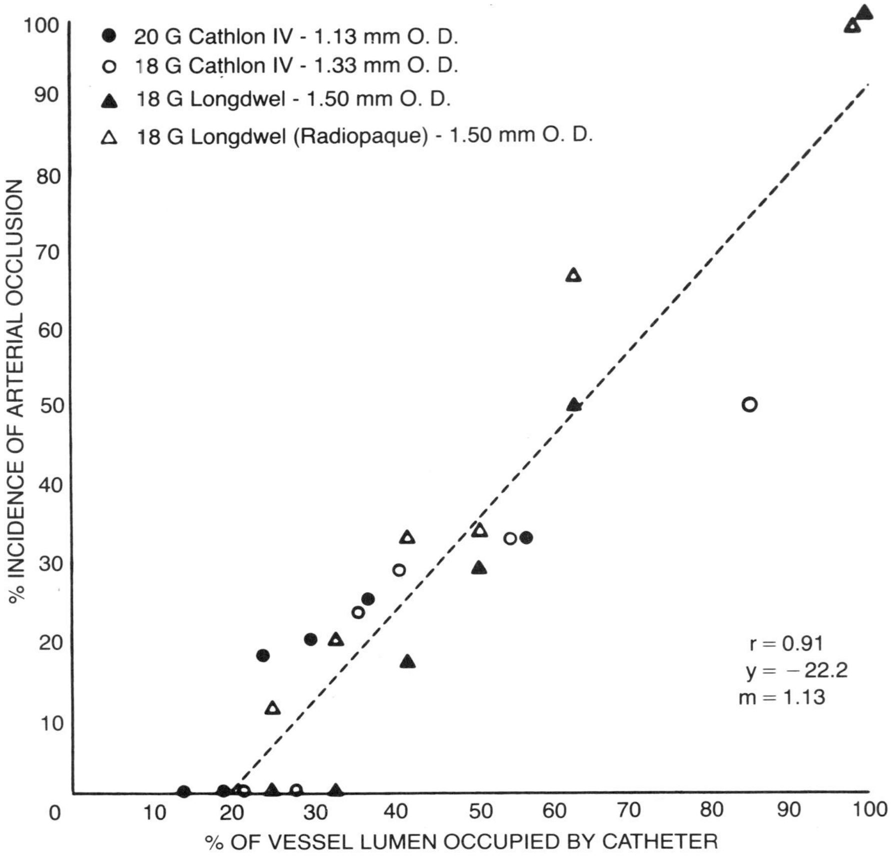

Figure 7–13. The incidence of occlusion of the radial artery after cannulation is increased by the use of 18-gauge, as opposed to 20-gauge, catheters. This results from the increased proportion of the vessel lumen that is occupied by the catheter. (From Bedford RF: Radial arterial function following percutaneous cannulation with 18- and 20-gauge catheters. Anesthesiology 1977; 47:39.)

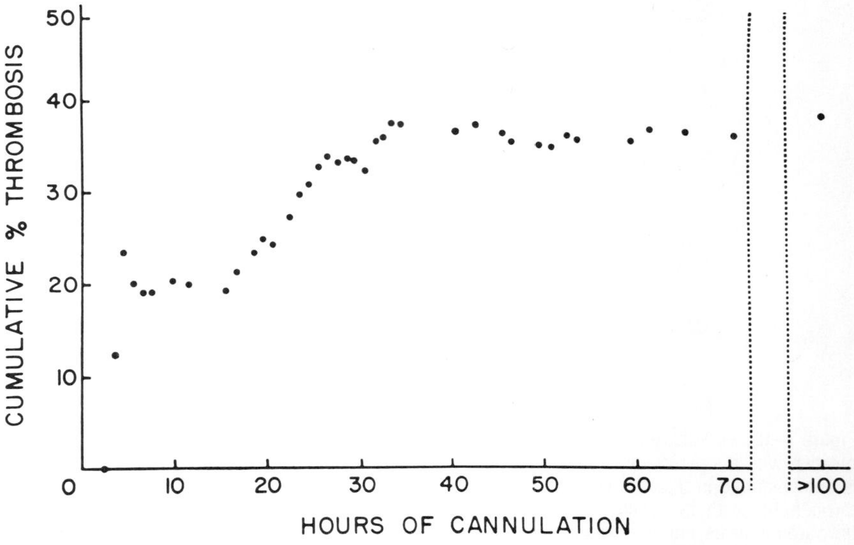

Figure 7–14. The incidence of radial artery thrombosis increases with the duration of cannulation, from no thrombosis with cannulations of less than 2 hours to a 38% incidence with more than 40 hours of cannulation. (From Bedford RF, Wollmann H: Complications of percutaneous radial-artery cannulation: An objective prospective study in man. Anesthesiology 1973; 38:231.)

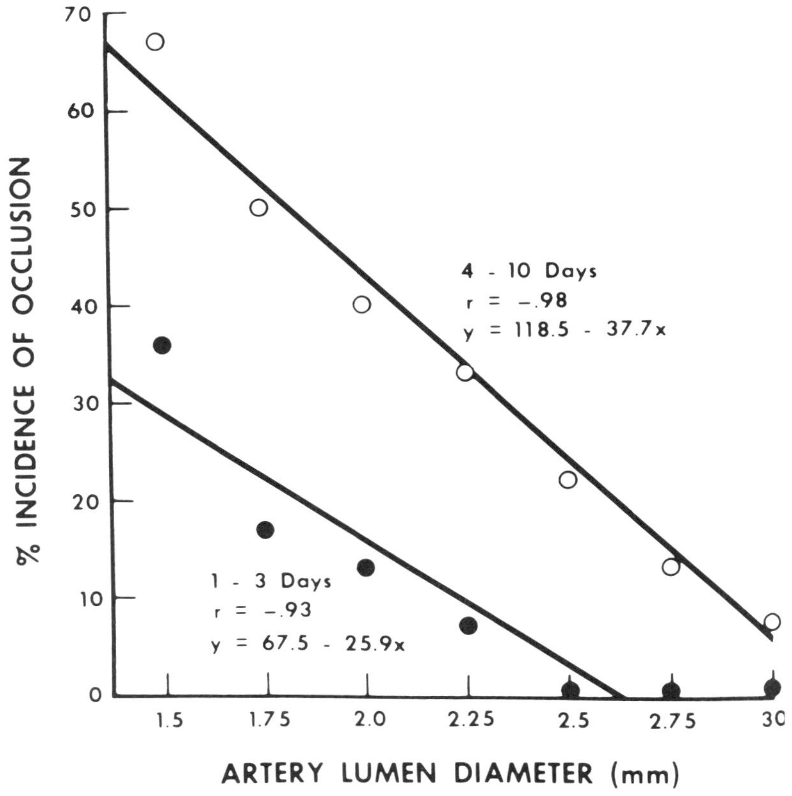

Figure 7–15. The incidence of thrombosis increases with duration of arterial cannulation. After 1–3 days, the incidence is 11%; after 4–10 days, it is 29%. Cannula dysfunction also increases after more than 3 days of cannulation. (From Bedford RF: Longterm radial artery cannulation. Effects on subsequent vessel function. Crit Care Med 1978; 6:66. © Williams & Wilkins, 1978.)

pressure measurement occur. Placement of self-retaining chest wall retractors for dissection of internal mammary arteries for use as coronary artery bypass grafts distorts normal arterial anatomy, resulting in damping of the arterial pressure waveform.[130, 131] However, the mean arterial pressure remains accurate.[132] Factors contributing to this problem include lateral tilt of the operating table, compression of the arm, and the position of the retractor. Although measurement of arterial pressure in the opposite extremity obviates the immediate problem, concern about the adequacy of blood flow to the arm warrants retractor repositioning. Similar problems have been noted with opening of sternal retractors, particularly in short, obese patients.[133] Retractor opening in these patients causes a condition similar to the thoracic outlet syndrome.[133]

Inaccurate radial artery pressure measurements immediately after discontinuation of cardiopulmonary bypass have been reported in both children and adults.[134–136] A gradient between the aortic and radial pressures develops when bypass is discontinued.[137] Both central aortic and femoral ar-

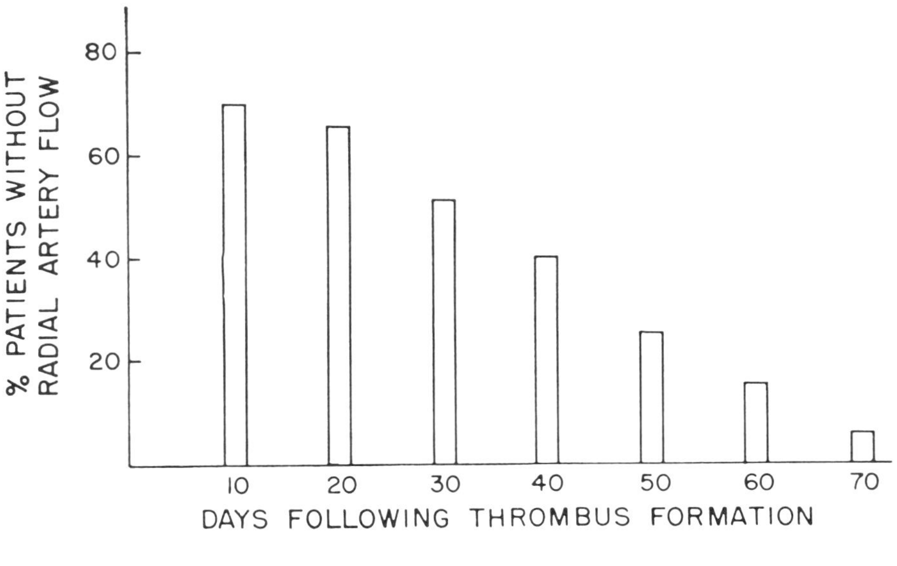

Figure 7–16. The time to recanalization of the radial artery after thrombosis ranges from 3 to 75 days; the majority are recanalized by 40 days after cannula removal. (From Bedford RF, Wollmann H: Complications of radial-artery cannulation: An objective prospective study in man. Anesthesiology 1973; 38:232.)

terial pressures are commonly higher than radial pressures for 45–60 minutes after termination of extracorporeal circulation in some patients. When vigorous cardiac contractility is directly observed, but peripherally measured pressures are disproportionately low, arterial pressure should be measured in the aorta, femoral artery, or axillary artery, or by using an automated oscillometric cuff on the brachial artery until the peripheral circulation returns to normal.[134, 137] Gradients usually resolve within 10–60 minutes after bypass is terminated.

The etiology of these gradients may be peripheral vasoconstriction,[136] decreased forearm vascular resistance during rewarming from bypass,[86, 136] hypothermia, hypovolemia, or proximal shunting.[86, 134–136] Additional volume replacement eliminated the gradient associated with decreased cardiac index and mixed venous oxygen saturation (previously abnormally increased) and increased systemic vascular resistance in Mohr's series of patients.[135] Patients without gradients between femoral and radial artery pressures did not demonstrate alteration in systemic resistance after discontinuation of bypass. Another possibility is previously unrecognized Raynaud's syndrome. Carter and colleagues associated a marked decrease or loss of finger systolic pressure with the sympathetic vasoconstriction induced by cooling.[138]

REFERENCES

1. Bruner JMR, Krenis LJ, Kunsman JM, Sherman AP: Comparison of direct and indirect methods of measuring arterial blood pressure. Med Instrum 1981; 15:11–21 (Part I); Med Instrum 15:97–101 (Part II); Med Instrum 15:182–188 (Part III).
2. O'Rourke MF, Yaginuma T: Wave reflections and the arterial pulse. Arch Intern Med 1984; 144:366–371.
3. Gerber MJ, Hines RL, Barash PG: Arterial waveforms and systemic vascular resistance: Is there a correlation? Anesthesiology 1987; 66:823–825.
4. Karamanoglu M, O'Rourke MF, Avolio AP, Kelly RP: An analysis of the relationship between central aortic and peripheral upper limb pressure waves in man. Eur Heart J 1993; 14:160–167.
5. Gravlee GP, Brockschmidt JK: Accuracy of four indirect methods of blood pressure measurement, with hemodynamic correlations. J Clin Monit 1990; 6:284–298.
6. Emergency Care Research Institute: Physiologic monitoring and the standard of care. Health Devices 1991; 20:104–105.
7. Kirkendall WN, Feinleib M, Freis ED, Mark AL: Recommendations for human blood pressure determination by sphygmomanometers. Circulation 1980; 62:1145A–1155A.
8. Wallace CT, Baker JD, Alpert CC, et al: Comparison of blood pressure measurement by Doppler and by pulse oximetry techniques. Anesth Analg 1987; 66:1018–1019.
9. Korotkoff NS: On the subject of methods of determining blood pressure. Bull Imperial Med Acad 1905; 11:365.
10. Ramsey M III: Noninvasive blood pressure monitoring methods and validation. In Gravenstein JS et al (eds): Essential Noninvasive Monitoring in Anesthesia. New York: Grune & Stratton, 1980;37–51.
11. Blank SG, West JE, Muller FB, et al: Wideband external pulse recording during cuff deflation: A new technique for evaluation of the arterial pressure pulse and measurement of blood pressure. Circulation 1988; 77:1297–1305.
12. Manning DM, Kuchirka C, Kamienski J: Miscuffing: Inappropriate blood pressure cuff application. Circulation 1983; 68:763–766.
13. Ragan C, Bordley J: The accuracy of clinical measurements of arterial blood pressure. Bull J Hopkins Hosp 1941; 69:504–528.
14. Holland WW, Humerfelt S: Measurement of blood pressure, comparison of intra-arterial and cuff values. Br Med J 1964; 2:1241–1243.
15. Simpson JA, Jamieson G, Dickhaus DW: Effect of size of cuff bladder on accuracy of measurements of indirect blood pressure. Am Heart J 1965; 70:208–215.
16. Breit SN, O'Rourke MF: Comparison of direct and indirect arterial pressure measurements in hospitalized patients. Austr N Z J Med 1974; 4:485–491.
17. Apple HP: Automatic noninvasive blood pressure monitors: What is available. In Gravenstein JS et al (eds): Essential Noninvasive Monitoring in Anesthesia. New York: Grune & Stratton, 1980;7–24.
18. Morgan JL, Kemmerer WT, Halber MD: Doppler shifted ultrasound. Minn Med 1969; 52:503–506.
19. Kirby RR, Kemmerer WT, Morgan JL: Transcutaneous doppler measurement of blood pressure. Anesthesiology 1969; 31:86–89.
20. Stegall HF, Kardon MB, Kemmerer WT: Indirect measurement of arterial blood pressure by Doppler ultrasonic sphygmomanometry. J Appl Physiol 1968; 25:793–798.
21. Hernandez A, Goldring D, Hartman AF: Measurement of blood pressure in infants and children by the Doppler ultrasound technique. Pediatrics 1971; 48:788.
22. Waltemath CL, Preuss DD: Determination of blood pressure in low-flow states by the Doppler technique. Anesthesiology 1971; 34:77–79.
23. Von Recklinghausen H: Neue Wege zur blutdruckmessung. Berlin: Springer-Verlag, 1931.
24. Hutton P, Prys-Roberts C: The oscillotonometer in theory and practice. Br J Anaesth 1982; 54:581–591.
25. Ramsey M III: Noninvasive automatic determination of mean arterial pressure. Med Biol Eng 1979; 17:11–18.
26. Borow KM, Newburger JW: Noninvasive estimation of central aortic pressure using the oscillometric method for analyzing systemic artery pulsatile blood flow: Comparative study of indirect systolic, diastolic, and mean brachial artery pressure with simultaneous direct ascending aortic pressure measurements. Am Heart J 1982; 103:879–896.
27. Yelderman M, Ream AK: Indirect measurement of mean blood pressure in anesthetized patient. Anesthesiology 1979; 50:253–256.
28. Hutton P, Dye J, Prys-Roberts C: An assessment of the dinamap 845. Anaesthesia 1984; 39: 261–267.
29. Nystrom E, Reid KH, Bennett R, et al: A comparison of two automated indirect arterial blood pressure meters: With recordings from a radial arterial catheter in anesthetized surgical patients. Anesthesiology 1985; 62:526–530.
30. Friesen RH, Lichtor JL: Indirect measurement of blood pressure in neonates and infants utilizing an automatic noninvasive oscillometric monitor. Anesth Analg 1981; 60:742–745.
31. Kimble KJ, Darnall RA, Yelderman M, Ariagno RL, Ream AK: An automated oscillometric technique for estimating mean arterial pressure in critically ill newborns. Anesthesiology 1981; 54:423–425.
32. Sesler JM, Munroe WP, McKenney JM: Clinical evaluation of a finger oscillometric blood pressure device. DICP Ann Pharmacother 1991;25:1310–1314.
33. Peñaz J: Photoelectric measurement of blood pressure volume and flow in the finger. Digest, 10th International Conference of Medical Biological Engineers 1973; 104.
34. Wesseling KH, de Wit B, Snoeck B, et al: An implementation of the Peñaz method for measuring arterial blood pressure in the finger and first results of an evaluation. Inst Med Physics TNO Prog Rep 1978; 6:168–173.
35. Wesseling KH, van Bemmel R, van Dieren A, et al: Two methods for the assessment of hemodynamic parameters of epidemiology. Acta Cardiol 1978; 33:84–87.
36. Imholz BPM, Langewouters GJ, Van Montfrancs GA, et al: Feasibility of ambulatory, continuous 24-hour finger arterial pressure recording. Hypertension 1993; 21:65–73.
37. Gorback MS, Quill TJ, Lavine ML: The relative accuracies of two automated noninvasive arterial pressure measurement devices. J Clin Monit 1991; 7:13–22.
38. Molhoek GP, Wesseling KH, Settels, JJ et al: Evaluation of the Peñaz servo-plethysmo-manometer for the continuous, noninvasive measurement of finger blood pressure. Basic Res Cardiol 1984; 79:598–609.
39. Kurki T, Smith NT, Head N, Dec-Silver H, Quinn A: Noninvasive continuous blood pressure measurement from the finger: Optimal measurement conditions and factors affecting reliability. J Clin Monit 1987; 3:6–13.
40. Smith NT, Wesseling KH, deWit B: Evaluation of two prototype

devices producing noninvasive, pulsatile, calibrated blood pressure measurement from a finger. J Clin Monit 1985; 1:17–29.
41. Gravenstein JS, Paulus DA, Feldman J, McLaughlin G: Tissue hypoxia distal to a penaz finger blood pressure cuff. J Clin Monit 1985; 1:120–125.
42. Imholz BP, Parati G, Mancia G, Wesseling KH: Effects of graded vasoconstriction upon the measurement of finger arterial pressure. J Hypertens 1992; 10:979–984.
43. Dorlas JC, Nijboer JA, Butijn T, et al: Effects of peripheral vasoconstriction on the blood pressure in the finger, measured continuously by a new noninvasive method (the Finapres). Anesthesiology 1985; 62:342–345.
44. Aitken HA, Todd JG, Kenny GN: Comparison of the Finapres and direct arterial pressure monitoring during profound hypotensive anaesthesia. Br J Anaesth 1991; 67:36–40.
45. Kemmotsu O, Ueda A, Otsuka H, et al: Arterial tonometry for noninvasive continuous blood pressure monitoring during anesthesia. Anesthesiology 1991; 75:333–340.
46. Kemmotsu O, Ueda M, Otsuka H, et al: Blood pressure measurement by arterial tonometry in controlled hypotension. Anesth Analg 1991; 73: 54–58.
47. Sato T, Nishinaga M, Kawamoto A, Ozawa T, Takatsuji H: Accuracy of a continuous blood pressure monitor based on arterial tonometry. Hypertension 1993; 21:866–874.
48. Sy WP: Ulnar nerve palsy possibly related to use of automatically cycled blood pressure cuff. Anesth Analg 1981; 60:687–688.
49. Noreng MF: Blood flow in the radial artery before and after arterial puncture. Acta Anaesthesiol Scand 1986; 30:281–282.
50. Pierson DJ, Hudson LD: Monitoring hemodynamics in the critically ill. Med Clin North Am 1983; 67:1343–1360.
51. Peterson LH, Dripps RD, Risman GC: A method for recording the arterial pressure pulse and blood pressure in man. Am Heart J 1949; 37:771–782.
52. Bedford RF: Percutaneous radial-artery cannulation. Increased safety using Teflon catheters. Anesthesiology 1975; 42:219–222.
53. Van Beck JO, White RD, Abenstein JP, Mullany CJ, Orszulak TA: Comparison of axillary artery or brachial artery pressure with aortic pressure after cardiopulmonary bypass using a long radial artery catheter. J Cardiothorac Vasc Anesth 1993; 7:312–315.
54. Gardner RM, Schwartz R, Wong JC, Burke JP: Percutaneous indwelling radial-artery catheters for monitoring cardiovascular function. N Engl J Med 1974; 290:1227–1231.
55. Talmage EA: Shearing hazard of intra-arterial teflon catheters. Anesth Analg 1976; 55:597–598.
56. Brodsky JB, Wong AL, Meyer JA: Percutaneous cannulation of weakly palpable arteries. Anesth Analg 1977; 56:448.
57. Buakham C, Kim JM: Cannulation of a nonpalpable artery with the aid of a Doppler monitor. Anesth Analg 1977; 56:125–126.
58. Chinyanga HM, Smith JM: A modified doppler flow detector probe—An aid to percutaneous radial arterial cannulation in infants and small children. Anesthesiology 1979; 50:256–258.
59. Introna RPS, Silverstein PI: A new use for the pulse oximeter. Anesthesiology 1986; 65:342.
60. Johnson RW: Complication of radial artery cannulation. Anesthesiology 1974; 40:353–355.
61. Gordon LH, Brown M, Brown OW, Brown EM: Alternative sites for continuous arterial monitoring. South Med J 1984; 77:1498–1500.
62. Pyles ST, Scher KS, Vega ET, Harrah JD, Rubis LJ: Cannulation of the dorsal radial artery: A new technique. Anesth Analg 1982; 61:876–878.
63. Paster SB, Middleton P: Roentgenographic evaluation of umbilical artery and vein catheters. JAMA 1975; 231:742–746.
64. Moorthy SS: Cannulation of the anterior peroneal artery in adults. Anesth Analg 1981; 60:360–361.
65. Prian GW: New proximal approach works well in temporal artery catheterization. JAMA 1976; 235:2693–2694.
66. Hegemann CO, Rappaport I, Berger WJ: Superficial temporal artery cannulation. Arch Surg 1969; 99:619–624.
67. Husum B, Palm T, Eriksen J: Percutaneous cannulation of the dorsalis pedis artery. Br J Anaesth 1979; 51:1055–1058.
68. Barnes RW, Foster EJ, Janssen GA, Boutros AR: Safety of brachial arterial catheters as monitors in the intensive care unit: Prospective evaluation with Doppler ultrasonic velocity detector. Anesthesiology 1976; 44:260–264.
69. Adler DC, Bryan-Brown CW: Use of the axillary artery for intravascular monitoring. Crit Care Med 1973; 1:148–150.
70. Rose SH: Ischemic complications of radial artery cannulation: An association with a calcinosis, Raynaud's phenomenon, esophageal dysmotility, sclerodactyly, and telangiectasia variant of scleroderma. Anesthesiology 1993; 78:587–589.
71. Mozersky DJ, Buckley CJ, Hagood C, et al: Ultrasonic evaluation of the palmar circulation. Am J Surg 1973; 126:810–812.
72. Allen EV: Thromboangiitis obliterans: Methods of diagnosis of chronic occlusive arterial lesions distal to the wrist with illustrative cases. Am J Med Sci 1929; 178:237–244.
73. Husum B, Berthelsen P: Allen's test and systolic arterial pressure in the thumb. Br J Anaesth 1981; 53:635.
74. Hirai M, Kawai S: False positive and negative results in Allen test. J Cardiovasc Surg 1980; 21:353–360.
75. Gandhi SK, Reynolds AC: A modification of Allen's test to detect aberrant ulnar collateral circulation. Anesthesiology 1983; 59:147–148.
76. Coleman SS, Anson BJ: Arterial patterns in the hand based upon a study of 650 specimens. Surg Gynecol Obstet 1961; 113:409–424.
77. Brodsky JB: A simple method to determine patency of the ulnar artery intraoperatively prior to radial artery cannulation. Anesthesiology 1975; 426–627.
78. Ramanathan S, Chalon J, Turndorf H: Determining patency of palmar arches by retrograde radial pulsation. Anesthesiology 1975; 42:756–758.
79. Nowak GS, McNiece WL: Use of pulse oximetry for assessment of collateral arterial flow. Anesthesiology 1986; 64:527.
80. Greenhow DE: Incorrect performance of Allen's test: Ulnar artery flow erroneously presumed inadequate. Anesthesiology 1972; 37:356–357.
81. Kamienski RW, Barnes RW: Critique of the Allen test for continuity of palmar arch assessed by Doppler ultrasound. Surg Gynecol Obstet 1976; 142:861–864.
82. Slogoff S, Keats AS, Arlund C: On the safety of radial artery cannulation. Anesthesiology 1983; 59:42–47.
83. Mandel MA, Dauchot PJ: Radial artery cannulation in 1000 patients: Precautions and complications. J Hand Surg 1977; 2:482–485.
84. Mangano DT, Hickey RF: Ischemic injury following uncomplicated radial artery catheterization. Anesth Analg 1979; 58:55–57.
85. Macon WL, Futrell JW: Median-nerve neuropathy after percutaneous puncture of the brachial artery in patients receiving anticoagulants. N Engl J Med 1973; 288:1296.
86. Pauca AL, Meredith JW: Possibility of A-V shunting upon cardiopulmonary bypass discontinuation. Anesthesiology 1987; 67:91–94.
87. Pascarelli EF, Bertrand CA: Comparison of blood pressures in the arms and legs. N Engl J Med 1964; 270:693–698.
88. Yacoub OF, Bacaling JH, Kelly M: Monitoring of axillary arterial pressure in a patient with Buerger's disease requiring clipping of an intracranial aneurysm. Br J Anaesth 1987; 59:1056–1058.
89. Christian CM, Naraghi M: A complication of femoral arterial cannulation in a patient undergoing cardiopulmonary bypass. Anesthesiology 1978; 49:436–437.
90. Glenski JA, Beynen FM, Brady J: A prospective evaluation of femoral artery monitoring in pediatric patients. Anesthesiology 1987; 66:227–229.
91. Rosenthal A, Anderson M, Thomson SJ, et al: Superficial femoral artery catheterization in infants and small children. Circulation 1977; 56:102–105.
92. Spoerel WE, Deimling P, Aitken R: Direct arterial pressure monitoring from the dorsalis pedis artery. Can Anaesth Soc J 1975; 22:91–99.
93. Huber JF: The arterial network supplying the dorsum of the foot. Anat Rec 1941; 80:373–391.
94. Youngberg JA, Miller ED: Evaluation of percutaneous cannulation of the dorsalis pedis artery. Anesthesiology 1976; 44:80–83.
95. Palm T, Husum B: Blood pressure in the great toe with simulated occlusion of the dorsalis pedis artery. Anesth Analg 1978; 57:453–456.
96. Johnstone RE, Greenhow DE: Catheterization of the dorsalis pedis artery. Anesthesiology 1973; 39:654–655.
97. Vidyasagar D, Downes JJ, Boggs TR: Respiratory distress syndrome of newborn infants: II—Technic of catheterization of umbilical artery and clinical results of treatment. Clin Pediatr 1970; 9:332–336.
98. Cole AFD, Rolbin SH: A technique for rapid catheterization of the umbilical artery. Anesthesiology 1980; 53:254–255.
99. McFadden PM, Ochsner JL: Neonatal aortic thrombosis: Complication of umbilical artery cannulation. J Cardiovasc Surg 1983; 24:1–4.

100. Marsh JL, Fonkalsrud EW: Serious complications after umbilical artery catheterization for neonatal monitoring. Arch Surg 1975; 110:1203–1208.
101. Feeley TW: Re-establishment of radial-artery patency for arterial monitoring. Anesthesiology 1977; 46:73–75.
102. Bedford RF: Removal of radial-artery thrombi following percutaneous cannulation for monitoring. Anesthesiology 1977; 46:430–432.
103. Lowenstein E, Little JW, Lo HH: Prevention of cerebral embolization from flushing radial-artery cannulas. N Engl J Med 1971; 285:1414–1415.
104. Chang C, Dughi J, Shitabata P, et al: Air embolism and the radial arterial line. Crit Care Med 1988; 16:141–143.
105. Edmonds JF, Barker GA, Conn AW: Current concepts in cardiovascular monitoring in children. Crit Care Med 1980; 8:548–553.
106. Gardner RM, Bond EL, Clark JS: Safety and efficacy of continuous flush systems for arterial and pulmonary artery catheters. Ann Thorac Surg 1977; 23:534–538.
107. Harbort RA, Dalgetty RG: Bubble formation in flush systems. Ann Thorac Surg 1978; 25:179–180.
108. Falk PS, Scuderi PE, Sherertz RJ, Motsinger SM: Infected radial artery pseudoaneurysms occurring after percutaneous cannulation. Chest 1992; 101:490–495.
109. Mathieu A, Dalton B, Fischer JE, Kumar A: Expanding aneurysm of the radial artery after frequent puncture. Anesthesiology 1973; 38:401–403.
110. Bright E, Baines DB, French FG, Cartmill TB: Upper limb amputation following radial artery cannulation. Anaesth Intens Care 1993; 21:351–353.
111. Cannon BW, Meshier WT: Extremity amputation following radial artery cannulation in a patient with hyperlipoproteinemia Type V. Anesthesiology 1982; 56:222–223.
112. Dalton B, Laver MB: Vasospasm with an indwelling radial artery cannula. Anesthesiology 1973; 34:194–197.
113. Bedford RF, Wollman H: Complications of percutaneous radial-artery cannulation: An objective prospective study in man. Anesthesiology 1973; 38:228–236.
114. Miyasaka K, Edmons JF, Conn AW: Complications of radial artery lines in the pediatric patient. Can Anesth Soc J 1976; 23:9–14.
115. Gauer PK, Downs JB: Complications of arterial catheterization. Respir Care 1982; 27:435–444.
116. Bedford RF: Radial artery function following cannulation with 18 and 20 gauge catheters. Anesthesiology 1977; 47:37–39.
117. Palm T: Evaluation of peripheral arterial pressure on the thumb following radial artery cannulation. Br J Anaesth 1977; 49:819–824.
118. Davis FM, Stewart JM: Radial artery cannulation. Br J Anaesth 1980; 52:674–684.
119. Downs JB, Rackstein AD, Klein EF, Hawkins IF: Hazards of radial-artery catheterization. Anesthesiology 1973; 38:283–286.
120. Bedford RF: Wrist circumference predicts the risk of radial-arterial occlusion after cannulation. Anesthesiology 1978; 48:377–378.
121. Jones RM, Hill AB, Nahrwold ML, Bolles RE: The effect of method of radial artery cannulation on postcannulation blood flow and thrombus formation. Anesthesiology 1981; 55:76–78.
122. Bedford RF, Ashford TP: Aspirin pretreatment prevents post-cannulation radial-artery thrombosis. Anesthesiology 1979; 51:176–178.
123. Kim JM, Arakawa K, Bliss J: Arterial cannulation: Factors in the development of occlusion. Anesth Analg 1975; 54:836–841.
124. Vender JS, Watts RD: Differential diagnosis of hand ischemia in the presence of an arterial cannula. Anesth Analg 1982; 61:465–468.
125. Band JD, Maki DG: Infection caused by arterial catheters used for hemodynamic monitoring. Am J Med 1979; 67:735–741.
126. Freeman R, King B: Analysis of results of catheter tip culture in open-heart surgery patients. Thorax 1975; 30:26–30.
127. Shinozaki T, Deane R, Mazuzan JE, Hamel AJ, Hazelton D: Bacterial contamination of arterial lines: A prospective study. JAMA 1983; 249:223–225.
128. Weinstein RA, Stamm WE, Kramer L: Pressure monitoring devices: Overlooked sources of nosocomial infection. JAMA 1976; 236:936–938.
129. Ducharme FM, Gauthier M, Lacroix J, Lafleur L: Incidence of infection related to arterial catheterization in children: A prospective study. Crit Care Med 1988; 16:272–276.
130. Kinzer JB, Lichtenthal PR, Wade LD: Loss of radial artery pressure trace during internal mammary artery dissection for coronary artery bypass graft surgery. Anesth Analg 1985; 64:1134–1136.
131. Daimant M, Arkin DB: False radial-artery blood-pressure readings [Letter]. Anesthesiology 1976; 44:273.
132. Nicolson SC, Jobes DR: Arterial pressure monitoring during internal mammary artery harvesting. Anesth Analg 1986; 65:821.
133. Saka D, Lin YT, Oka Y: An unusual cause of false radial-artery blood-pressure readings during cardiopulmonary bypass. Anesthesiology 1975; 43:487–489.
134. Stern DH, Gerson JI, Allen FB, Parker FB: Can we trust the direct radial artery pressure immediately following cardiopulmonary bypass? Anesthesiology 1985; 62:557–561.
135. Mohr R, Lavee J, Goor DA: Inaccuracy of radial artery pressure measurement after cardiac operations. J Thorac Cardiovasc Surg 1987; 94:286–290.
136. Gallagher JD, Moore RA, McNicholas KW, Jose AB: Comparison of radial and femoral arterial blood pressures in children after cardiopulmonary bypass. J Clin Monit 1985; 1:168–171.
137. Rich GF, Lubanski RE, McLoughlin TM: Differences between aortic and radial artery pressure associated with cardiopulmonary bypass. Anesthesiology 1992; 77:63–66.
138. Carter SA, Dean E, Kroeger EA: Apparent finger systolic pressures during cooling in patients with Raynaud's syndrome. Circulation 1988; 77:988–996.

CHAPTER 8

Venous and Pulmonary Pressures

KAREN J. SCHWENZER, M.D.

Access to the central venous circulation is widely used in the perioperative management of patients in order to administer fluids and vasoactive drugs, obtain blood samples, and monitor central vascular pressures. Central venous pressure (CVP) reflects left ventricular preload in healthy hearts. However, in many clinical situations, this relationship between CVP and left ventricular preload is not valid. With the flow-directed, balloon-tipped pulmonary artery catheter, left ventricular preload and function are better assessed by monitoring pulmonary artery pressure (PAP) and pulmonary capillary wedge pressure (PCWP). This chapter reviews the literature and discusses the indications, risks, and benefits of the important methods used to monitor CVP and PAP in the evaluation of hemodynamic function in patients in the operating room and critical care units.

MONITORING OF CENTRAL VENOUS PRESSURE

LEFT VENTRICULAR FUNCTION

The goal of hemodynamic management is to ensure that tissue perfusion meets aerobic metabolic needs. A balance among intravascular blood volume, cardiac output, and vascular resistance must be achieved. The vital component is the maintenance of an adequate cardiac output.

The Frank-Starling law of myocardial function states that as the initial myocardial fiber length increases, the force of contraction of that fiber increases. In the intact heart, myocardial fiber length is represented by left or right ventricular end-diastolic volume or preload (Fig. 8–1). Measurement of preload permits accurate assessment of intravascular volume in relation to myocardial performance. However, measurement of cardiac performance, which is accomplished by evaluation of stroke volume or cardiac output, urine output, capillary refill, and the patient's level of consciousness, is also required. In addition, the construction of a Frank-Starling myocardial function curve relating stroke volume to left ventricular preload is clinically useful in assessing therapeutic protocols in critically ill patients.

PRELOAD

It is technically difficult to repeatedly measure accurate, quantitative ventricular volumes. Therefore, left ventricular end-diastolic pressure (LVEDP) is used as an approximation of left ventricular preload. This relationship between ventricular volume and pressure is myocardial compliance.

In the normal heart, the thick, muscular left ventricle is relatively noncompliant as compared with the thin-walled right ventricle. The difference in compliance of the two ventricles, as a consequence of their anatomic structure, is responsible for the changes in the slopes of their corresponding Frank-Starling curves (Fig. 8–2). When compliance is normal, LVEDP is a good index of left ventricular preload. However, in a very stiff, noncompliant ventricle, LVEDP does not accurately reflect left ventricular end-diastolic volume.[1] In such situations, LVEDP may be increased, whereas end-diastolic volume is normal.

The relationship of LVEDP and other CVPs is diagrammed in Figure 8–3. The use of CVP to assess left ventricular preload has its limitations because CVP reflects right atrial pressure, which primarily reflects changes in right ventricular end-diastolic pressure (RVEDP) and only secondarily reflects changes in pulmonary venous pressure and LVEDP. However, if one recognizes that comparative changes in preload and stroke volume in response to therapy or disease are more important than absolute values of CVP or PCWP, the CVP can serve as a reliable indicator of intravascular blood volume. In addition, in patients with good ejection fractions, the CVP approximates LVEDP in absolute number as well as in change.[2, 3]

In an abnormal heart, the left and right ventricular function curves are markedly different from one another, and the CVP is a poor reflection of left-sided preload. In the

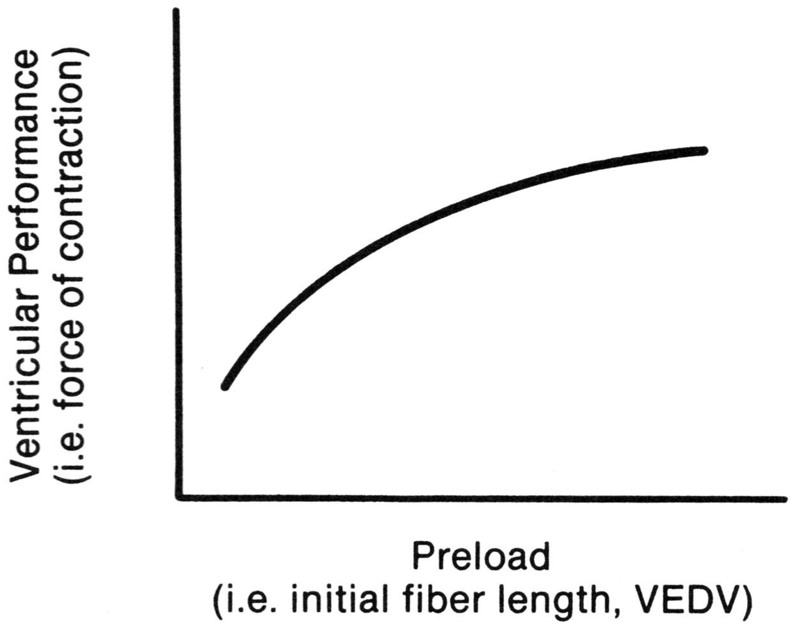

Figure 8–1. The Frank-Starling principle states that ventricular performance (i.e., force of contraction) is directly proportional to preload (i.e., ventricular end diastolic volume [VEDV]). (From Benumof JL: Anesthesia for Thoracic Surgery. Philadelphia: WB Saunders, 1987;181.)

presence of left ventricular failure, a higher LVEDP is needed to generate an adequate stroke volume (Fig. 8–4). In such situations, achieving a "normal" CVP results in a suboptimal intravascular volume, preload, and cardiac output. The CVP may not only be an inadequate index of intravascular volume but can also be quite misleading. For instance, the presence of tricuspid valvular stenosis interferes with the correlation between CVP (or mean right atrial pressure) and RVEDP. In this and similar situations, PCWP better reflects LVEDP.

At end-diastole the left ventricle, left atrium, pulmonary veins, pulmonary capillaries, and pulmonary artery function as a single, fluid-filled chamber. In the absence of mitral valve disease, left atrial pressure equals LVEDP. Bedside measurement of PCWP is obtained with a flow-directed, balloon-tipped pulmonary artery catheter. When the balloon is properly placed in a pulmonary artery, its inflation completely obstructs blood flow through the artery and forms a static column of blood distal to the catheter tip. This column of blood allows the catheter tip to measure pulmonary

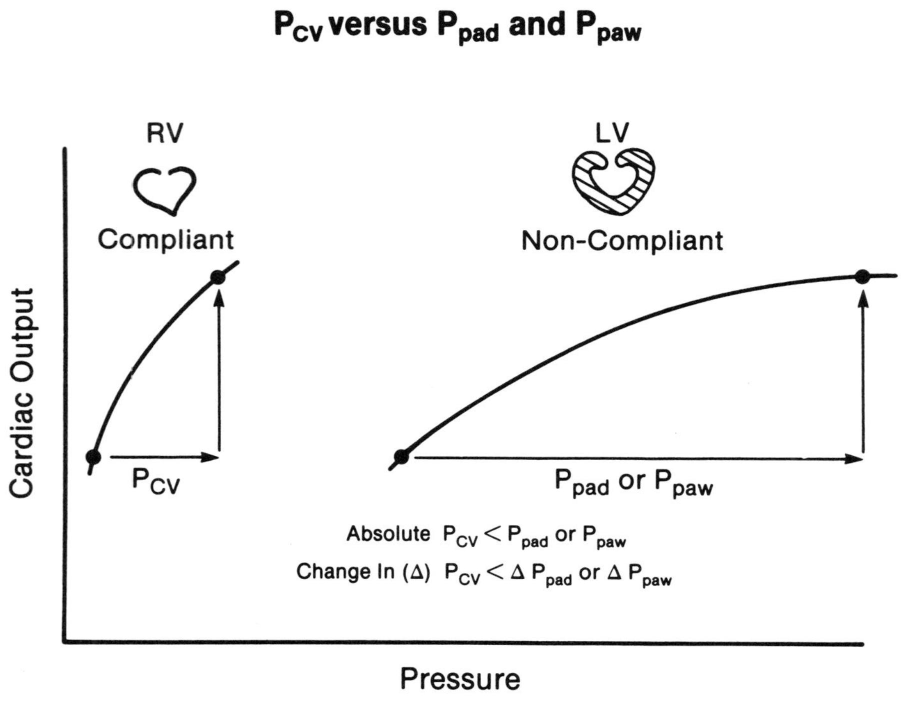

Figure 8–2. The relationship between central venous pressure (P_{CV}) and pulmonary artery wedge pressure (P_{paw}) and pulmonary artery diastolic pressure (P_{pad}) is normally based on the differences in compliance between the right ventricle (RV) and the left ventricle (LV). The right ventricle is relatively compliant because of its thin musculature, and the left ventricle is relatively noncompliant because of its thick musculature. Thus, when preload is changed in a normal heart, the P_{CV} (as a reflection of RVEDV) increases only a small amount for a given increase in cardiac output, whereas the P_{paw} and P_{pad} (as reflections of LVEDV) increase a large amount for the same increase in cardiac output. Thus, because of the differences in compliance between the two ventricles, the absolute P_{CV} is always less than the P_{paw} and P_{pad}, and the change in the P_{CV} is always less than the change in P_{paw} and P_{pad}. (From Benumof JL: Anesthesia for Thoracic Surgery. Philadelphia: WB Saunders, 1987;190.)

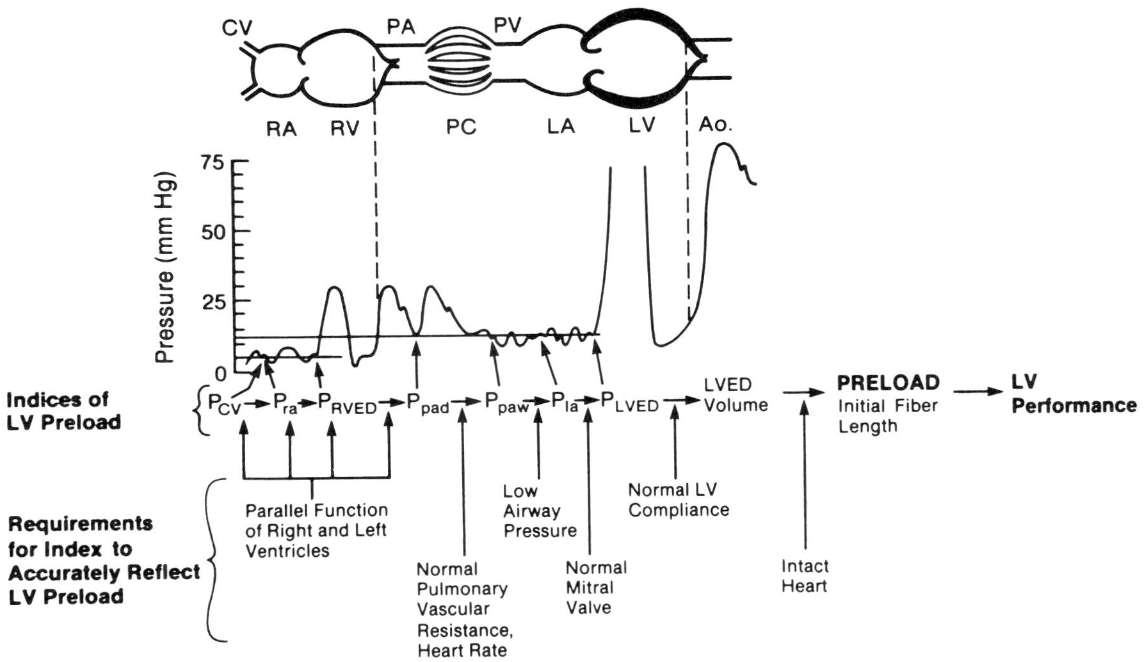

Figure 8–3. The relationship of LVEDP and other central venous pressures. In the top portion of the diagram, the various central vascular and cardiac chambers are portrayed in the sequence that blood flows through them. The cardiac valves portray the end-diastolic moment, the pulmonary and aortic valves are closed, and the mitral valve is open. The graph depicts the characteristic vascular pressure contours. Below this graph, the various indices of left ventricular preload are labeled. At the bottom of the diagram, the requirements for each of the indices to reflect accurately left ventricular preload are shown. (From Benumof JL: Anesthesia for Thoracic Surgery. Philadelphia: WB Saunders, 1987;182.)

venous circulation. Because there are normally no pressure gradients between the pulmonary veins and the left atrium, the pulmonary artery obstruction pressure or, more familiarly, the PCWP, reflects left atrial pressure and LVEDP. In the presence of mitral valve disease, however, the correlation between mean left atrial pressure (or PCWP) and LVEDP is distorted.

Another index of left ventricular preload is the pulmonary artery diastolic pressure (PADP), which is obtained with a flow-directed pulmonary artery catheter or a transthoracic pulmonary artery catheter. In the absence of elevated pulmonary vascular resistance, PADP is an excellent estimate of LVEDP.

CLINICAL USES

Assessment of Venous Return and Hypovolemia

The CVP monitors the adequacy of central venous return, intravascular blood volume, and right ventricular function. The CVP actually reflects the pressure in the great veins as blood returns to the heart. If blood return decreases, venous

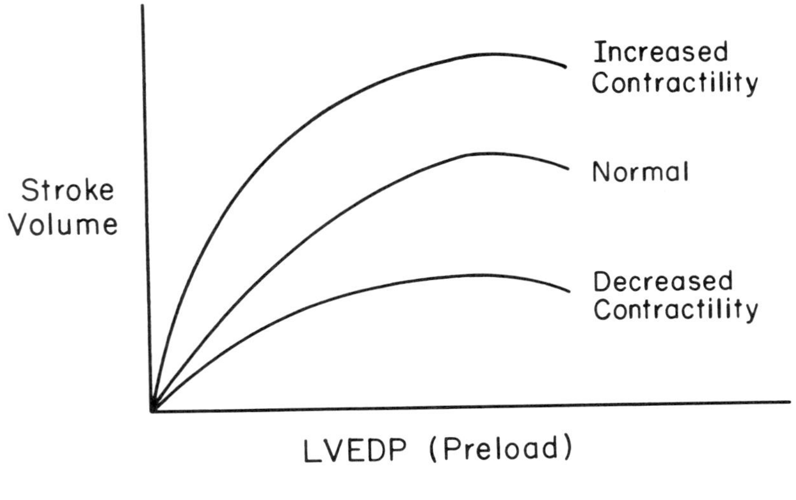

Figure 8–4. A family of Frank-Starling curves. The horizontal axis represents the preload of the heart, and the verticle axis represents the myocardial work.

pressure also decreases. In general, a decreased venous pressure reflects decreased blood volume and indicates the need for additional fluid or blood to expand the intravascular space. The administration of fluid in such situations increases CVP, indicating restoration of intravascular volume. No predetermined number for CVP should be used; instead, the goal of volume repletion is the restoration of tissue perfusion. For this reason, serial measurements, rather than single, absolute ones, are highly valued in the assessment of intravascular volume.

Surgical Indications for Monitoring CVP

During anesthesia and surgery, assessment of cardiovascular performance and intravascular volume is paramount to a patient's well-being. Failure to recognize inadequately replaced preoperative losses, hemorrhage, intraoperative fluid shifts, and faulty fluid management lead to hypovolemia. Depending on the clinical scenario, frequent assessment of pulse pressure, systolic pressure, heart rate, capillary refill, and urine output alerts the anesthesiologist to the presence of hypovolemia.

The decision to use invasive CVP monitoring during surgery is based on a patient's preoperative condition and intraoperative requirements. A patient with pre-existing cardiorespiratory disease or one who is undergoing surgical procedures causing further derangement in cardiorespiratory function during the perioperative period benefits from invasive measurement of CVP. Operative procedures involving anticipated massive blood and fluid transfusion (trauma), significant intravascular fluid shifts (hemicolectomy), or decreased venous return (performed in the lateral decubitus position), as well as those near the great vessels, heart, or other mediastinal structures (portacaval shunt), warrant the use of invasive monitoring to assess intravascular volume. Invasive hemodynamic monitoring is especially prudent if the surgical procedure is complicated by the presence of sepsis, heart disease, or respiratory failure.

Other Indications for Central Venous Catheterization

Central venous catheterization is often accomplished for the sole purpose of obtaining venous access when peripheral veins are unavailable. A central venous catheter (CVC) allows access to the central circulation for fluid and drug infusions during the perioperative period. At other times, intravenous administration of vasoactive drugs and other drugs likely to injure peripheral veins and tissues requires central venous access. Hypertonic parenteral hyperalimentation must be administered directly into the central venous circulation. CVCs are used in the diagnosis and aspiration of venous air emboli as well as in the transvenous insertion of temporary pacing leads. In all these cases, the precautions and risks discussed here are applicable. Blood samples may be obtained from a CVC as long as the intravenous fluids are aspirated from the catheter prior to sampling. Failure to do this can lead to abnormal values, which should be suspected when eccentric laboratory reports are received (see Chapters 27 and 28).

INSERTION OF CENTRAL VENOUS CATHETERS

Proper skills for insertion of CVCs are best learned from a tutor skilled in the procedure. Percutaneous insertion is the preferred technique, although venous cutdowns are occasionally necessary in infants and some adults.

PATIENT PREPARATION

Proper equipment is essential for central venous catheterization. Table 8–1 outlines the necessary supplies, although numerous prepackaged central venous catheterization kits containing the necessities are available. The assistance of a technician or nurse familiar with the procedure is also recommended. Patient sedation with any number of drugs such as the benzodiazepines or narcotics is helpful. Insertion into the internal jugular, external jugular, and subclavian veins is facilitated by placing the patient in the Trendelenburg position to distend the veins for ease of puncture and to prevent the entrainment of air during insertion. With these approaches, the patient's head is turned to the side opposite the insertion site to increase exposure.

Sterile technique and universal precautions, which must be maintained throughout the procedure, are facilitated with sterile gloves, sterile gown, face mask, and appropriate hair covering. Central venous catheter–related infections are minimized by proper preparation of the skin surface prior to catheter insertion. The skin site is shaved, if needed, and an iodine preparation, such as povidone-iodine (Betadine), or 2% chlorhexidine is applied and allowed to dry. A solution of 70% alcohol is then applied and allowed to dry. The area is draped with sterile towels. The insertion site is infiltrated with a local anesthetic, such as 0.5–1.0% lidocaine, without vasoconstrictor.

TABLE 8–1. EQUIPMENT NEEDED FOR PLACEMENT OF CENTRAL VENOUS CATHETERS

Povidone iodone or chlorhexidine solution
Sterile drape or towels
25-gauge needle for local anesthetic infiltration
Local anesthetic without vasoconstricter
Filtered needle to aspirate local anesthetic
22-gauge seeker needle
18-gauge 6.35-cm thin-walled needle with a radiopaque catheter
18-gauge 6.35-cm thin-walled needle
Two 5-ml syringes
Stainless steel guidewire with flexible tip on one end and a J-tip on the other
Scalpel
Venous dilator
Radiopaque polyurethane central venous catheter
Luer lock injection caps
Suture material with needle
Sterile gauze

CHOICE OF TECHNIQUE

There are three basic methods of gaining access to the central circulation: catheter-over-the-needle, catheter-through-the-needle, and catheter-over-a-guidewire (Seldinger) techniques.

Catheter-over-the-Needle Technique

With the catheter-over-the-needle technique, once the needle tip is located within the lumen of the vein, the CVC is advanced directly over the needle. The entire needle-catheter assembly must be of adequate length to reach the central circulation. There are a number of prepackaged catheter-over-the-needle products available to perform this direct approach to the central circulation. The most common length is 5.5–6 inches, which allows the catheter to reach the superior vena cava (SVC) from the jugular or subclavian vein. The entire insertion is relatively simple and done in one step. In addition, the catheter completely occupies the puncture made in the vessel wall by the needle, minimizing bleeding. However, many clinicians find the length of the device cumbersome, especially when a syringe is attached to the hub during insertion. Another disadvantage is that the needle tip may be within the vein while the leading edge of the catheter is still extraluminal. Consequently, the catheter cannot be successfully advanced.

Catheter-through-the-Needle Technique

Catheter-through-the-needle techniques also employ prepackaged devices, commonly 60 cm for the antecubital approach. With this technique, once the needle is within the lumen of the vein, the catheter is passed through it and advanced to its proper position. Because the needle cannot be removed past the hub of the catheter, a protective sheath must fix the needle to the catheter to ensure that the catheter is not cut by the sharp edge of the needle. Attempts to withdraw the catheter into the needle should be avoided, because shearing of the catheter with subsequent embolism can result. In addition, the catheter diameter is smaller than the needle puncture, so leakage of blood around the catheter is common.

Seldinger Technique

The preferred technique is the one described by Seldinger,[4] using a catheter-over-a-guidewire technique. Once the needle tip (18 or 20 gauge) is located in the lumen of the vein and venous blood is seen in the syringe, the syringe can be removed and a guidewire can be inserted through the needle. Guidewires are available in many diameters and lengths. One end of the guidewire is flexible, either with a straight configuration or with a J-tip to facilitate advancement of the wire into the central circulation. The guidewire is prepackaged with a short sheath that is used to straighten the J-tip in order to ease insertion into the needle. The outside diameter of the guidewire must be smaller than the inside of the needle or cannula through which it must pass (Table 8–2). The wire should be at least 10 cm longer than the central catheter, although a wire twice as long as the catheter is generally used. During catheterization of the central circulation, the guidewire should be firmly grasped to prevent embolism of the wire.

Once the wire is inserted 15–20 cm into the vein, the needle is removed over the wire, leaving the wire in the vein. The puncture site and vein are dilated to accommodate the central catheter by advancing a tapered obturator over the guidewire. A small skin incision using a scalpel may be necessary in order to accommodate larger catheters. The CVC is passed over the guidewire and advanced to the central circulation, with the guidewire always grasped. The guidewire is removed, and venous blood is aspirated from the catheter lumen. One modification of the Seldinger technique uses a short over-the-needle cannula, which is advanced off the needle into the vein after the initial venous puncture. The guidewire is then threaded through the cannula.

Either guidewire technique allows the initial venipuncture to be accomplished with a small needle or cannula, minimizing the risk of traumatizing adjacent structures. Either technique permits a wide variety of CVCs or vascular sheaths to be inserted over the guidewire.

DOPPLER ULTRASOUND GUIDANCE

Doppler ultrasound to assist cannulation of the internal jugular vein was reported as early as 1984.[5–7] Real-time, two-dimensional ultrasound can image the anatomy of the internal jugular vein and guide placement of needles, guidewires, and CVCs. Improved complication and success rates, as well as decreased time for cannulation and fewer needle passes, are reported both with bulky standard ultrasound equipment[8, 9] and smaller, portable ultrasound probes.[10, 11] These improvements, though significant, are small; the real clinical usefulness of ultrasound guidance is seen when venous cannulation using external landmark guidance

TABLE 8–2. RELATIVE SIZES OF ANGIOGRAPHIC WIRES, CANNULAS, AND NEEDLES

Outer Diameter of Wire (inches)*	Smallest Thin-Walled Needle Through Which Wire Fits (gauge)	Smallest Cannula Through Which Wire Fits (gauge)
0.018–0.021	21	22
0.022–0.025*	19	20
0.028	19	18
0.035	18	16
0.038	18	16

*A 0.025-inch or smaller wire will fit through the lumina of most pulmonary artery catheters.

From Blitt CD (ed): Monitoring in Anesthesia and Critical Care Medicine, 2nd Ed. New York: Churchill Livingstone, 1990; 184.

fails.[8, 10–12] Ultrasound can establish the reason for failure and safely guide wires and catheters. It may be especially helpful when anatomic landmarks are distorted, such as in patients with short necks, obesity, pregnancy, prior surgical interventions or radiation to the neck area, and young children.[9, 13] Reports of ultrasound guidance for cannulation of the subclavian vein are limited, and no recommendations can be made at this time.[6, 14]

CHOICE OF CATHETER

The choice of one type of CVC over another is based on the intended use. For instance, some catheters are designed to be flexible and nonirritating and are ideal for long-term central hyperalimentation. Others are easy to insert and are preferred for emergency fluid resuscitation.

CVCs are available in a variety of materials. The most common materials are polyvinylchloride, polypropylene, polyethylene, polyurethane, polytef (Teflon), and polymeric silicone (silastic). Most are chemically inert, although the risk of thrombus formation is variable (Table 8–3). Some polyvinylchloride pulmonary artery catheters are coated with heparin to reduce the incidence of thrombus formation on the catheter. Other catheters are coated by the manufacturer with antibiotics or can be coated by the physician prior to insertion to reduce the incidence of catheter-related infections.[15]

Multilumen CVCs are widely accepted in the operating room and intensive care units. These devices have two to four lumina, enabling simultaneous continuous CVP monitoring and fluid or drug administration. When multilumen CVCs are used the proximal lumina are flushed with heparinized saline solution (1 U/ml) prior to insertion and capped with syringes or Luer-Loks to prevent thrombus formation and air entrainment during insertion. The distal port is then threaded over the guidewire. Once the catheter is properly positioned within the central venous circulation, aspiration of blood from all the ports should be possible.

CHOICE OF SITE

A number of sites are available for central venous catheterization. The choice of a particular site is determined by the experience of the physician, accessibility, convenience, success rate in directing the catheter to the central venous circulation, risk to the patient, and probable duration of use.

Internal Jugular Vein

The internal jugular vein is often the site of choice because the site is clean, the incidence of thrombophlebitis is low, and the patient is allowed freedom of movement. It is a favored site for anesthesiologists because of its easy accessibility during surgery.

The highest success rate of localizing the catheter in the SVC or right atrium (RA) is achieved through the right internal jugular vein. This provides a straight path into the SVC. Disruption of anatomic relationships by tumor or trauma and the inability to position the patient's head properly are contraindications to this approach. Previous neck surgery, coagulopathy,[16] and systemic anticoagulation are relative contraindications. The potential success rate (using ultrasound guidance) after carotid endarterectomy is 79%.[17]

Despite the multiplicity of techniques that have been described for catheterization of the internal jugular vein, there are three basic approaches as determined by the vein's relation to the two heads of the sternocleidomastoid muscle—the posterior, central, and anterior routes (Fig. 8–5). From its origin at the jugular foramen, the internal jugular vein runs directly caudad, under the clavicle, to join the subclavian vein. The internal jugular vein, carotid artery, and vagus nerve run together within the carotid sheath. Initially in its course through the neck, the vein lies posterior to the carotid artery but then becomes lateral to it near the clavicle.

The most widely accepted route is the central approach to the right internal jugular vein. The patient is prepared, as described previously, with the head turned away from the site of catheterization. The triangle formed by the sternal and clavicular heads of the sternocleidomastoid muscle and the clavicle is identified. The course of the vein follows a line connecting the mastoid process and the clavicular head of the sternocleidomastoid muscle, which is the lateral wall of the triangle. The puncture site is made at the apex of the triangle, and the needle is directed along this line at a 45°

TABLE 8–3. COMPARISON OF CENTRAL VENOUS CATHETER MATERIALS

Type of Material	Chemical Inertness	Thrombogenicity	Flexibility	Transparent
Polyvinylchloride (PVC)	− − −	+ + +	+ + +	Yes
Siliconized PVC	−	+ +	+ +	Yes
Polyethylene	− −	+ + +	+ +	Yes
Polypropylene	− −	+ + +	+ +	Yes
Siliconized polypropylene	0	+	+ +	Sometimes
Teflon	−	+	+	No
Silastic	0	0	+ + + +	No
Polyurethane	− −	+	+ + +	No

Key: 0 = none, + = minimal, + + = moderate, + + + and + + + + = large, − = less, − − = much less, − − − = markedly less.
From Blitt CD (ed): Monitoring in Anesthesia and Critical Care Medicine, 2nd Ed. New York: Churchill Livingstone, 1990; 180.

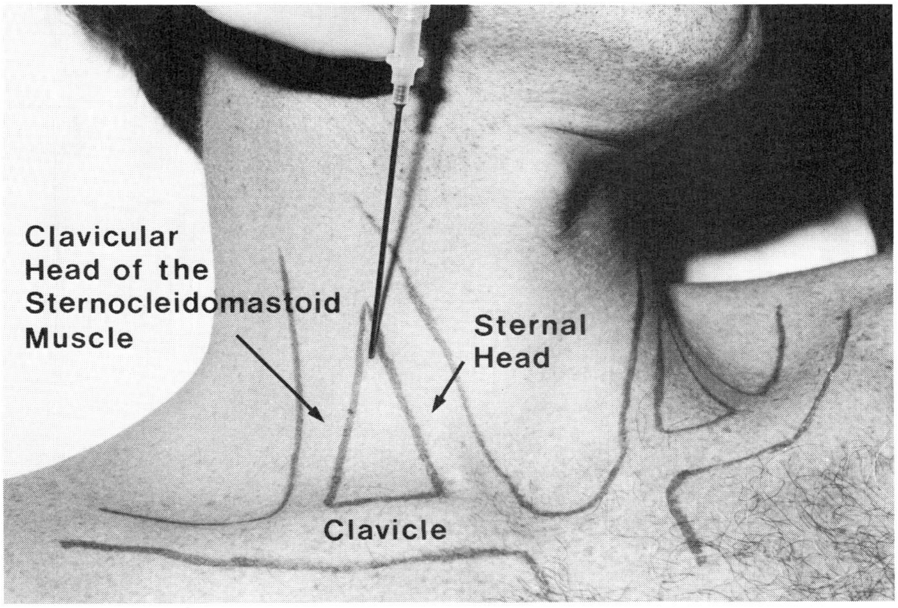

Figure 8–5. Anatomic landmarks and needle approach to the internal jugular vein.

angle to the skin. Prior to puncture, the carotid artery is palpated to ensure its medial location. Attempts to ''slide'' the artery out of the path of the needle are not recommended because the artery and vein lie in a common sheath. Rather, the risk of cannulating the carotid artery can be minimized by careful adherence to proven technique and use of a small-caliber needle or catheter (20–21 gauge) to localize the internal jugular vein prior to insertion of the large-bore needle and subsequent catheter or sheath introducer.

As the needle is passed, gentle negative pressure is applied to the syringe until venous blood is easily aspirated. If the vein is not entered, the needle is withdrawn slowly and completely with gentle aspiration. If, as occasionally occurs, the vein has been punctured through and through, blood returns to the syringe during withdrawal. The appearance of rapid, pulsatile, bright red blood flow from the needle may indicate arterial puncture. However, hypotension, hypoxia, sepsis, adult respiratory distress syndrome, and hepatic failure all can alter this observation, and its absence does not ensure venous puncture.[16, 18] If there is doubt or if the nature of the punctured blood vessel is critical, such as in a patient with a coagulopathy, additional maneuvers may be necessary prior to placement of a CVC. The inserted needle or catheter may be attached to a transducer with sterile tubing. Both the waveform and the pressure should confirm venous puncture.[19] Alternatively, sterile tubing may be attached to the inserted needle or catheter and positioned like a manometer. Venous insertion will exhibit a blood level within the tubing that reaches a constant level, and then fluctuates with the patient's respirations. Arterial insertion will exhibit a blood level that will continuously rise and flow out of the top of the tubing.[16, 20] Blood gases obtained from the needle and an arterial catheter can be analyzed simultaneously as well, but this is time-consuming. Once venous access is obtained, catheter placement proceeds as previously described.

Multiple variations on the landmarks and insertion point have been described, all with very good success rates. Nevertheless, carotid artery puncture remains the most frequent complication of the internal jugular approach, in spite of these techniques designed to avoid it. This usually is not a serious problem, except when a large catheter or introducer is inadvertently passed into the artery and/or the patient has a coagulopathy.

Subclavian Vein

Subclavian venipuncture as a venous access route was first described by Aubaniac over 40 years ago.[21] It offers the same advantages of the internal jugular approach, but the potential development of a pneumothorax must be considered.

The *infraclavicular approach* to the subclavian vein requires that the patient's head be turned slightly away from the side of catheterization and rested flat on the bed. A small, rolled towel placed longitudinally between the scapulae allows the shoulders to fall back onto the bed and brings the subclavian vein closer to the clavicle (Fig. 8–6). The clavicular head of the sternocleidomastoid muscle as it inserts on the clavicle and the anterior scalene muscle as it passes behind the clavicle are identified (Fig. 8–7). The location of the subclavian vein in this area is constant as it passes beneath the clavicle. If it is displaced, it is only more cephalad, as in the case of the patient with emphysema. It does not lie posterior to the scalene muscle.

After proper patient preparation, the skin is punctured just inferior to the clavicle at the junction of its middle and

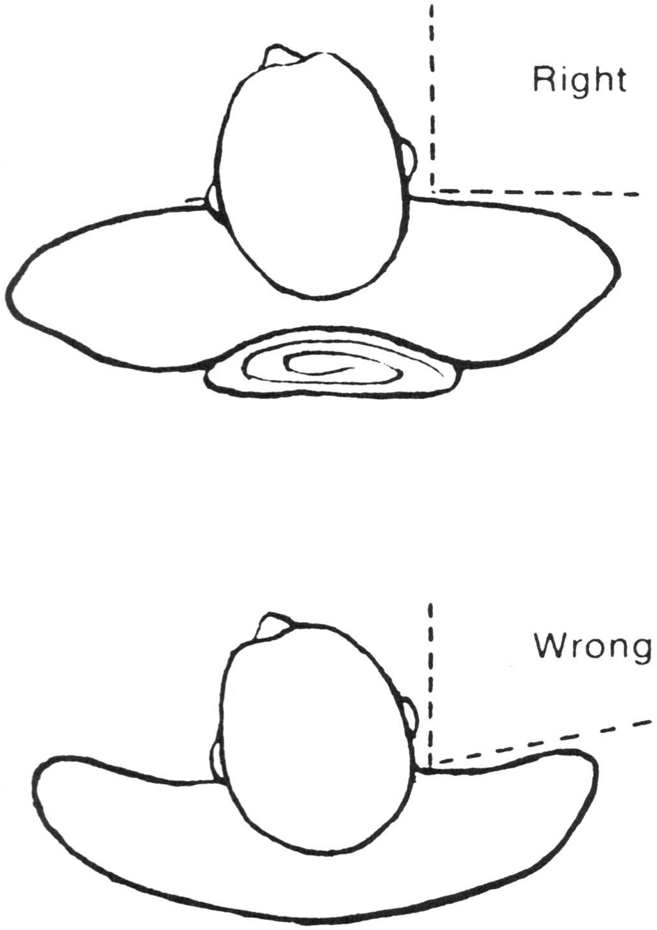

Figure 8–6. Correct position of the patient for insertion of subclavian catheter is the Trendelenburg position with the arms by the side, extended toward the feet. A rolled towel is placed along the thoracic spine to allow the shoulders to fall back into the bed. (From Grant JP: Handbook of Total Parenteral Nutrition. Philadelphia: WB Saunders, 1980;50.)

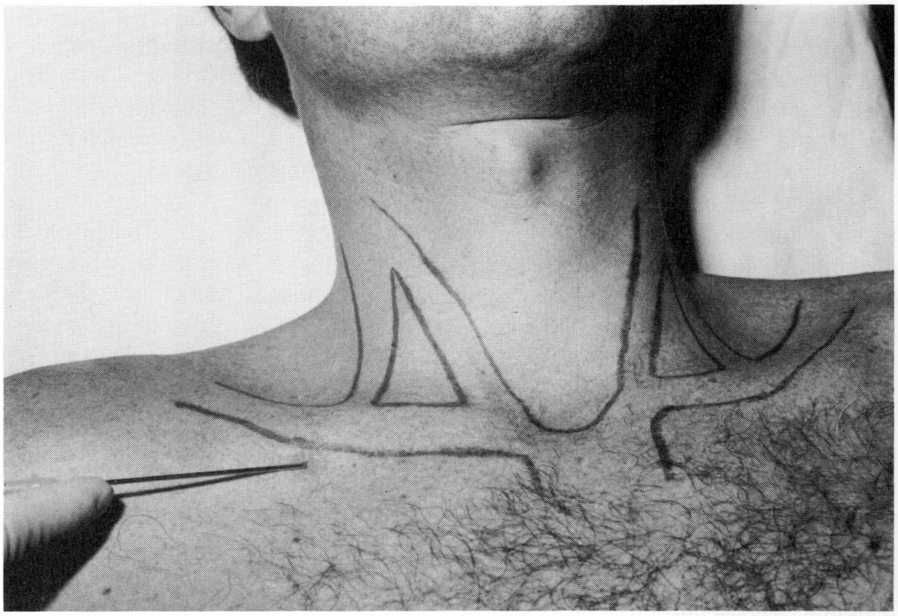

Figure 8–7. Infraclavicular approach to the subclavian vein.

outer thirds, with the needle aimed at a point behind the sternal manubrium. The puncture site should permit a horizontal approach to the vein, with the needle tip always anterior to the anterior scalene muscle. As the needle passes under the clavicle, gentle negative pressure is applied to the syringe until venous blood is easily aspirated. If the vein is not entered, the needle is withdrawn slowly and completely with gentle aspiration. If this procedure is unsuccessful, the landmarks are re-evaluated, and re-entry is directed slightly more cephalad or medially. The temptation to direct the needle more posteriorly should absolutely be avoided, because the vein does not lie behind the anterior scalene muscle, but the subclavian artery and the cupula of the lung do. Upon puncture of the subclavian vein and free return of blood into the syringe, the catheter is inserted as previously described.

In 1965, Yoffa described a supraclavicular approach to the subclavian vein.[22] He reported a decreased number of complications associated with inadvertent puncture of arterial and pulmonary structures, probably related to the experience of the operator. The important landmarks for the *supraclavicular approach* to the subclavian vein are the sternocleidomastoid muscle as it inserts on the clavicle, the anterior scalene muscle behind the clavicle, and the subclavian artery behind the anterior scalene muscle (Fig. 8–8). After proper patient preparation, skin puncture is directed just behind the clavicle at a 45° angle to the sagittal plane and pointed 15° forward of the coronal plane. While the syringe is aspirated gently, the needle is advanced, moving safely away from the structures of the subclavian artery and the lung. Once venous access is obtained, the syringe is lowered toward the shoulder to align the needle with the vein. Catheter placement then proceeds as previously described.

External Jugular Vein

The external jugular vein runs obliquely across the body of the sternocleidomastoid muscle toward the middle of the clavicle and into the subclavian vein. In spite of this vein's superficial location, successful placement of CVCs using this approach is often difficult owing to the two sets of valves within it and the acute angle with which it joins the subclavian vein. A guidewire with a flexible J-tip can be directed past the valves, bends, and branching vessels of the vein to increase the success rate of properly positioning CVCs.[23, 24]

Blitt and coworkers described external jugular vein cannulation with a 5.5- or 6-inch over-the-needle cannula.[23] However, a variation of this method using a modified Seldinger technique with a short over-the-needle cannula is less cumbersome and enables the clinician to insert a variety of catheters over the guidewire. Cannulation should only be attempted if the vein is easily visible or palpable. Applying pressure just above the clavicle may help to distend the vein. The patient's performance of a Valsalva maneuver or use of gentle hepatic pressure also distends the external jugular vein. After proper patient preparation, skin puncture is made slightly distal to the midpoint of the vein. The needle is advanced while the syringe is aspirated gently until free flow of venous blood is obtained. The short over-the-needle cannula is advanced off the needle into the vein, and the needle is then removed. Blood should be easily aspirated from the cannula prior to the insertion of the J-tipped guidewire. This may require some manipulation until free flow is obtained. Then the guidewire is advanced through the short cannula. If advancing the wire into the central circulation is difficult, the wire can be rolled between the thumb and the index finger while the wire is

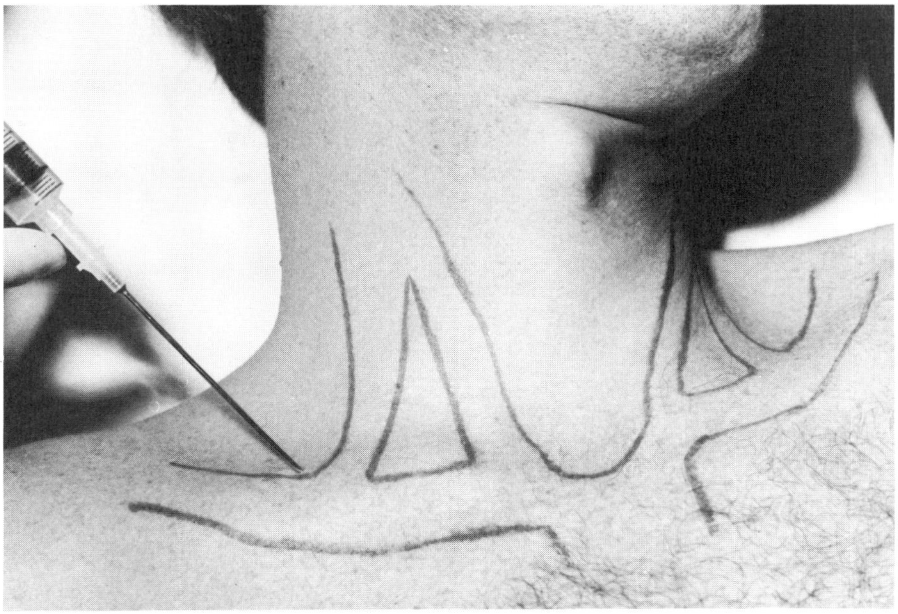

Figure 8–8. Supraclavicular approach to the subclavian vein.

moved in and out 1–2 cm. Once the guidewire is advanced into the central circulation, the short cannula is removed and the central catheter is inserted in the usual fashion.

The external jugular vein is a popular site for access to the central circulation, because it is associated with a low complication rate and a reasonably high success rate, and it is easily accessible to the anesthesiologist during an operation.[23, 25] Catheterization of the external jugular vein avoids the risks of inserting a needle deep into the neck and is safe for the patient with a bleeding diathesis or receiving anticoagulants. Pulmonary artery catheterization can be accomplished with this approach, although the large venous introducers occasionally cannot be successfully passed under the clavicle. At other times, the introducer cannot turn the acute angle as it enters the subclavian vein, causing kinking and precluding passage of the pulmonary artery catheter through it. One potential solution is to remove the introducer sheath slightly as the pulmonary artery catheter is advanced in the external jugular vein. Nevertheless, even in experienced hands, the rate of successful placement of CVCs and introducers is higher with the internal jugular and subclavian vein approaches than with the external jugular vein approach.

Femoral Vein

The femoral vein is used to gain access to the central circulation, provided the catheter is long enough to reach the mediastinal level of the vena cava. The femoral vein accompanies the femoral artery and becomes the external iliac vein, which flows into the inferior vena cava. The femoral vein is easily cannulated percutaneously in the femoral triangle just below the inguinal ligament. The major structures in the triangle, from lateral to medial, are the femoral nerve, femoral artery, femoral vein, and lymph tissue (Fig. 8–9). The structures are superficial, and the arterial pulse can be easily identified just below the inguinal ligament. Skin puncture is made about 1 cm medial to the arterial pulse with a straight thin-walled needle, directed slightly medially, parallel to the palpated pulse. Gentle aspiration is maintained with a syringe attached to the needle as it is advanced until free flow of venous blood is obtained. A guidewire is advanced through the needle. The chosen central catheter is then threaded over the wire in the usual fashion. The modified-Seldinger technique, consisting of a wire passed through a short over-the-needle cannula, can also be used for femoral vein access.

Catheterization of the femoral vein is simple and has a success rate of ≥90%.[26] However, femoral vein catheterization has been associated with a high incidence of complications. Deep vein thrombosis or thrombophlebitis occurs in 5–50% of cases, and pulmonary embolism occurs in approximately 2%.[27] Catheter-related infections have been reported in 0–20% of cases.[26–28] Therefore, it is recommended that catheterization of the femoral vein be avoided except for short-term use or in unusual circumstances.

Antecubital Veins

The antecubital veins are frequently cannulated owing to their size, ease of puncture, or limited access to the subclavian and jugular veins. In patients with increased intracra-

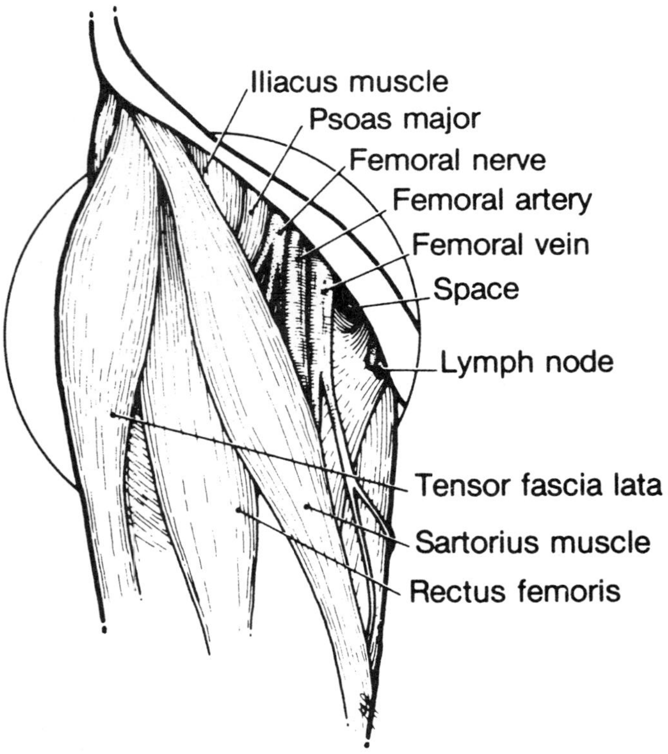

Figure 8–9. Anatomy of the femoral region. (From Otto CW: Central venous pressure monitoring. In Blitt CD (ed): Monitoring in Anesthesia and Critical Care Medicine, 2nd Ed. New York: Churchill Livingstone, 1990;205.)

nial pressure or severe coagulopathy, the antecubital veins may be the site of choice. In addition, the antecubital approach can be less stressful for the patient. However, the success rate for correct positioning within the central circulation is lower by this route than by other routes, though this will improve with the experience of the physician.[29]

The medial basilic vein is preferred over the more lateral cephalic vein because of the difficulty that may occur when the catheter is advanced through the shoulder region using the lateral cephalic vein (Fig. 8–10). A catheter-through-the-needle method is the common technique employed for basilic vein cannulation. Prepackaged, single-lumen devices, available in appropriate lengths, have a removable, flexible guidewire within the catheter for ease of insertion. The puncture site is prepared as described previously, a tourniquet is applied, and the needle puncture is made. Free flow of venous blood into the catheter is the best evidence that the needle is free within the vein. The tourniquet is removed, and the catheter is advanced through the needle. Any early resistance or early cessation of advancement suggests that the catheter is extraluminal or even located within the venous wall. The needle and catheter should be withdrawn, and a new puncture should be made. The catheter should not be withdrawn through the needle to avoid shearing and embolism of the catheter. Difficulty with continued advancement may occur at the shoulder region, particularly if the cephalic vein is used. Manipulating the arm by rotating, adducting, abducting, or straightening it often permits further advancement of the catheter tip. The catheter may also meet some resistance at the venous valves, which can be overcome with gentle manipulation of the catheter. Sometimes, the catheter passes into the ipsilateral internal jugular vein. The chance of this occurring can be reduced by turning the patient's head toward the side of the needle puncture.[30, 31] After insertion, care must be taken to fix the needle tip so that it cannot sever the catheter.

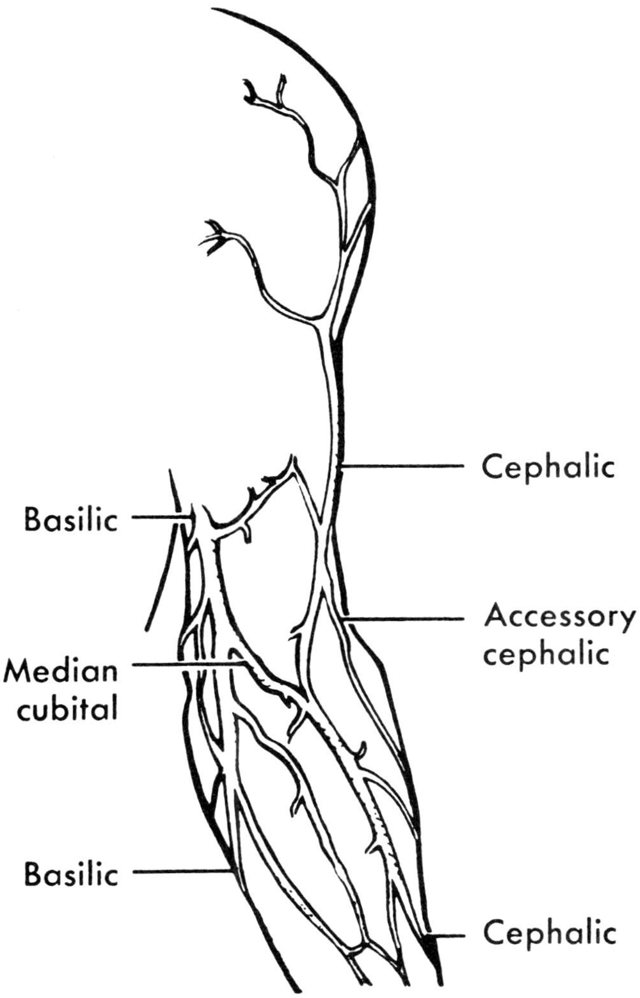

Figure 8–10. Anatomy of the antecubital fossa. (From Daily EK, Schroeder JS [eds]: Techniques in Bedside Hemodynamic Monitoring. St. Louis: CV Mosby, 1985;58.)

A modified Seldinger technique may also be utilized for inserting introducers when pulmonary artery catheterization is indicated. The site should be prepared as previously described, a tourniquet should be applied, and the vein should be punctured. Once free flow of blood is obtained in the syringe, the short cannula should be threaded off the needle and into the vein. A guidewire is passed and the introducer sheath is placed in the usual fashion.

Axillary Vein

The axillary vein can be catheterized in patients in whom other sites cannot be used. The patient is supine, the arm is abducted away from the patient's side, and the hand is placed behind the occiput. The axilla is shaved, if needed, and prepared as previously described. To avoid placement into the ipsilateral internal jugular vein, the head should face the puncture side during the procedure. The needle is inserted high in the axilla, 1 cm medial to the palpable axillary artery, at a 30° angle to the skin, and is directed parallel to the course of the artery toward the chest wall. Once venous access is obtained, catheter placement proceeds as previously described.

The axillary vein approach has a lower success rate and a higher incidence of catheter malpositioning and arterial puncture than the internal jugular and subclavian routes.[32–35] On the other hand, it carries a lower risk of pneumothorax than the internal jugular and subclavian routes. To limit the complications associated with axillary artery puncture, venous placement should be verified as previously described prior to placement of CVCs (''Internal Jugular Vein''). The axillary approach can be less stressful for the patient, and successful placement in the central circulation will improve with the experience of the operator.

CATHETER CARE AND POSITION

To prevent inadvertent removal or advancement of the catheter, it is sutured in place and taped securely. A sterile dressing with antimicrobial ointment is applied. Catheters intended for monitoring of central venous pressure should have a constant infusion source to maintain catheter patency. However, using a high-pressure bag with a continuous flush device risks fluid overload, particularly in children. It is recommended that a syringe or Harvard pump system be used to maintain catheter patency in infants and small children and that fluid infusions be controlled at 1 ml/hour. When pulmonary hypertension is present, a constant infusion of 2 ml/hour is recommended to maintain catheter patency. Anticoagulation of flush solutions with heparin is a personal decision, although an hourly infusion of 1 U of heparin should not cause coagulopathy.

A chest radiograph is always obtained following central venous catheterization to ascertain the position of the catheter tip and to check for pneumothorax and other complications. The proper position of a CVC depends on its purpose. For measurement of right ventricular filling pressures, a right atrial placement would be theoretically ideal. However, owing to the thinness of the atrial wall and its contractile movement, the risk of perforation and cardiac tamponade precludes long-term placement of catheters within the RA. Because the venous pressure in any of the intrathoracic veins reflects RA pressure,[36] the ideal location of a CVC placed for monitoring of CVP is within the SVC, just proximal to its entry into the RA. Locating this point on chest radiographs is difficult because the relationship between the SVC-RA junction and bony landmarks (clavicles, ribs, vertebral bodies) is not consistent. Rather, the SVC-RA junction can be identified on chest radiograph by the characteristic widening of the right mediastinal border at this point. In the operating room and other situations in which a chest radiograph is not practical, catheter position is verified by observation of the waveform and aspiration of blood through the lumen(s). RA placement can be minimized by estimating the correct length of catheter needed to reach the SVC-RA junction. Using a right internal jugular, right external jugular, and left subclavian approach, 15–20 cm of catheter is usually necessary to reach the SVC-RA junction. Using the left internal or external jugular approach requires 20–25 cm. Alternatively, patient height and site of placement can be correlated to ensure proper placement.[37]

Aspiration of air from a catheter placed in the RA establishes the diagnosis of venous air emboli (VAE) during surgical procedures. The ability to treat VAE and prevent cardiovascular collapse by aspirating large quantities of air is not as widely accepted, although multiorificed catheters are available for this purpose. Whether a catheter is intended to diagnose or to treat VAE, proper placement high in the RA at the SVC junction, where air tends to collect, is of paramount importance.[38, 39] Proper placement can be achieved by ECG control, radiographs, or pressure recordings. Using ECG control, single-orificed catheters can be placed relative to the SA node.[40] The catheters should be filled with a bicarbonate solution,[41] and the V lead should be attached to the proximal end of the catheter via a metal stopcock, hub, or guidewire. The other leads are attached at the standard four limb sites. The ECG derived from the distal tip of the catheter is observed as the catheter is advanced. The P wave develops a progressively more negative deflection as the catheter tip approaches the SA node, which is near the SVC-RA junction (Fig. 8–11).[42] The ECG recorded from a multiorificed catheter originates from a location proximal to the catheter tip, although controversial.[43–45] A multiorificed catheter should be advanced until the negative P wave develops a small positive deflection. The catheter is then withdrawn slightly to obtain a negative P wave again. This procedure ensures that most of the orifices are near the SVC-RA junction.[46]

MONITORING OF CVP IN PEDIATRIC PATIENTS

General Considerations

Invasive hemodynamic monitoring with central venous and pulmonary artery catheters has become routine in critically ill children for the diagnosis and management of hemodynamic problems. However, pediatric patients who require hemodynamic monitoring present a wide range of problems that are absent in the adult patient. The clinician must recognize the unique physiologic characteristics of children that make them different from adults (Table 8–4). These differences influence the choice of monitoring used, whether noninvasive or invasive. In addition, certain basic considerations should be understood. A child's small vascular lumen makes cannulation difficult. The quality of pressure tracings from small catheters inserted into these lumina are less than ideal. Blood loss occurring during the insertion procedure and during the sampling of central venous blood may account for a significant portion of a small infant's total blood volume. Fluid overload can occur quite insidiously in small children when continuous flush devices are used. Children are also more susceptible to infection, and sterile technique must be strictly maintained. The potential for paradoxical air embolus is real in children with

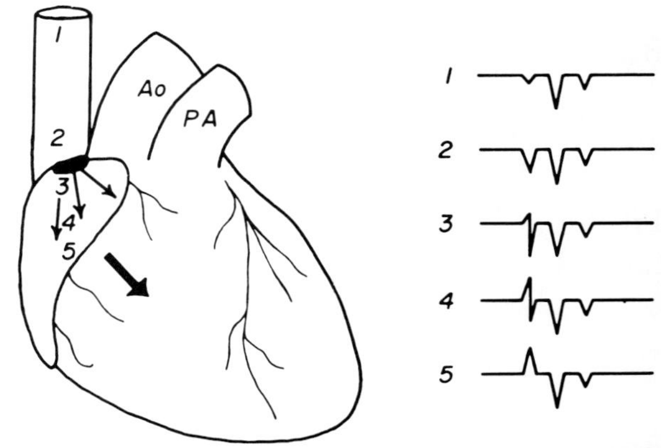

Figure 8–11. ECG tracings from the catheter tip in various locations. The P wave is initially negative and small (1). As the catheter tip approaches the SVC-RA junction, the P wave becomes progressively more negative (2). When the tip enters the RA, a small positive deflection can be seen (3). The P wave is large and biphasic in midatrium (4). A large positive P wave indicates low RA placement (5). (From Cucchiara RF, Messick JM, Gronert GG, Michenfelder JD: Time required and success rate of percutaneous right atrial catheterization. Can Anaesth Soc J 1980; 27:572.)

TABLE 8–4. COMPARISON OF PEDIATRIC AND ADULT HEMODYNAMIC VARIABLES

	Pediatric	Adult
Estimated Blood Volume	80 ml/kg	65 ml/kg
Heart Rate (Age-related)		
Infants	120–160 beats/minute	
	50–80 beats/minute	
Toddlers	90–140	
Preschoolers	80–110	
School-age children	75–100	
Adolescents	60–90	
Systemic Arterial Pressure (Age-related)		
Neonates	60–90/20–60 mmHg	
	90–140/60–90 mmHg	
Infants	74–100/50–70	
Toddlers	80–112/50–80	
Preschoolers	82–100/50–78	
School-age children	84–120/54–80	
Adolescents	94–140/62–80	
Stroke Volume		
Neonates	5 ml/beat	50–120 ml/beat
Preschoolers	15 ml/beat	
School-age children	35 ml/beat	
Cardiac Index	3.5–4 l/minute/m^2	2.5–4/minute/m^2
SVR	800–1600	
PVR	80–240	
RA Pressure	3 mmHg	5 mmHg
RA Pressure	30/3 mmHg	25/4 mmHg
RA Pressure	30/10 mmHg	25/12 mmHg
PCWP/LAP	8 mmHg	10 mmHg
LV Pressure	100/6 mm Hg	120/10 mmHg
Aortic Pressure	100/6 mmHg	120/80 mmHg

From Daily EK, Schroeder JS (eds): Techniques in Bedside Hemodynamic Monitoring. St. Louis: CV Mosby, 1985.

right-to-left shunts, and strict adherence to proven technique is necessary. Finally, children are usually unable to cooperate with central venous catheterization and require physical and pharmacologic restraints in order to maintain safe and sterile technique.

Physiology

As with normal adults, there is good correlation among CVP, PADP, and LVEDP in children. However, many situations invalidate this relationship. Severe pulmonary disease—such as neonatal respiratory distress syndrome and other forms of respiratory failure, the use of positive pressure ventilation at high pressures, cardiopulmonary bypass, hypothermia, and massive blood transfusion—alter the relationship between CVP and LVEDP. In addition, sepsis, hypoxemia, and acidosis increase pulmonary vascular resistance, which poses additional difficulties in monitoring left ventricular function. Although CVCs can be used for infusion of large volumes of fluid and vasoactive drugs, for the measurement of right-sided filling pressures, for parenteral alimentation, and for venous access, the use of pulmonary artery catheters for evaluation of LVEDP and cardiac function in small children and infants has gained wide acceptance.

Technique

Central venous access in pediatric patients is obtained by cutdown or percutaneously after induction of general anesthesia or administration of sedation. The most commonly used insertion sites are the femoral, internal jugular, subclavian, antecubital, and axillary veins, although CVCs can be placed in the umbilical vein in the newborn infant (Fig. 8–12). A wide variety of CVCs (including pulmonary artery catheters) can be inserted using the traditional or modified Seldinger technique.[47] The site is often determined by the experience of the physician.

Anatomic studies at autopsy in pediatric patients less than 1 year of age and 6 kg of weight suggest that the internal and external jugular veins should be considered for access into the central venous system because they enter the SVC with a straight course. The right and left subclavian veins appear to enter the central venous system at acute angles, which become less acute as the child grows.[48] Percutaneous access to the internal jugular vein can be obtained by either a high or a low approach.[49, 50] Success in either approach to the internal jugular vein is probably related more to the experience of the physician than to the choice of technique.

Some physicians prefer access to the central circulation of the child through an easily visualized external jugular vein. This avoids blind needle puncture in the neck and decreases the risk of pneumothorax from a subclavian vein approach. However, this must be weighed against the significant occurrence of improper positioning of the tip of the catheter within the central venous circulation. Success of proper intrathoracic position increases with the experience of the physician and the age of the child.[51, 52]

The infraclavicular approach to the subclavian vein is often preferred for long-term catheterization in children, although there is significant risk of pneumothorax, hydrothorax, and hemothorax.[52–54] The basilic vein has the advantages of being peripheral and easily visible or palpable. However, the success rate in reaching a central venous location is limited in small children. In children weighing over 20 kg, a removable guidewire within the prepackaged catheter, using a direct through-the-needle approach, can increase the rate of successful placement from the antecubital veins. Alternatively, the femoral vein provides a large vein that is easily identified in the femoral triangle. The axillary vein can also be used as an alternative access site in critically ill infants and children.[55]

COMPLICATIONS

The number of CVC-related problems is conservatively estimated to be as high as 10% of the approximately 3 million CVCs performed annually in the United States. Central venous catheterization should be performed only when the potential benefits appear to outweigh the risks of the procedure. Catheterization must be performed by

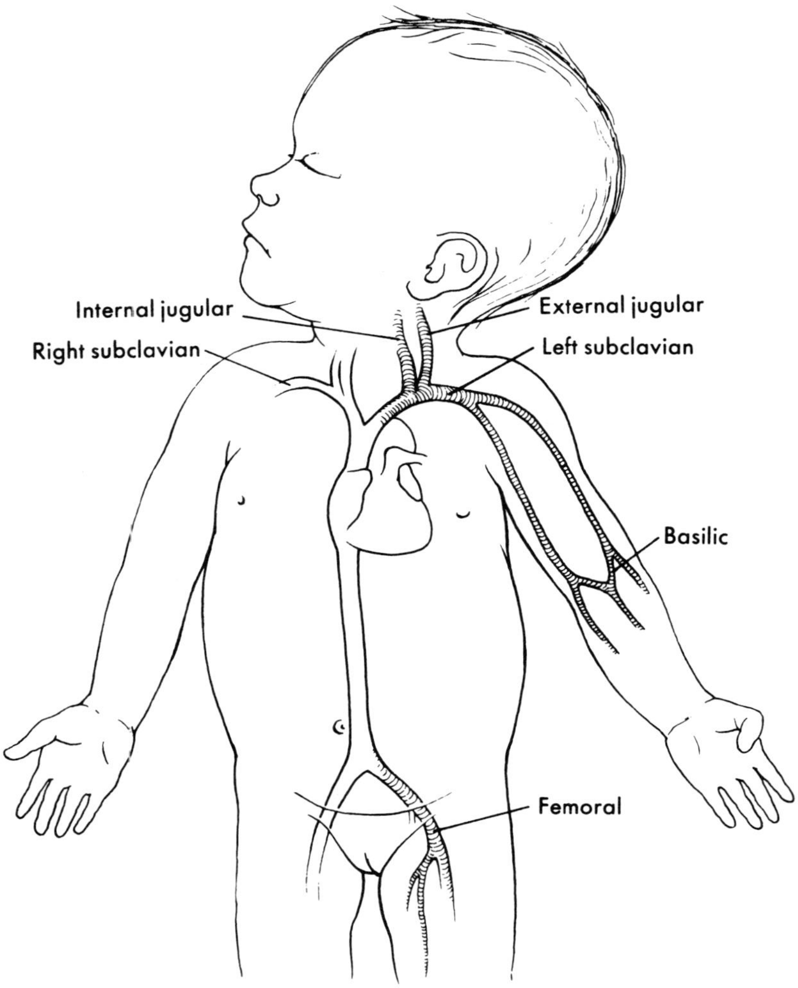

Figure 8–12. Commonly used sites for access to the central venous circulation in infants. (From Daily EK, Schroeder JS (eds): Techniques in Hemodynamic Monitoring. St. Louis: CV Mosby, 1985;146.)

trained personnel who are well versed in anatomic landmarks, safe technique, and potential complications. Users-in-training must be closely supervised by qualified personnel to ensure their technical expertise prior to independent performance of these procedures. Those placing CVCs should be familiar with the specific equipment used as well as the proper selection of insertion site and catheter type, size, and length. Those caring for patients with indwelling CVCs should be well informed of the appropriate care and associated complications of CVCs.

Erroneous Data

Calibrated Transducer Versus Water Manometer

Measurement of CVP can be done with a simple manometer filled with an isotonic aqueous solution or with a pressure transducer system having a high-frequency response. The saline manometers are more commonly reported in centimeters of water, which is converted to millimeters of mercury by dividing by 1.36 (1 mmHg = 1.36 cmH_2O). The zero point of the manometer or transducer must be positioned exactly if low venous pressures are to be measured accurately. The RA is usually considered the zero level, and it corresponds to the midaxillary line in the supine patient who has normal anatomy of the spine and thorax.

Although simple, water manometers have been replaced by more accurate, calibrated pressure transducers in the operating room and the intensive care unit. To obtain accurate CVP measurements, proper interpretation of the waveform must be made. Central venous waveforms obtained by electronic transducers show respiratory and cardiovascular fluctuations (Fig. 8–13). A digital display averages these fluctuations and gives inaccurate information if there are large intrapleural pressure changes with spontaneous or mechanical ventilation. Therefore, it is recommended that CVP waveforms be interpreted using a strip-chart recorder rather than a digital display.[56]

Alterations of the Central Venous Waveform

The normal central venous waveform is diagrammed in Figure 8–14. The best way to recognize waves is to look for descents or collapses. The first phase of the CVP waveform is the a wave. It corresponds to atrial contraction and comes just before the systolic collapse or x′ descent. A

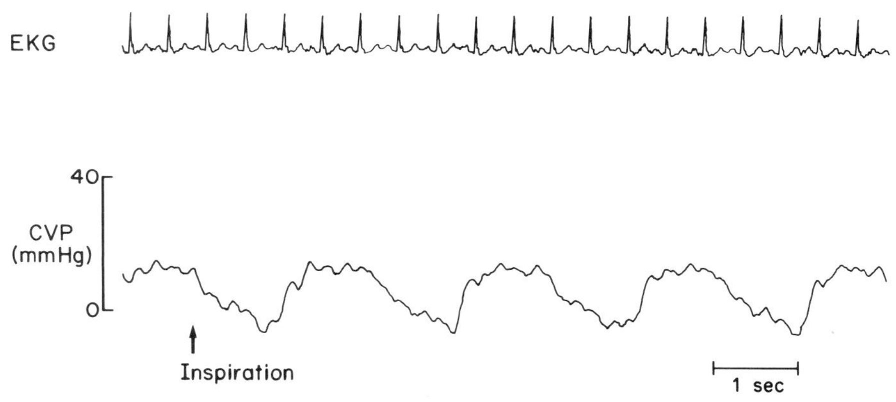

Figure 8–13. Large negative deflection in central venous pressure waveform with inspiration.

large a wave in sinus rhythm implies the presence of a stronger-than-normal right atrial contraction such as occurs with an obstruction at the tricuspid valve or with a stiff, noncompliant right ventricle. If the atrium contracts when the tricuspid valve is closed, atrial pressure is transmitted backward into the vena cava to form a large a wave, called a "cannon wave." Cannon waves occur with early p waves, such as with premature atrial depolarization, a junctional pacemaker, or atrioventricular dissociation. In atrial fibrillation, there is no atrial contraction and, therefore, no a wave.

The systolic collapse, or the x′ descent, is produced at midsystole as the right ventricle draws down the floor of the atrium. A poor right ventricular contraction, such as with right ventricular infarction or failure, may attenuate or even eliminate the x′ descent. Atrial fibrillation decreases the x′ descent owing to loss of the atrial kick and subsequent decreased ventricular volume. In the presence of tricuspid regurgitation, the RA fills during systole, and the regurgitant flow encroaches on the x′ descent. This is seen as a higher-than-normal v wave. Normally, the v wave occurs during late systole as the ventricular contraction is waning. The tricuspid valve is still closed, and flow from the vena cava into the RA is unimpeded. This increased flow is seen as the v wave. Therefore, any increased flow into the RA during ventricular systole, such as with atrial septal defects and tricuspid regurgitation, increases the size of the v wave. The v wave begins earlier in atrial fibrillation, and only a prominent y descent is seen on the CVP waveform. The final phase of the CVP trace is the diastolic collapse, or y descent. The y descent occurs with opening of the atrioventricular valves and ventricular filling.[57, 58]

Effects of Intrathoracic Pressure

Changes in the CVP occur with ventilation because changes in intrathoracic pressure are readily transmitted through the pericardium and relatively thin-walled atria and venae cavae. During spontaneous ventilation, inspiration lowers the CVP. All forms of positive pressure ventilation increase CVP, as does coughing or any Valsalva maneuver. To minimize the effects of respiration, CVP measurements are made at end-expiration using a calibrated pressure transducer and a strip-chart recorder.

Positive End-Expiratory Pressure

Positive end-expiratory pressure (PEEP) presents additional problems in interpreting CVP in critically ill patients. The application of PEEP to a patient's airway is transmitted to the central vascular structures and increases right atrial pressure, measured CVP, and intrapleural pressure. The increase in right atrial pressure decreases venous return, resulting in a decreased cardiac output, making interpretation of a high CVP and cardiac function difficult. Ideally, transmural right atrial pressure (intravascular right atrial pressure minus intrathoracic pressure) reflects the true filling pressure. PEEP causes a decreased true filling pressure with an increase in measured CVP.[59]

A possible solution is to temporarily remove the patient from PEEP to make hemodynamic measurements. However, the beneficial effects on gas exchange that PEEP pro-

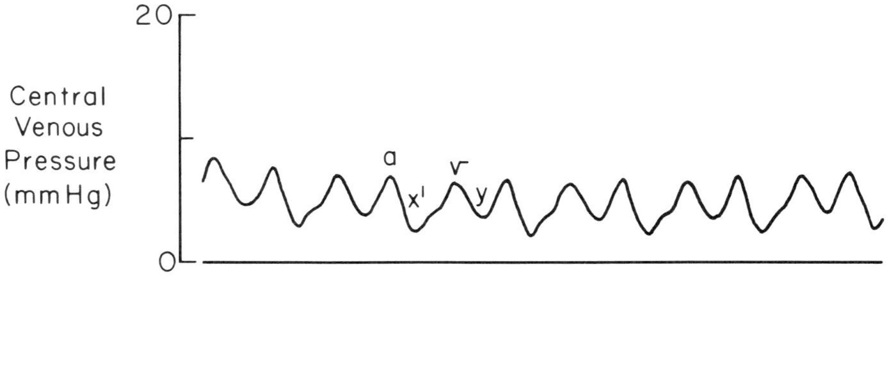

Figure 8–14. A normal central venous pressure waveform.

vides are quickly lost. When PEEP is reapplied, recovery of these benefits is prolonged. If PEEP is compromising cardiac output, temporary removal increases venous return and alters the patient's cardiovascular condition. Monitoring the patient in this way does not reflect his or her true hemodynamic state when PEEP is present. Therefore, it is recommended that the patient's cardiovascular performance be monitored when PEEP is present, recognizing that the CVP measurements obtained are slightly higher than those obtained without PEEP. It is important to emphasize that no predetermined number for CVP should be used in these situations, and that serial measurements combined with other signs of intravascular volume status should be used to assess the adequacy of tissue perfusion.

Physical Damage During Insertion of the Catheter

The potential for complications when inserting CVCs is related to needle injury of adjacent tissues and vessels. The most common injury is inadvertent arterial puncture, which carries an incidence of approximately 2%.[60] The potential for vascular injury is decreased with the initial use of a small (22-gauge) needle to locate the internal jugular vein. Few complications follow arterial puncture if the needle is immediately withdrawn and local pressure is applied. Inadvertent arterial puncture and some venous punctures can lead to localized hematoma formation. Observing the patient's vital signs should indicate more serious sequelae, such as pericardial tamponade from a subclavian artery puncture. The needle may also damage nerves at multiple sites, particularly the brachial plexus, stellate ganglion, and phrenic nerve. Inexperience with central venous catheterization procedures and poor attention to proper technique can lead to such complications.

Complications associated with the needle puncturing the pleura include pneumothoraces, hemothoraces, and chylothoraces. Mediastinal structures can be injured as well from the subclavian approach, resulting in pneumomediastinum, hemomediastinum, pneumopericardium, and pericardial tamponade.

Entry of a bolus of air into the venous system is a potentially fatal event associated with insertion of CVCs if the site of cannulation is above the level of the right atrium. Air embolism can also occur when intravenous tubing is changed or accidentally disconnected, or when the subcutaneous track fails to close immediately following removal of a catheter.[61] Even though introducer sheaths have one-way valves, these valves will become incompetent with time as catheters are left in place through them. In such situations, air can be entrained through the introducer if the indwelling catheter is removed. Proper attention to detail at insertion and meticulous care of CVCs prevent air embolism.

Plastic catheters are easily sheared off into the central circulation by traction on the beveled tip of the inserting needle. There are numerous reports of catheter shearing and inevitable cardiac embolization.[62–65] To avoid this complication, plastic catheters should be inserted with the distal beveled tip of the needle introducer facing the patient. Unsuccessful catheterization necessitates simultaneous withdrawal of the catheter and needle to avoid shearing. No attempts should be made to manipulate the catheter in and out through the insertion needle during catheter placement. If embolization to the heart occurs, the retained catheter fragments must be removed because of the problems of myocardial thrombi, recurrent episodes of sepsis, and cardiac arrhythmias. Catheter fragments can be removed by a variety of percutaneous transvenous techniques. If transvenous techniques using fluoroscopy are unsuccessful, a simple incision may suffice. For some heart fragments, cardiopulmonary bypass occasionally becomes necessary.[66, 67]

Improper Position of the Catheter

It is very important that the CVC tip be located properly at the SVC-RA junction for routine use. Catheters that enter small venous tributaries or the contralateral internal jugular or subclavian vein should be repositioned. Catheter tips located in the RA or right ventricle have been reported to perforate these chambers[68, 69] or cause arrhythmias.[70] Extravascular catheter tips can lead to hydrothorax, hemothorax, and hemomediastinum. Checking for free flow of venous blood from the catheter lumen aids early detection of extravascular locations.

Long-Term Complications

Late complications associated with central venous catheterization include infection, thrombosis, and perforation of vascular or cardiac structures.

Local and Systemic Infections

CVCs are important causes of nosocomial infections and sepsis. Contamination can occur at the time of insertion owing to poor sterile technique with secondary bacterial migration from the skin after catheter placement, from hematogenous spread from distant infected foci, or from infected intravenous fluids, tubings, or transducers. Once the catheter is colonized, it may become a nidus for disseminated infection, particularly in the seriously ill and immunocompromised. Identifying microbial colonization is a sensitive index of CVC-related infection, although historic, standard broth culture methods lack specificity. The specificity of CVC cultures improved when Maki and colleagues[71] developed a semiquantitative blood agar culture technique that distinguishes colonized catheters from contaminated catheters. The tip of a catheter is rolled on the agar. A positive semiquantitative culture ($>$15 colonies) denotes that the catheter is colonized. If the same organism is isolated from the blood, CVC-related bacteremia can be diagnosed. Other methods for the diagnosis of intravascular catheter-related infection include Gram's staining of the catheter[72] and an impression smear.[73] Scanning electron microscopy also reveals bacterial colonization.[74] These other techniques do not enjoy the widespread popularity of Maki's semiquantitiative technique.

The risk of CVC-related bacteremia is approximately 4%, as compared with the 1% risk for Teflon peripheral venous catheters.[75] Previous studies have suggested that most bloodstream infections related to intravascular devices originate from the patient's flora or from organisms on the hands of the personnel inserting the catheter.[76] At least two studies have demonstrated an association between the organisms present on the skin at the cannula insertion site and the organisms causing the bloodstream infection.[76, 77] Although rigorous aseptic measures preclude the introduction of organisms at the time of catheter insertion, additional measures, such as careful maintenance of sterile technique during dressing changes and the prudent use of an appropriate antimicrobial ointment, are needed to prevent the invasion of organisms into the wound site after catheter insertion. Coating CVCs with antibiotics has helped to reduce catheter-related infections.[16] A silver impregnated collagen cuff placed at the time of catheter insertion can significantly delay colonization and reduce the incidence of CVC-related bacteremia.[78]

Single-lumen catheters maintained for parenteral hyperalimentation have a low incidence of infection and are not regarded as requiring routine replacement.[79, 80] However, multilumen catheters used for monitoring and other purposes are controversial. The incidence of infection has been linked with the duration of catheterization, and many physicians routinely change CVCs every 3–4 days in spite of the fact that controlled, randomized trials have failed to demonstrate that scheduled replacements have any benefit in reducing catheter-related infections.[81, 82] Therefore, it is recommended that CVCs be placed with the use of aseptic procedures and remain in place until there is a clinical indication for change, such as fever without a known source or a catheter malfunction. Whether to replace a catheter with guidewire assistance or a new puncture site remains unclear. Certainly, when replacing malfunctioning catheters, guidewire assistance with semiquantitative culture of the initial catheter seems reasonable. In the presence of obvious site infection or when semiquantitative cultures are positive, a new puncture site is indicated.[82, 83]

Thrombophlebitis

Complications associated with the presence of CVCs include venous thrombosis and thrombophlebitis. Most patients with thrombosis display edema of the involved arm, neck, and face. Infrequently, the first sign of central vein thrombosis is inability to catheterize a previously cannulated vein. No other symptoms may be present. An unknown source of sepsis may be the presenting sign of central vein thrombosis after secondary colonization with bacteria or fungi.

When there is central vein thrombosis, microembolization and significant pulmonary embolization can occur.[84, 85] If the clinical situation indicates pulmonary embolism, thrombosis of the central veins should be suspected, and venograms should be considered. Treatment of central vein thrombosis requires removal of the catheter, culturing of the tip, and initiation of intravenous heparin therapy. Local symptoms should resolve in 24–48 hours, although eventual recannulation of the vein is difficult to document.

MONITORING OF PULMONARY ARTERY AND CAPILLARY WEDGE PRESSURES

When used judiciously, pulmonary artery catheters assist in the management of critically ill patients by allowing bedside determination of left ventricular filling pressure and cardiac output. However, the enthusiasm for invasive central monitoring that arose in the 1970s and early 1980s has been tempered by the recognition of multiple associated complications, such as ventricular arrhythmias, pulmonary artery rupture, pulmonary infarction, and systemic or local infections. Therefore, a pulmonary artery catheter is only indicated when the data obtained will improve therapeutic decision making without unnecessary risk.

The pulmonary artery catheter measures CVP, PAP, and PCWP. It is balloon-tipped, allowing bedside placement without the aid of fluoroscopy. Pulmonary artery systolic, diastolic, and mean pressures are easily determined with pulmonary artery catheters. Measurement of PADP is used to estimate LVEDP. At the end of diastole, the pulmonary arteries, pulmonary veins, left atrium, and left ventricle form a single chamber with a small pressure gradient in the direction of flow. When the pulmonary vascular bed, mitral valve, and left ventricle function normally, PADP, PCWP, mean left atrial pressure, and LVEDP are approximately equal.[86–88]

The distal thermistor can be utilized for the rapid determination of cardiac output using the thermodilution method. Numerous other parameters, such as cardiac index, systemic and pulmonary vascular resistances, and ventricular function curves, can be derived from these data. The catheter can be used to sample mixed venous blood, allowing determination of physiologic intrapulmonary shunting, oxygen consumption, and lactate levels. Finally, the pulmonary artery can be used for the administration of medications likely to cause phlebitis in the peripheral vasculature or that must be directed in a concentrated form into the heart or great vessels.

PCWP

Although measurement of CVP is valuable in determining right ventricular preload, in evaluating right ventricular dysfunction in right ventricular infarcts, and in diagnosing cardiac tamponade, CVP has limited value in assessing left ventricular hemodynamics. Studies in a variety of clinical settings have demonstrated a poor correlation between right and left atrial filling pressures.[89, 90] In order to look at LVEDP, one of its correlates, PCWP[91] or PADP,[92] is used as a better estimate of left-sided preload.

Equating PCWP with left atrial pressure assumes an open circuit from the catheter tip to the left atrium with minimal pressure gradients. This is not the case if the catheter is located in West's zone I or II in the pulmonary vascular tree, where alveolar pressure is greater than arterial pressure (zone I) or venous pressure (zones I and II) (Fig. 8–15).[93]

In zone III, where both pulmonary arterial and venous pressures exceed alveolar pressure, there is continuous flow, and conditions are met for accurate measurement of PCWP. Fortunately, most of the lung enters zone III when the patient is supine, and most pulmonary artery catheters float into zone III because most of the blood is flowing into this zone.[94] However, during low-flow states, such as hypovolemia[95] or when PEEP increases alveolar pressure above pulmonary venous pressure, zone III may be converted to zone II. If the tip of the catheter is at or below the left atrium, the conditions in zone III exist even if PEEP values are as high as 30 cm H_2O.[96] A cross-table lateral chest radiograph will aid in confirming the location of the catheter tip relative to the left atrium when its position is in doubt.[96, 97] If the tip is above the atrium, the catheter should be repositioned to ensure zone III placement.

Effects of Ventilatory Mode

Transmural distending pressure determines ventricular inflow and stroke volume and is equal to the difference between intravascular pressure and extravascular pressure. In the majority of pulmonary blood vessels, extravascular pressure is atmospheric; therefore, when a measurement from a pulmonary artery catheter is referenced to atmospheric pressure, the recorded intravascular pressure equals the transmural pressure. If the extravascular pressure becomes positive, as with positive pressure ventilation, transmural pressure is reduced by the amount of extravascular pressure. Negative extravascular pressure, as with spontaneous ventilation, increases transmural pressure and tends to dilate the pulmonary blood vessels and to increase flow. In both situations, transmural pressure is not reflected by the measured intravascular pressure. The solution is to measure the PADP and PCWP at end-expiration when extravascular pressure is closest to atmospheric pressure. This ensures that pulmonary vascular pressures are not influenced by changes in pleural pressure. Measurements are made manually using a strip-chart recorder or from a calibrated screen so that the expiratory phase can be identified.

There are additional problems due to PEEP-induced changes in vascular and pleural pressures. As discussed previously, when positive pressure is applied to the airway at end-expiration, the increased alveolar pressure can convert a zone III to a zone II or I. In addition, PEEP alters pleural pressure and intravascular pressures.[59] The amount of pressure transmitted to the pleural space and intrathoracic vessels depends on the level of PEEP and the compliance of the lungs and chest wall. A stiff, noncompliant lung does not transmit as much airway pressure to intrathoracic vessels as a noncompliant lung. As long as the pulmonary artery catheter is maintained at zone III, the measured intravascular PCWP approximates left atrial pressure. In fact, one study reports that PEEP up to 30 cmH_2O does not markedly affect intravascular pressures in patients with very poor lung compliance.[98] The understanding is that the stiffer

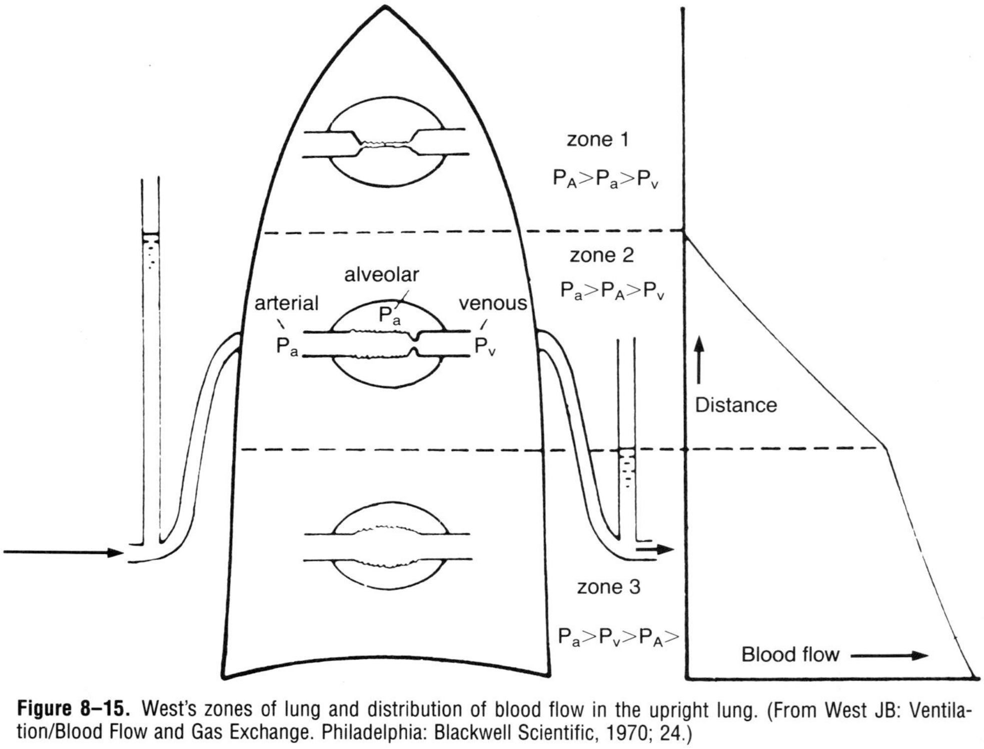

Figure 8–15. West's zones of lung and distribution of blood flow in the upright lung. (From West JB: Ventilation/Blood Flow and Gas Exchange. Philadelphia: Blackwell Scientific, 1970; 24.)

the lungs, the less the transmitted pressure. When high levels of PEEP are used in compliant lungs, more pressure is transmitted to the vessels, making interpretation of pressure measurements quite difficult.

One potential solution to this problem is to disconnect the patient from the ventilator and measure all the pressures referenced to atmospheric pressure at end-expiration. This is not always safe and is not recommended. The second solution is to place a pulmonary artery catheter in zone III of the lung and to keep the level of PEEP below 10 cmH_2O. If the PEEP level is higher, the measured vascular pressures may increase 1–2 mmHg for every 5 cm of PEEP applied above 10 cmH_2O.[94] Thus, although a PCWP of 20 mmHg in a patient breathing spontaneously would be associated with interstitial pulmonary edema, it may be an acceptable value in a patient receiving PEEP at 20 cmH_2O. The third alternative is to directly measure intrapleural pressure as a means of assessing the transmural pressure gradient.[99] This can be accomplished by inserting a catheter into the pleural space or by using an esophageal balloon. See Chapter 12.

Effects of Cardiac Pathology

Left atrial pressure and PCWP is not equal to LVEDP in the presence of mitral valve disease or markedly reduced ventricular compliance.[86, 92, 93] Additionally, LVEDP itself does not always reflect left ventricular end-diastolic volume.[1] Increased LVEDP in a normal ventricle may be associated with a normal end-diastolic volume in a stiff, noncompliant ventricle. This poor correlation between PCWP and left ventricular end-diastolic volume is present in many critically ill patients, demonstrating the heterogeneity of myocardial compliance in the septic shock syndrome, ischemic heart disease, and hemorrhagic shock.[100–102] In such settings, the absolute measurement of PCWP is less helpful and construction of ventricular function curves and the trending of data better assess tissue perfusion.

Pulmonary Hypertension

Jenkins and coworkers[103] and Scheinman and coworkers[104] correlated PADP to left atrial pressure in patients with heart disease but normal pulmonary vascular resistance. When pulmonary vascular resistance is abnormal, as with pulmonary hypertension, this correlation is lost. Increased pulmonary vascular resistance is usually associated with increased PAP and right ventricular afterload. This contributes to right ventricular failure and an increase in CVP as well. Despite these changes, left atrial pressure remains in the normal range. Thus, in the presence of pulmonary hypertension, one must determine PCWP and not use PADP as an approximation of LVEDP.[88, 92]

The pulmonary artery catheter can aid in diagnosing pulmonary hypertension and evaluating intracardiac pressures. The administration of vasoactive drugs directly into the right-sided heart chamber or pulmonary vasculature can be guided by the hemodynamic information obtained during pharmacologic intervention.

CLINICAL USES

Cardiac Surgery

Pulmonary artery catheters are used in the perioperative management of patients with compromised ventricular function undergoing valve replacement, coronary artery bypass grafting, resection of ventricular aneurysms, and repair of congenital heart defects. The accurate reflection of left- and right-sided preload and the rapid determination of cardiac output by the thermodilution technique permit mechanical and pharmacologic therapy to optimize cardiac function and tissue perfusion in the perioperative period. Balloon-tipped 7-, 7.5-, or 8-F thermodilution catheters are inserted percutaneously in adults and advanced into the pulmonary artery by continuous pressure monitoring preoperatively. In the presence of mitral regurgitation, large v waves are seen (Fig. 8–16).

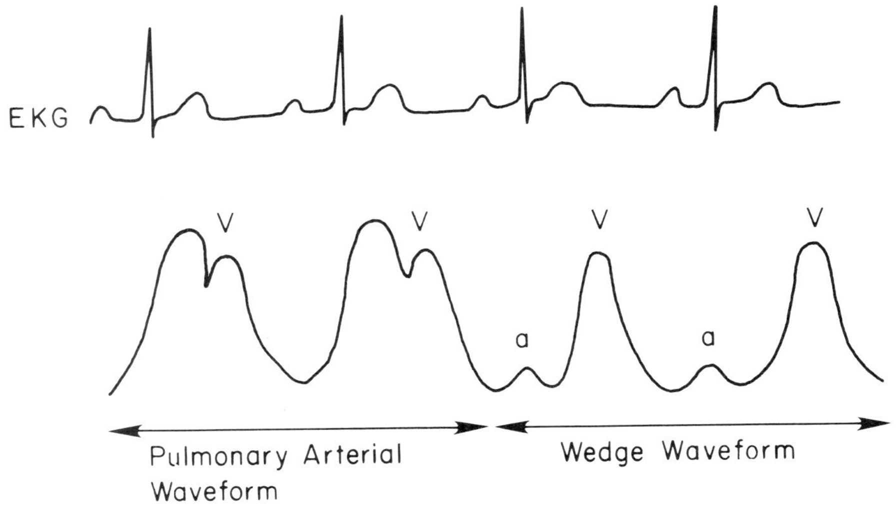

Figure 8–16. Presence of a large V wave with mitral regurgitation. (From Nadeau S, Noble WH: Misinterpretation of pressure measurements from the pulmonary artery catheter. Can Anaesth Soc J 1986; 33:352.)

Thermodilution catheters without balloon tips may be inserted directly into the RA during cardiac surgical procedures. This technique is applicable to pediatric patients or to patients with disease of tricuspid or pulmonic valves.

General Surgery

Induction of anesthesia, endotracheal intubation, and other circumstances associated with marked alteration in left ventricular afterload or blood volume represent periods of intense stress to the surgical patient. Extensive surgical procedures, such as large abdominal resections and transurethral prostatic resections, are associated with changes in blood volume that may be poorly tolerated in patients with prior myocardial infarction, angina pectoris, or pulmonary hypertension. Accurate assessment of volume status and cardiac performance is especially helpful in elderly patients or in patients with severe cardiac or pulmonary disease. Vascular procedures, such as surgery for resection of thoracic or abdominal aortic aneurysms and hepatic transplantation, are facilitated by perioperative control of preload and cardiac output to limit the cardiac and renal complications associated with these procedures. Prolonged orthopedic procedures, debridement and grafting of severe burns, and surgery for multitrauma may indicate the need for invasive hemodynamic monitoring with a pulmonary artery catheter.

Intensive Care Units

Hemodynamic Monitoring

The flow-directed, balloon-tipped catheter is commonly employed in intensive care units for patients with septic shock, multisystem organ failure, instability during hemodialysis, intra-aortic balloon counterpulsation, and vasoactive drug therapy. Pulmonary artery catheterization has not been shown to decrease mortality in the critically ill, although it provides data useful for diagnosis and therapy. Pulmonary artery catheters distinguish cardiogenic from noncardiogenic pulmonary edema and guide treatment in patients with adult respiratory distress syndrome, pulmonary embolus, cor pulmonale, fat embolism syndrome, and acute renal failure.

A pulmonary artery catheter guides preload and afterload therapy in patients with severe congestive heart failure or unstable angina. Constrictive pericarditis or cardiac tamponade due to a variety of causes is effectively recognized by the near equality of right atrial pressure, right ventricular diastolic pressure, PADP, and PCWP. Acute bacterial endocarditis and congestive cardiomyopathy are additional indications for hemodynamic monitoring in the intensive care unit.

Patients with acute myocardial infarction complicated by perforated ventricular septum, mitral regurgitation, severe pulmonary congestion, or cardiogenic shock benefit from invasive hemodynamic monitoring.[105, 106] When clinical shock follows acute myocardial infarction, the short-term mortality and morbidity rates are reduced from 85–90% to 50% or less with measurement of PAPs.[107] In contrast to these findings, a community-wide study of patients with acute myocardial infarction failed to demonstrate a decrease in hospital stay or mortality rate when a pulmonary artery catheter was used to manage patients with congestive heart failure, hypotension, or cardiogenic shock.[108] The question of whether or not pulmonary artery catheterization benefits patients with acute myocardial infarction remains unresolved.[109]

Sampling of Mixed Venous Blood

The capability of obtaining true mixed venous blood from the distal port of the pulmonary artery catheter for analysis of oxygen consumption, intrapulmonary shunt fraction, arterial minus mixed venous oxygen content difference, and lactate levels is an advantage of the pulmonary artery catheter over simple CVCs. Although the partial pressure of oxygen in the SVC of normal persons is close to the true mixed venous partial pressure, it is much higher in patients in shock because blood flow is redistributed away from the renal and splanchnic beds. Blood from the inferior vena cava is also a poor reflection of true mixed venous oxygen tension ($P\bar{v}O_2$) because of the large nonmetabolic blood flow from the kidneys. Use of blood from the RA for determination of $P\bar{v}O_2$ also may yield an inaccurate measurement because there may be inadequate mixing of the three sources of mixed venous blood (the inferior vena cava, SVC, and coronary sinus) in the atrium.

Because the true $P\bar{v}O_2$ reflects the difference between the oxygen delivered and the oxygen consumed, it is important to obtain an accurate sample in the critically ill patient to assess the adequacy of perfusion. The normal $P\bar{v}O_2$ is 40 mmHg. Because of regional difference in blood flow, a normal $P\bar{v}O_2$ does not necessarily indicate adequate perfusion in each organ system. This is especially evident in patients with multisystem organ failure associated with adult respiratory distress syndrome,[110] although it is safe to say that the finding of a reduction in mixed venous oxygen does suggest poor tissue oxygenation. A decreased $P\bar{v}O_2$ is found whenever the oxygen delivery system fails, whether from decreased arterial oxygen saturation, decreased hemoglobin, or decreased cardiac output. For instance, in patients with congestive heart failure, the mixed venous oxygen content declines and decreases further with the onset of cardiogenic shock as the myocardial pump fails.[111] A reduction in $P\bar{v}O_2$ also occurs when there are increased tissue requirements for oxygen, such as with sepsis, severe burns, and seizures.

A fiberoptic flow-directed thermal dilution pulmonary artery catheter capable of continuously monitoring the mixed venous saturation is available. These catheters have gained acceptance for the management of hemodynamically unstable patients.[112]

Myocardial Ischemia

Left ventricular ischemia decreases left ventricular compliance, increasing LVEDP, left atrial pressure, PCWP, and PADP. When the myocardium is ischemic and noncompliant, the PCWP waveform reveals a large a wave during atrial contraction. Although an increase in PCWP once was considered an indication of myocardial ischemia, later studies failed to document an association between increased PCWP and myocardial ischemia noted by ECG or wall motion abnormalities.[113, 114] Elevated PCWP is relatively insensitive and may be *either* impaired diastolic relaxation or impaired systolic contraction. Haggmark and coworkers confirmed that an elevated PCWP with a normal waveform did not predict intraoperative ischemia as determined by ECG or cardiokymography. However, there was an association between elevated PCWPs and an abnormal waveform. Only 13% of recorded PCWPs were associated with an abnormal waveform, and these coincided with only 19% of the intraoperative ischemic events.[113] In 98 patients undergoing coronary grafting, Van Daele and coworkers noted very low sensitivity and positive predictive value for increased PCWP.[114] The usefulness of PCWP was not increased by testing different increments of PCWP change. Although ischemia impairs diastolic ventricular relaxation and increases LVEDP, it is not reflected in the mean diastolic pressure of PCWP.

Finally, Kaul and coworkers determined that ischemic mitral regurgitation causing V waves on PCWP is not due to either papillary muscle dysfunction or dysfunction of peripapillary muscle myocardium.[115] Mitral regurgitation occurs only with global left ventricular dysfunction rather than papillary muscle dysfunction, and its severity is inversely related to ventricular function.[115]

Measurement of Thermodilution Cardiac Output

The modification of the pulmonary artery catheter by Forrester and associates permits multiple and rapid determinations of cardiac output in the operating room and intensive care unit via the thermodilution technique.[116] The technique employs a known amount of sterile solution of known temperature, usually 3–10 ml of 0°C or room temperature 5% dextrose. The indicator is injected into the RA, and the resultant change in blood temperature is measured in the pulmonary artery by the distal thermistor. By integrating the temperature change over time, cardiac output is computed. Care must be taken to assure rapid injection, complete indicator mixing, and no indicator loss. Once cardiac output data are determined, ventricular function curves can be made and used to assess ventricular performance while evaluating therapies. If intracardiac shunts and tricuspid regurgitation are present, the method is not accurate, in which case indicator dye dilution or other techniques must be used. Refer to the appropriate cardiac output computer manual for specific instructions on the use of thermodilution catheters for cardiac output determination (see also Chapter 10). In addition to cardiac output, systemic and pulmonary vascular resistance and other hemodynamic variables are easily calculated (see Table 10–3).

INSERTION TECHNIQUE

Choice of Catheter

The standard no. 7-F thermodilution pulmonary artery catheter is 110 cm in length and contains four lumina: a distal pulmonary artery port, a proximal central venous port, a balloon inflation port, and a thermistor connector (Fig. 8–17). It is constructed of flexible, radiopaque polyvinylchloride.

The quadruple-lumen catheter comes in two sizes: nos. 5 and 7 F. The no. 5-F size is suitable for children under 18 kg, whereas the no. 7-F size is suitable for larger children and adults.[117] Both have proximal and distal ports and an inflatable balloon of 1.5-ml capacity. The fourth lumen supports the wiring to the thermistor located near the tip. Proper use of the 5-F catheter requires an understanding of the differences between the two sizes. The smaller catheter does not allow rapid infusion of fluids, which would falsely elevate pressure readings. Its use in small infants is difficult because of the distance between the proximal and the distal ports. Although the tip may be placed appropriately in the pulmonary artery, the proximal port may lie outside the internal jugular vein. For such infants, nos. 2.5- and 3.5-F double-lumen thermodilution catheters, consisting of a vascular lumen and thermistor, are available. (Fig. 8–18). They can be used in children under 10 kg of weight for the measurement of cardiac output, with the separate insertion of a right atrial catheter for cardiac output injectates.[118, 119] These nonballoon thermodilution catheters are inserted directly into the RA and pulmonary artery at the time of cardiac surgery.[120] Such catheters are also used in adults who have disease of tricuspid or pulmonic valves.

In addition to the standard no. 7-F thermodilution pulmonary artery catheter, no. 7.5-F catheters with one or two extra venous infusion ports are available. These catheters are helpful when managing critically ill patients who are receiving numerous vasoactive infusions or parenteral hyperalimentation, though their small lumen size can limit the rate of infusion. Pulmonary artery catheters with an oximeter are available with an extra venous infusion port.

Choice of Site

Catheterization of the pulmonary circulation is accomplished from subclavian, internal jugular, external jugular, femoral, antecubital, or axillary veins. In general, insertion into the internal jugular vein is preferred, because this approach is associated with a lower incidence of pneumothorax than insertion into the subclavian vein.[110, 111] The internal jugular vein is readily available to the anesthesiologist, allowing intraoperative manipulation of the catheter if necessary. Pulmonary artery catheters are easier to secure in the neck or subclavian area than in the antecubital fossa

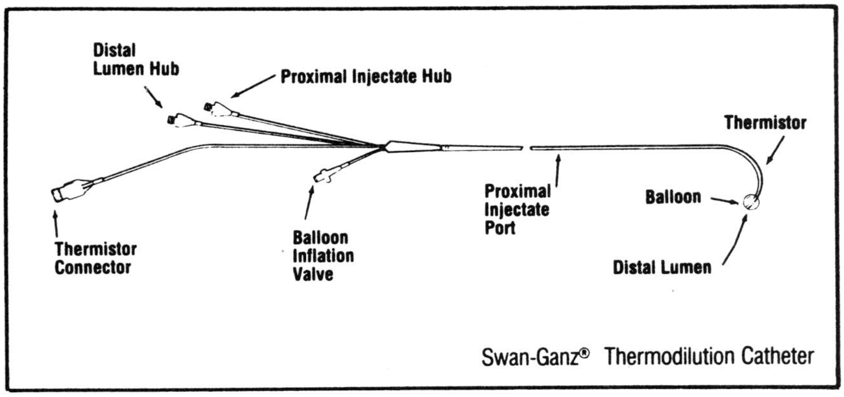

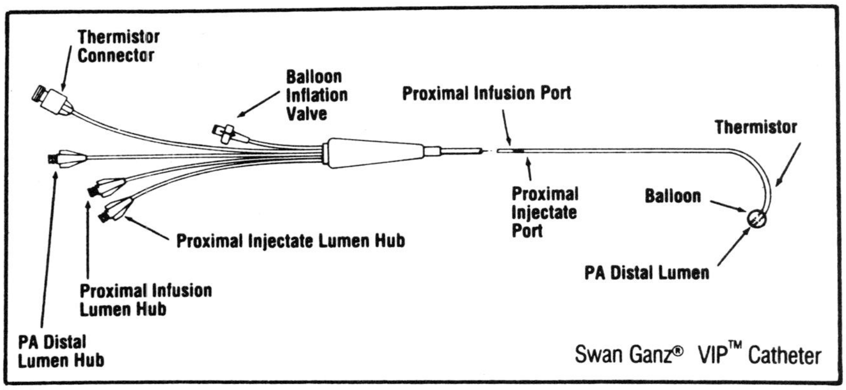

Figure 8–17. Four- and five-lumen balloon-tipped pulmonary artery catheters. (Courtesy of Baxter Healthcare Corp., Edwards Critical Care Division, Irvine, CA.)

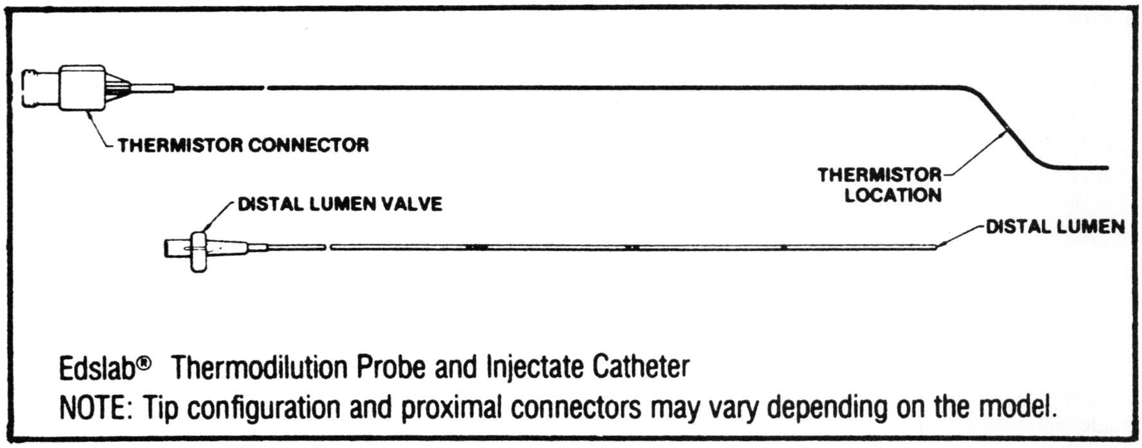

Figure 8–18. Non–balloon-tipped pulmonary artery catheter and separate injectate catheter. (Courtesy of Baxter Healthcare Corp., Edwards Critical Care Division, Irvine, CA.)

and are less likely to become malpositioned by patient movement. The antecubital fossa or femoral vein are preferred sites in patients with a bleeding diathesis in order to avoid hemorrhage associated with accidental carotid or subclavian artery puncture. The use of the external jugular vein is limited by the sharp angle the vein makes with the subclavian vein, which can lead to kinking of the introducer sheath or catheter.

Placement Technique

Pulmonary artery catheters can be inserted after preparation of the patient as previously described for CVC placement. It is essential to decrease the patient's pain, anxiety, and myocardial stimulation with appropriate sedatives and analgesics. Pressure transducers are zeroed and calibrated. The catheter's injectate and pressure monitoring lumina are debubbled and connected to the flush system and pressure transducers. The patency of the balloon is checked prior to insertion. Continuous ECG monitoring is used to evaluate any arrhythmias that occur during insertion. Antiarrhythmic drugs, defibrillating equipment, and respiratory-assist equipment should be readily available. Catheters should not be bent, stretched, or wiped excessively (which can remove the heparin coating) during preparation.

The catheter is usually inserted through an introducer sheath that is one size larger than the pulmonary artery catheter. Prepackaged trays containing the necessary supplies for both venous cannulation and placement of nos. 8-, 8.5-, and 9-F introducers are available. After successful catheterization of the central veins, the pulmonary artery catheter is inserted into the introducer and advanced while the pressure and waveform of the distal port are observed (Fig. 8–19). After the catheter enters the central circulation (usually a distance of 20–30 cm from jugular or subclavian entry), the balloon is fully inflated and advanced into the RA. Venous entry at the right arm requires about 40 cm, at the left arm 50 cm, and at the femoral vein 60 cm to reach the RA. Only the recommended volume of air, never liquid, should be used for balloon inflation. The catheter length necessary to reach the RA can be initially measured by noting the length from the insertion site to the sternal manubrium.

The catheter floats across the tricuspid valve through the right ventricle, across the pulmonic valve, and into the pulmonary artery, verified by the waveform. The catheter is advanced into the pulmonary artery with the balloon inflated until the pressure waveform appears "damped" and the numeric display records a pressure that is less than the PAP. This represents the PCWP. If deflation of the balloon does not restore the pulmonary artery waveform, the catheter has been inserted too far and should be withdrawn slowly until a pulmonary artery waveform returns. The catheter is then secured in place at the insertion site and protected by a sterile dressing. A chest radiograph confirms proper placement of the catheter.

It is important not to use an excessive length of pulmonary artery catheter during insertion. If the right ventricle pressure waveform is still observed after advancing the catheter 15 cm beyond the point that the initial right ventricle pressure was observed, the catheter may be looping in the ventricle, which can result in kinking or knotting of the catheter. If insertion is unsuccessful initially, the balloon is deflated, the catheter is withdrawn to the right atrial position, and insertion begins anew. Failure of a balloon-tipped pulmonary artery catheter to enter the right ventricle or pulmonary artery is rare but can occur in patients with an enlarged RA or ventricle, low cardiac output, tricuspid insufficiency, or pulmonary hypertension. Deep inspiration by the patient during advancement may facilitate passage. Fluoroscopic guidance for placement should be required only rarely. At no time should force be used during insertion, because this may damage the catheter lumina.

PEDIATRIC PULMONARY ARTERY CATHETERIZATION

Flow-directed pulmonary artery catheters are employed in critically ill pediatric patients to monitor left and right ventricular preload.[117, 121–123] Measurement of cardiac output by the thermodilution technique is reliable in children over a wide range of flow values.[124, 125]

Indications for pulmonary artery catheters in infants and children include (1) assessment of right ventricular preload and tricuspid valve adequacy by monitoring the CVP, (2) assessment of left ventricular function and adequacy of

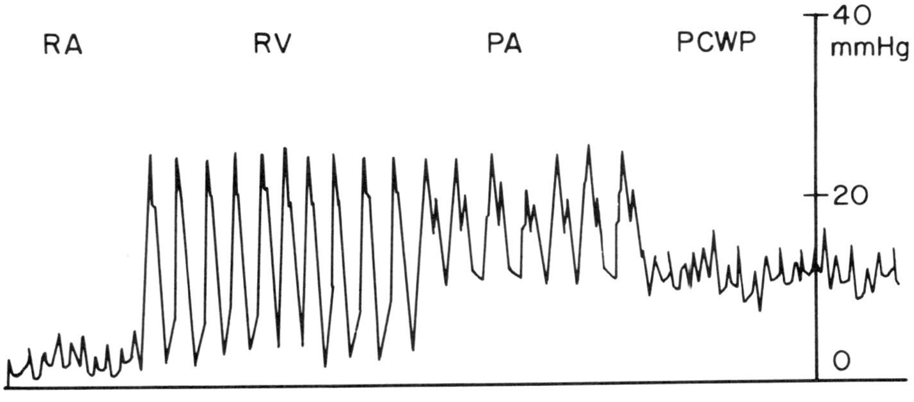

Figure 8–19. Pressure tracing obtained from a balloon-tipped pulmonary artery catheter during insertion. (From Wiedemann HP, Matthay MA, Matthay RA: Cardiovascular-pulmonary monitoring in the intensive care unit (Part I). Chest 1984; 85:540.)

mitral valve function by monitoring the PADP and PCWP, (3) assessment of pulmonary blood flow and resistance, (4) measurement of cardiac output, (5) assessment of systemic vascular resistance, and (6) measurement of mixed venous oxygen tension.

Cannulating the central circulation in infants and children is difficult and requires a high degree of vigilance to maintain catheter position and patency. As in CVCs, pulmonary artery catheters require only 1 ml/hour delivery of fluid to maintain patency that should be delivered by syringe or Holter pump. If pulmonary pressures exceed 50 mmHg, a constant infusion of 2 ml/hour maintains patency. If the pulmonary artery pressures are greater than 100 mmHg, an infusion rate of 3 ml/hour is needed.[126]

The same sterile technique and precautions (e.g., continuous ECG and pressure monitoring) employed in adult patients are employed in children. Common insertion sites include the internal and external jugular veins, subclavian vein, basilic vein, and femoral vein. After the introducer is inserted, the pulmonary artery catheter is passed. Air is normally used to inflate the balloon, but the risk of air embolism in patients with intracardiac shunts may be reduced by the use of carbon dioxide.

COMPLICATIONS OF PULMONARY ARTERY CATHETERIZATION

Since the introduction of the pulmonary artery catheter for continuous monitoring of hemodynamic function, numerous complications related to both insertion and the presence of the catheter in the pulmonary artery have been reported.

Erroneous Data

Equipment

The pressure transducer must be calibrated in the range of PAPs rather than systemic pressures and zeroed at the level of the mid left atrium. If the patient's position changes, the transducer should be repositioned to obtain accurate data.

The discrepancy between automated digital and analog (strip-chart) recording systems may be therapeutically misleading because of the unselective nature of averaging values with digital readout (see Chapter 6).[127] In a patient with respiratory variability (as in asthma, chronic obstructive pulmonary disease, or positive-pressure ventilation with high-peak inspiratory pressures), the pulmonary pressures are subject to considerable alteration. The errors in automated pressure measurement believed to be clinically important vary with the ventilatory mode used. Patients breathing spontaneously have the largest measurement error: 42% of these patients have a clinically important error in PADP. Patients on assist/control modes have the fewest errors in automated pressure measurements.[128]

Because graphic data can be correlated to changes in intrathoracic pressure and end-expiration can be identified, it is prudent to measure pulmonary vascular pressures with an analog recording system. Pressures are read directly from a calibrated screen or printout rather than from a digital readout.[129] In a patient with rapid respiration, identifying the end-expiratory point may be difficult, and a simultaneous tracing of airway pressures may be helpful.

Overwedging

Serious complications are related to peripheral migration of the catheter tip as a result of cardiac contractions, catheter softening, or cardiac manipulation. The catheter should initially be positioned so that full balloon inflation is required to obtain a wedge waveform. When the pulmonary artery catheter has migrated too far peripherally, a PCWP waveform is obtained spontaneously without inflation of the balloon. The permanent wedge position must be recognized and corrected before any attempts are made to inflate the balloon. Other times, a PCWP waveform is obtained without complete inflation of the balloon, and full inflation causes "overwedging," giving falsely elevated values. These complications of pulmonary artery catheterization can be minimized by meticulous attention to detail. One should anticipate this migration and continuously monitor the waveform as well as obtain daily chest radiographs. Balloon inflation should be performed gradually with constant monitoring and should be stopped as soon as the PCWP waveform is seen.

Physical Damage during Insertion of the Catheter

Complications from Passage of the Catheter

Central venous access must be obtained prior to passage of a pulmonary artery catheter. The complications of this procedure—arterial puncture, pneumothorax, air embolization, hematoma formation, and nerve injury—were discussed earlier. Complications reported with passage of the pulmonary artery catheter include dysrhythmias, valvular damage, and knotting of the catheter.

Dysrhythmias. Serious ventricular dysrhythmias during pulmonary artery catheterization are common in the critically ill patient and are usually self-limited, but they may be sustained and may require therapeutic intervention.[130, 131–134] Premature ventricular contractions usually stop once the tip of the catheter has left the ventricle. If they are sustained, or deteriorate to ventricular tachycardia, the absence of effective cardiac output prevents flotation of the catheter from the ventricle. In such cases, the pulmonary artery catheter should be pulled back to the RA until the dysrhythmia ceases.

Administration of lidocaine has been advocated prior to the flotation of the catheter tip through the right side of the heart to electrically stabilize the myocardium.[131] However, in a double-blind comparison, lidocaine, 1 mg/kg, was no more effective than saline solution in suppressing catheter-induced ventricular ectopy.[135]

Dysrhythmias related to catheterization may also occur long after insertion. They are usually associated with looping of the catheter in the RA or ventricle.[136] The catheter tip may also become displaced from the pulmonary artery and become withdrawn into the right ventricle. These arrhythmias are highly resistant to antiarrhythmic therapy and require removal or repositioning of the catheter.

The pulmonary artery catheter can affect the cardiac conduction pathways. Up to 5% of patients develop new right bundle-branch block with passage of the catheter through the heart.[130, 133, 137, 138] Although it is usually hemodynamically insignificant, the pre-existence of a left bundle-branch block may predispose the patient to complete heart block, and the capability for artificial pacing should be available prior to inserting the catheter. Alternatively, pacemaker pulmonary artery catheters are available, but these may be unreliable pacemakers during insertion attempts.

Valvular Damage and Intracardiac Knotting. Pulmonary artery catheters have also been associated with tricuspid and pulmonary valve damage, particularly with prolonged catheterization.[130, 139–141]

Intracardiac knotting of the catheter has been reported.[142, 143] Knots occur during insertion when the catheter coils in the right ventricle. This can be suspected when excessive length is used to float the catheter out of the right ventricle, although it is usually not recognized until a chest radiograph is obtained after placement of the catheter. The coiled catheter can be removed through the introducer, but this approach should be abandoned when resistance is encountered. Sometimes the knot can be resolved by insertion of a suitable guidewire and manipulation of the catheter.[144] More often, it becomes necessary to utilize fluoroscopy to untie the knot. If the knot does not include any intracardiac structures, it can be gently tightened and the catheter can be withdrawn through the site of entry.[142, 144, 145] Occasionally, operative intervention becomes necessary.

Rupture of the Balloon. Rupture of the balloon has been reported rarely.[90] Air is not recommended for balloon inflation in any pediatric patient or adults with suspected right-to-left intracardiac shunts.[94] Instead, carbon dioxide (passed through a bacterial filter) should be used because of its rapid absorption. No more than the recommended volume of 1.5 ml of air is used to inflate the balloon. Passive balloon deflation prolongs balloon lifespan.

Complications from Improper Position of the Catheter

Pulmonary Infarction. Thromboembolism in the pulmonary vascular bed occurs with pulmonary artery catheters, resulting in pulmonary infarction.[130, 146, 147] Prolonged balloon inflation while the catheter is in a wedge position should be avoided because it occludes the pulmonary artery and leads to pulmonary infarctions.

Pulmonary Artery Rupture. The most serious of all complications when utilizing pulmonary artery catheters is rupture of the pulmonary artery, leading to massive pulmonary hemorrhage or death.[147–150] Several significant risk factors have been identified. Serious injury to the pulmonary artery is more likely in patients with pulmonary hypertension, hypothermia, and advanced age. Imminent rupture may be preceded by small amounts of hemoptysis. A fatal outcome may be more likely in patients given anticoagulants. Usually the episode of bleeding is associated with distal migration of the catheter and subsequent balloon inflation, although hemoptysis has been reported after flushing a catheter in the wedge position.[151]

Extreme caution should be exercised during the measurement of PCWP in patients with pulmonary hypertension. It is recommended that the period during which the balloon remains inflated and wedged in these patients should be limited to two respiratory cycles, or 10–15 seconds. If PADP and PCWP are nearly identical, PADP is substituted for PCWP, obviating the need for repeated balloon inflation.

Long-Term Complications

Local and Systemic Infections

The incidence of catheter-related sepsis is low but averages about 2% in most series. However, an incidence as high as 35% has been reported.[130, 152, 153, 154] The presence of bacteremia at the time of insertion has been associated with catheter-related infections.[153] The need to change introducer sheaths and pulmonary artery catheters on a routine basis is controversial, although a recent study failed to show a reduction in catheter-related infections using scheduled changes.[82, 153, 155] The diagnosis of catheter colonization and bacteremia is guided by the use of semiquantitative cultures of the pulmonary artery catheter and introducer tips as described by Maki and colleagues.[71]

Endocardial Vegetations

Intravascular catheters traumatize the intimal vascular surface and may produce intramural thrombosis or hemorrhage. Asymptomatic thrombotic complications are frequent with the routine use of pulmonary artery catheters and may be more likely with a diminished cardiac output.[130, 156]

Review of autopsies documented the presence of petechial hemorrhages on the pulmonary valve leaflets and thrombotic vegetations on the endocardial surface of the RA as well as on the tricuspid and pulmonic valves.[130, 157–160] Evidence suggests that both septic and aseptic vegetations occur and that these vegetations may embolize.[157, 159, 161]

MONITORING OF LEFT ATRIAL PRESSURE

Normally, left atrial pressure corresponds to the PCWP and PADP. In the presence of increased pulmonary vascular resistance, this relationship is altered, and the information obtained with routine central venous and pulmonary artery catheters fails to permit estimation of LVEDP. In such situations, directly measured left atrial pressure guides fluid and drug therapy during the postoperative period.

USE IN CARDIAC SURGERY

At the time of cardiothoracic surgery, the catheter is inserted through the chest wall, through the right superior pulmonary vein, and threaded into the left atrium (Fig. 8–20). Left atrial catheters are indicated when the pulmonary circulation cannot be cannulated because of congenital anomalies or pulmonary hypertension. Direct atrial cannulation is also warranted when pulmonary pressures provide inaccurate reflection of left ventricular pressure, as in mitral stenosis. These catheters ensure continuous, accurate assessment of left filling pressure during the separation of the patient from cardiopulmonary bypass and throughout the postoperative period. Similar catheters are available for infants and children.[124]

COMPLICATIONS

Problems related to transthoracic intracardiac monitoring catheters include bleeding, retained catheter fragments, catheter malposition, and dysrhythmias. In a series of 100 adult patients with transthoracic left atrial catheters undergoing open heart surgery for acquired valvular disease of the heart, no fatal complications occurred, although one patient required re-exploration for uncontrolled bleeding after the catheter needle inadvertently damaged the internal mammary artery.[162]

A study of pediatric patients undergoing cardiac surgical procedures who had transthoracic intracardiac monitoring catheters inserted in the pulmonary artery, left atrium, and RA demonstrated an overall complication rate of 0.59%.[163] The complications were divided into two general types. The first group included patients with catheters that could not be removed at the time desired. These patients required various procedures, including surgical exploration, to remove the retained catheter fragments. The second group was composed of patients in whom intrapericardial bleeding occurred after catheter removal. It is recommended that patients be monitored closely for bleeding after catheter removal, and the physician should be prepared to rapidly resuscitate and re-explore the patient if hemodynamic compromise occurs.

Most complications of transthoracic intracardiac monitoring catheters can be safely managed if recognized early and treated aggressively. The hemodynamic information obtained with these catheters is highly valued, and their use is a routine practice for many cardiac surgeons performing valve replacement and congenital heart surgery.

DETERMINATION OF BLOOD VOLUME

The end result of an inadequate blood volume is organ failure leading to immediate or delayed patient death. The normal blood volume of an adult human is about 5000 ml, about 3000 ml of which is plasma; the remaining 2000 ml is erythrocytes. Age, sex, weight, antidiuretic hormone, atrial stretch receptors, sympathetic nervous system activ-

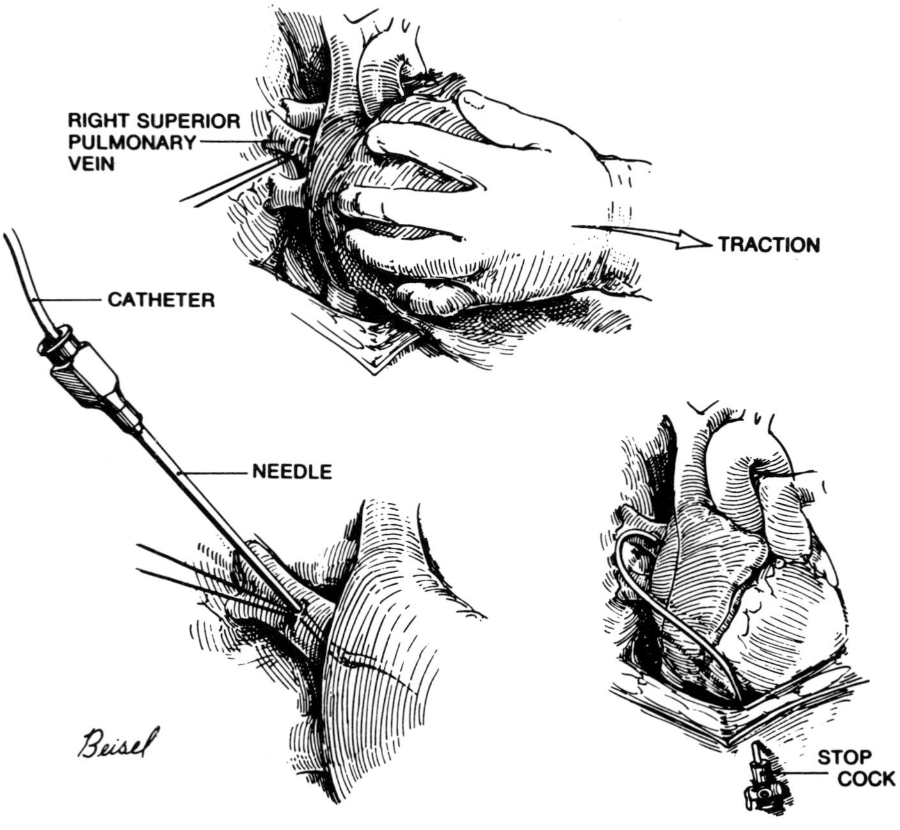

Figure 8–20. Insertion of a transthoracic left atrial catheter during cardiac surgery. (From Waldausen JA, et al: Pump oxygenators, techniques of cardiopulmonary bypass. *In* Johnson's Surgery of the Chest, 5th Ed. Chicago: Yearbook Medical, 1985;257.)

ity, and other factors affect blood volume. Plasma volume is determined by dilution techniques using Evans blue dye or radiolabeled albumin (^{131}I albumin). Alternatively, labeled erythrocytes (^{51}Cr) are used to determine blood volume by a dilution technique. Because the greater the blood volume, the less concentrated the labeled erythrocytes are after dissemination in the circulation, blood volume is calculated as

$$\text{Blood volume (ml)} = \frac{\text{Quantity of radiolabeled test substance}}{\text{Concentration of radiolabel/ml blood}}$$

These techniques for the determination of blood volume are not routinely used in clinical practice. The physician instead depends on clinical skills to assess intravascular volume. During the initial assessment of blood volume, vital signs, urinary output, level of consciousness, and capillary refill are important. If hypovolemia is suggested by the history and physical examination, fluid therapy is started initially. Treatment is directed toward restoring cellular and organ perfusion with adequately oxygenated blood. Further therapeutic and diagnostic decisions are based on the observed response. In general, return of blood pressure, pulse pressure, and pulse rate toward normal is a positive sign and indicates stabilization of the circulation. However, these observations give no information regarding organ perfusion. Improvements in the neurologic status and skin circulation are important evidence of enhanced perfusion but are difficult to quantitate. The urinary output can quantitate the renal response to restoration of perfusion and is reasonably sensitive (if not modified by diuretics). Adequate blood volume should produce a urinary output of approximately 0.5–1 ml/kg/hour. Inability to obtain such an output suggests an inadequate blood volume. This situation calls for further fluid replacement and diagnosis.

Changes in CVP can provide valuable information in the more complex patient. CVP monitoring is used as a guide to the ability of the right side of the heart to accept a fluid load. Properly interpreted, the response of the CVP to fluid administration is helpful in evaluating volume replacement. However, CVP and actual blood volume are not necessarily related. The initial CVP is sometimes increased, even with a significant volume deficit, especially in patients with generalized vasoconstriction and rapid fluid replacement. A minimal increase in an initially low CVP with fluid therapy suggests the need for further volume expansion. A decreasing CVP suggests ongoing fluid loss and the need for additional fluid or blood replacement. Abrupt or persistent elevation in the CVP suggests adequate volume replacement, too-rapid replacement, or compromised cardiac function. A flow-directed pulmonary artery catheter is then indicated to monitor the PADP and PCWP and to assess cardiac output.

REFERENCES

1. Alderman EL, Glantz SA: Acute hemodynamic interventions shift the diastolic pressure-volume curve in man. Circulation 1976; 54:662–671.
2. Risk C, Rudo N, Falltrick R, et al: Comparison of right atrial and pulmonary capillary wedge pressures. Crit Care Med 1978; 6:172–175.
3. Mangano DT: Monitoring pulmonary arterial pressure in coronary-artery disease. Anesthesiology 1981; 53:364–370.
4. Seldinger SI: Catheter replacement of the needle in percutaneous arteriography. Acta Radiol 1953; 39:368–376.
5. Legler D, Nugent M: Doppler localization of the internal jugular vein facilitates central venous cannulation. Anesthesiology 1984; 60:481–482.
6. Machi J, Takeda J, Kakegawa T: Safe jugular and subclavian venipuncture under ultrasonographic guidance. Am J Surg 1987; 153:321–323.
7. Yonei A, Nonoue T, Sari A: Real-time ultrasonic guidance for percutaneous puncture of the internal jugular vein. Anesthesiology 1986; 64:830–831.
8. Mallory DL, McGee WT, Shawker TH, et al: Ultrasound guidance improves the success rate of internal jugular vein cannulation: A prospective, randomized trial. Chest 1990; 98:157–160.
9. Lee W, Leduc L, Cotton DB: Ultrasonographic guidance for central venous access during pregnancy. Am J Obstet Gynecol 1989; 161:1012–1013.
10. Troianos CA, Jobes DR, Ellison N: Ultrasound-guided cannulation of the internal jugular vein: A prospective, randomized study. Anesth Analg 1991; 72:823–826.
11. Denys BG, Uretsky BF, Reddy PS: Ultrasound-assisted cannulation of the internal jugular vein. Circulation 1993; 87:1557–1562.
12. Denys BG, Uretsky BF: Anatomical variations of internal jugular vein location: Impact on central venous access. Crit Care Med 1991; 19:1516–1519.
13. Alderson PJ, Burrows FA, Stemp LI, Holtby HM: Use of ultrasound to evaluate internal jugular vein anatomy and to facilitate central venous cannulation in paediatric patients. J Anaesth 1993; 70:145–148.
14. Nolsoe C, Nielsen L. Karstrup S, Lauritsen K: Ultrasonically guided subclavian vein catheterization. Acta Radiol 1989; 30:108–109.
15. Kamal GD, Pfaller M, Rempe LE, Jebson PJR: Reduced intravascular catheter infection by antibiotic bonding. JAMA 1991; 265:2364–2368.
16. Foster PF, Moore LR, Sankary HN, Hart ME, Ashmann MK, Williams JW: Central venous catheterization in patients with coagulopathy. Arch Surg 1992; 127:273–275.
17. Horrow JC, Metz S, Thickman D, Frederic MW: Prior carotid surgery does not affect the reliability of landmarks for location of internal jugular vein. Anesth Analg 1987; 66:452–456.
18. Polos PG, Rinaldo FE, Bhalla M, Sahn SA: Arterial or venous? You make the call. Chest 1992; 101:591.
19. Jobes DR, Schwartz AJ, Greenhow DE, et al: Safer jugular vein cannulation: Recognition of arterial puncture and preferential use of the external jugular route. Anesthesiology 1983; 59:353–355.
20. Todd MR, Barone JE: Recognition of accidental arterial cannulation after attempted central venipuncture. Crit Care Med 1991; 19:1081–1083.
21. Aubaniac R: L'injection intraveineuse sous-claviculaire. Avantages et technique. Presse Med 1952; 60:1456.
22. Yoffa D: Supraclavicular subclavian venipuncture and catheterization. Lancet 1965; 2:614–617.
23. Blitt CD, Wright WA, Petty WC, et al: Central venous catheterization via the external jugular vein: A technique employing the J-wire. JAMA 1974; 229:817–818.
24. Blitt CD, Carlson GL, Wright WA, et al: J-wire versus straight wire for central venous system cannulation via the external jugular vein. Anesth Analg 1982; 61:536–537.
25. Belani KG, Buckley JJ, Gordon JR, Castenada W: Percutaneous cervical central venous line placement: A comparison of the internal and external jugular vein routes. Anesth Analg 1980; 59:40–44.
26. Williams JF, Seneff MG, Friedman BC, et al: Use of femoral venous catheters in critically ill adults: Prospective study. Crit Care Med 1991; 19:550–553.
27. Bonner CD: Experience with plastic tubing in prolonged intravenous therapy. N Engl J Med 1951; 245:97–98.
28. Bansmer G, Keith D, Tesluk H: Complications following use of indwelling catheters of inferior vena cava. JAMA 1958; 167:1606–1611.
29. Webre DR, Arens JF: Use of cephalic and basilic veins for introduction of central venous catheters. Anesthesiology 1973; 38:389–392.

30. Burgess GE, Marino RJ, Peuler MJ: Effect of head position in the location of venous catheters inserted via basilic veins. Anesthesiology 1977; 46:212–213.
31. Langston CS: The aberrant central venous catheter and its complications. Radiology 1971; 100:55–59.
32. Spracklen FA, Niesche F, Lord PW, et al: Percutaneous catheterization for the axillary vein. Cardiovasc Res 1967; 1:297–300.
33. Ayim EN: Percutaneous catheterization of the axillary vein and proximal basilic vein. Anaesthesia 1977; 32:753–759.
34. Martin C, Auffray JP, Saux P: The axillary vein: An alternative approach for percutaneous pulmonary artery catheterization. Chest 1986; 90:694–697.
35. Martin C, Eon B, Auffray J, Saux P, Gouin F: Axillary or internal jugular central venous catheterization. Crit Care Med 1990; 18:400–402.
36. Guyton AC, Jones CE: Central venous pressure: Physiological significance and clinical implications. Am Heart J 1973; 86:431–437.
37. Peres PW: Positioning central venous catheters—A prospective survey. Anaesth Intens Care 1990; 18:536–539.
38. Bunegin L, Albin M, Helsel P, et al: Positioning the right atrial catheter: A model for reappraisal. Anesthesiology 1981; 55:343–348.
39. Cucchiara RF, Black S, Steinkeler JA: Anesthesia for intracranial procedures. *In* Barash PG, Cullen BF, Stoelting RK (eds): Clinical Anesthesia. Philadelphia: JB Lippincott, 1989; 849.
40. Martin JT: Neuroanesthetic adjuncts for patients in the sitting position, part III. Intravascular electrocardiogram. Anesth Analg 1970; 49:793–808.
41. Colley PS, Artru AA: ECG-guided placement of Sorensen CVP catheters via arm veins. Anesth Analg 1984; 63:953–956.
42. Cucchiara RF, Messick JM, Gronert GG, Michenfelder JD: Time required and success rate of percutaneous right atrial catheterization: Description of a technique. Can Anaesth Soc J 1980; 27:572–573.
43. Johans TG: Multiorificed catheter placement with an intravascular electrocardiographic technique. Anesthesiology 1986; 64:411–413.
44. Warner DO, Cucchiara RF: Position of proximal orifice determines electrocardiogram recorded from multiorificed catheter. Anesthesiology 1986; 65:235–236.
45. Artru AA, Colley PS: The site of origin of the intravascular electrocardiogram recorded from multiorificed intravascular catheters. Anesthesiology 1988; 69:44–48.
46. Black S, Cucchiara RF: Tumor surgery. *In* Cucchiara RF, Michenfelder JD (eds): Clinical Neuroanesthesia. New York: Churchill Livingstone, 1990; 296.
47. Gauderer MW: Vascular access techniques and devices in the pediatric patient. Surg Clin North Am 1992; 72:1267–1284.
48. Cobb LM, Vinocur CD, Wagner CW, Weintraub WH: The central venous anatomy in infants. Surg Gynecol Obstet 1987; 165:230–234.
49. Cote CJ, Jobes DR, Schwartz AJ, Ellison N: Two approaches to cannulation of a child's internal jugular vein. Anesthesiology 1979; 50:371–373.
50. Prince SR, Sullivan RL, Hackel A: Percutaneous catheterization of the internal jugular vein in infants and children. Anesthesiology 1976; 44 170–174.
51. Humphrey MJ, Blitt CD: Central venous access in children via the external jugular vein. Anesthesiology 1982; 57:50–51.
52. Eichelberger MR, Rous PG, Hoelzer DJ, et al: Percutaneous subclavian venous catheters in neonates and children. J Pediatr Surg 1981; 16:547–553.
53. Pybus DA, Poole JL, Crawford MC: Subclavian venous catheterization in small children using the Seldinger technique. Anaesthesia 1982; 37 451–453.
54. Kron IL, Rheuban K, Miller ED, et al: Subclavian vein catheterization for central line placement in children under 2 years of age. Am Surg 1985; 51:272–273.
55. Metz RI, Lucking SE, Chaten FC, Williams TM, Mickell JJ: Percutaneous catheterization of the axillary vein in infants and children. Pediatrics 1990; 85:531–533.
56. Verweij J, Kester A, Stroes W, et al: Comparison of three methods for measuring central venous pressure. Crit Care Med 1986; 14:288–290.
57. Constant J: The bedside recognition of abnormal jugular contours. Resident Staff Physician 1987; 33:51–58.
58. Mark JB. Central venous pressure monitoring: Clinical insights beyond the numbers. J Cardiothorac Vasc Anesth 1991; 5:163–173.
59. Qvist J, Pontoppidan H, Wilson RS, et al: Hemodynamic responses to mechanical ventilation with PEEP: The effect of hypervolemia. Anesthesiology 1975; 42:54–55.
60. Shah KB, Rao TLK, Laughlin S, El-Etr AA: A review of pulmonary artery catheterization in 6245 patients. Anesthesiology 1984; 61:271–275.
61. Paskin DL, Hoffman WS, Tuddenham WJ: A new complication of subclavian vein catheterization. Ann Surg 1974; 179:266–268.
62. Steiner ML, Bartley TD, Byers FM, Krovetz LJ: Polyethylene catheter in the heart. Report of a case with successful removal. JAMA 1965; 193:1054–1056.
63. Massumi RA, Ross AM: Atraumatic, nonsurgical technique for removal of broken catheters from cardiac cavities. N Engl J Med 1967; 277:195–196.
64. McSweeney WJ, Schwartz DC: Retrieval of a catheter foreign body from the right heart using a guide wire deflector system. Radiology 1971; 100:61–62.
65. Edelstein J: Atraumatic removal of a polyethylene catheter from the superior vena cava. Chest 1970; 57:381–383.
66. Lillehei CW, Bonnabeau RC Jr, Grossling S: Removal of iatrogenic foreign bodies within cardiac chambers and great vessels. Circulation 1965; 32:782–787.
67. Block PC: Transvenous retrieval of foreign bodies in the cardiac circulation. JAMA 1973; 224:241–242.
68. Johnson CE: Perforation of right atrium by a polyethylene catheter. JAMA 1966; 195:584–586.
69. Friedman BA, Jurgeleit HC: Perforation of atrium by polyethylene central venous catheter. JAMA 1968; 203:1141–1142.
70. Brady RE, Weinberg PM: Atrioventricular conduction disturbance during total parenteral nutrition. J Pediatr 1976; 88:113–114.
71. Maki DG, Weise CE, Sarafin HW: A semiquantitative culture method for identifying intravenous-catheter-related infection. N Engl J Med 1977; 296: 1305–1309.
72. Cooper GL, Hopkins CC: Rapid diagnosis of intravascular catheter-associated infection by direct Gram staining of catheter segments. N Engl J Med 1985; 312:1142–1147.
73. Collignon P, Chan R, Munro R: Rapid diagnosis of intravascular catheter-related sepsis. Arch Intern Med 1987; 147:1609–1612.
74. Passerini L, Phang PT, Jackson FL, et al: Biofilms of right heart flow-directed catheters. Chest 1987; 92:440–446.
75. Maki DG, Ringer M: Evaluation of dressing regimens for prevention of infection with peripheral intravenous catheters. Gauze, a transparent polyurethane dressing, and an iodophor-transparant dressing. JAMA 1987; 258:2396–2403.
76. Snydman DR, Pober BR, Murray SA, et al: Predictive value of surveillance skin cultures in total-parenteral nutrition-related infection. Lancet 1982; 2:1385–1388.
77. Bjornson HS, Colley R, Bower RH, et al: Association between microorganism growth at the catheter insertion site and colonization of the catheter in patients receiving total parenteral nutrition. Surgery 1982; 92:720–727.
78. Flowers RH, Schwenzer KJ, Kopel RF, Fisch MJ, Tucker SI, Farr BM: Efficacy of an attachable subcutaneous cuff for the prevention of intravascular catheter-related infection: A randomized, controlled trial. JAMA 1989; 261:878–883.
79. Ryan JA, Abel, Abbott WM, et al: Catheter complications in total parenteral nutrition: A prospective study of 200 consecutive patients. N Engl J Med 1974; 290:757–761.
80. Sitzmann JV, Townsend TR, Siler MC, Bartlett JG: Septic and technical complications of central venous catheterization: A prospective study of 200 consecutive patients. Ann Surg 1985; 202:766–770.
81. Eyer S, Brummitt C, Crossley K, Siegel R, Cerra F: Catheter-related sepsis: A prospective, randomized study of three methods of long-term catheter maintenance. Crit Care Med 1990; 18:1073–1079.
82. Cobb DK, High KP, Sawyer RG, Sable CA, Adams RB, Lindley DA, Pruett TL, Schwenzer KJ, Farr BM: A controlled trial of scheduled replacement of central venous and pulmonary artery catheters. N Engl J Med 1992; 327:1062–1068.
83. Hagley MT, Martin B, Gast P, Traeger SM: Infections and mechanical complications of central venous catheters placed by percutaneous venipuncture and over guidelines. Crit Care Med 1992; 20:1426–1430.
84. Peters WR, Bush HW Jr, McIntyre RD, Hill LD: The development of fibrin sheath on indwelling venous catheters. Surg Gynecol Obstet 1973; 137:43–47.
85. Ryan JA Jr, Abel RM, Abbott WM, et al: Catheter complications in

total parenteral nutrition: A prospective study of 200 consecutive patients. N Engl J Med 1974; 290:757–761.
86. Bouchard RJ, Gault JH, Ross J Jr: Evaluation of pulmonary arterial end-diastolic pressure as an estimate of left ventricular end-diastolic pressure in patients with normal and abnormal left ventricular performance. Circulation 1971; 44:1072–1079.
87. Falicov RE, Resnekov L: Relationship of the pulmonary artery end-diastolic pressure to the left ventricular end-diastolic and mean filling pressures in patients with and without left ventricular dysfunction. Circulation 1970; 42:65–73.
88. Lappas D, Lell WA, Gabel JC, et al: Indirect measurement of left-atrial pressure in surgical patients-pulmonary capillary wedge and pulmonary artery diastolic pressures compared with left atrial pressure. Anesthesiology 1973:38:394–397.
89. Forrester JS, Diamond G, McHugh TJ, Swan HJC: Filling pressures in the right and left sides of the heart in acute myocardial infarction: A reappraisal of central-venous-pressure monitoring. N Engl J Med 1971; 285:190–193.
90. Archer G, Cobb LA: Long-term pulmonary artery pressure monitoring in the management of the critically ill. Ann Surg 1974; 180:747–752.
91. Forrester J, Diamond G, Ganz W, et al: Right and left heart pressures in the acutely ill patient. Clin Res 1970; 18:306.
92. Rahimtoola SH, Loeb HS, Ehsani A, et al: Relationship of pulmonary artery to left ventricular diastolic pressures in acute myocardial infarction. Circulation 1972; 46:283–290.
93. West JB, Dollery CT, Naimark A: Distribution of blood flow in isolated lung: Relation to vascular and alveolar pressures. J Appl Physiol 1964; 19:713–724.
94. Goldenheim PD, Kazemi H: Cardiopulmonary monitoring of critically ill patients, part 2. N Engl J Med 1984; 311:776–778.
95. Todd TR, Baile EM, Hogg JC: Pulmonary arterial wedge pressure in hemorrhagic shock. Am Rev Respir Dis 1978; 118:613–616.
96. Shasby DM, Daube IM, Pfister S, et al: Swan-Ganz catheter location and left atrial pressure determine the accuracy of the wedge pressure when positive end-expiratory pressure is used. Chest 1981; 80:666–670.
97. Roy R, Powers SR Jr, Feustel PJ, Dutton RE: Pulmonary wedge catheterization during positive end-expiratory pressure ventilation in the dog. Anesthesiology 1977; 46:385–390.
98. Zapol WM, Snider MT: Pulmonary hypertension in severe acute respiratory failure. N Engl J Med 1977; 296:476–480.
99. Downs JB: A technique for direct measurement of intrapleural pressure. Crit Care Med 1976; 4:207–210.
100. McCans JL, Parker JO: Left ventricular pressure-volume relationship during myocardial ischemia in man. Circulation 1973; 48:775–785.
101. Mann T, Mann R, Goldberg S, et al: Factors contributing to altered left ventricular diastolic properties during angina pectoris. Circulation 1979; 59:14–20.
102. Calvin JE, Driedger AA, Sibbald WJ: Does the pulmonary capillary wedge pressure predict left ventricular preload in critically ill patients? Crit Care Med 1981; 9:437–443.
103. Jenkins BS, Bradley RD, Branthwaite MA: Evaluation of pulmonary arterial end-diastolic as an indirect estimate of left atrial mean pressure. Circulation 1970; 42:75–90.
104. Scheinman M, Evans GT, Weiss A, et al: Relationship between pulmonary artery end-diastolic pressure and left ventricular filling pressure in patients in shock. Circulation 1973; 47:317–324.
105. Chatterjee K, Parmley WW, Ganz W, et al: Hemodynamic and metabolic responses to vasodilator therapy in acute myocardial infarction. Circulation 1973; 48:1183–1193.
106. Dalen JE: Bedside hemodynamic monitoring. N Engl J Med 1979; 301:1176–1178.
107. Chatterjee K, Swan HJ, Kaushik VS, et al: Effects of vasodilator therapy for severe pump failure in acute myocardial infarction on short-term and long-term prognosis. Circulation 1976; 53:797–802.
108. Zion MM, Balkin J, Rosenmann D, et al: Use of pulmonary artery catheter in patients with acute myocardial infarction. Analysis of experience in 5841 patients in the Sprint Registry. Chest 1990; 98:1331–1335.
109. Gore JM, Goldberg RJ, Spodick DH, et al: A community-wide assessment of the use of pulmonary artery catheters in patients with acute myocardial infarction. Chest 1987; 92:721–731.
110. Danek SJ, Lynch JP, Weg JG, Dantsker DR: The dependence of oxygen uptake on oxygen delivery in the adult respiratory distress syndrome. Am Rev Respir Dis 1980; 122:387–395.
111. Goldman RH, Klughaupt M, Metcalf T, et al: Measurement of central venous oxygen saturation in patients with myocardial infarction. Circulation 1968; 38:941–946.
112. Pond CG, Blessios G, Bowlin J, McCawley C, Lappas DG: Perioperative evaluation of a new mixed venous oxygen saturation catheter in cardiac surgery patients. J Cardiothorac Vasc Anesth 1992; 6: 280–282.
113. Haggmark S, Hohner P, Ostman M, et al: Comparison of hemodynamic, electrocardiographic, mechanical, and metabolic indicators of intraoperative myocardial ischemia in vascular surgical patients with coronary artery disease. Anesthesiology 1989; 70:19–25.
114. Van Daele MERM, Sutherland GR, Mitchell MM, et al: Do changes in PCWP adequately reflect myocardial ischemia during anesthesia? Circulation 1990; 81:865–871.
115. Kaul S, Spotnitz WD, Glasheen WP, Touchstone DA: Mechanism of ischemic mitral regurgitation. Circulation 1991; 84:2167–2180.
116. Forrester JS, Ganz W, Diamond G, et al: Thermodilution cardiac output determination with a single flow-directed catheter. Am Heart J 1972; 83:306–311.
117. Katz RW, Pollack M, Weibley R: Pulmonary artery catheterization in pediatric intensive care. Adv Pediatr 1983; 30:169–190.
118. Alfieri O, Agosti J, Subramanian S: Thermodilution cardiac output measurement in infants and small children following intracardiac surgery. J Pediatr Surg 1975; 10:649–656.
119. Mathur M, Harris EA, Yarrow S, Baratt-Boyes BG: Measurement of cardiac output by thermodilution in infants and children after open-heart operations. J Thorac Cardiovasc Surg 1976; 72:221–225.
120. Rah KH, Dunwiddle WC, Lower RR: A method of continuous post-operative monitoring of mixing venous oxygen saturation in infants and children after open heart procedures. Anesth Analg 1984; 63:873–881.
121. Freed MD, Keane JF: Cardiac output measured by thermodilution in infants and children. J Pediatr 1978; 92:39–42.
122. Pollack MM, Reed TP, Holbrook PR, et al: Bedside pulmonary artery catheterization in pediatrics. J Pediatr 1980; 96:274–276.
123. Swan HJ, Ganz W: Measurement of right atrial and pulmonary arterial pressures and cardiac output: Clinical application of hemodynamic monitoring. Adv Intern Med 1982; 27:453–473.
124. Wyse SD, Pfitzner J, Rees A, et al: Measurement of cardiac output by thermodilution in infants and children. Thorax 1975; 30:262–265.
125. Moodie DS, Feldt RH, Kaye MP, et al: Measurement of cardiac output by thermodilution: Development of accurate measurement at flow applicable to the pediatric patient. J Surg Res 1978; 25:305–311.
126. Webster H: Hemodynamic monitoring in children. *In* Daily EK, Schroeder JS (eds): Techniques of Hemodynamic Monitoring. St. Louis: CV Mosby, 1985; 138–179.
127. Maran AG: Variables in pulmonary capillary wedge pressure: Variation with intrathoracic pressure, graphic and digital recorders. Crit Care Med 1980:102–105.
128. Cengiz M, Crapo RO, Gardner RM: The effect of ventilation on the accuracy of pulmonary artery and wedge pressure measurements. Crit Care Med 1983; 11:502–507.
129. Berryhill RE, Benumof JL, Rauscher LA: Pulmonary vascular pressure reading at the end of exhalation. Anesthesiology 1978; 49:365–368.
130. Elliot CG, Zimmerman GA, Clemmer TP: Complications of pulmonary artery catheterization in the care of critically ill patients. Chest 1979; 76:647–652.
131. Swan HJC, Ganz W, Forrester J, et al: Catheterization of the heart in man—Use of a flow-directed balloon-tipped catheter. N Engl J Med 1979; 283:447–451.
132. Sprung CL, Jacobs LJ, Caralis PV, et al: Ventricular arrhythmias during Swan Ganz catheterization of the critically ill. Chest 1981; 79:413–415.
133. Sprung CL, Poizen RG, Rozanski JJ, et al: Advanced ventricular arrhythmias during bedside pulmonary artery catheterization. Am J Med 1982; 72:203–208.
134. Geha DG, Davis NJ, Lappas DG: Persistent atrial arrhythmias associated with placement of a Swan-Ganz catheter. Anesthesiology 1973; 39:651–653.
135. Salmenpera M, Peltola K, Rosenberg P: Does prophylactic lidocaine control cardiac arrhythmias associated with pulmonary artery catheterization? Anesthesiology 1982; 56:210–212.
136. Voukydis PC, Cohen SI: Catheter-induced arrhythmias. Am Heart J 1974; 88:588–592.

137. Abernathy WS: Complete heart block caused by the Swan-Ganz catheter. Chest 1974; 65:349.
138. Thomson IR, Dalton BC, Lappas DG, Lowenstein E: Right bundle branch block and complete heart block caused by the Swan-Ganz catheter. Anesthesiology 1979; 51:359–362.
139. O'Toole JD, Wurtzbacher JJ, Wearer NE, et al: Pulmonary valve injury and insufficiency during pulmonary-artery catheterization. N Engl J Med 1979; 301:1167–1168.
140. Boscoe MJ, Delange S: Damage of the tricuspid valve with a Swan-Ganz catheter. Br Med J 1981; 283:346–347.
141. Smith WR, Glauser FL, Jemison P: Ruptured chordae of the tricuspid valve: The consequence of flow directed Swan-Ganz catheterization. Chest 1976; 70: 790–792.
142. Lipp H, O'Donoghue K, Resnekov L: Intracardiac knotting of a flow-directed balloon catheter. N Engl J Med 1971; 284:220.
143. Iberti TJ, Jayagopal SG: Knotting of a Swan-Ganz catheter in pulmonary artery [Letter]. Chest 1983; 83:711.
144. Mond HG, Dwight WC, Nesbitt SJ, et al: A technique for unknotting an intracardiac flow-directed balloon. Chest 1975; 67:731–732.
145. Dach JL, Galbut DL, Lepage JR: The knotted Swan-Ganz catheter: New solution to a vexing problem. Am J Radiol 1981; 137:1274–1275.
146. Foote GA, Schabel SI, Hodges M: Pulmonary complications of the flow-directed balloon-tipped catheter. N Engl J Med 1974; 290:927–931.
147. Pape LA, Haffajee CI, Markis JE, et al: Fatal pulmonary hemorrhage after use of the flow-directed balloon-tipped catheter. Ann Intern Med 1979; 90:344–347.
148. Rosenbaum L, Rosenbaum SH, Askanazi J, Hyman AI: Small amounts of hemoptysis as an early warning sign of pulmonary artery rupture by a pulmonary arterial catheter. Crit Care Med 1981; 9:319–320.
149. Hart U, Ward DR, Gillilian R, Brawley RK: Fatal pulmonary hemorrhage complicating Swan-Ganz catheterization. Surgery 1982; 91:24–27.
150. Chun GMH, Ellested MH: Perforation of the pulmonary artery by Swan-Ganz catheter. N Engl J Med 1971; 295: 1356–1362.
151. Meltzer R, Kint PP, Simmons M: Hemoptysis after flushing Swan-Ganz catheters in the wedge position [Letter]. N Engl J Med 1981, 304:1171.
152. Puri VK, Carlson RW, Bander JJ, Weil MH: Complications of vascular catheterization in the critically ill: A prospective study. Crit Care Med 1980; 8:495–499.
153. Applefeld JJ, Caruthers TE, Reno DJ, Civetta JM: Assessment of the sterility of long-term cardiac catheterization using the thermodilution Swan-Ganz catheter. Chest 1978; 74:377–380.
154. Lange HW, Galliani CA, Edwards JE: Local complications associated with indwelling Swan-Ganz catheters. Am J Cardiol 1983; 52:1108–1111.
155. Senagore A, Waller JD, Bonnell BW, et al: Pulmonary artery catheterization: A prospective study of internal jugular and subclavian approaches. Crit Care Med 1987; 15:35–37.
156. Chastre J, Comud F, Bouchama A, et al: Thrombosis as a complication of pulmonary-artery catheterization via the internal jugular vein: Prospective evaluation by phlebography. N Engl J Med 1982; 306:278–281.
157. Greene JF Jr, Cummings KC: Aseptic thrombotic endocardial vegetations: A complication of indwelling pulmonary artery catheters. JAMA 1973; 225:1525–1526.
158. Pace NL, Horton W: Indwelling pulmonary artery catheters: Their relationship to aseptic thrombotic endocardial vegetations. JAMA 1974; 233:893–894.
159. Greene JF Jr, Fitzwater JE, Clemmer TP: Septic endocarditis and indwelling pulmonary artery catheters. JAMA 1976; 233:891–892.
160. Katz JD, Cronau LH, Barash PG, et al: Pulmonary artery flow-guided catheters in the perioperative period. JAMA 1977; 237:2832–2834.
161. Rowley KM, Clubb KS, Smith GJW, Cabin HS: Right-sided infective endocarditis as a consequence of flow-directed pulmonary-artery catheterization. N Engl J Med 1984; 311:1152–1156.
162. Sarin CL, Yalav E, Clement AJ, Braimbridge MV: The necessity for measurement of left atrial pressure after cardiac valve surgery. Thorax 25:185–189.
163. Gold JP, Jonas RA, Lang P, et al: Transthoracic intracardiac monitoring in pediatric surgical patients: A ten year experience. Ann Thorac Surg 1986; 42:185–191.

CHAPTER 9

Perioperative Echocardiography

DANIEL M. THYS, M.D., STEVEN KONSTADT, M.D., and ZAK HILLEL, M.D., Ph.D.

Since the first edition of this book was published in 1990, the role of intraoperative echocardiography (IOE) has significantly expanded.[1] In a survey published in 1988, only 20% of the responders reported the use of IOE at their institution.[2] At that time, there were about 50 transesophageal echocardiography (TEE) probes in use. Since then, approximately 700 TEE systems for the operating room have been sold in the United States, and IOE now is nearly the standard of care in certain procedures. Based on a combination of technologic advancement and scientific investigation, countless applications of IOE have been developed. Studies have also demonstrated the ability of IOE to alter surgical management and to predict outcome.[3–5]

PROPERTIES OF ULTRASOUND

In echocardiography, the heart and great vessels are probed with ultrasound, which is sound above the human audible range. The ultrasound is sent into the thoracic cavity and is partially reflected by the cardiac structures. From these reflections, information on distance, velocity, and density of objects within the chest is derived.[6, 7]

WAVELENGTH, FREQUENCY, VELOCITY

An ultrasound beam is a continuous or intermittent train of waves emitted by a transducer or wave generator. It is composed of density or pressure waves and can exist in any medium with the exception of a vacuum. Ultrasound waves are characterized by their wavelength, frequency, and velocity. *Wavelength* is the distance between the two nearest points of equal pressure or density in an ultrasound beam, whereas *velocity* is the speed at which the waves propagate through a medium. As the waves travel by any fixed point in an ultrasound beam, the pressure cycles regularly and continuously between a high and a low value. The number of cycles per second (Hertz) is called the *frequency* of the wave. Ultrasound is sound with frequencies above 20,000 Hz, which is the upper limit of the human audible range. The relationship among the frequency (f), wavelength (l), and velocity (v) of a sound wave is defined by the formula:

$$v = f \times l \qquad 9\text{–}1$$

The velocity of sound varies with the properties of the medium through which it travels. For soft tissues, this velocity approximates 1540 m/second. Because the frequency of an ultrasound beam is determined by the properties of the emitting transducer, and because the velocity is a function of the tissues through which the sound travels, wavelengths vary to maintain the relation $v = f \times l$.

ATTENUATION, REFLECTION, SCATTER

Waves interact with the medium in which they travel and with one another. Interaction among waves is called interference. The manner in which waves interact with a medium is determined by the medium's density and homogeneity. When a wave is propagating through an inhomogeneous medium—and all living tissue is essentially inhomogeneous—it is partly absorbed, partly reflected, and partly scattered. Reflected echoes, also called specular echoes, are usually much stronger than scattered echoes. A grossly inhomogeneous medium, such as a stone in a water bucket or a cardiac valve in a blood-filled heart chamber, produces strong specular reflections at the water-stone or blood-valve interface. Conversely, media that are inhomogeneous at the microscopic level, such as muscle, produce more scatter than specular reflection. Specular reflections are obtained when the width of the reflecting object is larger

TABLE 9–1. HALF-POWER DISTANCES FOR TISSUES AND SUBSTANCES IMPORTANT IN ECHOCARDIOGRAPHY

Material	Half-Power Distance (cm)
Water	380
Blood	15
Soft tissue (except muscle)	5–1
Muscle	1–0.6
Bone	0.7–0.2
Air	0.08
Lung	0.05

than one fourth of the wavelength of the ultrasound. It is clear that to visualize smaller objects, ultrasound of shorter wavelength must be used. Because the velocity of sound in soft tissue is approximately constant, shorter wavelengths are obtained by increasing the frequency of the ultrasound beam (Equation 9–1). Although smaller objects can be visualized with higher frequencies, more scatter is produced by insignificant inhomogeneities in the medium, and confusing signals are generated.

Any ultrasound beam traveling through tissues will be weakened or attenuated as it progresses. Table 9–1 gives the distance in various tissues at which the intensity or amplitude of an ultrasound wave of 2 MHz is halved (the half-power distance). Clearly, echo studies across lung or other gas-containing tissues are not feasible. Nor are they feasible across dense structures such as bone or across strongly scattering tissues such as thick muscle.

Modern ultrasound transducers employ piezoelectric crystals to transmit ultrasound and receive echoes. A high-frequency electric signal stimulates the crystal, which emits ultrasound. Conversely, reflected ultrasound echoes striking the crystal's surface generate vibrations that are converted to electrical impulses, amplified, processed, and then imaged on a television screen. Electronic circuits measure the delay between the emitted and received echo and, using the known speed of ultrasound in tissue, convert this delay into the precise distance between transducer and tissue.

The commonly used transducer spends a small amount of time, typically on the order of 1 μsec (10^{-6} seconds), emitting a pulse of ultrasound waves. The transducer then "listens" for the returning echoes for about 0.25 msec and pauses for 0.75 msec or less before repeating the cycle. Ultrasound takes about 0.1 msec to travel through 10 cm of human tissue and to be reflected or echoed back to the transducer. There is no time loss in the reflection process.

IMAGING TECHNIQUES

M-MODE

The most basic form of ultrasound imaging is *M-mode* echocardiography. In this mode, the density and position of all tissues in the path of a narrow ultrasound beam (i.e., *along a single line*) are displayed as a scroll on a video screen. The scrolling produces an updated, continuously changing time plot of the studied tissue section, several seconds in duration. Because this is a timed *motion display* (normal cardiac tissue is always in motion), it is called M-mode. Because only a very limited part of the heart is being observed at any one time and because the image requires considerable interpretation, M-mode is not currently used as a primary imaging technique. This mode is useful for the precise timing of events within the cardiac cycle, however, and is often used in combination with color flow Doppler for the timing of abnormal flows (see later section on color flow mapping).

Quantitative measurements of size, distance, and velocity are also easily performed in the M-mode without the need for sophisticated analysis systems (Fig. 9–1). Whenever a measurement includes a temporal component, the M-mode image is more advantageous than a 2D image because it is updated a thousand times each second. Thus, more subtle changes in motion or dimension can be appreciated.

TWO-DIMENSIONAL (2D) MODE

By rapid, repetitive scanning along many different radii within an area in the shape of a fan (sector), echocardiography generates a 2D image of a section of the heart. This image, which resembles an anatomic section and thus can be more easily interpreted, is called a 2D scan. Information on structures and motion in the plane of a 2D scan is updated 30–60 times per second. This produces a "live" (real-time) image of the heart. Scanning 2D echo devices image the heart either by using a mechanically steered transducer or, as is common in many of the newer devices, by using an electronically steered ultrasound beam (phased-array transducer). Probes with two transducers scanning in two orthogonal planes (biplane) also exist.

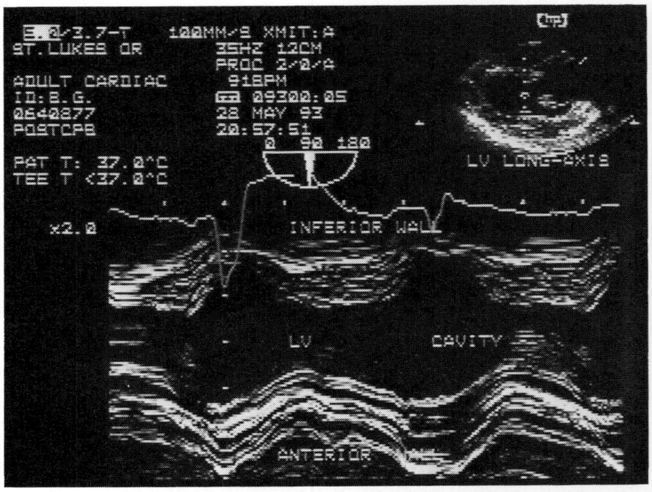

Figure 9–1. M-mode display of regional left ventricular function near the base of the papillary muscles *(bottom image)* obtained from a transesophageal long-axis image *(upper right corner inset)*. The fractional shortening in LV cavity inferior-anterior diameter from diastole to systole exceeds 50% in this hyperdynamic ventricle.

DOPPLER TECHNIQUES

Most modern echo scanners combine Doppler capabilities with their 2D imaging capabilities. After the desired view of the heart has been obtained by 2D echocardiography, the Doppler beam, represented by a cursor, is superimposed on the 2D image. The operator positions the cursor as parallel as possible to the assumed direction of blood flow and then empirically adjusts the direction of the beam to optimize the audio and visual representations of the reflected Doppler signal. At present, Doppler technology can be utilized in at least four different ways to measure blood velocities: pulsed, high-repetition frequency, continuous wave, and color flow Doppler. Although each of these methods has specific applications, they are seldom concurrently available and then only on the most sophisticated and expensive echocardiographic devices.

DOPPLER EFFECT

Information on blood flow dynamics can be obtained by applying Doppler frequency shift analysis to echoes reflected by the moving red blood cells.[8, 9] Blood flow velocity, direction, and acceleration can be instantaneously determined. This information is different from that obtained in 2D imaging and, hence, complements it.

The Doppler principle as applied in echocardiography states that the frequency of ultrasound reflected by a moving target (red blood cells) will be different from the frequency of the transmitted ultrasound. The magnitude and direction of the frequency shift is related to the velocity and direction of the moving target. The velocity of the target is calculated with the Doppler equation:

$$v = \frac{c \times f_d}{2\, f_o \times \cos \theta} \qquad 9\text{–}2$$

where v = the flow velocity, f_d = the frequency shift, f_o = the frequency of the emitted ultrasound, and θ = the angle between the ultrasound beam and the direction of blood flow.

The only ambiguity in the Doppler equation is that, theoretically, the direction of the ultrasonic signal could refer either to the transmitted or to the received beam. By convention, however, Doppler displays are made with reference to the received beam; thus, if the blood flow and the reflected beam travel in the same direction, the incidence angle is 0° and the cosine is +1. As a result, the frequency of the reflected signal will be higher than the frequency of the emitted signal.

Equipment currently used in clinical practice displays blood flow velocities as waveforms. The waveforms consist of a spectral analysis of velocities on the ordinate over time on the abscissa. On such a display, blood flow toward the transducer is by convention represented above the baseline. If the blood flows away from the transducer, the incidence angle will be 180°, the cosine will equal −1, and the waveform will be displayed below the baseline. When the blood flow is perpendicular to the ultrasonic beam, the incidence angle will be 90° or 270°, the cosine of either angle being zero, and no frequency shift will be detected. The inclusion of the cosine of the incidence angle in the Doppler equation results in the observation that blood flow velocities will be most accurately measured when the ultrasonic beam is, as nearly as possible, parallel (or antiparallel) to the direction of blood flow. In clinical practice, a deviation from parallel of up to 20° can be tolerated, because this results in an error of only 6% or less.

PULSED WAVE DOPPLER

In pulsed wave (PW) Doppler, blood flow parameters can be determined at precise locations within the heart by emitting repetitive, short bursts of ultrasound at a specific frequency (pulse-repetition frequency, or PRF) and analyzing the frequency shift of the reflected echoes at an identical sampling frequency (f_s). A delay between the emission of the ultrasound signal burst and the sampling of the reflected signal determines the depth at which the velocities are sampled. The delay is proportional to the distance between the transducer and the location of the velocity measurements. To sample at a given depth (D), sufficient time must be allowed for the signal to travel a distance of 2 × D (from the transducer to the sample volume and back). The time delay (Td) between the emission of the signal and the reception of the reflected signal is related to D and to the speed of sound in tissues (c) by the following formula:

$$D = \frac{cTd}{2} \qquad 9\text{–}3$$

The operator varies the depth of sampling by varying the delay between the emission of the ultrasonic signal and the sampling of the reflected wave. In practice, the sampling location, or *sample volume*, is represented by a small marker, which can be positioned at any point along the Doppler beam by moving it up or down the Doppler cursor. On some devices, it is also possible to vary the width and height of the sample volume.

The trade-off for the ability to measure flow at precise locations is that ambiguous information is obtained when flow velocity is very high. A simple reference to Western movies will clearly illustrate this point. When a stagecoach gets underway, its wheel spokes are observed as rotating in the correct direction. As soon as a certain speed is attained, however, the wheel spokes appear to rotate in the opposite direction. This is because the camera frame rate is too slow to correctly observe the motion of the wheel spokes. In PW Doppler, the ambiguity exists because the measured Doppler frequencies (f_d) and the sampling frequency (f_s) are in the same frequency (kilohertz) range. Ambiguity will only be avoided if the f_d is less than half the sampling frequency:

$$f_d < \frac{f_s}{2} \qquad 9\text{–}4$$

The expression, $f_s/2$, is also known as the Nyquist limit.

Doppler shifts above the Nyquist limit will create artifacts described as "aliasing" or "wraparound," and blood flow velocities will appear in a direction opposite to the conventional one. Blood flowing with high velocity toward the transducer will result in a display of velocities above and below the baseline. This artifact can be avoided by increasing the f_s, but this then limits the time available for a pulse to travel to the sample volume and back, thus limiting the range. The relationship between the maximal detectable velocity and the range at which it can be detected is known as the range velocity product, or V_mR:

$$V_mR = \frac{c^2}{8f_o} \qquad 9\text{–}5$$

where V_m = the maximal velocity that can be unambiguously measured and R = the range or distance from the transducer at which the measurement is to be made. PW Doppler measurements are performed with the same transducer as the one used for imaging.

CONTINUOUS WAVE DOPPLER

The continuous wave (CW) Doppler technique uses continuous, rather than discrete, pulses of ultrasound waves. As a result, the region in which flow dynamics are measured cannot be precisely localized. Blood flow velocity is measured with great accuracy even at high flow, however.

Although many echo scanners have both PW and CW Doppler capabilities, not all transesophageal echocardiography (TEE) probes can perform CW measurements. Dedicated CW probes have two transducers, one of which continuously transmits ultrasound while the other continuously receives echoes. CW Doppler is particularly useful for the evaluation of patients with valvular or congenital lesions. It is also the preferred technique when attempting to derive hemodynamic information from Doppler signals (Fig. 9–2*A*, see color plate).

COLOR FLOW MAPPING

Advances in electronics and computer technology have led to the development of color flow Doppler (CFD) ultrasound scanners capable of displaying blood flow within the heart in colors, in real time, while showing 2D images in black and white. In addition to showing the location, direction, and velocity of cardiac blood flow, the images produced by these devices allow estimation of flow acceleration and differentiation of laminar and turbulent blood flow. CFD echocardiography is based on the principle of multigated, PW Doppler.[10] According to this principle, blood flow velocity is sampled at many locations, along many lines covering the entire imaging sector. At the same time, the sector is also scanned to generate a 2D image.

Doppler color flow imaging uses the three primary colors (red, cyan, and green) from standard color television. Each picture element (pixel) on the video monitor screen displays the color red, cyan, green, or any combination of these. Any location in the heart where the scanner has detected flow towards the transducer (the top of the image sector) is assigned the color red. Flow away from the direction of the top is assigned the color cyan (Fig. 9–3, see color plate). This color assignment is completely arbitrary and determined by the equipment's manufacturer.

In the most common color flow coding scheme, the faster the velocity (up to a limit), the more intense the color. Flow velocities that change by more than a preset value within a brief interval (flow variance) have the color green added to either the red or the blue. Thus, they are mapped in brighter hues of red or blue. Both rapidly accelerating laminar flow (change in flow speed) and turbulent flow (change in flow direction) satisfy the criteria for rapid changes in velocity. Color Doppler aliasing, like PW Doppler aliasing, occurs at velocities in excess of the Nyquist limit and is frequently observed during imaging (Fig. 9–2*B*). In summary, the intensity of the red or cyan colors at any location and time is usually proportional to the corresponding flow velocity, whereas the hue is proportional to the temporal rate of change of the velocity.

CONTRAST ECHOCARDIOGRAPHY

Contrast echocardiography is a recently developed clinical diagnostic tool for assessing myocardial perfusion. It employs injected contrast agents, typically nontoxic solutions containing gaseous microbubbles, which reflect the ultrasonic beam emitted by the echo transducer. Thus, the "tracer" microbubbles imaged by ultrasonic backscatter represent blood flow within the tissue or organ on which the ultrasound beam is focused. Areas of impaired perfusion or no perfusion are therefore visualized.

Contrast echocardiography was originally reported in 1968 by Gramiak and Shah,[11] who described visualization of aortic valve incompetence at the time of left heart catheterization. Subsequently, contrast echocardiography has been used to image intracardiac shunts,[12–15] right and left heart valvular incompetence,[10, 16–19] and pericardial effusions. In addition, left ventricular injections of hand-agitated microbubble solutions have been used to identify left ventricular endocardial edges, cardiac output, and valvular regurgitation (semiquantitative), as shown in Figure 9–4.[10–18]

Initially, contrast agents consisted of various solutions that had been agitated by hand to produce microbubbles that would serve as ultrasonic reflectors. Hand-agitated microbubbles, however, are relatively large and unstable (40–50 μm in diameter) and therefore preclude quantitative analysis of contrast-enhanced images.[20]

Microbubbles produced by ultrasonic cavitation (sonication) have been shown to be superior to the hand-agitated microbubbles. Specifically, sonicated microbubbles have been shown to be smaller than hand-agitated microbubbles and, in fact, smaller than red blood cells. Indeed, sonicated microbubbles have been shown to be capable of both pass-

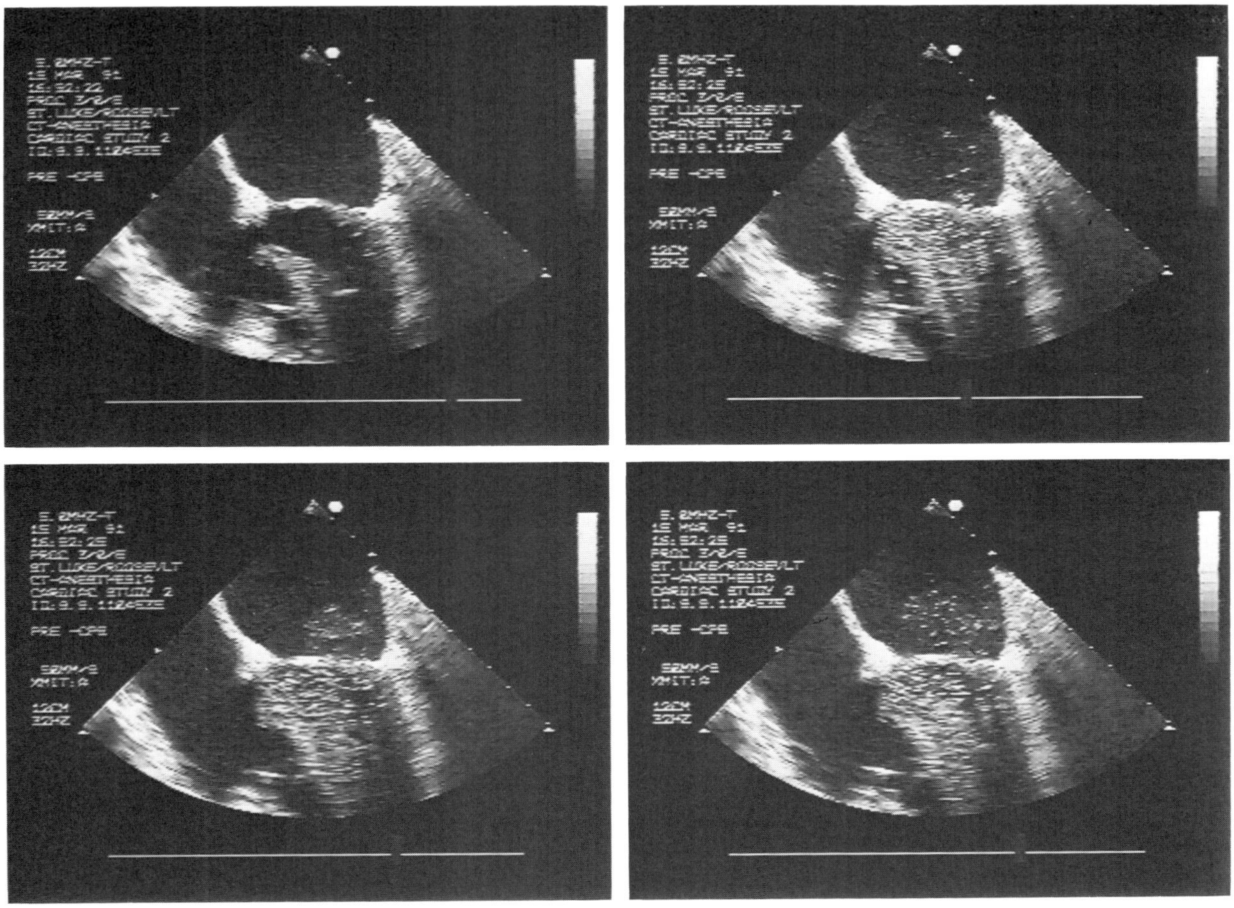

Figure 9–4. Intraoperative assessment of mitral valve regurgitation using hand-agitated microbubble contrast solution. The heart was imaged in the standard four-chamber view. *Top left,* Before contrast injection, enlarged LA, PA catheter in the RV, and injection needle in the LV are demonstrated. *Top right, bottom left, and bottom right,* Sequential systolic frames after contrast injection showing near-complete contrast opacification of the LV and increasing but relatively small amounts of contrast in the LA due to back flow across the valve consistent with mild MR. (Figure prepared with the assistance of B.P. Mindich, MD.)

ing along with the red blood cells through the microcapillary vascular bed and reflecting the echo beam. These smaller sonicated microbubbles thus permit direct ultrasonic imaging of tissue perfusion and detection of valvular abnormalities.[21]

In addition to small size, the sonicated microbubbles have been shown to exhibit intracavitary velocities comparable to those of red blood cells as observed by Doppler.[22] Numerous investigations have postulated that by controlling the size and stability of the microbubbles, quantitative measurements could be made. Contrast ultrasonography can be used for calculating absolute blood flow and volume *in vitro* and *in vivo*.[23–25] Clinical contrast echo studies have safely used a commercially prepared, air-filled albumin microsphere with known concentrations and size to visualize left heart structures following intravenous injections.[26] These studies suggest the possibility of noninvasive perfusion evaluation using contrast echocardiography; however, the ultimate quantitation of perfusion with contrast echo will require further development of ultrasound contrast agents (tracers) and ultrasound machines (detectors), along with application of mathematical models such as classic dye dilution theory.[27]

ECHOSCANNERS

BASIC PRINCIPLES

The conversion of reflected ultrasound echoes into 2D video images is a complicated process involving numerous electronic and digital manipulations. A 2D echo image is generated by scanning the heart every 17 msec, or about 60 times each second. The image generated from a single 1/60th of a second scan is called a *field*. A process called *interlacing* combines two scans or fields into a frame of 1/30th of a second. Because the eye cannot capture an image lasting 1/30th of a second, microprocessors further process the frame electronically in real time. The intrinsic persistence of the television screen enhances image quality, and the result is a fairly smooth picture.

RESOLUTION

Resolution is the ability of ultrasound to distinguish fine detail. The resolution of an echo system is the minimum distance that must separate two distinct reflectors so that they can be imaged as separate entities. Image resolution depends significantly on two major image axes: axial and lateral. Along the direction of the beam, the axial resolution of a pulsed instrument is approximately equal to:

$$0.77 \times \text{number of cycles in one pulse per frequency} \qquad 9\text{–}6$$

Typically, for a 2.5-MHz transducer with a narrow, three-cycle pulse duration, the axial transducer resolution is calculated at:

$$\frac{0.77 \times 3}{2.5} = 1 \text{ mm}$$

Lateral resolution is the minimum distance perpendicular to the ultrasound beam at which two objects can be imaged as distinct. It is determined almost entirely by the beam diameter; the narrower the beam, the better the lateral resolution. Typical values for lateral resolution range from 2 to 3 mm. Axial resolution is better than lateral resolution, because along the axis of the beam, image data are used as detected. In the lateral direction, the image is formed by the juxtaposition of many line scans.

IMAGE STORAGE

All modern echoscanners allow the operator to store or ''freeze'' a single echo image on the display screen. This allows the scrutiny of any unusual transient anatomic or physiologic observations. Once frozen, an image can also be subjected to some simple quantitative measurements. With the continuous motion of the cardiac structures, it is often difficult, however, to capture the exact frame that is to be analyzed. For this reason, techniques to acquire several consecutive frames have been developed.

CINE MEMORY

One of the widely used techniques for information storage is cine memory. When activated, this mode captures a sequence of several echo images in digital memory. Because of the digital storage technique, the quality of the stored images is high. They can be displayed again in several different ways. In one method, the frames are displayed one by one as the operator manually controls the transition from one frame to the next using a trackball. Any amount of time can be spent on a single frame. The images can also be replayed continuously in repeated endless-loop fashion, at the same or at a different speed than the original recording speed.

VIDEOTAPE

The video recorder is the most common long-term, mass-storage medium used in echocardiography. Most echoscanners are equipped with 1/2″ VHS, ''super'' VHS, or 3/4″ video cassette recorders (VCRs). Because VCRs store images in analog format, the quality of videotaped images is currently inferior to the real-time display or the digital cine memory replay.

OTHER STORAGE MEDIA

Photographic or digital paper chart recorders are available for most devices and are used to record the continuously scrolled information of M-mode and PW Doppler. The scrolls can subsequently be used for quantitative analysis of these types of data. These devices can also provide prints of single-frame 2D images.

Prints with color flow information can be obtained with instant Polaroid-type cameras, 35mm cameras, or color video printers. The latter images, although expensive, are of higher quality than those acquired by more conventional techniques.

Digital image storage is possible on magnetic disk. Standard floppy disks have a very limited storage capability, because the amount of information in a single video frame can be of the order of 1 megabyte (MB). Furthermore, neither storage nor retrieval can be achieved in an expeditious manner. A new digital mass storage medium uses ''write-once, read-many'' digitally encoded laser disks. Using a large 810-MB memory, it can store 24,000 frames or 800 different cine loops, each 30 frames long.

TRANSESOPHAGEAL TRANSDUCERS

Because fat, bone, and air-containing lung interfere with sound wave penetration, clear transthoracic echocardiogram views are particularly difficult to obtain in patients with obesity, emphysema, or abnormal chest wall anatomy. To avoid these problems, esophageal transducers were developed. Sound waves emitted from an esophageal transducer only have to pass through the esophageal wall and the pericardium to reach the heart; thus, there is less likelihood of image distortion, and there are potentially new echocardiographic windows. Other advantages of TEE include the stability of the transducer position and the possibility of obtaining continuous recordings of cardiac activity for extended periods.

The first TEE examination was performed in 1975. The probe used allowed only M-mode imaging and had limited control of direction. Two-dimensional TEE was first performed with a mechanical system,[28] consisting of a vertical and a horizontal mechanical scanner connected to a 3.5-MHz ultrasonic transducer contained in a 12 × 20 × 6 mm oil bag. The transducer were rotated by a single phase commutator motor via flexible shafts.

Subsequently, phased array transducers were mounted into gastroscope housings.[29, 30] With their greater flexibility and control, these probes allowed 2D scanning of the heart through many planes, and the probes became the prototypes of the currently used models. Recently, annular array probes have been introduced. Phased and annular array systems offer a multitude of imaging capabilities: (1) M-mode, (2) 2D (gray scale and B color, in which the typical gray scale is replaced by range of colors), (3) high-resolution modes, (4) PW Doppler, (5) CW Doppler, (6) color flow mapping, and (7) computerized data processing for measurements and cine loop display.

All TEE probes share several common features. All of the currently available transducers employ a 5-MHz transducer that is mounted on the tip of a gastroscope housing. The tip can be directed by the adjustment of knobs placed at the proximal handle. In most adult probes, there are two knobs: one allows anterior and posterior movement, and the other permits side-to-side motion. Thus, in combination with the ability to advance, withdraw, and rotate the probe, many echocardiographic windows are possible. Another feature common to most probes is the inclusion of a temperature sensor to warn of possible thermal injury to the esophagus.

Currently there are five types of TEE commercially available: adult single plane (transverse orientation: perpendicular to the shaft), adult biplane (transverse and longitudinal orientation, parallel to the shaft), adult multiplane (variable orientation of the scanning plane—Fig. 9–5), single plane pediatric, and biplane pediatric. The adult probes usually have a shaft length of 100 cm and are between 9 and 12 mm in diameter. The tips of the probe vary slightly in shape and size, but are generally 1–2 mm wider than the shaft. The size of these probes requires the patient to weigh at least 20 kg. Depending on the manufacturer, the adult probes contain between 32 and 64 elements per scanning orientation. In general, the image quality is directly related to the number of elements used.

The pediatric probes are mounted on a narrower, shorter shaft with smaller transducers. These probes may be used in patients as small as 1 kg. Because of size limitations, these probes may not possess a lateral control knob. The question has been asked, Why not use the pediatric probe on all patients to decrease the risk of esophageal injury? The answer is that the smaller probes provide less diagnostic information. The number of elements is reduced, the aperture is smaller, there is less control of the tip, and the smaller transducer tip does not usually make good contact in the adult esophagus. These factors combine to significantly reduce image quality.

In the near future, several important new features will be available. Most probe handles are not sealed, and accidental wetting results in ruining the probe; newer probe handles will be immersible. Another feature that will soon be available is the ability to alter the scanning frequency among 3.5 MHz, 5 MHz, and 7 MHz. A lower frequency, such as 3.5 MHz, has greater penetration and is more suited for the transgastric view. It also increases the Doppler velocity limits. Conversely, the higher frequencies yield better resolution for detailed imaging. One of the limitations of TEE is that structures very close to the probe are seen only in a very narrow sector. Newer probes may also allow a broader near field view. Finally, newer probes may be able to scan simultaneously in more than one plane.

With more than 12 models from at least 7 manufacturers, choosing a system is extremely difficult. Price, image quality, features, size, training, and service are the key considerations. One additional point to consider is that none of the TEE probes uses more than 64 elements, and that technical limitations will probably prevent an increase in the number of elements used. If only TEE is planned, it is only necessary to obtain a 64-element ultrasonograph, which can result in substantial savings.

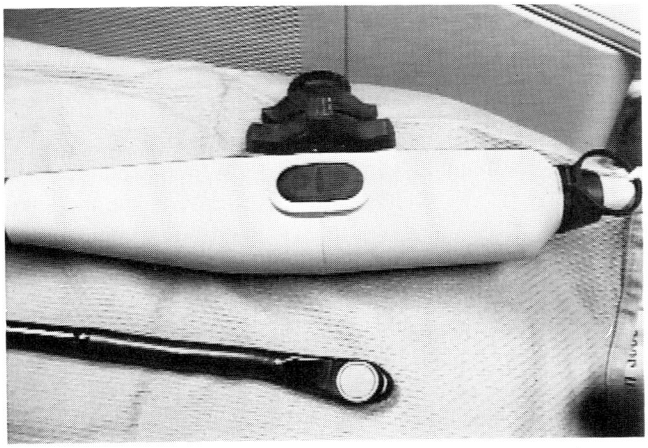

Figure 9–5. An advanced design TEE probe capable of multiple-plane imaging between the transverse and longitudinal orientations of the transducer and the probe shaft. The two buttons shown under the positioning knobs in the probe's handle activate a motor that rotates the round phased array at the tip of the probe below the handle. The angle between the image scanning plane and the probe shaft varies between 0° and 180° and is displayed on the video screen (see Figs. 9–1 and 9–7).

INDICATIONS

GLOBAL VENTRICULAR FUNCTION

The development of quantitative analysis techniques for TEE applications has been fairly rapid because many of the mathematical models had already been used for transthoracic or epicardial echocardiography. The practical applications of quantitative TEE analysis have been limited by the necessity for time-consuming tracings and the meticulous attention to detail that is essential to avoid errors. Thus, the best quantitative TEE analyses are performed some time after the images have been acquired, or "off-line." In addition, the well-trained echocardiographer may be capable of qualitatively grading myocardial performance in a clinically useful way during the actual examination, or "on-line." The impending development of accurate, reliable, on-line automated endocardial border detection is the factor that will probably bring quantitative analysis to the forefront of TEE analysis techniques.

Visual Estimation of Function

In routine clinical use, the anesthesiologist-echocardiographer must make visual estimates of ventricular wall motion and overall function. These depend on the ability of the individual to interpret the images and correctly ''quantify'' subjective assessments of ventricular function. The clinician may be aided by video recordings of prior function or video images displayed on split screens. These estimations of global ventricular function are usually performed in the short-axis view of the left ventricle (LV) but additional information can be gained by assessing the long-axis view of the LV. In this assessment, the observer examines the end-diastolic image and compares it to the end-systolic frame to determine the degree of ejection. The rate of ejection is also estimated.

Clements et al demonstrated that segmental wall motion abnormalities (SWMAs) may be identified on visual inspection of echo images by anesthesiologists.[31] However, later work by Hillel et al[32] and Saada et al[33] has shown that ejection fraction (EF) and wall motion changes may not be adequately detected by visual inspection alone. The preliminary data in these two studies are further supported by Lazar et al,[34] who found that qualitative scoring did not detect improvements in regional LV function that were detected by off-line quantitative wall thickening analysis. In contrast, several recent studies have documented that an educated visual analysis of echocardiographic images provides a better estimation of left ventricular ejection fraction (LVEF) than more sophisticated and time-consuming computer techniques.[35, 36]

Echocardiographic Tracings

Consistency in the acquisition and analysis of 2D TEE images is required if meaningful data are to be obtained from a 2D view of a 3D heart. For the purposes of LV wall motion analysis, the midpapillary view of the LV has become the standard view because maximal ventricular excursion is seen in this view. The ''true'' short-axis view is somewhat difficult to maintain, however, because slight anteflexion or retroflexion of the probe leads to multiple oblique views that are similar in appearance but yield widely varying information.[37] Thus, the papillary muscle morphology must be continually observed to maintain a consistent short-axis view.

Other issues that are essential to the consistency of quantitative analysis are stability of cardiac rhythm, surgical manipulations, and the respiratory cycle. Ectopic and post-extrasystolic beats will yield abnormal values when compared to normal sinus rhythm. Irregular cardiac rhythms such as atrial fibrillation are problematic because the derived parameters vary from beat to beat. Averaging of information from several beats may be necessary. Surgical manipulations may alter loading conditions (e.g., vena caval obstruction, aortic retraction), temporarily alter cardiac function (e.g., pericardial irritation with hot solutions), or change the echocardiographic image (e.g., retraction or lifting of the heart). The respiratory cycle also results in cyclic changes in loading conditions and the anatomic relationship of the heart to the esophagus.

Once the echocardiographic image has been acquired, the method of tracing the endocardial and/or epicardial borders becomes important. Echocardiographic images may be traced using software that is included in most echocardiography machines or by using a separate work station. The ability to identify borders is aided by viewing the moving echocardiographic image just prior to tracing. Cine loops and videotape playback help the operator to determine what represents the actual border and to ''fill in'' missing or unclear regions using the operator's knowledge of the shape of the border.

The tracing of endocardial borders is complicated by trabeculation of the ventricular wall and the observed ''thickness'' of the endocardial border. On an echo image, the endocardial border appears thicker at the anterior and posterior walls where the border runs perpendicular to the ultrasound transmission. This perceived thickness has a leading edge and a trailing edge. The accepted method of tracing endocardial borders uses the ''leading edge–leading edge'' outline. Wyatt et al found that this technique led to acceptable correlations with *in vitro* measurements.[38] For all quantitative echocardiographic measurements, it is recommended that at least four consecutive contractions be averaged because of the considerable beat-to-beat variation.

Preload/Diastolic Function

End-Diastolic Dimensions

Although preload is often estimated by measuring left heart filling pressures (pulmonary capillary wedge pressure [PCWP], left atrial pressure [LAP], or left ventricular end-diastolic pressure [LVEDP]), in echocardiography it can be determined by measuring LV end-diastolic dimensions. In M-mode echocardiography, a single ventricular diameter is obtained, whereas in 2D echocardiography one or multiple tomographic cuts are recorded. It has been proposed that end-diastolic dimensions provide a better index of preload than the PCWP does. In one study, PCWP and end-diastolic volumes (EDVs), derived from short-axis areas at the level of the papillary muscles, were compared as predictors of cardiac index (CI) in patients undergoing coronary artery surgery.[39] Strong correlations were observed between end-diastolic areas, or EDV, and CI, whereas no significant correlation was found between PCWP and CI. The ongoing debate as to the number of planes required to accurately represent ventricular volumes is beyond the scope of this discussion.[40, 41]

TEE is often, for practical reasons, limited to a single short-axis view at the level of the papillary muscles. Some evidence suggests that end-diastolic short-axis areas (EDA) measured at this level correlate reasonably well with measurements obtained by on-heart echocardiography[42] and with

EDV measured simultaneously using radionuclides.[43] Other investigators disagreed with these conclusions, however. Using a combined radionuclide and thermodilution technique, Urbanowicz and coworkers found that the correlation coefficient between the LV EDA by TEE and the LV end-diastolic volume index (LVEDVI) was only 0.74. In addition, they noted discordant changes in four of nine patients.[44]

Transmitral Blood Flow

Another approach to the evaluation of left ventricular filling is to examine the flow across the mitral valve. This approach adds information on the entire diastolic period, not just end-diastole. After valvular dysfunction has been excluded, the sample volume of the PW Doppler system is placed in the mitral inflow. The best location for the sample volume is in the center of the mitral flow, just slightly to the ventricular side of the mitral valve. Flow velocity measured with the sample volume in this location will result in a typical flow velocity pattern. After opening of the mitral valve, the early inflow into the left ventricle will be recognized as a large velocity peak (E peak). It is followed by a period of diastasis and a second, smaller velocity peak (A peak) representing the flow produced by the atrial contraction. Analysis of the diastolic inflow includes the measurement of peak E and A velocities and their ratio (E:A), the derivation of acceleration and deceleration for each peak, calculation of various intervals, and integration of the total area (time-velocity integral) under the velocity display (Fig. 9–6, see color plate).

Deviations from the normal diastolic velocity pattern have been described under various circumstances. With tachycardia, fusion of the E and A peaks occurs, whereas the A peak is absent during atrial fibrillation. In mitral regurgitation, the E peak is much larger than the A peak, and the E peak velocity exceeds values observed in normal persons. The diastolic inflow of the patient with mitral stenosis is marked by high E peak velocity, prolonged deceleration from the peak velocity, and continuous flow throughout diastole. The most commonly observed abnormality is a reversal of the E:A ratio indicating impaired early LV filling. This has been noted with advanced age, ischemic heart disease, hypertrophic cardiomyopathy, secondary LV hypertrophy, dilated cardiomyopathy, and in patients with right ventricular pressure overload.

The determinants of E peak velocity have been investigated in animal and human studies. Variables that have been clearly recognized as determinants of E peak velocity include the left atrial pressure, the LV relaxation rate, and the systemic arterial pressure. The E peak velocity varies directly with increasing LAP and inversely with increases in the time constant of relaxation or systemic arterial pressure.[45]

Other factors that have not been directly associated with the E peak velocity but are nonetheless important for the onset of diastolic flow include the ventricular suction effect and mitral ring recoil. Interpretation of diastolic peak velocity is further confounded by changes in heart rate (HR) and loading conditions. In one study, Nishimura et al observed that fluid infusion that which increased PCWP also increased E peak velocity, whereas phenylephrine infusions had the opposite effect.[46]

Acceleration and Deceleration

Acceleration of flow in early diastole is the result of the pressure gradient between the left atrium and the LV, whereas deceleration coincides with the reversal of the pressure gradient between these chambers.[47] Under normal circumstances, the average forward gradient associated with acceleration is significantly greater than the reverse gradient associated with deceleration. The determinants of E wave deceleration are similar to those of E peak velocity.

Area Integration

Integration of *partial* areas under the flow velocity curve has been suggested for the assessment of ventricular filling and diastolic function.[48] Areas that have been studied include the areas for the first 33% of diastole, the first 50% of diastole, the area under the E peak (Ei), and the area under the A peak (Ai). Using the ratio of Ei/Ai, Pearson et al observed an inverse linear relationship between age and early diastolic filling.[49] This observation suggests that, with increasing age, the filling of the LV becomes more dependent on atrial contraction. In children, Snider et al found that the ratio of the area under the first 33% of diastole over the total area was larger in normal than in hypertensive children.[50] Conversely, the ratio of Ai over total area was larger in hypertensive patients.

Intraoperative Applications

Diastolic function has been assessed intraoperatively by PW Doppler echocardiography in only a few studies. It was observed that some cardiac surgery patients with normal mitral inflow patterns before cardiopulmonary bypass (CPB) had signs of impaired ventricular filling after bypass.[51] More recently, Rinder et al reported that diastolic filling was significantly impaired 2 hours after CPB.[52] They noted a trend toward recovery by 4 hours and a return to baseline by 18 hours. Other potential intraoperative applications of the determination of diastolic mitral flow by PW Doppler echocardiography include the assessment of the atrial contribution to stroke volume and the detection of ischemia.

The contribution of the atrial contraction to ventricular filling is ideally studied by the measurement of mitral flow velocity. The Ai will be directly proportional to the fraction of the stroke volume (SV) contributed by the atrial contraction. In cardiac surgery patients, it has been demonstrated that the decrease in CI occurring as a result of the loss of the atrial contraction will be greater in patients with lower E/A ratios.[53] Others have used PW Doppler echocardiography to document increased CI with atrioventricular versus ventricular pacing or to optimize atrioventricular delay intervals during atrioventricular sequential pacing.[54–56]

Ventricular relaxation requires energy; one of the early consequences of myocardial ischemia is impaired ventricular relaxation and early ventricular filling. When myocardial ischemia is produced by transient occlusion of a coronary artery, as occurs during angioplasty, the observation of a rapid reduction in E peak velocity suggests impaired relaxation. In one study, diastolic LV dysfunction was the earliest change noted after coronary occlusion, and it often preceded the development of abnormal systolic function.[57] In another study, it was observed that acute ischemia not only altered early ventricular filling but also produced marked abnormalities in late ventricular filling.[58]

Afterload

Although afterload cannot be determined by echocardiography alone, the combination of ventricular dimensions with ventricular wall thickness and systolic arterial pressure yields end-systolic wall stress. Ventricular wall thickness is derived by calculating the difference between the epicardial and endocardial areas, whereas the ventricular dimension corresponds to the endocardial area.[59]

The formula to calculate wall stress was derived by Sandler and Dodge from the Laplace equation:

$$\text{Wall stress} = \frac{(1.33 \times P \times \text{LVEDd})}{4\text{WT}\ (1 + \text{WT/LVEDd})} \qquad 9\text{–}7$$

where P = the systolic arterial pressure, WT = wall thickness, LVEDd = the left ventricular end-diastolic cavity dimension, and 1.33 converts mmHg to dynes-cm^{-2}.[60]

A simplified version of the wall stress equation states that:

$$\text{Wall stress} = \frac{P \times \text{LVEDd}}{\text{WT}} \qquad 9\text{–}8$$

Diastolic dimensions are selected because it is assumed that peak-systolic wall stress occurs during isovolumic ventricular contraction while the ventricle still possesses its diastolic anatomic configuration.

Elevations in wall stress have been observed in patients with LV enlargement due to systemic hypertension, aortic stenosis, or aortic regurgitation.[61] Wall stress certainly provides a better index of afterload than systemic vascular resistance (SVR) when forward SV is not equal to the total ventricular ejection, such as in mitral regurgitation or in the presence of a ventricular septal defect. Whether the same is true in patients without such lesions is unclear. In one animal study, it was observed that SVR and wall stress did not correlate well during pharmacologic interventions and occasionally varied in opposite directions.[62]

In cardiac surgical patients, similarly poor correlations between SVR and end-systolic wall stress were observed.[63] In patients undergoing carotid artery surgery, Smith et al studied wall stress under various anesthetic regimens.[64] Patients receiving higher concentrations of volatile anesthetics plus phenylephrine had significantly greater wall stress than those receiving lower concentrations without phenylephrine.

Contractility

Echocardiography has been utilized to estimate contractility in a variety of ways. It is best suited for the evaluation of contractility during the ejection phase of contraction, but other approaches also have been explored.

Ejection Phase Indices

With echocardiography, contractility has most frequently been estimated with ejection phase indices. A wide array of ejection phase indices have been described, but all require measurement of end-diastolic and end-systolic dimensions. In M-mode echocardiography, these dimensions will often be simple linear, internal dimensions of the LV cavity. The ratio of

$$\text{FS} = \frac{\text{LVIDd} - \text{LVISd}}{\text{LVIDd}} \qquad 9\text{–}9$$

where LVIDd = LV internal diastolic dimension and LVISd = LV internal systolic dimension will yield fractional shortening (FS), a basic ejection phase index of contractility.

With 2D echocardiography, multiple tomographic cuts can be obtained and utilized to calculate ventricular volumes using a variety of formulas such as Simpson's Rules.[65] Using the ventricular volumes, EF can then be calculated with the standard formula:

$$\text{EF} = \frac{\text{LVEDV} - \text{LVESV}}{\text{LVEDV}} \qquad 9\text{–}10$$

where LVEDV = LV end-diastolic volume and LVESV = LV end-systolic volume.

During intraoperative TEE, it is most convenient to monitor a single, short-axis view at the level of the midpapillary muscles. Once the end-diastolic and end-systolic endocardial areas have been delineated with the help of tracing software, the contractility may be estimated using the fractional area of contraction (FAC) or the ejection fraction area (EFA):

$$\text{EFA} = \frac{\text{LVEDA} - \text{LVESA}}{\text{LVEDA}} \qquad 9\text{–}11$$

where LVEDA = end-diastolic area and LVESA = the end-systolic area (Fig. 9–7).

Isovolumic Phase Indices

The standard isovolumic phase index, dP/dt, cannot be obtained using TEE. Some information on the isovolumic phase can, however, be gathered by measuring the length of the pre-ejection period (PEP). The PEP is the time between the onset of the Q wave on the ECG and the opening of the aortic valve on M-mode echocardiography. The usefulness and limitations of the PEP, as well as of the other

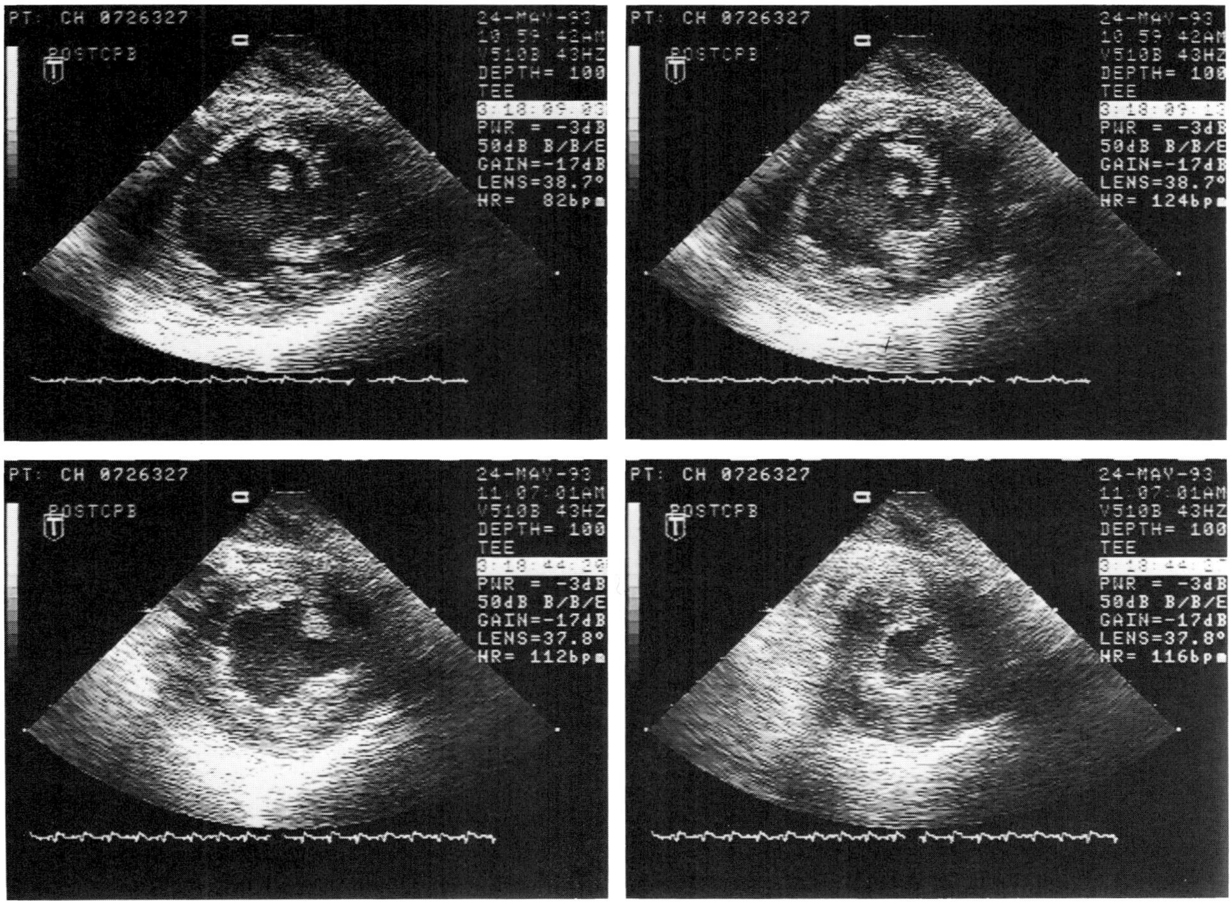

Figure 9–7. Global systolic left ventricular function at the mid-papillary muscle level in a patient after myocardial revascularization and cardiopulmonary bypass. The top two panels demonstrate depressed LV function immediately following bypass: the LV end-diastolic cavity *(top left)* changes little at end-systole *(top right)*, indicating a low ejection fraction area. The bottom two panels show normal systolic LV function in the same patient in a similar imaging plane approximately 7 minutes later after starting IV infusion of dopamine and increasing the arterial blood pressure: the end-diastolic cavity *(bottom left)* empties dramatically at end-systole *(bottom right)*. Note also that during depressed systolic function, the LV cavity also is dilated notably in diastole compared to the diastolic size during normal LV function (top left vs. bottom left panels).

systolic intervals, have been more extensively reviewed elsewhere.[66, 67]

The maximal acceleration of blood flow in the aorta is another measurement related to the isovolumic phase of the contraction.[68] Maximal blood flow acceleration occurs in the early part of the LV ejection and can be measured by Doppler echocardiography. It is determined by placing a Doppler transducer in the suprasternal notch and aiming the ultrasound beam at the aortic valve. A variety of studies have demonstrated that maximum blood flow acceleration sampled in this manner provides information on LV contractility.[69–71] The currently available TEE imaging planes are not suitable for this type of measurement.

End-Systolic Pressure/Volume Relationship

An important limitation of isovolumic and ejection phase indices of contractility is their significant sensitivity to ventricular loading conditions. Load-independent indices have been explored in order to circumvent this problem. One such index is the LV end-systolic pressure/volume relationship (ESPVR) or end-systolic elastance.[72] Multiple end-systolic pressures and volumes need to be measured during rapid alterations in LV preload (e.g., vena caval occlusion) in order to calculate the ESPVR.

On a pressure/volume diagram, points defined by the end-systolic pressures and volumes of several cardiac cycles will be positioned on a single line. The slope of this line is relatively independent of loading conditions and proportional to contractility—the steeper the slope, the greater the contractility. The intraoperative determination of contractility by this technique has been hampered by difficulties in obtaining accurate ventricular volumes and pressures in sufficiently varying preload. Nonetheless, using single short-axis views and radial arterial pressures, the linearity of the ESPVR has been confirmed.[73] In addition, predicted changes in the direction of the slope have been demonstrated after the administration of known positive and negative inotropic agents.[74]

Other Techniques

Because of the difficulties in measuring ESPVR, alternative approaches have been attempted. One such alternative is the use of the end-systolic stress/end-systolic area (ESS/ESA) relationship.[74] Initial work demonstrates that the relationship is linear over a wide range of systolic pressures and shifts in an appropriate fashion during postextrasystolic potentiation. Further work to define the effects of positive and negative inotropes on the ESS/ESA is needed to determine the applicability of this relationship. Simonson and Schiller proposed an interesting, alternative approach to the determination of LV function.[75] They studied the systolic excursion of the mitral annulus in a quantitative manner, and compared it to LVEF. They found that the excursion of the ventricular base was always at least 8 mm in normal humans, whereas it was less in patients with decreased ventricular function. Simonson and Schiller also observed that the relationship between this variable and LVEF was linear.

Cardiac Output

M-Mode

Early in the development of echocardiography, Feigenbaum et al compared echocardiographic and angiographic volumes in an attempt to relate M-mode echo measurements to actual ventricular sizes.[76] Cubed, single M-mode echocardiographic dimensions correlated with angiographic equivalents.

Nevertheless, the good correlations between echo and angiographic volumes prompted other investigators to develop several methods for deriving ventricular volumes from single M-mode dimensions.[77–81] Kronik et al calculated SV from M-mode echocardiography using a number of these methods and compared their findings to thermodilution measurements in patients with and without symmetric ventricular contractions.[82] They concluded that clinically useful SV could be obtained using the Teichholz formula if the ventricular contraction was symmetric or nearly symmetric. Other formulae were unsatisfactory even in patients with a similar contraction pattern, whereas all formulae failed in patients with asymmetric contractions.

Using the Teichholz equation, ventricular volumes are calculated as:

$$\text{Volume} = \frac{7D^3}{2.4 + D} \qquad 9\text{–}12$$

where D = the ventricular internal dimension. SV is calculated as the difference between EDV and ESV. The American Society of Echocardiography has recommended that internal dimensions be measured from leading edge to leading edge and that the end-diastolic dimension coincide with the Q wave on the ECG. The end-systolic dimension is best measured at the time of the peak downward motion of the posterior endocardium.[83] When TEE was utilized to obtain these ventricular dimensions, correlations between SV obtained by echo and indicator dilution varied from r = 0.72 in patients undergoing cardiac surgery[84] to r = 0.97 in critically ill patients.[85]

Two-Dimensional

In patients undergoing coronary artery bypass surgery (CABG), SV was derived from 2D short-axis views using epicardial echocardiography.[54] Comparisons of echo-derived CI with simultaneous thermodilution CI yielded a correlation coefficient of 0.80.

Doppler

Integration of the *total* area under the transmitral Doppler flow velocity display has been used for the measurement of SV. The flow velocity integral is multiplied by the cross-sectional area (CSA) of the mitral valve to determine SV. There are different models for the calculation of mitral valve CSA, however.[86, 87] Using TEE, Roewer et al calculated SV in 27 surgical patients.[88] A comparison of Doppler-determined cardiac output (CO) with those obtained by thermodilution yielded an excellent correlation (r = 0.95). LaMantia et al found only a modest correlation (r = 0.68) in 13 cardiac surgical patients.[89]

When the results of various studies are compared, it is important to know the method of calculating the flow velocity integral and the CSA of the mitral valve as well as the location of the Doppler sampling volume. Because PW Doppler provides a spectral display of instantaneous velocities, different areas would be obtained if peak velocities, mean velocities, or the mode of the velocities was utilized for the integration. The measurement of the mitral orifice diameter should probably be repeated at various COs. It has been well established that the size of the mitral orifice varies with varying flows. The importance of the sample volume location was demonstrated by Dittmann et al, who noted that SV was underestimated when the sampling volume was placed at the mitral leaflet tips and overestimated at the mitral annulus.[90]

Investigations have used PA Doppler flow-velocity integrals and estimations of the vessel area to perform off-line calculations of SV and CO. Muhiudeen et al found that transmitral Doppler CO did not correlate with thermodilution, and that pulmonary artery (PA) Doppler CO correlated only weakly (r = 0.65) with thermodilution.[91] They concluded that transesophageal Doppler has significant limitations as an off-line monitor of CO. In contrast, Savino et al found good agreement and correlation (r = 0.93) between transesophageal PA Doppler and thermodilution CO.[92] They were, however, unable to visualize the main PA in 24% of patients. In addition, the method was tedious and not suitable for on-line analysis with current equipment and software.

Determination of Intravascular Pressures

In an interesting application of echocardiography, various echocardiographic techniques have been utilized to

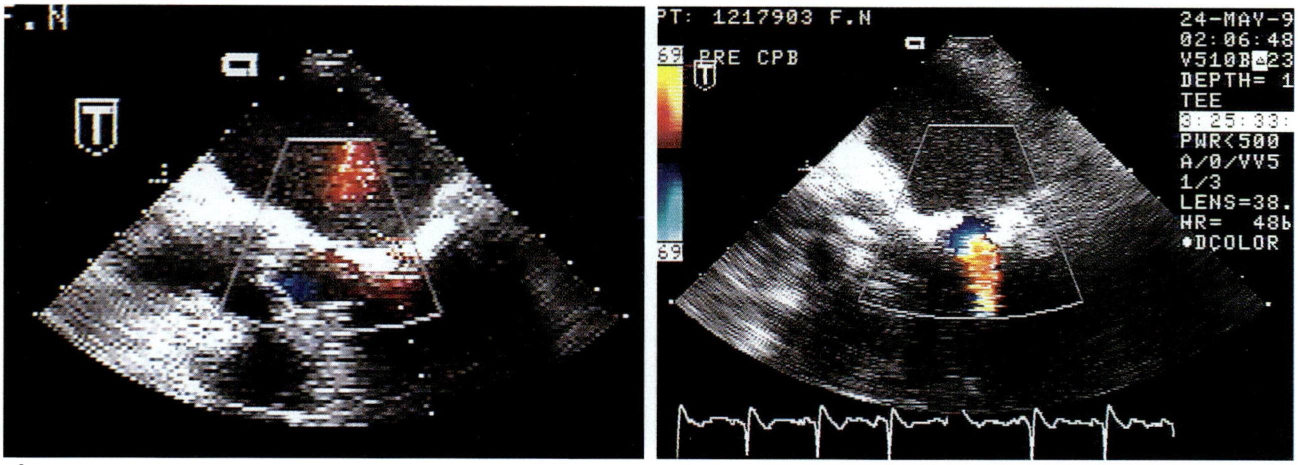

A — B

Figure 9–2. *A*, Continuous wave Doppler spectrum *(bottom image)* of the velocities of blood flow across the mitral valve in a patient with mitral valve stenosis *(top insert)* in sinus rhythm. The peak flow velocity of nearly 2m/second corresponds to a transvalvular pressure gradient of 16 mmHg, which is abnormally high and indicates a significant degree of stenosis. At slow heart rates, fusion of the two inflow waves in diastole due to delayed deceleration of the early peak is typical of mitral stenosis. *B*, 2D color flow Doppler image of a four-chamber view of the heart demonstrating color aliasing (blue to red change) in the narrow diastolic LV inflow jet in mitral valve stenosis.

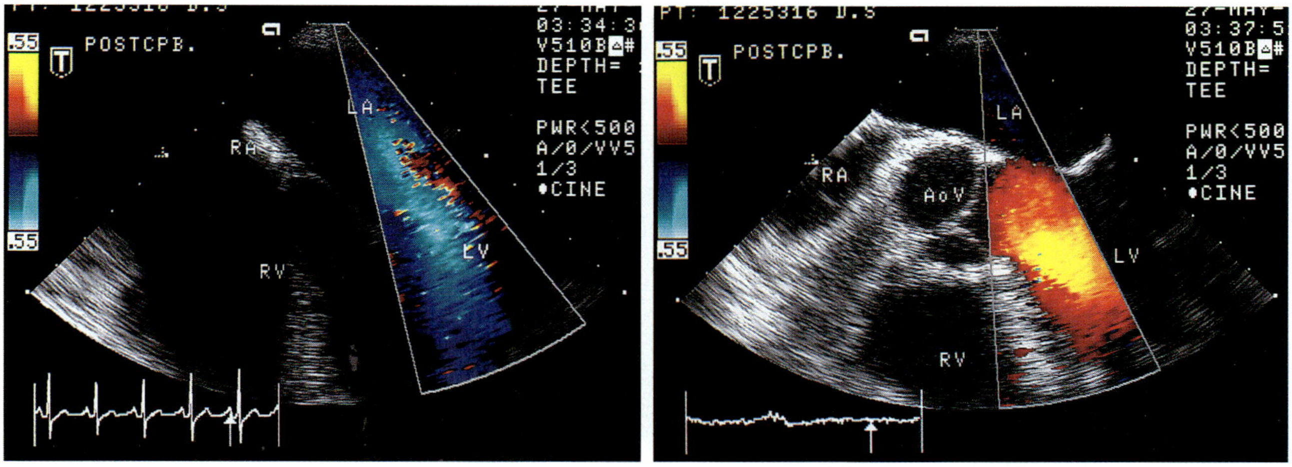

A — B

Figure 9–3. Color flow Doppler maps of normal blood flow during a cardiac cycle demonstrated in the four-chamber and five-chamber views: *A*, Late ventricular diastolic filling of the LV during LA systole demonstrating blood flow away from the transducer color coded in blue. *B*, LV ejection during systole from the LV outflow tract toward the aortic valve and toward the transducer color coded in bright red, orange, and yellow.

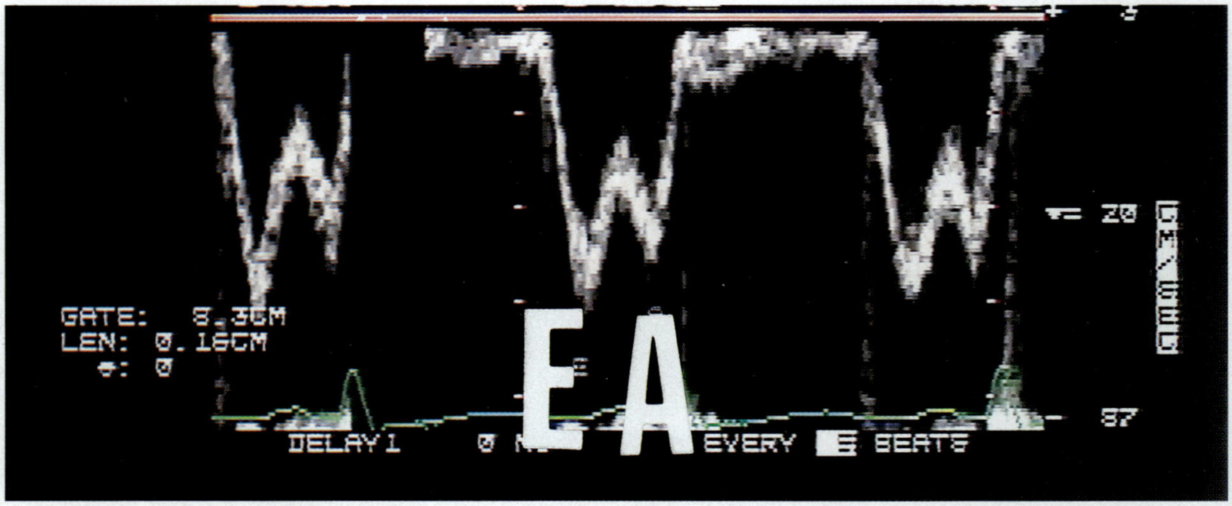

Figure 9–6. Pulsed-wave Doppler velocity profile at the level of the mitral valve. The early diastolic filling peak (E peak) and the atrial filling peak (A peak) are merged because of a rapid heart rate.

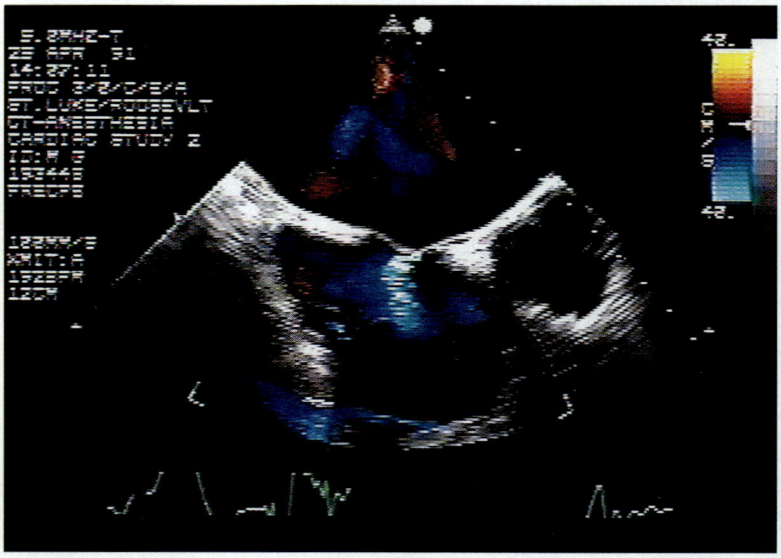

Figure 9–10. Left-to-right shunt across a patent foramen ovale demonstrated by CFD in a partial five-chamber view of a patient with mitral and aortic valve disease. The top of the scan sector is the enlarged left atrium; below it, in the center, is the right atrium. The interatrial septum is seen to bulge toward the RA, indicating elevated LA pressure. Blood flow (mapped in blue colors) originating at the atrial septum into the RA is consistent with flow across a patent foramen ovale. The small black cavity near the right edge of the image sector is the aortic root.

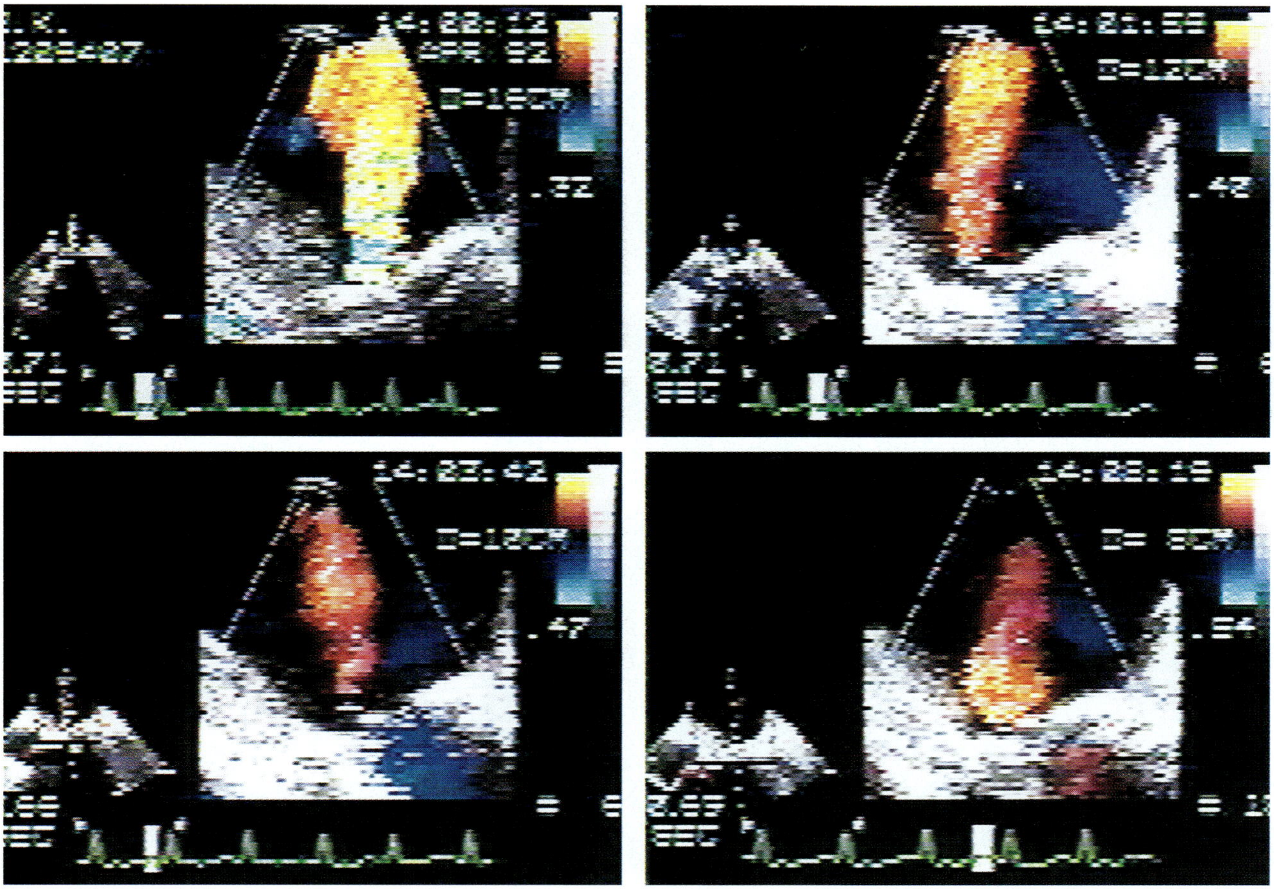

Figure 9–11. The effect of the Nyquist limit on the Doppler color flow map of an MR jet. Hemodynamic conditions and imaging planes were the same in each of the four panels. The same enhanced color maps were used in each panel; they differ only in their Nyquist limits. The MR jet into the left atrial cavity is seen in yellow, orange, and red. *Top left*, Color Nyquist limit of 0.32 m/second produces the brightest and largest jet size because bright hues are assigned to the entire jet. *Top right*, At a Nyquist limit of 0.42 m/second, the brightest colors are assigned to less than the entire jet, making it appear smaller. *Bottom left*, At a Nyquist limit of 0.47 m/second, the MR jet appears yet smaller because of dimmer color assignment, especially at the jet's edges. *Bottom right*, The smallest MR jet map is produced at the highest Nyquist limit of 0.54 m/second.

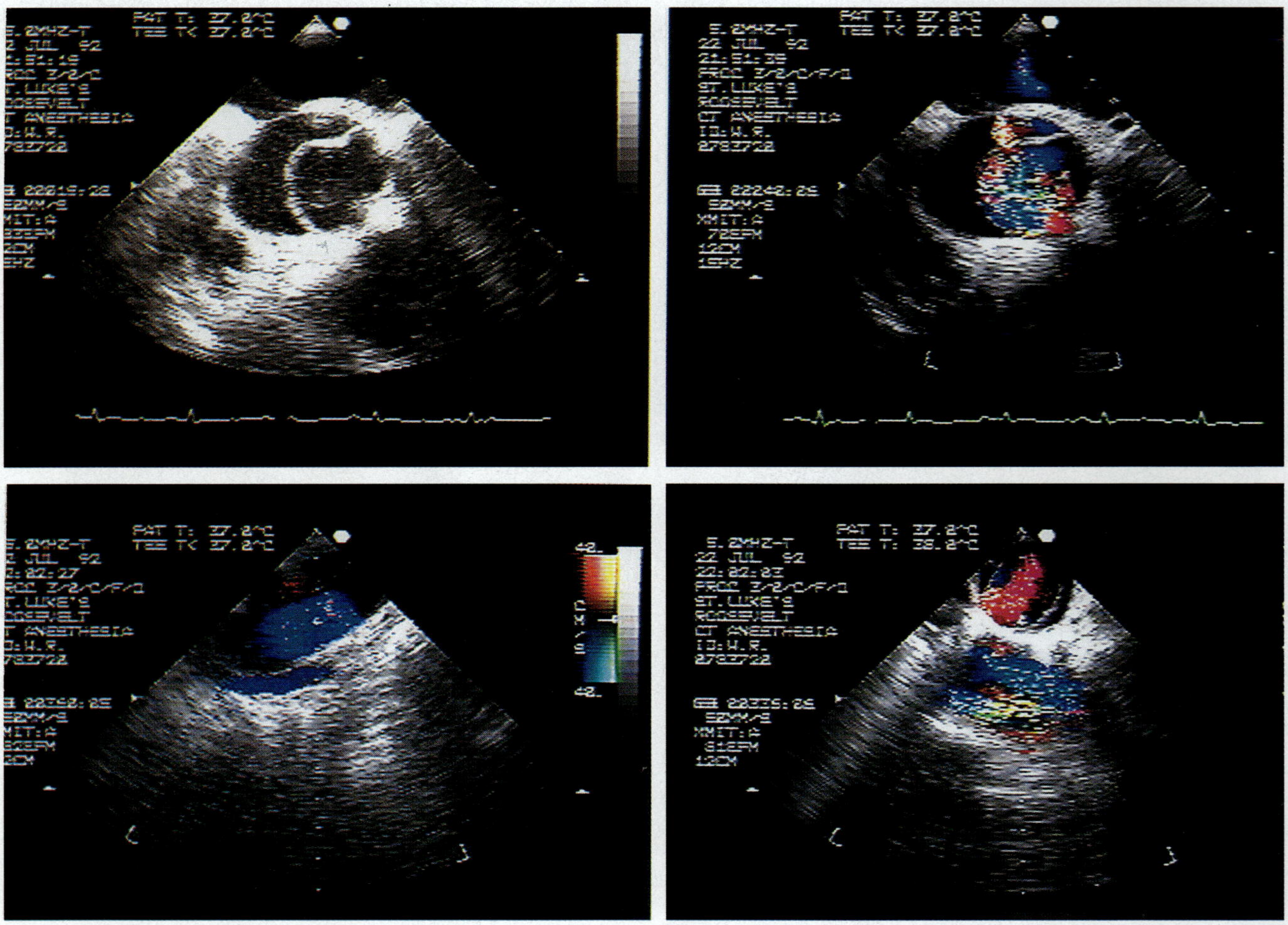

Figure 9–12. TEE assessment of a thoracic aortic dissection at different anatomic levels of the aorta. *Top left,* The aorta just above the aortic valve demonstrates two lumens and the dissection flap, and shows that the dissection extends into the aortic root. *Top right,* The same imaging plane of the aortic root with added color Doppler mapping demonstrates blood flow in the true lumen and a communication with the false lumen through a small, brightly colored jet near the top of the dissection flap. *Bottom left,* Partial view of the aortic arch shows blue color mapped blood flow in the true lumen and very little flow in the false lumen, which is above the true lumen, closer to the esophagus. *Bottom right,* Cross-sectional view of the descending thoracic aorta demonstrates blood flow in red in the true lumen, the dissection flap toward the right, and the partially collapsed false lumen.

gauge intracardiac or intravascular pressures. Stevenson recently compared six different echocardiographic techniques to measure pulmonary artery pressure (PAP).[93] When compared with direct measurements, some of these techniques yielded highly accurate correlations ($r = 0.97$), but were not always applicable in all patients. Using TEE, several investigators have attempted to derive PCWP or LAP from pulmonary venous Doppler velocity signals.[94, 95] In one study, the LAP correlated best with the systolic forward flow in the left upper pulmonary vein; in the other study, the LAP correlated best with flow velocity reversal in that vein during atrial contraction.

MYOCARDIAL ISCHEMIA MONITORING

Regional Wall Motion and Systolic Wall Thickness

The relationship of echocardiographic indices of regional myocardial function to ischemia has been compared to changes that occur with surface electrocardiography, PCWP, and the onset of chest pain. As early as 1935 it was recognized that acute myocardial ischemia results in abnormal inward motion and thickening of the affected myocardial region.[96] Since then, wall motion abnormalities have been shown to occur within seconds of inadequate blood flow or oxygen supply.[97] These abnormal contraction patterns typically occur at the same time as regional lactate production.[98, 99]

Diagnosis of Ischemia

The precise sequence of regional functional changes that occur in the myocardium after interruption of flow has been studied in models of acute ischemia, including percutaneous transluminal coronary angioplasty (PTCA).[100–102] Abnormalities in diastolic function usually precede abnormal changes in systolic function. Normal diastolic function is critical for LV filling and depends on ventricular relaxation and compliance and on atrial contraction. Diastolic ventricular function can be assessed by monitoring the rate of filling associated with changes in chamber dimensions as described earlier. Regional systolic function can be estimated by echocardiographic determination of wall thickening and wall motion during systole in both long- and short-axis views of the ventricle. The short-axis view of the LV at the papillary muscle level displays myocardium perfused by the three major coronary arteries (Fig. 9–8). However, because the short-axis view does not image the ventricular apex, which is a very common location of ischemia, the long-axis and longitudinal ventricular views are also clinically important.[103]

In the clinical assessment of regional function with the short-axis view, the ventricle is usually subdivided into four quadrants: posterior, anterior, septal, and lateral. Regional function can be evaluated by wall motion and/or wall thickening. Wall thickening can be assessed qualitatively or it can be quantitatively evaluated by calculating systolic wall thickening from the following equation:

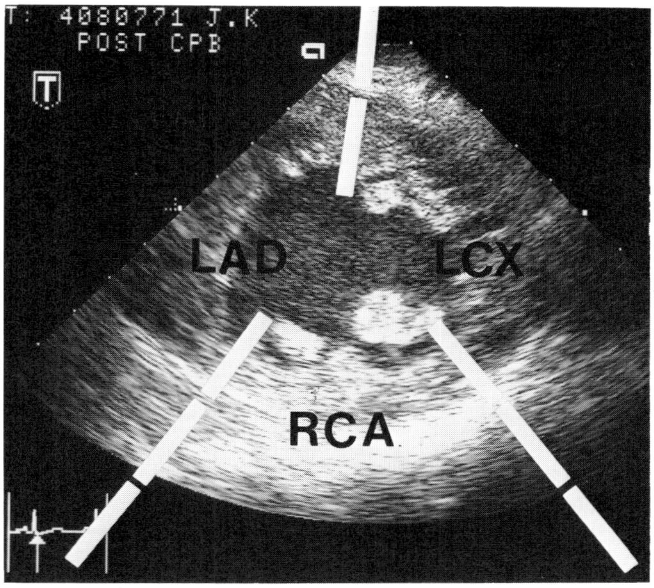

Figure 9–8. Short-axis view of the left ventricle at the level of the papillary muscles. The areas perfused by the three major coronary arteries are indicated on the image. LAD = Left anterior descending coronary artery; RCA = Right coronary artery; LCX = Left circumflex coronary artery.

$$\text{PSWT} = \frac{\text{SWT} - \text{DWT}}{\text{SWT} \times 100} \qquad 9\text{–}13$$

where PSWT = percentage of systolic wall thickening, SWT = end-systolic wall thickness, and DWT = end-diastolic wall thickness. Although wall thickening is probably a more specific marker of ischemia than wall motion, its measurement requires visualization of the epicardium, which is not always possible. Alternatively, by observing the movement of the endocardium toward the center of the cavity during systole, segmental wall motion can almost always be assessed. As the myocardial oxygen supply to demand balance worsens, systolic wall motion changes from mild hypokinesia to severe hypokinesia, akinesia, and finally dyskinesia.[104]

Normal contraction is defined as >30% shortening of the radius from the center to the endocardial border. Mild hypokinesia refers to inward contraction that is slower and less vigorous than normal during systole with radial shortening of 10–30%. Severe hypokinesia is defined as <10% radial shortening. The precise distinction between varying degrees of hypokinesia can be difficult. Akinesia refers to the absence of wall motion or no inward movement of the endocardium during systole. Dyskinesia refers to paradoxical wall motion or movement outward during ventricular systole. These measurements of regional wall motion are obviously based on the determination of the center of the ventricular cavity. Unfortunately, because of cardiac translation, this center may move during the cardiac cycle. Two reference systems have been employed: fixed reference and floating reference. Because of its relative simplicity and the fact that in most situations the impact of translation is minimal, the fixed reference system is generally used. In conditions of significant translation such as after cardiopulmonary bypass, the more cumbersome floating system may be more appropriate.[105]

Limitations

Although TEE appears to have many advantages over traditional intraoperative monitors of myocardial ischemia, there remain limitations. The most obvious is the fact that ischemia cannot be detected during critical periods such as induction, laryngoscopy, intubation, emergence, and extubation. In addition, the adequacy of SWMA analysis may be influenced by artifact.[106] Artifacts can be produced by the ultrasound system itself or by the particular tangential section being imaged.

Another potential problem of SWMA assessment is evaluation of the discoordinated contraction that occurs from a bundle-branch block or ventricular pacing. In these situations, the system used to assess SWMAs must compensate for global motion of the heart (usually done with a floating frame of reference) and evaluate not only regional endocardial wall motion but myocardial thickening as well.

Not all SWMAs indicate myocardial ischemia or infarction. Clearly, under normal conditions, all hearts do not contract in a homogeneous and consistent manner.[107] It is reasonable to assume, however, that most acute changes in regional cardiac contraction patterns are attributable to myocardial ischemia. An important exception to this rule may apply in models of acute coronary artery occlusion. In these models, it has been established that myocardial function becomes abnormal in the center of an ischemic zone, but it is also true that the myocardial regions adjacent to the ischemic zone become dysfunctional as well.

Several studies have reported that the total area of dysfunctional myocardium commonly exceeds the area of ischemic or infarcted myocardium.[108, 109] The impairment of function in nonischemic tissue has been linked to a tethering effect. Tethering, or the attachment of noncontracting tissue that mechanically impairs contraction in normally perfused adjacent tissue, probably accounts for the consistent overestimation of infarct size by echocardiography when compared to postmortem studies.[110]

Another limitation of SWMA analysis during surgery is that it does not differentiate stunned or hibernating myocardium from acute ischemia,[111] nor does it differentiate between causes of ischemia such as increased oxygen demand and decreased oxygen supply. Finally, it should be noted that areas of previous ischemia or scarring may become unmasked by changes in afterload and appear as new SWMAs or wall thickening abnormalities.[112] This is particularly important in vascular surgery, which involves major abrupt changes in afterload.

DIAGNOSTIC APPLICATIONS

Intraoperative TEE initially was focused on monitoring applications such as the detection of ischemia and the assessment of global function. Improved 2D resolution and Doppler echocardiography coupled with greater experience in echocardiography has increased the use of TEE as a diagnostic tool in the operating room. These diagnostic capabilities permit rapid assessment of emergency surgery patients who have not had adequate prior evaluation and complement the routine preoperative studies. In many cases, TEE is either the gold standard or provides a unique means to obtain the information. The diagnostic information obtained has been shown to alter surgical decision making and to predict patient outcome.[3] TEE may also be used to evaluate the positioning of intravascular devices.[113] Other diagnostic applications include the assessment of cardiac structures, cavities, and their contents.

INTRACARDIAC CONTRAST

Because air has a different density than blood and is easily visualized by echocardiography, TEE has been used in the detection of venous and arterial air embolism. Patients undergoing surgical procedures such as sitting craniotomies or pelvic exenteration, where there may be open veins in which the pressure is subatmospheric, are at significant risk of air embolism. Animal studies have shown that 2D TEE can detect smaller amounts of air than transthoracic Doppler echocardiography can.[114, 115] Furthermore, both TEE and transthoracic Doppler techniques have been shown to be far superior to PA pressure and end-tidal carbon dioxide monitoring for the detection of venous air emboli.[115] Similar results have been obtained in human studies.[115] Additionally, 2D echocardiography can be used to localize the position of the air and thus is the only technique able to detect paradoxical emboli.

Air may also enter the heart during cardiac surgery. M-mode echocardiography detected air in 11% of patients without cardiotomy and in 79% of patients with cardiotomy.[116] Similar results have been obtained using 2D scanning, but the presence of air in the left side of the heart did not correlate with neurologic outcome.[117] Despite the inability to clearly show a relationship between the presence of echo contrast and neurologic outcome, TEE may still prove valuable in assessing the adequacy of air removal techniques following open left-sided procedures (Fig. 9–9).

ATRIA

TEE is an extremely effective means to image both atria, the interatrial septum, and catheter and surgical treatment of atrial pathology. Echodensities in the atria may indicate the presence of clot, tumor, foreign body, or an anatomic variant. Intra-atrial clot is most often located in the left-atrial (LA) appendage, but can also be seen in the right-atrial (RA) appendage or other parts of the atria. The clot is usually highly echogenic, irregular in shape, and almost always associated with stasis secondary to atrial enlargement, valvular disease, and/or atrial fibrillation. TEE is su-

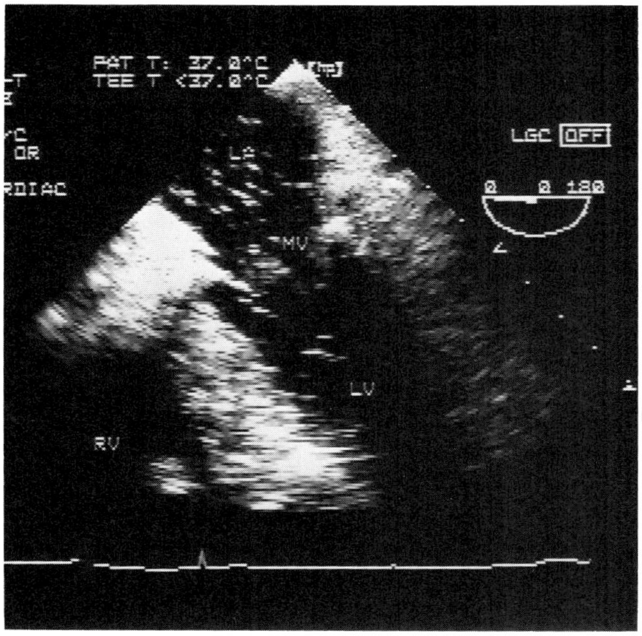

Figure 9–9. Four-chamber image after aortic valve replacement shows residual microbubble intracardiac contrast in the left atrium just prior to weaning from cardiopulmonary bypass. This intraoperative TEE observation has not been associated with any postoperative clinical events.

perior to transthoracic echocardiography in the detection of clot.[118]

Tumors seen within the atria are usually myxomas, but may be other primary cardiac lesions or metastatic lesions. Myxomas usually involve the left atrium, but may also occur in the right atrium or, even more rarely, in the ventricles.[119] The characteristic appearance of a myxoma is a pedunculated homogeneous mass that is attached to the interatrial septum. In addition to merely identifying the tumor, TEE is able to precisely define the attachment site and the extent of the tumor.[120]

Normal variants may create atrial echodensities. In the LA, the muscle band between the LA appendage and the left upper pulmonary vein may be confused with a mass.[121] In the RA, eustachian valves, remnants of Chiari network, and thickened atrial septa may appear as masses.[122]

Competence of the interatrial septum is an important function that can be evaluated by TEE. Incompetence may be due to either an atrial septal defect (ASD) or a patent foramen ovale (PFO). Depending on the location, ASDs can be divided into primum, secundum, and sinus venosus types. The defect is seen as an area of echo dropout, and flow across the defect is seen by either PW or color Doppler (Fig. 9–10, see color plate). TEE is extremely sensitive at diagnosing all three types, and it can define the pulmonary vein anatomy to detect associated anomalous pulmonary venous drainage.[123] Echocardiographic measurement of the defect size has also been shown to closely correlate with surgical measurement (horizontal width r = 0.92, vertical length r = 0.85).[124]

PFO is an anatomic variant that is found in autopsy studies in approximately 25% of the population and that may be a risk factor for stroke.[125] In anesthetized patients with venous air embolism, a PFO is also a risk factor for paradoxical air embolism with potentially grave effects.[126] Although initial attempts to diagnose PFO intraoperatively did not approximate results of the autopsy studies[127] and two instances of failed detection were reported,[128] more recent work demonstrated that contrast TEE can detect PFOs about as well as the autopsy studies could.[129] The keys to successful diagnosis include the use of the biatrial view and the complete opacification of the RA with contrast. Although some patients will demonstrate interatrial flow spontaneously during the cardiac cycle, in others it is necessary to apply sustained positive airway pressure and then release it so that the right atrial pressure (RAP) transiently exceeds the LAP to drive the contrast from the RA to the LA.[130] If possible, it is best to monitor the central venous pressure (CVP) and PCWP during the study to ensure that the pressure reversal occurs. In addition to diagnosing a PFO, TEE can also be used to guide balloon catheter closure of the defect.[131]

VENTRICLES

TEE diagnostic applications include assessment of the LV outflow tract and myocardial mass, the detection of clot, and the interrogation of the intraventricular septum. The echocardiographic findings of obstructive cardiomyopathy are readily visualized in the five-chamber long-axis view of the heart. There is thickening of the proximal septum resulting in a narrow LV outflow tract; the resulting flow disturbance causes systolic anterior motion (SAM) of the anterior mitral valve leaflet. The severity of the obstruction is related to the extent of the SAM; when the anterior leaflet actually touches the septum, this usually indicates severe obstruction. It is likely that SAM is caused by Venturi forces created by the narrow outflow tract. Because of the nearly perpendicular relationship between the direction of the blood flow and the Doppler cursor, quantitative measurement of the gradient is not usually possible.

Clot within the LV is generally found in a noncontractile aneurysmal segment, which is frequently located in the apex. Unfortunately, because of the distance from the transducer to the ventricular apex, it is difficult to image this portion of the heart; thus, TEE is not optimal for detecting ventricular clot. If clot is detected, the information is valuable because it may limit surgical manipulation of the LV prior to cross-clamp application during cardiopulmonary bypass.

Congenital and acquired postmyocardial infarct ventricular septal defects (VSDs) can be visualized by TEE, and thus TEE may be useful in the intraoperative assessment of the closure of the defect. This application, however, is limited by the inability to visualize the distal septum and by the nearly perpendicular angle between the Doppler beam and blood flow across the septum.

VALVE ANATOMY AND PHYSIOLOGY

Although it is possible to obtain images of all of the cardiac valves, TEE is most suited for the evaluation of the aortic and mitral valves. The three leaflets of the aortic valve are easily visualized, and vegetations or calcifications can be identified. Care is needed to differentiate tangential cuts through the valve cusps that look like valve nodules from actual masses on the valve. This differentiation can usually be performed by examining the tissue density of the presumed nodule (calcified nodules are more echogenic) and by slightly moving the probe (masses will generally persist). True masses will also be present throughout the cardiac cycle, but tangential cuts will disappear with movement of the valve. Finally, nodules will frequently create some aortic regurgitation that can be seen by Doppler echocardiography. Because of the orientation of the scan planes and aortic flow, TEE is not an optimal technique for the quantification of aortic insufficiency. However, several methods for its quantification have been described.[132]

Mitral valve anatomy is also easily visualized by transverse TEE, but to truly evaluate posterior leaflet structure and motion, longitudinal scanning is necessary. The mitral valve is a complex structure consisting of the two leaflets, the fibrous annulus, chordae tendineae, two papillary muscles, and their attachment sites to the ventricular wall. The annulus is composed of fibroelastic tissue and completely encircles the orifice in a cone-like shape. The anteromedial leaflet is triangular and is continuous with the aortic valve. This leaflet is more mobile than the posterolateral leaflet, but it encircles only one third of the annulus. The posterolateral leaflet is quadrangular; consists of a medial, a center, and a lateral scallop; and covers the remaining two thirds of the annulus.

Proper mitral valve function depends on the normal function of each of these components. There are numerous etiologies of mitral regurgitation, and the distinction is frequently made intraoperatively. The defects of mitral valve function can be divided into four categories: excessive leaflet motion, restricted leaflet motion, perforated leaflet, and annular dilatation. Examples of excessive leaflet motion are mitral valve prolapse, ruptured chordae, and ruptured papillary muscle(s). Restricted motion examples are chordal sclerosis/calcification, papillary muscle or ventricular wall ischemia, and vegetation- or mass-obstructed coaptation of the leaflets. Valvular incompetence is graded by a variety of measures including the location, width, and total size of the jet. Though at first glance, the use of color flow appears to be extremely simple because of its logical representation, this technique is subject to a host of technical and physiologic variables that can significantly alter the image. Technical variables include transducer frequency, color gain, color scale, sector width, depth, and transducer angle (Fig. 9–11, see color plate).

Because each echocardiograph is different, the operator must be acquainted with the specific controls and the default settings employed. Physiologic variables that can significantly alter the image include blood volume, blood viscosity, cardiac chamber pressures, heart rate, and inotropic state of the myocardium. Ideally the examination should be performed under the patient's usual hemodynamic conditions, but intraoperatively this is rarely possible. Thus, the findings must be interpreted carefully.

To assess the physiologic impact of mitral regurgitation, one can examine the pulmonary venous flow pattern by pulsed-wave Doppler. The normal flow pattern in sinus rhythm is triphasic. Following atrial contraction, a small negative deflection called atrial reversal occurs. Then, with the onset of ventricular systole, there is a large positive wave that relates to the preponderance of LA filling. During diastole, there is additional flow into the LA. In patients with severe mitral regurgitation, however, the systolic flow is significantly decreased, eliminated, or even reversed.[133]

THORACIC AORTA

Prior to the advent of TEE, echocardiography was of minimal value in the evaluation of aortic pathology. Because of the intimate anatomic relationship of the aorta and the esophagus, TEE has proven useful in the diagnosis of aortic dissection and aneurysm.[134] It is particularly useful in defining the entrance intimal flap, in defining the true and false lumen, and in detecting associated problems such as pericardial effusion and aortic insufficiency (Fig. 9–12, see color plate).

Manipulation and instrumentation of the thoracic aorta that results in embolization of atheroma is a leading cause of perioperative stroke.[135] It is possible that detecting the location of the atheroma and modifying the surgical technique may reduce the incidence of stroke.[136, 137] One major limitation is that the distal ascending and transverse aorta are not well visualized by TEE.[138] Instead, this region should be scanned by placing a sterilely wrapped probe directly on the aorta.

NEW DEVELOPMENTS

TISSUE CHARACTERIZATION

Another important goal of cardiac diagnosis that remains to be achieved is the direct identification of myocardial tissue composition. Currently, only endomyocardial biopsy, with its inherent limitations, permits direct identification of myocardial composition.

An ultrasound beam that travels through tissue is attenuated as a result of the absorption and scatter of its energy. Scattering is a multidirectional phenomenon that is due to the interaction between tissue inhomogeneities and the incident ultrasound beam. The wavelength of the ultrasound beam is always larger than the boundaries between the various components that make up the tissue.[139] The scatter that is directed toward the transmitting transducer is called backscatter. Backscattered echoes originate from within a tissue and characterize the tissue from which they originate. In quantitative tissue characterization, the backscatter reflected from specific tissues is analyzed and quantitated.

There has been increasing interest in quantitative analysis of ultrasonic characterization of myocardial tissue. Experimental and preliminary clinical investigations have demonstrated that ultrasound interacts differently with abnormal and with normal tissue.[140–142] The rationale for ultrasonic cardiac tissue characterization is that the acoustic properties of normal myocardium, ischemic myocardium, and infarcted myocardium differ quantitatively, making differentiation of these regions possible on the basis of tissue characterization. Conventional imaging techniques such as x-ray ventriculography, 2D echocardiography, and radionuclide ventriculography cannot differentiate viable but stunned myocardium from irreversibly damaged myocardium, because segmental function (wall motion or wall thickening) is impaired in both entities. Tissue characterization with ultrasound, on the other hand, has been used to determine whether SWMAs are a consequence of ischemia or of infarction.

Initial qualitative observations with conventional echocardiograms have demonstrated increases in regional myocardial echo amplitude within 15 minutes of coronary occlusion.[143] These increases correlated with infarct size in experimental animals as determined by histochemical techniques. Further efforts to facilitate identification of the ultrasound characteristics of ischemia have utilized the quantitative analysis of ultrasonic radio frequency signals.

In experiments that used ultrasonic radio frequency signal analysis, it has been reported that regional myocardial tissue acoustic impedance decreases within 15 minutes of coronary occlusion in dogs. This change has been noted to persist for up to 24 hours. Thereafter, this decreased attenuation has been replaced by an increase in attenuation.[144] These early experimental results indicate that ultrasonic tissue characterization techniques may allow estimation of the temporal staging of an acute injury. In addition to attenuation measurements for ultrasonic tissue characterization, other techniques have been used—for example, assessment of integrated backscatter,[145] calculation of the ratio of mean regional echo amplitude to the standard deviation of echo amplitudes,[146] assessment of cyclic variation of ultrasound backscatter with cardiac contraction,[147] and assessment of echocardiographic image gray level characteristics.[148]

Data suggest that echocardiographic tissue characterization techniques may aid in the identification of potentially viable myocardium despite temporary contraction abnormalities. Using a canine preparation, Rasmussen et al demonstrated that alterations in ultrasound backscatter that occurred following 20 minutes of coronary artery occlusion were reversed following 30 minutes of reperfusion.[149] Similar changes have been observed with respect to regional echo amplitude data[150] and cardiac cycle–dependent variations in backscatter.[151] It has been demonstrated in patients that cyclic variation of backscatter may recover following reperfusion before wall motion and wall thickening abnormalities are reversed.[151] Thus, viable but stunned myocardium may be differentiated from necrotic dysfunctional tissue. Radio frequency data may enable the differentiation of subacute from chronic infarcted myocardial tissue. Mimbs et al have noted that attenuation through infarcted tissue was greater than attenuation in normal tissue, beginning approximately 3 days after coronary occlusion.[144] In contrast, measurements made 15 minutes to 24 hours after occlusion demonstrated decreased attenuation compared to normal.

The characteristic acoustic changes are thought to represent histologic stages of infarction before the deposition of collagen. These early changes in the acoustic properties are thought to be due to changes in myocardial perfusion, alterations in the formed elements of blood within the affected tissue, and edema. The changes in acoustic properties 2 or more days after coronary occlusion have been thought to be due to early cellular infiltration and other features of the necrotic process. Hoyt et al analyzed specimens of fibrotic human myocardium and demonstrated a correlation between collagen content and integrated ultrasound backscatter.[152] Other studies have confirmed that the deposition of collagen appears to be responsible for acoustic alterations manifested as increased attenuation, lack of cyclic variation of integrated backscatter, and increased background backscatter of abnormal tissue.

In one developed application of tissue characterization, differences in backscatter between myocardial tissue and blood are utilized to automatically delineate the endocardial edge. Further processing allows the automatic and continuous quantification of endocardial cavity size and the calculation of FAC.

TISSUE PERFUSION

Intraoperative monitors, such as those that assess ECG current of injury or repolarization abnormalities, hemodynamic or LV compliance changes, and wall motion changes, do not directly measure tissue viability. These monitors are limited because they rely on the detection of dysfunctional myocardium as an index of underlying tissue ischemia and do not provide a true measurement of nonviable myocardial tissue. See Chapters 4, 8, and 10.

The emergence of contrast 2D IOE has permitted real-time assessment of regional myocardial perfusion patterns during coronary bypass surgery. Spontaneous contrast effect was first observed after infusion of cardioplegia solution during CABG.[153] These observations probably resulted from microcavitations in the cardioplegia solution. Subsequent attempts to use contrast ultrasonography to delineate myocardial blood flow during surgery were limited by contrast agents, injection techniques, and methods of analyzing the ultrasound signal. Since then, other investigators have evaluated myocardial perfusion with smaller, sonicated microbubbles that more efficiently pass through the microcirculation.[154]

The first experience with contrast ultrasonography for

evaluating myocardial revascularization during surgery was reported by Kabbas et al in 1990.[155] They safely used sonicated Renografin-76 (Squibb) microbubbles to assess the immediate results of CABG in 29 saphenous vein grafts. Because of the technique and the low volume of contrast used, however, they could not visualize contrast enhancement from aortic root injections. Assessment of myocardial perfusion from aortic root injections was later reported by Spotnitz and Kaul.[156] They injected sonicated albumin at the time of cardioplegia delivery and used a hand-held epicardial ultrasound transducer to obtain myocardial images.

Subsequently, TEE was used to image the heart before, during, and after CPB.[157] Contrast was injected into the cardioplegia catheter in the aortic root to identify myocardial regions with compromised flow before CABG. Next, selective injections of contrast were made into the proximal end of the saphenous veins after completion of the distal anastomosis. Injections directly into the saphenous veins provided useful information about the magnitude and geometric distribution of new vessel flow into the heart. Finally, after the completion of all CABGs, contrast was again injected into the aortic root during warm blood reperfusion through the cardioplegia line. These latter injections allowed the identification of myocardial regions that remained poorly perfused after grafting. Areas with perfusion deficits before termination of CPB correlated with regions with SWMAs after separation from CPB. When predicted myocardial perfusion patterns (based on preoperative angiograms) were compared to actual perfusion patterns assessed from intraoperative contrast studies, predicted patterns were actualized 84% of the time. These results suggest that intraoperative contrast ultrasound during CABG surgery could improve results in up to 16% of grafted vessels.

The infusion of cold potassium cardioplegia solution has been instrumental in reducing the morbidity and mortality associated with cardiac surgery. Optimal myocardial protection during CPB is predicated on complete distribution of cardioplegia solution to all myocardial segments. Coronary artery stenosis may impair antegrade delivery of cardioplegic solutions through the aortic root and contribute to perioperative ischemia and infarction. Traditionally, the efficacy of cardioplegia perfusion has been assessed by quiescence of electrical activity on the ECG, a decrease in myocardial temperature, and direct visualization. Recently, contrast echocardiography has been used to indicate the adequacy of cardioplegia distribution within the myocardium by means of antegrade and retrograde (coronary sinus) delivery techniques.[158, 159]

Retrograde delivery of cardioplegia solution has been shown to provide complete myocardial distribution (including the intraventricular septum) in humans despite varying degrees of coronary artery stenosis.[160] The segmental and transmural distribution of retrograde cardioplegia delivery was assessed with videodensitometry to analyze the peak ultrasound pixel intensity within the endocardium and epicardium in the LV free wall and intraventricular septum. The endocardium/epicardium ratio was 1.39 ± 0.33 and 1.42 ± 0.27 for the intraventricular septum and free wall, respectively, following retrograde cardioplegia. The monitoring of cardioplegia delivery with contrast ultrasound, therefore, is a direct, real-time intraoperative technique that enables the surgeon and anesthesiologist to assess the adequacy of cardioplegia distribution to all myocardial segments.

The development of coronary artery collaterization that occurs in obstructive coronary artery disease significantly influences the preservation of myocardial blood flow and LV function. Until recently, the methods available to assess collateral blood vessels in patients were limited to coronary angiography or nuclear methods. Unfortunately, both methods have limitations for intraoperative use. Spotnitz et al, using contrast ultrasonography during CABG, reported evidence of collateral flow in six patients.[161] After comparing these results to those predicted from preoperative coronary angiography, they found that no collateral flow was noted angiographically in three of the six patients.

Despite its attractive possibilities, contrast echocardiography currently has two major limitations. First, to obtain myocardial perfusion data, one must make injections into the left side of the heart, which limits applicability. Second, the currently available echo equipment is not configured to provide easy access to the video intensity data.

MULTIPLANE THREE-DIMENSIONAL RECONSTRUCTION

Three-dimensional echocardiography requires a reconstruction of the 3D image of the LV from multiple 2D planes using complex computer software. These planes may be acquired by several short-axis views at different levels of the esophagus, using multiple oblique views from one point in the esophagus,[162] or by biplane imaging. The tedious nature of manual endocardial border tracings and the extended time required for off-line computer reconstruction of the 3D image have thus far limited this technique to research applications.

Using a transesophageal transducer with a precision micromanipulator at its tip, Martin and Bashein demonstrated that 3D TEE-derived SV compared favorably ($r = 0.92$) with thermodilution measurements in dogs.[163] A subsequent animal investigation demonstrated that radionuclide-determined EF and ventricular volumes agreed more closely with 3D echocardiographic measurements than did 2D measurements.[164]

COMPLICATIONS

Complications resulting from intraoperative TEE can be separated into two groups: injury from direct trauma to the airway and esophagus and indirect effects of TEE. In the first group, potential complications include laryngeal discomfort and esophageal bleeding, burning, tearing, and dysphagia. Many of these complications could result from pressure exerted by the tip of the probe on the esophagus and the airway. Although in most patients, even maximal flexion of the probe will not result in pressures greater than 17 mmHg, occasionally, even in the absence of esophageal disease, pressures greater than 60 mmHg will result.[165] To look more closely at the effects on the esophagus, animal autopsy studies have been performed. In dogs as small as 5 kg on cardiopulmonary bypass with full heparinization, researchers noted no evidence of macroscopic or microscopic injury to the esophageal mucosa following 6 hours of maximally flexed probe positioning.[166]

Further confirmation of the low incidence of esophageal injury from TEE is apparent in the few case reports of complications. In the world's literature, there is only one report of a fatal esophageal perforation (this occurred in a patient with unsuspected esophageal cancer)[167] and one report of a benign Mallory-Weiss tear following intraoperative TEE.[168]

Another possible complication of esophageal trauma is bacteremia. Studies have shown that the incidence of positive blood cultures in patients undergoing upper gastrointestinal endoscopy is 4–13%[169, 170] and 0–17% in patients undergoing TEE.[171–173] Even though bacteremia may occur, it does not always cause endocarditis. Antibiotic prophylaxis in accordance with the American Heart Association guidelines is recommended in patients with prosthetic or abnormal valves or who are otherwise at significant risk for endocarditis.[174]

In one of the earliest studies using TEE, transient vocal cord paralysis was reported in two patients undergoing neurosurgery in the sitting position with the head maximally flexed and in the presence of an armored endotracheal tube.[175] This complication was believed to be due to the pressure the TEE probe exerted against the larynx. Since this initial report, no further problems of this kind have been reported with the use of the newer equipment.

The second group of complications that result from TEE include hemodynamic and pulmonary effects and, particularly for new TEE operators, distraction from patient care. Fortunately, in the anesthetized patient, there are rarely hemodynamic consequences to esophageal placement of the probe, and there are no studies that specifically address this question. One potential hemodynamic effect of TEE, even in the well-anesthetized patient, is direct cardiac irritation from the probe with resultant atrial and ventricular dysrhythmias. More important for the anesthesiologist are the problems of distraction from patient care. Although these reports have not appeared in the literature, we have heard of several endotracheal tube disconnections that went unnoticed to the point of desaturation during TEE. Additionally, severe hemodynamic abnormalities have been missed because of fascination with the images or the controls of the echocardiograph. Clearly, new echo operators should enlist the assistance of an associate to watch the patient during the echo examination. This second anesthesiologist will become unnecessary after the novice gains sufficient experience. It is also important to be sure that all the respiratory and hemodynamic alarms are activated during the echo examinations. One report that did appear in the literature was that during TEE, an esophageal stethoscope was inadvertently pushed into the patient's stomach and was only noticed to be missing when the patient developed a small bowel obstruction.[176]

SAFETY GUIDELINES AND CONTRAINDICATIONS

To ensure the continued safety of TEE, we offer the following recommendations. Inspect the probe prior to each insertion for cleanliness and structural integrity. If possible, the electrical isolation should also be checked. Insert the probe gently; if resistance is met, abort the procedure. Use minimal transducer energy and freeze the image when not in use. Finally, when not imaging, leave the probe in the neutral unlocked position to avoid prolonged pressure on the esophageal mucosa.

Absolute contraindications to TEE in intubated patients include esophageal stricture, diverticulae, tumor, recent suture lines, and known esophageal interruption. Relative contraindications include symptomatic hiatal hernia, esophagitis, coagulopathy, esophageal varices, and unexplained upper gastrointestinal bleeding. It should be noted that despite these relative contraindications, TEE has been used in patients undergoing hepatic transplantation without reported sequelae.[177]

TRAINING/QUALITY ASSURANCE

At present, no absolute minimum training criteria to perform intraoperative TEE have been established, nor is there any organization that grants certification. The one established set of guidelines was created by a task force from the American Society of Echocardiography.[178] These guidelines are not specific for IOE and were created by a group without representation by anesthesiologists. The publication describes several recommended training components and the skills needed to perform TEE.

Unfortunately, these guidelines are not based on achievement. Obviously, different individuals learn at different rates, and thus meeting these guidelines does not ensure competence, nor does failure to meet these guidelines preclude competence. Furthermore, gaining proficiency in a limited number of areas such as interpreting wall motion, global function, and even mitral regurgitation can be more rapidly achieved.

Despite the problems with defining competence, it is clear that intraoperative TEE is a new field to anesthesiologists and that specific training is needed. Ideally, this training should begin with a dedicated training period. This is most easily accomplished during a cardiac anesthesia fellowship but can be done by postgraduate physicians as well. The subject is best approached through a combination of tutorials, scientific review courses, self-instruction using teaching tapes and interactive computer-assisted learning programs, and participation in echo reading sessions. Frequently, a symbiotic relationship with the cardiology division can be established in which the anesthesiologists can teach the fundamentals of airway management, operating room physiology, and the use of local anesthetics, while learning the principles of echocardiography from the cardiologists.

Quality assurance is another area for which no specific guidelines currently exist. It is clear that each intraoperative study should be recorded in a standardized fashion and accompanied by a written report that becomes part of the patient's chart. Furthermore, key images should also be copied and included in the chart, and careful records of any complications should be maintained. To ensure that the proper images are being obtained and that the interpretations are correct, studies should be reviewed periodically. This is another area in which the relationship between cardiology and anesthesiology can be productive.

Although there have been warnings and objections to anesthesiologists making diagnoses and aiding in surgical decision making,[179] there is no inherent reason that an anesthesiologist cannot provide this valuable service to the patient. The key factors are proper training, extensive experience with IOE, and available backup by a recognized echocardiographer.

REFERENCES

1. Konstadt SN, Reich DL, Thys DM, Aronson S: Transesophageal echocardiography. *In* Kaplan JA (ed): Cardiac Anesthesia, 3rd Ed. Philadelphia: WB Saunders, 1993; 342–385.
2. Hillel Z, Mikula S, Thys D: The current state of IOE in North America: Results of a survey. J Cardiothor Anesth 1988; 2:803–811.
3. Kyo SK, Takamoto S, Matsumura M, et al: Immediate and early postoperative evaluation of results of cardiac surgery by transesophageal two-dimensional Doppler echocardiography. Circulation 1987; 76:113–121.
4. Sheikh KH, Bengston JR, Rankin J, et al: Intraoperative transesophageal Doppler color-flow imaging used to guide patient selection and operative treatment of ischemic mitral regurgitation. Circulation 1991; 84:594–604.
5. Goldman M, Guarino T, Lazar S, et al: Impact of intraoperative echocardiography: The first 1000 patients [Abstract]. J Am Coll Cardiol [Am] 1989; 13:23.
6. Thys DM, Hillel Z, Konstadt SN, Goldman ME: Intraoperative echocardiography. *In* Kaplan JA (ed): Cardiac Anesthesia, 2nd Ed. Orlando, FL: Grune & Stratton, 1987; 255–318.
7. Thys DM, Hillel Z: How it works: Basic concepts in echocardiography. *In* Bruijn NP, Clements F (eds): Intraoperative Use of Echocardiography. Philadelphia: JB Lippincott, 1991; 13–44.
8. Hatle L, Angelsen B: Doppler Ultrasound in Cardiology, 2nd Ed. Philadelphia: Lea & Febiger, 1984.
9. Kisslo J, Adams D, Mark DB: Basic Doppler Echocardiography. New York: Churchill Livingstone, 1986.
10. Kisslo J, Adams DB, Belkin RN: Doppler Color-Flow Imaging. New York: Churchill Livingstone, 1988.
11. Gramiak R, Shah PM: Echocardiography of the aortic root. Invest Radiol 1968; 3:356.
12. Sahn DJ, Allen HD, George W, et al: The utility of contrast echocardiographic techniques in the care of critically ill infants with cardiac and pulmonary disease. Circulation 1977; 56:959–968.
13. Allen HD, Sahn DJ, Goldberg SJ: New serial contrast technique for assessment of left-to-right shunting patent ductus arteriosus in the neonate. Am J Cardiol 1978; 41:288–294.
14. Ryssing E: Contrast echocardiography: The descending thoracic aorta and the left atrial posterior wall in neonates. Acta Paediatr Scand 1981; 70:735–738.
15. Zednikova M, Bayen MG, Yoshida Y, Emmanouilides GC: Precordial contrast echocardiographic detection of patent ductus arteriosus in small preterm infants. Pediatr Cardiol 1982; 2:271–275.
16. Roelandt J, Meltzer RS, Serruys PW: Contrast echocardiography of the left ventricle. *In* Rÿsferborgh M (ed): Echocardiology. Amsterdam, The Netherlands: Martinus Nijhoff, 1981; 219–232.
17. Roelandt J: Contrast echocardiography. Ultrasound Med Biol 1982; 8:471–492.
18. Feigenbaum H, Stone JM, Lee DA, et al: Identification of ultrasound echoes from the left ventricle by use of intracardiac injections of indocyanine green. Circulation 1970; 41:615–621.
19. Reid CL, Kawanishi DT, McKay CR, et al: Accuracy of evaluation of the presence and severity of aortic and mitral regurgitation by contrast two-dimensional echocardiography. Am J Cardiol 1983; 52:519–524.
20. Meltzer RS, Vered Z, Roelandt J, Neufeld HN: Systematic analysis of contrast echocardiograms. Am J Cardiol 1983; 52:375–380.
21. Feinstein SB, TenCate FJ, Zwehl W, et al: Two-dimensional contrast echocardiography: In vitro development and quantitative analysis of echo contrast agents. J Am Coll Cardiol 1984; 3:6–13.
22. Levine RA, Teichholz LE, Goldman ME, et al: Microbubbles have intracardiac velocities similar to those of red blood cells. J Am Coll Cardiol 1984; 3:28–33.
23. Heidenreich PA, Wiencek JG, Zaroff JG, et al: Contrast echo: In vitro flow calculations [Abstract]. Circulation 1989; 80:370.
24. Aronson S, Wiencek JG, Zaroff JG, et al: Assessment of renal blood flow in the dog with contrast ultrasound. Anesth Analg 1990; 70:S10.
25. Heidenreich PA, Wiencek JG, Zaroff JG, et al: Measurement of renal blood flow/volume with digital ultrasonography [Abstract]. Circulation 1989; 80:568.
26. Feinstein SB, Cheirif J, TenCate FJ, et al: Safety and efficacy of a new transpulmonary ultrasound contrast agent: Initial multicenter clinical results. J Am Coll Cardiol 1990; 16:316–324.
27. Walker R, Wiencek JG, Zaroff JG, et al: Pitfalls in quantitation of contrast echo: Threshold effects [Abstract]. J Am Soc Echocardiogr 1991; 4:301.
28. Hisanaga K, Hisanaga A, Nagata K, Yoshida S: A new transesophageal real-time two-dimensional echocardiographic system using a flexible tube and its clinical application. Proc Jpn J Med Ultrason 1977; 32:43–44.
29. Matsumoto M, Oka Y, Strom J, et al: Application of transesophageal echocardiography to continuous intraoperative monitoring of left ventricular performance. Am J Cardiol 1980; 46:95–105.
30. Schluter M, Langenstein B, Polster J, et al: Transesophageal cross-sectional echocardiography with a phased array transducer system. Technique and initial clinical results. Br Heart J 1982; 48:68–72.
31. Clements FM, Hill R, Kisslo J, et al: How easily can we learn to recognize regional wall motion abnormalities with 2D-transesophageal echocardiographic images? Society of Cardiovascular Anesthesiologists, 11th Annual Meeting, Seattle, 1989.
32. Hillel Z, Thys D, Ali J: Can left ventricular ejection fraction be estimated by visual inspection of 2D-echocardiographic images? Society of Cardiovascular Anesthesiologists, 11th Annual Meeting, Seattle, 1989.
33. Saada M, Cahalan MK, Lee E, et al: Real-time evaluation of segmental wall motion abnormalities [Abstract]. Anesth Analg 1989; 68:242.
34. Lazar HL, Plehn J, Schick EM, et al: Effects of coronary revascularization on regional wall motion. J Thorac Cardiovasc Surg 1989; 98:498–505.
35. Amico AF, Lichtenberg GS, Reisner SA, et al: Superiority of visual versus computerized echocardiographic estimation of radionuclide left ventricular ejection fraction. Am Heart J 1989; 118:1259–1265.
36. Stauffer JC, Mueller X, Homsi L, et al: Echocardiographic determination of ejection fraction with various methods: Comparison with contrast angiography [Abstract]. J Am Soc Echocardiogr 1990; 3:215.
37. Haendchen RV, Wyatt HL, Maurer G, et al: Quantitation of regional cardiac function by two-dimensional echocardiography. I. Patterns

of contraction of the normal left ventricle. Circulation 1983; 67:1234–1245.

38. Wyatt HL, Haendchen RV, Meerbaum S, et al: Assessment of quantitative methods for 2-dimensional echocardiography. Am J Cardiol 1983; 52:396–401.
39. Thys DM, Hillel Z, Goldman ME, et al: A comparison of hemodynamic indices by invasive monitoring and two-dimensional echocardiography. Anesthesiology 1987; 67:630–634.
40. Thys D, Hillel Z: Difference between M-mode and two-dimensional echocardiography. Anesthesiology 1988; 68:645–646.
41. Schiller NB, Shah PM, Crawford M, et al: Recommendations for quantitation of the left ventricle by two-dimensional echocardiography. J Am Soc Echocardiogr 1989; 2:358–367.
42. Konstadt SN, Thys D, Mindich BP, et al: Validation of quantitative intraoperative transesophageal echocardiography. Anesthesiology 1986; 65:418–421.
43. Clements FM, Harpole D, Quill T, et al: Simultaneous measurements of cardiac volumes, areas and ejection fractions by transesophageal echocardiography and first-pass radionuclide angiography. Anesthesiology 1988; 69:4.
44. Urbanowicz JH, Shaaban MJ, Cohen NH, et al: Comparison of transesophageal echocardiographic and scintigraphic estimates of left ventricular end-diastolic volume index and ejection fraction in patients following coronary artery bypass grafting. Anesthesiology 1990; 72:607–612.
45. Choong CY, Abascal V, Thomas JD, et al: Combined influence of ventricular loading and relaxation on the transmitral flow velocity profile in dogs measured by Doppler echocardiography. Circulation 1988; 78:672–683.
46. Nishimura RA, Abel MD, Housmans PR, et al: Mitral flow velocity curves as a function of different loading conditions: Evaluation by intraoperative transesophageal Doppler echocardiography. J Am Soc Echocardiogr 1989; 2:79–87.
47. Courtois M, Kovacs SJ, Ludbrook PA: Transmitral pressure-flow velocity relation. Circulation 1988; 78:661–671.
48. Kuo LC, Quinones MA, Rokey R, et al: Quantification of atrial contribution to left ventricular filling by pulsed Doppler echocardiography and the effects of age in the normal and diseased hearts. Am J Cardiol 1987; 59:1174–1178.
49. Pearson AC, Labovitz AJ, Mrosek D, et al: Assessment of diastolic function in normal and hypertrophied hearts: Comparison of Doppler echocardiography and M-mode echocardiography. Am Heart J 1987; 113:1417–1425.
50. Snider AR, Gidding SS, Rocchini AP, et al: Doppler evaluation of left ventricular diastolic filling in children with systemic hypertension. Am J Cardiol 1985; 56:921–926.
51. Thys DM, Hillel Z, Konstadt S, et al: The intraoperative evaluation of left ventricular filling by esophageal Doppler echocardiography. Society of Cardiovascular Anesthesiologists Eighth Annual Meeting, Montreal, 1986; 80.
52. Rinder CS, Wheeler LR, Alpern WD: Pulsed Doppler assessment of diastolic function before and after cardiopulmonary bypass. Anesthesiology 1988; 69:2.
53. Konstadt S, Reich D, Thys D, et al: Importance of atrial systole to ventricular filling predicted by transesophageal echocardiography. Anesthesiology 1990; 72:971–976.
54. Stewart WJ, Dicola VC, Harthorne W, et al: Doppler ultrasound measurement of cardiac output in patients with physiologic pacemakers. Am J Cardiol 1984; 54:308–312.
55. Haskell RJ, French WJ: Optimum AV interval in dual chamber pacemakers. PACE 1986; 9:670–675.
56. Pearson AC, Janosik DL, Redd RM, et al: Prediction of hemodynamic benefit of physiologic pacing from baseline Doppler-echocardiographic parameters [Abstract]. PACE 1987; 10:127.
57. Labovitz AJ, Lewen MK, Kern M, et al: Evaluation of left ventricular systolic and diastolic dysfunction during transient myocardial ischemia produced by angioplasty. J Am Coll Cardiol 1987; 10:748–755.
58. Bowman LK, Cleman MW, Cabin HS, et al: Dynamics of early and late left ventricular filling determined by Doppler two-dimensional echocardiography during percutaneous transluminal coronary angioplasty. Am J Cardiol 1988; 61:541–545.
59. Reichek N, Wilson J, St John Sutton M, et al: Noninvasive determination of left ventricular end-systolic stress: Validation of the method and initial application. Circulation 1982; 65:99–108.
60. Sandler H, Dodge HT: Left ventricular tension and stress in man. Circ Res 1963; 13:91–104.
61. Hartford M, Wilstand JCM, Wallentin I, et al: Left ventricular wall stress and systolic function in untreated primary hypertension. Hypertension 1985; 7:97–104.
62. Lang RL, Borow KM, Newman A, et al: Systemic vascular resistance: An unreliable index of afterload. Circulation 1986; 74:1114–1123.
63. O'Kelly BF, Tubau JF, Knight AA, et al: Measurement of left ventricular contractility using transesophageal echocardiography in patients undergoing coronary bypass grafting. Am Heart J 1991; 122:1041–1048.
64. Smith JS, Roizen MF, Cahalan MK, et al: Does anesthetic technique make a difference? Augmentation of systolic blood pressure during carotid endarterectomy: Effects of phenylephrine versus light anesthesia and of isoflurane versus halothane on the incidence of myocardial ischemia. Anesthesiology 1988; 69:846–853.
65. Folland ED, Parisi AF, Moynihan PF, et al: Assessment of left ventricular ejection fraction and volumes by real-time, two dimensional echocardiography. Circulation 1979; 60:760–766.
66. Weissler AM: Systolic time intervals. N Engl J Med 1977; 296:321–324.
67. Lewis RP, Rittgers SE, Forester WF, et al: A critical review of the systolic time intervals. Circulation 1977; 56:146–158.
68. Noble MIM, Trenchard D, Guz A: Left ventricular ejection in conscious dogs: 1. Measurement and significance of the maximum acceleration of blood from the left ventricle. Circ Res 1966: 19:139–147.
69. Bennett ED, Else W, Miller GAH, et al: Maximum acceleration of blood from the left ventricle in patients with ischaemic heart disease. Clin Sci Mol Med 1974; 46:49–59.
70. Mehta N, Bennett DE: Impaired left ventricular function in acute myocardial infarction assessed by Doppler measurement of ascending aortic blood velocity and maximum acceleration. Am J Cardiol 1986; 57:1052–1058.
71. Sabbah HN, Khaja F, Brymer JF, et al: Noninvasive evaluation of left ventricular performance based on peak aortic blood acceleration measured with a continuous-wave Doppler velocity meter. Circulation 1986; 74:323–329.
72. Suga H, Sagawa K: Instantaneous pressure-volume relationships and their ratio in the excised, supported canine left ventricle. Circ Res 1974; 35:117–126.
73. Hillel Z, Thys DM, Mindich BP, et al: A new method for the intraoperative determination of contractility. Anesth Analg 1986; 65:S72.
74. Hillel Z, Thys DM, Mindich BP, et al: Intraoperative measurement of the effects of dopamine on left ventricular contractility. Anesthesiology 1985; 63:A25.
75. Simonson JS, Schiller NB. Descent of the base of the left ventricle: An echocardiographic index of left ventricular function. J Am Soc Echocardiogr 1989; 2:25–35.
76. Feigenbaum H, Popp RL, Wolfe SB, et al: Ultrasound measurements of the left ventricle: A correlative study with angiocardiography. Arch Intern Med 1972; 129:461.
77. Gibson DG: Estimation of left ventricular size by echocardiography. Br Heart J 1973; 35:128–134.
78. Popp RL, Harrison DC: Ultrasonic cardiac echography for determining stroke volume and valvular regurgitation. Circulation 1970; 41:493–502.
79. Pombo JF, Troy BL, Russell RO: Left ventricular volumes and ejection fraction by echocardiography. Circulation 1971; 43:480–490.
80. Fortuin NJ, Hood WP, Sherman E, et al: Determinations of left ventricular volumes by ultrasound. Circulation 1971; 44:575–584.
81. Teichholz LE, Kreulen T, Herman MV, et al: Problems in echocardiographic volume determinations: Echocardiographic-angiographic correlations in the presence or absence of asynergy. Am J Cardiol 1976; 37:7–11.
82. Kronik G, Slany J, Mösslacher H: Comparative value of eight M-mode echocardiographic formulas for determining left ventricular stroke volume. Circulation 1979; 60:1308–1316.
83. Sahn DJ, De Maria A, Kisslo J, et al: Recommendations regarding quantitation in M-mode echocardiography: Results of echocardiographic measurements. Circulation 1978; 58:1072–1083.
84. Matsumoto M, Oka Y, Strom J, et al: Application of transesophageal

echocardiography to continuous intraoperative monitoring of left ventricular performance. Am J Cardiol 1980; 46:95–105.
85. Terai C, Venishi M, Sugimoto H, et al: Transesophageal echocardiographic dimensional analysis of four cardiac chambers during positive end-expiratory pressure. Anesthesiology 1985; 63:640–646.
86. Fisher DC, Sahn DJ, Allen HD, et al: The mitral valve orifice method for noninvasive two-dimensional echo Doppler determinations of cardiac output. Circulation 1983; 67:872–877.
87. Lewis JF, Kuo LC, Nelson JG, et al: Pulsed Doppler echocardiographic determination of stroke volume and cardiac output: Clinical validation of two new methods using the apical window. Circulation 1984; 70:425–431.
88. Roewer N, Bednarz F, Dziadka A, et al: Intraoperative cardiac output determination from transmitral and pulmonary blood flow measurements using transesophageal pulsed Doppler. J Cardiothorac Anesth 1987; 1:418–428.
89. LaMantia K, Harris S, Mortimore K, et al: Transesophageal pulse-wave Doppler assessment of cardiac output. Anesthesiology 1988; 69:A1.
90. Dittmann H, Voelker W, Karsch KR, et al: Influence of the sampling site and flow area on cardiac output measurements by Doppler echocardiography. J Am Coll Cardiol 1987; 10:818–823.
91. Muhiudeen IA, Kuecherer HF, Lee E, et al: Intraoperative estimation of cardiac output by transesophageal pulsed Doppler echocardiography. Anesthesiology 1991; 74:9–14.
92. Savino JS, Troianos CA, Aukburg S, et al: Measurement of pulmonary blood flow with two-dimensional echocardiography and Doppler echocardiography. Anesthesiology 1991; 75:445–451.
93. Stevenson JG: Comparison of several noninvasive methods for estimation of pulmonary artery pressure. J Am Soc Echocardiogr 1989; 2:157–171.
94. Kuecherer HF, Muhiudeen IA, Lee E, et al: Estimation of left atrial pressure by Doppler interrogation of phasic pulmonary venous flow: An intraoperative transesophageal study [Abstract]. Circulation 1989; 80:567.
95. Nishimura RA, Abel MD, Hatle LK, et al: Relation of pulmonary vein to mitral flow velocities by transesophageal Doppler echocardiography. Circulation 1990; 81:1488–1497.
96. Tennant R, Wiggers CJ: The effect of coronary occlusion on myocardial infarction. Am J Physiol 1935; 112:351–361.
97. Vatner SF: Correlation between acute reductions in myocardial blood flow and function in conscious dogs. Circ Res 1980; 47:201–207.
98. Waters DD, Luz PD, Wyatt HL, et al: Early changes in regional and global left ventricular function induced by graded reductions in regional coronary perfusion. Am J Cardiol 1977; 39:537–543.
99. Hauser AM, Gangadharan V, Ramos R, et al: Sequence of mechanical, electrocardiographic and clinical effects of repeated coronary artery occlusion in human beings: Echocardiographic observations during coronary angioplasty. J Am Coll Cardiol 1985; 5:193–197.
100. Massie BM, Botvinick EH, Brundage BH, et al: Relationship of regional myocardial perfusion to segmental wall motion: A physiological basis for understanding the presence of reversibility of asynergy. Circulation 1978; 58:1154–1163.
101. Alam M, Khaja F, Brymer J, et al: Echocardiographic evaluation of left ventricular function during coronary angioplasty. Am J Cardiol 1986; 57:20–25.
102. Labovitz AJ, Lewen MK, Kern M, et al: Evaluation of left ventricular systolic and diastolic dysfunction during transient myocardial ischemia by angioplasty. J Am Coll Cardiol 1988; 10:748–755.
103. Shah PM, Shunei K, Matsumura M, et al: Utility of biplane transesophageal echocardiography in left ventricular wall motion analysis. J Cardiothorac Vasc Anesth, 1991; 5:316–319.
104. Pandian NG, Kerber RE: Two-dimensional echocardiography in experimental coronary stenosis. I. Sensitivity and specificity in detecting transient myocardial dyskinesis: Comparison with sonomicrometers. Circulation 1982; 66:597–602.
105. Thys DM. The intraoperative assessment of regional myocardial performance: Is the cart before the horse? J Cardiothorac Anesth 1987; 1:273–275.
106. Clements FM, de Bruijn NP: Perioperative evaluation of regional wall motion by transesophageal two-dimensional echocardiography. Anesth Analg 1987; 66:249–261.
107. Pandian NG, Skorton DJ, Collins SM, et al: Heterogeneity of left ventricular segmental wall motion thickening and excursion in 2-dimensional echocardiograms of normal human subjects. Am J Cardiol 1983; 51:1667–1673.
108. Liberman AN, Weiss JL, Judutt BD, et al: Two-dimensional echocardiography and infarct size: Relationship of regional wall motion and thickening to the extent of myocardial infarction in the dog. Circulation 1981; 63:739–746.
109. Luma JAC, Becker LA, Melin JA, et al: Impaired thickening of nonischemic myocardium during acute regional ischemia in the dog. Circulation 1985; 71:1048–1059.
110. Force T, Kemper A, Perkins L, et al: Overestimation of infarct size by quantitative two-dimensional echocardiography: The role of tethering and of analytic procedures. Circulation 1986; 73:1360–1368.
111. Braunwald E, Kloner RA: The stunned myocardium: Prolonged, postischemic ventricular dysfunction. Circulation 1982; 66:1146–1149.
112. Buffington CW, Coyle RJ: Altered load dependence of postischemic myocardium. Anesthesiology 1991; 75:464–474.
113. Orihashi K, Hong YW, Chung BA, et al: New applications of two-dimensional transesophageal echocardiography in cardiac surgery. J Cardiothorac Vasc Anesth 1991; 5:33–39.
114. Furuya H, Okumura F: Detection of paradoxical air embolism by transesophageal echocardiography. Anesthesiology 1984; 60:374–377.
115. Glenski JA, Cucchiara RF, Michenfelder JD: Transesophageal echocardiography and transcutaneous O_2 and CO_2 monitoring for detection of venous air embolism. Anesthesiology 1986; 64:541–545.
116. Oka Y, Boriwaki K, Hong Y, et al: Detection of air emboli in the left heart by M-mode transesophageal echocardiography following cardiopulmonary bypass. Anesthesiology 1985; 63:109–113.
117. Topol EH, Humphrey LS, Bashan M, et al: Value of intraoperative left ventricular microbubbles detected by transesophageal two-dimensional echocardiography in predicting neurologic outcome after cardiac operations. Am J Cardiol 1985; 56:773–775.
118. Mugge A, Daniel WG, Haverich A, Lichtlen PR: Diagnosis of noninfective cardiac mass lesions by two-dimensional echocardiography. Circulation 1991; 83:70–78.
119. Wrisley D, Rosenberg J, Giambartolmei A, et al: Left ventricular myxoma discovered incidentally by echocardiography. Am Heart J 1991; 121:1554–1555.
120. Obeid AI, Marvasti M, Parker F, Rosenberg J: Comparison of transthoracic and transesophageal echocardiography of left atrial myxoma. Am J Cardiol 1989; 63:1006–1008.
121. Alam M, Sun I: Transesophageal echocardiographic evaluation of left atrial mass lesions. J Am Soc Echocardiogr 1991; 4:323–330.
122. Alam M, Sun I, Smith S: Transesophageal echocardiographic evaluation of right atrial mass lesions. J Am Soc Echocardiogr 1991; 4:331–337.
123. Kronzon I, Tunick PA, Freedberg RS, et al: Transesophageal echocardiography is superior to transthoracic echocardiography in the diagnosis of sinus venosus atrial septal defect. J Am Coll Cardiol 1991; 17:537–542.
124. Morimoto K, Matsuzaki M, Tohma Y, et al: Diagnosis and quantitative evaluation of secundum-type atrial septal defect by transesophageal Doppler echocardiography. Am J Cardiol 1990; 66:85–91.
125. Lechat PH, Mas JL, Lascault G, et al: Prevalence of patent foramen ovale in patients with stroke. N Engl J Med 1988; 318:1148–1152.
126. Gronert GA, Messick JM, Cucchiara RF, Michenfelder JD: Paradoxical air embolism from a patent foramen ovale. Anesthesiology 1979; 50:548–549.
127. Black S, Muzzi DA, Nishimura RA, Cucchiara RF: Preoperative and intraoperative echocardiography to detect right-to-left shunt in patients undergoing neurosurgical procedures in the sitting position. Anesthesiology 1990; 72:436–438.
128. Cucchiara RF, Nishimura RA, Black S: Failure of preoperative echo testing to prevent paradoxical air embolism: Report of two cases. Anesthesiology 1989; 71:604–607.
129. Konstadt SN, Louie EK, Black S, et al: Intraoperative detection of patent foramen ovale by transesophageal echocardiography. Anesthesiology 1991; 74:212–216.
130. Langholz D, Louie EK, Konstadt SN, et al: Transesophageal echocardiographic demonstration of distinct mechanisms for right-to-left shunting across a patent foramen ovale in the absence of pulmonary hypertension. J Am Coll Cardiol 1991; 18:1112–1127.
131. Gudipati CV, Nagelhout DA, Serota H, et al: Transesophageal echocardiographic guidance for balloon catheter occlusion of patent foramen ovale complicating right ventricular infarction. Am Heart J 1991; 121:919–922.
132. Oka Y, Strom J: Aortic valve. *In* Oka Y, Goldiner P (eds): Trans-

esophageal Echocardiography. Philadelphia: JB Lippincott, 1992; 167–188.
133. Castello R, Pearson AC, Lenzen P, Labovitz AJ: Effect of mitral regurgitation on pulmonary venous velocities derived from transesophageal echocardiography color-guided pulsed Doppler imaging. J Am Coll Cardiol 1991; 17:499–506.
134. Hashimoto S, Kumada T, Osakada G: Assessment of transesophageal Doppler echography in dissecting aortic aneurysm. J Am Coll Cardiol 1989; 14:1253–1263.
135. Blauth CI, Cosgrove C, Webb BW, et al: Atheroembolism from the ascending aorta. J Thorac Cardiovasc Surg 1992; 103:1104–1112.
136. Davila-Roman VG, Barilai B, Wareing TH, et al: Intraoperative ultrasonic evaluation of the ascending aorta in 100 consecutive patients undergoing cardiac surgery. Circulation 1991; 3(Suppl):47–53.
137. Tunick PA, Kronzon I: Protruding atherosclerotic plaque in the aortic arch of patients with systemic embolization: A new finding seen by transesophageal echocardiography. Am Heart J 1990; 120:658–660.
138. Konstadt SK, Reich D, Quintana C, et al: Transesophageal echocardiography does not visualize the entire ascending aorta [Abstract]. Anesthesiology 1993; 79:A70.
139. Perez JE, Miller JG, Barilai B, et al: Progress in quantitative ultrasonic characterization of myocardium: From the laboratory to the bedside. J Am Soc Echocardiogr 1991; 1:294–305.
140. Linzer M (ed): Ultrasound Tissue Characterization. II. National Bureau of Standards Special Publication 525. Washington, DC: U.S. Government Printing Office, 1979.
141. Miller JG, Perez JE, Sobel BE: Ultrasound characterization of myocardium. Prog Cardiovasc Dis 1985; 28:85–110.
142. Skorton DJ, Collins SM: Characterization of myocardial structure with ultrasound. *In* Greenleaf J (ed): Tissue Characterization with Ultrasound, Vol II. Results and Applications. Boca Raton, FL: CRC Press, 1986; 123–146.
143. Fraker TD, Nelson AD, Arthur JA, Wilderson RD: Altered acoustic reflectance on two-dimensional echocardiography as an early predictor of myocardial infarct size. Am J Cardiol 1984; 53:1699–1702.
144. Mimbs JW, O'Donnell M, Milley JG, et al: Changes in ultrasonic attentuation indicative of early myocardial ischemic injury. Am J Physiol 1979; 236:H340–344.
145. Mimbs JW, Bauwens D, Cohen RD, et al: Effects of myocardial ischemia on quantitative ultrasonic backscatter and identification of responsible determinates. Circ Res 1985; 49:89–96.
146. Schmittger IA, Vieli A, Heiserman JE, et al: Ultrasonic tissue characterization: Detection of acute myocardial infarction in dogs. Circulation 1985; 72:193–199.
147. Sagar KB, Rhyne TL, Warltier DC, et al: Intramyocardial variability in integrated backscatter: Effects of coronary occlusion and reperfusion. Circulation 1987; 75:436–442.
148. McPherson DD, Aylward PE, Knosp BM, et al: Ultrasound characterization of acute myocardial ischemia by quantitative texture analysis. Ultrason Imaging 1986; 8:227–240.
149. Rasmussen S, Lovelace E, Knoebel SB, et al: Echocardiographic detection of ischemia and infarcted myocardium. J Am Coll Cardiol 1984; 3:733–743.
150. Haendchen RV, Ong K, Fishbein MC, et al: Early differentiation of infarcted and noninfarcted reperfused myocardium in dogs by quantitative analysis of regional myocardial echo amplitudes. Circ Res 1985; 57:718–728.
151. Milynski MR, Mohr GA, Perez JE, et al: Ultrasonic tissue characterization with integrated backscatter and acute myocardial ischemia reperfusion, and stunned myocardium in patients. Circulation 1989; 80:491–503.
152. Hoyt RH, Collins SM, Skorton DJ, et al: Assessment of fibrosis in infarcted human hearts by analysis of ultrasonic backscatter. Circulation 1985; 71:740–744.
153. Goldman ME, Mindich BP: Intraoperative cardioplegic contrast echocardiography for assessing myocardial perfusion during open heart surgery. J Am Coll Cardiol 1984; 4:1029–1034.
154. Aronson S, Bender E, Feinstein SB, et al: Contrast echocardiography: A method to visualize changes in regional myocardial perfusion in the dog model for CABG surgery. Anesthesiology 1990; 72:295–301.
155. Kabbas JS, Kisslo J, Flick CL, et al: Intraoperative perfusion contrast echocardiography: Initial experience during coronary artery bypass grafting. J Thorac Cardiovasc Surg 1990; 99:536–542.
156. Spotnitz WD, Kaul S: Intraoperative assessment of myocardial perfusion using contrast echocardiography. Echocardiography 1990; 7:209–227.
157. Aronson S, Lee BK, Wiencek JG, et al: Assessment of myocardial perfusion during CABG surgery with two-dimensional transesophageal contrast echocardiography. Anesthesiology 1991; 75:433–440.
158. Aronson S, Lee BK, Leddicoat J, et al: Assessment of retrograde cardioplegia distribution using contrast echocardiography. Ann Thorac Surg (in press).
159. Villanueva FS, Spotnitz WD, Glasheen WP, et al: Assessment of the intramyocardial distribution of coronary sinus retrograde cardiplegia using myocardial contrast echocardiography [Abstract]. Circulation 1990; 82(Suppl 3):26.
160. Aronson S, Lee BK, Feinstein SB, et al: Direct assessment of myocardial retrograde cardioplegia distribution during cardiac surgery. Anesthesiology 1991; 75:A68.
161. Spotnitz WD, Matthew TL, Keller MW, et al: Intraoperative demonstration of coronary collateral flow using myocardial contrast two-dimensional echocardiography. Am J Cardiol 1990; 65:1259–1261.
162. Martin RW, Graham MM, Kao R, et al: Measurement of left ventricular ejection fraction and volumes with three-dimensional reconstructed transesophageal ultrasound scans: Comparison to radionuclide and thermal dilution measurements. J Cardiothorac Anesth 1989; 3:260–268.
163. Martin RW, Bashein G: Measurement of stroke volume with three-dimensional transesophageal ultrasonic scanning: Comparison with thermodilution measurement. Anesthesiology 1989; 70:470–476.
164. Nessly ML, Bashein G, Detmer PR, et al: Left ventricular ejection fraction: Single-plane and multiplanar transesophageal echocardiography versus equilibrium gated-pool scintigraphy. J Cardiothorac Vasc Anesth 1991; 5:40–45.
165. Urbanowicz JH, Kernoff RS, Oppenheim G, et al: Transesophageal echocardiography and its potential for esophageal damage. Anesthesiology 1990; 72:40–43.
166. O'Shea JP, Southern JF, D'Ambra MN, et al: Effects of prolonged transesophageal echocardiographic imaging and probe manipulation on the esophagus—An echocardiographic-pathologic study. J Am Coll Cardiol 1991; 17:1426–1429.
167. Daniel WG, Erbel R, Kasper W, et al: Safety of transesophageal echocardiography: A multicenter survey of 10,419 examinations. Circulation 1991; 83:817–821.
168. Dewhurst WE, Stragand JJ, Fleming BM: Mallory-Weiss tear complicating intraoperative transesophageal echocardiography in a patient undergoing aortic valve replacement. Anesthesiology 1990; 73:777–778.
169. Everett ED, Hirschman JV: Transient bacteremia and endocarditis prophylaxis. Medicine 1977; 56:61–67.
170. Botoman VA, Surawicz CM: Bacteremia with gastrointestinal endoscopic procedures. Gastrointest Endosc 1986; 32:342–346.
171. Gorge G, Erbel R, Henrichs KJ, et al: Positive blood cultures during transesophageal echocardiography. Am J Cardiol 1990; 65:1404–1405.
172. Melendez LJ, Chan KL, Cheung PK, et al: Incidence of bacteremia in transesophageal echocardiography: A prospective study of 140 consecutive patients. J Am Coll Cardiol 1991; 18:1650–1654.
173. Steckelberg JM, Khandheria BK, Anhalt JP, et al: Prospective evaluation of the risk of bacteremia associated with transesophageal echocardiography. Circulation 1991; 84:177–180.
174. Dajani AS, Bisno AAL, Chung KJ, et al: Prevention of Bacterial Endocarditis. JAMA 1990; 264:2919–2922.
175. Cucchiara RF, Nugent M, Seward JB, Messick JM: Air embolism in upright neurosurgical patients: Detection and localization by two-dimensional transesophageal echocardiography. Anesthesiology 1984; 60:353–355.
176. Humphrey LS: Esophageal stethoscope loss complicating transesophageal echocardiography. J Cardiothorac Anesthes 1988; 3:356–358.
177. Ellis JE, Lichtor JL, Feinstein SB, et al: Right heart dysfunction, pulmonary embolism, and paradoxical embolization during liver transplantation. Anesth Analg 1989; 68:777–782.
178. Pearlman AS, Gardin JM, Martin RP, et al: Guidelines for physician training in transesophageal echocardiography: Recommendations of the American Society of Echocardiography Committee for Physician Training in Echocardiography. J Am Soc Echocardiogr 1992; 5:187–194.
179. Kaplan JA: Monitoring technology: Advances and restraints. J Cardiothorac Anesth 1989; 3:257–259.

CHAPTER

10

Monitoring of Ventricular Function

CAROL L. LAKE, M.D.

Ventricular function includes both the intrinsic inotropic and the lusitropic state of the myocardium. Both components can be assessed by invasive and by noninvasive methods. Ideally, a measure of contractility should be sensitive to changing inotropy, reproducible, easily measured, insensitive to preload or afterload, and correctable for body size, ventricular dimensions, and thickness. None of the methods described below, however, achieves this ideal.

Accurate assessment of cardiac performance requires measurement of both pressure and flow.[1] Cardiac work describes ventricular function by the load carried and the distance it is moved. Using cardiac work instead of cardiac output or stroke volume to describe ventricular function has several advantages: (1) the stroke work index defines the area of the pressure-volume loop (described below), (2) stroke work index measures both systolic and diastolic performance, and (3) calculation of cardiac work includes the major variables affecting cardiac function: heart rate, preload, and afterload. Cardiac output is often the best clinical index of cardiac performance, despite its lack of a statistically significant relationship with total hemodynamic power.[1] Experimental determinations of the ventricular power index using angiography are independent of preload.[2]

PHYSIOLOGY OF THE HEART

Another approach to the assessment of cardiovascular function is oxygen uptake kinetics. This method is based on the concept that a primary function of the circulatory system is oxygen transport between the cells and the lungs. Wasserman reviews four methods for assessing adequacy of oxygen delivery: anaerobic threshold, rate of rise of oxygen uptake related to work rate increase, magnitude of phase I oxygen uptake (first 20 seconds of exercise) to phase II (increase in cellular respiration), and the slope of carbon dioxide production to oxygen consumption.[3]

Cardiac output, the volume of blood pumped by the heart each minute, is the product of heart rate and stroke volume. It varies slightly with body position. During exercise, stroke volume increases in the upright position, but is unchanged in the supine position. Intracardiac pressures also vary with position, but reports conflict as to whether the right or the left lateral position has a greater effect.[4, 5] Lange and coworkers noted that right ventricular peak systolic and end-diastolic pressure and left ventricular end-diastolic pressure are greater in the left lateral than in the supine position.[4] Other investigators noted greater increases in right ventricular pressures in right lateral position than in left lateral position due to changes in hydrostatic pressure secondary to the height of the right ventricle relative to the inferior vena cava.[5] The increases in ventricular pressures may result from extrinsic compression from lungs, upper abdominal organs, pericardium, or a combination.[4]

MYOCARDIAL LOADING CONDITIONS

Preload is the end-diastolic stress on the ventricle (end-diastolic fiber length or end-diastolic volume). End-diastolic volume is not linearly related to, or synonymous with, end-diastolic pressure. It is determined by blood volume, ventricular compliance, ventricular afterload, venous tone, and myocardial contractility. Increased preload increases wall tension, end-diastolic volume, and work performed by the ventricle. The clinical substitution of pulmonary wedge pressure for preload is predicated on the observation that within the clinical range of ventricular volume, ventricular pressure increases almost linearly with increased volume.

Ventricular contraction occurs against the resistance of the peripheral vasculature or afterload. Although often used clinically to estimate afterload, systemic vascular resistance is a poor index of left ventricular afterload. Systemic vascular resistance reflects peripheral arteriolar tone, whereas ventricular afterload is the ventricular fiber load (force opposing ventricular fiber shortening) during systole. The ventricular fiber load or wall stress is inversely related to wall thickness and directly related to chamber dimensions (shape, size, and radius). Left ventricular afterload peaks during the first third of systole and declines throughout the rest of systole. Reductions in afterload cause the ventricle to shorten more completely and quickly. Increased afterload decreases the velocity and extent of shortening, but increases the active tension and the time to peak tension.

CARDIAC MUSCLE MECHANICS

Myocardial muscle contraction occurs in three phases: (1) resting phase, (2) isometric contraction, and (3) isotonic contraction. The resting phase exists prior to intrinsic or extrinsic stimulation when the muscle length depends on its preload. A detailed discussion of myocardial physiology and the mechanical properties of cardiac muscle, such as shortening deactivation, hyperactivation, Starling's law, and homeometric autoregulation, is beyond the scope of this chapter; the reader is referred to Baan and Bachmann.[6] With shortening deactivation, the force developed at end-systole is less (because of fiber shortening) than that generated during isometric contractions. A related phenomenon is hyperactivation, in which the end-systolic pressure-volume point after a small amount of ventricular ejection lies to the left of the isovolumic end-systolic pressure-volume relation.

Initial contraction is isometric (tension development without a change in muscle length). Isotonic contraction follows with the shortening of the muscle, depending on preload and afterload. Mechanical function in isotonic contraction is defined by shortening velocity, time after activation, force or tension, and instantaneous muscle length.

Myocardial contractile force depends on two factors: myocardial contractile state and initial myocardial fiber stretch. Greater stretch of the fibers occurs at high filling volumes or pressures, i.e., increased preload. This relationship is the Frank-Starling law (Fig. 10–1*A*). The primary determinant of active tension development in the ventricle is sarcomere length, not muscle length per se. Normal hearts operate on the ascending limb of the curve with peak output occurring at filling pressures of 10 mmHg. Both atrial and ventricular muscle obey Starling's law. However, the Starling curve for the right ventricle is upward and to the left of the curve for the left ventricle, indicating the sensitivity of the right ventricle to preload. Functionally, Starling's law adapts left ventricular output to right ventricular output.

A descending limb of Starling's curve is questionable because sarcomere length in mammalian myocardium never exceeds 2.3 μm.[7] Rather than a descending limb for cardiac decompensation, the heart probably moves to a different curve. Starling's curves are affected by both preload and afterload, which must be controlled for changes in contractility to be verified (Fig. 10–1*B*).

EVALUATION OF VENTRICULAR INOTROPY

Ventricular inotropy is studied using either (1) ejection phase indices or (2) isovolumetric phase indices (Table 10–1). The ejection phase indices are mean and peak velocity of circumferential fiber shortening at peak wall stress (Vcf), mean systolic ejection rate, ejection fraction (EF), and percentage of fractional shortening (FS). The isovolumetric phase indices are measurements made prior to the opening of the aortic valve and include the peak rate of left ventricular pressure development (peak dP/dt), max dP/dt, peak velocity of shortening of the contractile element (Vpm), velocity of shortening of the unloaded contractile element (Vce or Vmax), and dP/dt at a ventricular pressure of 40 mmHg (dP/dt40). Such isovolumetric phase indices are sensitive to acutely increased afterload. Vce and Vmax, the extrapolation of Vce to zero pressure, are least sensitive to mild degrees of ventricular dysfunction.[8] Vpm is less sensitive to preload but underestimates contractility if compliance is decreased. A comprehensive theoretic analysis of the contractility indices is beyond the scope of this chapter. The interested reader should consult the paper of Kass and coworkers for details.[9]

ISOVOLUMETRIC PHASE INDICES

Rate of Rise of Left Ventricular Pressure (dP/dt)

The rate of rise of intraventricular pressure during the isometric phase of ventricular contraction is dP/dt. Maximal force of tension developed during contraction is max dP/dt. Factors affecting dP/dt are contractile state, preload, afterload, and muscle mass. It is underestimated when aortic regurgitation is present because aortic diastolic pressure is below normal and maximal dP/dt occurs early during ventricular ejection. Using the quotient (max dP/dt)/P, the maximal dP/dt at a specific ventricular pressure, obviates the preload dependence. Normal dP/dt values are 800–1700 mmHg/second.

EVALUATION OF EJECTION FUNCTION

Ventricular function is measured noninvasively by echocardiography, cardiokymography, and bioimpedance cardiography. Invasive methods include radionuclide, Fick, indicator-dilution, transesophageal echocardiography, flowmeter, and strain gauge arch techniques. Highly invasive methods such as flowmeters and strain gauge arch techniques are used only in experimental animals and are discussed in detail by Reves and Pruett.[10] Cardiac output, EF, and ventricular volumes are commonly measured.

EJECTION FRACTION

Radionuclide Methods

Techniques

EF is the ratio of blood ejected by the ventricle (stroke volume) to the blood in the ventricle at the end of diastole.

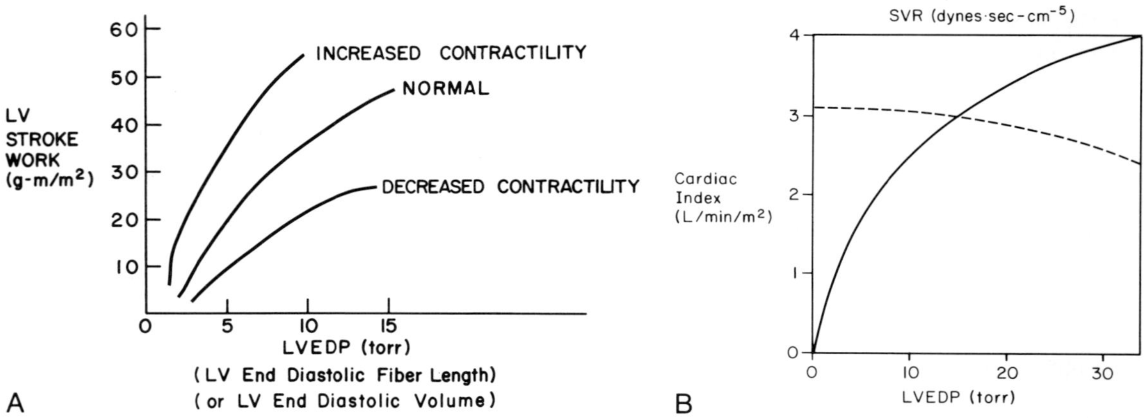

Figure 10–1. *A,* The Frank-Starling relationship, in which ventricular work is determined by end-diastolic fiber length *(solid lines).* (From Lake CL: Cardiovascular Anesthesia. New York: Springer-Verlag, 1985; 9, with permission.) *B,* The normal heart is affected more by preload *(solid line)* than by afterload *(dotted line).* (From Lake CL: Cardiovascular anatomy and physiology. *In* Barash PG, Stoelting RK, Cullen B [eds]: Clinical Anesthesia. Philadelphia: JB Lippincott, 1992; 1007, with permission.)

Two techniques are commonly used to assess EF from either ventricular volumes or radioactivity counts at end-systole and end-diastole: (1) gated blood pool imaging and (2) first-pass studies. First-pass techniques usually give slightly lower EFs than do gated blood pool images. EFs determined by radionuclide methods correlate well with those determined by angiography. Radionuclide determination of EF is relatively independent of ventricular geometry. A major limitation with radionuclide measurements is the inability to precisely determine onset and end of systole and diastole.

Intraoperative Use

Portable nuclear cardiac probes have been used to quantitate EF, end-systolic and end-diastolic ventricular volumes, filling velocities, and other parameters of ventricular performance.[11] Technetium-labeled human serum albumin or erythrocytes are injected intravenously. Electrocardiography (ECG)-synchronized, computer-processed recording of the radioactivity images the cardiac blood pool, providing views of ventricular wall motion throughout the cardiac cycle on nonportable devices. In portable devices, only regional and global ventricular time-activity curves are generated. Elimination of the capability to visualize ventricular wall motion in these devices permits determination of global ventricular function on a beat-to-beat basis. However, even the portable computer-camera device is expensive and cumbersome, and it requires operator practice for accurate positioning over the left ventricle. A 40° left anterior oblique projection with a 10–20° caudal tilt is used in supine, spontaneously breathing patients. The probe is slowly moved over the chest wall until the region of maximal counts is located. Background radioactivity is similarly determined and stored in the computer.

Variability of measurements with these instruments is about 6% in humans.[11] There is good correlation (r = 0.9) between EF measured with the nuclear stethoscope and EF measured with nonportable Anger scintillation camera-computer devices.[12] Positive pressure ventilation changes the measured ejection fractions about 3%.[11] Serial radionuclide monitoring is also useful to rapidly evaluate the effects of pharmacologic intervention in patients with poor ventricular function.[13]

TABLE 10–1. EVALUATION OF VENTRICULAR FUNCTION

Ejection Phase Indices
Mean velocity of circumferential fiber shortening
Peak velocity of circumferential fiber shortening
Mean systolic ejection rate
Mean normalized systolic ejection rate
Ejection fraction
Fractional shortening
Cardiac output
Left ventricular ejection time
Pressure-length loops
Pressure-volume loops
End-systolic pressure-volume relation
Isovolemic Phase Indexes
Peak dP/dt
Max dP/dt
dP/dt40
Peak velocity of shortening of contractile element
Velocity of shortening of the unloaded contractile element
Force-velocity curves
Pre-ejection period
Miscellaneous Methods
Ventricular pressures and volume
Pulse pressure and contour
Bioimpedance cardiography
Cardiokymography

Angiographic Methods

EF is commonly measured by angiography using biplane views. However, this technique is generally not applicable intraoperatively and is limited by the patient's exposure to radiation and contrast material. Dependence on preload, afterload, and heart rate causes EF to reflect mechanical ventricular performance but not actual myocardial contractility. Increased preload increases EF, whereas increased heart rate and afterload reduce it. The normal EF is 0.64 ± 0.08.

Left ventriculograms are also used to determine the mean normalized systolic ejection rate (MNSER) and the mean velocity of circumferential fiber shortening (Vcf).

$$\text{MNSER} = \text{EF/ET}$$

$$\text{Mean Vcf} = \text{Med} - \text{Mes/ET} \times \text{Med}$$

where ET = ejection time and Med and Mes = the ventricular short axis at end-diastole and end-systole in the right anterior oblique angiogram. MNSER and Vcf are affected by ejection time but generally provide information similar to that provided by EF.

CARDIOKYMOGRAPHY

Cardiokymography is a noninvasive method to determine regional wall motion in the closed chest. The cardiokymograph consists of a transducer that has a flat capacitive plate and a high-frequency oscillator. The transducer is strapped to the patient's chest, separated only by an air gap. Activation of the capacitive plate causes emission of a low-energy electromagnetic field that penetrates the chest. Motion within the electromagnetic field alters the capacitance and changes the frequency of oscillation. The change in frequency is converted to voltage proportional to the original motion, amplified, and recorded. Only the motion directly beneath the transducer can be recorded.

Normal cardiokymograms (Fig. 10–2) include an I point that occurs shortly after the beginning of ejection and a long period of inward motion during systole. Near the end of systole is the O point, where outward movement begins. In ventricular dyssynergy or dyskinesis, outward motion occurs during systole. Bellows and coworkers noted a 4% incidence of abnormal cardiokymograms indicative of ischemia during anesthetic induction.[14] These findings are confirmed with scintigraphy and M-mode echocardiography.[11]

ECHO-DOPPLER METHODS

Pulsed Doppler echocardiography assesses left ventricular filling dynamics and diastolic function by determining the percentage of left ventricular filling due to atrial systole or percentage of atrial contribution and the one-third filling fraction. Left ventricular systolic function (wall motion, chamber size, and cardiac output) is assessed by echocardiography as detailed in Chapter 9.

Theory

According to the Doppler principle, ultrasound waves are reflected by moving objects with a change in their frequency. The interrogating Doppler sound beam is produced when an electrical potential is applied to a piezoelectric crystal, changing its dimension. This process causes the crystal to emit and transmit sound through an acoustically coupled medium as a beam. Sound reflected from an object returns to the crystal and transducer as an electrical signal. Processing of the electrical signal produces either auditory or visual indication of the frequency shift. The change in frequency between the transmitted and reflected sound waves, the Doppler shift, is directly proportional to the velocity of the moving object and the angle at which the ultrasound strikes the object.

Two techniques, continuous wave (CW) and pulsed wave (PW) Doppler, are used in equipment for measurement of ventricular function. Only the velocity of flow and its rela-

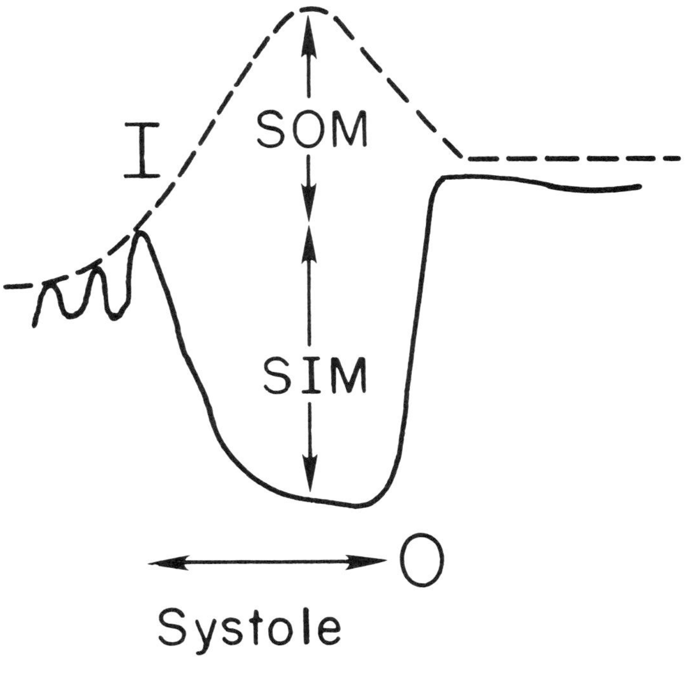

Figure 10–2. A normal cardiokymogram *(solid line)* has an I point indicating initial outward motion at the onset of ventricular ejection due to changes in the contour of the heart and an O point near the end of ejection. The majority of ventricular wall motion is inward during systole (SIM) with normal function. The *dashed line* indicates the alterations seen with ventricular dyskinesis in which much of the ventricular wall motion during systole is outward (SOM).

tive direction are determined with CW Doppler. CW Doppler transducers have two crystals, one continually transmitting and one continually receiving sound waves. The Doppler shift occurs only when blood moves relative to the transducer, so that an angle correction must be applied. Angle correction refers to the process of dividing the detected flow by the cosine of the angle between the blood flow and the beam. A disadvantage of CW Doppler is the inability to detect flow spatially because of a lack of range resolution.

Pulsed wave (PW) Doppler has only a single crystal to transmit and receive sound. Sound is transmitted intermittently at a specific number of sound pulses/second, the pulse repetition frequency. Because of the spatial localization of the source of sound reflection, PW Doppler is more informative.

Clinical Applications

Transesophageal and Transthoracic Devices

Doppler methods measure ascending and descending aortic flow using a suprasternal (noninvasive) probe or an esophageal (semi-invasive) probe. Cardiac outputs are initially measured with the suprasternal probe, which is then used to calibrate the no. 24-F, 5-MHz CW esophageal probe. The esophageal transducer is placed to a depth of 25–35 cm from the lips in a left lateral posterior position. Optimal position is achieved by slow rotation, insertion, and withdrawal until a clear, intense signal is present. The proportionality constant, K, relates the suprasternal to the esophageal velocity signal. Reproducibility of the K factor has been problematic in some patients. Alternatively, the initial value obtained with the esophageal probe is used to indicate subsequent trends. Calibration against cardiac output obtained by another method such as thermodilution is also feasible. Devices of this type include the older Ultracom and Accucom devices (Lawrence Medical Systems, Seattle, Washington) and the newer ODM (Doptek, Chichester, UK).

The ODM is a 4-MHz CW Doppler device in a 6-mm probe that must be precisely placed in the esophagus at 35–40 cm from the lips. Operator training is essential to ensure measurement of the proper waveform. In preliminary trials over a range of cardiac outputs from 1.5 to 11.4 L/minute, the coefficient of variation was 4.2% for this instrument.[15] Subsequent validation studies produced correlation coefficients of 0.86–0.93 compared to thermodilution.[16, 17] Long-term use has been reported without complications, although esophageal pathology is a relative contraindication.

In clinical applications, the cross-sectional aortic area is determined by two-dimensional echocardiography. Stroke volume (SV) is estimated from the product of mean aortic-root flow velocity, aortic cross-sectional area, and the R-R interval divided by the cosine 0, the angle between the ultrasound beam and the direction of blood flow summarized by the equation

$$SV = v \times ET \times CSA$$

where CSA = aortic cross-sectional area, v = average aortic systolic blood velocity, and ET = systolic ejection time.[18]

Practical Problems. Most clinical devices incorporate a nomogram into the monitor software to estimate aortic dimensions based on age, sex, height, and weight rather than measuring by echocardiographic techniques. Another problem is the assumption that ascending and descending aortic velocities are constant. Only blood flowing beyond the great vessels is included in the cardiac output measured by the esophageal probe. Accurate velocity determinations also depend on knowledge of the angle between the blood flow and the ultrasound beam. With these devices, the angle is assumed to be less than 20° and to remain constant during measurements. Nicolosi and colleagues studied the variability of six methods for Doppler flow and CSA and found more variability with measurement of flow across the mitral and tricuspid valves than across aorta or pulmonary trunk.[19] More error is introduced during recording of the Doppler flows and the cross-sectional echocardiograms than during subsequent analysis.[20] Perfect alignment of the transducer beam across the axis of flow is probably never achieved clinically. Thus, the correlation of echocardiographic measurement of aortic diameter with actual diameter is poor ($r = 0.31$).[21] Esophageal Doppler determinations of cardiac output are limited by intra-aortic balloon counterpulsation or aortic coarctation (causing turbulent flow) or aortic clamping (changing aortic dimensions).

Accuracy. The echo Doppler method correlates well with cardiac outputs measured by the Fick technique in infants and small children.[21] In adults, Doppler velocimeter measurements of cardiac output correlate well with both electromagnetic flow probes and thermodilution measurements.[22, 23] Crobson and coworkers reported a coefficient of variation of 8.8% for Doppler echocardiographic determination of cardiac output, with coefficients of variation of 4.1%, 6.4%, and 5.0% for aortic annular diameter, aortic velocity integral, and heart rate, respectively.[20] Differences of 0.41–0.9 L/minute between Doppler and thermodilution and a correlation coefficient of 0.68 have been reported.[22, 24, 25] Excellent correlation ($r = 0.91$) between thermodilution and transgastric CW Doppler assessment of both aortic valve flow velocity and area (measured at the aortic valve leaflet tips) was demonstrated by Katz and coworkers.[26] Doppler outputs do not include coronary blood flow, are inaccurate in the presence of turbulent aortic blood flow (aortic stenosis or left ventricular outflow track obstruction), and may be less reliable in the presence of left-to-right shunt through a patent ductus or in low-flow states.[18]

Limitations. Limitations of the Doppler output technique include esophageal pathology, abnormalities in the thoracic aorta, and, occasionally, inadequate acoustic windows. Averaging techniques create an additional source of error in patients with atrial fibrillation or frequent ventricular extrasystoles. Alterations in descending aortic flow secondary to aortic clamping also limit use of this technique. Even the newer, second-generation echo-Doppler cardiac output devices are useful only to monitor trends, not absolute values, in the perioperative period.[23, 27]

Other Echo-Doppler Devices

Doppler devices have also been attached to pulmonary artery catheters and endotracheal tubes[28] or have been placed directly on the aorta. The pulmonary artery flow velocity devices were not economically feasible and are no longer marketed. Advantages of the intratracheal position are measurements of the ascending aortic flow proximal to the great vessels, more constant anatomic position between aorta and trachea than between aorta and esophagus, and, in patients requiring intubation, the capability of cardiac output determination without additional invasive instrumentation.[28] The device is a 5-mm, 5-mHz transducer attached to an endotracheal tube beyond the tracheal cuff. The transducer itself is surrounded by a cuff to assure acoustic contact with the anterolateral tracheal wall. Essential requirements for satisfactory use include intratracheal positioning below the aortic arch but above the carina (suitable anatomy), adequate acoustic contact so the ultrasound beam intersects the ascending aorta, and measurement of ascending aortic dimensions and blood velocity. The correlation of outputs measured by transtracheal pulsed Doppler and thermodilution was 0.82 in a prototype device studied in dogs.[28] As with the esophageal devices, measurement of aortic diameter is a major source of error.

BIOIMPEDANCE CARDIOGRAPHY

Technique

Bioimpedance cardiography is a noninvasive technique measuring stroke volume on a beat-to-beat basis. A constant sinusoidal alternating current of 2.5–4 mA at 70–100 kHz is passed through the chest to sensing electrodes that detect the change in voltage due to transcardiac passage of the current. A total of eight electrodes is used, two sensing and two transmitting electrodes at the base of the neck and a similar set at the xiphoid process. The electrical conductivity of blood, varying in volume and velocity in the descending thoracic aorta, is the major source of the impedance change. The impedance, based on Ohm's law, is calculated from the current applied and the voltage produced. Stroke volume is determined from analysis of the impedance change over the cardiac cycle. An impedance cardiogram (ZCG), shown in Figure 10–3, is similar to an arterial pressure waveform. It is used to calculate stroke volume using the relationship

$$SV\ (ml) = (p)(L/Z_o)^2(dZ/dt\ max)(T)$$

where T = left ventricular ejection time in seconds, L = distance between electrodes, i.e., the length of the thorax from the root of the neck to the xiphoid, dZ/dt max = first derivative of the maximum rate of change of thoracic impedance in ohms/second, Z_o = total thoracic impedance in ohms, and p = resistivity of blood, 110–200 Ω • cm. The small, usually negative wave preceding the main systolic ejection wave is probably atrial in origin. Heart rate is simultaneously determined and multiplied by SV to give the cardiac output. Other parameters determined with this technique are ejection velocity index, thoracic fluid index, and ventricular ejection time.

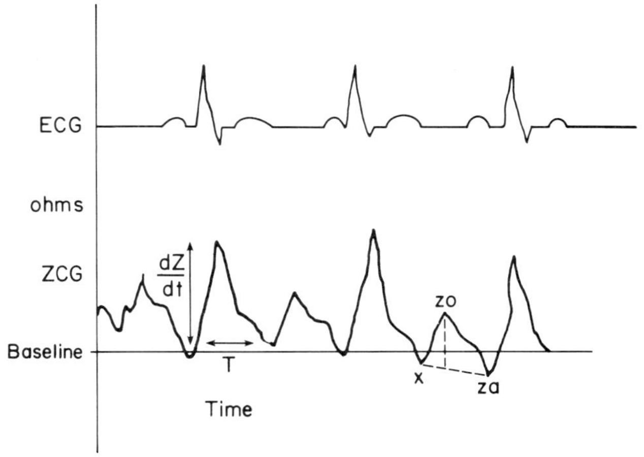

Figure 10–3. An impedance cardiogram is similar to an arterial pressure waveform. *T* is the ejection time in seconds, *dZ/dt* is the first derivative of the maximal rate of change of thoracic impedance (the vertical distance from the peak tracing to baseline), *x* is the x point of the impedance cardiogram, *za* is the vertical distance (ohms) from the nadir of za to baseline, *zo* is the peak height of zo measured from that peak to a line connecting x to za.

Pickett and Buell have combined bioimpedance cardiography with Doppler transmitral flow velocities to evaluate ventricular diastolic function.[29] They noted the preload dependence of the technique in both normal humans and patients with diastolic dysfunction.[30] The early diastolic bioimpedance wave Z_o was found to correlate well with Doppler early diastolic velocity (E wave).

Intracardiac Impedance Method

An intracardiac impedance method has also been developed in which the electrode bands are placed on a pulmonary artery catheter. Correct catheter position is essential and the technique must be calibrated against thermodilution-determined cardiac output.

Accuracy

In adults, impedance cardiographic measurements of cardiac output correlated well with the Fick method (≤ 5% difference).[31, 32] Correlation with Fick was further improved by comparison with SV or stroke index rather than cardiac output.[32, 33] Salandin and colleagues noted excellent repeatability of bioimpedance measurements in adults.[31] The accuracy of bioimpedance measurements to dye dilution outputs has also been confirmed.[34] Good correlation of bioimpedance with thermodilution cardiac output was reported by Pickett and Buell.[29] More recent investigations demonstrate poor correlation between bioimpedance and thermodilution measurements in adult patients.[35] The error increased with increasing cardiac index.[35]

Good correlation of cardiac output measured by bioimpedance in children was noted by Miles et al[36] and Introna et al.[37] However, in their studies, thoracic length (L) was adjusted until the measured bioimpedance output was within 10% of thermodilution outputs rather than using a nomogram or measured thoracic length. An error of 1 cm in thoracic length causes a 20% error in measured output. The assumption that L is 17% of patient height (as in adults) is inaccurate in children.[36] In children with systemic shunts (atrial septal defect, ventricular septal defect, or extracardiac shunts), Fick outputs were greater than systemic flow measured by bioimpedance.[37]

Practical Problems

Measurements are repeated easily without discomfort or risk to patients. However, the premise of the measurement—that the thorax is a homogeneous cylinder of blood during the cardiac cycle—is an extreme simplification and casts suspicion on the technique.[35] In children, the thorax more closely resembles a cylinder, whereas in adults, it may more closely resemble a truncated cone. However, modifications of the bioimpedance equation to compensate for differences in thoracic geometry underestimate cardiac output.[29]

Siegel et al, Weber et al, and Smith et al found poor correlation of impedance measurements with thermodilution ($r = 0.43$,[24] $r = 0.41$[38]) or between individual measurements using the Fick method.[32] However, Balestra et al showed that esophageal electrodes improve the accuracy of bioimpedance measurements.[39] Other problems occur in the presence of pulmonary edema or when hematocrit varies during major cardiac surgery. The bioimpedance method is also difficult to apply without infringement on the surgical field during many procedures. It is also unreliable to follow trends in cardiac function in the perioperative period,[24, 38] during dysrhythmias with widely variable R-R intervals, in aortic regurgitation, or in hyperdynamic septic shock.[31]

CONDUCTANCE CATHETER METHOD

A conductance catheter that measures the time-varying electrical conductances of five segments of left ventricular blood, proportional to the intraventricular volume of those segments, has been developed and studied in animals and humans by van der Velde and coworkers.[40] The catheter, with its eight electrodes, is positioned longitudinally between the ventricular apex (distal electrode) and the ascending aorta (proximal electrode) just above the valve. An electrical field develops in the ventricular cavity when a constant alternating current is applied through the proximal and distal electrodes of the catheter. The time-varying segment conductances of the segmental volumes defined by the remaining six electrodes are measured. The segmental (Vi (t)) and absolute (Vt) ventricular volumes are determined from the equations

$$Vi\,(t) = [1 / \alpha_i] \cdot [L^2 / o^{-b}] \cdot [Gi\,(t) - Gi^p]$$

$$Vt = [1 / \alpha_i] \cdot [L^2 / o^{-b}] \cdot [G\,(t) - G^p]$$

where Vi = segmental ventricular volume, Vt = total left ventricular volume, α_i = segmental slope constant, L = interelectrode distance, Gi^p = segmental parallel conductance, o^{-b} = conductivity of blood, G = conductance, Gi = segmental conductance, G (t) = total conductance or sum of conductances from six electrodes, and G^p = total parallel conductance.[40] Compared to computed tomographic measurements of overall left ventricular volume, conductance measurements correlate well with a coefficient of 0.965 in dogs. Only measurements from the uppermost segment of the ventricle correlated poorly with tomographic measurements.[40] In humans with normal or diseased hearts, conductance catheters permitted accurate, continuous measurements of left ventricular volume.[41] These measurements correlated closely with those obtained by angiography and can be used to determine end-systolic pressure volume relations under various physiologic conditions.[42, 43]

A principal advantage of conductance catheters is the avoidance of radioisotopes or radiocontrast. However, α_i (slope factor) shows considerable intersubject variability, and correction (calibration) for the offset in the relationship between measured conductance and intracavitary volume (parallel conductance) is also required. The calibration is usually performed by injection of hypertonic saline into the pulmonary artery, which alters the conductance of blood but not that of surrounding structures, and estimates the component of the signal due to non–blood-containing structures.

A modification that adds two electrodes at half of the distance between the proximal and distal electrodes allows passage of a secondary current to correct for the nonhomogeneous intracavitary electrical field.[44] This alteration increases the linearity between ventricular volume measurements and conductance over a larger range of volumes. Finally, Kass and coworkers suggest that conductance catheters work poorly in patients with reduced EFs because of the small differences in blood conductance between end-diastole and end-systole.[45]

PRESSURE/VOLUME LOOPS

The end-systolic pressure-volume relationship (ESPVR) is a clinically useful index of ventricular function because it is sensitive to changes in contractility. The slope of the ESPVR is a better technique to separate normal from abnormal ventricles than EF or end-systolic volume. A ventricular pressure-volume loop is constructed by relating intracavitary pressure on the y axis to the ventricular volume on the x axis over the entire cardiac cycle, providing information on both systolic and diastolic functions. The height of the loop is determined by ventricular systolic pressure, whereas the width of the loop is determined by SV. End-systolic pressure and volume are determined by afterload and ventricular inotropy. End-diastolic pressure and volume reflect preload and ventricular lusitropy (relaxation).[46]

An ideal loop for the left ventricle has four phases: phase I is the lower horizontal limb representing diastolic filling; phase II is the vertical limb of isovolumetric contraction; phase III is the upper horizontal limb of systolic ejection; and phase IV is the phase of isovolumetric relaxation. The slope of the ESPVR, generated by connecting the upper lefthand corners of pressure-volume loops generated at varying afterloads, is Emax, the maximal value of end-systolic elastance (Ees) (Fig. 10–4).

Calculation of the area within the loop is stroke work (pressure × volume). The systolic pressure-volume area (PVA) is linearly correlated with myocardial oxygen consumption in intact human and isolated canine hearts.[47] PVA correlates better with myocardial oxygen consumption ($M\dot{V}O_2$) than do rate pressure product, tension time index, and pressure-work index.[48] PVA reliably represents the total mechanical energy generated under different contractile states.[48]

Pressure-volume loops also indicate ventricular compliance. The normal relationship between diastolic pressure and volume is curvilinear. At low end-diastolic pressure the slope is gentle, with little change in pressure for large changes in volume. When end-diastolic pressures are abnormally increased, the curve becomes steeper, and pressure is almost exponentially related to end-diastolic volume.

Technique

Measurement of ventricular pressure using transducer-tipped catheters is possible, although the presence of a ventricular catheter increases ventricular ectopy. Likewise, ventricular volume can be measured using echocardiography or conductance catheters. Abrams and coworkers described a more clinically applicable method for determination of pressure-volume relations.[49] Using echo-Doppler continuous determination of cardiac output, transducer-tipped catheter measurements of left ventricular pressure, and the van der Pol oscillator model to describe changes occurring in the cardiac cycle, pressure-volume loops with a linear correlation to standard experimental techniques of 0.9 were found.[49]

Another limitation of pressure-volume relationships is that pressure may not accurately measure end-systolic afterload. However, the end-systolic pressure-volume relationship is only *relatively* load-independent, and its slope correlates with EF. It is, nevertheless, sensitive to end-diastolic volume, aortic impedance, and contractility.[6]

The use of the simple ratio between end-systolic pressure and volume to represent the ESPVR is an oversimplification, although it has been used as an index of ventricular contractility. It is more easily measured than ESPVR. However, changes in inotropy have variable effects on the slope of the relation of peak pressure and end-systolic dimension.

Right ventricular pressure-volume loops are similar to

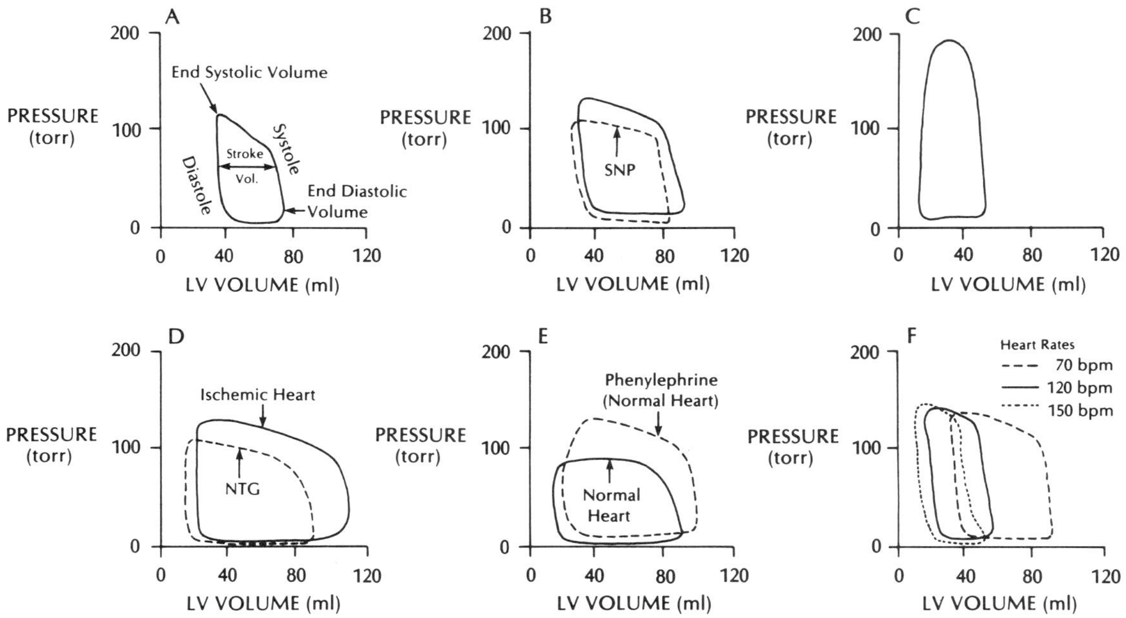

Figure 10–4. The normal pressure/volume loop is in *A*. The loop begins at the bottom left with opening of the mitral valve and initiation of ventricular filling. At the lower right portion of the loop is the end-diastolic volume point where the mitral valve closes and isovolumic contraction begins. At the upper right, aortic valvular opening and ejection begin, causing the loop to turn to the left. As the aortic valve closes at the upper left of the loop (the end-systolic pressure-volume relation), isovolumetric relaxation begins. Connection of the end-diastolic volume points at different afterloads gives a diastolic pressure/volume curve. Cardiac work is the area of the pressure-volume loop, whereas the width of the loop is stroke volume. Alterations in various states are shown in *B* through *E*. *B*, Afterload reduction. *C*, Aortic stenosis. *D*, Ischemia and relief of ischemia. *E*, Increased afterload in a normal heart. *F*, Tachycardia. (From Barash PG, et al [eds]: Clinical Anesthesia. Philadelphia: JB Lippincott, 1992; 1008, with permission.)

those of the left ventricle. Compared with left ventricular loops, right ventricular loops are more triangular in shape, with early peaking of pressure.[50] Right ventricular volume often continues to decrease beyond end-systole. Although Emax reflects contractile state in the right ventricle, right ventricular Emax has a wide range in normal hearts.[50]

Pathophysiologic Changes

Alterations in pressure-volume loops occur in response to drugs and disease (Fig. 10–4*B–E*). The end-systolic point is determined by contractility and afterload. End-systolic elastance is altered by chamber volume and mass. Positive inotropic interventions shift the end-systolic pressure-volume relation upward and leftward, whereas negative inotropic interventions shift the relation downward and to the right (Fig. 10–5). Decreased venous return reduces end-diastolic pressure and volume. Increased preload moves the point of end-diastole to the right and upward along the end-diastolic pressure-volume relation. Positive lusitropic interventions (e.g., relief of ischemia) enhance ventricular filling so that the loop begins at a higher end-diastolic volume and a lower end-diastolic pressure. Patients with primarily systolic heart failure demonstrate increased ventricular volume at end-diastole and reduced extent of shortening but normal developed systolic pressure. With primary diastolic dysfunction, a decrease in diastolic distensibility occurs so that a higher diastolic pressure is required to achieve the same diastolic volume.

PRESSURE-LENGTH LOOPS

Measurement of a pressure-length loop requires placement of a length gauge directly on the myocardium and thus is primarily applicable to animal studies. However, it is a sensitive and reproducible method to assess total cardiac and regional myocardial function during both systole and diastole (Fig. 10–6).[51] A series of pressure-length loops at different preloads or afterloads permits determination of the slope of the end-systolic pressure-length relationship.[52]

Pressure-length loops are indices of regional ventricular work. They lean rightward when contraction is asynchronous, as in the presence of ischemia. Ischemia of a small portion of the ventricle may not be visible on a pressure-length loop if the remaining ventricle compensates to maintain function. Increased preload increases the area of the loop. As afterload increases, the loop becomes taller at a similar preload. With ischemia, ventricular segment lengthening occurs after the end of diastole. Postsystolic shortening is ventricular contraction occurring after aortic valve closure that does not effectively contribute to the work of the heart.

FORCE-VELOCITY CURVES

Force-velocity curves evaluate the velocity of shortening at a constant fiber length in a preloaded (passively stretched) muscle that is stimulated to contract against either no load or an afterload. A Walton-Brodie strain gauge placed directly on the myocardium is used to measure the muscle contraction. As afterload is increased, the initial rate of shortening is hyperbolic (Fig. 10–7). The point at which no shortening occurs, although the muscle is developing maximal force, is Po. Vmax is the maximal velocity of shortening at zero pressure, determined by extrapolation of the curve back to zero load. It is sensitive to preload, although less so than dP/dt. Increased myocardial contractility shifts the force-velocity curve upward and to

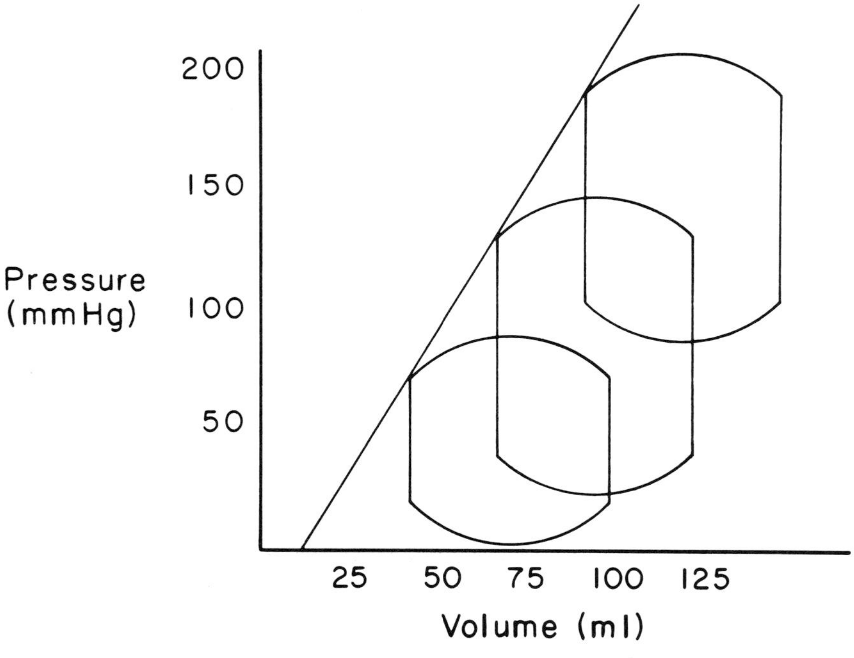

Figure 10–5. A series of pressure-volume loops is created from different preload and afterloads to define the end-systolic pressure-volume relation (ESPVR). The end-systolic points are connected to define the contractile state of the ventricle. A shift to the right of the normal relation indicates decreased contractility, whereas a leftward shift shows increased contractility.

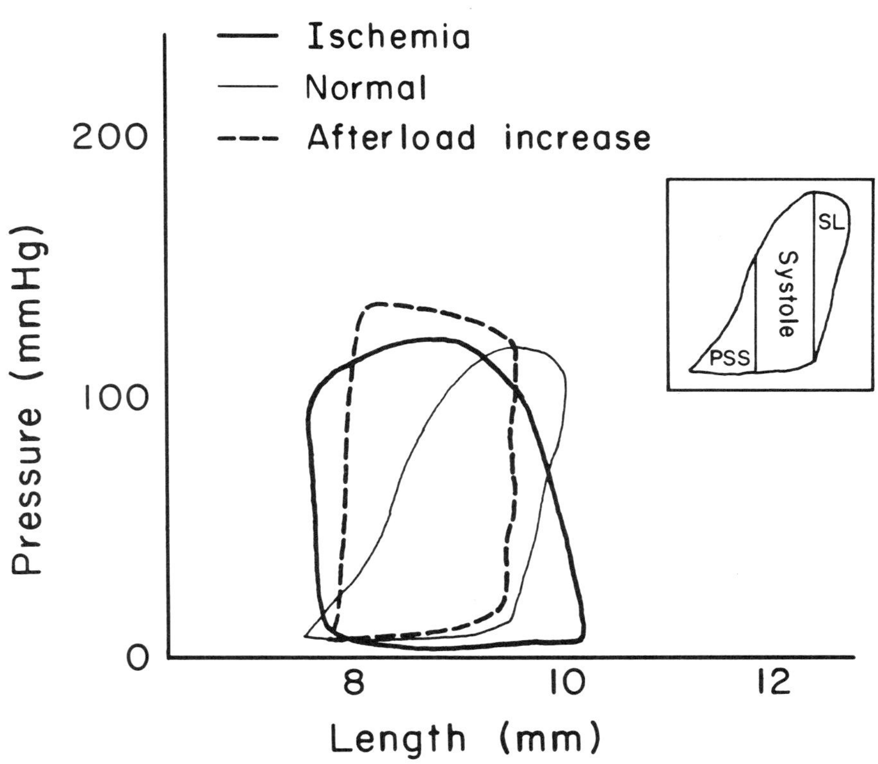

Figure 10–6. The normal pressure-length loop and alterations caused by ischemia and increased afterload are similar to those seen in pressure-volume loops. In a pressure-length loop, ventricular pressure is plotted on the y axis, whereas ventricular segment length appears on the x axis. Pressure-length loops, usually rectangular, have four segments: (1) Isovolumic contraction, (2) ejection, (3) isovolumic relaxation, and (4) ventricular filling. The end-systolic pressure-length relationship is the point at the upper left of the loop. The insert demonstrates specific alterations during ischemia, including development of post-systolic shortening (PSS) and systolic lengthening (SL). Only during systole does ventricular segment shortening contribute to effective cardiac work. *Thick solid line,* ischemia; *Thin solid line,* normal; *Dotted line,* afterload increase.

the right, increasing both developed tension and maximal velocity of shortening.

CARDIAC OUTPUT

Fick Method

The Fick principle uses the following relation to determine cardiac output:

$$\text{Cardiac output (ml/minute)} = \frac{\dot{V}O_2}{CaO_2 - C\bar{v}O_2} \times 100$$

because the size of a fluid stream can be calculated if the amount of a substance entering or leaving the stream and the concentration difference resulting from entry and removal are known. Oxygen is the traditional indicator substance in clinical determinations of cardiac output by the Fick method. Oxygen uptake or consumption is $\dot{V}O_2$ (milliliters per minute) which is the product of the volume of expired air and the difference between the oxygen content in the inspired and expired air (determined by gas analysis). Arterial and venous oxygen content differences ($CaO_2 - C\bar{v}O_2$) are determined from blood samples. Oxygen content is calculated as the solubility of oxygen in whole blood (0.0031 ml/100 ml/mmHg) plus 1.34 hemoglobin (gm/100 ml) times percentage of oxyhemoglobin saturation.

Although the Fick technique is often referred to as the gold standard for cardiac output measurement, it has numerous inherent difficulties.[53] The Fick equation assumes that the pulmonary oxygen consumption is negligible and that the rate of oxygen removal from the blood (tissue oxygen uptake) equals the rate of oxygen uptake at the mouth (lung oxygen uptake). The major disadvantage of the Fick technique is the necessity for maintaining steady state conditions (unchanged right and left ventricular outputs, constant oxygen saturation and arterial PO_2) for several minutes during the measurement. Values will be inaccurate if cardiac or pulmonary shunts are present. Inaccuracy also results from errors in sampling of mixed venous blood or inspired/expired gases and in other measurements as detailed by Taylor and Silke.[53] Widespread use of mass spectrometry has rekindled interest in the perioperative measurement of cardiac output using the Fick method.

Rebreathing Fick Method

Morton described a rebreathing maneuver to estimate the oxygenated mixed venous PCO_2, which when combined with end-tidal PCO_2 and CO_2 production, allows noninvasive assessment of cardiac output using the Fick method.[54] Carbon dioxide production was determined using the Siemens 930 carbon dioxide analyzer by integrating the product of instantaneous expiratory flow and instantaneous expired PCO_2. Mixed venous PCO_2 was determined by allowing the patient to rebreathe a test mixture of 6–9% carbon dioxide in oxygen with the ventilator's rate and volume approximated manually. Expired PCO_2 is recorded after the second, third, and fourth breaths. The rebreathing maneuver is repeated three or four times with different test gases, and a plot of inspired PCO_2 against the difference of expired and inspired PCO_2 is created. The x intercept (where expired PCO_2 equals inspired PCO_2) is mixed venous carbon dioxide.

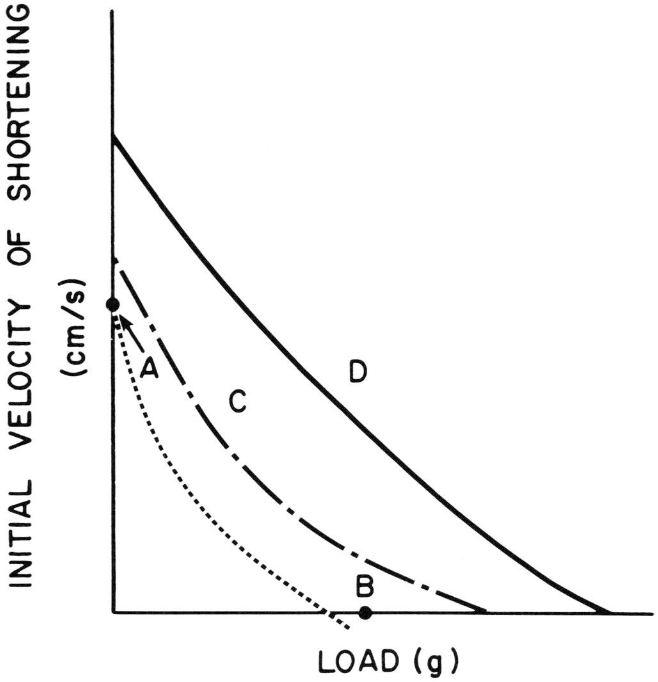

Figure 10–7. Force-velocity curve for cardiac muscle. Point A is Vmax, the point of maximal velocity of shortening with no load. Point B is Po, where tension development is maximal but no shortening occurs. The effect of increased preload is seen in curve C; on any curve, afterload increases from left to right. Curve D demonstrates the effect of increased contractility. (From Lake CL: Cardiovascular Anesthesia. New York: Springer Verlag, 1985; 10, with permission.)

Arteriovenous oxygen content difference is shown at bottom of page; where $Pvco_2$ = oxygenated partial pressure of carbon dioxide in mixed venous blood, $Paco_2$ = partial pressure of carbon dioxide in arterial blood, and Hb = hemoglobin. The calculated value is used in the classic Fick equation. This method has a correlation coefficient of 0.9 with dye-dilution methods.[54]

Continuous Fick Method

A continuous method for determination of cardiac output by the Fick technique is described by Davies and coworkers.[55] The components of the Fick equation were measured using a gas exchange analyzer to determine inspired/expired gas content and volumes with pulse and mixed venous catheter oximetry to determine oxygen contents. A computer calculates the output from these parameters every 20 seconds. Correlation between this method and thermodilution was 0.86, but outputs measured by thermodilution are always higher. Advantages of the continuous Fick method over the thermodilution method are its rapid repetition, the contribution of each of the individual components to the patient's overall cardiorespiratory status, and the validity of the Fick principle to measure cardiac output.

Indicator-Dilution Method

The major difference between the indicator-dilution and the Fick methods is that the concentration gradient of a nontoxic dye, rather than oxygen, is measured. The usual indicator dye is indocyanine green, which is rapidly mixed with blood, is bound to plasma protein, is rapidly metabolized in the liver, is nondiffusible in the lungs, and is easily measured with a photodensitometer. A bolus of dye is injected into the central venous or peripheral circulation. Blood is withdrawn from an artery continuously into a photoelectric curvette densitometer, where the concentration of the dye is measured. The curve relating the dye concentration to elapsed time is plotted. Figure 10–8 shows the normal indicator dilution curve in which there is an uninterrupted build-up slope, a sharp concentration, a steep disappearance slope, and a prominent recirculation peak. Total curve area does not indicate the total concentration of dye for the measured interval because some dye recirculates early and is measured twice. For this reason, the downslope of the curve is extrapolated to near zero to eliminate recirculation effects.

The following equation (termed the Stewart-Hamilton equation for the two investigators who described it) indicates the relationship between dye concentration and cardiac output (L/minute):

$$\frac{60 \times \text{indicator dose (mg)}}{\text{average concentration} \times \text{time (seconds)}}$$

Cardiac output equals the amount of indicator injected divided by the area under the curve.

The efficacy of the dye-dilution method in the evaluation and management of infants and children during and after cardiac surgery was demonstrated by Truccone and coworkers.[56] Right-to-left shunting causes an abnormal early-appearing hump in the build-up slope because the dye reaches the arterial circulation early. With left-to-right shunts, there is a decreased peak concentration of dye, disappearance of dye is prolonged, and recirculation is absent. In shock states, recirculation may occur so early that its recognition is impossible.

Limitations of the indicator-dilution method include the need to withdraw as much as 50 ml of blood (which can be returned to the patient if drawn into sterile tubing), the need for arterial catheterization, measurement of only mean flow, and the need for a steady state for 30–40 seconds. As little as 4–5 ml of arterial blood can be withdrawn in children without decreasing the accuracy of measurement.[56] Cardiopulmonary bypass significantly decreases clearance of indocyanine green because of decreased hepatic blood flow.[57]

Because of these limitations, dye dilution has been refined by using a thermal indicator, the thermodilution method. Common to both dye dilution and thermal dilution are the need for constant flow, constant blood volume,

$$11.02\,(Pvco_2^{0.396} - Paco_2^{0.396}) - 0.015\,(Pvco_2 - Paco_2)\,(15 - Hb) - 0.064\,(95 - Sao_2)$$

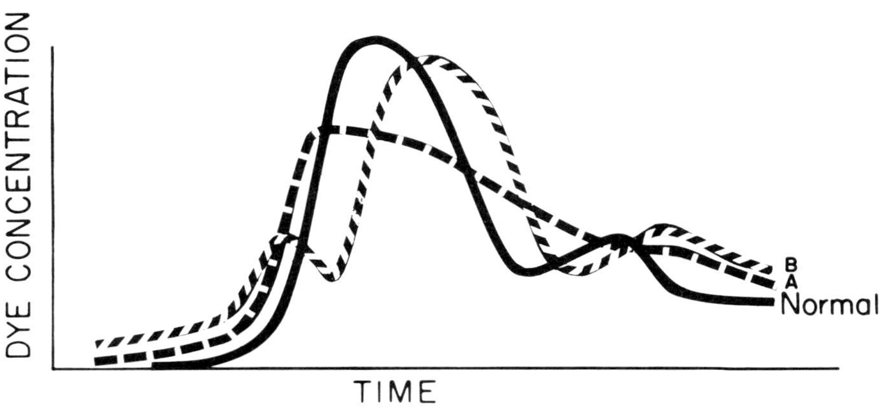

Figure 10–8. A normal indicator (dye)–dilution curve. Curve A demonstrates the effects of left-to-right shunting. Curve B shows right-to-left shunting. (From Lake CL: Cardiovascular Anesthesia. New York: Springer-Verlag, 1985; 70, with permission.)

absence of recirculation, constant indicator distribution times, and measured flow representative of total flow.[58]

Thermodilution Method

The thermal indicator was introduced by Fegler in 1954.[59] However, Ganz and colleagues introduced the thermodilution technique for cardiac output determination in 1971.[60] Advantages of the thermodilution technique are simplicity, reproducibility, lack of recirculation, rapid repetition, safe indicator, rapid indicator mixing with blood, and no requirements for blood withdrawal. Thermodilution has been accepted as a de facto gold standard of cardiac output measurement.

Technique

Thermodilution is a modification of the indicator-dilution technique in which cooled dextrose is injected into the right atrium or central vein through the proximal lumen of a pulmonary artery catheter or a central venous pressure catheter. A thermistor in the pulmonary artery, balanced through a Wheatstone bridge, records the change in temperature as a resistance change. The current in the thermistor is small and does not significantly heat the blood. Theoretically, if a known amount of cold indicator (i.e., "negative" heat) is injected into the circulation, calculation of the cardiac output from the resultant cooling curve recorded downstream of the injection is possible. Passage through two cardiac valves (tricuspid and pulmonic) and one cardiac chamber (right ventricle) allows adequate mixing of injectate with blood.

The equation for calculation of cardiac output by thermodilution is

$$\text{Cardiac output} = \frac{V_I \times (Tb - T_I) \times S_I \times C_I \times 60}{S_B \times C_B \int_0^\infty \Delta T_B\,(t)dt}$$

where Tb is initial blood temperature, T_I is time from start to termination of percentage of integration at 30% of peak of thermodilution curve, S_I and S_B are the specific gravities of indicator and blood, respectively, C_I and C_B are the specific heats of indicator and blood, respectively, V_I is volume of injectate in liters, and integral from 0 to infinity of $\Delta T_B(t)dt$ is the area under the blood temperature change curve in degrees Celsius multiplied by time in seconds. Correction factors for the increase in injectate temperature during passage through the catheter, injectate volume, the area lost by cutoff of the curve at 30% of peak, and 60 are often entered as a constant into commercially available thermodilution computers. The operator's manual for the specific computer used should be consulted for details.

Equipment

Thermodilution cardiac output determinations in adults are performed using a multilumen pulmonary artery catheter with injectate administered through a proximal lumen placed in the right atrium or central vein and the thermistor located in the pulmonary artery. Alternatively, in patients undergoing surgery of the tricuspid or pulmonic valves or those in whom size precludes accurate placement of the injection site and thermistor (pediatric patients), separate central venous and pulmonary artery thermistors can be placed.[61] The thermistor is placed through a purse-string suture in the right ventricular outflow tract and threaded into the main pulmonary artery, and its position is verified by palpation. The central venous catheter is placed either directly or percutaneously. The injectate catheter must be accurately calibrated for the thermal exchange occurring between the catheter and the tissue during injection.[62] Either the precalibrated catheter supplied with the thermistor or any central venous catheter with known volume and thermal characteristics is used.

Cardiac Output Curves

The thermal curve should be visually inspected or recorded before accepting the measured cardiac output value. A normal cardiac output curve (Fig. 10–9) is smooth with a rapid rise to peak and slow return to baseline.

Accuracy

Close correlation ($r = 0.94$) of thermodilution with Fick and dye dilution is demonstrable (Fig. 10–10).[63, 64] However, the bronchial blood flow component of cardiac output is not included in thermodilution measurements. In adult patients, cardiac outputs determined with separate thermis-

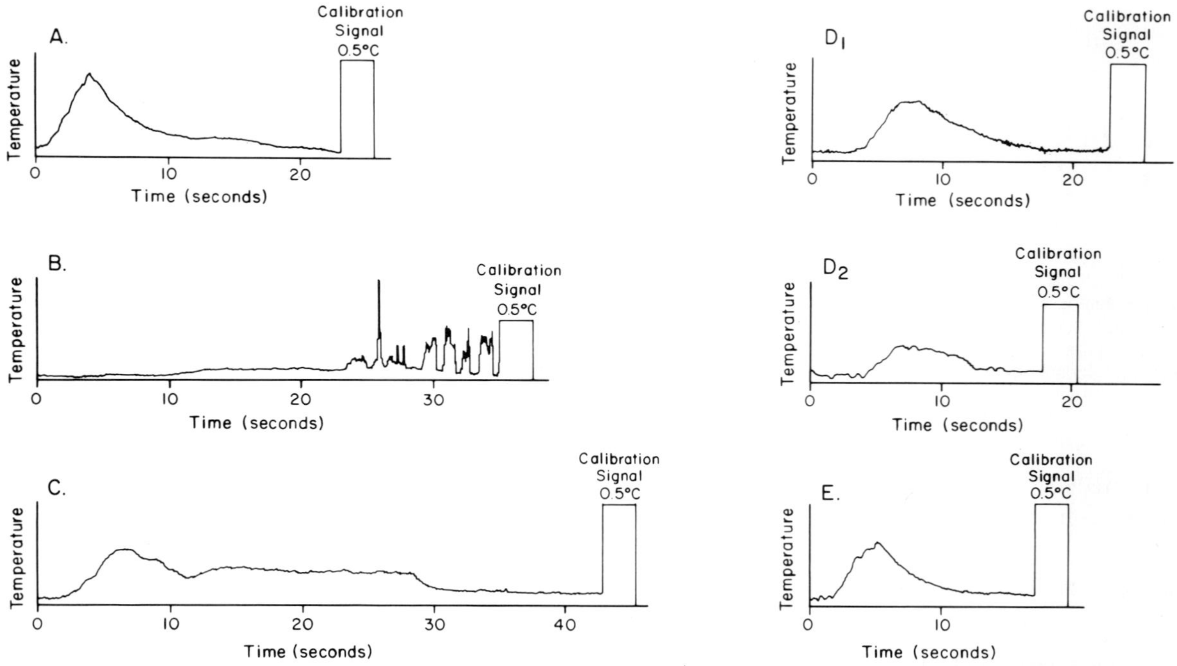

Figure 10–9. Types of cardiac output curves. *A,* Normal thermodilution cardiac output curve. The 0.5°C calibration signal appears after the termination of the curve. *B,* The thermodilution curve is delayed and of low amplitude when injectate is administered slowly over 15 seconds. *C,* The thermistor is against the vessel wall in a wedge position, causing an irregular, low-amplitude curve. D_1, The type of curve resulting from injection of 10 ml of injectate. D_2, The curve in the same patient when only 5 ml of injectate is given, erroneously increasing the measured output. *E,* An irregular curve with an unsteady baseline results from patient motion during injection.

tor probes and with standard pulmonary artery catheters are almost identical.[65] McCormick and coworkers used two identical computers to compute values for cardiac outputs from a single injection sensed by both the separate and the catheter-mounted thermistor.[65] Variation of the position of the injection catheter in the vena cava did not influence measurement.

Similar excellent correlations between separate thermis-

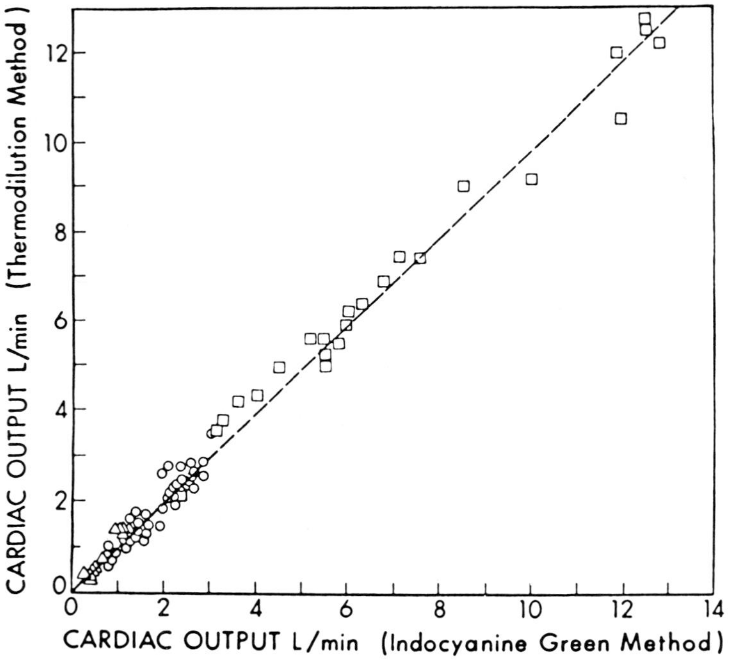

Figure 10–10. There is excellent correlation between cardiac output measured by dye dilution and that measured by thermodilution in monkeys *(triangles),* dogs *(circles),* and humans *(squares).* (From Weisel RD, et al: Measurement of cardiac output by thermodilution. N Engl J Med 1975; 292:682–684, with permission.)

tors and pediatric pulmonary artery catheters are reported in pediatric patients.[62, 66, 67] Kohanna and Cunningham compared 125 thermodilution and dye dilution outputs in 10 postoperative patients.[66] Except in extremely low-output states, in which dye-dilution outputs were always smaller, results were similar with both techniques. Thermodilution outputs always exceeded dye dilution measurements by 1.6% even in normal circulatory states. Reproducibility of the dye dilution outputs was always less than thermodilution. Maruschak and colleagues recommended prefilling of the central venous injectate catheter with 1 ml of injectate-temperature fluid 20 seconds prior to bolus injection to prevent thermal injectate loss and overestimation of cardiac output.[68]

Standard errors of the mean of thermodilution determinations vary from 2–5% for three measurements per determination to 3–8% for single measurements.[69, 70] Thus, clinical significance should not be attributed to values differing by less than 12–15%.[70]

Sources of Inaccuracy

There are numerous sources of inaccuracy in the thermodilution technique, which have been reviewed recently by Nishikawa and Dohi.[71] Variation between cardiac outputs performed in the clinical setting results from inconsistent technical performance, catheter or computer malfunction, respiratory effects on right ventricular filling, cardiac shunting or valvular regurgitation, and hemodynamic instability (Table 10–2).

Most computers contain internal verification systems giving error messages when baseline drift is present, the thermistor is against the vessel wall, or the catheter is too distal in the pulmonary artery. Figure 10–9*B–E* demonstrates common types of anomalous curves.[63] Both respiratory and cardiac cycles alter baselines. The thermal curve rises slowly when the thermistor is positioned too distally in the pulmonary artery.[63, 72] Irregularities in thermal curves result from rapid changes in heart rate or blood pressure, patient movement, inadequate indicator mixing with blood, or contact between vessel wall and thermistor.[63, 72] Low-amplitude curves occur when the injectate volume is too small, the thermistor is within the right ventricle or is too distal in the pulmonary artery, or the temperature differential between injectate and patient is too small.[72] Immediately after discontinuation of cardiopulmonary bypass, the thermal baseline may be so unstable as to preclude accurate measurements. Bazaral et al reported underestimation of thermodilution outputs during the first 10 minutes following bypass.[73]

TABLE 10–2. THERMODILUTION METHOD: SOURCES OF ERROR

Patient Variables
Motion (shivering, extremity movement)
Respiration (panting, Valsalva maneuver, sighing)
Alterations in ventricular performance/dysrhythmias
Valvular regurgitation
Intracardiac shunts
Inaccurate temperature measurement
Injectate Factors
Wrong substance
Wrong temperature or rewarming of injectate
Wrong volume of injectate
Rapid repetition of measurements
Insufficient mixing with blood
Thermistor Factors
Thermistor malposition
Thermistor thrombus
Intracatheter shunts
Rapid volume effusion
Concurrent electrocautery use
Improper constants

Injectate. Both room temperature and iced injectates are used. Variability among outputs is about 5.5% with room temperature injectate.[63] However, the signal of temperature change is two to three times smaller with room temperature injectates than with iced injectate. Several investigators have demonstrated similar results with either room temperature or ice (Fig. 10–11).[74, 75] Although the temperature differential between room temperature injectate and blood temperature in a hypothermic (31–33°C) patient is small, correlation coefficients of 0.951 for 10-ml volumes and 0.925 for 5-ml volumes of injectate were demonstrated in mechanically ventilated adults.[75, 76] Volume of injectate is an important factor in accuracy because volumes of 5 ml or less cause significant variability (as much as 1.5 L/minute).

Closed injectate systems obviate the need to prepare individual syringes for injectate, minimizing infection risk[77] and equilibration time.[72] Repeated aspiration of injectate from a rubber-stoppered intravenous bottle immersed in an ice bath and connection/disconnection from the injection port of the pulmonary artery catheter are sources of bacterial contamination.[77] However, if the tubing of such systems is not maintained at the same temperature as that of the injectate as it enters the catheter, measured cardiac output is inaccurate.[78] Prefilled refrigerated syringes offer an alternative to closed injectate systems. Rewarming of iced injectate begins within 30 seconds of its removal from an iced bath, particularly with application of firm manual pressure on the syringe by the person making the injection.[72, 79] A 1°C error in injectate temperature causes an error in measured output of 2.7% with iced injectate and a 7.7% error with room temperature injectate in a normothermic patient.[72] Measurement of the injectate temperature as it enters the circulation is optimal.[79]

Timing of Injection. Measurement of pulmonary artery diastolic pressures is timed to the apneic period at the end of expiration because of the respiratory effects on right heart and pulmonary pressures. Performance of thermodilution outputs at random times in the respiratory cycle causes marked variability in results because pulmonary artery temperature decreases during inspiration, particularly in mechanically ventilated patients (Fig. 10–12).[63, 80–82] Maximum variability in outputs was 70% for the right heart and 40% for the left heart in random measurements during the respiratory cycle.[82] Pulmonary artery temperature vari-

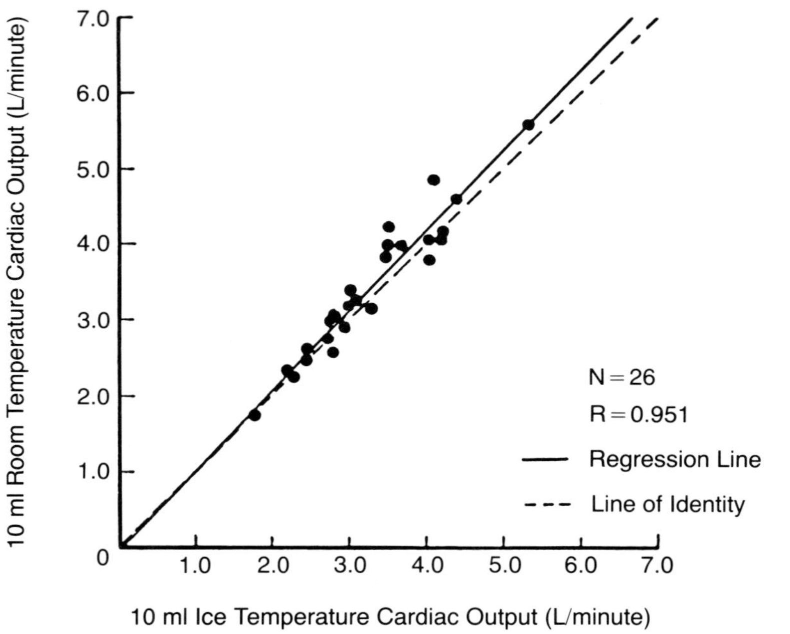

Figure 10–11. Thermodilution cardiac output determinations using either room temperature or iced injectate yield similar results. (From Shellock FG et al: Thermodilution cardiac output determination in hypothermic postcardiac surgery patients: Room vs ice temperature injectate. Crit Care Med 1983; 11:669, with permission.)

ation with the phase of the respiratory cycle results from right ventricular surface cooling from overlying lung and changes in vena caval flows.[72] Measurements at peak inspiration or end-expiration have less variability and smaller standard deviations.[83] For convenience, end-expiration is often used, because cessation of respirator noise and chest wall movement permit easy detection of the optimal time.

Marked variation in pulmonary artery temperatures may preclude the use of room temperature injectate for thermodilution output determinations. Such changes occur with panting, shivering, deep spontaneous respiration, performance of the Valsalva maneuver, or elevation of the extremities.[72]

Disease Process. Structural cardiac disease impairs or

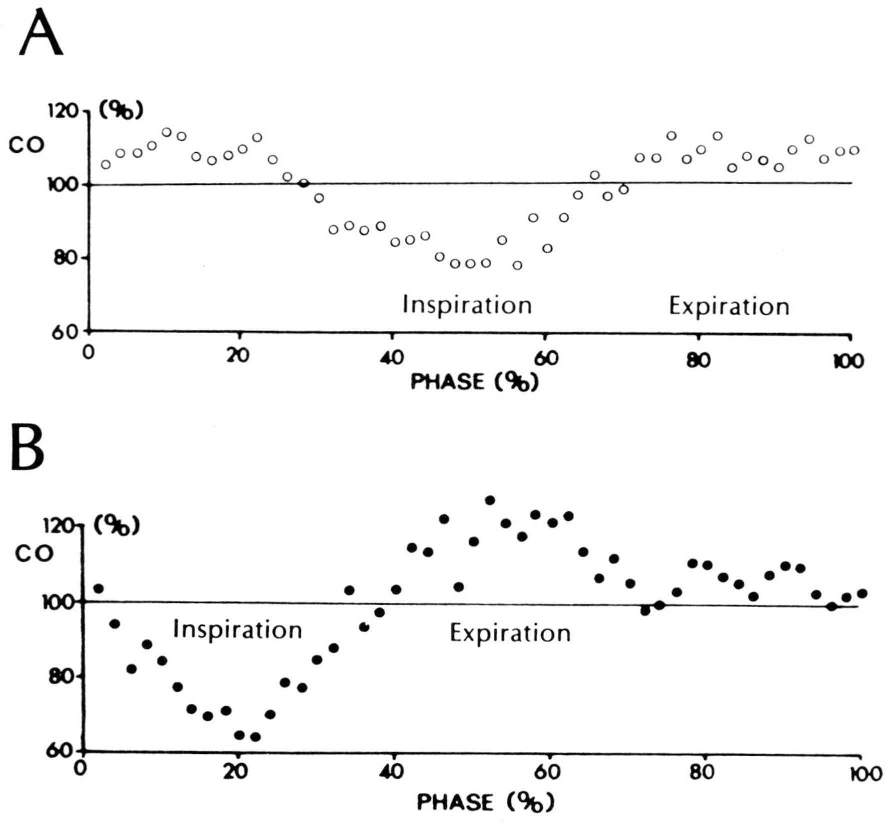

Figure 10–12. Alterations in left heart output *(A)* and right heart output *(B)* during a single respiratory cycle. Flow decreases during inspiration, increasing and reaching a plateau during expiration. For this reason, thermodilution outputs should be determined at end-expiration. (From Jansen JRC, et al: Thermodilution technique for measurement of cardiac output during artificial ventilation. J Appl Physiol 1981; 50:584–591, with permission.)

prevents measurement of cardiac output by thermodilution. Theoretically, tricuspid regurgitation should produce significant recirculation of blood in the right heart such that accurate output measurements are unlikely because of the resulting broad, low-amplitude curves and increased amount of artifact.[84] In patients with left heart regurgitant lesions, the thermodilution technique produces curves with less recirculation-induced distortion than the dye-dilution method does with right-sided injection and left-sided sampling.[64] Boerboom et al suggest that cardiac output is underestimated in acute tricuspid regurgitation in proportion to the amount of regurgitation and the cardiac output.[85] Artifacts in the thermal curve are less likely to be rejected by thermodilution computers. However, Konishi and coworkers noted acceptable correlation between Fick and thermodilution measurements in humans with mild, moderate, and severe tricuspid regurgitation.[86]

The downslope of the curve is also affected to an unknown extent by recirculation of indicator through intracardiac or extracardiac shunts.[63, 72] The direction and volume of the shunt as well as speed of injectate injection influence the accuracy of the resultant measurements.[87] Morady and coworkers reported a method for determining the magnitude of left-to-right shunt by extrapolation of the curve to baseline just before early recirculation.[88] The area under the extrapolated portion and entire curve are measured by planimetry. Shunt size is the ratio of the total area to the area prior to recirculation ([A + B]/A), which correlates well with shunt ratios determined using the Fick equation.[88] Erroneously high outputs were measured in a patient in cardiogenic shock with an aortopulmonary fistula.[89]

The thermodilution method can be satisfactorily used to measured cardiac output in patients with residual left-to-right shunts.[90] Placement of right and left atrial catheters and a pulmonary artery thermistor allows measurement of output after injection through either catheter. When a computer that stops integrating the thermal curve at 30% of baseline is used to avoid recirculation, systemic flow ($\dot{Q}s$) is determined by the equation

$$\dot{Q}s = D_{rai}\,(1 - D_{rai}/D_{lai})$$

where rai and lai = thermodilution outputs determined after right and left atrial injections, respectively.[90]

Finally, during moderate exercise at outputs between 2 and 13 L/minute, both thermodilution and Fick methods accurately measure cardiac output.[91] However, during maximal exercise, thermodilution cardiac outputs are less than those measured using the Fick technique.[92] At outputs of 15–23 L, thermodilution and Fick correlate well, but may be subject to inaccuracy due to alterations in mixed venous oxygen saturation, hematocrit, fluctuation in pulmonary artery temperature during hyperventilation, and increased heat exchange.

Injectate Factors. Because the specific gravity and specific heat of dextrose and saline are similar (specific gravity = 1.018 for dextrose vs. 1.005 for saline; specific heat = 0.965 for dextrose vs. 0.997 for saline), the product of the specific heat and specific gravity for either substance is similar, and either substance can be used. If multiple determinations must be made, saline may be preferable to minimize hyperglycemia. The volume of injectate varies according to the type of syringe used, but this error is small. However, if the syringe volume is less than the value entered into the computer, the area under the thermal curve is proportionately smaller, causing overestimation of cardiac output.[93] Recirculation of the cold injectate causes the thermal curve to have a diminished peak and longer tail than a dye-dilution curve. The "cold" radiates from the catheter after injection and arrives at the thermistor about 5–35 seconds after the bolus injection.

Repetition of injections must be delayed at least 90 seconds to permit resumption of steady blood temperature. Automatic injectors are helpful to maintain consistency of injection rate.[94] Speed of injection affects the constants in the thermodilution equation, which are based on a rate of 10 ml injected within 4 seconds or less in most computer systems.[95] The increase in injectate temperature (injectate at 0–1°C) during passage through a catheter inserted to 45 cm is 6–7°C.[69]

Mixing and Thermistor Factors. A distance of 20 cm or more is necessary for adequate mixing of the injectate with blood. The thermistor must also be located in the center of the flowing blood, at least 2 mm from the vessel wall for reproducibility of the outputs, because a thermal gradient exists between the central and lateral portions of a flowing stream.[96] An undamped pulmonary artery waveform usually assures acceptable thermistor position.

Bjoraker and coworkers reported that the presence of thrombus on the catheter prolongs warming and cooling of the thermistor after the cool bolus, overestimating the area under the curve and decreasing cardiac output.[97] The error is proportional to the size of the thrombus, with underestimation of flow as thrombus size increases.

The presence of a defect in the septum of the catheter between the proximal and distal lumens decreases measured cardiac output. Such defects decrease the temperature at the thermistor because the injectate is channeled into the distal lumen and emerges distal to the thermistor.[98–100] Rapid volume infusions during determinations also artifactually reduce measured outputs.[101]

Complications

The major complication, cardiac dysrhythmia, relates to the temperature of the injectate. Iced injectate has been associated with atrial fibrillation,[102] bradycardia,[103] and other transient dysrhythmias such as slowing of the intrinsic sinus rhythm,[104] which results from cooling of the sinoatrial node.[105] Ventricular fibrillation after injection of room temperature injectate was reported by Katz and coworkers.[106]

Semicontinuous Thermodilution Method

Thermal indicator can also be produced using a 10-cm thermal filament that introduces an average of 7.5 W of heat into right ventricular blood (Fig. 10–13). With heat infusion of less than 7.5 W, the surface of the catheter remains less than 44°C, a temperature that does not adversely affect blood or myocardium.[107] The computer also continually measures the filament temperature and adjusts it automatically to safe ranges. The surface temperature over the filament is determined by blood flow and velocity, filament surface area, and heat flux. However, the actual thermal contact by blood is brief and limited by the blood velocity and the thin boundary layer of blood at the catheter surface. From the pulses of heat, a thermal curve is detected and correlated with the input of thermal energy, and cardiac output is calculated from the area under the curve.[108] The displayed cardiac output results from an averaging technique that represents the cardiac output of the previous 3–6 minutes and is thus semicontinuous.

Compared to bolus injections of room temperature indicator, the semicontinuous method demonstrates correlation coefficients of 0.94 in critical care patients.[107, 109] No user calibration, catheter positioning, or other special protocol is required beyond catheter insertion techniques, which are described in Chapter 8. However, signal processing enhancement, using the principle of stochastic system identification, is required because of thermal noise due to changes in venous return associated with patient movement, respiration, or hemodynamic changes in the pulmonary artery.

The indications for semicontinuous cardiac output determinations are less clear than are those for intermittent measurements. Yelderman et al suggest its use for monitoring volume infusion, titration of vasoactive drugs, early detection of adverse trends, and adjustment of ventilatory variables.[110]

Pulse Contour and Pressure Methods

The area under the arterial waveform indicates cardiac output. Numerous techniques for the determination of stroke volume from central aortic pressure waveform have been described.[111, 112] Common to all methods is the equation

$$\text{Stroke volume} = K \int_0^{\infty} \{P(t) - PED\}dt$$

where K = a constant and $\{P(t) - PED\}dt$ = the difference between the actual pressure (P[t]) and the end-diastolic pressure (PED) over time (d[t]).[113]

In the Warner method, pressure waveforms from a central aortic catheter are sampled by computer 200 samples/second for 45 seconds. Computer analysis of the waveform using the following equation allows determination of stroke volume:

$$\text{Stroke volume} = K\,(pmd)\,(1 + Sa/Da)$$

where K = a calibration constant equal to F(1 + Ts/Td), F = the factor relating calculated stroke volume to stroke volume measured with another technique (thermodilution, dye dilution), Ts = duration of systolic ejection, Td = duration of diastole, pmd = the difference between average aortic pressures during the last 80 msec of systole and diastole, Sa = the systolic area of the curve, and Da = the diastolic area. The calibration constant varies significantly.[114]

Disadvantages of the pulse contour method are the requirement for calibration against thermodilution or another measurement technique, the need to use a central aortic waveform because of the variability of pressure patterns in central and peripheral arteries, and alterations in pulse wave velocity.[115] Because of these disadvantages, other pulse contour methods have been described by Wesseling et al[116] and Gratz et al.[117] Their equations derive the admittance (the reciprocal of impedance) by computer algorithm from the pulse contour curve modified by factors for wave reflection and age. Wesseling's formula also corrects for changes in blood pressure and heart rate.[116]

English and colleagues found good correlation of cardiac outputs measured by thermodilution, flowmeter, and pulse contour during halothane (0.5–2%) administration in

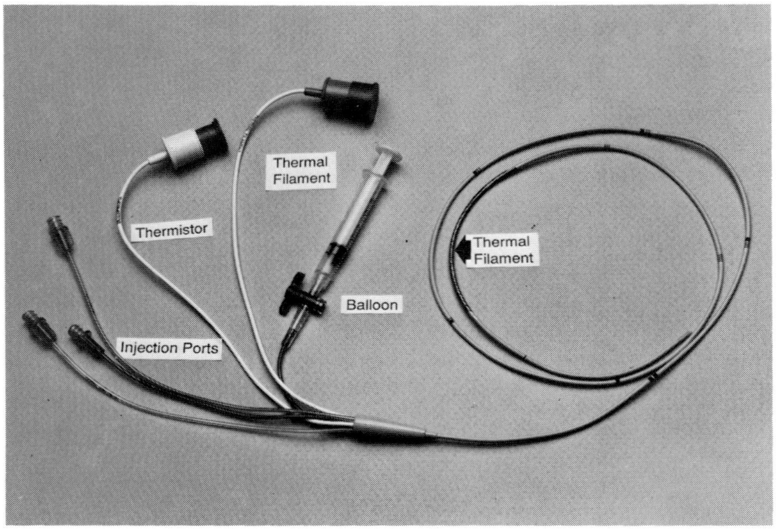

Figure 10–13. A pulmonary artery catheter with a thermal filament for semicontinuous measurement of cardiac output.

dogs.[118] However, changes in systemic vascular resistance greater than 30–50% of control reduced the correlation.[118] Cundick and colleagues noted poor correlation of Warner (r = 0.58) and Bourgeois (r = 0.50) pressure-pulse cardiac output determinations with those obtained with the Fick method in cardiac surgical patients.[114] In these studies, arterial compliance was inconstant and varied inversely with mean pressure, causing the calibration constant K to vary. Frequent recalibration improves the correlation to 0.68.[119] Gratz and coworkers demonstrated a correlation coefficient of 0.78 between pulse contour and thermodilution in cardiac surgical patients with radial arterial catheters.[115]

MONITORING OF RIGHT VENTRICULAR FUNCTION

The right ventricle has limited functional significance during normal circulatory states. Although the spiral muscles of the right ventricle contract during systole, the right ventricular free wall is pulled toward the interventricular septum by alignment of septal fibers and the left ventricular pressure. Right ventricular stroke volume is more sensitive to increased afterload than the left ventricle. Other factors determining right ventricular function include its contractility, its filling volume, its sympathetic tone, its myocardial structural integrity, and the chemical content of the coronary perfusate.[120] Compliance of the right ventricle is greater than that of the left ventricle.

Monitoring of right ventricular function is indicated in patients with pulmonary hypertension, pulmonary parenchymal disease, sepsis, heart-lung transplantation, or right ventricular infarction, as well as in patients receiving ventilation with positive end-expiratory pressure. Evaluation of right ventricular function includes the measurement of both pressure and volume. Central venous or right atrial pressure, discussed in Chapter 8, is most commonly used to assess right ventricular pressure. Normal right ventricular systolic pressures are 30–40 mmHg with diastolic pressures of 0–5 mmHg. Many of the techniques described previously for measurement of left ventricular volume have been applied with limited success to the right ventricle. However, the anatomic shape of the right ventricle is variable, appearing as an ellipse, a tetrahedron, a crescent, or a pyramid, depending on the viewpoint.

Radionuclide Techniques

Both the first-pass and equilibrium-gated blood pool scan have been used successfully to determine right ventricular EF, systolic ejection time, peak filling rates, peak EF, and rate of contractility. Problems with the first-pass technique include invalidation of results by artifacts such as arrhythmias and the need to inject radioactive tracers for each determination. Gated scans permit repeated measurements with a single bolus injection of radioactive tracer and scanning in the left anterior oblique position.[121] One problem with this technique is the superimposition of the right atrium over the right ventricle.[122] For this reason, first-pass studies are preferred for determination of right ventricular EF.

Echocardiographic Techniques

Either two-dimensional or M-mode echocardiography provides information about right ventricular dimensions, interventricular septal motion, and right ventricular free wall thickness. The apical four-chamber view permits calculation of right ventricular short and long axes and systolic shortening. From the echocardiographic data, Simpson's rule is used to determine right ventricular volume. However, these methods often overestimate right ventricular volume and fail to allow for alterations in right ventricular size and geometry under various clinical conditions.

Another echocardiographic measurement to determine right ventricular function is tricuspid annular plane systolic excursion (TAPSE).[123] The tricuspid valve moves toward the right ventricular apex during systole; thus, TAPSE measures the integrity of both right ventricular walls in a simple, reproducible method independent of geometric assumptions.

Thermodilution Techniques

Right ventricular EF is measured by the thermodilution technique using a rapid response thermistor pulmonary artery catheter.[124, 125] This technique has the advantages of costing less than echocardiography, bedside applicability, no risk of indicator accumulation with repeated measurements, and a degree of invasiveness similar to that of standard pulmonary artery catheters. Kay and colleagues compared thermodilution measurements of right ventricular EF with radionuclide studies in both animal models and humans.[126] The rapid response thermistor has a response time of 50 msec compared with the usual thermodilution thermistor response of 300–1000 msec and detects 80–90% of the actual temperature change, depending on heart rate. Increased response time permits observation of beat-to-beat variations in pulmonary artery temperature in response to atrial injection of cold injectate indicator (just proximal to the tricuspid valve) through a multiorificed catheter. The injectate mixes with right ventricular blood and equilibrates within two beats.[125] During subsequent ventricular ejections, the indicator is ejected in an exponentially decreasing fashion. Pulmonary artery concentrations of indicator during each systole reflect ventricular end-diastolic concentrations. The changes in temperature associated with successive diastolic plateaus can be measured. However, the plateaus in the indicator decay curve may not always be well defined because of fibrin deposition around the thermistor. The distance of the thermistor from the pulmonary valve does not affect measured right ventricular EF (Fig. 10–14).[127] Calculation of the EF, stroke volume, and right ventricular end-systolic and end-diastolic volumes is possible using the following formulas:

$$EF = 1 - RF$$

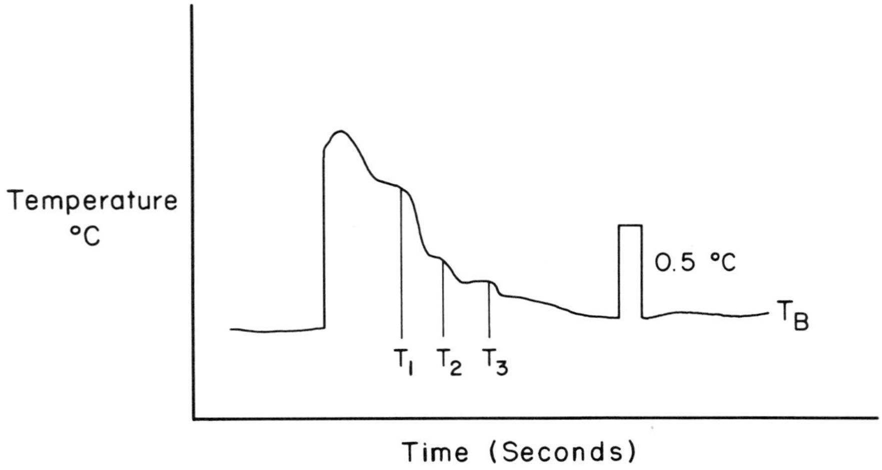

Figure 10–14. A right ventricular thermodilution curve demonstrates the plateaus on the downslope during diastole when temperature change is minimal. The standard 0.5°C is shown after the curve. T_1, T_2, and T_3 are the differences between each diastolic temperature and T_B, the baseline temperature.

where EF = ejection fraction and RF = mean residual fraction. RF is determined as

$$RF = \frac{RF_1 + RF_2}{2} \text{ and}$$

$$RF_1 = \frac{T_2 - T_B}{T_1 - T_B} \text{ and}$$

$$RF_2 = \frac{T_3 - T_B}{T_2 - T_B}$$

Either intracardiac or surface electrodes measure the R-R interval of the ECG to allow calculation of the stroke volume. Normal right ventricular EF = 0.4.

Limitations of this technique arise when regurgitant lesions of the tricuspid or pulmonic valve, cardiac dysfunction, and cardiac dysrhythmias are present. Reproducibility of measurements decreases at larger EFs.[125] Right ventricular EF is decreased by tricuspid regurgitation. If the injectate port is located 5–7 cm from the tricuspid valve, measured EF is erroneously low.[127] Only forward flow is measured, but placement of a thermistor in the right atrium allows calculation of the regurgitant fraction resulting from tricuspid insufficiency. The problem with dysrhythmias is overcome by averaging the thermal curves obtained over five beats. Likewise, averaging of four determinations over various phases of the respiratory cycle at respiratory rates > 15/minute or apnea produces greatest reproducibility.[128] Finally, it is unclear whether equipment algorithms to fit an exponential to the slope of the decay curve can compensate for dampened frequency responses of catheter-mounted thermistors and fibrin deposition on the thermistors.

Determinations of right ventricular EF vary about 12%.[129] Correlations between right ventricular EFs measured by thermodilution and nuclear techniques are 0.8–0.9.[129, 130] Thermodilution underestimates right ventricular EF compared with angiography.[129] Weaker correlations with two-dimensional echocardiographic measurements (0.74) were noted by Jardin and colleagues.[131]

Changes in right ventricular function occur with ischemia, infarction, application of positive end-expiratory pressure to the airway, chronic obstructive lung disease, and with pulmonary vasoconstriction of any etiology. In septic patients, Diebel and coworkers suggested that right ventricular end-diastolic volume determined by thermodilution was a better indicator of preload-recruitable increases in cardiac output than was pulmonary wedge pressure.[131] The reader is referred to reviews by Hines and Barash[133] and by Hines[134] for the details of pathologic alterations in right ventricular function.

EVALUATION OF VENTRICULAR LUSITROPY

Ventricular lusitropy (relaxation) and diastolic function are assessed using echocardiography (described in Chapter 9) or pressure-volume relations as described earlier. Except for these techniques, there are no devices that specifically measure ventricular diastolic function.

DETERMINATION OF DERIVED PARAMETERS

Monitoring of isolated parameters leads to erroneous conclusions about a patient's general status. For this reason, profiles including data on hemodynamic, respiratory, renal, and metabolic function are often used.[135] The basis of most profiles is calculated hemodynamic variables. Systemic and pulmonary vascular resistance, right and left ventricular stroke volume and work, and cardiac index are calculated from directly measured intravascular pressures and systemic and pulmonary flows (Table 10–3). Cardiac index is calculated by normalizing cardiac output for body surface area (determined from a nomogram of height and weight). The usefulness of these measures of ventricular performance is enhanced by construction of a ventricular function curve that relates stroke work or stroke power to end-diastolic fiber length (end-diastolic volume or pressure is usually substituted clinically). These curves can be replot-

TABLE 10–3. CALCULATION OF HEMODYNAMIC VARIABLES

Variables	Formula	Normal Values
Cardiac index	$\frac{\text{cardiac output (L/minute)}}{\text{body surface area (M)}}$	2.8–4.2 L/minute/m²
Stroke index	$\frac{\text{stroke volume (ml/beat)}}{\text{body surface area (M)}}$	30–65 ml/beat/m²
Stroke volume	$\frac{\text{cardiac output (L/minute)} \times 1000}{\text{heart rate (beats/minute)}}$	60–90 ml/minute
Right ventricular stroke work index	0.0136 (mean pulmonary artery pressure* − central venous pressure) × stroke index	5–10 gm-m/beat/m²
Left ventricular stroke work index	0.0136 (mean arterial pressure − mean pulmonary artery pressure) × stroke index	45–60 gm-m/beat/m²
Systemic vascular resistance	$\frac{\text{mean arterial pressure} - \text{central venous pressure}}{\text{cardiac output (L/minute)}} \times 79.9$	1200–1500 dynes · sec · cm^{-5}
Pulmonary vascular resistance	$\frac{\text{mean pulmonary artery pressure} - \text{mean pulmonary capillary wedge pressure}}{\text{cardiac output (L/minute)}} \times 79.9$	100–300 dynes · sec · cm^{-5}

*All pressures are measured in mmHg.

ted after interventions such as administration of drugs, exercise, diuresis, relief of ischemia, or volume loading.

Values of systemic and pulmonary vascular resistance are expressed in hybrid (Wood) units or in an absolute resistance unit (dynes · sec · cm^{-5}). Absolute resistance units are converted to Wood units by dividing by 79.9. Systemic and pulmonary vascular resistance are also normalized for body surface area by using cardiac index in place of cardiac output in the formula. Mohr and coworkers report a continuous on-line method to measure systemic vascular resistance using the peripheral arterial waveform.[136] Computer solution of the following equation is utilized:

$$SVR = F \times \frac{P'}{dP/dt} - a$$

where dP/dt = the peak dP/dt of the peripheral arterial waveform, P′ = the pressure at peak dP/dt, and F and a = calibration constants. This method requires determination of these calibration constants against thermodilution or other independent methods. However, because pulmonary vascular resistance varies with pulmonary blood flow, pulmonary tone, and left atrial pressure, the effects of therapeutic intervention should be monitored by pulmonary pressure-flow curves, direct measurement of pulmonary flow, or the pulmonary diastolic-pulmonary wedge pressure gradient.[137]

MEASUREMENT OF PERIPHERAL FLOW

Doppler output techniques measure blood flow velocity in meters or centimeters per second rather than flow in traditional liters per minute. Doppler flow velocity is measured across a heart valve (mitral) or great vessel such as the aorta using either PW or CW techniques. The product of the area under the flow velocity curve and the cross-sectional area of the structure where the flow velocity was measured is the stroke volume. Laser techniques are also used to measure flow.

In addition to flow velocity, the acceleration of the moving blood and the flow time (usually corrected for heart rate–corrected flow time [FTc]) are also measured. These Doppler indices can be used to study various hemodynamic states. However, contractility is not directly measured by these techniques. Peak velocity, but not flow time, correlates with systemic vascular resistance.[15] Normal FTc is 330–360 msec. Peak flow velocity is age-dependent, varying from 90–120 cm/second in 20-year-old persons to 50–80 cm/second in 70-year-old persons. Mean acceleration is about 15 m/second/second.[15]

NORMAL ALTERATIONS IN VENTRICULAR FUNCTION

Cardiac output is increased by increased load, either pressure or volume, a process termed heterometric autoregulation. It also increases because of the treppe phenomenon and the Anrep effect. The staircase effect (treppe or Bowditch phenomenon) is a progressive increase in contractile force in response to sudden increases in heart rate. The reverse, or negative, staircase effect is an increased force of contraction after a long pause between heartbeats. Abrupt increases in aortic or left ventricular pressure cause the Anrep effect, a response of increased contractility resulting from more rapid activation of the contractile process, increased velocity of shortening, or increased developed force. The Anrep effect is transient because the initially increased ventricular end-diastolic volume and circumference decrease as stroke work recovers.

Alterations of volume and pressure in one ventricle affect these parameters in the other because of the phenomenon of ventricular interdependence. Although interdependence depends somewhat on the presence of the pericardium, it exists after pericardiotomy. The transseptal pressure gradient, septal position and deformability, and ventricular distensibility affect ventricular interdependence. Distention of either ventricle alters the geometry and compliance of the opposite ventricle. Ventricular hypertrophy, particularly of the interventricular septum, limits interdependence by decreasing the transfer of pressure and volume changes. Increased left ventricular pressure decreases right ventricular systolic function and diastolic compliance.

REFERENCES

1. Wright G, Sum Ping JST, Campbell CS, Tobias MA: Assessment of cardiovascular function in patients undergoing coronary artery bypass grafting. J Thorac Cardiovasc Surg 1988; 96:400–407.
2. Unterberg RH, Korfer R, Politz B, et al: Assessment of left ventricular function by a power index: An intraoperative study. Basic Res Cardiol 1984; 79:423–431.
3. Wasserman K: New concepts in assessing cardiovascular function. Circulation 1988; 78:1060–1071.
4. Lange RA, Katz J, McBride W, et al: Effects of supine and lateral positions on cardiac output and intracardiac pressures. Am J Cardiol 1988; 62:330–333.
5. Nakao S, Come PC, Miller MJ, et al: Effects of supine and lateral positions on cardiac output and intracardiac pressures: An experimental study. Circulation 1986; 73:579–585.
6. Baan J, Bachmann K: Ventricular function and pressure-volume analysis. Eur Heart J 1992; 13(Suppl E):1–79.
7. Spotnitz HM, Sonnenblick EH, Spiro D: Relation of ultrastructure to function in the intact heart: Sarcomere structure relative to pressure-volume curves of intact left ventricles of dog and cat. Circ Res 1966; 18:49–66.
8. Kreulen TH, Bove AA, McDonough MT, et al: The evaluation of left ventricular function in man. Circulation 1975; 51:677–688.
9. Kass DA, Maughan WL, Guo ZM, et al: Comparative influence of load versus inotropic states on indexes of ventricular contractility: Experimental and theoretical analysis based on pressure-volume relationships. Circulation 1987; 76:1422–1436.
10. Reves JG, Pruett JK: Use of the Walton-Brodie strain gauge arch to measure contractile force during anesthesia. Br J Anaesth 1988; 60:78S–84S.
11. Giles RW, Berger HJ, Barash PG, et al: Continuous monitoring of left ventricular performance with the computerized nuclear probe during laryngoscopy and intubation before coronary artery bypass surgery. Am J Cardiol 1982; 50:735–741.
12. Wagner HN, Rigo P, Baxter RH, et al: Monitoring ventricular function at rest and during exercise with a nonimaging nuclear detector. Am J Cardiol 1979; 43:975–979.
13. Breisblatt WM, Vita NA, Armuchastegui M, et al: Usefulness of serial radionuclide monitoring during graded nitroglycerin infusion for unstable angina pectoris for determining left ventricular function and individualized therapeutic dose. Am J Cardiol 1988; 61:685–690.
14. Bellows WH, Bode RH, Levy JH, et al: Noninvasive detection of periinduction ischemic ventricular dysfunction by cardiokymography in humans: Preliminary experience. Anesthesiology 1984; 60:155–158.
15. Singer M: Esophageal Doppler monitoring of aortic blood flow: Beat by beat cardiac output monitoring. *In* Royston D, Feeley TW (eds): Monitoring in Anesthesiology: Current Standards and Newer Techniques. Int Anesth Clin 1993; 31:99–125.
16. Lefrant JY, Aya G, de la Coussaye JE, et al: Comparison of cardiac output measured by esophageal Doppler versus thermodilution [Abstract]. Intens Care Med 1992; 18(Suppl 2):238.
17. Belot JP, Valtier B, de la Coussaye JE, et al: Continuous estimation of cardiac output in critically ill mechanically ventilated patients by a new transoesophageal Doppler probe [Abstract]. Intens Care Med 1992; 18(Suppl 2):241.
18. Alverson DC, Eldridge M, Dillon T, et al: Noninvasive pulsed Doppler determination of cardiac output in neonates and children. J Pediatr 1982; 101:46–50.
19. Nicolosi GL, Pungercic E, Cervesato E, et al: Feasibility and variability of six methods for the echocardiographic and Doppler determination of cardiac output. Br Heart J 1988; 59:299–303.
20. Crobson S, Murray A, Peart I, et al: Reproducibility of cardiac output measurement by cross sectional and Doppler echocardiography. Br Heart J 1988; 59:680–684.
21. Lees MH: Cardiac output determination in the neonate. J Pediatr 1983; 102:709–711.
22. Bojanowski LMR, Timmis AD, Najm YC, Gosling RG: Pulsed doppler ultrasound compared with thermodilution for monitoring cardiac output responses to changing left ventricular function. Cardiovasc Res 1987; 21:260–268.
23. Mark JB, Steinbrook RA, Gugino LD et al: Continuous noninvasive monitoring of cardiac output with esophageal doppler ultrasound during cardiac surgery. Anesth Analg 1986; 65:1013–1020.
24. Siegel LC, Shafer SL, Martinez GM, et al: Simultaneous measurements of cardiac output by thermodilution, esophageal Doppler, and electrical impedance in anaesthetized patients. J Cardiothorac Anesth 1988; 2:590–595.
25. Freund PR: Transesophageal doppler scanning versus thermodilution during general anesthesia. Am J Surg 1987; 153:490–494.
26. Katz WE, Gasior TA, Quinlan JJ, Gorcsan J: Transgastric continuous-wave doppler to determine cardiac output. Am J Cardiol 1993; 71:853–857.
27. Schmid ER, Spahn DR, Tornic M: Reliability of a new generation transesophageal Doppler device for cardiac output monitoring. Anesth Analg 1993; 77:971–979.
28. Abrams JH, Weber RE, Holman KD: Transtracheal Doppler: A new procedure for continuous cardiac output measurement. Anesthesiology 1989; 70:134–138.
29. Pickett BR, Buell JC: Validity of cardiac output measurement by computer-averaged impedance cardiography, and comparison with simultaneous thermodilution determination. Am J Cardiol 1992; 69:1354–1358.
30. Pickett BR, Buell JC: Usefulness of the impedance cardiogram to reflect left ventricular diastolic function. Am J Cardiol 1993; 71:1099–1103.
31. Salandin V, Zussa C, Risica G, et al: Comparison of cardiac output estimation by thoracic electrical bioimpedance, thermodilution, and Fick methods. Crit Care Med 1988; 16:1157–1158.
32. Smith SA, Russell AE, West MJ, et al: Automated non-invasive measurement of cardiac output: Comparison of electrical bioimpedance and carbon dioxide rebreathing techniques. Br Heart J 1988; 59:292–298.
33. Naggar CZ, Dobnik DB, Flessas AP, et al: Accuracy of the stroke index as determined by the transthoracic electrical impedance method. Anesthesiology 1975; 42:201–205.
34. Russell AE, Smith SA, West MJ, et al: Automated noninvasive measurement of CO by the CO_2 rebreathing method: Comparisons with dye dilution and thermodilution. Br Heart J 1990; 63:1195–1199.
35. Young JD, McQuillan P: Comparison of thoracic electrical bioimpedance and thermodilution for the measurement of cardiac index in patients with severe sepsis. Br J Anaesth 1993; 70:58–62.
36. Miles DS, Gotshall RW, Golden JC, et al: Accuracy of electrical impedance cardiography for measuring cardiac output in children with congenital heart defects. Am J Cardiol 1988; 61:612–616.
37. Introna RPS, Pruett JK, Crumrine RC, Cuadrado AR: Use of transthoracic bioimpedance to determine cardiac output in pediatric patients. Crit Care Med 1988; 16:1101–1105.
38. Weber J, Heidelmeyer CF, Kubatz E, Bruckner JB: Measuring cardiac output under positive end-expiratory pressure with the noninvasive continuous cardiac output monitor "NCCOM 3" by bioimpedance as compared with thermodilution measurements. A study in anaesthetized dogs. Anaesthesist 1986; 35:744–747.
39. Balestra B, Malacrida R, Leonardi L, et al: Esophageal electrodes allow precise assessment of cardiac output by bioimpedance. Crit Care Med 1992; 20:62–67.
40. Van der Velde ET, van Duk AD, Steenduk P, et al: Left ventricular segmental volume by conductance catheter and Cine-CT. Eur Heart J 1992; 12(Suppl E):15–21.
41. Odake M, Takeuchi M, Takaoka H, et al: Determination of left ventricular volume using a conductance catheter in the diseased human heart. Eur Heart J 1992; 13(Suppl E):22–27.
42. Kass DA, Yamazaki T, Burkhoff D, et al: Determination of left ventricular end-systolic pressure-volume relationships by the con-

ductance (volume) catheter technique. Circulation 1986; 73:586–595.
43. Burkhoff D, Van der Velde E, Kass D, et al: Accuracy of volume measurement by conductance catheter in isolated, ejecting canine hearts. Circulation 1985; 72:440–447.
44. Steenduk P, van der Velde ET, Baan J: Single and dual excitation of the conductance-volume catheter analysed in a spheroidal mathematical model of the canine left ventricle. Eur Heart J 1992; 13:(Suppl E):28–34.
45. Kass DA, Midei M, Graves W, et al: Use of a conductance (volume) catheter and transient inferior venal caval occlusion for rapid determination of pressure-volume relationships in man. Cathet Cardiovasc Diagn 1988; 15:192–202.
46. Katz AM: Influence of altered inotropy and lusitropy on ventricular pressure-volume loops. J Am Coll Cardiol 1988; 11:438–445.
47. Takaoka H, Takeuchi M, Odake M, Yokoyama M: Assessment of myocardial oxygen consumption(Vo_2) and systolic pressure-volume (PVA) in human hearts. Eur Heart J 1992; 13(Suppl E):85–90.
48. Takaoka H, Takeuchi M, Odake M, et al: Comparison of hemodynamic determinants for myocardial oxygen consumption under different contractile states in human ventricle. Circulation 1993; 87:59–69.
49. Abrams JH, Irwin ED, Walvatne CS, et al: Use of a modified van der Pol's oscillator to construct ventricular pressure-volume relations. J Cardiothorac Vasc Anesth 1993; 7:195–199.
50. Brown KA, Ditchey RV: Human right ventricular end-systolic pressure-volume relation defined by maximal elastance. Circulation 1988; 78:81–91.
51. Forrester JS, Tyberg JV, Wyatt HL, et al: Pressure-length loop: A new method for simultaneous measurement of segmental and total cardiac function. J Appl Physiol 1974; 37:771–775.
52. Foex P, Francis CM, Cutfield GR, Leone B: The pressure-length loop. Br J Anaesth 1988; 60:65S–71S.
53. Taylor SH, Silke B: Is the measurement of cardiac output useful in clinical practice? Br J Anaesth 1988; 60:90S–98S.
54. Morton WD: The non-invasive determination of cardiac output in children. Anesthesiology 1988; 69:223–226.
55. Davies GG, Jebson PJR, Glasgow BM, Hess DR: Continuous Fick cardiac output compared to thermodilution cardiac output. Crit Care Med 1986; 14:881–885.
56. Truccone NJ, Spotnitz HM, Gersony WM, et al: Cardiac output in infants and children after open-heart surgery. J Thorac Cardiovasc Surg 1976; 71:410–414.
57. Kramer WG, Romagnoli A: Effect of surgery and cardiopulmonary bypass on indocyanine green pharmacokinetics. Tex Heart Inst J 1986; 13:77–82.
58. Bilfinger TV, Lin CY, Anagnostopoulos CE: In vitro determination of accuracy of cardiac output measurements by thermal dilution. J Surg Res 1982; 33:409–414.
59. Fegler G: Measurement of cardiac output in anesthetized animals by a thermodilution method. Q J Exp Physiol 1954; 39:153–164.
60. Ganz W, Donoso R, Marcus HS, et al: A new technique for measurement of cardiac output by thermodilution in man. Am J Cardiol 1971; 27:392–396.
61. Rah KH, Dunwiddie WC, Lower RR: A method of continuous postoperative measurement of mixed venous oxygen saturation in infants and children after open heart procedures. Anesth Analg 1984; 63:873–881.
62. Mathur M, Harris EA, Yarrow S, Barratt-Boyes BG: Measurement of cardiac output by thermodilution in infants and children after open-heart operations. J Thorac Cardiovasc Surg 1976; 72:221–225.
63. Fischer AP, Benis AM, Jurado RA, et al: Analysis of errors in measurement of cardiac output by simultaneous dye and thermal dilution in cardiothoracic surgical patients. Cardiovasc Res 1978; 12:190–199.
64. Hillis LD, Firth BG, Winniford MD: Comparison of thermodilution and indocyanine green dye in low cardiac output or left-sided regurgitation. Am J Cardiol 1986; 57:1201–1202.
65. McCormick JR, Dobnik DB, Mieszala JR, Berger RL: Simple method for measurement of cardiac output by thermodilution after cardiac operation. J Thorac Cardiovasc Surg 1979; 78:792–795.
66. Kohanna FH, Cunningham JN: Monitoring of cardiac output by thermodilution after open heart surgery. J Thorac Cardiovasc Surg 1977; 73:451–457.
67. Moodie DS, Feldt RH, Kaye MP, et al: Measurement of postoperative cardiac output by thermodilution in pediatric and adult patients. J Thorac Cardiovasc Surg 1979; 78:796–798.
68. Maruschak GF, Potter AM, Schauble JF, Rogers MC: Overestimating pediatric cardiac output by thermal indicator loss. Circulation 1982; 65:380–383.
69. Forrester JS, Ganz W, Diamond G, et al: Thermodilution cardiac output determination with a single flow-directed catheter. Am Heart J 1972; 83:306–311.
70. Stetz CW, Miller RG, Kelly GE, Raffin TA: Reliability of the thermodilution method in the determination of cardiac output in clinical practice. Am Rev Respir Dis 1982; 126:1001–1004.
71. Nishikawa T, Dohi S: Errors in the measurement of cardiac output by thermodilution. Can J Anaesth 1993; 40:142–153.
72. Levett JM, Replogle RL: Thermodilution cardiac output: A critical analysis and review of the literature. J Surg Res 1979; 27:392–404.
73. Bazaral MG, Petre J, Novoa R: Errors in thermodilution cardiac output measurements caused by rapid pulmonary artery temperature decreases after cardiopulmonary bypass. Anesthesiology 1992; 77:31–37.
74. Vennix CV, Nelson DH, Pierpoint GL: Thermodilution cardiac output in critically ill patients: Comparison of room-temperature and iced injectate. Heart Lung 1984; 13:574–578.
75. Shellock FG, Riedinger MS, Bateman TM, Gray RJ: Thermodilution cardiac output determination in hypothermic postcardiac surgery patients: Room vs ice temperature injectate. Crit Care Med 1983; 11:668–670.
76. Merrick SH, Hessel EA, Dillard DH: Determination of cardiac output by thermodilution during hypothermia. Am J Cardiol 1980; 46:419–422.
77. Stiles GM, Imazaki G, Stiles QR: Thermodilution cardiac output studies as a cause of prosthetic valve bacterial endocarditis. J Thorac Cardiovasc Surg 1984; 88:1035–1037.
78. Plachetka JR, Larson DF, Salomon NW, Copeland JG: Comparison of two closed systems for thermodilution cardiac outputs. Crit Care Med 1981; 9:487–489.
79. Meissner H, Glanert G, Stackmeier B, et al: Indicator loss during injection in the thermodilution system. Res Exp Med 1973; 159:183–196.
80. Buchbinder N, Ganz W: Hemodynamic monitoring: Invasive techniques. Anesthesiology 1976; 45:146–155.
81. Woods M, Scott RN, Harken AH: Practical considerations for the use of pulmonary artery thermistor catheter. Surgery 1976; 79:469–475.
82. Jansen JRC, Schreuder JJ, Bogaard JM, et al: Thermodilution technique for measurement of cardiac output during artificial ventilation. J Appl Physiol 1981; 584–591.
83. Stevens JH, Raffin TA, Mihm FG, et al: Thermodilution cardiac output measurement. JAMA 1985; 253:2240–2242.
84. Heerdt PM, Pond CG, Blessios GA, Rosenbloom M: Inaccuracy of cardiac output by thermodilution during acute tricuspid regurgitation. Ann Thorac Surg 1992; 53:706–708.
85. Boerboom LE, Kinney TE, Olinger GN, Hoffman RG: Validity of CO measurement by the thermodilution method in the presence of acute tricuspid regurgitation. J Thorac Cardiovasc Surg 1993; 106:636–642.
86. Konishi T, Nakamura Y, Morii I, et al: Comparison of thermodilution and Fick methods for measurements of cardiac output in tricuspid regurgitation. Am J Cardiol 1992; 70:538–539.
87. Pearl RG, Siegel LC: Thermodilution cardiac output measurement with a large left-to-right shunt. J Clin Monit 1991; 7:146–153.
88. Morady F, Brundage BH, Gelberg HJ: Rapid method for determination of shunt ratio using a thermodilution technique. Am Heart J 1983; 106:369–373.
89. Kahan F, Profeta J, Thys DM: High cardiac output measurements in a patient with congestive heart failure. J Cardiothorac Anesth 1987; 1:234–236.
90. Sade RM, Richi AA, Dearing JP: Calculation of systemic blood flow with pulmonary artery thermistor probe. J Thorac Cardiovasc Surg 1979; 78:576–578.
91. Lipkin DP, Poole-Wilson PA: Measurement of cardiac output during exercise by the thermodilution and direct Fick techniques in patients with chronic congestive heart failure. Am J Cardiol 1985; 56:321–324.
92. Kubo SH, Burchenal JEB, Cody RJ: Comparison of direct Fick and thermodilution cardiac output techniques at high flow rates. Am J Cardiol 1987; 59:384–386.

93. Reininger EJ, Troy BL: Error in thermodilution cardiac output measurement caused by variation in syringe volume. Cathet Cardiovasc Diag 1976; 2:415–417.
94. Nelson LD, Houtchens BA: Automatic versus manual injections for thermodilution cardiac output determination. Crit Care Med 1982; 10:190–192.
95. Dizon CT, Gezari WA, Barash PG, Crittenden JF: Hand held thermodilution cardiac output injector. Crit Care Med 1977; 5:210–212.
96. Wessel HU, Paul MH, James GW, Grahn AR: Limitations of thermal dilution curves for cardiac output determination. J Appl Physiol 1971; 30:643–652.
97. Bjoraker DG, Ketcham TR: Catheter thrombus artifactually decreases thermodilution cardiac output measurements. Anesth Analg 1983; 62:1031–1034.
98. Spackman TN: Thermodilution cardiac output due to an intracatheter septal defect. Anesth Analg 1984; 63:962–963.
99. Kiggins CM, Lake CL, Ross WT: The case of the shunting Swan. J Cardiothorac Anesth 1989; 3:229–234.
100. Paulsen AW, Valek TR: Actifactually low cardiac outputs resulting from a communication between the proximal and distal lumens of an Edwards pacing thermodilution Swan-Ganz catheter. Anesthesiology 1988; 68:308–309.
101. Wetzel RC, Latson TW: Major errors in thermodilution cardiac output measurement during rapid volume infusion. Anesthesiology 1985; 62:684–687.
102. Todd MM: Atrial fibrillation induced by the right atrial injection of cold fluids during thermodilution cardiac output determination. A case report. Anesthesiology 1983; 59:253–255.
103. Nishikawa T, Dohi S: Slowing of heart rate during cardiac output measurement by thermodilution. Anesthesiology 1982; 57:538–539.
104. Harris AP, Miller CF, Beattie C, et al: The slowing of sinus rhythm during thermodilution cardiac output determination and the effect of altering injectate temperature. Anesthesiology 1985; 63:540–541.
105. Nishikawa T, Namiki A: Mechanisms for slowing of heart rate and associated changes in pulmonary circulation elicited by cold injectate during thermodilution cardiac output determination in dogs. Anesthesiology 1988; 68:221–225.
106. Katz RI, Teller ED, Poppers PJ: Ventricular fibrillation during thermodilution cardiac output determination. Anesthesiology 1985; 62:376–377.
107. Yelderman M, Quinn MD, McKown RC: Thermal safety of a filamented pulmonary artery catheter. J Clin Monit 1992; 8:147–149.
108. Yelderman M, Quinn MD, McKown RC: Continuous thermodilution cardiac output measurement in sheep. J Thorac Cardiovasc Surg 1992; 104:315–320.
109. Yelderman M: Continuous cardiac output by thermodilution. *In* Royston D, Feeley TW (eds): Monitoring in Anesthesiology: Current Standards and Newer Techniques. Int Anesth Clin 1993; 31:127–140.
110. Yelderman ML, Ramsay MA, Quinn MD, et al: Continuous thermodilution cardiac output measurement in intensive care unit patients. J Cardiothorac Vasc Anesth 1992; 6:270–274.
111. Warner HR, Swan HJC, Connolly DC, et al: Quantitation of beat-to-beat changes in stroke volume from the aortic pulse contour in man. J Appl Physiol 1953; 5:495–507.
112. Bourgeois MJ, Gilbert BK, von Bernuth G, Wood EH: Continuous determination of beat-to-beat stroke volume from aortic pressure pulses in the dog. Circ Res 1976; 39:15–24.
113. Prys-Roberts C: Monitoring of the cardiovascular system. *In* Saidman LJ, Smith NT (eds): Monitoring in Anesthesia. New York: John Wiley and Sons, 1978; 62.
114. Cundick RM, Gardner RM: Clinical comparison of pressure-pulse and indicator-dilution cardiac output determination. Circulation 1980; 62:371–376.
115. Gratz I, Kraidin J, Afshar M: Continuous cardiac output by pulse waveform. *In* Royston D, Feeley TW (eds): Monitoring in Anesthesiology: Current Standards and Newer Techniques. Int Anesth Clin 1993; 31:87–98.
116. Wesseling KH, de Wit B, Weber AP, Smith NT: A simple device for the continuous measurement of cardiac output. Adv Cardiovasc Phys 1983; 5:16–52.
117. Gratz I, Kraidin J, Jacobi AG, et al: Continuous noninvasive cardiac output as estimated from the pulse contour curve. J Clin Monit 1992; 8:20–27.
118. English JB, Hodges MR, Sentker C, et al: Comparison of aortic pulse-wave contour analysis and thermodilution methods of measuring cardiac output during anesthesia in the dog. Anesthesiology 1980; 52:56–61.
119. Rutherford BD, Gardner RM, Warner HR: Comparison of dye dilution curve and arterial pulse contour analyses for determination of stroke volume in critically ill patients [Abstract]. Chest 1972; 62:376.
120. Weber KT, Janicki JS, Shroff SG, et al: The right ventricle: Physiologic and pathophysiologic considerations. Crit Care Med 1983; 11:323–328.
121. Maddahi J, Berman DS, Matsuoka DT, et al: Technique for assessing right ventricular ejection fraction using rapid multiple-gated equilibrium cardiac blood pool scintigraphy: Description, validation and finding in coronary artery disease. Circulation 1979; 60:581–589.
122. Dehmer GJ, Firth BG, Hills LO, et al: Nongeometric determination of RV volume from equilibrium blood pool scans. Am J Cardiol 1982; 49:78–84.
123. Kaul S, Tei C, Hopkins JM, Shah PM: Assessment of right ventricular function using two-dimensional echocardiography. Am Heart J 1984; 107:526–531.
124. Bing R, Heimbecker R, Falholt W: An estimation of the residual volume of blood in the right ventricle of normal and diseased human hearts in vivo. Am Heart J 1951; 42:483–502.
125. Hines R, Rafferty T, Schauble JF: Right ventricular ejection fraction catheter: Toy or tool? J Cardiothorac Vasc Anesth 1993; 7:236–242.
126. Kay H, Afshari M, Barash PG, et al: Measurement of ejection fraction by thermal dilution techniques. J Surg Res 1983; 34:337–346.
127. Spinale FG, Zellner JL, Mukherjee R, Crawford FA: Placement considerations for measuring thermodilution right ventricular ejection fractions. Crit Care Med 1991; 19:417–421.
128. Assman R, Heidelmeyer CF, Trampisch H-J, et al: Right ventricular function assessed by thermodilution techniques during apnea and mechanical ventilation. Crit Care Med 1991; 19:810–817.
129. Urban P, Scheidegger D, Gabathuler J, Rutishauser W: Thermodilution determination of right ventricular volume and ejection fraction: A comparison with biplane angiography. Crit Care Med 1987; 15:652–655.
130. Dhainaut J-F, Brunet F, Monsallier JF, et al: Bedside evaluation of right ventricular performance using a rapid computerized thermodilution method. Crit Care Med 1987; 15:148–152.
131. Jardin F, Gueret P, Dubourg O, et al: Right ventricular volumes by thermodilution in ARDS. Chest 1985; 88:34–39.
132. Diebel LN, Wilson RF, Tagett MZG, Kline RA: End-diastolic volume. Arch Surg 1992; 127:817–822.
133. Hines R, Barash PG: Right ventricular function in the perioperative period. Mt Sinai J Med 1985; 52:529–533.
134. Hines R: Monitoring right ventricular function. *In* Barash PG (ed): Cardiac Monitoring. Philadelphia: WB Saunders, 1988; 851–863.
135. Savino JA, Vo N, Agarwal N, et al: Systemic organ assessment using computerized profiles. Med Instrum 1983; 17:433–436.
136. Mohr R, Meir O, Smolinsky A, Goor DA: A method for continuous on-line monitoring of systemic vascular resistance (COMS) after open heart procedures. J Cardiovasc Surg 1987; 28:558–565.
137. Hilgenberg JC: Pulmonary vascular impedance: Resistance versus pulmonary artery diastolic-pulmonary artery occluded pressure gradient. Anesthesiology 1983; 58:484–485.

SECTION

THREE

Monitoring Respiratory Function

CHAPTER

11

Monitoring of Oxygen

KEVIN K. TREMPER, Ph.D., M.D., and
STEVEN J. BARKER, Ph.D., M.D.

While reading this sentence you are consuming approximately 100 million trillion molecules of oxygen per second. This phenomenal oxygen transport to the tissues is required to maintain aerobic metabolism in the average 70-kg adult at rest. As single-celled animals evolved to multicelled organisms and eventually to large mammals, an immense problem of oxygen distribution had to be solved.

There are two limitations on oxygen delivery in cellular life in an aqueous environment. First, molecular diffusion of gases in liquids is an extremely slow process. Second, the solubility of oxygen in water is very low. The diffusion constant (diffusivity) of oxygen in water is approximately 10^{-5} cm^2/second. For single-celled creatures, oxygen can diffuse rapidly from the cell wall to the mitochondria because the diffusion distance is so short. As the number of cells grows and the diffusion distance increases, the rate of oxygen transport limits aerobic metabolism. It would take nearly a day for an oxygen molecule to diffuse 1 cm in water by pure molecular diffusion. Consequently, as multicellular organisms evolved, they developed a more efficient transport system to distribute oxygen by bulk flow to each cell. Because the solubility of oxygen in water is low, the transport system also needed a mechanism to increase the oxygen-carrying capacity of an aqueous medium. The result in vertebrate life is the cardiovascular system and blood, using hemoglobin as a carrier to increase the oxygen capacity of the transport medium.

Over the past several decades, medicine has developed a number of oxygen transport variables to quantitate the effectiveness of the oxygen delivery system. Since the 1970s, both invasive and noninvasive continuous monitoring systems have been developed to assess the adequacy of oxygen transport. These devices monitor oxygenation by different means and at different points in the oxygen transport system. In this chapter, the commonly measured and calculated oxygen transport variables are described, and available oxygen monitoring techniques are reviewed in depth. For each technique, the physics and engineering behind the measurement as well as the physiologic interpretation of the measured variable are discussed. Each technique has its limitations in the detection of hypoxia.

ANALYSIS OF INSPIRED OXYGEN

Inspired oxygen in an anesthetic circuit can be measured by a mass spectrometer, a Raman spectrometer, or an analyzer that measures oxygen only. Mass and Raman spectrometers are discussed in Chapter 24. Several types of oxygen-only analyzers have been used in clinical practice, including polarographic, paramagnetic, and galvanic (fuel cell) devices. All present-generation machines have integrated inspired oxygen analyzers that are activated whenever the machine is turned on. Older machines have separate oxygen analyzers that often use battery powered supplies.

Monitoring the oxygen concentration in the anesthetic or ventilator circuit is mandatory (see Chapter 23). Although this does not ensure an adequate arterial oxygen tension ($Pa{O_2}$), it confirms that hypoxic oxygen concentrations are not delivered to the patient's airway.

POLAROGRAPHIC ANALYZERS

Polarographic analyzers are based on the principle of the Clark electrode (described in Chapters 27 and 28). The breakdown (reduction) of oxygen occurs at a charged metal cathode (a "rest" voltage of 0.5–0.8 V is applied) in the polarographic electrode, and the current produced by the reaction alters the conductivity of an electrolyte solution of potassium chloride. Essential components are a silver anode, a platinum or gold cathode, and a gas-permeable, polymeric membrane. The specific rest voltage causes only oxygen to react. When a gas sample contains oxygen, the current flow is proportional to the partial pressure of oxygen ($P{O_2}$) in the electrolyte solution. Response times for these analyzers are about 10–60 seconds.

If accuracy at concentrations of oxygen of less than 50% is desired, these analyzers are calibrated using room air.

Accuracy in the 90–100% range requires calibration on 100% oxygen. Several minutes are required for calibration. Because the analyzer depends on a battery (to operate the meter and to induce a voltage on the electrode) and the electrode has a limited lifespan, regular preventive maintenance (replacement of electrode membrane and electrolyte gel) is essential to ensure a functional analyzer.

PARAMAGNETIC ANALYZERS

Oxygen is a paramagnetic gas, whereas all other gases are diamagnetic. Paramagnetic gases are attracted to the strongest portion of a magnetic field. If the two glass spheres (containing nitrogen or other diamagnetic gas) in a "dumbbell" configuration are suspended on a quartz fiber in a chamber between two magnetic poles, introduction of oxygen into the chamber results in displacement of the spheres from between the magnetic poles. A mirror attached to the quartz fiber reflects a beam of light onto a translucent scale to measure the oxygen concentration. The number of oxygen molecules or PO_2 determines the degree of mirror displacement.

Paramagnetic analyzers have inherently long response times because of the washout time of the sample cell. Of the anesthetic agents, only nitrous oxide has a weak diamagnetic effect. Although these analyzers are highly accurate, their fragile suspension system, sensitivity to water vapor, and long response time have caused them to be replaced by sensors based on a magnetoacoustic device without moving parts.[1]

GALVANIC CELL ANALYZERS

These analyzers produce a current flow by the reduction of molecular oxygen, which releases electrons. An electrolyte solution in the galvanic cell is contained by a thin plastic membrane over the cathode through which oxygen diffuses to the anode. The percentage of oxygen is displayed on a scale when a microammeter senses the current produced, which is proportional to the PO_2. Because of their limited lifespan, galvanic analyzers have also been largely replaced by magnetoacoustic devices on anesthesia machines.

CLINICAL USE

Ideally, an inspired oxygen analyzer should be accurate to $\pm 2\%$ and capable of response within 2–10 seconds. It should be unaffected by the relative humidity within the 30–90% range. Studies have demonstrated that water vapor significantly affects (i.e., produces falsely low readings in) the Beckman OM-1 analyzer.[2] Analyzers should be compensated for both temperature and pressure. Exposure to anesthetic gases should not affect their accuracy. Westenskow and coworkers noted that Critikon model 800–021 and Teledyne microfuel cell class C-1 (Harris-Lake) sensors had higher rates of drift in halothane-air mixtures than in air alone.[2] Such effects may result from diffusion of halothane into the oxygen-permeable membrane. Calibration is best performed using dry 100% oxygen. After calibration, accuracy should be maintained for at least 8 hours.

High- and low-concentration alarms are essential features of most oxygen analyzers. Both visual and auditory alarms must be present and functional during use of an anesthesia machine or ventilator. Although oxygen analyzers can detect disconnections in fresh gas lines, they are unable to detect disconnection of the patient's endotracheal tube from the anesthetic breathing circuit unless the sensor is placed in the expiratory limb of the circle system.[3]

QUANTITATIVE OXYGEN TRANSPORT VARIABLES

OXYGEN CONTENT

Oxygen content is defined as the volume of oxygen (milliliters) carried in 100 ml of blood. It is a basic variable that is found in all oxygen transport calculations. Although oxygen content can be measured directly by the volumetric method of Van Slyke and Neill,[4] it is usually calculated from this equation:

$$CaO_2 = Hb \times 1.37 \times HbO_2 + 0.0034 \times PaO_2 \qquad 11\text{–}1$$

where: CaO_2 = arterial oxygen content (a denotes an arterial sample) in ml/100 ml (also called vol%)
Hb = hemoglobin concentration in gm/dl
1.37 = volume of oxygen (ml) carried by 1 gm of fully saturated hemoglobin
HbO_2 = fractional hemoglobin saturation (discussed later)
0.0034 = solubility coefficient of oxygen in plasma (ml of oxygen per 100 ml plasma per mmHg)
PaO_2 = arterial oxygen tension in mmHg

With a normal hemoglobin of 15 gm/dl and normal PaO_2 and HbO_2 values of 95 mmHg and 95%, respectively, the CaO_2 is 20 ml/100ml. Coincidentally, this is very similar to the oxygen content of room air at sea level. Thus, the cardiovascular system produces the same oxygen content near each cell that would exist if the cells were surrounded by room air. Methods of measuring both HbO_2 and PO_2 are discussed below.

In Equation 11–1, the oxygen content is very sensitive to the hemoglobin concentration and HbO_2, whereas it is relatively insensitive to the PO_2 because of the small solubility coefficient for oxygen in plasma. However, the oxygen saturation itself depends nonlinearly on PO_2. Because oxygen content is proportional to hemoglobin concentration, if the arterial hemoglobin is fully saturated, the content can be roughly estimated as equalling slightly less than half the hematocrit. The hematocrit equals approximately three times the hemoglobin concentration.

OXYGEN DELIVERY

The overall flow rate of oxygen to the tissues is called the oxygen delivery (O_2 del), determined as the CaO_2 times the cardiac output. At a cardiac output of 5 L/minute for a 70-kg adult, normal oxygen delivery is 1000 ml of oxygen/minute (20 ml of oxygen/100 ml or 200 ml of oxygen/L × 5 L/minute = 1000 ml of oxygen/minute). Because normal cardiac output depends on the size of the patient, cardiac output is indexed to body surface area: cardiac index (CI) = cardiac output/body surface area (m^2). The range for CI is 2.5–3.4 L/minute/m^2. The O_2 del index (Equation 11–2) is defined as the arterial oxygen content times the CI:

$$\begin{aligned} O_2 \text{ del index} &= Ca{O_2} \times CI \text{ (ml oxygen/minute/m}^2\text{)} \\ \text{Normal } O_2 \text{ del index} &= 20 \text{ ml/dl} \times 10 \text{ dl/L} \times 3 \text{ L/minute/m}^2 \\ &= 600 \text{ ml/minute/m}^2 \end{aligned} \qquad 11\text{–}2$$

O_2 del index is an overall assessment of oxygen transport to the tissues but does not ensure adequate oxygen supply to any specific organ. The oxygen delivery to each organ can be defined as the CaO_2 times the blood flow to the specific organ.

OXYGEN CONSUMPTION

Human tissues consume an average of 5 ml of oxygen from every 100 ml of blood flow. Because the normal CaO_2 is 20 ml/100 ml of blood, 75% of the oxygen remains in the venous blood. The oxygen consumption ($\dot{V}O_2$) of the body (Equation 11–3) can be calculated by subtracting the mixed venous blood oxygen content ($C\bar{v}O_2$) from the CaO_2 and multiplying this difference by the cardiac output:

$$\dot{V}O_2 = (CaO_2 - C\bar{v}O_2) \times \text{cardiac output} \qquad 11\text{–}3$$

As with oxygen delivery, oxygen consumption is indexed so that the normal value is independent of patient size:

$$\begin{aligned} \dot{V}O_2 \text{ index} &= \dot{V}O_2\ (CaO_2 - C\bar{v}O_2) \times CI \\ \dot{V}O_2 \text{ index} &= (20 \text{ ml/dl} - 15 \text{ ml/dl}) \\ &\quad \times 3 \text{ L/minute/m}^2 \times 10 \text{ dl/L} \\ \dot{V}O_2 \text{ index} &= 150 \text{ ml/minute/m}^2 \end{aligned}$$

The normal range of oxygen consumption index is 115–165 ml/minute/m^2. These values are for healthy resting humans and increase up to 10 times with exercise, shivering, hyperthermia, or sepsis. $\dot{V}O_2$ index decreases during anesthesia and hypothermia.

Mixed Venous Oxygen

Mixed venous blood is sampled from the pulmonary artery to ensure proper mixing. A mixed venous sample does not reflect the oxygen returned to the heart from any specific organ. The normal $C\bar{v}O_2$ is 15 ml/dl, which corresponds to a mixed venous saturation of 75% and an oxygen tension of 40 mmHg. Mixed venous blood oxygen tension ($P\bar{v}O_2$) should reflect tissue PO_2. Although tissue PO_2 values vary greatly, the mean PO_2 of interstitial fluid is the same as the $P\bar{v}O_2$, i.e., 40 mmHg.[5]

Oxygen Extraction

The oxygen extraction ratio (O_2 ext) is a supply-demand balance for oxygenation:

$$O_2 \text{ ext} = \frac{CaO_2 - C\bar{v}O_2}{CaO_2} \times 100\% \qquad 11\text{–}4$$

The O_2 ext is actually the ratio of oxygen consumption to oxygen delivery:

$$O_2 \text{ ext} = \frac{(CaO_2 - C\bar{v}O_2) \times CI}{CaO_2 \times CI} \times 100\%$$

Because CI appears in both the numerator and the denominator of the above equation, it need not be measured to calculate O_2 ext. For this reason, O_2 ext was an especially useful variable prior to the availability of thermodilution pulmonary artery catheters. The normal O_2 ext is only 25%, so there appears to be a wide margin of safety for oxygen transport. In fact, the body can easily extract up to 50% of the delivered oxygen without obligatory tissue hypoxia. When the O_2 ext exceeds 50%, there is an increasing incidence of tissue hypoxia because of the low PO_2 (the 50% hemoglobin saturation, or P_{50}, of adult hemoglobin is normally 26.7 mmHg).

HYPOXIA: DEFINITIONS

Hypoxia is defined as inadequate tissue oxygenation due to either inadequate blood flow or low CaO_2. Hypoxia due to inadequate blood flow is ischemic hypoxia. Hypoxia due to low oxygen content is hypoxemic hypoxia. CaO_2 can be reduced as a result of decreased hemoglobin (anemic hypoxemia), PaO_2 (hypoxemic hypoxemia), or HbO_2 (toxic hypoxemia). Toxic hypoxemia (decreased fractional hemoglobin saturation) results from increased methemoglobin or carboxyhemoglobin and is discussed later.

MEASUREMENT OF OXYGEN TENSION

CLARK PO_2 ELECTRODE

Oxygen partial pressure (or "tension") in a liquid is defined as the PO_2 in the equilibrium gas phase. When several phases are in contact at equilibrium (e.g., lipid, water, and gas), the PO_2 will be equal in all phases, but the oxygen concentration in each phase will be proportional to its solubility in that phase. In 1956, Leland Clark developed the polarographic oxygen electrode for measuring PO_2.[6] Before this invention, blood PO_2 was not measured. With the addition of the Severinghaus carbon dioxide electrode in 1958, the blood gas machine was developed, and critical patient care was revolutionized.[7]

The Clark electrode is an electrical cell composed of a platinum cathode and a silver anode (Fig. 11–1). In this electrochemical cell there is a plateau voltage range over which the current does not increase with voltage but does increase with oxygen tension in the cell. An oxygen-consuming electrochemical reaction takes place at the cathode, and the electric current in the circuit is directly proportional

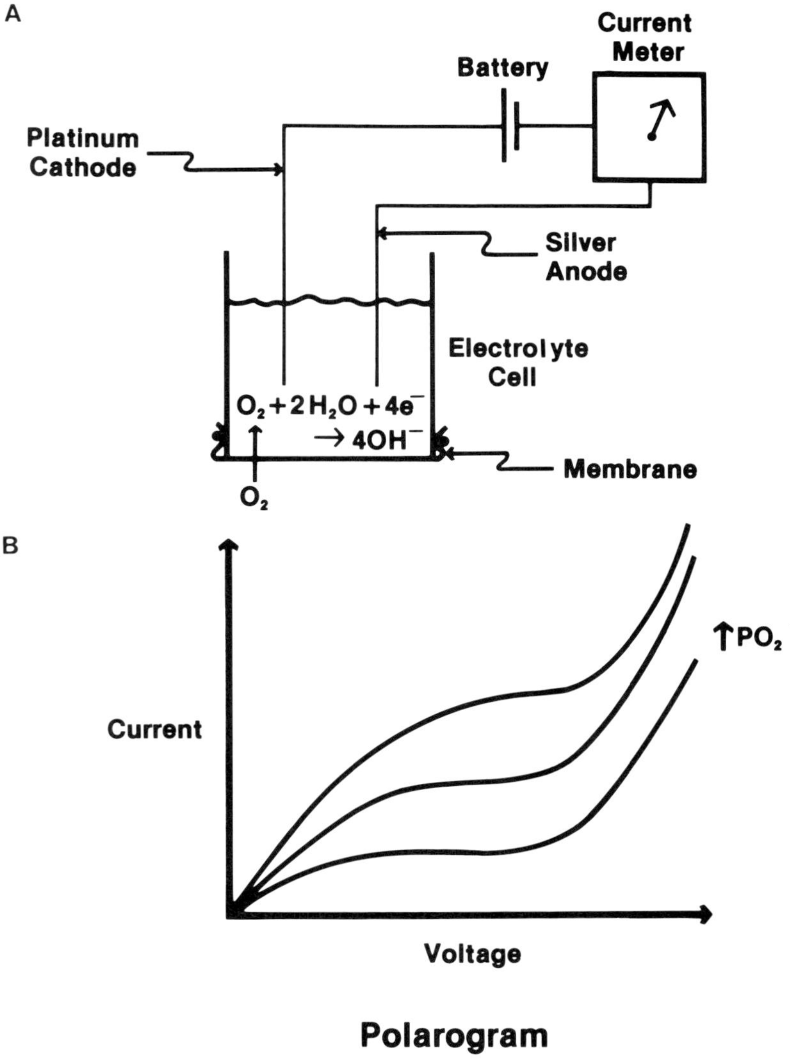

Figure 11–1. *A*, Schematic of a Clark polarographic oxygen electrode. The circuit consists of a voltage source (battery) and a current meter connecting platinum and silver electrodes. The electrodes are immersed in an electrolyte cell. A membrane permeable to oxygen, but not to the electrolyte, covers one surface of the cell. Oxygen diffuses through the membrane and reacts at the platinum cathode with water to produce hydroxyl ions. The ammeter measures the current produced by the electrons consumed in this reaction at the cathode. *B*, A plot of current produced as a function of the voltage between the two electrodes (polarizing voltage). This plot is called a polarogram. In the range near 660 mV there is a plateau in the polarogram. The plateau occurs at higher currents as the Po_2 in the cell is increased. Most polarographic oxygen electrodes use 600 to 800 mV polarizing voltage to obtain a stable current at each Po_2.

to the oxygen consumed at the cathode. This cell is covered h a membrane that is freely permeable to oxygen. Clark's polarographic oxygen electrode has been used for over 30 years to measure Po_2 in gases and liquids in both medicine and industry.

Po_2 OPTODE

The phenomenon of photoluminescence quenching has been used to develop a new sensor for measuring Po_2, called the "optode."[8,9] When light shines on a luminescent material, specific light frequencies are absorbed, exciting electrons to a higher energy state (Fig. 11–2). These electrons then fall spontaneously into a lower energy state by emitting a photon of a frequency different from that of the original light. In some luminescent dyes, this light emission is "quenched" by the presence of oxygen. When the excited electron falls into a lower energy state, its energy can be either emitted as a photon (luminescence) or absorbed by an oxygen molecule, thereby increasing the energy of the latter (see Fig. 11–2). For these photoluminescence quenching dyes, the amount of oxygen present can be related to the luminescent intensity. The empirical relationship governing this phenomenon is known at the Stern-Volmer equation.[8]

$$I\,(Po_2) = \frac{I_0}{(1 + K \times Po_2)} \qquad 11\text{–}5$$

where: I = intensity of the luminescent signal at the Po_2 being measured
I_0 = intensity of the luminescent signal in the absence of oxygen
Po_2 = oxygen partial pressure
K = quenching constant

The advantages of the optode as a Po_2 measuring device are its simplicity and size. The sensor consists of a small fiberoptic strand with a dye encapsulated at the tip, and it can be easily miniaturized. Figure 11–3 shows an optode that easily fits through a 22-gauge intravenous cannula.[9] Another advantage of optode technology is that pH-sensitive dyes are also available; therefore, a three-fiber optode

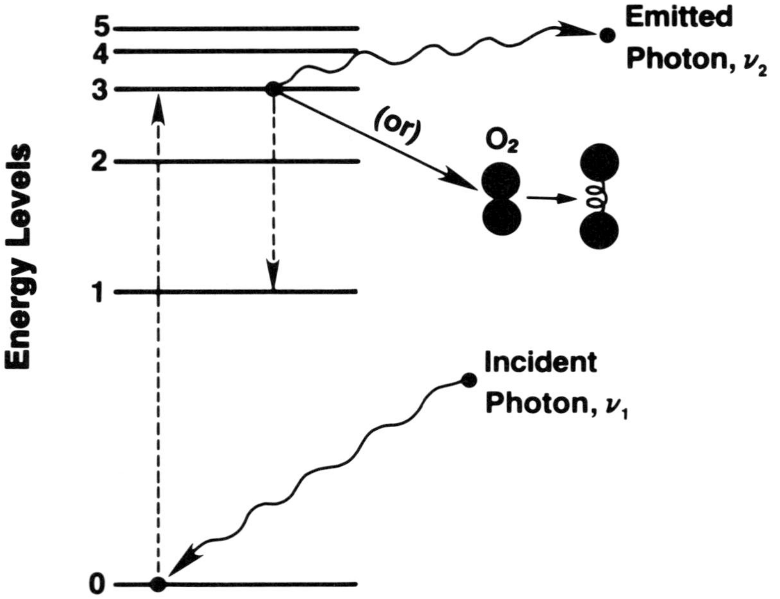

Figure 11–2. The photoluminescence-quenching phenomenon. An electron of the fluorescent dye is excited to a higher energy level by an incident photon (γ_1). This excited electron can return to a lower energy level either by emitting a photon (γ_2) or by interacting with and raising an oxygen molecule to a higher vibrational energy level. (From Barker SJ, Tremper KK, Hyatt J, et al: Continuous fiberoptic arterial oxygen tension measurements in dogs. J Clin Monit 1987; 3:48–52.)

sensor can measure Po_2, partial pressure of carbon dioxide (Pco_2), and pH simultaneously.[10]

CONTINUOUS OXYGEN TENSION MONITORING

INVASIVE Po_2 MONITORING

Clark Electrode

The primary problem in continuous invasive Pao_2 monitoring is miniaturization of the Clark electrode to fit through an arterial cannula. There are two approaches to this problem. One is to insert only the platinum cathode in the arterial cannula and place the reference anode on the skin surface. The platinum cathode is surrounded by a thin layer of electrolyte and covered with an oxygen-permeable membrane.[11, 12] The second approach involves miniaturization of the entire anode-cathode electrode for intra-arterial insertion.[13, 14]

Studies of intra-arterial Po_2 monitoring using Clark electrodes have yielded conflicting results. It is often difficult to compare such studies because the data are usually analyzed by linear regression and correlation coefficients. The correlation coefficient is extremely sensitive to the x and y range over which the data are collected. Furthermore, a high correlation coefficient (r close to 1.0) implies a high degree of association between the methods (i.e., when one goes up, the other will go up), but it does not imply that one method can replace the other.

As an alternative, Altman and Bland recommend using the mean and standard deviation of the difference between the two methods of measurement as an assessment of agreement.[15–18] The mean difference is called the ''bias,'' and the standard deviation is the ''precision.'' The bias indicates a consistent overestimate or underestimate of one method relative to the other, and the precision represents the scatter or random error.[15–18] Note that a larger precision implies a less precise measurement. For example, Figure 11–4 is a ''scattergram'' plot of data from an intra-arterial Clark electrode used in neonatal patients.[14] The abscissa of this plot is Pao_2 determined on arterial samples by a blood gas analyzer, and the ordinate is the intra-arterial electrode Pao_2. Although these data yield a correlation coefficient of 0.88, y varies greatly on x over the entire range of Pao_2. For example, at a Pao_2 of 40 mmHg, the intra-arterial probe Po_2 values vary from the mid 20s to 70 mmHg, with one data point as high as 100 mmHg.

Umbilical artery Clark electrodes in neonates have been associated with a number of complications, including thrombus formation, embolism, vascular perforation, infarction, lower extremity ischemia, and infection. Probe size has also caused problems in the use of Clark electrodes for both umbilical and radial arterial monitoring. Damping of the arterial pressure waveform and inaccurate blood pressure measurements are commonly reported.[13, 18] Other reported problems include calibration drift and systematic underestimation of Pao_2. The causes of these errors are not understood, but they may involve decreased blood flow around the electrode tip or clot formation on the electrode surface. The most recently developed electrodes have reportedly reduced these problems, but there are no confirmatory studies.[19]

Optode Po_2 Sensors

The above discussion of optode principles suggests that these sensors lend themselves to miniaturization more readily than the Clark electrode. In fact, three component optodes (pH, Pco_2, Po_2) have been incorporated into a probe with a diameter of 0.5–0.6 mm. Such a sensor will pass easily through a 20-gauge cannula without preventing the

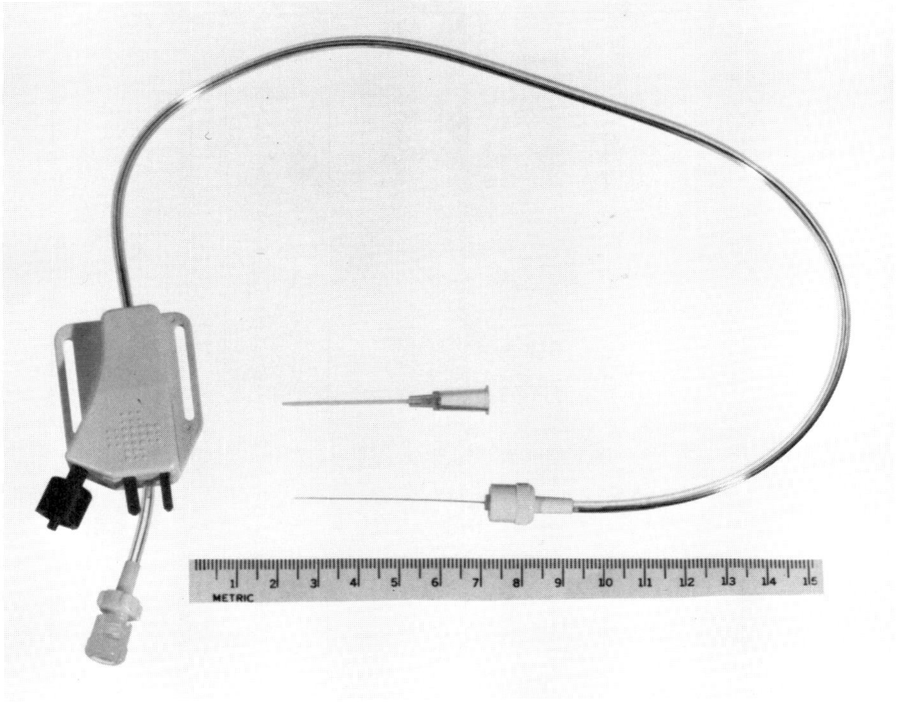

Figure 11–3. An optode probe and the 20-gauge cannula through which it is inserted. (From Barker SJ, Tremper KK, Hyatt J, et al: Continuous fiberoptic arterial oxygen tension measurements in dogs. J Clin Monit 1987; 3:48–52.)

aspiration of blood samples or monitoring of pressure waveforms. There have been several clinical and volunteer studies of three-component optodes inserted through intra-arterial cannulas in both the operating room and the intensive care unit.[20, 21] Figure 11–5 shows a scattergram plot of intra-arterial optode Po_2 versus Pao_2 in 15 patients undergoing surgery.[20] The accuracy shown here is within a clinically acceptable range, particularly at low Po_2 values

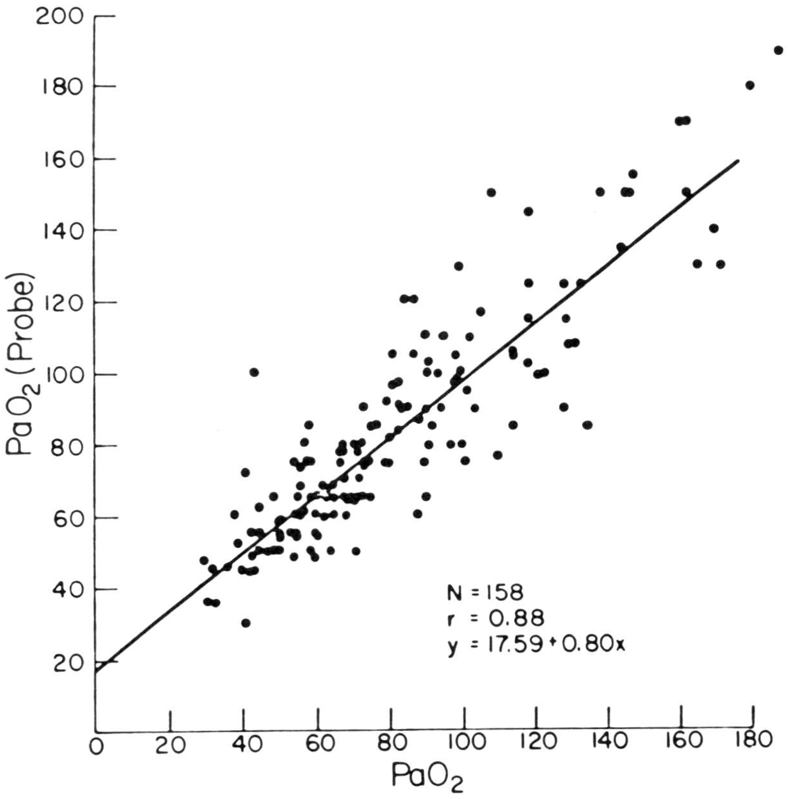

Figure 11–4. Relation between arterial oxygen tension (Pao_2) and intravascular oxygen tension (probe) measurements. (From Malalis L, Bhat R, Vidyasagar D: Comparison of intravascular Po_2 with transcutaneous and Pao_2 values. Crit Care Med 1983; 11(2):110–113, © Williams & Wilkins.)

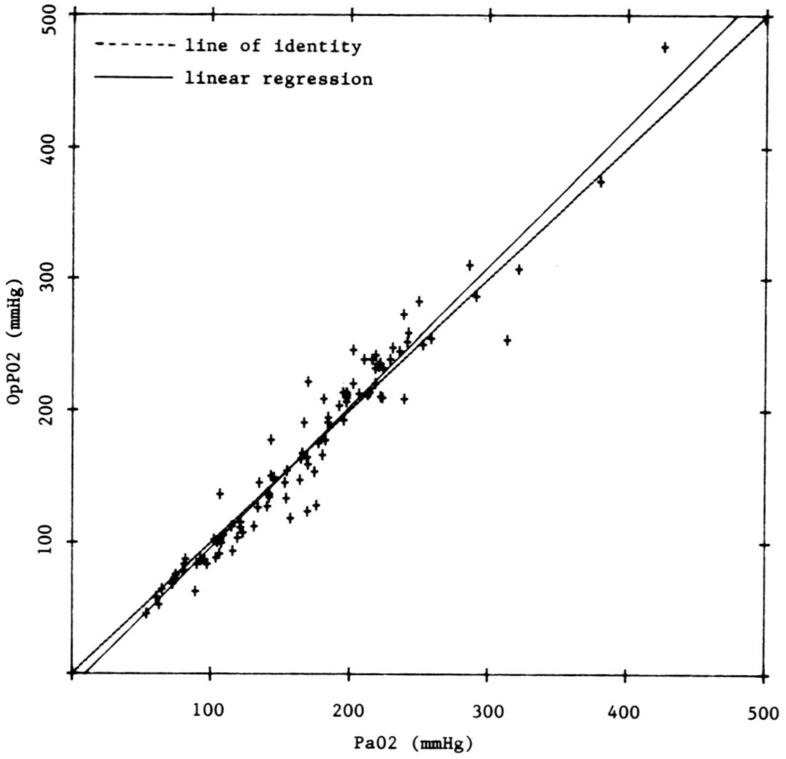

Figure 11–5. Arterial oxygen tension determined by optode ($OpPo_2$) versus arterial oxygen tension determined by blood-gas analysis (Pao_2). There are 96 data points. (From Barker SJ, Tremper KK: Intra-arterial PO_2 monitoring. *In* Tremper KK, Barker SJ [eds]: Advances in Oxygen Monitoring. Int Anesthesiol Clin 1987; 25:206.)

(Table 11–1). Case reports have also documented the usefulness of the optode in the early diagnosis of hypoxia and acid-base disorders.[22, 23] Although there have been apparent problems in biocompatibility (e.g., fibrin deposition on the sensor), optodes are now being used in many clinical trials and may soon be available to the medical community.

NONINVASIVE Po_2 MONITORING

Transcutaneous Po_2

In 1972, two researchers reported that Po_2 values similar to arterial Po_2 could be obtained by heating a Clark electrode and placing it on the skin surface of a newborn infant.[24, 25] Over the next decade, this technique—transcutaneous oxygen monitoring—became routine in the care of premature infants at risk of both hypoxia and hyperoxia.[26, 27] In the late 1970s, transcutaneous Po_2 values ($Ptco_2$) were found to be significantly lower than Pao_2 values during episodes of hemodynamic instability.[28, 29] Although this discovery lessened the usefulness of $Ptco_2$ as an arterial oxygen tension monitor, it did give the user a valuable indicator of peripheral perfusion.

$Ptco_2$ is the oxygen tension of heated skin. To obtain a measurable Po_2 at the skin surface with a fast response time, the skin must be heated to at least 43°C. The stratum corneum, composed of lipid in a protein matrix, is normally a very efficient barrier to gas transport. When heated above 41°C, the structural characteristics of this layer change, allowing oxygen to diffuse through it readily.[30, 31] In the epidermis, heating causes vasodilatation of the dermal capillaries, which is said to ''arterialize'' this capillary blood.

The perfusion of this hyperemic epidermal capillary bed depends on adequate blood flow to the dermal vasculature. Consequently, if the cardiac output decreases, skin blood flow and oxygen delivery to the transcutaneous sensor decrease. Figure 11–6 illustrates the relation between Pao_2 and $Ptco_2$ during induced hypoxemia (hypoxemic hypoxia) followed by hemorrhagic shock (ischemic hypoxia) in an animal study.[32] During the shock state, $Ptco_2$ decreased with decreasing cardiac output even though Pao_2 was relatively unchanged.

This effect of cardiac output on the $Ptco_2$-Pao_2 relationship can be quantitated in terms of a transcutaneous oxygen index:

TABLE 11–1. STATISTICAL COMPARISON OF ARTERIAL OXYGEN TENSIONS OBTAINED BY OPTODE AND BY BLOOD-GAS ANALYSIS IN 12 SURGICAL PATIENTS

Variable	0–700 mmHg	0–150 mmHg
n	96	38
r	0.970	0.923
Linear regression		
Slope	1.07	1.05
Intercept	−10.6	−8.5
Bias	−1.10	3.74
Precision	19.0	11.7

From Barker SJ, Tremper KK: Intra-arterial Po_2 monitoring. *In* Barker SJ, Tremper KK (eds): Advances in Oxygen Monitoring. Int Anesthesiol Clin 1987; 25:199–208, with permission.

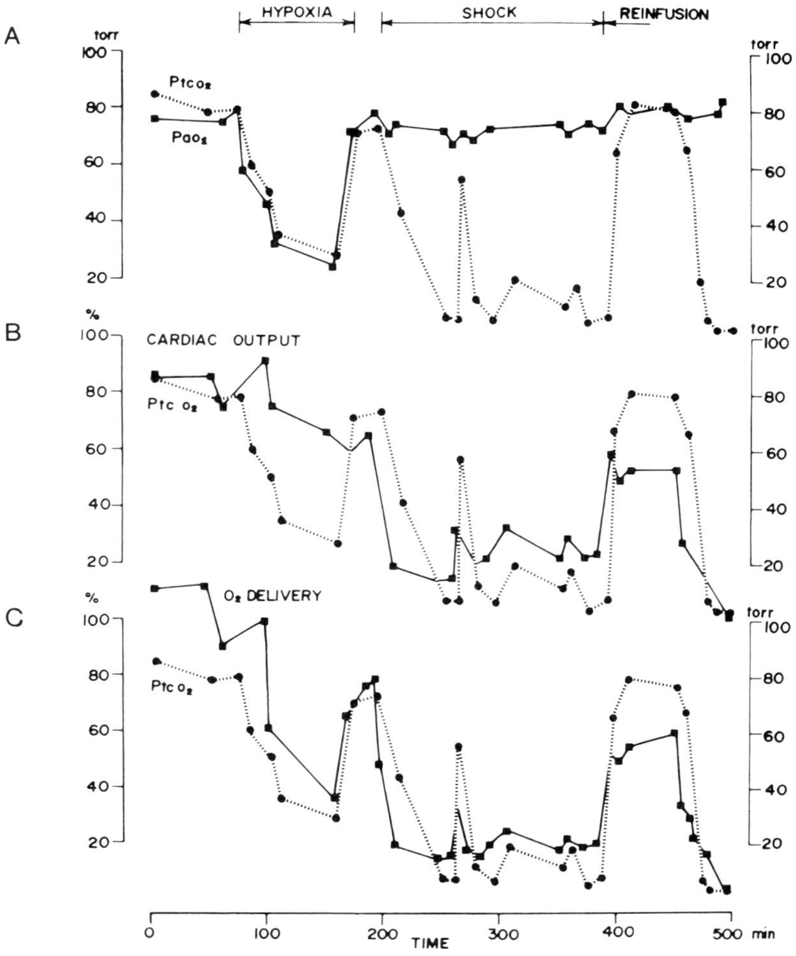

Figure 11–6. Hypoxia and hypovolemic shock study in dogs. *A*, Serial transcutaneous oxygen tension ($Ptco_2$) and arterial oxygen tension (Pao_2). *B*, $Ptco_2$ and cardiac output. *C*, $Ptco_2$ and oxygen delivery throughout a representative experiment. Note: $Ptco_2$ values follow the Pao_2 values during hypoxia, but not during shock; $Ptco_2$ values follow cardiac output during shock, but not during hypoxia; however, $Ptco_2$ values most closely follow oxygen delivery throughout the entire experiment. (From Tremper KK, Waxman K, Shoemaker WC: Effects of hypoxia and shock on transcutaneous Po_2 values in dogs. Crit Care Med 1979; 7:529–531, © Williams & Wilkins.)

$$Ptco_2 \text{ index} = \frac{Ptco_2}{Pao_2} \qquad 11\text{–}6$$

$Ptco_2$ index has been used as an indicator of peripheral perfusion analogous to the alveolar-arterial Po_2 gradient for the assessment of pulmonary function.[33] Table 11–2 shows the $Ptco_2$ index as a function of CI found in adult patients in critical care units. Under stable hemodynamic conditions, the normal $Ptco_2$ index for adult patients was 0.79, whereas this index fell to 0.49 when the cardiac index decreased below 2.2 L/minute/m^2.[33] A review of the published $Ptco_2$ values on hemodynamically stable patients in various age groups reveals that $Ptco_2$ index decreases progressively with age from premature infants to elderly patients (see Table 11–2). Glenski and Cucchiara also found that $Ptco_2$ index is relatively independent of probe location as long as the probe is on the central body rather than on an extremity.[34]

A study showed that $Ptco_2$ also depends on $Paco_2$, and that during hyperventilation both skin blood flow and $Ptco_2$ index are significantly decreased.[35] Voluntary hyperventilation in healthy subjects decreased $Ptco_2$ index to values as low as 0.1. $Ptco_2$ is thus a noninvasive monitor of peripheral tissue Po_2, and as such it depends on all parameters that affect oxygen delivery.

Practical Considerations and Limitations of $Ptco_2$ Monitoring

Probe Temperature and Skin Burn. Because the $Ptco_2$ electrode is heated above body temperature, small, electrode-sized skin burns can occur. No study has reported the incidence of burns from transcutaneous electrodes as a

TABLE 11–2. CHANGES IN $Ptco_2$ INDEX WITH AGE AND CARDIAC OUTPUT

$Ptco_2$ Index* ($Ptco_2$/Pao_2)	Age Group
1.14	Premature infants
1.0	Newborn
0.84	Pediatric
0.8	Adult
0.7	Older adult (>65 years old)
$Ptco_2$ Index†	**Cardiac Index (L/minute/m^2)**
0.8	> 2.2
0.5	1.5 to 2.2
0.1	< 1.5

*All of these $Ptco_2$ index values have a standard deviation of approximately 0.1.
†These data are from adult patients.

function of probe temperature and duration of application. From the experience of frequent users of the technique, the following guidelines are usually applied. For premature infants, an electrode temperature of 43.5°C is usually used, and the location is changed every 2–4 hours. For older children and adults, an electrode temperature of 44°C is used, and the site is changed every 4–6 hours. Although a 45°C temperature has been used in the past, this higher electrode temperature is unnecessary for adequate function and increases the incidence of skin burns.

Sensor Calibration and Drift. As with any Clark electrode, the transcutaneous Po_2 sensor must be properly calibrated and maintained. The zero O_2 tension point on the $Ptco_2$ electrode is usually stable and requires calibration on a monthly basis. The high Po_2 calibration uses room air, and should be rechecked prior to each application on the skin. Current $Ptco_2$ electrodes have miniaturized electrolyte reservoirs to bathe the electrode and 12- to 25-μm membranes on the surface. The electrolyte and membrane should be checked daily and usually require replacement at least once a week.

Effects of Anesthetic Agents on $Ptco_2$ Sensors. In 1971, John Severinghaus reported that halothane was reduced at the cathode of the Clark electrode, producing a dramatic upward drift of the Po_2 reading.[36] Because halothane exposure of the electrode in a blood gas analyzer is very low, little calibration drift is noted during intermittent blood gas analysis. On the other hand, the transcutaneous Po_2 sensor is applied directly and continously to the skin surface, where significant halothane interference can occur.

Measurements of the calibration drift after anesthetics involving halothane, enflurane, isoflurane, nitrous oxide, and local anesthesia revealed a drift of 0.7 mmHg/hour in the zero-point calibration in patients receiving halothane anesthesia.[37] This drift is clinically insignificant and within the manufacturer's specifications for the electrode, which was covered by a 25-μm Teflon membrane. Newer combination O_2 and CO_2 electrodes, in which the membrane is 12 ½-μm Teflon, exhibit significant upward drift in the presence of halothane anesthesia.

Sensor Location and Warm-Up. Site-to-site variation of $Ptco_2$ values is significant; approximately 10% variation occurs even with adjacent locations. Lower values are found on the extremities even in the absence of peripheral vascular disease. After being placed on the skin, a $Ptco_2$ sensor requires 8–15 minutes to equilibrate before yielding a steady value.

Another intraoperative limitation is that the sensor should be visible to the user. If the sensor becomes dislodged from the skin surface, it reads room air Po_2 (159 mmHg at sea level). Furthermore, external pressure on the sensor under the surgical drapes produces falsely low $Ptco_2$ values owing to compression of the dermal capillaries.

In summary, $Ptco_2$ values follow the trend of Pao_2 under conditions of adequate cardiac output and decrease relative to Pao_2 under conditions of low cardiac output states or hyperventilation. Thus, $Ptco_2$ aids in the diagnosis and treatment of low-flow shock conditions. The limitations of $Ptco_2$ monitoring include calibration and electrode maintenance, warm-up time, the possibility of skin burns, and potential interference by halothane.

Conjunctival Po_2

Equipment

When the eyes are closed, the cornea receives its oxygen supply from the palpebral conjunctiva. Therefore, this inner layer of the eyelid is well vascularized and has few cell layers between the capillaries and the mucous surface. The blood supply to the palpebral conjunctiva is derived from a branch of the ophthalmic artery, which in turn is a branch of the internal carotid artery. To measure Po_2 on this well-perfused surface, miniaturized Clark electrodes have been made to fit an ocular conformer ring. This conformer directly applies the Clark electrode to the inner surface of the palpebral conjunctiva. The electrode is not heated and therefore measures the surface oxygen directly from the tissue.

Advantages and Limitations

There are several advantages to this technique. First, because the probe is not heated, it requires only 60 seconds to equilibrate with the local tissue Po_2. Second, because the blood supply is from the carotid artery, conjunctival Po_2 ($Pcjo_2$) detects changes in carotid blood flow.[38] $Pcjo_2$ values are affected by both Pao_2 and perfusion as described previously for $Ptco_2$.[39–41] Therefore, $Pcjo_2$ values are also divided by Pao_2 to yield an index, which is then a measure of the relative perfusion of conjunctival tissue. The normal $Pcjo_2$ index is reported to be 0.6–0.7, with lower values in elderly patients.[42, 43] The index decreases with decreasing blood volume or cardiac output, again like $Ptco_2$.[39] Clinical studies have demonstrated that a $Pcjo_2$ index of less than 0.5 is associated with a blood volume deficit of at least 15%.[44]

Practical limitations of conjunctival oxygen monitoring are the same as those of transcutaneous monitoring: electrode maintenance, calibration, and anesthetic (halothane) interference. Unlike $Ptco_2$, the $Pcjo_2$ sensor does not produce burns or require prolonged warm-up, but eye injury can occur. Clinical studies to date have not reported serious eye problems.

MEASUREMENT OF HEMOGLOBIN SATURATION

HEMOGLOBIN SATURATION VERSUS OXYGEN SATURATION

Oxygen saturation is defined as the blood oxygen content divided by the oxygen capacity times 100%. Oxygen content was originally measured volumetrically by the method of Van Slyke and Neill.[4] The oxygen capacity is defined as the oxygen content of the blood after it has been equilibrated with room air (Po_2 = 159 mmHg). When this definition was formed, the maximum blood oxygen content clinically achieved occurred at room air Po_2 because increased inspired oxygen concentrations were not available. From the oxygen content formula (see Equation 11–1), we see that this definition of oxygen saturation includes contributions from both hemoglobin-bound and dissolved oxygen. Adult blood usually contains four species of hemoglobin: oxyhemoglobin (O_2Hb), reduced hemoglobin (Hb), methemoglobin (MetHb), and carboxyhemoglobin (COHb). COHb and MetHb are found in low concentrations except in pathologic states. Because these dyshemoglobins do not transport oxygen, they do not contribute to the oxygen content or to the definition of oxygen saturation given previously. When spectrophotometric methods for measuring hemoglobin species concentration became available, hemoglobin saturation could be more easily determined. The term "functional" hemoglobin saturation (Sao_2) is defined as

$$Sao_2 = \frac{[O_2Hb]}{[O_2Hb] + [Hb]} \times 100\% \qquad 11\text{–}7$$

where square brackets denote concentration. This definition of hemoglobin saturation does not include MetHb or COHb because they do not contribute to oxygen transport. Fractional hemoglobin saturation (Hbo_2), which is also called oxyhemoglobin fraction, is defined as

$$Hbo_2 = \frac{[O_2Hb]}{[O_2Hb] + [Hb] + [COHb] + [MetHb]} \times 100\% \qquad 11\text{–}8$$

This definition of hemoglobin saturation—that is, the ratio of oxyhemoglobin to total hemoglobin—is the saturation used in the calculation of oxygen content and delivery (see Equation 11–2). It is important to remember these definitions when evaluating the clinical utility and limitations of hemoglobin saturation monitors.

Hemoglobin Saturation Measurement: Beer's Law

Spectrophotometry was first used to determine the hemoglobin concentration of blood in the 1930s.[45] This method is based on the Lambert-Beer law (Equation 11–9), which relates the concentration of a solute to the intensity of light transmitted through the solution (Fig. 11–7).

$$I_{trans} = I_{in}\, e^{-DC\alpha\lambda} \qquad 11\text{–}9$$

where: I_{trans} = intensity of transmitted light
I_{in} = intensity of incident light
e = base of natural logarithm (2.718)
D = distance light is transmitted through the liquid
C = concentration of the solute (hemoglobin)
$\alpha\lambda$ = extinction coefficient of the solute (a constant for a given solute at a specific light wavelength λ)*

Thus, if a known solute is dissolved in a clear solvent in a cuvette of known dimensions, the solute concentration can be calculated if the incident and transmitted light intensity are measured (see Fig. 11–7). The extinction coefficient $\alpha\lambda$ is independent of the concentration, but is a function of the light wavelength used (Fig. 11–8).

Laboratory oximeters use this principle to determine hemoglobin concentration by measuring the intensity of light transmitted through a hemoglobin dispersion produced from lysed red blood cells.[46] For each wavelength of light used, an independent Lambert-Beer equation can be written. If the number of equations is equal to the number of solutes (i.e., hemoglobin species), we can solve for the concentration of each type. Therefore, at least four wavelengths of light are required to determine the concentrations of four species of hemoglobin (Fig. 11–9). For the Lambert-Beer law to be valid, both the solvent and the cuvette must be transparent at the light wavelengths used, the light path length must be known exactly, and no other absorbers can be present in the solution. It is difficult to fulfill all of these requirements in clinical devices. Consequently, although these devices are theoretically based on the Lambert-Beer law, empiric corrections are required to improve their accuracy.

INVASIVE HEMOGLOBIN SATURATION MONITORING

Mixed Venous Hemoglobin Saturation

Mixed venous oxygen tension ($P\bar{v}o_2$) and mixed venous hemoglobin saturation ($S\bar{v}o_2$) reflect global tissue oxygenation and the ability of the cardiopulmonary system to transport sufficient oxygen to meet body oxygen needs. Thus, continuous mixed venous oxygen monitoring should be useful clinically. In 1973, a fiberoptic system was reported to accurately measure $S\bar{v}o_2$ in humans.[47] This device used optical fibers incorporated into a pulmonary artery catheter to estimate the hemoglobin saturation from a reflected light signal. Light at red and infrared wavelengths was transmitted down one set of fiberoptic channels while the reflected signal from intact circulating red cells was transmitted back via other fibers to an external photodetector.[47] Although this first system appeared to work, it was not commercially produced because of the technical problems of inserting a pulmonary artery catheter that was made relatively stiff by the fiberoptic bundles.

In the late 1970s, Oximetrix, Inc. (Division of Abbott Laboratories) developed two fiberoptic reflectance systems for measuring hemoglobin saturation. The first system, introduced in 1977, employed a no. 7-F double-lumen umbilical artery catheter to be used in monitoring critically ill newborn infants.[48] The second system, introduced in 1981, used a no. 7.5-F pulmonary artery catheter with thermodilution capability for cardiac output measurement in addition to continuous mixed venous saturation monitoring.[49] These new systems used three wavelengths of light to calculate saturation. However, a minimum of four wavelengths are required to calculate hemoglobin saturation from Beer's

*This law further states that the absorbance from multiple solutes in solution is the sum of the absorbances of the various solutes times their respective concentrations, e.g., $C_1\alpha_{\lambda_1} + C_2\alpha_{\lambda_2} + C_3\alpha_{\lambda_3}$, etc.

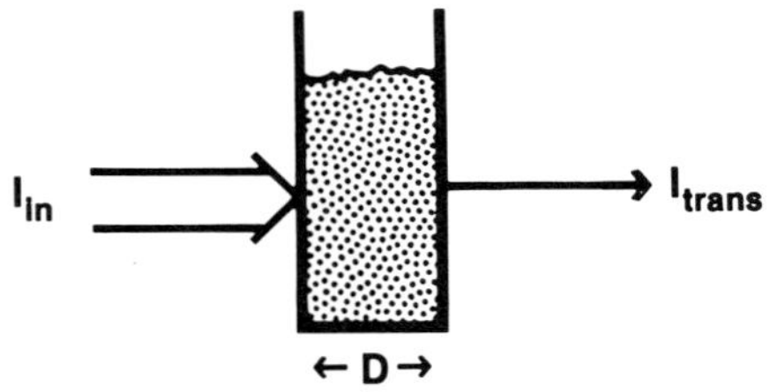

$I_{trans} = I_{in}e^{-(D \times C \times a_{\lambda})}$

I_{trans} = intensity of light transmitted
I_{in} = intensity of incident light
D = distance light is transmitted through the liquid
C = concentration of solute (oxyhemoglobin)
a_{λ} = extinction coefficient of the solute (a constant)

Figure 11–7. The concentration of a solute dissolved in a solvent can be calculated from the logarithmic relationship between the incident and transmitted light intensity and the solute concentration. (From Tremper KK, Barker SJ: Pulse oximetry and oxygen transport. *In* Payne JP, Severinghaus JW [eds]: Pulse Oximetry. Berlin: Springer-Verlag, 1986; 19–27.)

law in the presence of MetHb and COHb. The Oximetrix mixed venous saturation monitor can accurately measure functional hemoglobin saturation in the absence of significant dyshemoglobin concentrations.[49] However, an experimental study has shown that methemoglobinemia produces significant errors in the saturation measurement.[50] See the next section, Pulse Oximetry.

American Edwards Corporation has also produced a mixed venous saturation pulmonary artery catheter that uses two wavelengths of light. This device requires manual entry of the total hemoglobin to improve accuracy, whereas the Oximetrix system can accurately measure mixed venous saturation over a wide range of hematocrits.[51, 52]

Continuous $S\bar{v}O_2$ monitoring detects acute changes in the relationship of oxygen delivery to oxygen consumption (decreased supply, increased demand, or both). Three causes of reduced oxygen delivery decrease $S\bar{v}O_2$: decreased cardiac output, decreased hemoglobin, and decreased SaO_2. Abnormal hemoglobins also fail to deliver oxygen to tissue. Other factors decreasing $S\bar{v}O_2$ in clinical situations are shivering, malignant hyperthermia, exercise, agitation, fever, and thyroid storm. Monitoring $S\bar{v}O_2$ has been recommended in cardiac surgery patients and other critically ill patients at risk of acute cardiopulmonary decompensation.[53–55] It is an especially valuable adjunct in the management of ventilator-dependent patients on positive end-expiratory pressure (PEEP). As PEEP increases, arterial saturation improves. Eventually, PEEP decreases venous return and cardiac output, causing a decrease in $S\bar{v}O_2$.

$S\bar{v}O_2$ monitoring will not determine the source of an imbalance between oxygen delivery and oxygen consumption, nor does it detect regional ischemia. Monitoring of $S\bar{v}O_2$ requires the insertion of a pulmonary artery catheter and hence is inappropriate in many patients.

Pulse Oximetry

Only a few years after its introduction to the operating room, the pulse oximeter became an anesthetic standard of care.[56, 57] Several published studies also have strongly supported the routine use of pulse oximetry in the recovery room and intensive care unit.[58, 59] This technique was rapidly accepted by the anesthesia community because it continuously and noninvasively monitors arterial oxygenation with little user effort. This section discusses the theoretic principles on which pulse oximetry is based, its technical and physiologic limitations, and its clinical applications.

Technical Development of Pulse Oximetry

The term oximeter was coined by Millikan, who developed a lightweight device for noninvasively monitoring hemoglobin saturation in the 1940s.[60] This device estimated

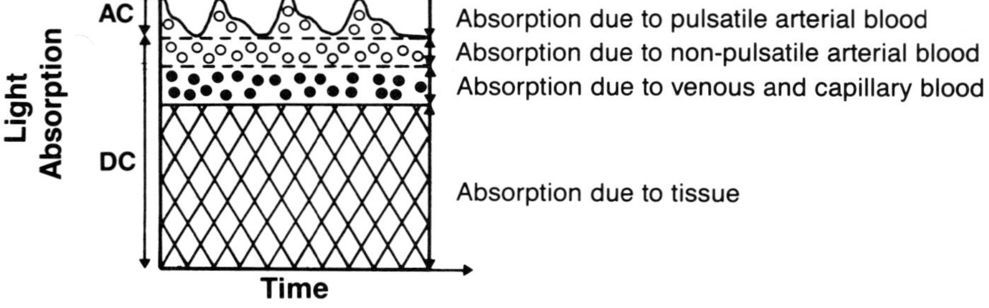

Figure 11–8. Light absorption through living tissue. The alternating current signal is due to the pulsatile component of the arterial blood; the direct current signal comprises all the nonpulsatile absorbers in the tissue: nonpulsatile arterial blood, nonpulsatile venous and capillary blood, and all other tissues. (Modified from Ohmeda Pulse Oximeter Model 3700 Service Manual, 1986; 22.)

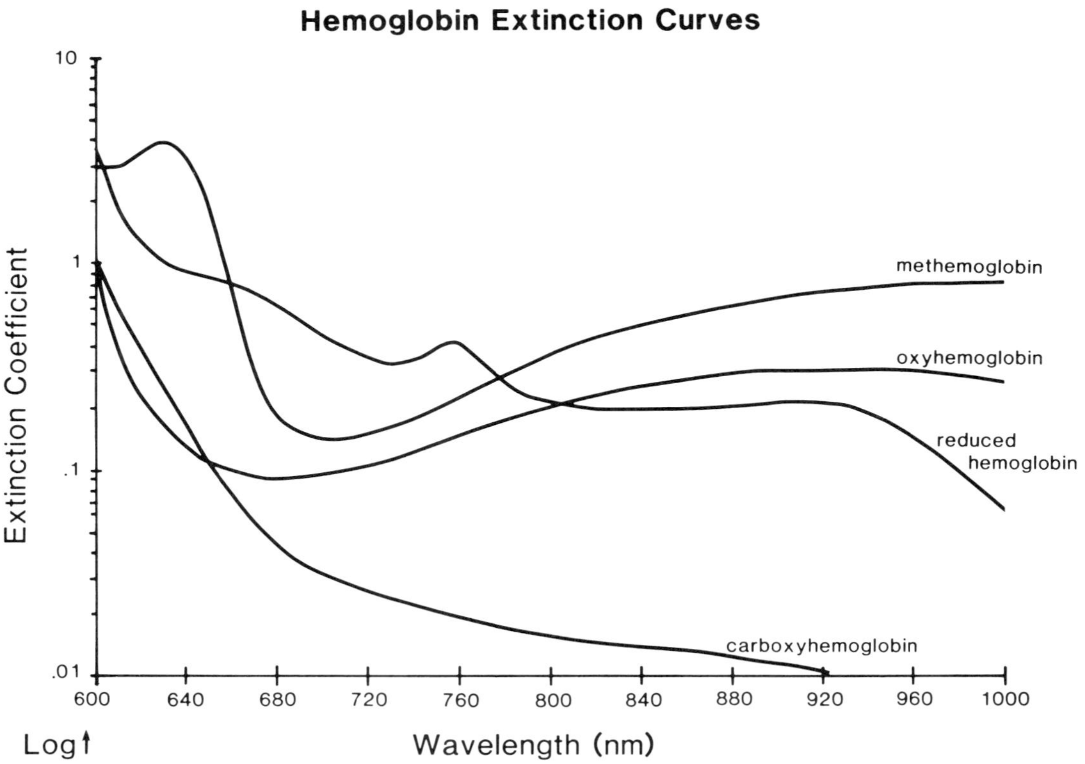

Figure 11–9. Transmitted light absorbance spectra of four hemoglobin species: oxyhemoglobin, reduced hemoglobin, carboxyhemoglobin, and methemoglobin. (From Barker SJ, Tremper KK: Pulse oximetry: Applications and limitations. *In* Barker SJ, Tremper KK [eds]: Advances in Oxygen Monitoring. Int Anesthesiol Clin 1987; 25:155–175.)

hemoglobin saturation by transilluminating the ear with light of two wavelengths, one in the red and one in the infrared range. The transmitted light was measured with a photodetector. This device effectively used the earlobe as a cuvette containing hemoglobin (Beer's Law) (see Fig. 11–7). Two major technical problems involved estimating arterial hemoglobin saturation in living tissue rather than *in vitro*. First, there are many light absorbers other than hemoglobin in the tissues. Second, the tissues contain not only arterial blood, but also venous and capillary blood. Millikan approached these problems by first measuring the absorbance of the ear while it was compressed to eliminate the blood. After this bloodless baseline measurement, the ear was heated to "arterialize" the blood. The difference between this absorbance and the baseline value was thus related to the arterial blood. This device was demonstrated to accurately detect intraoperative desaturations in the early 1950s, but was never adopted into routine clinical use.[61]

In the mid 1970s, Takuo Aoyagi made an ingenious discovery. He noted that the pulsatile components of the absorbances of red and infrared light transmitted through tissue were related to arterial hemoglobin saturation.[60] This eliminated the need to heat the tissue to obtain an arterial estimate. He used two wavelengths of light, one red (660 nm) and one infrared (940 nm). Such a device relies on the detection of a pulsatile signal and is referred to as a pulse oximeter.

Figure 11–9 schematically illustrates the absorbers in the living tissue. At the top of the figure is the pulsatile, or alternating current (AC), component, which is attributed to the pulsating arterial blood. The baseline, or direct current (DC), component represents the absorbance of the tissue bed including venous blood, capillary blood, and nonpulsatile arterial blood. All pulse oximeters assume that the only pulsatile absorbance between the light source and the photodetector is that of arterial blood. The pulse oximeter determines the AC component of the absorbance at each wavelength and divides this by the corresponding DC component to obtain a "pulse-added" absorbance that is independent of the incident light intensity. It then calculates the ratio of the pulse-added absorbances at the two wavelengths, which is then empirically related to $Sa{O_2}$ (Equation 11–10):

$$R = \frac{\text{AC red/DC red}}{\text{AC infrared/DC infrared}} \qquad 11\text{–}10$$

where R = absorbance ratio. Figure 11–10 is an example of a pulse oximeter calibration curve. These empirical curves are developed by measuring the R in human volunteers and simultaneously sampling arterial blood for *in vitro* saturation measurements. R varies from 0.4 to 3.4 over the saturation range of 0–100%. Note that an R of 1.0 corresponds to a pulse oximeter saturation ($Sp{O_2}$) of approximately 85%.

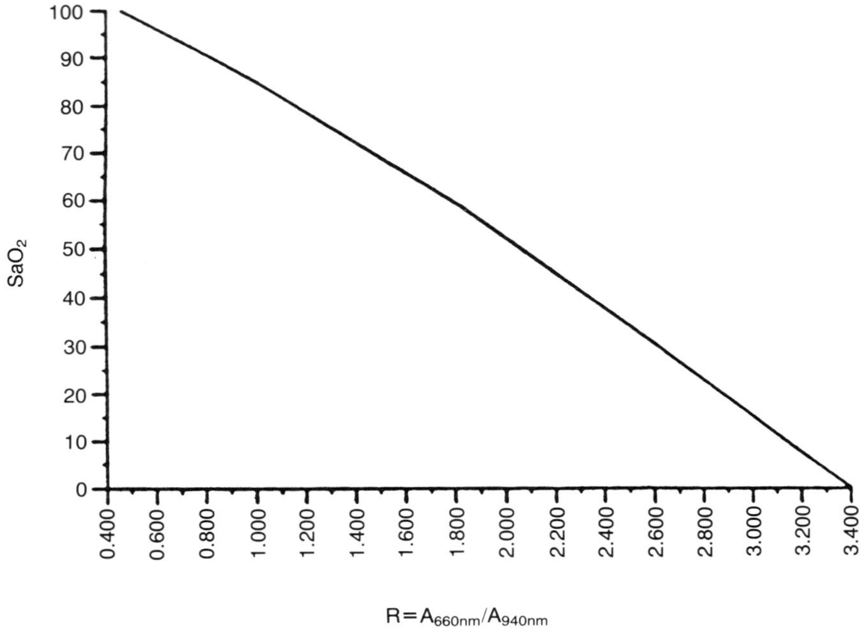

Figure 11–10. A typical pulse oximeter calibration curve. The Sao_2 estimate is determined from the ratio (R) of the pulse-added absorbance at 660 nm to the pulse-added absorbance at 940 nm. The ratios of red to infrared absorbances vary from approximately 0.4 at 100% saturation to 3.4 at 0% saturation. The ratio of red to infrared absorbance is 1.0 at a saturation of approximately 85%. This curve can be approximately determined from theory, but for accurate predictions of Spo_2, empirical modifications are required. (From Pologe JA: Pulse oximetry: Technical aspects of machine design. *In* Tremper KK, Barker SJ [eds]: Advances in Oxygen Monitoring. Int Anesthesiol Clin 1987; 25:142.)

Technical Application of Pulse Oximetry

Although the theory of the pulse oximeter is straightforward, application of this theory to a clinically useful device engenders technical problems and physiologic limitations. One of the limitations is a consequence of Beer's Law and the definitions of Sao_2 and Hbo_2. Because it is a two-wavelength device, the pulse oximeter calibration assumes that there are only two hemoglobin types in the bloodstream: O_2Hb and Hb. If MetHb or COHb is present, it contributes to the pulse-added absorbance signal and is interpreted as O_2Hb, Hb, or some combination of the two.

Carboxyhemoglobin. Some insight into the effects of dyshemoglobins on the pulse oximeter is gained by examining the absorbance spectra (see Fig. 11–9). COHb absorbs very little light at 940 nm (infrared), whereas it absorbs as much as does O_2Hb at 660 nm (red light). This is clinically illustrated by the fact that patients with carboxyhemoglobin toxemia appear red. The effects of COHb on Spo_2 values have been evaluated experimentally.[62] Spo_2 was roughly determined by $O_2Hb + 0.9 \times COHb$.

Methemoglobin. In the case of methemoglobin, the absorbance is high at both the red and infrared wavelengths (see Fig. 11–9). Consequently MetHb produces a large pulse-added absorbance at both wavelengths. Adding a large absorbance to both the numerator and denominator of the R tends to force this ratio toward unity. On the pulse oximeter calibration curve (see Fig. 11–10), a ratio of 1 corresponds to a saturation of 85%, as noted above. The effects of methemoglobinemia also have been evaluated experimentally, confirming the hypothesis that high MetHb levels will force Spo_2 toward 85% regardless of the Pao_2 and Sao_2 values.[50]

Dyes. Any substance that absorbs light at the red and infrared pulse oximeter wavelengths and is present in the pulsatile arterial blood may cause errors. A clinical example of this effect is intravenously injected dyes. In a volunteer study it was shown that intravenous methylene blue decreased Spo_2 to approximately 65% for 1–2 minutes, whereas indigo carmine produced a very slight decrease. Indocyanine green had an intermediate effect.[61–63]

Nail polish also adversely affects pulse oximeter accuracy. Blue, black, or green polish significantly decreased measured saturation. Greater reduction in saturation occurred with blue and green than with purple or red. These findings were unrelated to absorbance by the nail polish at wavelengths used by the oximeter to determine saturation.[62–64]

Fetal Hemoglobin

With the adoption of pulse oximetry in the neonatal intensive care unit, the accuracy of the pulse oximeter in the presence of fetal hemoglobin (HbF) must be established. Fetal hemoglobin has a greater affinity for oxygen (a lower P_{50}) than adult hemoglobin (HbA); thus it will become fully saturated at a lower Pao_2. However, the light absorption coefficients for HbF are no different than those of HbA, so the presence of fetal hemoglobin should not cause errors in pulse oximeters.[65, 66] Because the O_2Hb dissociation curve of HbF is shifted to the left from that of HbF, the Pao_2 at a given Sao_2 is lower for HbF. Thus, the presence of HbF affects treatment only if one plans to maintain a specific Pao_2 as opposed to a specific Sao_2.

Technical Limitations

Because the photodiode detectors in the pulse oximeter sensor respond to light of any wavelength, ambient light contaminates the light emitting diode (LED) signal.[67–69] The pulse oximeter designers have reduced this light interference by alternately turning on the red and infrared LEDs and then turning both LEDs off. The sensor first detects a signal from the red LED plus room light, followed by the infrared LED plus room light, and finally the ambient room light signal alone when both LEDs are turned off. This sequence is repeated rapidly in an effort to subtract the room light signal even in a quickly changing light background. Despite this clever design, room light interference can cause erroneous Spo_2 values or prevent the pulse oximeter from obtaining any Spo_2 value. This problem can be alleviated by an opaque covering on the sensor.[70]

The most difficult problem in the design of the pulse oximeter is management of low signal-to-noise ratios. This problem has two causes.

First, when there is a small absorbance signal due to a weak pulse, the device automatically increases signal amplification to produce a measurable pulse-added absorbance signal. Unfortunately, as the signal is amplified, the background noise is also amplified. In situations of a weak or nonexistent pulse signal, the noise can be amplified until it is interpreted by the oximeter as a pulse-added absorbance. New pulse oximeters have signal strength limits, below which they will display a "low signal-strength" error message. Most devices also display a pulse waveform that can be visually observed to monitor signal quality.

Because of its automatic gain control, the pulse oximeter can deal with both large and small pulse signals and is relatively insensitive to changes in peripheral pulse amplitude and flow. Lawson and coworkers objectively assessed the blood flow limits of Spo_2 estimation in the following experiment.[71] The peripheral blood flow at the finger was measured by a laser Doppler flow probe. A pulse oximeter was placed on the finger adjacent to the flow probe while a blood pressure cuff was progressively inflated on the upper arm. The pulse oximeter stopped estimating saturation and gave a "low perfusion" warning when the peripheral blood flow had decreased to 8.6% of the control value. As the blood pressure cuff was slowly deflated from full occlusion, the pulse oximeter again displayed a pulse and saturation estimate when the blood flow was only 4% of baseline. This study demonstrates the ability of the pulse oximeter to estimate saturation over an extreme range of peripheral blood flow. Other clinical experimental studies confirm that the pulse oximeter can estimate saturation over a wide range of cardiac outputs if an adequate pulse is detected.[72, 73]

Second, a serious signal-to-noise problem results from patient motion artifacts. For recovery room and intensive care unit applications, this may be the most troublesome problem in using pulse oximeters. Most pulse oximeters employ a variety of signal averaging modes to minimize motion effects. That is, the device averages multiple pulses to obtain its saturation estimate, thereby diminishing the effect of single spurious motion signals. However, increasing the signal averaging time has a deleterious effect on the time response of the pulse oximeter to acute saturation changes. The manufacturers can also incorporate more sophisticated algorithms to discriminate motion signals from arterial pulse signals by using the rate of change of Spo_2. For example, if the calculated Spo_2 changes from 95% to 50% in 0.1 seconds, this new and presumably spurious saturation estimate is either dropped from the averaging or given a lower weighting factor. One manufacturer (Nellcor) has attempted to minimize motion artifact by using an ECG signal to synchronize the pulse oximeter with the actual heart beat. Although these and other algorithms have improved performance when compared with early models, motion artifact remains a serious problem in the intensive care setting.

Another pulse oximeter error involves the variability of the wavelengths of light emitted by the LEDs. Although these diodes nominally radiate at either 660 nm or 940 nm, in reality each diode emits a slightly different wavelength. The peak or center wavelength of light from the LED can vary ± 10 nm from the specified value. As we see from the extinction coefficients in Figure 11–9, shifts in the LED wavelength change the extinction coefficient. Because the oximeter software assumes an extinction coefficient at a specified wavelength, an unknown change in that wavelength causes an error in the saturation estimate. Therefore, there is a probe-to-probe variability in accuracy. Some manufacturers minimize this error by narrowing the wavelength tolerance on the LEDs used in their sensors. Others compensate for the error by designing the sensor to identify its specific LED wavelengths to the pulse oximeter monitor, which then electronically corrects for shifted center wavelengths.

Accuracy and Response

Most pulse oximeters have a specified accuracy of ±2% from 100% down to 70% saturation, ±3% from 70% saturation to 50%, and no unspecified accuracy below 50% saturation.[74] This implies that the Spo_2 is within 2% above or below the actual Sao_2 67% of the time (±1 standard deviation around the mean). This corresponds to a 99% confidence interval of ±6% (i.e., ±3 standard deviations) from 100% to 70% saturation, and ±9% from 70% to 50% saturation. Although these manufacturer's specifications are based on volunteer data collected under optimal conditions, the accuracies found in clinical studies are comparable. It is difficult to compare clinical studies to manufacturer's specifications, because the studies usually report correlation coefficients and linear regression analysis rather than the more appropriate bias and precision. From the available studies, it appears that under steady-state conditions the Spo_2 value is usually within ±2–3 saturation points (±1 standard deviation).[75–80]

Two recent studies in adult volunteers evaluated the response time of pulse oximeters to sudden desaturation and resaturation.[79, 80] Kagle and colleagues measured the 50% recovery time for resaturation from a hypoxic state. They used a fast (3-second) time-averaging mode and found a 50% recovery time (T½) of 6 seconds for the ear probe and 24 seconds for the finger probe.[79] Severinghaus and Naifeh also found that the ear probe responds more quickly than the finger probe does during desaturation and resaturation.[80] Their T½ values for ear probes ranged from 9.6 to 19.8 seconds, whereas the T½ for finger probes ranged from 24 to 35.1 seconds.

The arterial hemoglobin saturation provides limited information on the oxygen transport status. Hemoglobin saturation does not imply oxygen content unless the total hemoglobin is known. Furthermore, saturation values do not inform us of the directional change of Pa_{O_2} until the latter drops below 75–80 mmHg. Intraoperatively, there may be large changes in Pa_{O_2} that are thus not detected by pulse oximetry. For example, the pulse oximeter is not a sensitive detector of inadvertent endobronchial intubation at the inspired oxygen fraction normally used in the operating room.[81] Finally, the pulse oximeter measures a pulse but not peripheral perfusion. The presence or absence of a pulse will be quickly detected, but the presence of a pulse does not ensure adequate blood flow.

Considering all the sources of possible error, pulse oximeters are impressively accurate clinical devices. Because the manufacturers' specified accuracy of $\pm$2–3% is for a confidence interval of only 68%, it is surprising that clinical studies have found accuracies similar to these.

Monitoring Oxygen Saturation by Pulse Oximetry

In 1947, Comroe and Botelho published a classic study showing the unreliability of direct observation for the detection of cyanosis.[82] This finding was confirmed intraoperatively for patients under general anesthesia in 1951.[61] With the advent of pulse oximetry, several perioperative studies again confirmed this fact during even routine anesthetics in healthy patients.[83–88] Coté and coworkers conducted a randomized, controlled study with anesthetized pediatric patients.[83] One hundred fifty-two surgical patients were continuously monitored with pulse oximeters. In half of these patients, the pulse oximeter data were unavailable to the anesthesia team. The study revealed 24 major desaturation events ($Sp_{O_2} \leq 85\%$ for 30 seconds) in the patients for which the pulse oximeter data were unavailable, and only 11 in the other group. Most of these major events occurred in patients 2 years of age or younger.[83] Raemer and colleagues conducted a similar study on healthy outpatients during gynecologic surgery.[84] They noted severe desaturations ($Sp_{O_2} < 85\%$) in 5% of their cases.

Two studies have evaluated oxygenation by pulse oximeter during transport from the operating room to the recovery room.[85, 86] Pullerits and coworkers monitored 71 healthy pediatric patients during transport and found that 28.1% had Sp_{O_2} values $\leq 90\%$, whereas cyanosis was clinically observed in only 45% of these patients.[85] In a similar study of adults, Tyler and colleagues found that saturation values fall to $\leq 85\%$ during transport in 12% of patients.[86] Both studies concluded that all patients should receive supplemental oxygen during transport to the recovery room.

Two studies on recovery room patients have again emphasized the fact that our clinical abilities to detect cyanosis are poor. Soliman and coworkers compared pulse oximeter Sp_{O_2} values to postanesthesia recovery scores in children.[87] These scores are based on motor activity, respiratory effort, blood pressure, level of consciousness, and skin color. They found no correlation between scores and Sp_{O_2} values in these healthy pediatric patients. Morris and colleagues evaluated adult patients in the recovery room by measuring Sp_{O_2} on admission to the recovery room, 5 minutes after admission, 30 minutes after admission, and finally just before discharge.[88] Of the 149 patients studied, 14% had episodes of desaturation ($Sp_{O_2} < 90\%$). Curiously, the highest incidence of desaturation was at the time of discharge from the recovery room. Both studies concluded that patients in the recovery room should either be continuously monitored with pulse oximeters or at least tested as part of the routine discharge criteria.

Pulse oximetry is a minimum standard of care in the operating room and is becoming a *de facto* standard in the recovery room and intensive care unit. Sp_{O_2} monitoring is becoming routine in most settings where supplemental oxygen is required or the possibility of cardiopulmonary compromise is significant. Because pulse oximeters are easy to use and noninvasive, it is difficult to find an argument not to use a pulse oximeter in an acute care setting. Sensors can be placed on fingers, toes, nose, ears, or tongue to assure continuous Sp_{O_2} values.[89]

REFERENCES

1. Merilainen PT: A differential paramagnetic sensor for breath-by-breath oximetry. J Clin Monit 1990; 6:65–73.
2. Westenskow DR, Jordan WS, Jordan R, Gillmor ST: Evaluation of oxygen monitors for use during anesthesia. Anesth Analg 1981; 60:53–56.
3. McGarrigle R, White S: Oxygen analyzers can detect disconnections. Anesth Analg 1985; 63:464–465.
4. Van Slyke DD, Neill JM: The determination of gases in blood and other solutions by vacuum extraction and manometric measurement. Int J Biol Chem 1924; 61:523–557.
5. Guyton AC: Transport of oxygen and carbon dioxide in the blood and body fluids. *In* Textbook of Medical Physiology. Philadelphia: WB Saunders, 1981; Chap 41.
6. Clark LC: Monitor and control of tissue O_2 tensions. Trans Am Soc Artif Intern Organs 1956; 2:41–48.
7. Severinghaus JW, Bradley AF: Electrodes for blood P_{O_2} and P_{CO_2} determination. J Appl Physiol 1958; 13:515–520.
8. Gehrich JL, Lubbers DW, Opitz N, et al: Optical fluorescence and its application to an intravascular blood gas monitoring system. IEEE Trans Biomed Eng 1986; 33:117–132.
9. Barker SJ, Tremper KK, Hyatt J, et al: Continuous fiberoptic arterial oxygen tension measurements in dogs. J Clin Monit 1987; 3:48–52.
10. Shapiro BA, Cane RD, Chomka CM, et al: Evaluation of a new intraarterial blood gas system in dogs [Abstract]. Crit Care Med 1987; 15:361.
11. Kollmeyer KR, Tsang RC: Complications of umbilical oxygen electrodes. J Pediatr 1974; 84:894–897.
12. Harris TR, Nugent M: Continuous arterial oxygen tension monitoring in the newborn infant. J Pediatr 1973; 82:929–939.
13. Bratanow N, Polk K, Bland R, et al: Continuous polarographic monitoring of intra-arterial oxygen in the perioperative period. Crit Care Med 1985; 13:859–860.
14. Malalis L, Bhat R, Vidyasagar D: Comparison of intravascular P_{O_2} with transcutaneous and Pa_{O_2} values. Crit Care Med 1983; 11:110–113.
15. Altman DG, Bland JM: Measurement in medicine: The analysis of method comparison studies. Statistician 1983; 32:307–317.
16. Bland JM, Altman DG: Statistical methods for assessing agreement

between two methods of clinical measurement. Lancet 1986; 1:307–310.
17. Altman DG: Statistics and ethics in medical research. Vol 6, Presentation of results. Br Med J 1980; 2:1542–1544.
18. Rithalia SVS, Bennett PJ, Tinker J: The performance characteristics of an intra-arterial oxygen electrode. Intens Care Med 1981; 7:305–307.
19. Stanley Frank, Ph.D.: Personal communication. Biomedical Sensors, Inc., Kansas City, Mo.
20. Barker SJ, Hyatt J: Continuous measurement of intraarterial pHa, Pa_{CO_2}, and Pa_{O_2} in the operating room. Anesth Analg 1991; 73:43–48.
21. Mahutte CK, Sassoon CS, Muro JR: Progress in the development of a fluorescent intravascular blood gas system. J Clin Monit 1990; 6:147–157.
22. Greenblott GB, Barker SJ, Tremper KK, et al: Detection of venous air embolism by continuous intraarterial oxygen monitoring. J Clin Monit 1990; 6:53–56.
23. Greenblott GB, Tremper KK, Barker SJ, et al: Continuous blood gas monitoring with an intraarterial optode during one-lung anesthesia. J Cardiothorac Anaesth 1991; 5:365–367.
24. Eberhard P, Hammacher K, Mindt W: Perkutane messung des sauerstoffpartialdruckes: Methodik und anwendugen [Abstract]. Stuttgart Proc Medizin-Technik 1972; 26.
25. Huch A, Huch R, Meinzer K, et al: Eine schuelle, behitze Ptoberflachenelektrode zur kontinuierlichen Uberwachung des P_{O_2} beim Menschen: Elektrodenaufbau und Eigenschaften [Abstract]. Stuttgart Proc Medizin-Technik 1972; 26.
26. Huch R, Huch A, Albani M, et al: Transcutaneous P_{O_2} monitoring in routine management of infants and children with cardiorespiratory problems. Pediatrics 1976; 57:681–688.
27. Peabody JL, Willis MM, Gregory GA, et al: Clinical limitations and advantages of transcutaneous oxygen electrodes. Acta Anaesthesiol Scand Suppl 1978; 68:76–81.
28. Marshall TA, Kattwinkel J, Berry FA, Shaw A: Transcutaneous oxygen monitoring of neonates during surgery. J Pediatr Surg 1980; 15:797–803.
29. Versmold HT, Linderkamp O, Holzman M, et al: Transcutaneous monitoring of P_{O_2} in newborn infants. Where are the limits? Influences of blood pressure, blood volume, blood flow, viscosity, and acid base state. Birth Defects 1979; 4:286–294.
30. Baumgardner JE, Graves DJ, Newfeld GR, Quinn JA: Gas flux through human skin: Effects of temperature, stripping and inspired tension. J Appl Physiol 1985; 5:1536–1545.
31. Van Duzee BF: Thermal analysis of human stratum corneum. J Invest Dermatol 1975; 65:404–408.
32. Tremper KK, Waxman K, Shoemaker WC. Effects of hypoxia and shock on transcutaneous P_{O_2} values in dogs. Crit Care Med 1979; 7:526–531.
33. Tremper KK, Shoemaker WC: Transcutaneous oxygen monitoring of critically ill adults, with and without low flow shock. Crit Care Med 1981; 9:706–709.
34. Glenski JA, Cucchiara RF: Transcutaneous O_2 and CO_2 monitoring of neurosurgical patient: Detection of air embolism. Anesthesiology 1986; 64:546–550.
35. Barker SJ, Hyatt J, Clark C, Tremper KK: Hyperventilation reduces transcutaneous oxygen tension and skin blood flow. Anesthesiology 1991; 75:619–624.
36. Severinghaus JW, Weiskopf RB, Nishimura M, Bradley AF: Oxygen electrode errors due to polarographic reduction of halothane. J Appl Physiol 1971; 31:640–642.
37. Tremper KK, Barker SJ, Blatt DH, Wender RH: Effects of anesthetic agents on the drift of a transcutaneous P_{O_2} sensor. J Clin Monit 1986; 2:234–236.
38. Shoemaker WC, Lawner P: Method for continuous conjunctival oxygen monitoring during carotid artery surgery. Crit Care Med 1983; 11:946–949.
39. Smith M, Abraham E: Conjunctival oxygen monitoring during hemorrhage. J Trauma 1986; 26:217–224.
40. Abraham E, Fink S: Conjunctival and cardiorespiratory monitoring during resuscitation from hemorrhage. Crit Care Med 1986; 12:1004–1009.
41. Abraham E: Continuous conjunctival and transcutaneous oxygen tension monitoring during resuscitation in a patient. Resuscitation 1984; 12:207–211.
42. Hess D, Evans C, Thomas K, et al: The relationship between conjunctival P_{O_2} and arterial P_{O_2} in 16 normal persons. Respir Care 1986; 31:191–198.
43. Chapman KR, Liu FLW, Watson RM, Rebuck AS: Conjunctival oxygen tension and its relationship to arterial oxygen tension. J Clin Monit 1986; 2:100–104.
44. Abraham E, Oye RK, Smith M: Detection of blood volume deficits through conjunctival oxygen tension monitoring. Crit Care Med 1985; 12:931–934.
45. Severinghaus JW: Historical development of oxygenation monitoring. *In* Payne JP, Severinghaus JW (eds): Pulse Oximetry. Berlin: Springer-Verlag, 1986.
46. Brown LJ: A new instrument for the simultaneous measurement of total hemoglobin, % oxyhemoglobin, % carboxyhemoglobin, % methemoglobin, and oxygen content in whole blood. IEEE Trans Biomed Eng 1980; 27:132–138.
47. Martin WE, Cheung PW, Johnson CC, Wong KC: Continuous monitoring of mixed venous oxygen saturation in man. Anesth Analg 1973; 52:784–793.
48. Wilkinson AR, Phibbs RH, Gregory GA: Continuous measurement of oxygen saturation in sick newborn infants. J Pediatr 1978; 93:1016–1019.
49. Beale PL, McMichan JC, Marsh HM, et al: Continuous monitoring of mixed venous oxygen saturation in critically ill patients. Anesth Analg 1982; 61:513–517.
50. Barker SJ, Tremper KK, Hyatt J, Zaccari J: Effects of methemoglobinemia on pulse oximetry and mixed venous oximetry. Anesthesiology 1989; 70:112–117.
51. Gettinger A, Detraglia MC, Glass DD: In vivo comparison of two mixed venous saturation catheters. Anesthesiology 1987; 66:373–375.
52. Lee SE, Tremper KK, Barker SJ: Effects of anemia on pulse oximetry and continuous mixed venous oxygen saturation monitoring in dogs. Anesth Analg 1988; 67:S130.
53. Jamieson WRE, Turnbull KW, Larrieu AJ, et al: Continuous monitoring of mixed venous oxygen saturation in cardiac surgery. Can J Surg 1982: 25(5):538–543.
54. Schmidt CR, Frank LP, Forsythe MJ, Estafanous FG: Continuous S_{VO_2} measurement and oxygen transport patterns in cardiac surgery patients. Crit Care Med 1984; 12:523–557.
55. Waller JL, Kaplan JA, Bauman DI, Craver JM: Clinical evaluation of a new fiberoptic catheter oximeter during cardiac surgery. Anesth Analg (Cleve) 1982; 61:676–679.
56. Eichorn JH, Cooper JB, Cullen BF, et al: Standards for patient monitoring during anesthesia at Harvard Medical School. JAMA 1986; 256:1017–1020.
57. American Society of Anesthesiologists: Standards for basic intra-operative monitoring. Anesthesia Patient Safety Foundation 1987; March 3.
58. Canet J, Ricos M, Vidal F: Early postoperative arterial desaturation: Determining factors and response to oxygen therapy. Anesth Analg 1989; 69:207–212.
59. Lampe GH, Wauk LZ, Whitendale P, et al: Postoperative hypoxemia after nonabdominal surgery: A frequent event not caused by nitrous oxide. Anesth Analg 1990; 71:597–601.
60. Severinghaus JW, Astrup PB: History of blood gas analysis. Anesth Clin 1987; 25:1–215.
61. Stephen CR, Slater HM, Johnson AL, Sekelj P: The oximeter—A technical aid for the anesthesiologist. Anesthesiology 1951; 12:541–555.
62. Barker SJ, Tremper KK: The effect of carbon monoxide inhalation on pulse oximeter signal detection. Anesthesiology 1987; 66:677–679.
63. Scheller MS, Unger RJ, Kelner MJ: Effects of intravenously administered dyes on pulse oximetry readings. Anesthesiology 1986; 65:550–552.
64. Coté CJ, Goldstein A, Fuschsman WH, Hoaglin DC: The effect of nail polish on pulse oximetry. Anesth Analg 1988; 67:683–686.
65. Pologe JA, Raley DM: Effects of fetal hemoglobin on pulse oximetry. J Perinatol 1987; 7:324–326.
66. Anderson JV: The accuracy of pulse oximetry in neonates. Effects of fetal hemoglobin and bilirubin. J Perinatol 1987; 7:323.
67. Brooks TD, Paulus DA, Winkle WE: Infrared heat lamps interfere with pulse oximeters [Letter]. Anesthesiology 1984; 61:630.
68. Costarino AT, Davis DA, Keon TP: Falsely normal saturation reading with the pulse oximeter. Anesthesiology 1987; 67:830–831.
69. Eisele JH, Downs D: Ambient light affects pulse oximeters. Anesthesiology 1987; 67:864–865.

70. Siegel MN, Gravenstein N: Preventing ambient light from affecting pulse oximetry [Letter]. Anesthesiology 1987; 67:280.
71. Lawson D, Norley I, Korbon G. Blood flow limits and pulse oximeter signal detection. Anesthesiology 1987; 67:599–603.
72. Tremper KK, Hufstedler S, Zaccari J, et al: Pulse oximetry and transcutaneous Po_2 during hemorrhagic and normotensive shock in dogs [Abstract]. Anesthesiology 1984; 61:A163.
73. Tremper KK, Hufstedler S, Barker SJ, et al: Accuracy of a pulse oximeter in the critically ill adult: Effect of temperature and hemodynamics [Abstract]. Anesthesiology 1985; 63:A175.
74. Nellcor N100 Technical Manual. Nellcor Corporation, Hayward, CA.
75. Mihm FG, Halperin DH: Noninvasive detection of profound arterial desaturations using pulse oximetry device. Anesthesiology 1985; 62:85–87.
76. Cecil WT, Thorpe JK, Fibuch EE, Tuohy GF: A clinical evaluation of the accuracy of the Nellcor N100 and the Ohmeda 3700 pulse oximeters. J Clin Monit 1988; 4:31–36.
77. Boxer RA, Gottesfeld I, Singh S, et al: Noninvasive pulse oximetry in children with cyanotic congenital heart disease. Crit Care Med 1987; 15:1062–1064.
78. Fait CD, Wetzel RC, Dean JM, et al: Pulse oximetry in critically ill children. J Clin Monit 1985; 1:232–235.
79. Kagle DM, Alexander CM, Berko RS, et al: Evaluation of the Ohmeda 3700 pulse oximeter: Steady-state and transient response characteristics. Anesthesiology 1987; 66:376–380.
80. Severinghaus JW, Naifeh KH: Accuracy of response of six pulse oximeters to profound hypoxia. Anesthesiology 1987; 67:551–558.
81. Barker SJ, Tremper KK, Hyatt J, Heitzmann H: Comparison of three oxygen monitors in detecting endobronchial intubation. J Clin Monit 1988; 4:240–243.
82. Comroe JH Jr, Botelho S: The reliability of cyanosis in the recognition of arterial anoxemia. Am J Med Sci 1947; 214:1–6.
83. Coté CJ, Goldstein EA, Coté MA, et al: A single blind study of pulse oximetry in children. Anesthesiology 1988; 68:184–188.
84. Raemer DB, Warren DL, Morris R, et al: Hypoxemia during ambulatory gynecologic surgery as evaluated by the pulse oximeter. J Clin Monit 1987; 3:244–248.
85. Pullerits J, Burrows FA, Roy WL: Arterial desaturation in healthy children during transfer to the recovery room. Can J Anesth 1987; 34:470–473.
86. Tyler IL, Tantisira B, Winter PM, Motoyama EK: Continuous monitoring of arterial oxygen saturation with pulse oximetry during transfer to the recovery room. Anesth Analg 1985; 64:1108–1112.
87. Soliman IE, Patel RI, Ehrenpreis MB, Hannallah RS: Recovery scores do not correlate with post-operative hypoxemia in children. Anesth Analg 1988; 67:53–56.
88. Morris RW, Buschman A, Warren DL, et al: The prevalence of hypoxemia detected by pulse oximetry during recovery from anesthesia. J Clin Monit 1988; 4:16–20.
89. Jobes DR, Nicolson SC: Monitoring of arterial hemoglobin oxygen saturation using a tongue sensor. Anesth Analg 1988; 67:186–188.

CHAPTER

12

Monitoring the Respiratory System

THOMAS J. GAL, M.D.

Monitoring the function of the respiratory system is of great importance to the anesthesiologist because the problems associated with inadequate ventilation, if unrecognized, can contribute significantly to anesthetic morbidity. Some monitoring techniques are sophisticated and invasive, whereas others rely on more simple clinical observation. This chapter considers the wide range of techniques available to monitor respiratory function and ventilation with an emphasis on the physiologic principles that form the basis of the measurements. The goal is to enhance the clinician's understanding of the indications, interpretations, and limitations of such respiratory measurements.

RESPIRATORY MECHANICS

Respiratory mechanics concerns the study of the respiratory system's function as an air pump and analyzes the forces that physically transport air into and back out of the alveoli. Contraction of the respiratory muscles produces the force necessary to move air in and out of the lungs. This force must in turn overcome three basic opposing forces: inertance, elastance, and resistance.

RESPIRATORY MUSCLES

Contraction of the inspiratory muscles produces expansion of the chest and fills the lungs with air. The principle muscle of inspiration, the diaphragm, contracts and descends to expand the chest longitudinally and to elevate the lower ribs. This action is responsible for more than two thirds of the air movement during quiet inspiration. The remaining volume is due to contraction of the external intercostals to further elevate the ribs and enlarge both the transverse and anteroposterior chest dimensions. Expiration during quiet breathing results essentially from the passive recoil of the lungs and chest wall. Only during higher levels of ventilation or when air movement is impeded do the internal intercostals and abdominal muscles contract to depress the ribs and compress the abdominal contents to provide active expiratory effort. The expiratory muscles, however, play important roles in other breathing-related activities, such as talking, singing, and coughing.

All measurements of pulmonary function that require patient effort are influenced by respiratory muscle strength. This can be evaluated specifically by measurements of maximal static respiratory pressures. These pressures are generated against an occluded airway during a maximal forced effort and can be measured with simple aneroid gauges.[1] The inspiratory muscles are at their optimal length near residual volume. Thus, maximal inspiratory pressure (PImax) is usually measured after a forced exhalation. Similarly, maximum expiratory pressure (PEmax) is measured at total lung capacity, at which expiratory muscles are stretched to their optimal length by a full inspiration. A typical value for PImax in healthy young males is about -125 cm H_2O, whereas PEmax may be as high as $+200$ cm H_2O.

Values for PEmax less than $+40$ cm H_2O suggest impaired coughing ability,[2] whereas PImax values of -25 cm H_2O or less indicate severe inability to take a deep breath. The latter value is often utilized as a criterion for extubation; however, observations in healthy volunteers during partial curarization suggest that this level of adequate ventilatory ability is too low to ensure adequate airway integrity.[3]

FORCES OPPOSING AIRFLOW

The movement of air in and out of the lungs is opposed by three basic forces—inertance, elastance, and resistance—which must be overcome. During most breathing activities, inertance, which is the impedance to acceleration of gas and tissue, is negligible. Elastance and its reciprocal force, compliance, are reflections of the relationships of pressure to volume when there is no airflow. Hence, such measurements are referred to as static. Resistance, on the other hand, is highly dependent on the rate of change of lung volume, i.e., flow. Such measurements during active breathing are referred to as dynamic.

STATIC FORCES

The respiratory system and its component lung and chest wall are elastic. That is, they tend to regain their original size and configuration following deformation when deforming forces are removed. Both lung and chest wall have positions of equilibrium. These are the volumes that they tend to assume in the absence of external forces acting on them and the volumes to which they continuously attempt to return when displaced. The equilibrium position of the lung is at residual volume (RV). To sustain any volume in the lung above RV, force must be applied to the lung, and the lung will recoil with an equal and opposite force. At all volumes above RV, the lung recoils inward. The equilibrium position of the chest wall is at a relatively large volume, about 60% of total lung capacity. To sustain any volume in the chest wall below this point, the wall must be contracted and it will tend to recoil outward, opposite in direction from the lung. To sustain any volume in the chest wall above its equilibrium point, the wall must be actively enlarged and it recoils inward, the same direction as the lung.

In the intact respiratory system, the lung and chest wall are coupled and work together. Behavior of the respiratory system is determined by the individual properties of the lung and chest wall. The equilibrium position of the respiratory system will be at that volume at which the tendency of the lung to recoil inward is balanced by the tendency of the wall to recoil outward (Fig. 12–1). To sustain any volume in the respiratory system other than this resting volume, which is the functional residual capacity (FRC), a force must be applied to displace both lung and chest wall. The recoil pressure of the respiratory system (Prs) that develops is the algebraic sum of the individual recoil pressure of the lung (PL) and the chest wall (Pw). Thus,

Prs = PL + Pw; at FRC, Prs = 0

The lung is a distensible elastic body enclosed in an elastic container, the thoracic cavity. Just as a spring is described by the force required to stretch it to a certain length, so can the respiratory system be described by the static pressure required to change its volume. This relation between changes in volume and changes in pressure is termed compliance ($\Delta V/\Delta P$). For the various components of the respiratory system, compliance is determined by relating the change in volume to the given distending pressure. These various pressures are

1. Transpulmonary pressure (PL) or pressure across lung:

   PL = Palv − Ppl

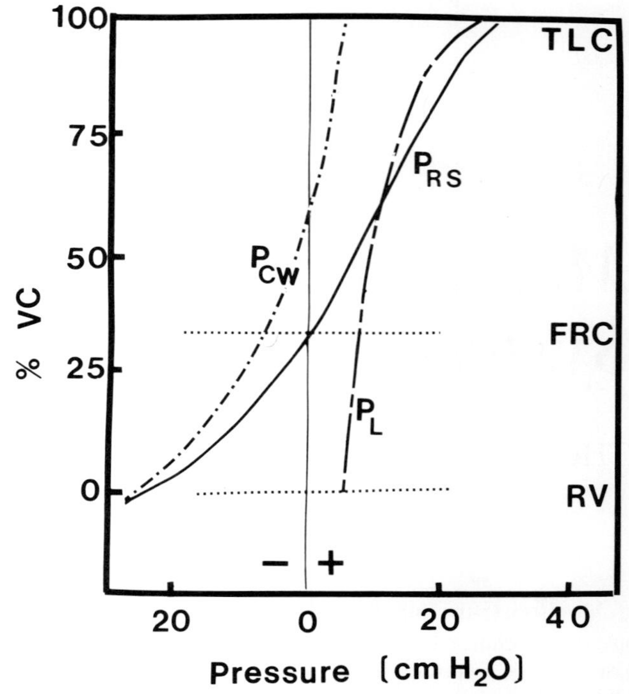

Figure 12–1. Recoil pressures for lung (PL), chest wall (Pcw), and total respiratory system (Prs) are plotted as a function of lung volume, in this case vital capacity (VC). (FRC = functional residual capacity, RV = residual volume, TLC = total lung capacity.)

   where Palv = alveolar pressure. It is the same as mouth pressure under condition of zero flow. Ppl = pleural pressure, usually estimated by esophageal pressure.

2. Pressure across chest wall (Pcw):

   Pcw = Ppl − Pbs

   where Pbs = pressure at body surface (atmospheric).

3. Transthoracic or pressure across respiratory system (Prs):

   Prs = Palv − Pbs

Because the pressure-volume curves for the respiratory system are curvilinear (see Fig. 12–1), compliance will vary from one portion of the curve to another, depending on the range of lung volume. Values, therefore, are usually obtained in the range of 1 L above FRC, where the P-V relationships are most linear.

The measurement of Ppl was previously estimated by a special thin-walled balloon in the midesophagus. The balloon was 10 cm long and was usually filled with 0.5 ml of air.[4] More recently, a 127-cm-long nasogastric tube incorporating a similar balloon became available commercially[5] and made the measurement more accessible to the clinician (Fig. 12–2). The PL is thus measured by connecting the balloon to one port of a differential pressure transducer while the other port of the transducer senses mouth pressure.

It is important to distinguish between the terms static and

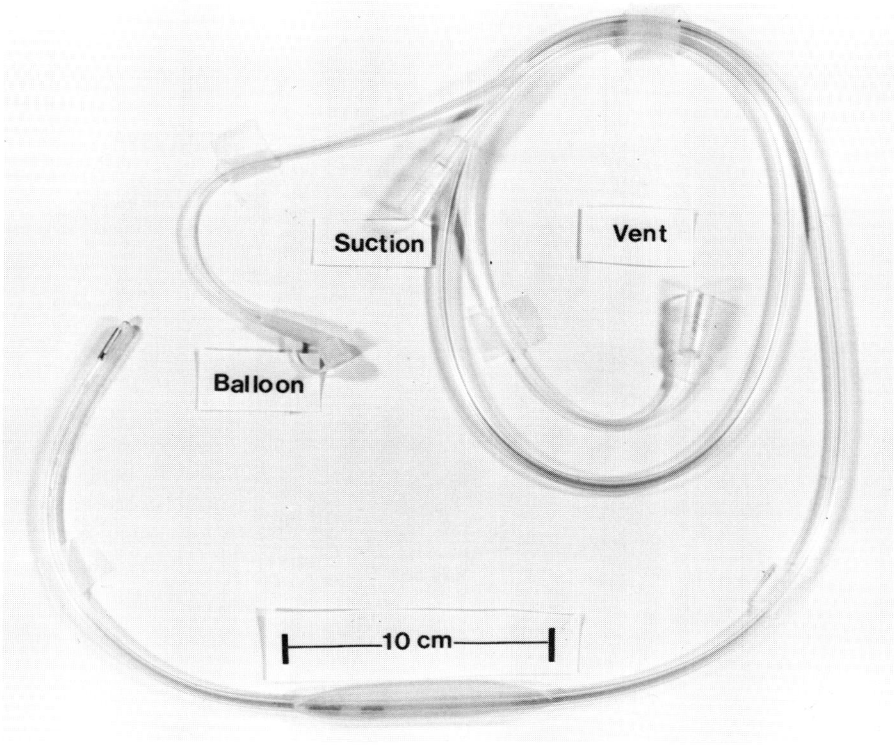

Figure 12–2. Commercially available nasogastric tube incorporating the 10-cm esophageal balloon used to measure pleural pressures. (Courtesy of NCC Division, Mallinkrodt, Argyle, NY.)

dynamic compliance. When no gas flow occurs and pressure and volume are kept constant, the measurement is termed static compliance. Such would be the case if the patient's lung were inflated and kept inflated by a device such as a super syringe. Dynamic compliance, on the other hand, relates pressure and tidal volume at the moment inspiration changes to expiration and flow ceases only momentarily. Ideally, these two compliance measurements are similar. However, if flow is impeded for some reason, such as by bronchoconstriction or a kink in the endotracheal tube, dynamic compliance is influenced by resistance to flow and does not reflect the true static compliance. The compliance figures differ by an amount related to flow resistance at end-inspiration. The difference in pressures (peak vs. plateau) can be readily appreciated in circuits utilizing a ventilator equipped with an inspiratory hold or pause with no flow or by merely clamping the expiratory tubing. The relationship between delivered volume and plateau pressure during this pause is often referred to as the quasi-static or effective compliance (Fig. 12–3).

DYNAMIC FORCES

Resistance

Resistance deals with conditions of airflow and describes the relationships between pressure and flow in the respiratory system. Resistance therefore is computed from pressure differences responsible for flow and the simultaneous measurement of airflow ($R = \Delta P/\dot{V}$).

Various components of the respiratory system contribute to the total resistance to airflow. These include an elastic component, the chest wall, and a nonelastic component, termed pulmonary resistance, which for practical purposes is synonymous with airway resistance (Raw). Approximately 60% of total respiratory resistance is Raw; the remaining 40% is accounted for by the chest wall. It is important to note that the chest wall in physiologic terms includes not only the bony thorax but the diaphragm and abdominal contents as well. Therefore, changes in muscle tone may affect measurements of total respiratory system resistance without actually altering Raw.

One other important factor to consider about Raw is the fact that resistance to airflow is determined by the size of the airways. Airways are largest at high lung volumes and smallest at low volumes, such as RV. Passive changes in Raw can thus occur with changes in lung volume in the absence of bronchodilation or constriction. Because the relationship of Raw to lung volume is not linear, the reciprocal of Raw, conductance (Gaw), is related to lung volume in linear fashion and is utilized to identify the presence of bronchoconstriction or bronchodilation. Such determinants of Raw are, by convention, made at FRC.

Methods of Measuring Resistance

Flow-Pressure-Volume Method. Simultaneous recordings of the three variables—flow, pressure, and tidal volume (Fig. 12–4)—provide the basis for this analysis. The change in pressure (ΔP) and change in flow ($\Delta\dot{V}$) between two points at which volume is identical are used to calculate resistance. This method of analysis is termed the isovolume technique. Another more complex technique relating pres-

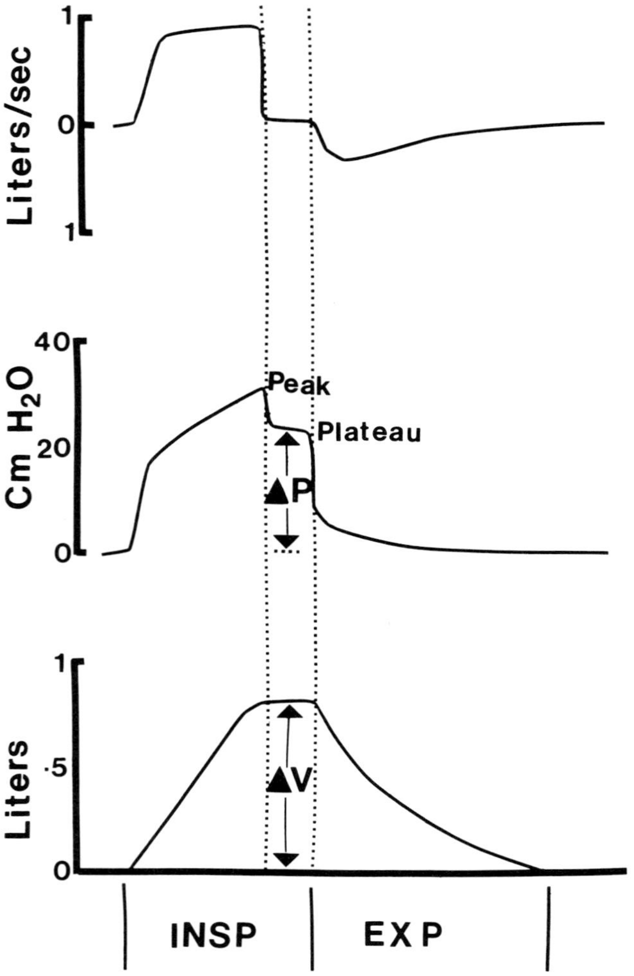

Figure 12–3. Flow (L/second), pressure (P), and tidal volume (V) typical of a cycle of mechanical ventilation incorporating an inspiratory pause (area enclosed between dotted lines).

sure flow and volume is termed the Comroe Nissel-Nims Technique.[6] With this method, static compliance is first calculated by dividing the total inspired volume by the pressure measured immediately prior to exhalation. Next, the point on the flow trace at which the expiratory flow is 0.5 L/second is noted, and the volume of gas remaining in the lungs at this point also is measured. Dividing this volume by the compliance value gives a pressure that is associated with a flow of 0.5 L/second and thus provides the calculation of resistance. In either of these cases, the use of airway or mouth pressure yields total respiratory system resistance, whereas the use of transpulmonary pressure (P_L) yields pulmonary resistance.

Passive Exhalation Method. The time it takes for the volume of the respiratory system to decrease to 37% of its initial pre-expiratory value is termed the time constant. This time constant (t) is essentially equal to the product of resistance and compliance. In this method, compliance is determined much as it is in the Comroe Nissel-Nims Technique, by relating $\Delta\dot{V}$ to ΔP prior to exhalation. If the interval to exhale to 370 ml (Fig. 12–5) is then measured and divided by this compliance value, another calculation of total respiratory system resistance is provided.

Forced Oscillation. Total respiratory resistance can be measured during quiet breathing by imposing rapid small sine wave oscillations at the mouth and recording the resultant sine wave flows and pressures. Such oscillations are produced by a loudspeaker or valveless pump. To measure the pressure change due to resistance, the components due to compliance and inertance must be eliminated. This is done by choosing the resonant frequency of the respiratory system (3–8 Hz) where compliance and inertance are 180° out of phase (i.e., equal magnitude and opposite sign) and cancel each other out. The oscillating pressure wave is then due to resistance alone.[7] One of the major advantages of this technique is that it requires very little patient cooperation. However, for this method to reflect changes in airway tone, lung volume changes must be taken into account.

Body Plethysmography. This technique, first described by DuBois et al,[8] has the advantage of specifically deter-

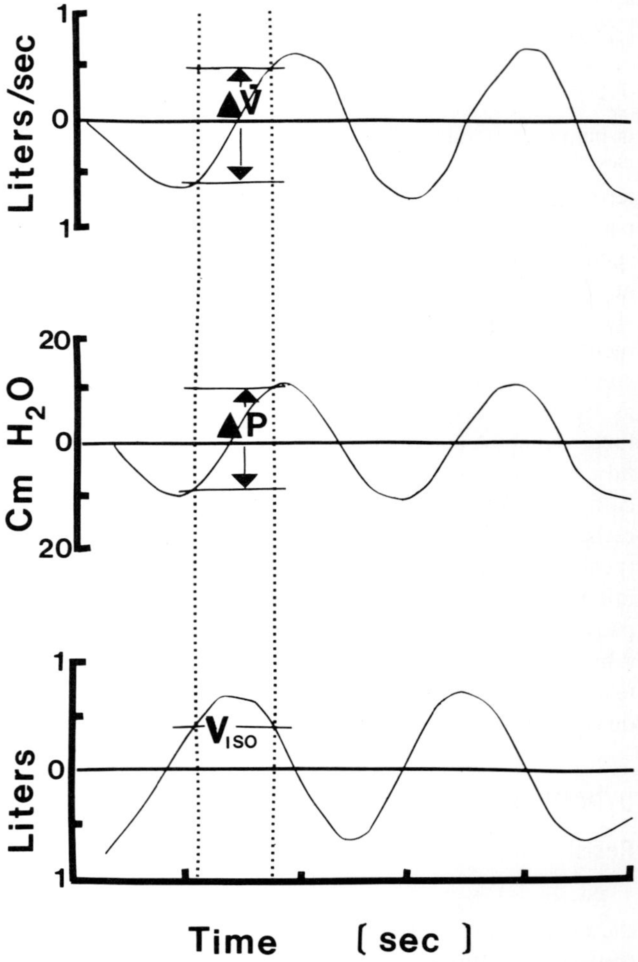

Figure 12–4. Simultaneous record of flow (V), pressure (P), and volume (V) for determination of resistance by the isovolume technique. Change in pressure (ΔP) and change in flow (ΔV) between two points at which volume is identical (V_{iso}) provide an estimate of resistance.

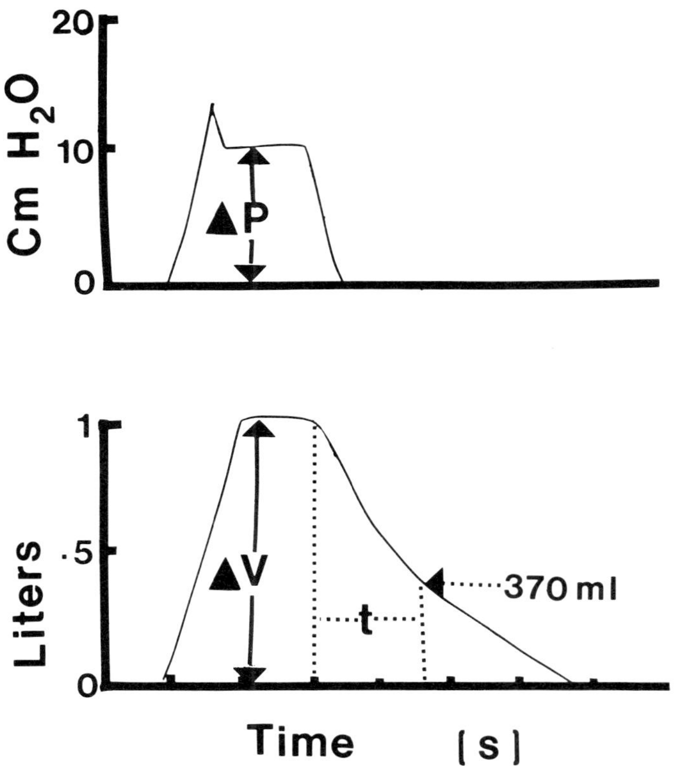

Figure 12–5. Passive exhalation method for estimating resistance. Compliance (C) is calculated as ΔV/ΔP prior to exhalation. (t = time required to exhale to 37% of pre-expiratory volume [i.e., 370 ml].) Resistance (R) is calculated from equation: R × C = t.

mining Raw and simultaneously providing a measurement of thoracic gas volume. The patient must sit in a closed box and breathe via a mouthpiece. As the patient takes panting-like breaths (2–3 breaths/second), flow at the mouth measured by a pneumotachograph is displayed on the y axis of an oscilloscope while box pressure is displayed on the x axis. The slope of this loop is usually measured between 0 and 5 L/second to compute resistance (Fig. 12–6*A*). When the airway is occluded during such panting, pressure at the mouth is displayed on the y axis and related to box pressure to estimate thoracic gas volume, which in most cases is the FRC (Fig. 12–6*B*).

Flow Interrupter Technique. A rapid, noninvasive, and convenient means of estimating respiratory system resistance utilizes rapid airway occlusion. The technique requires that pressure and flow at the mouth or airway opening be monitored while flow is suddenly interrupted at the end of an inspiration (Fig. 12–7). Such a condition occurs with the inspiratory pause phase on most anesthesia ventilators. A measure of total respiratory resistance (Rrs) is obtained by dividing the peak, or maximal, pressure (Pmax) by the flow ($\dot{V}$) immediately prior to the occlusion, or pause. The Pmax at end inspiration is the total dynamic pressure required for delivery of the set tidal volume at the set flow rate. As the end-inspiratory occlusion or pause takes place, Pmax immediately decreases to P_1 followed by a slower decay to a plateau value (P_2). The latter represents static elastic recoil pressure at the end-inspiratory lung volume and serves as the basis for calculating compliance. The immediate decrease in pressure from Pmax to P_1 with interruption of flow reflects the intrinsic flow resistance of the airways including the tracheal tube.

A calculation of this intrinsic airway resistance, or interrupter resistance (Rint), is obtained by subtracting P_1 from Pmax and dividing by flow (see Fig. 12–7). If one subtracts P_2 from P_1 and divides by flow the other component of Rrs, the effective additional resistance (ΔRrs) is estimated. The ΔRrs is also referred to as tissue resistance (Rti) and reflects the viscoelastic properties of lung tissue and inequalities in regional time constants.[9] The accuracy of estimating these components of flow resistance, and in particular ΔRrs, depends highly on a sufficiently long pause to allow pressure differences due to regional lung inhomogeneities to equilibrate at a stable P_2.

The intrinsic flow resistance (Rint) decreases with increasing inflation volumes because airway caliber is passively increased. On the other hand, tissue resistance, or ΔRrs, increases to a greater extent with inflation such that Rrs is greater also.

Conventional wisdom suggests that as inspiratory flow increases, Rrs should increase as well, especially in patients with obstructive airway disease. Actually, with inflation volumes of 0.5 L or more, Rrs was noted to decrease as flow was increased, and reached a value at a flow of 1.0 L/second, which was about half that at 0.25 L/second.[10] A comparable relationship between flow and Rrs was shown in 16 normal, anesthetized, paralyzed subjects[11] and in 8 patients with adult respiratory distress syndrome.[12] This decrease in Rrs with increasing flow is clinically relevant because it occurs in the flow range commonly used in the care of patients (0.75–1.0 L/second) and with commonly used tidal volumes (10 ml/kg). It appears that the increased airway resistance (Rint) with increased flow is offset by a greater decrease in ΔRrs, or Rti, than occurs as either flow rates or breathing frequencies increase.

Because total Rrs in chronic obstructive pulmonary disease (COPD) is nearly three times that of normal, it follows that both Rint, the airway resistance component, and ΔRrs, the tissue component, are increased. Time constant inequalities that affect ΔRrs play a greater role in COPD patients compared with healthy individuals and contribute considerably to the increased dynamic work of breathing. The magnitude of this tissue resistance is greatest with low inspiratory flows and large tidal volumes. Thus, the rapid shallow breathing pattern characteristic of COPD patients, especially with ventilatory failure, may be an attempt to reduce the work of breathing.

MEASUREMENT OF LUNG VOLUMES

In a clinical setting, only a few volumes are worth monitoring. The simplest of these is resting tidal volume. In

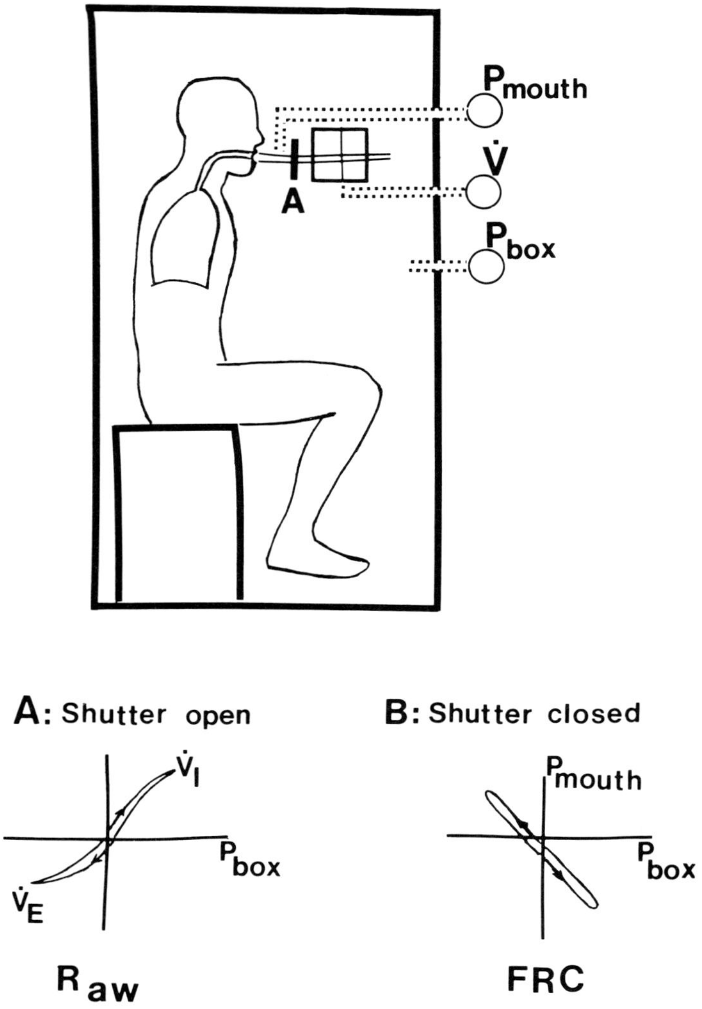

Figure 12–6. Constant volume body plethysmograph used to determine airway resistance (R_{aw}) and thoracic gas volume (FRC) by utilizing relationships of flow ($\dot{V}$), box pressure (P_{box}), and mouth pressure (P_{mouth}) during panting with shutter open *(A)* and closed *(B)*. ($\dot{V}_I$ = inspiratory flow, $\dot{V}_E$ = expiratory flow.)

patients connected to a ventilator or anesthetic circuit, it is important to place the measuring device (to be discussed later) on the expiratory side of the circuit and as close to the patient as possible. The latter is important to minimize the effects of added gas flow from continuous positive pressure circuits or fresh gas flow from the anesthesia machine.

VITAL CAPACITY

The vital capacity in the normal adult is basically a measure of stature, i.e., it strongly correlates with height. The volume represents the difference between the limits of maximum voluntary inspiration (total lung capacity) and voluntary expiration (Rv). Devices for measuring this volume will be discussed later.

Normally, vital capacity is more than 10 times the resting tidal volume. The relationship between the two is often used to estimate ventilatory reserve. In disease, the vital capacity is reduced by abnormalities of the bony thorax, increased lung stiffness, abdominal distension, muscle weakness, and loss of functional alveoli. Other factors, such as pain, fatigue, and poor effort, may prevent the maximum full inspiration and expiratory effort required for normal measured volumes.

FUNCTIONAL RESIDUAL CAPACITY

FRC refers to the gas remaining in the lungs at the end of a normal expiration or, more precisely, the volume at which the recoil of the lung and thorax oppose each other equally (see Fig. 12–1). In most clinical situations, a reduction in FRC is associated with increased lung recoil, i.e., decreased compliance.[13] Thus, there appears to be little advantage to measuring FRC in the usual clinical setting of the operating room or intensive care unit.

The techniques available for determining FRC are also somewhat difficult to apply in these areas. The most accurate technique utilizes the body plethysmograph as during Raw determinations. This technique is virtually impossible in the unconscious, artificially ventilated patient because of the need for confinement in an air-tight box. Lung volume by this technique is estimated by using Boyle's law to relate changes in box pressure to changes in mouth pressure during panting against a closed airway (see Fig. 12–6*B*).

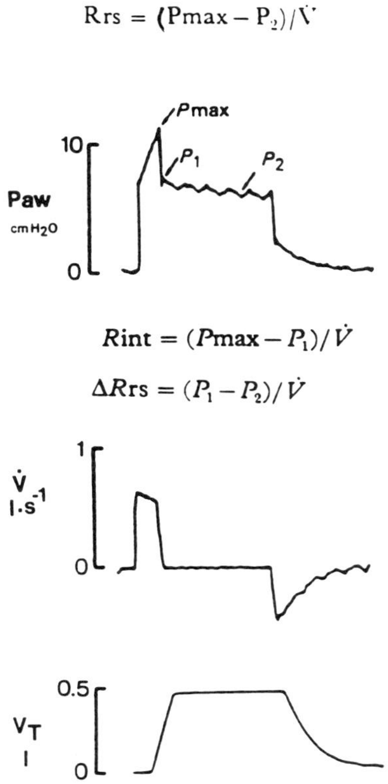

Figure 12–7. Tracing of flow (V̇), airway opening pressure, and changes in lung volume to illustrate rapid occlusion at end-inspiration during constant flow inflation. Pressure immediately decreases from its maximal value (Pmax) to an intermediate pressure (P_1) and then slowly decays to a plateau value (P_2). The various components of total respiratory resistance (Rrs) are calculated from these pressures and V̇. (See text for further explanation.)

Multiple Breath Nitrogen Washout

In this open circuit technique the washout of nitrogen (N_2) from the lungs after a switch from air breathing to 100% O_2 is measured. Although the volume of the lungs (FRC) is unknown, the gas content is 80% N_2. Thus, if the total volume of N_2 in the lungs could be measured, the volume of the alveolar gas (FRC) could be calculated. The expired gas can be collected into a large spirometer and its final N_2 content can be determined or, as is now more common, N_2 concentration and volume are continuously measured until expired N_2 concentration is 1.5% or less. This concentration can be achieved in 2–3 minutes in some healthy subjects, but in patients with obstructive lung disease, it may take 7–10 minutes or even longer. As a consequence of the slower N_2 washout, FRC is usually underestimated in such patients in contrast to values obtained for the true thoracic gas volume with the body plethysmograph.

Helium Dilution

This closed circuit technique is most frequently used during anesthesia and in other clinical settings. Essentially, the patient's alveolar gas is allowed to equilibrate with a closed circuit (e.g., a bag) containing a known amount of helium (He_I). At the beginning of rebreathing, there is no helium in the lung (He_I = 0). All helium is in the circuit or bag. At the end of a period of rebreathing, helium concentration is equal in both. Because initial (He_I) and final (He_F) helium concentrations are measured and volume of the bag or circuit is known, the volume of the lungs (FRC) can be calculated:

$$\text{FRC}(He_I) = \text{bag vol}(He_I) = He_F(\text{FRC} + \text{bag volumes})$$

Much like N_2 washout, the completeness of helium dilution requires communication of all lung areas with the circuit. In disease states, particularly when there is airway obstruction, this technique also underestimates the true FRC.

EFFECTS OF GENERAL ANESTHESIA ON RESPIRATORY MECHANICS

This section briefly discusses the effects of general anesthesia on lung volumes (FRC), pressure-volume, and pressure-flow behavior of the respiratory system. In normal recumbent humans, FRC is reduced by about 500 ml after the induction of general anesthesia. The changes occur within a minute and are not further affected by muscle paralysis. Although the exact mechanism is uncertain, simultaneous determination by N_2 washout and body plethysmography agree and suggest that the changes are probably not due simply to gas trapped in closed distal airways.[14] The degree of change appears to be related to body habitus and shape of the chest wall, which allow for differing degrees of diaphragmatic displacement.

The pressure-volume curve of the respiratory system tends to shift to the right 20–30 minutes after induction of anesthesia. Thus, compliance is decreased. The decrease in lung compliance is due to the decreased FRC. The changes can be likened to tightly strapping the chest. The altered function of the chest wall, therefore, secondarily affects the mechanical properties of the lungs.

The changes in pressure-flow relationships of the respiratory system with anesthesia are much less understood. Pulmonary resistance increases owing largely to placement of the endotracheal tube, reflex changes in airway smooth muscle tone, airway secretions, and increased lung recoil.

MEASUREMENTS OF VENTILATION

FLOW AND VOLUME

Peak Flow Meter

A measurement widely used in the management of variable airflow limitation is the peak expiratory flow rate (PEFR). PEFR is the maximal flow generated during a forced expiration begun at the position of full inspiration. This flow can be measured conveniently with hand-held flowmeters (Fig. 12–8) and is markedly affected by changes in the caliber of large airways. Because repeat measure-

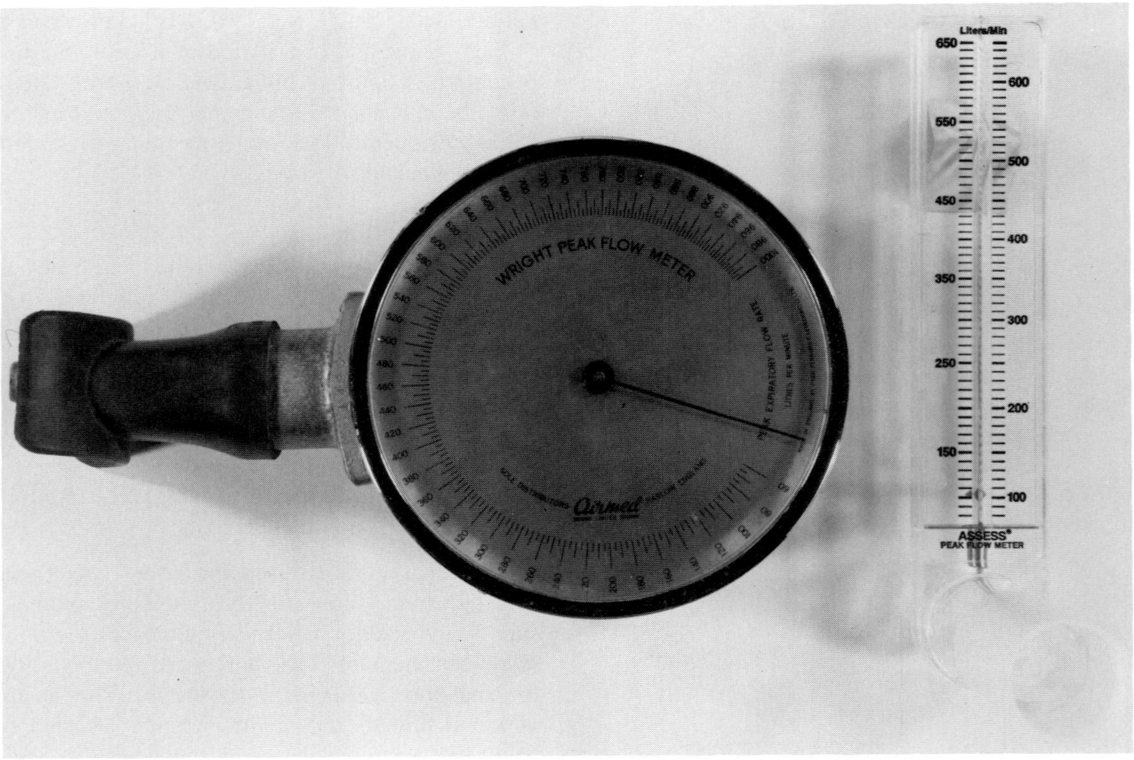

Figure 12–8. Hand-held peak flowmeters for bedside measurement. The original Wright meter is on the left. An inexpensive model is on the right. (Courtesy of Health Scan Products, Cedar Grove, NJ.)

ments are relatively easy to obtain, peak flow rates are often used to monitor responses to bronchodilator therapy in patients with bronchospasm.[15]

The original instrument, the Wright Peak Flow Meter, and all subsequent devices essentially measure a pressure drop that is directly related to flow in the presence of a fixed resistance. Normal peak flow values in young healthy males are greater than 500 L/minute.[16] Values less than 200 L/minute in the surgical candidate suggest impaired cough efficiency and the increased likelihood of postoperative complications.[17] The test is much less unpleasant and exhausting than the full forced vital capacity (FVC) maneuver; therefore, it is a valuable tool to identify gross pulmonary disability at the bedside. It is important, however, to understand that the measurement depends on effort and thus can be influenced by patient cooperation and other factors such as muscle weakness.

Pneumotachography

Of the devices available to measure flow, the pneumotachograph is perhaps the best known. A low mechanical resistance, usually in the form of a screen, is placed directly in the stream of gas flow. The pressure gradient across this resistance is sensed by a differential pressure transducer. This pressure drop is linearly related to flows as long as flow is laminar. To assure such linearity, it is important to select the pneumotachograph that is linear in the flow rates likely to be experienced (e.g., for forced expiration, 6–10 L/second; for quiet adult tidal volumes, 0–1 L/second).

The pressure gradient not only depends on flow rate but also on the density and viscosity of the gas mixture, as well as its temperature. Furthermore, condensation of moisture increases screen resistance and may cause turbulence. The latter is usually eliminated by electrically heating the screen. Despite these limitations, the rapid response, small dead space, and low resistance of the pneumotachograph render it useful for many flow measurement applications. Also, by integrating this flow electronically with respect to time, a measurement of volume can be derived.

Hot Wire Spirometers

A heated wire or thermistor will be cooled by a gas stream to an extent dependent on the flow rate and thermal conductivity of the gas. Such devices tend to be robust and easily sterilized and are suitable for applications not requiring a high degree of accuracy. They do, however, rapidly diminish in sensitivity if coated with foreign debris, such as airway secretions.

Ultrasonic Flowmeters

The velocity of gas flow can be measured with ultrasound. The basis for such ultrasonic flow meters is the measurement of the change in the speed of sound. Two piezoelectric crystals aligned at angles to the gas flow alternately transmit and receive bursts of oscillations at a frequency of 100 kHz. Such flowmeters have advantages over pneumotachographs in certain situations because of their low resistance. They also lack problems with moisture, positive pressure, or motion artifact, and they tend to be more stable, i.e., exhibit less drift over long periods of use.

Thoracoabdominal Movement

Konno and Mead measured movements of the chest wall and abdomen and demonstrated their relationship to tidal volume during unobstructed respiration.[18] Various transducers and devices have measured the changes in physical shape and, hence, electric properties of the chest and abdomen during respiration. These devices have consisted of mercury in rubber strain gauges, magnetometers, impedance electrodes, and, most recently, the inductance plethysmograph (Respitrace, Ambulatory Monitoring Inc., Ardsley, NY).[19] The device consists of two insulated coils: one encircles the abdomen and the other the rib cage. The coils are contained within a net-like garment and are excited by a high-frequency oscillation. The inductance of the coils changes with respiration as a function of changes in cross-sectional area of the compartment enclosed within. The instrument can detect apnea and eliminates the need for mouthpieces or masks. For measurement of volumes, however, devices such as the Respitrace must be regarded as semiquantitative unless rigorous calibrations with a spirometer are repeatedly performed.

Collection Devices

Gas Meters

Dry gas meters (Parkinson-Cowan) have been used to measure minute ventilation for extended periods. The meters have large internal volumes and have an intolerable amount of dead space, which allows rebreathing. Thus, gas must be collected via a one-way valve on the expiratory limb or in a Douglas bag and then emptied into the meters. The gas volumes are collected at ambient temperature and pressure saturated with H_2O vapor (ATPS); but for precision, respiratory volumes are expressed at body temperature and pressure saturated with H_2O vapor (BTPS). Many tables are available for such conversion factors, which are calculated as follows:

$$\text{BTPS vol} = \frac{\text{ATPS vol} \times (273 \times \text{Tb°C})}{(273 \times \text{Tatm°C})} \times \frac{(\text{Patm} - \text{PH}_2\text{O Tb})}{(\text{Patm} - \text{PH}_2\text{O Tatm})}$$

where:

Tb = body temperature
Tatm = atmospheric temperature
PH_2O = vapor pressure of H_2O at Tb or Tatm
Patm = atmospheric or barometric pressure

Spirometers

The classic Collins water seal spirometers are reliable and accurate, and they are the reference standard for volume measurements. However, they are cumbersome and poorly suited for use in the operating room or intensive care unit. Dry spirometers, such as the rolling seal or wedge types, have similar problems of bulk but have better frequency responses that render them more useful for forced respiratory maneuvers. In addition, they often have electrical circuitry capable of differentiating the volume signal to obtain flow. The principle shortcoming of such spirometers lies in the difficulty of applying them to systems in which rebreathing takes place or additional fresh gas is added to the volume inspired.

Mechanical Respirometers

In contrast to the limitations of conventional spirometers, mechanical respirometers provide less expensive, more convenient access to the breathing circuit. Such devices estimate volume from rotation of a low-friction inertia vane. The widely used Wright respirometer contains a geared system that converts rotation of the vane into movements of hands over a dial. Tangential slots around the vane ensure that flow is recorded in only one direction. Thus, the respirometer may be inserted between the endotracheal tube and breathing circuit. The small dead space (20–25 ml) and relatively low resistance render it suitable for spontaneously breathing patients. The instrument is more accurate at flows of about 20 L/minute. These flows are typical of quiet expiration in adults. Because of inertia, resistance, and momentum of the vane, the Wright respirometer tends to overread at higher flows and underread at lower flows. Although changes in gas composition have relatively little effect, water condensation is often a problem after extended use, as is accumulation of foreign material.

These problems of the Wright respirometer are shared by a number of similar devices. Such is the case of the larger, widely used Drager respirometer. The latter senses flow in either direction and must be placed in an area of unidirectional flow—hence, its conventional location on the expiratory limb of an anesthesia circuit. Such placement of the respirometer renders it prone to overreading because of increases in fresh gas delivery to the system, particularly when such delivered flows are large (e.g., 10 L/minute).[20]

PRESSURE MONITORING

Airway pressures (Paw) may be simply measured with the aneroid gauges present in anesthesia or ventilator circuits. These simple measurements are usually sufficiently accurate to make some assessment of patient or system mechanics. However, for most accurate assessment of patient mechanics, pressures should be sensed as close to the patient as possible and ideally at the inlet to an endotracheal tube. Automated measurement of Paw from the same sites can be obtained with simple strain gauge transducers such as those used to measure blood pressure. If an esophageal balloon is used to measure intrapleural pressure, a differential pressure transducer, i.e., one with two ports, will be needed. The negative or subambient intrapleural pressure

(Ppl) must be referenced to mouth pressure (Pm) to derive the transpulmonary (P_L) pressure. Thus,

$$P_L = Pm - Ppl$$

MEAN AIRWAY PRESSURE

The instantaneous positive pressure applied to the airway varies during each respiratory cycle. The physiologic effects of such pressure depend not only on the instantaneous magnitude of the pressure but also on the length of time it is applied to the airway. A clinically useful composite of all the pressures transmitted to the airway during mechanical ventilation is the mean airway pressure ($\overline{Paw}$), or the average pressure present in the airways. The $\overline{Paw}$ can be thought of simply as the area under the pressure curve. This can be estimated graphically or by electronic integration of the signal from a pressure transducer. In either case, $\overline{Paw}$ is computed by dividing the area under the pressure curve by the total time for each entire respiratory cycle (i.e., inspiration plus expiration).

Many factors influence the values of $\overline{Paw}$. Perhaps the most obvious is the deliberate use of high driving pressures or excessive volumes to ventilate. Prolongation of the inspiratory time also increases $\overline{Paw}$ because the inspiratory portion of the pressure curve has the largest area per unit time.

Essentially, the area under the pressure curve varies directly with the duration of inspiration and inversely with the length of expiration. Thus, any increase in the ratio of inspiratory time to expiratory time (I:E ratio) will increase $\overline{Paw}$ if the total respiratory cycle is unchanged. One such prolongation of inspiration occurs with an end-inspiratory pause in which the lungs are held inflated at a fixed level of pressure or volume for a time. The longer this time, the greater the area under the pressure curve and the higher the $\overline{Paw}$.

Expiratory resistance or ''retard'' has been employed in mechanical ventilation to mimic breathing with pursed-lips in the hope of allowing more uniform lung emptying. The technique involves placement of a variable resistance in the exhalation circuit to slow expiratory flow. Thus, expiratory pressures decrease more slowly and contribute to increasing $\overline{Paw}$.

Positive end-expiratory pressure (PEEP) is a maneuver in which airway pressure is not allowed to decrease to atmospheric pressure at the end of exhalation. The elevated baseline pressure that results with PEEP also contributes to an increased $\overline{Paw}$. Conversely, if negative pressure were applied during exhalation to produce negative end-expiratory pressure, $\overline{Paw}$ would decrease.

For the most part, $\overline{Paw}$ is considered synonymous with mean alveolar pressure ($\overline{Palv}$). Thus, $\overline{Palv}$ is closely related to the efficiency of ventilation, oxygenation, and cardiovascular effects of mechanical ventilation as well as to lung distention and barotrauma. For the most part, $\overline{Paw}$ can be assumed to equal $\overline{Palv}$ unless differences arise because of inspiratory or expiratory flow or resistance losses.[21] The same $\overline{Palv}$ may be achieved with the application of PEEP or by extending the inspiratory time with an end-inspiratory pause. However, these two methods of achieving the same $\overline{Palv}$ have different effects on gas exchange. PEEP predictably increases dead space, whereas the inspiratory pause appears to improve the efficiency of alveolar ventilation by producing a lower maximal $\overline{Palv}$ for a greater portion of the total respiratory cycle. This appears to promote recruitment of refractory, but potentially functional, lung areas.[22]

PRESSURE-VOLUME RELATIONSHIPS

The effects of circuit distensibility or compliance in reducing the actual amount of delivered volume are well recognized. This distension of tubing can be minimized with stiffer circuit material. However, another factor, compression of gases with the tubing, is not prevented. The latter is a function of circuit size (including humidifier) and the pressure at end-inspiration. The discrepancies due to gas compression become important when small tidal volumes are used, particularly in the face of high inflation pressures. This gas, which is compressed during inspiration, is added to the measured expired volume to overestimate volume. The gas composition is also diluted by the same added gas, resulting in decreased tension from expired gases such as CO_2.

Figure 12–3 illustrates typical flow, volume, and pressure relationships in the patient circuit during cycling of a mechanical ventilator. Maximum (peak) airway pressure and plateau or static pressures can be readily measured and, in conjunction with VT measurements, can be used to estimate dynamic compliance (Cdyn) and static compliance (Cst):

$$Cdyn = V_T/\text{peak pressure}$$
$$Cst = V_T/\text{plateau pressure}$$

Plateau pressure can be estimated during the period of no flow, i.e., of inspiratory pause, available on most ventilators. If this is not available, the expiratory limb of the circuit may be clamped. The value is often referred to as quasistatic because it is not truly a static measurement such as might be obtained by inflation with a super syringe or passive deflation against an occlusion.

Another useful form of quasistatic compliance measurement applicable to ventilator patients receiving constant inspiratory flow is based on the pressure rise per unit of time during such flow.[23] This pulse method is based on the principle that when a constant flow is introduced to the respiratory system, the rate of increase in pressure is inversely related to the compliance of the system.[24]

$$\text{Compliance} = \frac{\text{flow}}{\Delta\ \text{pressure/time}}$$

Because flow $= \Delta$ volume/time,

$$\text{Compliance} = \frac{\Delta\ \text{volume}}{\Delta\ \text{pressure}}$$

Values for compliance estimated by this method in all patients were nearly identical to those obtained by relating delivered VT to the plateau pressure and are considered quasistatic. The estimation of compliance by this pulse method is illustrated in Figure 12–9.

Compliance can also be estimated from pressure-volume loops provided by a new pressure-based flow sensor and respiratory gas monitor (Capnomac Ultima, Datex Inc., Helsinki, Finland). The pressure on the x-axis at the delivery of a VT on the y-axis (Fig. 12–10*A*) can be used to calculate compliance, whereas Δ volume/time approximates dynamic compliance. Changes in flow resistance can be estimated by the character of the flow-volume curves (Fig. 12–10*B*). Both of these measurements can help to subjectively assess the adequacy of ventilation in the anesthetized patient.

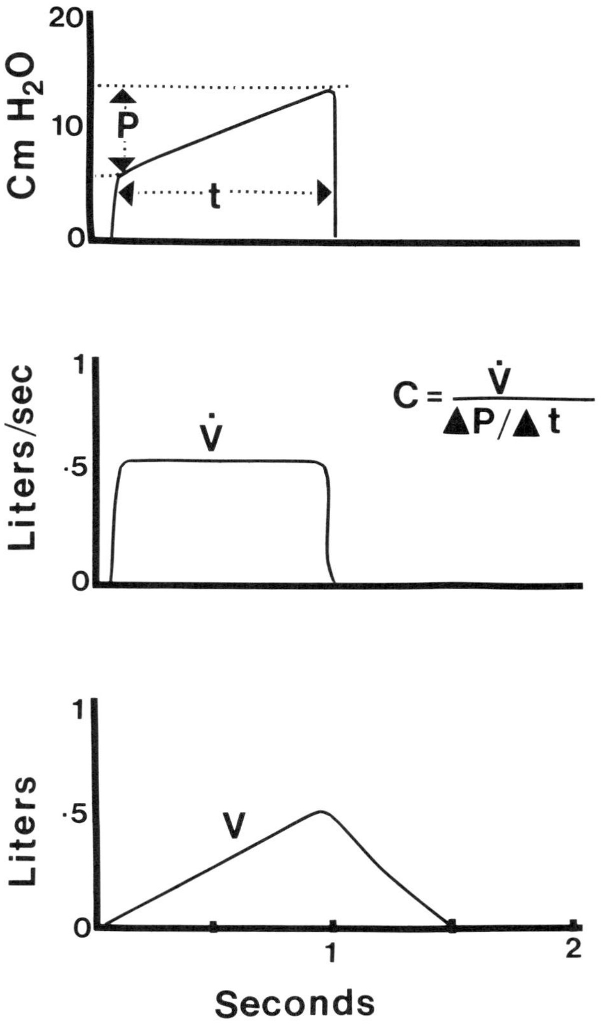

Figure 12–9. Pulse method for estimating compliance (C) by dividing the constant flow ($\dot{V}$) by the rate of rise of pressure (ΔP/Δt).

MONITORING GAS EXCHANGE

CAPNOMETRY AND CAPNOGRAPHY

Analysis of carbon dioxide (CO_2) in the respired gases has become commonplace in the operating room setting. The actual measurement of CO_2 concentration is termed capnometry. Capnography, on the other hand, refers to the display of this concentration on a screen or recording chart, usually as a function of time. This latter ability to actually see the CO_2 waveforms enhances their interpretations in contrast to the simple digital readout of CO_2 concentrations (capnometry).

Methods of Analysis

The most common systems available for breath-by-breath CO_2 analysis utilize the infrared absorption of gases. Infrared light of a certain wave length (2600 or 4300 nm) passes through a reference gas sample containing no CO_2 or a known amount. The light also passes through the gas sample to be analyzed. The CO_2 absorbs the infrared energy in proportion to its concentration. Photocells sense a difference in intensity between light transmitted through the reference chamber and that transmitted through the sample gas which is related to the CO_2 concentration in the sample chamber.

Instruments monitor CO_2 either by direct in-line measurement at the sample site by a flow-through device or by aspiration of the gas sample into a separate monitor. The in-line sensors, such as are available from Siemens Corporation and Hewlett-Packard, are placed directly in the breathing system with a special adapter and are ideally as close to the patient as possible. Such sensors are fragile, expensive, and somewhat cumbersome, and they have relatively large dead space. On the other hand, moisture is not a problem, and there is no limitation on where the actual monitor console need be placed. Such monitors also do not require standard gases for calibration.

Analyzers that continually withdraw gas samples are more common. It is important to realize that this sample gas (up to 250 ml/minute) must be returned to the anesthesia system or scavenger to avoid pollution due to anesthetic gases. Such analyzers are plagued by excess moisture and require that the small-diameter sampling tube be as short as possible in order to improve response time. The response time is inherently shorter with in-line sensors, which analyze gas directly in the airway and thus lack the delay and mixing of gases associated with suction and transport to a remote infrared analyzer.

Capnograms

Normally, CO_2 concentrations are displayed with respect to time (Fig. 12–11). However, the expired volume may also substitute for time on the abscissa. Such curves require more effort and equipment but may yield more information regarding respiratory dead space.[25]

During each breath, gases emerge sequentially from the

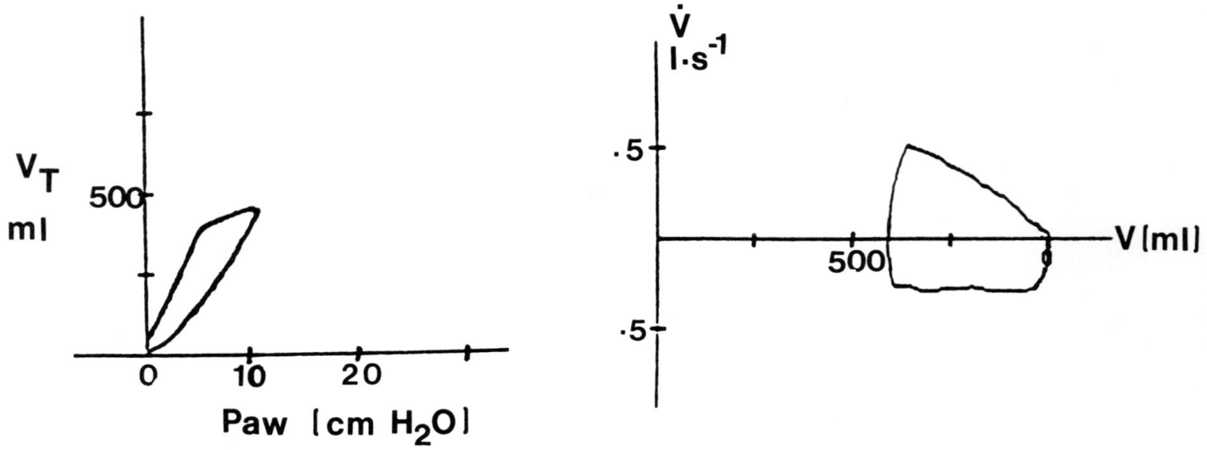

Figure 12–10. Typical normal pressure-volume *(A)* and flow volume *(B)* curves recorded in a paralyzed, mechanically ventilated patient with the pressure-based flow sensor of the capnomac ultima. (Courtesy of Date, Helsinki, Finland.)

conducting airways that compose the anatomic dead space and finally from the alveoli. The characteristic CO_2 waveform displayed in Figure 12–11 exhibits three basic phases during expiration that are followed by an abrupt decrease in CO_2 concentration during inspiration. During the initial phase (A), the CO_2 concentration remains near the previous inspiratory concentration and reflects gas cleared from the anatomic dead space. In phase B, which follows, there is an admixture of residual dead space gas and alveolar gas that is beginning to emerge from lung areas having relatively short conducting airways. The CO_2 concentration increases rapidly in phase B to approach alveolar levels. The final phase C is often referred to as the alveolar plateau because it represents gas washed out of the alveoli. The slope of this phase is increased when there is nonhomogeneous mixing of gas, such as with airway obstruction. It also increases with exercise and hypermetabolic states. Because of this upward slope of the alveolar plateau, end-tidal CO_2 tension ($PETCO_2$) exceeds the mean alveolar CO_2 ($PACO_2$). Normally, however, there is sufficient mixing with dead space gas such that $PETCO_2$ is somewhat less than arterial CO_2 tension ($PaCO_2$).

Clinically, $PETCO_2$ is used to provide a noninvasive estimate of $PaCO_2$. Under ideal conditions, even in the presence of general anesthesia, the difference between them is negligible.[26] The most significant determinant of a gradient between $PaCO_2$ and $PETCO_2$ is the presence of lung disease characterized by the extremes of high relationships between ventilation and blood flow ($\dot{V}/\dot{Q}$), which behave functionally as dead space areas. These poorly or nonperfused lung units have a $PaCO_2$ of nearly zero. Thus, the weighted average of all lung units will yield a low $PETCO_2$.

The other major sources of abnormally low $PETCO_2$ values involve sampling errors. The most obvious is a system leak such that some of the exhaled volume is lost and not subjected to sampling. Most leaks are obvious, but some, such as a poorly sealed endotracheal tube cuff, may require more intense scrutiny. The other sampling problem relates solely to aspirating devices and the relationship of sampling volume to patient VT. In adults, the expired VTs are usually sufficient to supply the aspirated sample. Dilution of this sample with CO_2 free fresh gas can occur if the sample site is far from the patient's airway, or if exhaled volumes decrease (as with shallow breathing). The implications of this problem in pediatric systems with high fresh gas flows are obvious.

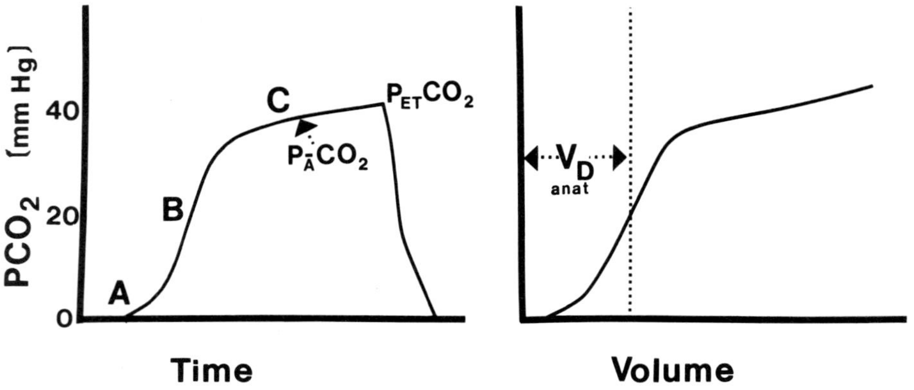

Figure 12–11. Characteristic waveform of exhaled CO_2 plotted as a function of time and of volume. ($PACO_2$ = mean alveolar CO_2 tension, $PETCO_2$ = end-tidal CO_2 tension, VDanat = anatomic deadspace.)

DEAD SPACE

Respiratory deadspace is most often considered in physiologic terms, i.e., the volume of inspired and expired gas that does not partake of gas exchange in the alveoli. The physiologic dead space (VDphys) has two components: the conducting airways or anatomic dead space (VDanat) and the alveolar dead space (VDalv). In most instances, VDanat among different individuals relates to factors affecting lung volume and airway size, such as posture, tracheal intubation, bronchodilators, and pneumonectomy. The capnograph allows estimation of VDanat (see Fig. 12–11) by what is often referred to as the equal area method first described by Aitken and Clark Kennedy.[27] Essentially, VDanat is identified by the vertical line that subdivides phase B into two equal portions by assuming this volume represents the abrupt transition between the conducting dead space and the alveolar gas component. Unfortunately, this technique tends to overestimate VDanat when the slope of the alveolar phase (phase C) is increased (i.e., hypermetabolic states and asynchronous alveolar emptying with lung diseases).

The alveolar component of physiologic dead space is not measured directly but is determined from simultaneous measurements of VDanat and VDphys. The latter, which exceeds VDanat by inclusion of VDalv, is now usually defined by the mixing equation originally devised by Bohr but later modified by Enghoff, who substituted arterial CO_2 tension ($Paco_2$) for alveolar CO_2 tension ($PAco_2$) in the equation:

$$\text{VDphys} = \text{VT} \times \frac{(Paco_2 - P\bar{E}co_2)}{(Paco_2 - PIco_2)}$$

Clinical measurement of VDphys requires a sample of arterial blood for $Paco_2$. Mixed expired gases are collected over several minutes in a large bag or spirometer to measure mixed expired CO_2 tension ($P\bar{E}co_2$). VT can be conveniently measured with a Wright respirometer. Because no rebreathing usually is involved, inspired CO_2 tension ($PIco_2$) is usually assumed to be zero. It is also important to subtract apparatus deadspace (facemask, valves, tubing) to obtain accurate measurements of VDphys.

In normal patients, this VD accounts for less than one third of VT (i.e., $VD/VT \leq 0.33$). The calculation of VD/VT helps to estimate the relationship between alveolar ventilation and minute ventilation, or more specifically the efficiency of ventilation. Such information can be very useful in determining whether to institute or discontinue mechanical ventilation.

CLINICAL APPLICATIONS AND LIMITATIONS

The useful information presented by capnography provides particular insight into the mechanical and gas exchange function of the patient's lung. However, changes in metabolic and cardiovascular function are also detectable. For example, malignant hyperthermia with its increased CO_2 production may be detected early by the increase in $PETco_2$ and particularly by the more prominent slope of the alveolar plateau. Capnography can also indicate the quality of the circulation. A sudden decrease in $PETco_2$ could be the result of decreased blood flow to the lungs secondary to hypovolemia, embolism, or myocardial dysfunction.

Perhaps the greatest emphasis on capnography concerns its potential for identifying malfunction of breathing systems such as the anesthesia circuit (Fig. 12–12). For example, incompetent unidirectional valves, exhausted or bypassed CO_2 absorber, or inadequate fresh gas flows may all result in increased $PETco_2$. This is usually due to rebreathing and, therefore, will be accompanied by increased inspired CO_2 (i.e., above zero). The same rise in CO_2 without breathing may be due either to addition of exogenous or endogenous CO_2 or to hypoventilation as a result of leaks in the system.

Sudden drops in $PETco_2$ to near zero generally signal major problems. These include extubation, esophageal intubation, total airway obstruction, and complete disconnection. Numerous reports have emphasized the utility of capnography in detecting these phenomena. However, it is important to recognize that the capnogram associated with any of these events is nonspecific and provides no clue to diagnosis. It simply indicates that there is a major problem. This may be due to instrument malfunction (e.g., clogged sample tube) and may provide false information or divert attention from the patient. It is prudent to rule out any of the above problems before troubleshooting the CO_2 analyzer. In summary, capnography appears to be approaching the status of a standard-of-care item in anesthesia. Nevertheless, it is important that the anesthetist realize its limitations as an early warning device.

ASSESSING ADEQUACY OF OXYGENATION

Techniques for measuring and sampling delivered oxygen concentrations are discussed elsewhere (see Chapter 11). The end result, the arterial O_2 tension (Pao_2), requires, of course, analysis of arterial blood (see Chapter 27). To fully understand the implications of a given value of Pao_2, one must examine its relationship to the alveolar O_2 tension (PAo_2) by utilizing the alveolar air equation. This equation describes the gas content in lung alveoli and, in particular, the alveolar partial pressure for oxygen (PAo_2). PAo_2 can be calculated beginning with the Po_2 in the trachea (PIo_2). The partial pressure of water vapor at body temperature (PH_2O Tb), which is 47 mmHg, must be included in the calculation because, as dry gas enters the airway, it is warmed to body temperature and humidified prior to reaching the alveoli:

$$PIo_2 = FIo_2\,(Pb - 47)$$

where PIo_2 = partial pressure of O_2 in trachea, FIo_2 = fractional O_2 concentration in inspired air, Pb = atmos-

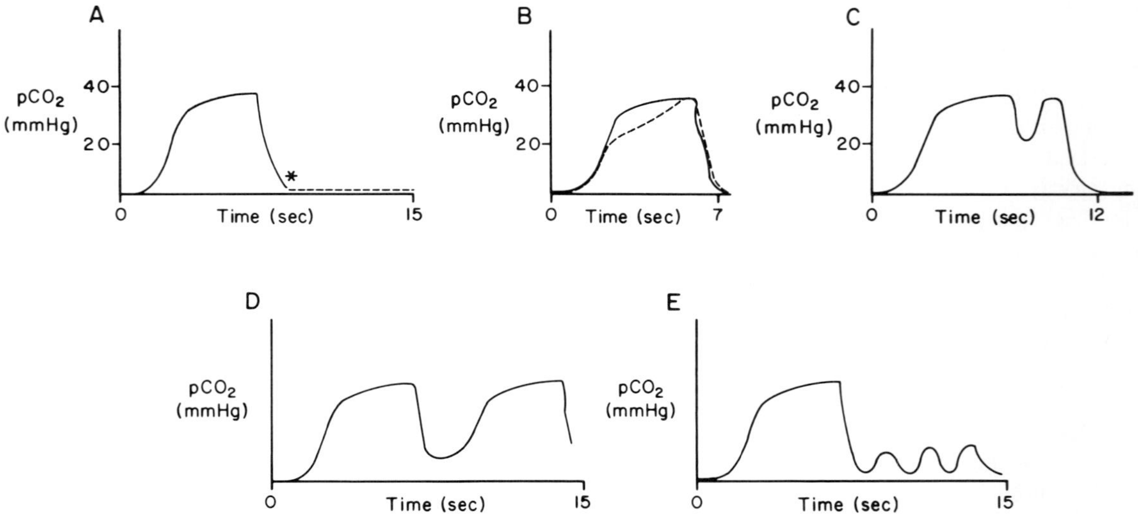

Figure 12–12. Exhaled carbon dioxide waveforms in clinical situations. *A*, Breathing circuit disconnection (*) or esophageal intubation that produces no carbon dioxide at sampling site. The specific cause can be differentiated by clinical findings. *B*, The normal waveform is compared with that occurring during airway obstruction (endotracheal tube kinking or obstructive lung disease). The expiratory ascent to the alveolar plateau is slowed, and the inspiratory portion is unaffected. *C*, Spontaneous ventilation during controlled mechanical ventilation. *D*, Rebreathing within a breathing circuit causes elevation of the baseline of the capnogram owing to inspiration of exhaled CO_2. *E*, Normal breath followed by panting. The sine waves do not reflect alveolar gas because of the rapid respiratory rate with limited inspiratory time.

pheric pressure (760 mmHg at sea level), and 47 mmHg = partial pressure of H_2O vapor at 37°C.

Because carbon dioxide is added to the alveolar gas from the blood, the $PACO_2$ must be subtracted. The $PaCO_2$ is usually substituted because the $PACO_2$ cannot easily be measured. The $PaCO_2$ must be corrected by the respiratory exchange ratio (R) because less carbon dioxide is produced than oxygen is consumed (normally R = 0.8). Thus, in a normal subject breathing ambient air at sea level, the PAO_2 can be estimated assuming a normal $PaCO_2$ of 40 mmHg:

$$PAO_2 = PIO_2 - PaCO_2/R$$
$$PAO_2 = 0.21\ (760 - 47) - 40/0.8 = 100\ \text{mmHg}$$

This shortened form of the equation produces a small (5%) underestimation of PAO_2 when R = 0.8. If R = 1.0, there is no error.

If ventilation and pulmonary blood flow were matched perfectly, the PaO_2 would be the same as the PAO_2. However, regional variation in both prevents the development of this ideal situation. Thus, even in healthy individuals, the PaO_2 is 10–15 mmHg less than PAO_2. This difference is referred to as the A-a gradient, i.e., the alveolar-arterial gradient for oxygen (A-aO_2). Its magnitude reflects the degree of inefficient gas exchange on the part of the lung. Because this gradient is exaggerated by disease, the interpretation of a value of PaO_2 is only valid when the PAO_2 is considered as well.

This is illustrated by an example of two patients, both of whom have identical PaO_2 values while breathing room air:

Patient A	Patient B
PaO_2 65 mmHg	PaO_2 65 mmHg
$PaCO_2$ 56 mmHg	$PaCO_2$ 28 mmHg

The PAO_2 value in patient A is calculated as:

$$0.21\ (760 - 47) - 56/0.8 = 80\ \text{mmHg}$$

The A-aO_2 is thus 15 mmHg, which is still within the normal range and does not indicate lung disease. The specimen was drawn from a healthy young patient following a large dose of a narcotic. In patient B, the PAO_2 value is

$$0.21\ (760 - 47) - 28/0.8 = 115$$

The A-aO_2 in this case is 50 mmHg, nearly four times the normal value, which clearly indicates abnormal oxygen transfer. The patient in this example was breathing very rapidly with signs of marked dyspnea and had pneumonia.

The normal A-aO_2 tends to increase in normal humans and in patients with pulmonary disease as FIO_2 is increased. This finding tends to limit the usefulness in assessing gas exchange in patients when FIO_2 is changed. One attempt to standardize PaO_2 values was suggested by dividing PaO_2 by FIO_2,[28] the oxygenation ratio. This ratio produces rather confusing units and fails to account for differences in $PaCO_2$. Another index of gas exchange less affected by the FIO_2 is the ratio of arterial to alveolar O_2 (a/APO_2).[29] Although not as stable as originally suggested, a/APO_2 is still far more constant than the A-aO_2. It is most stable above PAO_2 values of 200 mmHg, i.e., when FIO_2 exceeds 0.3.[30] In normal persons the a/A values are about 0.7–0.8.

Estimation of Shunt ($\dot{Q}s/\dot{Q}t$)

The most common causes of arterial hypoxemia are low or decreased ventilation-perfusion relationships ($\dot{V}/\dot{Q}$) in numerous regional lung units. Because these regional units are underventilated and normally perfused, there is a low PAO_2 and a decreased PaO_2 in the blood leaving to enter the systemic circulation. If increasing the FIO_2 has little or no effect in increasing PaO_2, right-to-left shunting is assumed to be the cause of the low PaO_2. A regional lung unit is the site of shunting when it has essentially zero ventilation and relatively persistent perfusion, such that $\dot{V}/\dot{Q}$ approaches zero. Blood flows past an alveolus whose PAO_2 is zero and retains its low venous O_2 tension prior to entering the systemic circulation.

The calculation of this shunt ($\dot{Q}s/\dot{Q}t$) has been utilized as an indicator of the ability of the lungs to oxygenate blood. To calculate shunt, one must know barometric pressure, PAO_2, $PaCO_2$, hemoglobin concentration, and mixed venous O_2 tension ($P\bar{v}O_2$). Thus, equipment consists of barometer, blood gas analyzer, blood sampling devices, and either pulmonary artery or central venous catheter to obtain $P\bar{v}O_2$. It is also necessary to ensure that the patient is breathing 100% O_2 for at least 20 minutes.

The formula used to calculate shunt is

$$\dot{Q}s/\dot{Q}t = \frac{Cco_2 - CaO_2}{Cco_2 - C\bar{v}O_2}$$

where Cco_2 = O_2 content of ventilated and perfused pulmonary capillaries, CaO_2 = O_2 content of arterial blood, and $C\bar{v}O_2$ = O_2 content of mixed venous blood.

Because perfused capillaries ventilated with O_2 are exposed to the PAO_2, the latter must be calculated from the alveolar air equation. The PAO_2 is multiplied by the solubility coefficient (0.003) to calculate dissolved O_2. Because each gram of hemoglobin also holds 1.39 ml of O_2 when fully saturated,

$$Cco_2 = (Hb \times 1.39) + (PAO_2 \times 0.003)$$

The Cco_2 represents an ideal O_2 content in the pulmonary end capillaries, which assumes that hemoglobin concentration in that vascular bed is equal to that of arterial blood and that the O_2 tension of the capillary blood is equal to the ideal PAO_2 calculated from the alveolar air equation. This ideal PAO_2 is not always achieved in all lung areas, and the variable inaccuracies that arise from this assumption may result in larger-than-expected calculations of $\dot{Q}s/\dot{Q}t$.[31]

Arterial Hb is not fully saturated; therefore,

$$CaO_2 = (Hb \times 1.39 \times \%saturation) + (PaO_2 \times 0.003)$$

$C\bar{v}O_2$ is calculated in similar fashion except that $P\bar{v}O_2$ is multiplied by 0.003 to estimate dissolved O_2. Thus,

$$C\bar{v}O_2 = (Hb \times 1.39 \times \%saturation) + (P\bar{v}O_2 \times 0.003)$$

The accuracy of the $\dot{Q}s/\dot{Q}t$ calculation also depends on many other variables, such as cardiac output, respiratory quotient, the quality of the mixed venous sample, or an assumed arterial venous O_2 content difference. Thus, many clinicians prefer to use the simpler $A\text{-}aO_2$ rather than shunt to assess adequacy of oxygenation. Others have proposed shortcut methods for calculating % shunt, assuming unchanged cardiac output and FIO_2 of 1.0.[32]

$$\%\ shunt = \frac{A\text{-}aO_2}{10}$$

The importance of cardiac output must be emphasized in patients with acute respiratory failure who often experience a reduction in cardiac output secondary to continuous positive pressure breathing. Cardiac output profoundly affects PaO_2 for a given level of shunting. Wide variation in a patient's PaO_2 can occur because of changes in cardiac output without an actual change in pulmonary status. The same increases and decreases in cardiac output can raise or lower the calculated $\dot{Q}s/\dot{Q}t$ values. Thus, neither $\dot{Q}s/\dot{Q}t$ nor $A\text{-}aO_2$ can be meaningfully interpreted unless cardiac output changes are considered.

Diffusion

The role of diffusion in producing abnormalities in gas exchange is of little importance and for practical purposes can be ignored under resting conditions.[26] Limitation of diffusion would consist of an oxygen gradient between alveolar and end-capillary O_2 tensions. This is normally zero. Only if cardiac output is increased and FIO_2 is decreased does such a gradient develop. Examples of such situations would be vigorous exercise and breathing at altitudes above 10,000 feet.

Diffusing capacity of the lungs (D_L) is defined as the rate at which a gas enters the blood divided by its driving pressure. The driving pressure is the gradient between alveolar and end-capillary tensions. D_L is expressed in milliliters per minute per millimeter of Hg. Measurement of D_L provides information about the amount of functioning capillaries in contact with ventilated air spaces such as may occur in certain pulmonary vascular and parenchymal disease states. The brief inhalation of nontoxic low concentrations of carbon monoxide (CO) has become standard for this purpose in most pulmonary function laboratories. The equipment requirements and the large variations in normal values for each of the techniques (single breath, steady state, rebreathing) render the measurement well outside the usual clinical realm and well beyond the scope of this discussion. For a comprehensive discussion of the interpretation and significance of such testing, the reader is referred to an excellent review.[33]

Carbon monoxide has several features that make it useful to measure D_L. It has 200 times the affinity for hemoglobin that oxygen does. Thus, CO will not build up rapidly in plasma. Most important, however, is the low CO concentration in the blood under normal conditions, such that pulmonary capillary tension can be assumed to be zero. Of the techniques utilizing CO, the rebreathing method is least influenced by changes in $\dot{V}/\dot{Q}$ distributions.

To measure D_L with CO, three values must be obtained. These are the milliliters of CO transferred from alveoli to blood per minute, the mean alveolar CO tension ($P\bar{A}CO$), and the pulmonary capillary CO tension ($PcCO$).

$$D_LCO = \frac{CO\ ml/minute/mmHg}{P\bar{A}CO - PcCO}$$

In the *single breath method*, the patient inspires a dilute mixture of CO and holds his or her breath for 10 seconds. During this period, CO leaves alveolar gas to enter the blood in proportion to the diffusing capacity. The milliliters of CO transferred is calculated from the percentage of CO in alveolar gas at the beginning and end of the breath hold by infrared analysis. To do this, FRC must be calculated from the helium dilution and then added to the inspiratory volume. The Pcco is essentially zero and can be ignored, but Pcco is not the simple average of PCO at the beginning and end of the breath hold and must be calculated by a special equation that considers alveolar volume as reflected by the ratio of inspired to expired helium concentrations.[34]

The single breath method requires very little patient cooperation, and is relatively simple to perform because it requires no blood samples. It is relatively insensitive to the back pressure of CO in the blood and is only mildly affected by ventilation-perfusion inequalities. Disadvantages include the extensive mathematical computations and the requirement for a 1.3-L or greater inspired volume with a breath hold. The latter may not be feasible in the dyspneic patient or in the exercising subject.

The *steady state method* is regarded as more physiologic than the single breath test because it can be measured in dyspneic or exercising patients. The patient breathes a low (0.1%) concentration of CO for about 30 seconds or until a steady state is established. The rate of CO disappearance from alveoli to blood is measured along with $P\bar{A}_{CO}$. Unfortunately, with steady state methods, $P\bar{A}_{CO}$ is again difficult to measure and must be estimated using an assumed value for arterial blood samples. The measurement is sensitive to maldistributions of ventilation and perfusion, which may lead to a small error in estimates of $P\bar{A}_{CO}$ and VD/VT but large variations in $D_{L}CO$. On the other hand, the steady state technique requires less equipment and fewer calculations. Little patient cooperation is needed because measurements are made during normal tidal breathing. Therefore, steady state $D_{L}CO$ can be measured during many activities, including general anesthesia.

Another technique for measuring $D_{L}CO$ is the *rebreathing method*. Here the patient exhales either to RV or to FRC. Then, a known volume of test gas is breathed at a rate of about 1 breath/second for 30 seconds while gas concentrations (He, O_2, CO) are monitored continuously. The rate of CO uptake is calculated from the known system volume and the rate of CO disappearance. The pressure gradient for CO is calculated from the exponential disappearance, assuming Pcco is zero. This measurement can be performed in patients with small VCs (1.3 L) and in most clinical settings. It appears to be the method least sensitive to inequalities of ventilation and perfusion. Although some patients have difficulty breathing at the fixed rate required, rebreathing appears to be the technique of choice when the single breath method cannot be used.[35]

In general, however, rebreathing steady state and single breath techniques give rather similar results. Normal values, depending on individual laboratories, range from 20 to 30 ml/minute/mmHg. Increases in $D_{L}CO$ occur with body size, age, lung volume, exercise, body position, and alveolar CO_2 and O_2 tensions. Therefore, changes in these variables must be considered when interpreting $D_{L}CO$ values.

Oxygen Cost of Breathing

During normal quiet breathing, the oxygen cost of breathing ($\dot{V}O_2R$) accounts for only a small amount (< 5%) of total O_2 consumption. As levels of ventilation increase, the power output of the respiratory muscles increases and $\dot{V}O_2R$ assumes a greater magnitude.[36] Such increases in $\dot{V}O_2R$ are common in patients who require mechanical ventilation and have been attributed to the increased ventilation required by the catabolic states as well as the increased work of breathing and inefficiency of respiratory muscles. A reasonable estimate of the increase in $\dot{V}O_2R$ can be made by measuring the difference in O_2 consumption ($\dot{V}O_2$) during spontaneous ventilation and that of the relaxed patient receiving mechanical ventilation.

The measurement of $\dot{V}O_2$ in ventilated patients has proven rather difficult. As a result, in many critical care unit patients, studies have calculated $\dot{V}O_2$ from the Fick equation:

$$\dot{V}O_2 = (\text{cardiac output}) \times (\text{arteriovenous } O_2 \text{ content difference})$$

This method has significant limitations because of the coupling that may occur between O_2 delivery and consumption.[37]

Prior clinical determinations of $\dot{V}O_2$ have utilized measurements of inspired and expired gas concentrations (O_2, CO_2, N_2). Collection of expired gas required a spirometer[38] or meteorologic balloon.[39] More recently, metabolic carts with rapid analyses of inspired and expired gases have made such clinical measurements of $\dot{V}O_2$ more feasible (see Chapter 20). Similarly rapid anesthetic gas analyzers that are presently available render similar, albeit approximate, calculations in anesthetized patients.

The O_2 consumed by aerobic metabolism entirely depends on the O_2 uptake from inspired gas. For a normal person at rest, this O_2 uptake ($\dot{V}O_2$) is usually about 250 ml/minute. This volume inspired per unit of time is equal to the volume of inspired gas times the fractional concentration of O_2 (i.e., VI × FIO_2). Likewise, the exhaled oxygen volume equals the product of exhaled volume and fractional expired O_2 concentration (VE × FEO_2). The $\dot{V}O_2$ equals the difference between the inspired and expired O_2:

$$\dot{V}O_2 = (VI \times FIO_2) - (VE \times FEO_2)$$

The measurement of both VI and VE at the same time is somewhat impractical. Therefore, VE, which is more easily measured, is utilized in the equation to calculate $\dot{V}O_2$:

$$\dot{V}O_2 = VE\ (STPD) \times \frac{FIO_2\ (1 - FEO_2 - FECO_2)}{1 - FIO_2 - FICO_2} \times FEO_2$$

Because variations in the relationship of VE to VI may be produced by changes in the respiratory quotient (i.e., the ratio of CO_2 production to O_2 consumption), another calculation that utilizes the rate of N_2 exchange in the lungs is utilized. Because no uptake or elimination of N_2 occurs in a steady state, the inhaled N_2 volume (VI × FIN_2) is equal to the exhaled N_2 volume (VE × FEN_2). The equation utilizing expired nitrogen (FEN_2) and inspired nitrogen (FIN_2) concentrations can serve as a check on the validity of the above calculation with O_2 and CO_2:

$$\dot{V}O_2 = VE\ (STPD) \left[\frac{FEN_2 \times FIO_2}{FIN_2} \right] - FEO_2$$

It is important to note that both calculations report $\dot{V}O_2$ in terms of VE defined at standard temperature, pressure dry (STPD). This normalization for temperature and pressure allows comparisons to be made for $\dot{V}O_2$ at different altitudes and hence barometric pressures because the volume occupied by any gas depends on temperature and pressure.

$$\dot{V}STPD = \dot{V}ATPS \times \frac{PB - PH_2O}{760} \times \frac{273}{273 + T}$$

where: $\dot{V}STPD$ = volume of gas at standard temperature and pressure, dry
$\dot{V}ATPS$ = volume of gas at ambient temperature and pressure, saturated with water vapor
PB = barometric pressure
PH_2O = vapor pressure of water at T
273 = absolute O°C
T = ambient or room temperature

A similar formula can be utilized to correct to $\dot{V}STPD$ from the volume of gas measured at ambient temperature and pressure, dry ($\dot{V}ATPD$). The latter is merely substituted in the equation for $\dot{V}ATPS$.

SIMPLE MONITORING OF VENTILATION WITHOUT INSTRUMENTATION

In the early days of anesthesia with diethyl ether, most patients breathed spontaneously, and ventilation was monitored by simple inspection of neck, chest, and abdomen. The data were correlated with gas movement by observation of the rebreathing bag. Normal quiet breathing in the supine position is primarily abdominal, i.e., consisting of diaphragmatic descent. Rib cage movement is nonexistent until higher levels of breathing occur or when mechanical ventilation is utilized. In the presence of respiratory obstruction, diaphragmatic power overcomes the action of the rib cage, and the rib cage may be drawn in paradoxically. This phenomenon is particularly evident in an infant or child whose thorax is far more flexible than that of an adult. The same paradoxical chest movement occurs with respiratory muscle weakness and is most evident in high levels of spinal cord injury.

In addition to simple patient observation, the adequacy of ventilation can be estimated by listening to breath sounds through esophageal or precordial stethoscopes. When placed on the precordium, the stethoscope can provide adequate transmission of heart sounds, but breath sounds may be inaudible, especially during spontaneous breathing. In this case, the relatively low flow rates (< 0.2 L/second) are difficult to hear. When placed over the jugular notch, however, the turbulent flows around the larynx are easily heard and can provide clear evidence of laryngeal spasm even when mild. Without question, the simplest and most reliable of the respiratory monitors is the esophageal stethoscope, which conveys both heart and breath sounds clearly. Wheezing, leaks, and accumulation of secretions can be readily identified. In addition, the absence of breath sounds is a simple, reliable monitor of circuit disconnection in the presence of mechanical ventilation and should trigger a response to check out other components of the breathing circuit, such as ventilator bellow and pressure gauges.

Monitoring movement of the breathing bag has been a mainstay of simple monitoring practice during spontaneous or manually controlled ventilation. One must be careful not to be deceived by errors produced by excessively high fresh gas flows or aspiration of gas from the circuit either for analysis or by the scavenging system. Thus, regardless of how simple such respiratory monitoring methods are, each has the potential for misinterpretation; therefore, a sound understanding of physiologic and mechanical concepts is as important for simple monitors as it is for the more sophisticated techniques.

REFERENCES

1. Black LF, Hyatt RE: Maximal static respiratory pressures in generalized neuromuscular disease. Am Rev Respir Dis 1971; 103:641–650.
2. O'Donoghue WJ, Baker JP, Bell F, et al: Respiratory failure in neuromuscular disease management in a respiratory intensive care unit. JAMA 1971; 235:733–735.
3. Pavlin EG, Holle RH, Schoene R: Recovery of airway protection compared to ventilation in humans after paralysis with curare. Anesthesiology 1989; 70:379–380.
4. Milic-Emili J, Mead J, Turner JM, et al: Improved technique for estimating pleural pressure from esophageal balloons. J Appl Physiol 1964; 19:207–211.
5. Leatherman NE: An improved balloon system for monitoring intraesophageal pressure in acutely ill patients. Crit Care Med 1978; 6:189–192.
6. Comroe JH, Nissell OL, Nims RG: A simple method for concurrent measurement of compliance and resistance to breathing in anesthetized animals and man. J Appl Physiol 1954; 7:225–228.
7. Fisher AB, DuBois AB, Hyde RW: Evaluation of the oscillation technique for the determination of resistance to breathing. J Clin Invest 1968; 47:2045–2057.
8. DuBois AB, Botelho SY, Comroe JH: A new method for measuring airway resistance in man using a body plethysmograph: Values in normal subjects and in patients with respiratory disease. J Clin Invest 1956; 35:326–335.
9. Bates JHT, Milic-Emili J: The flow interruption technique for measuring respiratory resistance. J Crit Care 1991; 6:227–238.
10. Tantucci C, Corbeil C, Chasse M, et al: Flow resistance in patients with chronic obstructive pulmonary disease in acute respiratory failure. Am Rev Respir Dis 1991; 144:384–389.
11. D'Angelo E, Robatto FM, Calerinin E, et al: Pulmonary and chest wall mechanics in anesthetized paralyzed humans. J Appl Physiol 1991; 70:2602–2610.
12. Eissa NT, Ranieri VM, Corbeil C, et al: Analysis of behavior of the respiratory system in ARDS: Effects of flow, volume, and time. J Appl Physiol 1991; 70:2719–2729.
13. Katz JA, Zinn SE, Ozanne GM, Fairley HB: Pulmonary chest wall

and lung-thorax elastance in acute respiratory failure. Chest 1981; 80:304–311.
14. Westbrook PR, Stubbs SE, Sessler AD, et al: Effects of anesthesia and muscle paralysis on respiratory mechanics in normal man. J Appl Physiol 1973; 34:81–86.
15. Banner AS, Shah RS, Addington WW: Rapid prediction of need for hospitalization in acute asthma. JAMA 1976; 235:1337–1338.
16. Leiner GC, Abramowitz S, Small MJ, et al: Expiratory peak flow rate, standard values for normal subjects, use as a clinical test of ventilatory function. Am Rev Respir Dis 1963; 88:644–651.
17. Stein M, Koota GM, Simon M, et al: Pulmonary evaluation of surgical patients. JAMA 1962; 181:765–770.
18. Konno K, Mead J: Measurement of the separate volume changes of the rib cage and abdomen during breathing. J Appl Physiol 1967; 22:407–422.
19. Cohn MA, Rao ASV, Broudy M, et al: The respiratory inductive plethysmograph: A new noninvasive monitor of respiration. Bull Eur Physiopathol Respir 1982; 18:643–658.
20. Mapleson WW: Physical aspects of automatic ventilators; some application of basic principles. *In* Mushin MA, Rendell-Baker L, Thompson PW, Mapleson WW (eds): Automatic Ventilation of the Lungs, 3rd Ed. Oxford: Blackwell Scientific, 1980; 132–151.
21. Marini JJ: Positive end expiratory pressure and adult respiratory distress syndrome. J Crit Care 1992; 7:137–141.
22. Marcy TW, Marini JJ: Inverse ratio ventilation in ARDS: Rationale and implementation. Chest 1991; 100:494–504.
23. Surratt PM, Owens O: A pulse method of measuring respiratory system compliance in ventilated patients. Chest 1981; 80:34–38.
24. Rattenborg CC, Holaday DA: Constant flow inflation of the lungs, theoretical analysis. Acta Anesthesiol Scand 1967; 23:211–223.
25. Fletcher R: Deadspace, invasive and noninvasive. Br J Anaesth 1985; 57:245–249.
26. Whitesall R, Assidao C, Gollman D, Jablonski J: Relationship between arterial and peak expired carbon dioxide pressure during anesthesia and factors influencing the difference. Anesth Analg 1981; 60:508–512.
27. Aitken RS, Clark Kennedy AE: On the fluctuation in the composition of the alveolar air during the respiratory cycle in muscular exercise. J Physiol (Lond) 1928; 65:389–411.
28. Model JH, Graves SA, Ketover A: Clinical course of 91 consecutive near-drowning victims. Chest 1976; 70:231.
29. Gilbert R, Keighley JF: The arterial-alveolar oxygen tension ratio. An index of gas exchange applicable to varying inspired oxygen concentrations. Am Rev Respir Dis 1974; 109:142–145.
30. Gilbert R, Auchinsloss JH, Kuppinger M, Thomas MV: Stability of the arterial-alveolar oxygen partial pressure ratio. Effects of low ventilation-perfusion ratios. Crit Care Med 1979; 7:267–272.
31. Marshall BE: Anesthesia for one lung ventilation. Anesthesiology 1988; 69:630–631.
32. Chiang ST: A nomogram for venous shunt (Q_S/Q_T) calculation. Thorax 1968; 23:563.
33. Staub NC: Alveolar-arterial oxygen tension gradient due to diffusion. J Appl Physiol 1963; 18:673–680.
34. Forster RE, DuBois AB, Briscoe WE, Fisher AB: The Lung, Physiologic Basis of Pulmonary Function Tests, 3rd Ed. Chicago: Yearbook, 1986; 295.
35. Davies NJH: Does the lung work? 4. What does the transfer of carbon-monoxide mean? Br J Dis Chest 1982; 76:105–124.
36. Bradley ME, Leith DE: Ventilatory muscle training and oxygen cost of sustained hyperventilation. J Appl Physiol 1978; 45:885–892.
37. Stock MC: The oxygen cost of breathing. Chest 1992; 101:1486–1487.
38. Wilson RS, Sullivan SF, Malm JR, Bowman FO: Oxygen cost of breathing following anesthesia and cardiac surgery. Anesthesiology 1973; 39:387–393.
39. Field S, Kelly SM, Macklem PT: The oxygen cost of breathing in patients with cardiorespiratory disease. Am Rev Respir Dis 1982; 129:9–13.

SECTION FOUR

Monitoring the Central and Peripheral Nervous System

CHAPTER

13

Monitoring of Intracranial Pressure

WAYNE K. MARSHALL, M.D.

Brain function directly depends on oxygen supply and blood flow. Cerebral blood flow (CBF) and metabolism are affected by intracranial pressure (ICP), anesthesia, and blood partial pressures of oxygen, carbon dioxide, and hydrogen ion. Preoperative neurologic function can be determined with a routine neurologic examination including level of consciousness, memory, cognition, sensation, motor strength, and cranial nerve evaluation, as well as cerebellar tests. Except during certain forms of regional anesthesia, such tests are impossible intraoperatively and in the early portions of the recovery period.

Various methods to monitor intraoperative cerebral function, such as measurement of ICP or of regional CBF and recording of cellular electrical activity using electroencephalography (see Chapter 15) or evoked potentials (see Chapter 16), have therefore evolved. Of these techniques, intraoperative measurement of regional CBF using ^{133}xenon washout is limited to only a few medical centers because it is invasive (inhalation, intravenous or intracarotid administration of radioactive tracer is required), it requires radiation exposure, and it provides only an intermittent measurement of blood flow. ICP, however, is more easily evaluated. This chapter discusses the origin and importance of normal cerebrospinal fluid (CSF) pressure and intracranial hypertension, the effects of commonly used drugs and anesthetics on ICP, the rationale for clinical measurement of ICP, and the common devices used for measurement of ICP.

PHYSIOLOGY OF CEREBRAL CIRCULATION

NORMAL CEREBRAL BLOOD FLOW

Normal CBF in awake humans averages 50 ml · gm^{-1} · min^{-1} for whole brain.[1,2] Blood flow to the brain provides nutrients (glucose) and oxygen and removes the waste products of cellular metabolism (carbon dioxide, lactic acid, and so on). Brain cells acutely depend on adequate blood flow to accomplish these tasks. As CBF decreases, both the delivery of glucose and oxygen and the removal of waste products decrease.

At levels of CBF under 25 ml · gm^{-1} · min^{-1}, early changes in cerebral electrical activity become apparent.[3] These electroencephalographic changes represent ischemia of brain cells. CBF of 25 ml · gm^{-1} · min^{-1} corresponds to a cerebral perfusion pressure (CPP) of 45 mmHg (Fig. 13–1).[4] This correlation of CPP to level of CBF provides a readily available, objective clinical indication of adequacy of cerebral perfusion.

CBF is directly responsible for delivery of glucose and oxygen to, and removal of carbon dioxide, lactic acid, and other waste products from, the actively metabolizing cells of the brain. In normal individuals, blood flow is regulated by several factors broadly categorized as either metabolic or neurogenic.[5] These various factors interact to produce an effect known as autoregulation of CBF. Cerebral autoregulation is the maintenance of cerebral blood flow over a pressure range of 60–150 mmHg. Metabolic, neurogenic, and autoregulatory effects are all ultimately mediated through changes in cerebral vessel size and, therefore, changes in the relative resistance to blood flow.

Metabolic Control

Four metabolic mechanisms affect CBF: hydrogen ion concentration, oxygen, carbon dioxide, and basic cerebral metabolic rate.

pH Effect

The concentration of hydrogen ions in the tissues surrounding the vessels in the brain affects blood flow. This is known as the pH effect. The relationship of pH to hydrogen ion concentration is illustrated in the following equation:

$$pH = -\log [H^+]$$

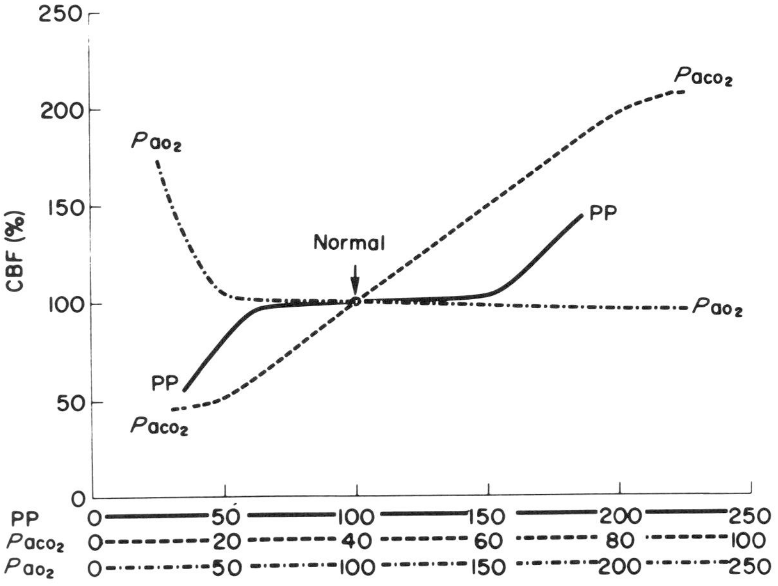

Figure 13–1. The effects on cerebral blood flow (CBF) of arterial oxygen tension (Pao_2 [torr]), arterial carbon dioxide tension (Pao_2 [torr]), as a percentage of control, and cerebral perfusion pressure (PP [torr]). Cerebral blood flow is little affected by Po_2 except during hypoxia. Autoregulation of CBF occurs between perfusion pressures of about 60–150 torr. CBF is quite sensitive to changes in $Paco_2$. (From Michenfelder, JD: The cerebral circulation. *In* Prys-Roberts C [ed]. The Circulation in Anaesthesia. London, Blackwell, 1980; 212.)

Therefore, increased hydrogen ion concentration produces a lower pH (acidosis), and decreased hydrogen ion concentration produces a higher pH (alkalosis).[6] An increased extracellular fluid hydrogen ion concentration decreases pH, and the resulting acidosis produces vasodilatation and increases blood flow.[7] Likewise, decreased extracellular fluid hydrogen ion concentration increases pH, and this alkalosis produces vasoconstriction and a decrease in blood flow.[7] Substances that affect pH by changing the hydrogen ion concentration are given in Table 13–1. The pH effect, although functional, usually plays a secondary role in regulation of cerebral blood flow when compared with other factors.[8]

Oxygen and Carbon Dioxide Effects

The effects of the respiratory gases oxygen and carbon dioxide are usually considered in relation to the arterial partial pressure of each gas (Pao_2 and $Paco_2$).

Pao_2 Effect. Insufficient oxygen supply to the brain, whether due to inadequate volume of blood or to inadequate oxygen tension in the blood, increases CBF through vasodilation of the cerebral vessels.[9] This occurs when the Pao_2 falls below 60 mmHg (Fig. 13–1).[9] High arterial oxygen tensions only minimally affect the cerebral vessels by vasoconstriction (see Fig. 13–1).[10]

$Paco_2$ Effect. The arterial tension of carbon dioxide exerts a vasoactive effect through two mechanisms. The direct effects of $Paco_2$ are progressive vasoconstriction and decreased blood flow in response to a decreased $Paco_2$,[11] and progressive vasodilatation and increased blood flow in response to an increased $Paco_2$ (see Fig. 13–1).[12] These effects are independent of changes in hydrogen ion concentration.[13–15]

The indirect effect of $Paco_2$ operates through the pH effect. Both arterial and tissue carbon dioxide combine with water to produce carbonic acid, which in turn dissociates to increase hydrogen ion concentration.[7] Therefore, increased $Paco_2$ produces increased hydrogen ion concentration, decreased pH, and resultant vasodilation and increased blood flow.[7, 9] Decreased $Paco_2$ produces decreased hydrogen ion concentration, increased pH, and resultant vasoconstriction and decreased cerebral blood flow.[16]

The duration of the vasoconstrictive effect of decreased $Paco_2$ through hyperventilation may also be limited. After an unpredictable period (as long as 72 hours), the effect of continuous hyperventilation begins to decrease. This is thought to be due to the buffering of the induced pH changes by the cerebrospinal fluid and renal compensatory mechanisms.

Metabolic Rate Effect

Finally, the overall basic rate of metabolism of brain cells also affects blood flow.[17] An increase in cerebral metabolic rate results in vasodilatation and increased blood flow.[18, 19] A decrease in cerebral metabolic rate results in vasoconstriction and decreased blood flow.[19]

TABLE 13–1. SUBSTANCES AFFECTING CEREBRAL VASCULATURE

Substance Affecting (H^+)	Effect on pH	Effect on Cerebral Vessels
Increased arterial Pco_2	Acidosis	Vasodilation
Decreased arterial Pco_2	Alkalosis	Vasoconstriction
Increased bicarbonate ion	Alkalosis	Vasoconstriction
Decreased bicarbonate ion	Acidosis	Vasodilation
Increased metabolic acid (lactic, pyruvic)	Acidosis	Vasodilation
Decreased metabolic acid	Alkalosis	Vasoconstriction

Neurogenic Control

Cerebral vessels are also under the control of the autonomic nervous system. The effects of neurogenic influences on cerebral blood flow are usually masked by the powerful metabolic mechanisms previously described.[7] However, the intracranial vessels are innervated by both sympathetic and parasympathetic fibers.[20] Under certain circumstances (e.g., severe exercise, intracranial hemorrhage, stroke), strong sympathetic outflow produces cerebral vasoconstriction and decreased cerebral blood flow.[17, 21]

Autoregulation

The multiple mechanisms described previously interact through control of cerebral vessel size to produce CBF levels that closely match the metabolic needs of the brain. Normally, this system of autoregulation operates over a range of mean CPPs from 60 to 150 mmHg (see Fig. 13–1).[4] Pressures below a mean of 60 mmHg decrease blood flow because vessels are maximally dilated and flow depends directly on pressure (see Fig. 13–1).[4] Conversely, at mean pressures above 150 mmHg, blood flow is again pressure-dependent because of maximal vessel constriction, and flow increases with pressure (see Fig. 13–1).[4] Within the normal range of mean CPP (60–150 mmHg), blood flow is held constant (see Fig. 13–1).[4]

The effects of the respiratory gases oxygen and carbon dioxide can defeat normal autoregulation.[10, 22] Thus, at any given perfusion pressure, a PaO_2 less than 60 mmHg or an increase in $PaCO_2$ produces vasodilatation and increases CBF; a decrease in $PaCO_2$ produces vasoconstriction and decreases blood flow.[4]

PHYSIOLOGY OF INTRACRANIAL PRESSURE

CEREBROSPINAL FLUID PHYSIOLOGY

CSF is the body's shock absorber for the central nervous system. It bathes and surrounds the entire brain and spinal cord to act as a natural cushion for those very delicate structures.

The normal intracranial-intraspinal volume of the central nervous system is approximately 1650 ml, of which 150 ml is CSF.[7] The normal rate of CSF production is approximately 500 ml/day.[23]

CSF is mainly produced by the choroid plexus in all four ventricles of the brain,[7, 23, 24] with the major portion coming from the lateral ventricles. It flows from the lateral ventricles through the foramen of Monro to the third ventricle, through the aqueduct of Sylvius to the fourth ventricle, through the foramen of Luschka and foramen of Magendie to the cisterna magna, and thence to the subarachnoid space surrounding the brain and spinal cord (Fig. 13–2).[7] Absorption (into the venous blood) occurs through the arachnoid villi in the sagittal venous sinus. In the absence of pathology, the rate of absorption is equal to the rate of production.[7] The fact that production is largely active (pressure-independent) and absorption is largely passive (pressure-dependent) produces a measurable CSF pressure (ICP) that is normally less than 15 mmHg.[7, 22]

DETERMINANTS OF INTRACRANIAL PRESSURE

The intracranial cavity is bordered by the cranium, a rigid structure of bone with only one real outlet for the intracra-

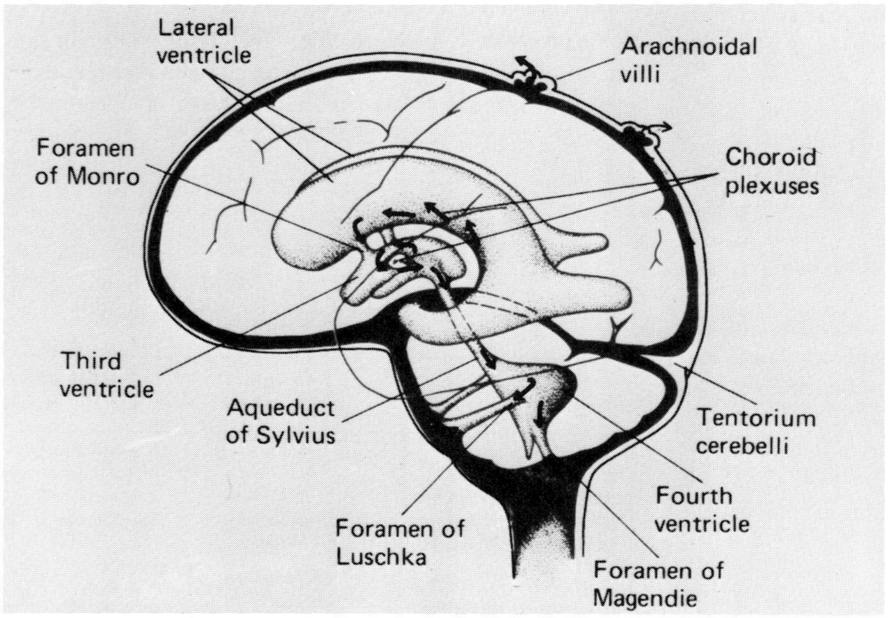

Figure 13–2. In the normal brain, cerebrospinal fluid flows from the lateral ventricles through the foramen of Monro to the third ventricle, through the aqueduct of Sylvius to the fourth ventricle, through the foramina of Magendie and Luschka to the cisterna magna, and finally to the cerebral and spinal subarachnoid spaces. (From Guyton AC: Textbook of Medical Physiology, 7th ed. Philadelphia: WB Saunders, 1986; 374.)

nial contents, the foramen magnum. CSF is only one of several substances contained in this cavity, the normal contents of which are listed in Figure 13–3.[25]

An increase in the volume of one or more of the normal constituents of the intracranial cavity produces a concomitant and compensating decrease in the volume of other intracranial contents to partially maintain volume and pressure at a constant level.[25] Glial cells, neurons, and extracellular fluid are noncompressible, have no ready avenue to exit the cranial vault, and are usually not part of this compensatory mechanism.[25] Thus, volume compensation results from the decrease of either intracranial intravascular blood volume or CSF volume, or both.[25] An overwhelming pathologic increase in intracranial volume exhausts this mechanism for compliance compensation, and ICP increases.[25] Any further increase in intracranial volume produces a concomitant increase in ICP.[25] This pressure-volume (intracranial compliance) relationship is illustrated in Figure 13–4.[26]

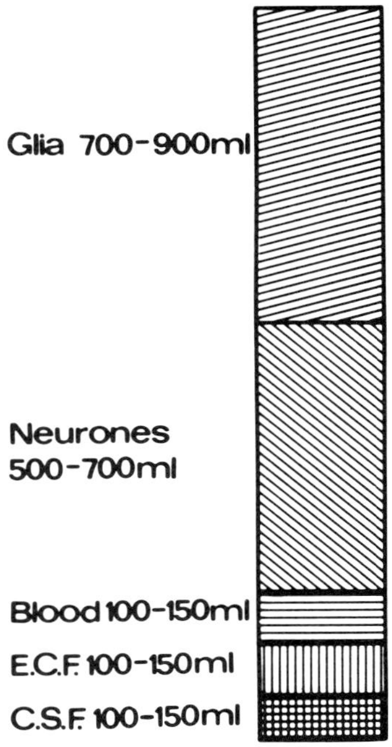

Figure 13–3. Intracranial contents and volume in an average adult human. Total intracranial volume is 1500–2050 ml. ECF = extracellular fluid; CSF = cerebrospinal fluid. (From Jennett B, Teasdale G: Management of Head Injuries. Philadelphia: FA Davis, 1981; 60.)

Intracranial Pressure-Volume Curve

Utilizing this pressure-volume relationship another way allows for the determination of intracranial pressure-volume status in individual patients. By injecting very small increments (0.1 ml—0.5 ml—1.0 ml) of sterile preservative-free saline into the CSF space and measuring the concomitant change in CSF pressure produced, relatively accurate determinations can be made about the position of an individual patient on the pressure-volume curve. The higher on the sharp limb of the curve, the tighter the brain is, and the more dramatic the increase in ICP with each increment in intracranial volume (see Fig. 13–4).

The effect of intracranial volume on ICP also depends on the rate of volume increase. Compensatory mechanisms respond more readily to slower increases in intracranial volume, and in this circumstance, acute changes in ICP in response to volume changes are less profound.[27] A very rapid increase in volume rapidly increases ICP.[27] However, there is an absolute limit to the volume compensatory mechanisms, and when that limit is exceeded, the rate of volume expansion becomes irrelevant.[27]

Causes of Intracranial Hypertension

Abnormal increases in ICP are produced by many different pathologic conditions.[7] The mechanisms of production of increased ICP include an expanding intracranial mass, cerebral edema formation, increased intracranial CSF volume, and increased intracranial blood volume.[7] Some conditions are caused by more than one mechanism.

Figure 13–4. Three possible intracranial pressure/volume curves. The most widely accepted is curve C. As the volume of intracranial (IC) mass increases, the intracranial pressure (ICP) increases. In curve C, the flat portion represents the volume compensation of normal brain. Once this compensation is exhausted, further increases in volume produce greater and greater increases in ICP. A patient with an elevation of ICP to point X is on the steep portion of the curve. Any further increase in volume (Y) produces a large increase in ICP in curve C, but smaller increases in curves A and B. The relative position of any patient on the curve (intracranial compliance) can be determined by injecting small increments of volume into the CSF *(arrows)* and observing the concomitant change in pressure (see text). (From Leech P, Miller JD: Intracranial volume-pressure relationships during experimental brain compression in primates. Pressure responses to changes in ventricular volume. J Neurol Neurosurg Psychiatry 1974; 37:1093–1098.)

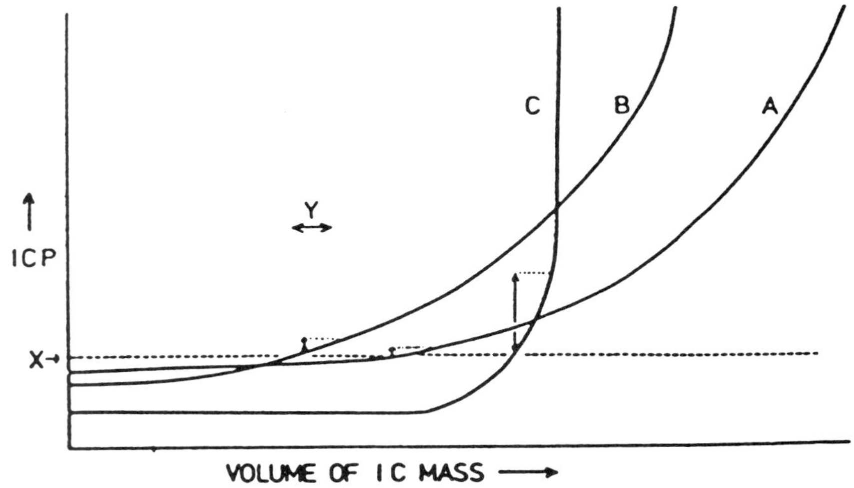

Intracranial Masses

Expanding intracranial masses include intracranial tumors and intracranial hematomas. These are conditions in which an abnormal constituent of increasing size is added to the intracranial contents. Although intravascular blood is a normal intracranial substance, extravascular collections of blood are not.

Cerebral Edema

Cerebral edema represents an increase in cellular volume and possibly an increase in extracellular fluid volume as well. Cerebral edema may be classified as either global or regional. Conditions producing global edema include closed head injury, cerebral anoxic damage, Reye's syndrome,[28] and severe systemic hypertension. Some examples of conditions producing regional cerebral edema are edema surrounding an intracranial tumor,[29] localized cerebral trauma, and stroke.

Increased CSF Volume

Intracranial CSF volume increases because of decreased absorption of CSF or obstruction of venous outflow from the head. Decreased absorption of CSF produces hydrocephalus. Communicating hydrocephalus occurs when the CSF is not normally absorbed through the arachnoid villi. Noncommunicating hydrocephalus is produced by an obstruction to CSF flow through the ventricles to the subarachnoid space. Usually, this obstruction occurs in the aqueduct of Sylvius between the third and fourth ventricles.

Venous outflow obstruction decreases CSF absorption probably by increasing the passive filtration pressure across the arachnoid villi through an increase in sagittal sinus venous pressure. Venous outflow obstruction can occur intracranially secondary to traumatic disruption of the venous sinus tract or extracranially from jugular venous compression or even assumption of the supine position, removing the negative venous hydrostatic pressure gradient present in the upright position.

Increased Intracranial Blood Volume

Increased intracranial blood volume is a consequence of venous outflow obstruction as well as a consequence of cerebral vasodilation. Cerebral vasodilation in turn can be caused by severe systemic hypertension, direct vasodilator drugs, and acute respiratory failure. It is also produced by a decrease in Pa_{O_2} (hypoxia), an increase in Pa_{CO_2} (hypercarbia), and a decrease in arterial pH (acidosis). Cerebral vasodilation increases cerebral blood volume.[7, 9, 11–15]

Intracranial Pressure Waveforms

When measured and displayed on an oscilloscope, the CSF pressure normally exhibits a characteristic pulsatile waveform.[27] The amplitude varies with the cardiac cycle, owing to transient changes in blood volume, and with respiration, probably owing to transient changes in intrathoracic pressure that are transmitted via the venous system to the venous sinus in the cranium. These pulsatile variations are superimposed on a steady-state volume level of cerebrospinal fluid (Fig. 13–5).

Normal CSF pressures are less than 15 mmHg. In cases of abnormally increased ICP, the amplitude of the pulsatile component increases. Abnormal waveforms seen in cases of pathologically increased ICP are usually intermittent and of two basic types: A waves, or plateau waves, lasting for several minutes, acutely exhibit ICP of 50–100 mmHg and usually denote very poor neurologic outcome; B waves are of lower amplitude with shorter duration than A waves (Fig. 13–6).[30]

Anesthetic Effects on Intracranial Pressure

The effects of various drugs on the ICP are summarized in Table 13–2. The potent anesthetic agents desflurane, enflurane, halothane, isoflurane, and sevoflurane increase ICP primarily by direct cerebral vasodilatation and resultant increased cerebral blood volume.[31–41] Uncompensated respiratory depression from these agents may also cause cerebral vasodilation secondary to an increase in Pa_{CO_2}.[12]

Although nitrous oxide (N_2O) does not clinically affect ICP, there is some evidence that it increases ICP under certain circumstances.[42–45] However, N_2O is still very

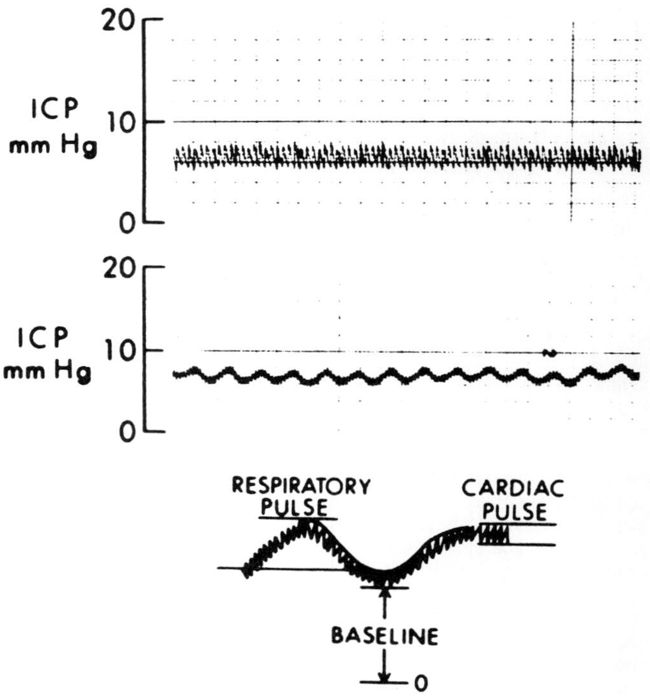

Figure 13–5. Normal intracranial pressure (ICP) is a pulsatile waveform with pressures of 5–7 torr. On this pressure are superimposed the effects of the cardiac and respiratory cycles. The top graph is at high paper speed to illustrate the cardiac effect; the middle graph represents the respiratory effect; the bottom graph illustrates the basic components of an ICP waveform during one respiratory cycle. (From Marmarou A, Tabaddor K: Intracranial pressure: Physiology and Pathophysiology. *In* Cooper PR [ed]: Head Injury. Baltimore: Williams & Wilkins, 1982; 115–127.)

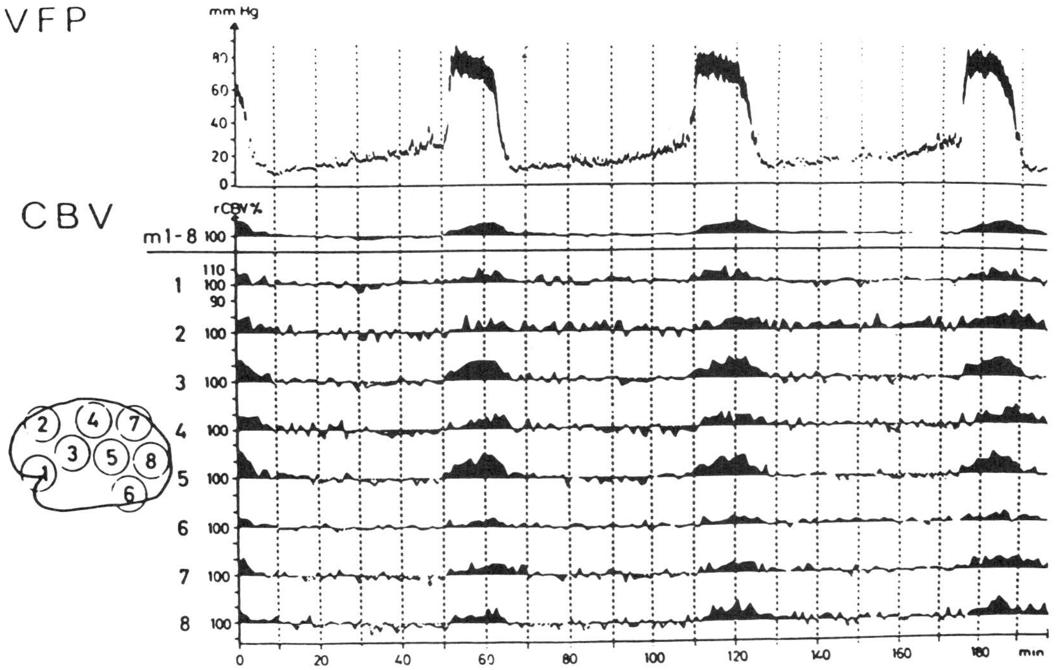

Figure 13–6. Simultaneous recordings of intracranial pressure (ventricular fluid pressure [VFP]) and cerebral blood volume (CBV) regionally in eight separate areas of the left hemisphere in a single patient. The Y-axis represents time in minutes during the measurement. The top graph illustrates VFP (ICP) A waves or plateau waves. The second graph represents average CBV from the eight areas. Note the similar course of VFP (ICP) and CBV; the A waves are accompanied by increases in CBV. (From Risberg J, Lundberg N, Ingvar DH: Regional cerebral blood volume during acute transient rises of the intracranial pressure [plateau waves]. J Neurosurg 1969; 31:303–310.)

widely used in patients with intracranial hypertension without deleterious effects. The one exception to this occurs when air is inside the cranium, as after pneumoencephalography.

The barbiturate drugs, of which thiopental sodium is commonly used in anesthesia, decrease ICP by direct cerebral vasoconstriction and decreased cerebral blood volume.[46, 47] Narcotic agents such as morphine and fentanyl either do not affect CSF pressure or may even decrease ICP by primarily decreasing cerebral metabolic rate and CBF.[48–54] However, like the potent anesthetic agents, narcotics also depress respiration; unless ventilation is supported when necessary, increased arterial P_{CO_2} may increase ICP.[12] The newer synthetic narcotics sufentanil and alfentanil, however, have demonstrated variable effects on ICP in different studies.[53, 54] These drugs should be used with care and the knowledge that some question of their efficacy may yet exist in patients with increased ICP.

Ketamine produces an increase in ICP owing to an increase in cerebral blood flow from cerebral vasodilation.[55–57] The benzodiazepines (diazepam, lorazepam, midazolam) decrease ICP by cerebral vasoconstriction.[58–60] Etomidate decreases ICP by decreasing CBF.[57]

A more recent drug used in neuroanesthesia and neurologic intensive care is propofol, an intravenous anesthetic agent. Propofol decreases ICP secondary to a decrease in the cerebral metabolic rate for oxygen, a decrease in CBF, and an increase in cerebral vascular resistance.[62] Although there is agreement on the effect of propofol on ICP, there is some evidence that propofol may decrease CBF and CPP because of a decrease in arterial blood pressure.[63]

The muscle relaxants commonly used in anesthesia vary in their effects on ICP. Pancuronium, vecuronium, and atracurium have all been shown to have no effect on ICP.[64–69] d-Tubocurarine, however, may increase ICP secondary to histamine release and cerebral vasodilation.[64] Succinylcholine is the most controversial member of this group because evidence shows that, although the drug causes increases in ICP, this effect may be attenuated by pretreatment with a nondepolarizing relaxant drug.[70–72]

Diuretic agents, including furosemide and mannitol, are commonly used to treat intracranial hypertension. Furosemide is a loop diuretic that decreases ICP by producing a fluid diuresis through the kidney.[73] The resultant fluid shifts effectively reduce cerebral edema. Mannitol, an osmotic diuretic, also produces this effect through diuresis, although it may also increase ICP transiently through an osmotic effect on brain water.[74, 75] Both drugs ultimately depend on normal renal function for their effect.

Hypotensive agents, such as primary vasodilators, trimethaphan, and beta-adrenergic blockers, are occasionally needed to control systemic hypertension or to produce deliberate hypotension (e.g., in cerebral aneurysm surgery). The primary vasodilator agents nitroprusside, hydralazine,

TABLE 13–2. DRUG EFFECTS ON INTRACRANIAL PRESSURE

Drug	Primary	Secondary	Reference
Potent anesthetic agents			
Halothane	++		31–33
Enflurane	++		34–36
Isoflurane	++		37–39
Desflurane	++		40
Sevoflurane	++		41
Barbiturates			
Thiopental sodium	−−		46, 47
Propofol	−		62, 63
Narcotics			
Morphine	0	+	48–52
Fentanyl citrate	0	+	48–52
Alfentanil	+−	+	54
Sufentanil	+−	+	53
Ketamine hydrochloride	+		55–57
Benzodiazepines			
Diazepam	−		58–60
Lorazepam	−		58–60
Midazolam	−		58–60
Neuromuscular-blocking drugs			
Succinylcholine chloride	+	0	70–72
d-tubocurarine	0	+	64
Pancuronium bromide	0		64, 65
Vecuronium bromide	0		66, 67
Atracurium besylate	0		68, 69
Etomidate	−		61
Diuretics			
Mannitol	−		74, 75
Furosemide	−		73
Vasodilators			
Sodium nitroprusside	+		76
Hydralazine hydrochloride	+		77
Nitroglycerin	+		78
Trimethaphan camsylate	0	+	76, 79
Calcium channel blocking drugs			
Nimodipine	0		83
Nicardipine	++		84
Beta-adrenergic blocking drugs			
Propranolol	0		80
Labetalol	0		81
Esmolol	0		82
Nitrous oxide	0	+	42–45

++ = major increase; + = moderate increase; 0 = no effect; −− = major decrease; − = moderate decrease; +− = positive *or* negative change may occur.

and nitroglycerin produce dose-related increases in ICP by dilating cerebral vessels and increasing CBF and cerebral blood volume.[76–78] Trimethaphan, a ganglionic blocking agent, may also increase ICP through vasodilation secondary to histamine release, although this effect is still debated.[76, 79] The beta-adrenergic blocking drugs propranolol, labetalol, and esmolol do not primarily affect ICP.[80–82]

Calcium channel blocking drugs, specifically nimodipine, are useful in the treatment of vasospasm secondary to subarachnoid blood. Nimodipine reduces vasospasm, increases CBF, and decreases cerebral vascular resistance without increasing ICP.[83] However, care should be used with this drug because decreases in arterial blood pressure may result in deterioration of CPP. Nicardipine has been shown to increase ICP, decrease CPP, and decrease arterial pressure in normal subjects and therefore is not a drug of choice in neuroanesthesia.[84]

PATHOPHYSIOLOGY OF INTRACRANIAL HYPERTENSION

CEREBRAL PERFUSION PRESSURE

To understand why increased ICP is a problem, it is necessary to understand the concept of cerebral perfusion pressure (CPP).[25] CPP is defined as the pressure gradient across the cerebral capillary bed, which perfuses blood through the brain. The CPP is calculated according to the following formula:

$$CPP = MAP - ICP$$

where MAP = mean arterial inflow pressure and ICP = the mean resistance of blood to outflow. For accuracy, the MAP should be measured at the level of the external auditory meatus. Under some circumstances, the central venous pressure measured at the level of the external auditory meatus may be used in place of the ICP.

Intracranial hypertension produces pathologic insults through two basic mechanisms: ischemia of brain tissue and mechanical damage due to bulk shifts of brain tissue.

Cerebral Ischemia

The final common pathway leading to cell damage from intracranial hypertension is ischemia of the cells in the brain.[85] As stated previously, CBF delivers oxygen and glucose and removes carbon dioxide and waste products from metabolizing brain cells. Ischemia of these cells produces hypoxia and acidosis of brain tissue. When CPP decreases below approximately 45 mmHg, CBF decreases to ischemic levels (see Fig. 13–1).[3]

From the preceding formula, it can be seen that CPP decreases as the MAP decreases and/or ICP increases. Normal CPP is between 60 and 150 mmHg. This corresponds to a CBF of 50 ml · gm^{-1} · min^{-1} (see Fig. 13–1).[3] As the CPP decreases below 60 mmHg, autoregulation is defeated and CBF decreases with pressure. At a CPP of 45 mmHg, CBF is approximately 50% of normal, i.e., 25 ml · gm^{-1} · min^{-1} (see Fig. 13–1). At this point, the first electrical evidence of ischemia appears.[3] Further reduction in CBF produces more profound changes. An absolute safe level of CBF during low-flow states that does not produce permanent cell damage is not known. However, in addition to the level of CBF achieved, the duration of time spent at that level plays an important role in determining the survival of cells. Pre-existing abnormal cerebral vessels reduce the margin for decreased CBF (as in chronic hypertension).[86] Therefore, when possible, every attempt should be made to maintain CPP at or near normal levels.

Herniation

In addition to brain cell ischemia, bulk shifts of brain tissue can produce mechanical damage to brain cells through the process known as herniation.[25, 27] Although herniation through a craniotomy is possible, brain herniation in the intact cranium occurs through the foramen magnum (cerebellum), the tentorium (temporal lobe or uncus), and the falx (cingulate gyrus and cerebral hemisphere). Herniation occurs with increases in ICP owing to mass effects from intracranial tumor or hematoma. The type of herniation that occurs depends on the location of the mass.[27] Supratentorial masses include temporal masses, which produce severe midbrain herniation, and frontal or occipital masses, which affect the brain stem less severely for the same size mass and same ICP level.[27] In addition to location, rapidly increasing masses produce a greater effect on the ICP and herniation than do more slowly growing masses.[27]

INTRACRANIAL PRESSURE MONITORING TECHNIQUES

GENERAL CONSIDERATIONS

Historically, many different techniques and devices have been used to measure ICP. Several are presently in common clinical use. In deciding which technique or device to use in a given clinical situation, several aspects of placement should be considered.[87] First, an ICP monitor should be reliable and stable during long-term use. In general, the simplier the device, the more reliable it is.[87] Second, the placement procedure should be as innocuous to the patient and the patient's central nervous system as possible. The risks of bleeding and infection should be minimal.[87] Third, the technique should allow for continuous measurement and recording of ICP while allowing adequate comfort and nursing care for the patient.[87] Finally, the technique chosen should be within the realm of expertise of the operator and as inexpensive as possible. Tables 13–3 and 13–4 list available products and manufacturers.

TABLE 13–3. MANUFACTURERS OF ICP MONITORING DEVICES

Manufacturer	Address	Telephone
Camino Laboratories Inc.	5955 Pacific Center Blvd. San Diego, CA 92121	619-455-1115
Cordis Corporation	POB 025700 Miami, FL 33102	800-327-2490
FiberOptic Sensor Technologies	501 Avis Drive Ann Arbor, MI 48108	313-665-6707
InnerSpace Medical	1923 South East Main Street Irvine, CA 92714	800-447-0304
Ladd Research Industries Inc.	POB 1005 Burlington, VT 05402	800-451-3406
Medical Measurements Inc.	53 Main Street Hackensack, NJ 07601	800-833-8031
Pudenz-Schulte Medical	125 B Cremona Drive Goleta, CA 93117	805-968-1546

TABLE 13–4. ICP MONITORING DEVICES AND THEIR MANUFACTURERS

Device Type	Manufacturer
Intraventricular devices	
Catheter	Cordis Corporation; Pudenz-Schulte Medical
Fiberoptic transducer	Camino Laboratories Inc.; InnerSpace Medical
Intraparenchymal devices	
Fiberoptic transducer	Camino Laboratories Inc.; InnerSpace Medical
Subarachnoid devices	
Bolt	Pudenz-Schulte Medical
Cup catheter	Cordis Corporation
Fiberoptic transducer	Camino Laboratories Inc.; InnerSpace Medical
Epidural devices	
Strain-gauge transducer	Medical Measurements Inc.
Fiberoptic transducer	Camino Laboratories Inc.; InnerSpace Medical
Pneumatic transducer	Ladd Research Industries Inc.

MONITORING INDICATIONS

Indications for monitoring ICP clinically, then, are based on the fact that ischemia or a decrease in CBF owing to a decrease in CPP is the primary common pathway for secondary brain injury after the initial insult has occurred.[85] Prevention of this secondary injury is where therapy may help, because no therapy can reverse the damage already produced by the primary insult.

ICP should be monitored whenever secondary injury is of concern:

1. In patients with head injuries with a Glasgow coma score of 7 or less.[78]
2. In patients with Reye's syndrome, because uncontrolled increases in ICP are a major factor in mortality.[28]
3. In patients with intracranial tumors, especially during induction of anesthesia when peritumoral edema is present.[29]
4. In any patient with intracranial pathology when the clinical neurologic examination cannot be followed—i.e., (a) intraoperatively (this becomes ineffective once the dura is opened), (b) during barbiturate-induced coma, and (c) when neuromuscular-blocking agents are used in neurosurgical patients in the intensive care unit.
5. Whenever therapeutic maneuvers adversely affect CPP and ICP.[85]

CLASSIFICATION OF DEVICES

The devices and techniques now available for monitoring ICP can be classified into groups by location of the device in the central nervous system, inherent invasiveness of the device, and method of measuring ICP. All of the devices outlined in this chapter require placement through surgical entry into the skull and, therefore, should be inserted only by an experienced operator.

The location of the device can vary among the lumbar spine, the cervical spine, the posterior fossa, and the supratentorial area of the cranium. Supratentorial placement is almost always preferred because of pathologically decreased flow of CSF around the tentorium in the subarachnoid space and subsequent intracranial herniation.[87] In patients with increased ICP, invasion of the subarachnoid space in the spinal canal and subsequent loss of CSF below the tentorium and/or the foramen magnum may even produce herniation.

ICP monitoring devices also can be described by method of measurement. Devices that place the pressure-measuring transducer at a site remote from the patient utilize a column of fluid in tubing to transmit the pressure wave from the CSF to the transducer. These devices are said to be fluid-coupled. The fluid and fluid path must be sterile, nonirritating to tissues, and free of leaks and air bubbles. The transducer should usually be placed at the level of the external auditory meatus for accuracy. Care must be taken to prevent any inadvertent injection of drugs or volume into this system. This has been a problem and is a continuing risk owing to the close resemblance of this system to other physiologic pressure monitoring equipment, i.e., arterial pressure apparatus.

Another necessary precaution is preventing the use of continuous flush systems in this setting. Nursing personnel and physicians caring for patients with fluid-coupled monitoring devices must be trained in the differences between other physiologic monitoring equipment and ICP monitors. Experienced operators, however, can safely perform clinical intracranial pressure-volume determinations on patients with this apparatus.

Newer devices utilize light transmission (fiberoptics) or a column of gas (pneumatics) instead of fluid-coupling to transmit the CSF pressure wave to the pressure-measuring electronic device. At least one device places the transducer directly in contact with the dura. There are also several experimental devices that attempt to implant the pressure transducer directly into the cerebrospinal fluid. The major problems with newer devices are reliability and miniaturization of the electronics or power supplies. Another development in ICP measurement is the implantation of devices into brain parenchyma. Pressures obtained in this way are reliable and compare well with conventionally measured pressures.[88] Intraparenchymal placement precludes CSF drainage or flushing of the device.

Intraventricular Devices

Classification according to the invasive nature of the device distinguishes among intraventricular devices, subarachnoid devices, epidural devices, and surface devices.

The intraventricular catheter is one of the oldest and simplest devices used to measure ICP.[89–91] It is classified as a fluid-coupled device; ICP waves are transmitted via an uninterrupted fluid path to a pressure sensor, usually a strain-gauge transducer outside of the cranium. This is accomplished by directly placing a hollow fluid-filled catheter into one of the lateral ventricles through a cranial burr hole and intact brain tissue. A typical arrangement of the tubing and transducer is shown in Figures 13–7 and 13–8. With this device, although it is very invasive, long-term ICP measurements can be made, pressure-volume determinations can be performed, intrathecal drugs (antibiotics) can be injected, and CSF can be withdrawn for both diagnostic studies and therapeutic needs (e.g., to decrease ICP). To achieve accurate ICP measurements with this device, the external transducer should be located at the level of the external auditory meatus (see Chapter 6).

Because the tubing arrangement for this device closely resembles that of other intravascular pressure monitoring devices, care must be taken to remove any continuous flush system from the apparatus. Flushing of the tubing and catheter are occasionally necessary but should be done carefully, only with preservative-free saline and only by an experienced operator. Because this technique requires invasion of tissue and violation of the dura, infection is possible and carries an estimated incidence of less than 6.3%.[92–94] Likewise, if the ventricular system is collapsed or relatively small, the operator may be unable to accurately place a catheter into the lateral ventricle (Fig. 13–9). Computed tomography facilitates location of the lateral ventricles and intraventricular catheter placement.

Subarachnoid Devices

Subarachnoid Bolt

In an effort to circumvent brain tissue perforation, as with a ventricular catheter, yet still directly interface with CSF, the subarachnoid bolt was developed (Fig. 13–10). Sometimes referred to as the Richmond bolt because of pioneering work done by Becker, Vires, Young, and others at the Medical College of Virginia, this device is also placed via a burr hole in the supratentorial area of the skull, with the tip placed below the arachnoid membrane.[80, 86] Figure 13–11 compares optimum insertion sites with undesirable locations. Like the intraventricular catheter, the bolt is fluid-coupled to an external pressure transducer, which should be placed at the level of the external meatus. Continuous flushing systems should be excluded from the fluid path (see Fig. 13–7). Regular flushing of the bolt should be performed manually but only with very small amounts of preservative-free saline. Because the tip of the bolt actually rests close to or on the brain surface, withdrawal of CSF is impossible. Pressure-volume determinations are possible; however, drugs cannot be reliably injected. Potential for infection does exist but is considered to be less likely than with a ventricular catheter.[94, 95] Because of the relative ease of placement and the relative accuracy of the pressure measurement, the subarachnoid bolt is widely used for measuring ICP.[95]

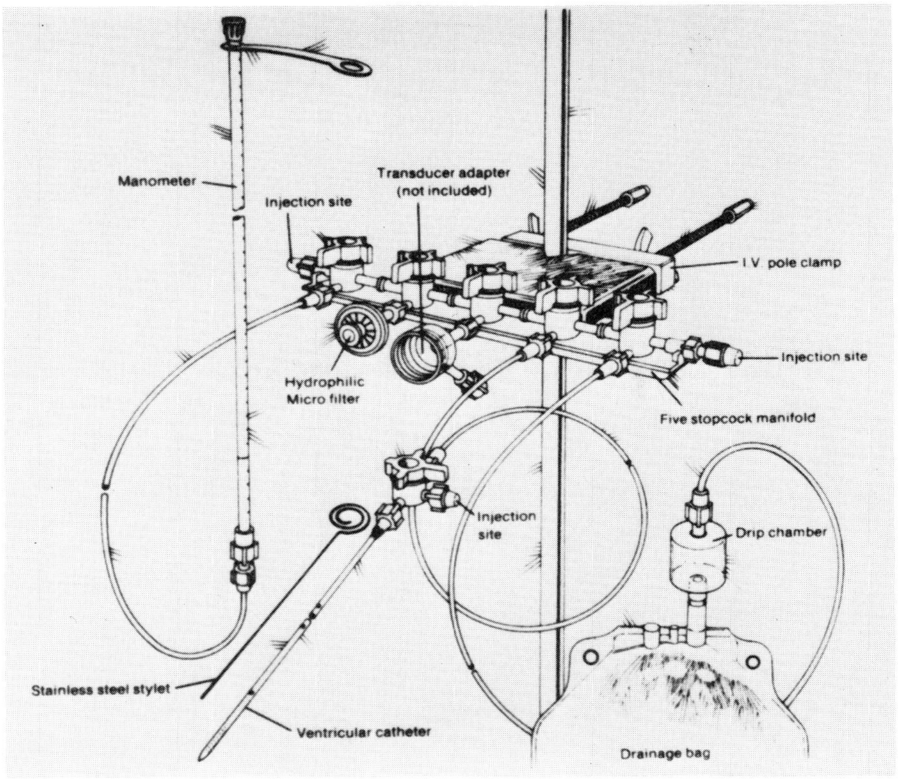

Figure 13–7. One arrangement of tubing, transducer, and drainage bag originally proposed by Becker. Note the transducer dome in the center, the absence of a continuous flush system, and ports for injection and drainage of cerebrospinal fluid. The transducer should be positioned at the level of the external auditory meatus. This apparatus may be used for measurement of either intraventricular or subarachnoid pressures. (From Wilkinson HA; Intracranial pressure monitoring: Techniques and pitfalls. *In* Cooper PR [ed]: Head Injury. Philadelphia: Williams & Wilkins, 1982; 155.)

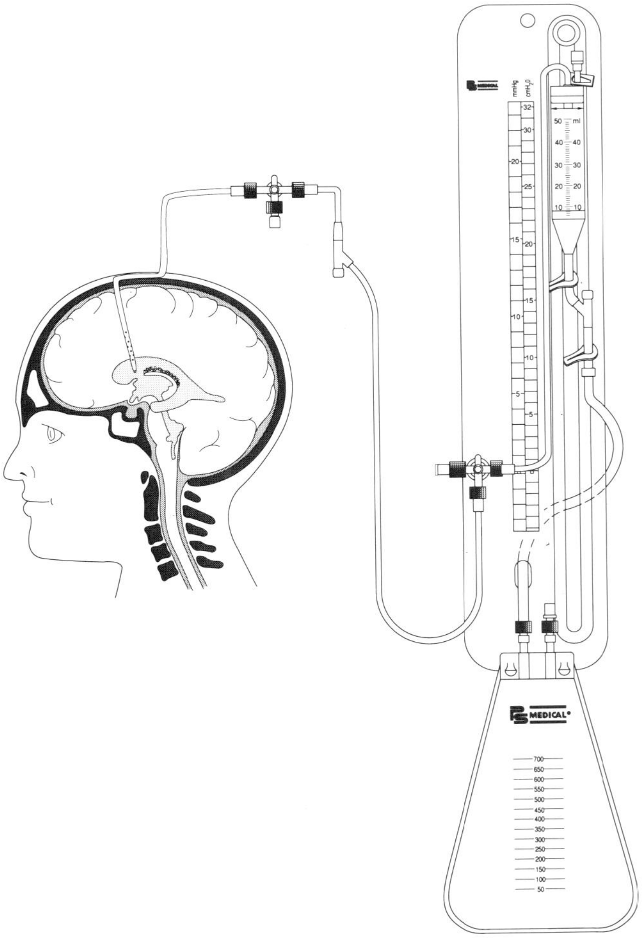

Figure 13–8. A new ICP measurement and drainage system. (Courtesy of Pudenz-Schulte Medical Corporation.)

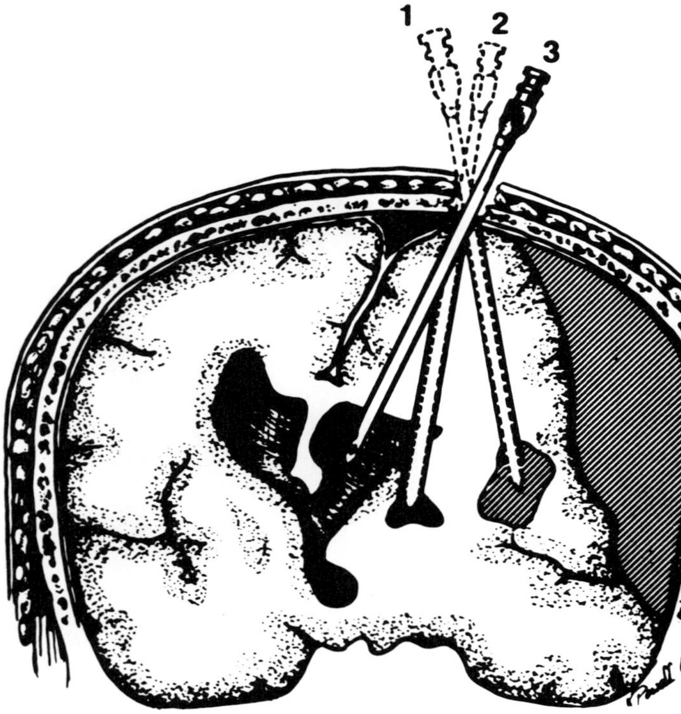

Figure 13–9. Potential problems encountered in placing an intraventricular catheter. The subdural hematoma has shifted the brain to the contralateral side and compressed the ipsilateral ventricle. Needle position 3 is the appropriate placement in this case and was achieved after blind passage, as in 1 and 2. With the ready availablity of computed tomography, needle placement is much more precise. (From Wilkinson HA: Intracranial pressure monitoring: Techniques and pitfalls. In Cooper PR [ed]: Head Injury. Baltimore: Williams & Wilkins, 1982; 158.)

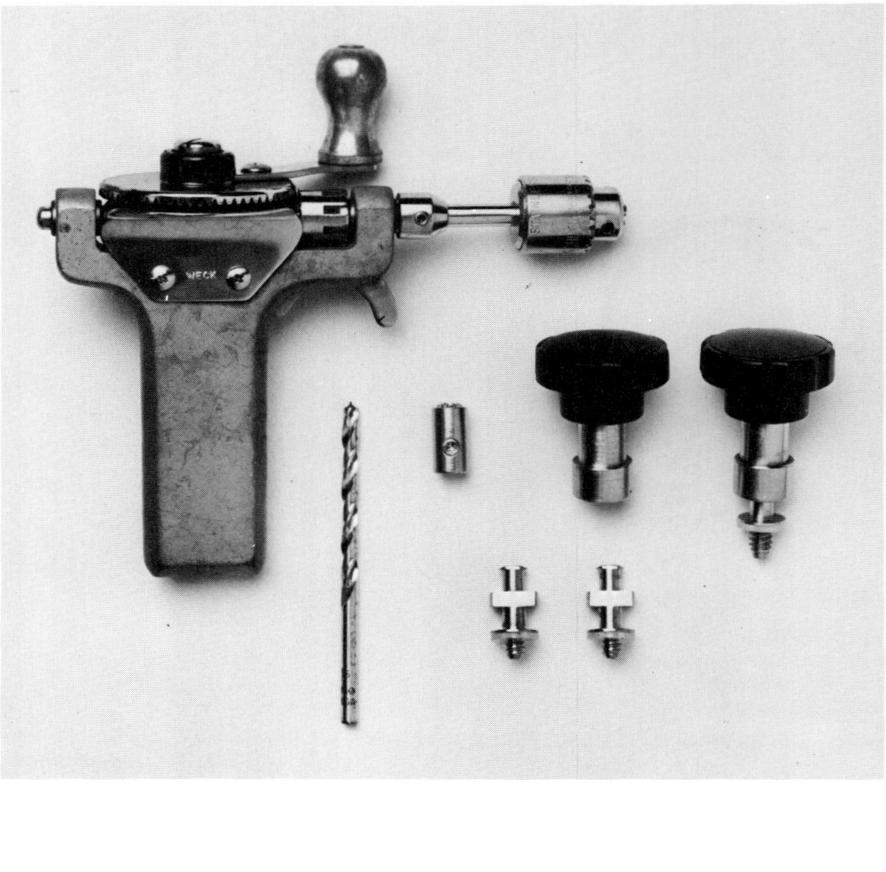

Figure 13–10. A subarachnoid bolt and the equipment for its insertion. The twist drill has a movable collar that produces a well in the outer table of the skull to allow accurate depth of placement. The black handles are for insertion of the bolt itself.

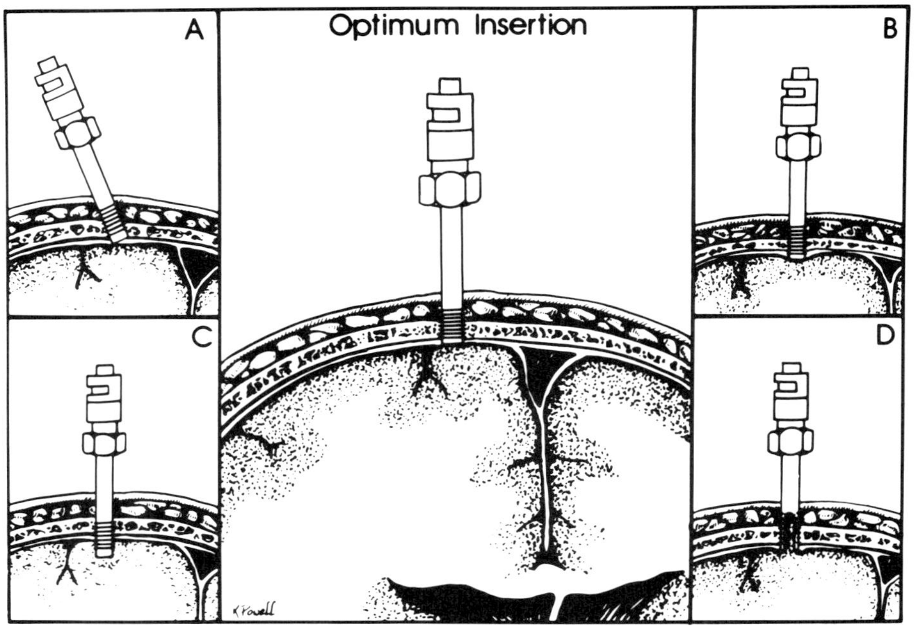

Figure 13–11. Optimum placement of the subarachnoid bolt is seen in the center of the figure. Potential problems with bolt placement: *A*, Oblique placement does not allow full approximation to the subarachnoid space. *B*, A thin cranium allows movement of the bolt and occlusion; *C*, Bolt placed too deep damages brain tissue; *D*, Herniation of brain tissue into the bolt and subsequent occlusion. (From Wilkinson HA: Intracranial pressure monitoring: Techniques and pitfalls. *In* Cooper PR [ed]: Head Injury. Philadelphia: Williams & Wilkins, 1982; 161.)

Cup Catheter

Another available subarachnoid device is the cup catheter, which operates similarly to the subarachnoid bolt (Fig. 13–12). This device is a ribbon-shaped catheter passed into the cerebral subarachnoid space through a burr hole, with the skin incision remote from the craniotomy site, thus possibly decreasing the incidence of infection.[96] The cup catheter is also fluid-coupled to ensure filling of the cup. This catheter is somewhat more difficult to place than the bolt and is less widely used.

Epidural Devices

Three devices are currently available for epidural ICP measurement: epidural transducer, fiberoptic transducer, and pneumatic transducer. All three devices measure ICP through the intact dura and avoid the use of a fluid path (i.e., they are not fluid-coupled). Because the dura is not opened, the risk of infection is thought to be less than with intraventricular or subarachnoid devices.

Epidural Transducer

The epidural transducer is produced and marketed by NV Phillips, The Netherlands. It is designed to be threaded into a burr hole in the skull far enough to stretch the intact dura across the flat sensor at the tip (Fig. 13–13).[97] The measurement of ICP with this device depends on the principle of coplanarity[98]—that is, the flat sensor must be exactly parallel to the plane of the dura and in intimate contact with it. The CSF pressure waves are transmitted across the intact dura to the transducer surface. Therefore, accuracy of placement is critical. When properly placed, however, the pressure measurements correspond well with those obtained with an intraventricular catheter.[97] Because there is no fluid-coupling, injection of drugs and intracranial pressure-volume measurement are impossible. The device does not need to be flushed periodically, as do fluid-coupled devices. However, the transducer is nondisposable and relatively expensive.[97]

Epidural Catheter Tip Pressure Transducer

This catheter differs from other catheters in that the pressure transducer is located at the catheter tip and is covered by a thin membrane (Figs. 13–14 and 13–15).[99, 100] No fluid-couple is needed because the thin membrane rests directly on the strain-gauge pressure measuring device during measurement. The device connects to existing pressure measuring modules via an adapter.

Usually used as an epidural sensor (Fig. 13–16), this device has been used in subdural space and even intraventricularly. Manufactured by Gaeltec and marketed by Medical Measurements Inc., the catheter is designed to allow *in vivo* calibration and zero checks.

Pneumatic Epidural Monitor

The Ladd-Steritek ICP monitoring system utilizes a disposable pneumatic sensor, which is placed in either epidural or subdural space through a burr hole in the skull (Figs. 13–17 through 13–19). The sensor membrane is placed toward the dura or brain surface. The sensor is designed to self-calibrate *in vivo*.

The Ladd-Steritek base unit (containing an air pump, transducer, and microprocessor) provides a constant flow of air at 40 ml/minute into the sensor chamber through the air inlet tube (see Figs. 13–18 and 13–19). The metal disk membrane occludes the air exhaust port when acted on by pressure outside the sensor. The pressure inside the chamber is measured constantly by the transducer. Air is pumped

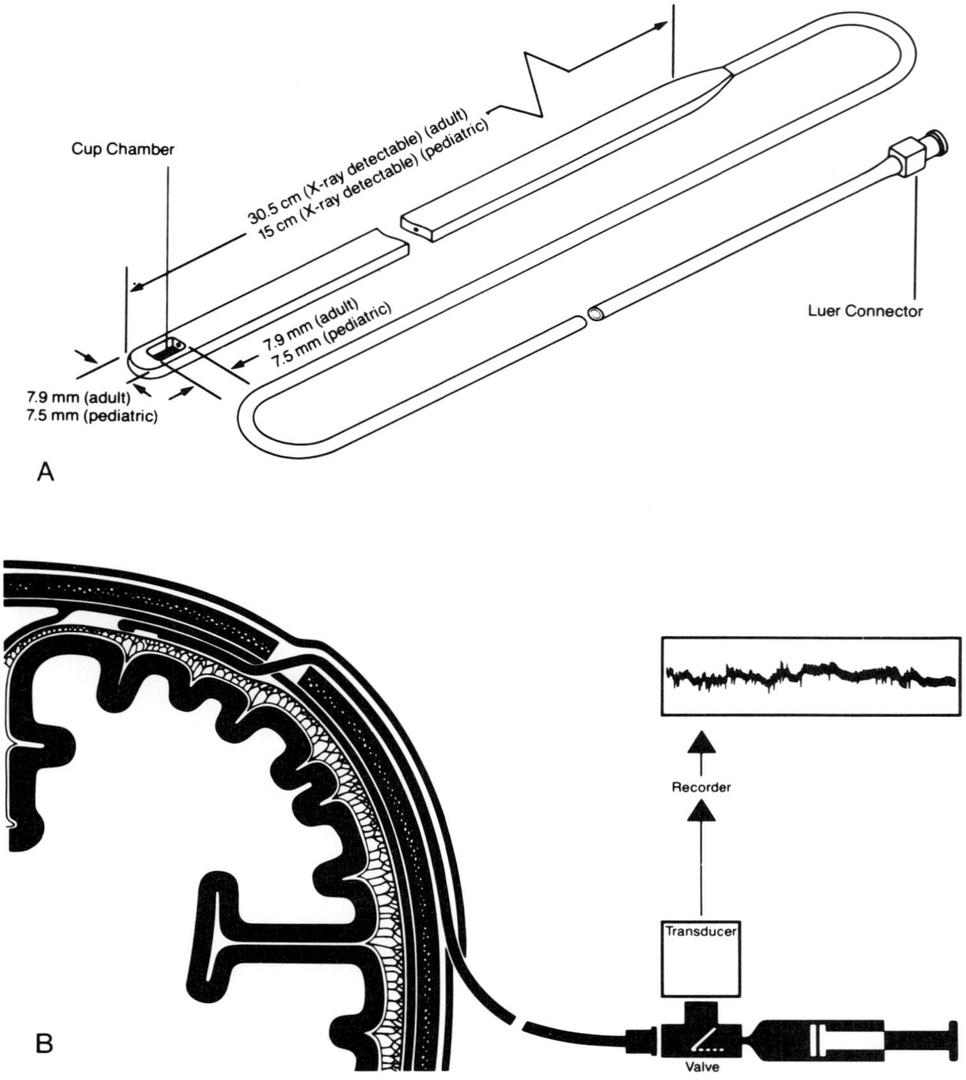

Figure 13–12. The cup catheter *(A)* is ribbon-shaped, and has a cup formed in its end. It is designed as a surface-monitoring device to be placed so that the open cup rests on the brain surface *(B)*. This device is also fluid-coupled and must be flushed periodically. (Courtesy of Cordis Corporation.)

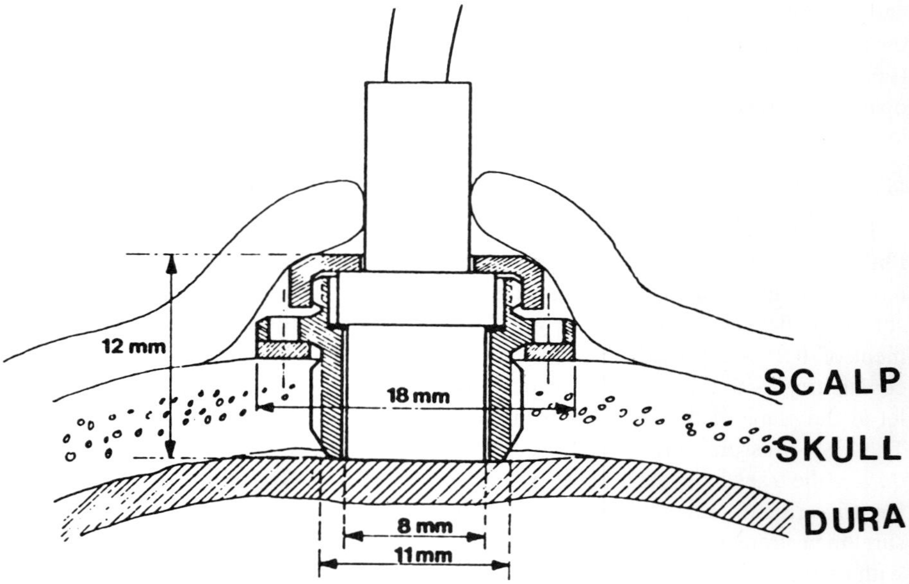

Figure 13–13. A schematic diagram of the epidural transducer. The clear layer overlapping the top edge of the device is scalp. The transducer is threaded into a burr hole in the skull, and the transducer surface adheres directly to the dura. (From Koster WG, Kuypers MH: Intracranial pressure and its epidural measurement. Med Prog Technol 1980; 7:21–27.)

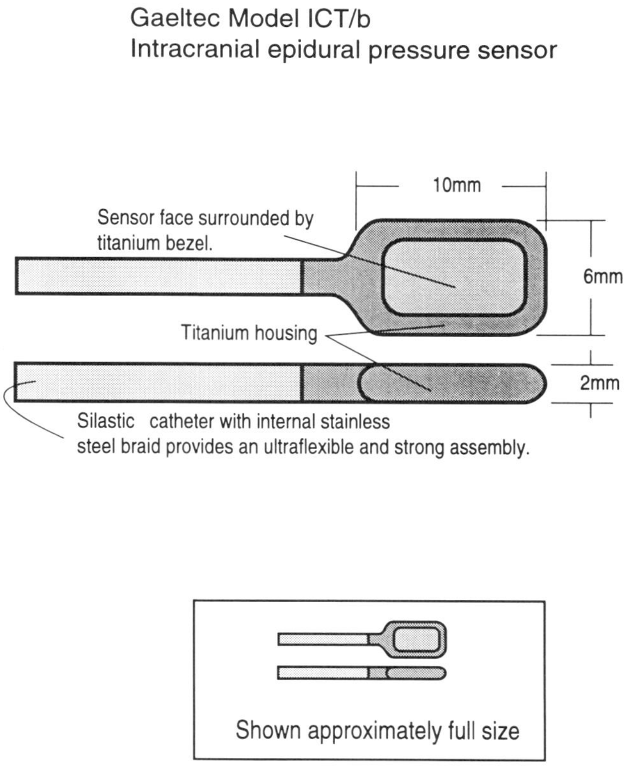

Figure 13–14. The Gaeltec catheter is made up of a dual-channel catheter with an electronic strain gauge pressure measuring device at the tip. A thin membrane covers the pressure sensor and lies in contact with it during measurement. (Courtesy of Medical Measurements Inc., Hackensack, NJ 07601.)

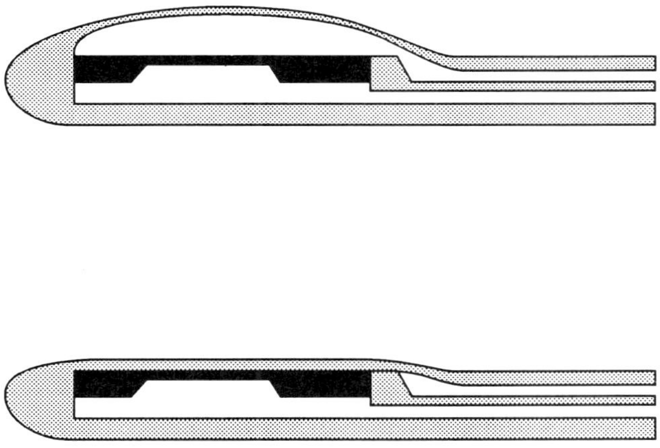

Figure 13–15. The Gaeltec dual-channel catheter allows for in vivo zero calibration of the device. One channel allows atmospheric pressure to the reverse side of the transducer during measurement; the membrane is in contact with the transducer during this phase *(bottom)*. To calibrate the unit in vivo, equal pressure is applied to both sides of the transducer via the first and second channels *(top)*. (Courtesy of Medical Measurements Inc., Hackensack, NJ 07601.)

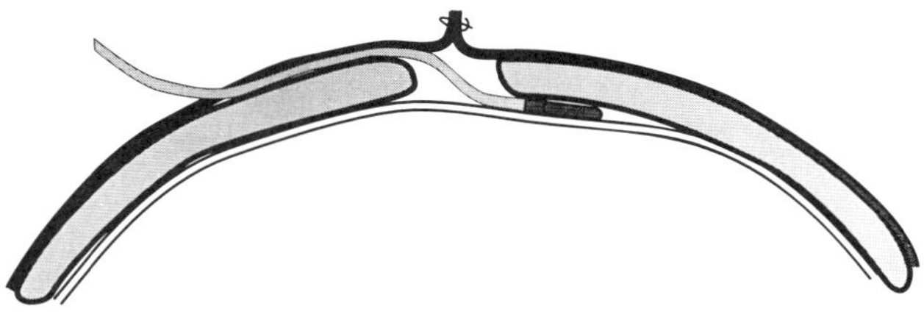

Figure 13–16. The Gaeltec catheter placed epidurally. (Courtesy of Medical Measurements Inc., Hackensack, NJ 07601.)

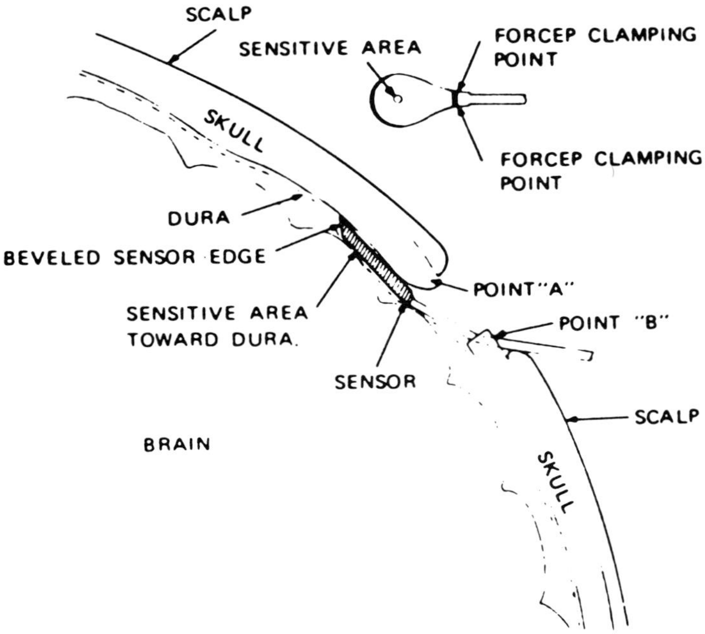

Figure 13–17. Placement of the Ladd sensor. The membrane surface is placed against the dura through a burr hole in the skull. (From Levin AB: The use of a fiberoptic intracranial pressure monitor in clinical practice. Neurosurgery 1977; 1:266–271.)

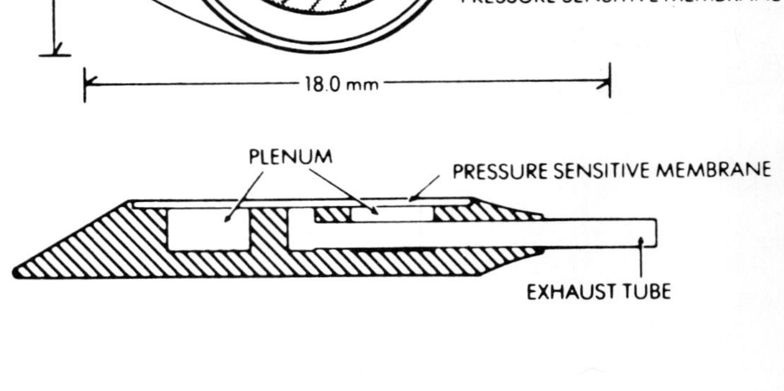

Figure 13–18. The disposable sensor for the Ladd-Steritek ICP monitoring system. The pressure-sensitive membrane is a thin metal disk that can occlude the exhaust gas port. Gas enters the sensor through the inlet port at 40 ml/minute. (Courtesy of Ladd Research Industries, Burlington, VT.)

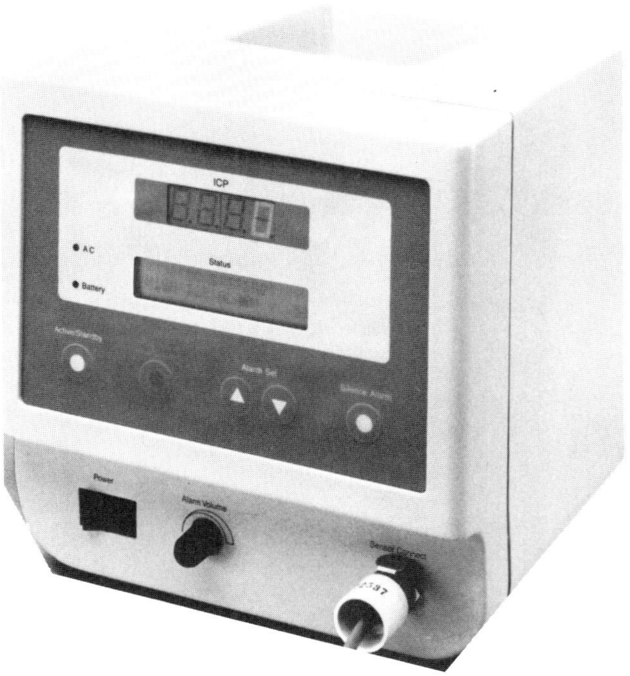

Figure 13–19. The microprocessor-based Ladd-Steritek ICP monitor base unit. The unit houses the microprocessor, transducer, and pneumatic pump. This device can be used for only one patient at a time. (Courtesy of Ladd Research Industries, Burlington, VT.)

into the chamber until the pressure is sufficient to lift the membrane and open the exhaust port again. This pressure is the ICP. Advantages of the Ladd-Steritek unit are disposability, lower cost, and less fragile sensors. However, it is a dedicated monitor that can be used on only one patient at a time, and it has no other uses.

All of the epidural devices presented here eliminate the need for fluid couples and the inherent problems of fluid systems (e.g., leakage and sterility). They are, however, more expensive and more difficult to place, and they are dedicated instruments with only one use.

FIBEROPTIC MONITOR

The most recent advance in ICP monitoring devices is the use of fiberoptics. Camino Laboratories manufactures a system utilizing a fiberoptic catheter (Fig. 13–20). This device requires the use of the manufacturer's monitor and recorder (Fig. 13–21). The catheter may be used as an epidural, subdural, intraventricular, or intraparenchymal monitor (Fig. 13–22).[101–104] The device measures ICP by the use of fiberoptic light paths in the catheter. One path transmits light generated in the monitor itself to the tip of the catheter. This light reflects off a flat reflecting surface, the other side of which is in contact with CSF or brain tissue. The second fiberoptic pathway transmits reflected light back to the monitor unit, where it is quantitatively measured and compared to the level of generated light. As pressure in the CSF increases, the reflecting surface is displaced at an ever increasing angle. As a result, less and less of the reflected light is captured by the return fiberoptic pathway and less light gets back to the monitor. The difference in the generated light and returned light gives a measure of the pressure at the catheter tip and therefore ICP. The fiberoptic catheter compares favorably to other methods of measuring ICP but cannot be zeroed or recalibrated *in vivo*. The only major fault with the catheter appears to be breakage of the fiber bundles with prolonged use. This can be remedied by replacing the catheter through the insertion device, which remains in situ (see Fig. 13–22).

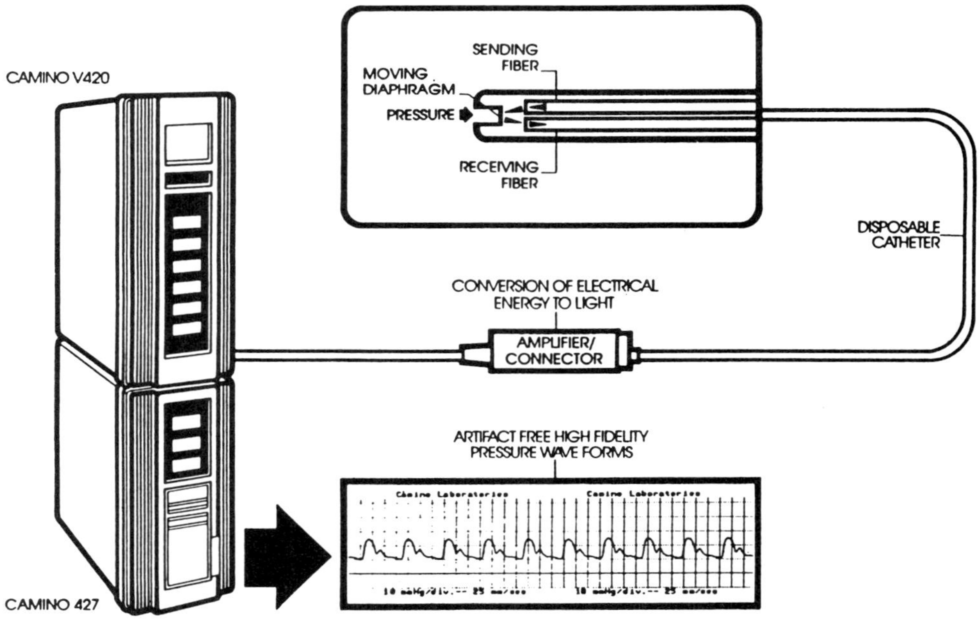

Figure 13–20. The Camino fiberoptic catheter utilizes dual fiberoptic light fibers and a moving diaphragm. As the diaphragm moves, light transmitted from the unit is deflected so that a smaller proportion is returned to the unit from the sensor. This differential is used to calculate the pressure needed to deflect the diaphragm and displayed as ICP on the unit. Wave forms generated from this device compare very favorably to direct intraventricular waves. (Courtesy of Camino Laboratories.)

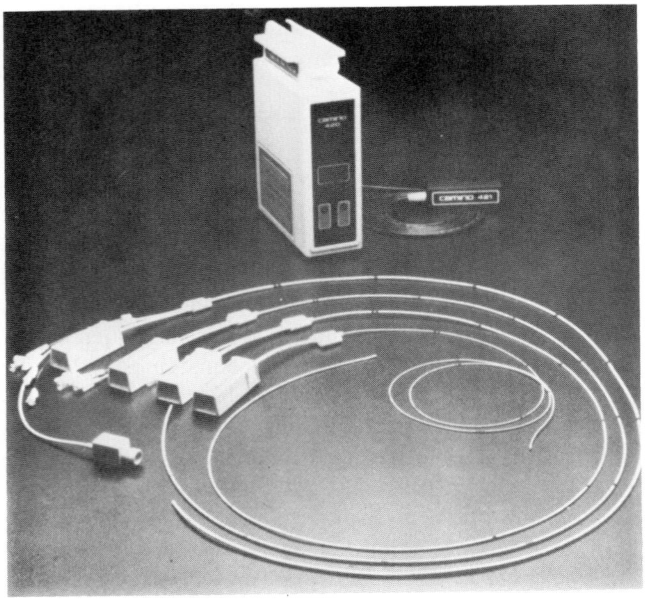

Figure 13–21. The Camino Laboratories ICP fiberoptic system.

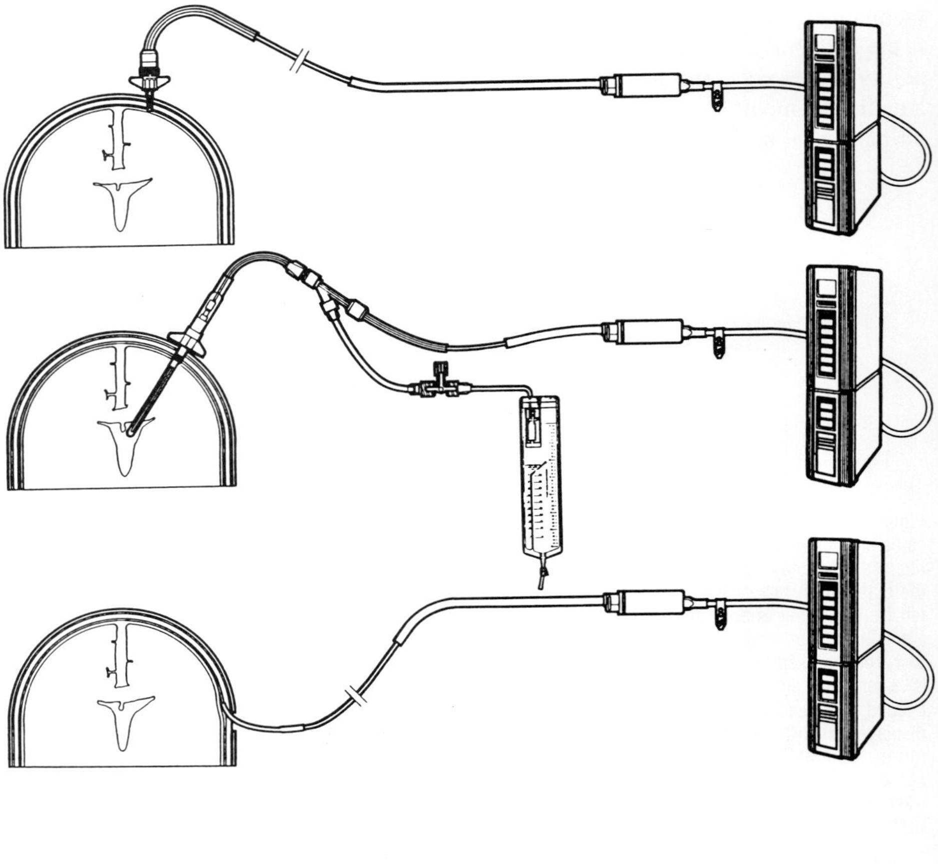

Figure 13–22. The fiberoptic system from Camino Labs can be used epidurally, subdurally, intraventricularly, and intraparenchymaly. In most applications, the sensor is placed via a stable cranial bolt and can be replaced as needed without removing the bolt.

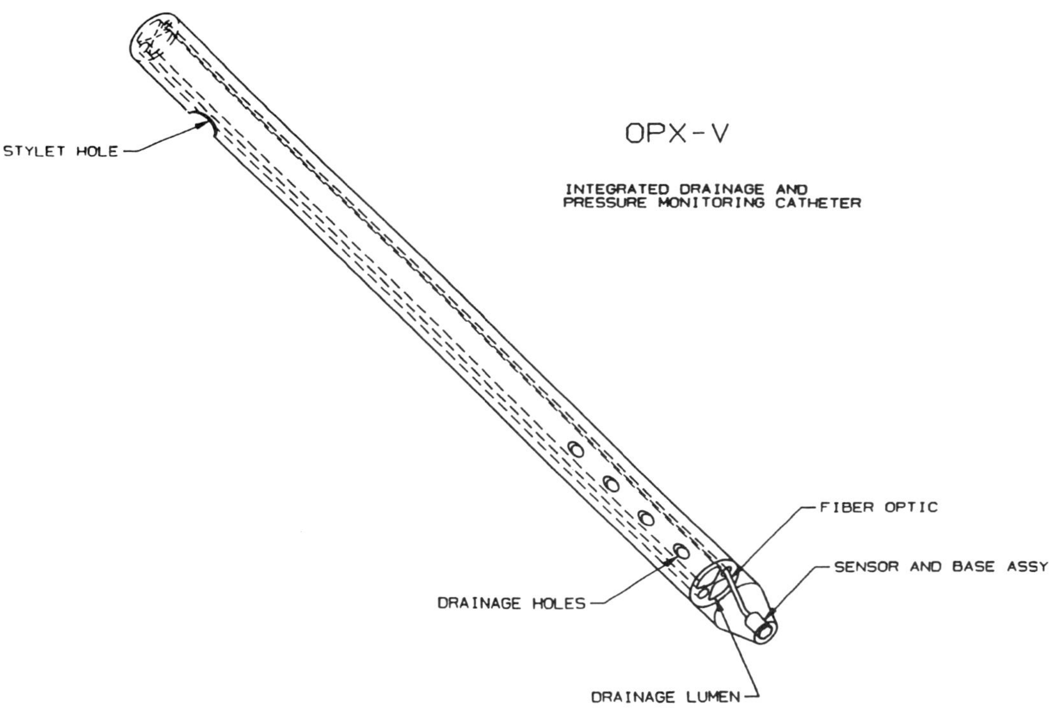

Figure 13–23. The OPX-V catheter from Innerspace Medical. The integration of catheter and miniature sensor allows for CSF drainage when placed intraventricularly. The sensor is a fiberoptic unit. (Courtesy of Innerspace Medical.)

Another similar fiberoptic device is the OPX catheter marketed by Innerspace Medical (Fig. 13–23). This device again requires the use of the manufacturer's monitoring technology (Fig. 13–24) but does allow drainage of CSF when used in the intraventricular mode.

THERAPY OF INCREASED INTRACRANIAL PRESSURE

The therapy of increased ICP is based on the contents of the intracranial cavity. Of the various structures and substances contained in the cranial vault, only the blood and CSF volumes can be readily affected by common therapeutic modalities.

Therefore, a decrease in ICP can be achieved by (1) decreasing the volume of CSF through ventriculostomy drainage, (2) decreasing intracranial blood volume through hyperventilation, barbiturate therapy, prevention of hypoxia, improving venous drainage (head-up position), avoiding jugular venous compression, maintaining normal CPP by avoiding hypotension, and avoiding cerebral vasodilator drugs, (3) decreasing cerebral edema and extracellular fluid with diuretics and avoidance of fluid overload, and (4) surgical removal of any existing intracranial mass such as a hematoma or tumor.[25, 85]

The need to measure ICP to guide therapy in pathologic conditions and the significance of elevated ICP in those circumstances stem from a sound knowledge base of the physiology of the cerebral circulation and the dynamics of the CSF. All clinical monitoring techniques available today require surgical procedures for placement. Of the various systems available, the older techniques of intraventricular and subarachnoid fluid-coupled devices are still the simplest, most reliable, and most cost-effective. The choice of technique depends on many factors, one of the most important of which is the expertise and preference of the operator.

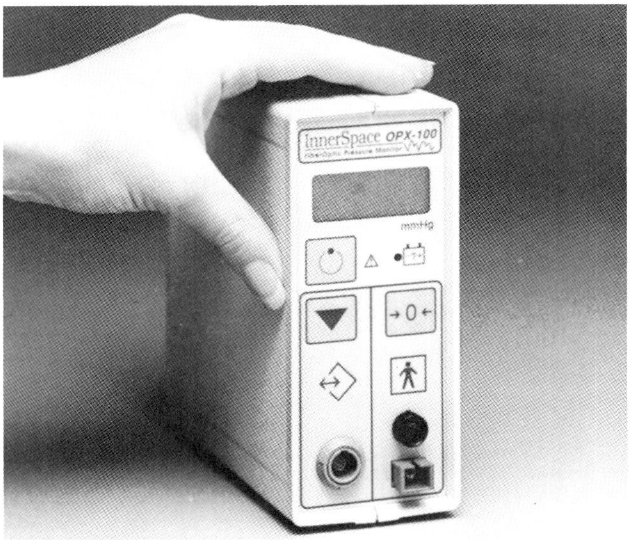

Figure 13–24. The OPX base unit. (Courtesy of Innerspace Medical.)

REFERENCES

1. Lassen NA, Ingvar DH: Radioisotopic assessment of regional cerebral blood flow. Prog Nucl Med 1972; 1:376–409.
2. Obrist WD, Thompson HK, Wand HS, Wilkinson WE: Regional cerebral blood flow estimated by ^{133}xenon inhalation. Stroke 1975; 6:245–256.
3. McKay RD, Sundt TM, Michenfelder JD: Internal carotid artery stump pressure and cerebral blood flow during carotid endarterectomy: Modification by halothane, enflurane and innovar. Anesthesiology 1976; 45:390–399.
4. Michenfelder JD: The cerebral circulation. *In* Prys-Roberts C (ed): The Circulation in Anesthesia. London: Blackwell Scientific, 1980; 212.
5. Halsey JH, McFarland S: Oxygen cycles and metabolic autoregulation. Stroke 1974; 5:219–225.
6. Shapiro BA, Harrison RD, Walton JR: Clinical Application of Blood Gases, 3rd Ed. Chicago: Year Book Medical, 1982; 14.
7. Guyton AC: Textbook of Medical Physiology, 7th Ed. Philadelphia: WB Saunders, 1986; 339.
8. Siesjo BK: Cerebral circulation and metabolism. J Neurosurg 1984; 60:883–908.
9. Seymour SS, Kety S, Schmidt CF: The effects of altered arterial tensions of carbon dioxide and oxygen on cerebral blood flow and cerebral oxygen consumption of normal young men. J Clin Invest 1948; 27:484–492.
10. Turner J, Lambertsen CJ, Owen SG, et al: Effects of .08 and .8 atmospheres of inspired PO_2 upon cerebral hemodynamics at a constant alveolar PCO_2 of 43 mmHg [Abstract]. Fed Proc 1967; 16:130.
11. Raichle ME, Posner JB, Plum F: Cerebral blood flow during and after hyperventilation. Arch Neurol 1970; 23:394–403.
12. Raichle ME, Stone HL: Cerebral blood flow autoregulation and graded hypercapnia. Eur Neurol 1971–72; 6:1–5.
13. Lambertsen CJ, Smyth SM, Gelfand R: H^+ and PCO_2 as chemical factors in respiratory and cerebral circulatory control. J Appl Physiol 1961; 16:473–484.
14. Harper AM, Bell RA: The effect of metabolic acidosis and alkalosis on the blood flow through the cerebral cortex. J Neurol Neurosurg Psychiatry 1963; 26:341–344.
15. Sokoloff L: The effect of carbon dioxide on the cerebral circulation. Anesthesiology 1960; 21:664–673.
16. Reivich M: Arterial PCO_2 and cerebral hemodynamics. Am J Physiol 1964; 206:25–35.
17. Lassen NA: Control of cerebral circulation in health and disease. Circ Res 1974; 34:749–760.
18. Olesen J: Contralateral focal increase of cerebral blood flow in man during arm work. Brain 1971, 94:635–646.
19. Lassen NA, Christensen MS: Physiology of cerebral blood flow. Br J Anaesth 1976; 48:719–734.
20. Wolfgang K, Wahl M: Local chemical and neurogenic regulation of cerebral vascular resistance. Physiol Rev 1978; 58:656–689.
21. Bevegard BS, Shepherd JT: Regulation of the circulation during exercise in man. Physiol Rev 1967; 47:178–213.
22. Michenfelder JD, Gronert GA, Rehder K: Neuroanesthesia. Anesthesiology 1969; 30:65–100.
23. Cutler RWP, Page L, Galicich J, Watters JV: Formation and absorption of cerebrospinal fluid in man. Brain 1968; 91:707–720.
24. Cserr HF: Physiology of the choroid plexus. Physiol Rev 1971; 51:273–311.
25. Jennett B, Teasdale G: Management of Head Injuries. Philadelphia: FA Davis, 1981.
26. Leech P, Miller JD: Intracranial volume-pressure relationships during experimental brain compression in primates. Pressure responses to changes in ventricular volume. J Neurol Neurosurg Psychiatry 1974; 37:1093–1098.
27. Marmarou A, Tabaddor K: Intracranial pressure: Physiology and pathophysiology. *In* Cooper PR (ed): Head Injury. Baltimore: Williams & Wilkins, 1982; 115–127.
28. Venes JL, Shaywitz BA, Spender DD: Management of severe cerebral edema in the metabolic encephalopathy of Reye-Johnson syndrome. J Neurosurg 1978; 48:903–915.
29. Bedford RF, Morris L, Jane JA: Intracranial hypertension during surgery for supratentorial tumor: Correlation with preoperative computed tomography scans. Anesth Analg 1982; 61:430–433.
30. Risberg J, Lundberg N, Ingvar DH: Regional cerebral blood volume during acute transient rises of the intracranial pressure (plateau waves). J Neurosurg 1969; 31:303–310.
31. McDowall DG: The effects of clinical concentrations of halothane on the blood flow and oxygen uptake of the cerebral cortex. Br J Anaesth 1967; 39:186–196.
32. Marx GF, Andrews IC, Orkin JR: Cerebrospinal fluid pressures during halothane anaesthesia. Can Anaesth Soc J 1962; 9:239–245.
33. Alexander SC, Wollman H, Cohen PJ, et al: Cerebrovascular response to $PaCO_2$ during halothane anesthesia in man. J Appl Physiol 1964; 19:561–565.
34. Manohar M, Parks CM: Porcine brain and myocardial perfusion during enflurane anesthesia without and with nitrous oxide. J Cardiovasc Pharmacol 1984; 6:1092–1101.
35. Artru AA: Relationship between cerebral blood volume and CSF pressure during anesthesia with halothane or enflurane in dogs. Anesthesiology 1983; 58:533–539.
36. Miletich DJ, Ivankovich AD, Albrecht RF, et al: Absence of autoregulation of cerebral blood flow during halothane and enflurane anesthesia. Anesth Analg 1976; 55:100–109.
37. Cucchiara RF, Theye RA, Michenfelder JD: The effects of isoflurane on canine cerebral metabolism and blood flow. Anesthesiology 1974; 40:571–574.
38. Artru AA: Relationship between cerebral blood volume and CSF pressure during anesthesia with isoflurane or fentanyl in dogs. Anesthesiology 1984; 60:575–579.
39. Eger EI: Isoflurane: A review. Anesthesiology 1981; 55:559–576.
40. Muzzi DA, Losasso TJ, Dietz NM, et al: The effect of desflurane and isoflurane on cerebrospinal fluid pressure in humans with supratentorial mass lesions. Anesthesiology 1992; 76:720–724.
41. Scheller MS, Tateishi A, Drummond JC, et al: The effects of sevoflurane on cerebral blood flow, cerebral metabolic rate for oxygen, intracranial pressure, and the electroencephalogram are similar to those of isoflurane in the rabbit. Anesthesiology 1988; 68:548–551.
42. Henriksen HT, Jorgensen PB: The effect of nitrous oxide on intracranial pressure in patients with intracranial disorders. Br J Anaesth 1973; 45:486–492.
43. Laitinen LV, Johansson GG, Tarkkanen L: The effect of nitrous oxide on pulsatile cerebral impedance and cerebral blood flow. Br J Anaesth 1967; 39:781–785.
44. Sokoloff L: The action of drugs on the cerebral circulation. Pharmacol Rev 1959; 11:1–85.
45. Smith AL, Wollman H: Cerebral blood flow and metabolism: Effects of anesthetic drugs and techniques. Anesthesiology 1972; 36:378–400.
46. Pierce ED, Lambertsen CJ, Deutsch S, et al: Cerebral circulation and metabolism during thiopental anesthesia and hyperventilation in man. J Clin Invest 1962; 41:1664–1671.
47. Shapiro HM, Galindo A, Wyte SR, Harris AB: Rapid intraoperative reduction of intracranial pressure with thiopentone. Br J Anaesth 1973; 45:1057–1062.
48. Jobes DR, Kennell E, Bitner R, et al: Effects of morphine-nitrous oxide anesthesia on cerebral autoregulation. Anesthesiology 1975; 42:30–34.
49. Jobes DR, Kennell EM, Bush GL, et al: Cerebral blood flow and metabolism during morphine-nitrous oxide anesthesia in man. Anesthesiology 1977; 47:16–18.
50. Keats AS, Mithoefer JC: The mechanism of increased intracranial pressure induced by morphine. N Engl J Med 1955; 30:1110–1113.
51. Moss E, Powell D, Gibson RM, McDowall DG: Effects of fentanyl on intracranial pressure and cerebral perfusion pressure during hypocapnia. Br J Anaesth 1978; 59:779–784.
52. Carlsson C, Smith DS, Keykhah MM, et al: The effects of high-dose fentanyl on cerebral circulation and metabolism in rats. Anesthesiology 1985; 57:375–380.
53. Milde LN, Milde JH, Gallagher WJ: Effects of sufentanil on cerebral circulation and metabolism in dogs. Anesth Analg 1990; 70:138–146.
54. Jung R, Shah N, Reinsel R, et al: Cerebrospinal fluid pressure in patients with brain tumors: Impact of fentanyl versus alfentanil during nitrous oxide-oxygen anesthesia. Anesth Analg 1990; 71:419–422.
55. Gibbs JM: The effect of intravenous ketamine on cerebrospinal fluid pressure. Br J Anaesth 1971; 44:1298–1302.
56. Shapiro HM, Wyte SR, Harris AB: Ketamine anaesthesia in patients with intracranial pathology. Br J Anaesth 1972; 44:1200–1204.

57. Sari A, Okuda Y, Takeshita H: The effect of ketamine on cerebrospinal fluid pressure. Anesth Analg 1972; 51:560–565.
58. Carlsson C, Chapman AG: The effect of diazepam on the cerebral metabolic state in rats and its interaction with nitrous oxide. Anesthesiology 1981; 54:488–495.
59. Foster A, Juge O, Morel D: Effects of midazolam on cerebral blood flow in human volunteers. Anesthesiology 1982; 56:453–455.
60. Rockoff MA, Naughton KVH, Shapiro HM, et al: Cerebral circulatory and metabolic responses to intravenously administered lorazepam. Anesthesiology 1980; 53:215–218.
61. Milde LN, Milde JH, Michenfelder JD: Cerebral functional, metabolic, and hemodynamic effects of etomidate in dogs. Anesthesiology 1985; 63:371–377.
62. Sebel PS, Lowdon JD: Propofol: A new intravenous anesthetic. Anesthesiology 1989; 71:260–277.
63. Pinaud M, Lelausque JN, Chetanneau A, et al: Effects of propofol on cerebral hemodynamics and metabolism in patients with brain trauma. Anesthesiology 1990; 73:404–409.
64. Varma YS, Sharma PL, Minocha KB: Comparative evaluation of cerebral and hepatic blood flow under d-tubocurarine and pancuronium in dogs. Indian J Med Res 1977; 66:317–322.
65. Belik J, Wagerle LC, Delivoria-Papadopoulos M: Cerebral blood flow and metabolism following pancuronium bromide in newborn lambs. Pediatr Res 1984; 18:1305–1308.
66. Griffin JP, Hartung J, Cottrell JE, et al: Effect of vecuronium on intracranial pressure, mean arterial pressure and heart rate in cats. Br J Anaesth 1986; 58:441–443.
67. Rosa G, Sanfilippo M, Vilardi M, et al: Effects of vecuronium bromide on intracranial pressure and cerebral perfusion pressure. Br J Anaesth 1986; 58:437–440.
68. Minton MD, Stirt JA, Bedford RF, Haworth C: Intracranial pressure after atracurium in neurosurgical patients. Anesth Analg 1985; 64:1113–1116.
69. Lanier WL, Milde JH, Michenfelder JD: The cerebral effects of pancuronium and atracurium in halothane-anesthetized dogs. Anesthesiology 1985; 63:589–597.
70. Lanier WL, Milde JM, Michenfelder JD: Cerebral stimulation following succinylcholine in dogs. Anesthesiology 1986; 64:551–559.
71. Minton MD, Grosslight K, Stirt JA, Bedford RF: Increases in intracranial pressure from succinylcholine: Prevention by prior nondepolarizing blockade. Anesthesiology 1986; 65:165–169.
72. Stirt JA, Grosslight KR, Bedford RF, Vollmer D: "Defasciculation" with metocurine prevents succinylcholine-induced increases in intracranial pressure. Anesthesiology 1987; 67:50–53.
73. Cottrell JE, Robustelli A, Post K, Turndorf H: Furosemide- and mannitol-induced changes in intracranial pressure and serum osmolality and electrolytes. Anesthesiology 1977; 47:28–30.
74. Leech P, Miller JD: Intracranial volume-pressure relationships during experimental brain compression in primates. J Neurol Neurosurg Psychiatry 1974; 37:1105–1111.
75. Johnston IH, Harper AM: The effect of mannitol on cerebral blood flow: An experimental study. J Neurosurg 1973; 38:461–471.
76. Turner JM, Powell D, Gibson RM, McDowall DG: Intracranial pressure changes in neurosurgical patients during hypotension induced with sodium nitroprusside or trimetaphan. Br J Anaesth 1977; 49:419–424.
77. James DJ, Bedford RF: Hydralazine for controlled hypotension during neurosurgical operations. Anesth Analg 1982; 61:1016–1019.
78. Ghani GA, Sung YF, Weinstein MS, et al: Effects of intravenous nitroglycerin on the intracranial pressure and volume pressure response. J Neurosurg 1983; 58:562–565.
79. Fahmy NR, Soter NA: Effects of trimethaphan on arterial blood histamine and systemic hemodynamics in humans. Anesthesiology 1985; 62:562–566.
80. Berntman L, Carlsson C, Siesjo BK: Influence of propranolol on cerebral metabolism and blood flow in the rat brain. Brain Res 1978; 151:220–224.
81. Aken HV, Puchstein C, Schweppe ML, Heinecke A: Effect of labetalol on intracranial pressure in dogs with and without intracranial hypertension. Acta Anaesthiol Scand 1982; 26:615–619.
82. Benfield P, Sorkin EM: Esmolol. A preliminary review of pharmacodynamic and pharmacokinetic properties, and therapeutic efficacy. Drugs 1987; 33:392–412.
83. Hadley MN, Spetzler RF, Fifield MS, et al: The effect of nimodipine on intracranial pressure. J Neurosurg 1987; 66:387–393.
84. Nishikawa T, Omote K, Namiki A, et al: The effects of nicardipine on cerebrospinal fluid pressure in humans. Anesth Analg 1986; 65:507–510.
85. Marshall LF, Bowers SA: Medical management of intracranial pressure. *In* Cooper PR (ed): Head Injury. Baltimore: Williams & Wilkins, 1982; 129–146.
86. Strandgaard S: Autoregulation of cerebral blood flow in hypertensive patients. Circulation 1975; 53:720–727.
87. Wilkinson HA: Intracranial pressure monitoring: Techniques and pitfalls. *In* Cooper PR (ed): Head Injury. Baltimore: Williams & Wilkins, 1982; 147–184.
88. Sundbarg G, Nordstrom CH, Messeter K, et al: A comparison of intraparenchymatous and intraventricular pressure recording in clinical practice. J Neurosurg 1987; 67:841–845.
89. Mendelow AD, Rowan JO, Murray L, Kerr AE: A clinical comparison of subdural screw pressure measurements with ventricular pressure. J Neurosurg 1983; 58:45–50.
90. Jorgensen PB, Riishede J: Comparative clinical studies of epidural and ventricular pressure. *In* Brock M, Dietz H (eds): Intracranial Pressure: Experimental and Clinical Aspects. Berlin: Springer-Verlag, 1972; 41–45.
91. Friedman WA, Vries JK: Percutaneous tunnel ventriculostomy. J Neurosurg 1980; 53:662–665.
92. Narayan RK, Kishore PR, Becker DP, et al: Intracranial pressure: To monitor or not to monitor? J Neurosurg 1982; 56:650–659.
93. Langfitt TW: Clinical methods for monitoring intracranial pressure and measuring cerebral blood flow. Clin Neurosurg 1976; 23:302–320.
94. Rosner MJ, Becker DP: ICP monitoring: Complications and associated factors. Clin Neurosurg 1976; 23:494–519.
95. Vries JK, Becker DP, Young HF: A subarachnoid screw for monitoring intracranial pressure. J Neurosurg 1973; 39:416–419.
96. Wilkinson HA: The intracranial pressure-monitoring cup catheter: Technical note. Neurosurgery 1977; 1:139–141.
97. Koster WG, Kuypers MH: Intracranial pressure and its epidural measurement. Med Prog Technol 1980; 7:21–27.
98. Kleiber M: Physical instruments for the biologist. Rev Sci Instr 1945; 15:79–81.
99. Barlow P, Mendelow AD, Lawrence AE, et al: Clinical evaluation of two methods of subdural pressure monitoring. J Neurosurg 1985; 63:578–582.
100. Allen R: Intracranial pressure: A review of clinical problems, measurement techniques and monitoring methods. J Med Eng Tech 1986; 10:299–320.
101. Crutchfield JS, Narayan RK, Robertson CS, et al: Evaluation of a fiberoptic intracranial pressure monitor. J Neurosurg 1990; 72:482–487.
102. Ostrup RC, Luerssen TG, Marshall LF, et al: Continuous monitoring of intracranial pressure with a miniaturized fiberoptic device. J Neurosurg 1987; 67:206–209.
103. Rabow L, Bergenheim T, Balfors E: Intraparenchymal and conventional monitoring of intracranial pressure. J Clin Monit 1990; 6:163.
104. Chambers IR, Mendelow AD, Sinar EJ, et al: A clinical evaluation of the camino subdural screw and ventricular monitoring kits. Neurosurgery 1990; 26:421–423.

CHAPTER

14

Specialized Neurophysiologic Monitoring

DAVID S. SMITH, M.D., Ph.D.,
and ERIC PERSILY, M.D.

Monitoring of brain function during surgery and in the intensive care unit continues to evolve. Three evolving modalities—transcranial Doppler ultrasound, jugular venous oximetry, and transcranial measurement of vascular hemoglobin saturation—appear promising. Transcranial measurement of hemoglobin saturation is in the development stage and has seen little clinical use, but it has significant potential for providing long-needed information about brain oxygenation. Transcranial Doppler is a more mature monitoring modality whose indications are beginning to emerge. Jugular venous oxygen measurements date back at least 80 years, but new indications are being explored that may result in more widespread use. An overview of the technology of each monitoring technique is presented, followed by a discussion of its perioperative or intensive care utility in humans.

TRANSCRANIAL DOPPLER

The transcranial Doppler (TCD) device enables the user to obtain real-time information about blood flow velocity (BFV) from the cerebral vasculature. Miller has reviewed most of the available equipment.[1] Using a low-frequency (2 MHz), pulsed, range-gated probe, it is possible to interrogate the anterior, middle, and posterior cerebral arteries, as well as the vertebral and basilar arteries (Table 14–1).[2] Newer instruments can perform bilateral measurements. Probes that can be fixed in place have been developed for long-term recording. Indications (Table 14–2) include diagnosis of cerebral artery stenosis, detection of embolic events, and measurement of changes in cerebral blood flow (CBF) and intracranial pressure (ICP). TCD has been used during carotid endarterectomy to detect perfusion changes during clamping of the internal carotid artery. The technique has been used to detect the onset of intracranial vasospasm after subarachnoid hemorrhage (SAH). Detailed reviews of TCD have been published.[4–6]

MEASUREMENT

TCD examinations of the cerebral vasculature are based on the same principles as other types of ultrasonic instruments. The signal is generated when the low-frequency waves bounce off the moving red blood cells. The shift in the frequency of the reflected signal compared with the original signal is directly proportional to the velocity of the red blood cells (Doppler principle). There are three main routes (windows) through which the TCD probe can be directed to obtain a signal from the cerebral vasculature: the temporal bone window, a transorbital window, and the foramen magnum.[4]

The temporal window is located above the zygomatic arch, between the ear and the orbit (Fig. 14–1). Here the bone is thin enough for passage of the signal. Signals from the middle cerebral artery (MCA), anterior cerebral artery (ACA), and posterior cerebral artery (PCA), as well as the internal carotid artery (ICA), can usually be obtained through this window. Occasionally, the anterior and posterior communicating arteries can also be insonated. When using this window, MCA and proximal PCA flow are normally directed toward the probe, terminal ICA flow is often bidirectional, and ACA flow is usually directed away from the probe.

The transorbital approach is used for insonating the ophthalmic artery (OA) and the carotid siphon. The probe is placed over the closed eyelid; blood flow can be detected from the OA at a depth of 40–50 mm.

The BFV detected by TCD as a function of time from an awake, normal volunteer is shown in Figure 14–2. Normal values for peak and mean BFV in the MCA, ACA, and PCA are 62 ± 12, 51 ± 12, and 44 ± 11 cm/second (mean ± 1 SD), respectively.[2, 3, 8] Aging decreases BFV

TABLE 14–1. CHARACTERISTICS OF THE TRANSCRANIAL DOPPLER INSTRUMENT

1. Emitting frequency—2 MHz
2. Total emitted ultrasonic power—350 mW reducible to 7 mW
3. Pulse repetition frequency—6.8–18 kHz
4. Pulse length—10 μsec
5. High-pass filter—100 Hz; low-pass filter—3.4–9 kHz
6. The position of a sample volume can be varied within a range of 3–8.5 cm in steps of 0.5 cm
7. Transducer—emitting area of 1.5 cm^3; polystyrene acoustic lens; focal length of approximately 5 cm; resolution of sample volume at focal length—axial 0.5 cm, lateral 0.8 cm

From Arnolds BJ, von Reutern G-M: Transcranial dopplersonography. Examination technique and normal reference valves. Ultrasound Med Biol 1986; 12:115–123. With kind permission from Pergamon Press Ltd., Headington Hill Hall, Oxford OX3 OBW, UK.

(Table 14–3).[8] In Aaslid et al's study, MCA signals were obtained in 100% of subjects.[2] The failure rate for PCA signals was 40%, and the failure rate for ACA signals was 20%. Hennerici et al had success rates that were slightly higher, but they excluded patients with small ultrasonic bone windows.[8] Aaslid and colleagues also determined that BFVs in the MCA, PCA, and ACA were higher than those in the extracranial ICA, suggesting that the highest velocities in the cerebral circulation are found in the basal cerebral arteries.[2] Peak systolic velocities in the ACA and MCA are comparable to that found in the aorta, despite the fact that the aorta is several times greater in size.[2] Schoning and Walter reported on a series of 49 patients in whom they studied the posterior cerebral circulation using TCD.[9] Signals were obtained from the posterior cerebral artery in 100% of subjects, from the basilar artery in 92%, and from the vertebral arteries in 89%. Mean systolic peak BFV was about 46 cm/second.

Some important considerations in using TCD include the angle of the probe and the stability of the measurements over time. The angle between the ultrasonic beam and the vessel is very important because the accuracy of the BFV measurements is improved as the angle approaches 0°, meaning that blood flow is directly toward the probe. This situation is most closely approximated in the MCA when using the temporal window. Changes in the angle from 0° to 30° ensure that the results will be accurate to within 15%. Another important factor is the stability of the measurement probe over time. For serial or continuous measurements, the probe should remain focused on the same segment. The diameter of the vessel is an important factor in BFV measurements; focusing on different segments of artery may give confusing or inaccurate results. In some elderly patients, temporal or suboccipital bone thickening may preclude TCD measurement.[6] The energy generated by the TCD probe appears to be below the threshold for tissue damage. However, reduction of signal intensity by 90% has been recommended when insonating through the orbit because of the potential for retinal injury.[6]

TABLE 14–2. INDICATIONS FOR USE OF TRANSCRANIAL DOPPLER

1. Detection of changes in cerebral blood flow velocity during carotid endarterectomy
2. Detection of embolic phenomena
3. Determination of stroke mechanism
4. Detection of cerebral vasospasm after subarachnoid hemorrhage or cranial surgery
5. Measurement of intracranial pressure
6. Detection of arteriovenous malformations
7. Detection of intracranial stenoses and collateral flow
8. Assessment of pharmacodynamic effects of anesthetics on the cerebral vasculature

RELATIONSHIP TO CEREBRAL BLOOD FLOW

Much of the research surrounding TCD attempts to quantify the relationship between cerebral BFV and actual CBF. Ideally, the linkage of these two variables would allow TCD to provide noninvasive estimates of CBF. Current CBF methods using various radioactive tracers (for example, ^{133}xenon or ^{15}oxygen) are invasive, expensive, and noncontinuous. Thus, TCD, which is both noninvasive and continuous, has potential advantages.

The relationship between BFV through an artery (in centimeters per second) and flow (in milliliters per minute) is

$$\dot{Q} = V \times A \qquad 14\text{–}1$$

where $\dot{Q}$ = blood flow, V = BFV, and A = arterial lumen area.[10] The volume of flow ($\dot{Q}'$) in the perfusion territory of an artery is

$$\dot{Q}' = rCBF \times T \qquad 14\text{–}2$$

where T = the weight of the perfusion territory (100 gm), rCBF = the blood flow through that region (ml/100 gm brain tissue/minute), and $\dot{Q}' = \dot{Q} \times 60$. Combining these two equations, the following relationship is obtained:

$$rCBF \times T = V \times A \times 60 \qquad 14\text{–}3$$

or

$$V = rCBF \times 1/60 \times T/A \qquad 14\text{–}4$$

This equation shows that BFV (as measured by TCD) will reflect changes in actual CBF provided that the luminal area of the artery (A) and the size of the perfusion territory (T) remain constant. Thus, if an intervention is performed that does not affect CBF, but cerebral BFV changes, the intervention must be changing arterial diameter or the territory served by the artery.[10]

Other indices have been derived from TCD signals. The pulsatility index (PI) is supposed to reflect changes in cerebral vascular resistance, although this relationship is being debated. It is calculated as the difference between the systolic and diastolic peak BFV divided by the mean BFV. However, the most accepted data formulation is BFV, which forms the bulk of the published data.

Dahl and colleagues performed a study comparing TCD with ^{133}xenon inhalation and single photon emission computed tomography (SPECT) to determine changes in response to acetazolamide (a vasodilatory stimulus).[10] They demonstrated a positive correlation between the absolute increase in CBF and the percentage of increase in BFV measured by the TCD. The TCD change correlated with

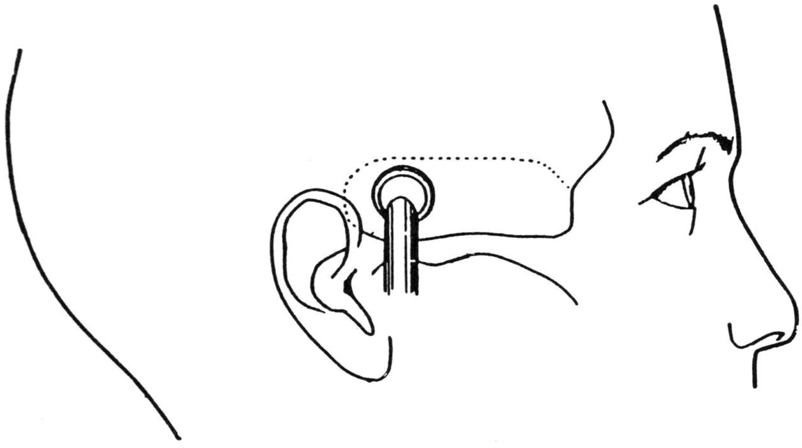

Figure 14–1. Diagram of the area *(dotted line)* where Doppler signals from intracranial arteries can be obtained. The zygomatic arch is indicated. The most likely location to obtain signals is shown by the position of the probe. (From Aaslid R, et al: Noninvasive transcranial Doppler ultrasound recording of flow velocity in basal cerebral arteries. J Neurosurg 1982; 57:769–774.)

changes in CBF 86% of the time and detected decreased cerebrovascular reactivity (potentially a sign of increased risk of injury during episodes of hypoxemia or hypotension).

Others have examined the effects of different perturbations of the cerebral vasculature to try to correlate TCD data with changes in CBF. Werner[5] and DeWitt and Wechsler[4] have reviewed this literature and present conflicting interpretations. Werner suggests that some studies have shown that larger cerebral vessels can and do change their diameter in response to physiologic (CO_2) and pharmacologic (vasoactive drugs) challenges.[5] DeWitt and Wechsler state that the larger vessels maintain their diameter unchanged in the face of changes in the partial pressure of CO_2 (PCO_2) and that changes in resistance are at the level of the arteriole.[4] If DeWitt and Wechsler are correct, changes in CBF caused by PCO_2 should be proportional to changes in cerebral BFV in the larger vessels.

Many variables affect CBF and cerebral BFV, including length and cross-sectional area of the vessel, ICP, PCO_2, and hemoglobin concentration. For example, a relationship between arterial diameter and BFV has been demonstrated in patients with SAH due to aneurysms or arteriovenous malformations (AVMs).[11] All patients with angiographic evidence of vasospasm had TCD BFV of 120 cm/second or more. Martin and colleagues compared TCD results with [133]xenon measurements of CBF in post-trauma patients with cerebral vasospasm.[12] They found a significant correlation between the lowest CBF and the highest MCA BFV, indicating that arterial narrowing can lead to impaired CBF. However, an increase in ICP may lead to decreased BFV even when vasospasm is present.[13] Brass and colleagues showed an inverse relationship between hematocrit (viscosity) and blood velocity, suggesting that increased BFV alone is insufficient to confirm vasospasm.[14] In the presence of anemia, BFV may be increased because of decreased viscosity.

Anesthetics affect TCD BFV. Trindle et al recently showed that both fentanyl and sufentanil, in equianesthetic doses, caused an increase in MCA BFV.[15] Ketamine has been shown to increase BFV and reduce the PI.[16] Propofol decreases BFV,[17] but there is no additional decrease when nitrous oxide is administered.

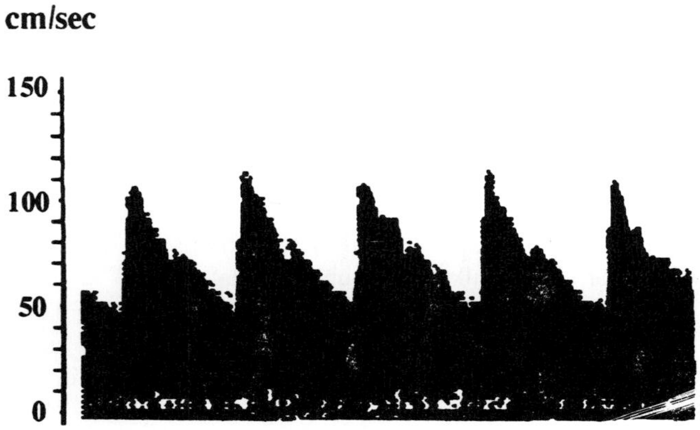

Figure 14–2. Blood flow velocity (ordinate) as a function of time (abscissa) obtained from the middle cerebral artery of a normal, awake volunteer. (From Werner C, et al: Transcranial doppler sonography as a supplement in the detection of cerebral circulatory arrest. J Neurosurg Anesth 1990; 2:159–165.)

CLINICAL USES

Carotid Endarterectomy (CEA)

TCD has been used to monitor the adequacy of cerebral circulation during carotid endarterectomy.[4, 5] Halsey and colleagues used TCD to measure MCA BFV in 31 patients undergoing CEA.[18] The electroencephalogram (EEG) and rCBF were also measured. BFV and rCBF measurements were made before, during, and after carotid clamping. If rCBF was increased, there was no correlation between rCBF and MCA BFV. However, with lower rCBF (< 20 ml/100 gm/minute), there was a positive correlation between rCBF and mean BFV. At extremely low rCBF (< 12 ml/100 gm/minute), there was almost always, at least momentarily, disappearance of the organized pulsatile BFV waveform. EEG changes correlated better with rCBF than with mean BFV, which may represent the biggest problem with using TCD as an estimate of CBF. rCBF is measured predominantly from the cortical convexity, whereas BFV is measured in vessels near the base of the brain. The authors

TABLE 14–3. NORMAL AGE-ADJUSTED CALCULATED (MEAN ± SD) VALUES OF TC DOPPLER FLOW VELOCITY WITHIN THE BASAL CEREBRAL ARTERIES

Arteries (Depth in mm)	Systolic Peak Velocity (cm/second)		Averaged Mean Velocity (cm/second)		Diastolic Peak Velocity (cm/second)		Age (Years)
MCA (50 mm)	94.5 ± 13.6	n.s.	58.4 ± 8.4	n.s.	45.6 ± 6.6	n.s.	<40
	91.0 ± 16.9		57.7 ± 11.5		44.3 ± 9.5		40–60
	78.1 ± 15.0	*	44.7 ± 11.1	*	31.9 ± 9.1	*	>60
ACA (70 mm)	76.4 ± 16.9	n.s.	47.3 ± 13.6	n.s.	36.0 ± 9.0	n.s.	<40
	86.4 ± 20.1		53.1 ± 10.5		41.1 ± 7.4		40–60
	73.3 ± 20.3	n.s.	45.3 ± 13.5	n.s.	34.2 ± 8.8	*	>60
PCA (60 mm)	53.2 ± 11.3	n.s.	34.2 ± 7.8	n.s.	25.9 ± 6.5	n.s.	<40
	60.1 ± 20.6		36.6 ± 9.8		28.7 ± 7.5		40–60
	51.0 ± 11.9	n.s.	29.9 ± 9.3	n.s.	22.0 ± 6.9	*	>60
VA/BA (75 mm)	56.3 ± 7.8	n.s.	34.9 ± 7.8	n.s.	27.0 ± 5.3	n.s.	<40
	59.5 ± 17.0		36.4 ± 11.7		29.2 ± 8.4		40–60
	50.9 ± 18.7	n.s.	30.5 ± 12.4	n.s.	21.2 ± 9.2	*	>60

MCA, middle cerebral artery; ACA, anterior cerebral artery; PCA, posterior cerebral artery; VA, vertebral artery; BA, basilar artery; n.s., not significant.
*Significantly different.
From Hennerici M, et al: Transcranial Doppler ultrasound for the assessment of intracranial arterial flow capacity—Part 1. Examination technique and normal values. Surg Neurol 1987; 27:439–448. Reprinted by permission of the publisher. Copyright 1987 by Elsevier Science Publishing Co., Inc.

state that because of these anatomic differences, one method cannot be validated by the other, nor should one replace the other. These methods measure different parameters and have different, complementary capabilities.

The International Transcranial Doppler Collaborators conducted a multi-institutional, retrospective study of 1495 patients and demonstrated that selective shunting reduced intraoperative stroke in patients whose BFV decreased to 0–15% during the first minute after cross clamping and that stroke risk may be increased in patients receiving carotid shunts, despite a first-minute cross-clamped BFV greater than 40% of that measured in control conditions.[19] These data suggest that TCD may play a role in the intraoperative monitoring of patients undergoing carotid endarterectomy.

Detection of Emboli

Another emerging clinical use of TCD is the detection of embolic phenomena, either during CEA or cardiac surgery (for a review, see Markus[20]). It has been suspected that neurologic deficits after cardiopulmonary bypass were due to embolism of air or of particulate matter. Padayachee and colleagues described the use of TCD to measure embolic events in the MCA during cardiopulmonary bypass with membrane or bubble oxygenators.[21] Harrison and colleagues were able to show that an extra arterial filter in the bypass circuit decreased TCD evidence of embolic events.[22] They also showed that patients in the group with the extra filter had fewer recorded embolic events and were less likely to show a postoperative deterioration in performance on neuropsychologic testing. Emboli have also been detected after reestablishment of blood flow in the common carotid artery during CEA.[23]

Stroke

TCD can be useful in the evaluation of patients with stroke. For instance, Teague and Sharma used TCD to detect paradoxical echo contrast in the cerebral vasculature.[24] The presence of intravascularly injected contrast in the arterial system implies a right-to-left shunt at the level of the heart (patent foramen ovale). They compared contrast echocardiography with TCD in 46 patients with stroke. TCD detected evidence of paradoxical echo contrast (altered signal) in 41% of these patients at rest and during the strain phase of a Valsalva maneuver. Transthoracic echocardiography detected shunting in only 26% of these patients at rest and in 15% during Valsalva maneuver. All patients with evidence of intracardiac shunting (microbubbles in left ventricle) were also detected by TCD. Discordant studies almost always had evidence of paradoxical embolization by TCD and indeterminate findings by two-dimensional (2D) echocardiography. In addition, six transthoracic echo studies were considered inadequate, whereas only one of the TCD studies was considered difficult (but adequate). Siebler and colleagues used TCD to detect silent intracranial embolism in patients with symptomatic carotid artery disease.[25]

Cerebral vascular insufficiency may also be detectable with TCD. Head and neck movements that cause cerebrovascular compression may cause reductions in BFV. In patients with symptoms of cerebrovascular deficiency as a function of head position, compromised blood flow can be confirmed with TCD measurements.[26]

Cerebrovascular Reactivity

Cerebral vasospasm is responsible for much of the morbidity and mortality associated with SAH both before and after surgery. The current method of measuring vasospasm, angiography, is expensive and invasive, and it cannot be used as a continuous monitor or repeated at frequent intervals. TCD detects cerebral vasospasm in patients who have suffered SAH or trauma. Increased BFV has been found in patients with SAH, and a rapid increase to high BFV has been shown to herald the onset of deficits caused by delayed ischemia.[11]

Grosset and colleagues studied 121 patients with SAH.[27] They performed TCD examinations every 2 days (or more frequently if symptoms of a neurologic deficit were developing) and were able to identify 20 patients who experienced a rapid increase in BFV in the MCA or ACA. These patients were asymptomatic when the change in velocity was noted. rCBF was determined in the 20 identified patients; 15 patients were studied prior to the onset of neurologic deficits, and 5 were studied after the onset of neurologic deficits. Of the first group of 15 patients, 14 had abnormal CBF measurements, and 10 eventually developed a neurologic deficit. Thus, TCD was able to detect a change in MCA BFV before the onset of neurologic symptoms in 10 patients. Four patients without clinical deficit had abnormal scan results. The importance of this latter finding is unknown, but it may represent patients with reversible ischemia.

TCD measurements alone will tend to overestimate the number of patients at risk for a neurologic deficit because the TCD cannot take into account compensatory changes such as increased oxygen extraction and blood flow redistribution. Of the five patients studied after onset of deficits, all had abnormal CBF in the areas supplied by the ACA or MCA, although the correlation for the ACA was not as strong, probably because of the capacity for collateral flow from the anterior communicating artery. The authors concluded that TCD may be useful in early detection of patients at risk for delayed ischemia. This may allow the clinician to begin treatment sooner and to improve outcome. Monitoring TCD during aneurysm surgery allowed Eng et al to detect aneurysm rupture by an abrupt change from the normal velocity flow pattern to an oscillating flow pattern of antegrade flow during systole and retrograde flow during diastole, which was consistent with a high ICP.[28]

Intracranial Pressure

Another area where TCD may prove useful is in patients with increased ICP. Pople measured BFV in the MCA of 248 children with ventriculoperitoneal shunts.[29] From these measurements, which were performed in asymptomatic children, a table of age-referenced normal values was generated. During his follow-up period, 20 children developed shunt malfunction, 11 of whom subsequently needed shunt revision. Nine of the eleven had abnormal TCD results upon their admission to the hospital. Changes in BFV have been recently correlated with B waves in the ICP waveform, suggesting that changes in BFV can be reflected in the ICP in patients with reduced intracranial compliance (see Chapter 13).[30]

CEREBRAL OXIMETRY

Sampling of internal jugular venous blood as a source of blood draining the brain dates to 1927 when Myerson et al reported venipuncture of the internal jugular vein at the level of the tip of mastoid.[31] In 1942, the technique was used to determine arterial-venous differences in oxygen, pH, lactic acid, and glucose in human volunteers.[32] The technique became central to the quantitative cerebral blood flow technique developed by Kety and Schmidt,[33] because a measure of the diffusible tracer in the blood draining the tissue of interest was a central part of this technique. Internal jugular venous sampling became less important with the introduction of radioactive tracers and external detection of tissue radioactivity levels that allowed calculation of blood flow (for a review see Obrist and Wilkinson[34]). However, the determination of cerebral metabolic rate for oxygen and brain extraction of various compounds still requires measurements in cerebral venous blood.

Despite the long availability of internal jugular venous blood sampling, it has seen little use except in research. Measurements of venous oxygen extraction and lactate production appear to be gaining importance in the initial therapy of patients with severe head injury. Estimates of oxygen extraction may improve the titration of hyperventilation to maximize its effects on reducing ICP while minimizing the risk of therapy-induced ischemia. In addition, measurements of venous oxygen extraction in patients undergoing cardiopulmonary bypass have identified a period of potential ischemia during rewarming, which may lead to changes in the clinical approach to rewarming.

TECHNIQUE

Placement of the Internal Jugular Venous Catheter

The initial techniques involved venipuncture near the jugular bulb using external landmarks. Most investigators insert a catheter into the jugular bulb either from the antecubital fossa with manipulation of the catheter into the jugular bulb with fluoroscopic guidance[35, 36] or by retrograde catheterization of the internal jugular vein (for a review and recent experience, see Goetting and Preston[37]). Regardless of the technique, precise localization of the catheter within the jugular bulb using radiographic confirmation of placement is important. Small errors in placement greatly increase the risk of contamination from noncerebral blood (Fig. 14–3). Typically, the tip of the catheter should lie between the base of the skull and the top of the second cervical vertebrae (C2).[38] A catheter lying below the level of C2 may have significant extracranial contamination.[38] Miller et al also note that a single internal jugular vein may contain most of the blood flow and suggest determining the dominant vein for cannulation, at least for patients with head injury.[38] In contrast, Robertson et al suggest catheter placement on the side with the greatest evidence of injury as determined by the computed tomography scan.[39] Others believe that although one internal jugular vein may drain the bulk of the brain, samples from either vessel are representative of the entire brain (for discussion, see Chan et al[40]).

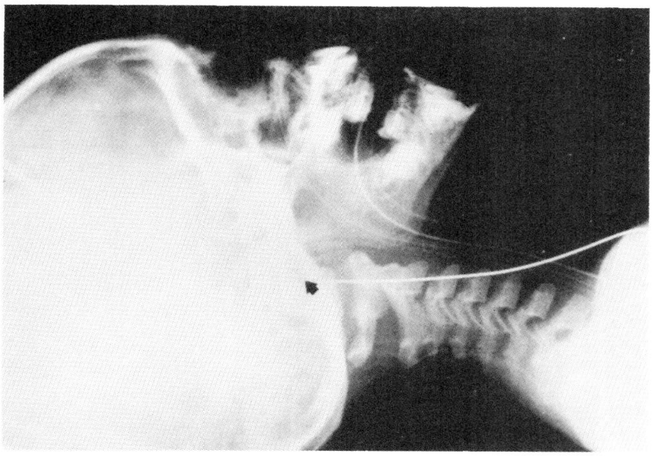

Figure 14–3. Radiograph demonstrating proper catheter tip position within the jugular bulb *(arrow)*. (From Goetting MG, Preston G: Jugular bulb catheterization: Experience with 123 patients. Crit Care Med 1990; 18:1220–1223.)

Determination of Oxygen

The most common use of internal jugular venous catheters is to determine oxygen extraction. When CBF is known, oxygen extraction is used to determine the cerebral metabolic rate for oxygen. In addition, changes in oxygen content in internal jugular venous blood relative to arterial blood provide an estimate of cerebral perfusion adequacy. Increasing oxygen extraction despite constant metabolic demand suggests inadequate oxygen delivery. However, in very low-flow states, jugular venous hemoglobin saturations (Sjo_2) may be high because of extracranial contamination. When catheters are used, the internal jugular venous blood is withdrawn simultaneously with an arterial sample and both are analyzed.

Fiberoptic catheters that measure hemoglobin saturation *in situ* have been developed.[41–43] These catheters can be inserted into the jugular bulb to allow continuous measurement of hemoglobin saturation.[44] In at least one study, fiberoptic catheters were used in both the internal jugular vein and an artery,[45] allowing simultaneous, continuous measurement of both arterial and venous hemoglobin saturations. Fiberoptic catheters use the ratio of light absorption at two or three wavelengths to provide values of hemoglobin saturation. They measure the light reflected from the red blood cells so that clot on the catheter tip, failure to have the catheter in the center of the vessel lumen, or severe anemia can lead to erroneous readings. Periodic calibration against sampled blood is recommended.

Normal levels of Sjo_2 as determined by Gibbs et al are 65% (Table 14–4).[32] Critical levels of Sjo_2 also have been determined. In anesthetized cats (ketamine infusion) subjected to increasing levels of intracranial hypertension induced by infusion of saline into the cisterna magna, energy failure, as determined by decreased brain phosphocreatine, or PCr (measured by ^{31}phosphorus magnetic resonance spectroscopy), occurred at a sagittal sinus oxygen content of 1.4 ± 0.6 vol% (mean ± 1 S.D.) (Table 14–5).[46] Sagittal sinus blood in animal studies is the equivalent of jugular bulb blood in humans. In unanesthetized volunteers, EEG slowing occurs at an Sjo_2 of 40%,[47] mental confusion at 33%, and loss of consciousness at 26%[48] (see Schell et al for a review[49]). Miller et al have defined cerebral ischemia in patients with head injury as Sjo_2 values less than 40% (difference between arterial and internal jugular vein oxygen contents [$AVDo_2$] > 9 ml/dl). They have found values in this range in patients suffering from seizures, systemic hypotension, or arterial hypoxemia. Table 14–6 lists many of the causes of abnormal $AVDo_2$.

A variety of approaches have been used to express the data obtained from internal jugular venous sampling. The simplest but perhaps least useful is the partial pressure of oxygen (Po_2). Most investigators express the data as hemoglobin saturation, either measured directly using an *in situ* fiberoptic catheter or determined from a blood sample by direct measurement or calculation. Oxygen content (hemoglobin concentration × 1.39 × % saturation + Po_2 × 0.003) is also widely used and compensates for changes in hemoglobin concentration and the carrying capacity of plasma.[44] $AVDo_2$ is the difference between the arterial and internal jugular vein oxygen contents ($Cao_2 - Cjo_2$), and the cerebral oxygen extraction ratio (OER) is the $AVDo_2$ divided by the Cao_2. The cerebral metabolic rate for oxygen ($CMRo_2 = AVDo_2 \times CBF$) is also used as is the cerebral extraction of oxygen (CEo_2), which has been defined as the difference between arterial and internal jugular vein hemoglobin saturations ($Sao_2 - Sjo_2$).

Determination of Lactate

The interpretation of lactate levels is more complex in that the brain can take up or excrete lactate. Thus arteriovenous concentration differences can be positive or nega-

TABLE 14–4. ARTERIAL AND INTERNAL JUGULAR VENOUS OXYGEN AND LACTIC ACID LEVELS FROM 50 HEALTHY YOUNG MEN AT REST

	Arterial Blood		Internal Jugular Blood		Arterial-Venous Difference	
Compound	*Mean ± S.D.*	*Range*	*Mean ± S.D.*	*Range*	*Mean ± S.D.*	*Range*
O_2 content (vol%)	19.6 ± 1.2	17.3–22.3	12.9 ± 1.3	11.0–16.1	6.7 ± 0.8	4.5–8.5
O_2 saturation (%)	93.9 ± 1	91.2–95.8	61.8 ± 3.7	55.3–70.7	31.7 ± 3.9	21.9–39.1
Lactic acid (mg/dl)	9.9 ± 2.6	5.9–19.1	11.5 ± 2.7	7.7–22.0	1.6 ± 0.9	0.3–3.8

Data from Gibbs EL, et al: Arterial and cerebral venous blood arterial-venous differences in man. J Biol Chem 1942; 144:325–332.

TABLE 14–5. ARTERIAL AND SAGITTAL SINUS OXYGEN CONTENTS BEFORE AND AFTER METABOLIC FAILURE* INDUCED BY INCREASING ICP IN SIX CATS

	Arterial Blood Oxygen Content (vol %)		Sagittal Sinus Blood Oxygen Content (vol %)		Arterial-Venous Difference	
Compound	*Mean ± S.D.*	*Range*	*Mean ± S.D.*	*Range*	*Mean ± S.D.*	*Range*
Normal PCr	12.8 ± 2.3	9.2–16.1	8.4 ± 1.6	5.9–10.4	4.4 ± 1.5	2.6–7.2
Reduced PCr (ICP: 84 ± 11.3 mmHg)	9.8 ± 3.8	5.7–17.6	1.4 ± 0.6	1.0–2.9	8.4 ± 3.2	4.7–14.7

*Metabolic failure was defined as a significant decrease in brain phosphocreatine (PCr).

Data from Sutton LN, et al: Cerebral venous oxygen content as a measure of brain energy metabolism with increased intracranial pressure and hyperventilation. J Neurosurg 1990; 73:927–932.

tive. Normal cerebral metabolic rates for lactate (CMRL) are −0.023 μmol/gm/minute, which is consistent with low baseline lactate production.[39] Increasing lactate levels in venous blood relative to arterial blood (increasing anaerobic glycolysis) are thought to reflect metabolic stress and inadequate oxygen delivery.

CLINICAL APPLICATION

Neuroanesthesia

Engberg and colleagues measured Cjo_2 during craniotomy with two different anesthetics: (1) halothane, fentanyl, and nitrous oxide, or (2) droperidol, fentanyl, and nitrous oxide.[51] With both techniques, the $AVDo_2$ decreased with incision and extubation. During the operation, the $AVDo_2$ in patients receiving droperidol was greater than that in patients receiving halothane.

Sanchez et al used changes in Cjo_2 to monitor the embolization of arteriovenous malformations (AVMs).[52] With the malformation intact, CBF is high and $AVDo_2$ is low. As the AVM is obliterated, CBF decreases and $AVDo_2$ increases toward normal values.

TABLE 14–6. POSSIBLE CAUSES OF CHANGES IN $AVDo_2$

Low $AVDo_2$ (Cerebral O_2 Supply > Demand)	High $AVDo_2$ (Cerebral O_2 Demand > Supply)
Increased CBF	Decreased CBF
Polycythemia	Anemia
Alkalemia	Decreased hemoglobin saturation
Temperature	Acidemia
Decreased 2,3-DPG levels	Pyrexia
Increased CPP	Decreased CPP
Decreased blood viscosity	Increased blood viscosity
Nondeformability of red cells	Increased cerebral metabolic function
Decreased cerebral metabolic function	Seizure activity
Sedative drugs	Use of analeptic drugs
Cyanide poisoning	
Contamination from extracerebral blood source	

$AVDo_2$ = arterial-jugular venous oxygen difference: CBF = cerebral blood flow; 2,3-DPG = 2,3-diphosphoglycerate; CPP = cerebral perfusion pressure.

From Gilbert J: Estimation of CBF by cerebral venous oxygen difference [Letter]. J Neurosurg 1989; 71:790.

Carotid Endarterectomy

Several groups have measured cerebral oxygen extraction during carotid endarterectomy.[53, 54] Sjo_2 values greater than 60% correlate with adequate brain perfusion. Cerebral dysfunction was found with Sjo_2 values less than 50%. However, Sjo_2 is, by its nature, a global measure and should be less sensitive than multichannel EEG. A direct comparison of EEG and Sjo_2 has not been performed.

Cardiopulmonary Bypass

Two groups have measured brain oxygen extraction during cardiopulmonary bypass.[55, 56] One group reported prebypass Sjo_2 values of 64.2 ± 5.7 (mean ± S.D.), whereas during rewarming, Sjo_2 decreased to 57.1 ± 7.6.[56] In the other study, 31 of 133 patients (23%) showed decrease in Sjo_2 to < 50% during rewarming.[55] The decrease in Sjo_2 was related to the speed of rewarming (Fig. 14–4). Of interest was the fact that one group used a fiberoptic oximeter catheter that allowed continuous Sjo_2 monitoring.[56] Both groups of investigators believed that the decrease in Sjo_2 during rewarming suggested the possibility of relative ischemia. Observation of hemoglobin desaturation during rewarming after cardiopulmonary bypass has also been made using noninvasive transcranial measurements of brain vascular hemoglobin saturation (discussed later). These observations suggest that ischemic damage seen after bypass may not only be related to emboli released into the cerebral circulation during bypass and decannulation but also a mismatch between oxygen supply and demand with a potential for ischemic brain damage. These initial studies failed to demonstrate increased neurologic damage in patients with increased oxygen extraction compared to those who did not; however, the numbers of patients in these studies were small.

Measurements of Sjo_2 are also used in infants undergoing heart surgery. van der Linden et al demonstrated that Sjo_2 remained adequate with pump flows reduced to 0.5 L/minute/m in profoundly hypothermic infants.[57] During rewarming, Sjo_2 decreased. Kern et al found that during cooling there were variations in the Sjo_2 and suggested that in some patients, brain cooling may not be uniform and areas of higher metabolism may exist just prior to the onset

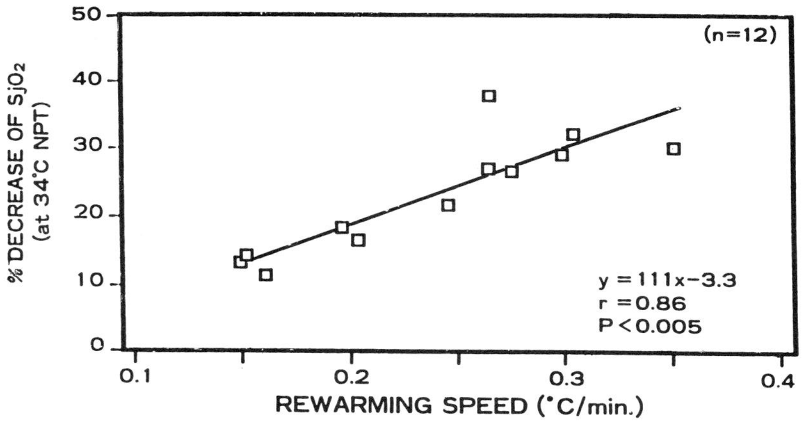

Figure 14–4. The relationship between rewarming speed and percentage of decrease of jugular venous hemoglobin saturation (Sjo_2). "Rewarming speed" was defined as an average increase in temperature per minute from initiation of rewarming to a nasopharyngeal temperature (NPT) 34°C. Percentage of decrease of Sjo_2 is (Sjo_2 before rewarming − Sjo_2 at 34°C NPT) × 100 / Sjo_2 before rewarming. (From Nakajima T, et al: Clinical evaluation of cerebral oxygen balance during cardiopulmonary bypass: On-line continuous monitoring of jugular venous oxyhemoglobin saturation. Anesth Analg 1992; 74:630–635.)

of complete cardiac arrest.[58] Whether or not internal jugular venous monitoring will become common in patients undergoing cardiopulmonary bypass is still not clear.

Head Injury

Experience with internal jugular bulb oxygen monitoring in the care of patients with head injury suggests that Sjo_2 or OER may be very helpful in maximizing brain perfusion. Cerebral ischemia not identifiable from measures of ICP or CPP may be detected. Miller et al noted Sjo_2 values ($<$ 40%) in patients with head injury and convulsions, systemic hypotension, arterial hypoxemia, and severe hyperventilation ($<$ 23 mmHg) and during elevations of ICP.

Several groups emphasize the benefits of continuous Sjo_2 monitoring.[40, 44, 59–61] Garlick and Bihari noted that during a 24-hour period, Sjo_2 may fluctuate as much as 30% and that transient changes may be missed with intermittent sampling.[44] Sheinberg et al used continuous Sjo_2 monitoring in 45 patients and found 60 episodes of Sjo_2 desaturation ($<$ 50% for 15 minutes).[59] Thirty-three of these episodes in 20 patients were confirmed by co-oximetry and included 12 episodes related to intracranial hypertension, 10 due to hypocarbia, 6 due to arterial hypoxemia, 6 due to combinations of these three, and 1 each due to systemic hypotension and to cerebral vasospasm. Cruz identified episodes of jugular vein desaturation unassociated with changes in CPP in patients with head injury.[62] The use of jugular vein oxygen monitoring allowed earlier recognition and treatment of the cerebral hypoxia. Gopinath et al reported worse neurologic outcome in patients with head injury, with multiple episodes of Sjo_2 desaturation to less than 50% for more than 10 minutes, compared with none or only one episode of desaturation.[63]

The use of hyperventilation to control ICP in patients with head injury is still a topic of intense debate (for a discussion see Miller et al[38] and Cruz et al[45]). Animal studies suggest that hyperventilation added to decreased CPP can produce brain metabolic failure and a decrease in Sjo_2.[46] Several groups avoid hyperventilation in the belief that any beneficial effects of hyperventilation are short-lived and that hyperventilation itself may place the injured brain at risk for ischemic damage. Other groups titrate the degree of hyperventilation to control the ICP, whereas others suggest that the best approach is measurement of the adequacy of oxygen delivery (Sjo_2 or CEo_2) to allow titration of the degree of hyperventilation with respect to both ICP and adequacy of oxygen delivery (optimized hyperventilation[45]). Cruz et al demonstrated that with Sjo_2 monitoring, a reduced amount of mannitol is needed and control of ICP with hyperventilation is improved.[60] This same group has also tried to combine measures of CEo_2 and CPP to arrive at an overall estimator of intracranial elastance during the initial stages of treatment after severe head injury.[61]

Roberston et al used CMRL together with $CMRo_2$ to predict the presence of infarction in patients with head injury.[39] They found that in patients with computed tomographic evidence of infarction, CMRL during the initial 2 post-injury days was considerably higher than CMRL in patients without infarction.

Gilbert provided an example of the use of $AVDo_2$ in clinical decision making.[50] He described a patient with an acute subdural hematoma who, after evacuation of the hematoma, had persistent intracranial hypertension despite hyperventilation. The $AVDo_2$ was high (8.7%), suggesting inadequate oxygen supply for the demand. The $AVDo_2$ was decreased by reducing the degree of hyperventilation, administering a diuretic, and using hypothermia.

In summary, measurement of jugular venous oxygen to determine brain oxygen extraction as an estimate of the balance of oxygen supply and demand is an old technique. Technical advances, particularly the use of fiberoptic oximeters inserted into the jugular bulb via retrograde internal jugular vein cannulation, have simplified the collection of data. Studies in patients undergoing cardiopulmonary bypass have identified the potential for brain ischemia during bypass. Ongoing investigations in patients with head injury suggest that jugular bulb oxygen measurements may be of value in determining the appropriate level of hyperventilation and allow better control of ICP without compromise of cerebral perfusion during the first 48 hours after injury.

NEAR INFRARED MEASUREMENT OF TISSUE OXYGEN

There is interest in improved monitoring of the adequacy of cerebral perfusion during anesthesia because of the exquisite sensitivity of the brain to even relatively brief periods of ischemia. In addition, there are situations in which brain perfusion is compromised but oxygen delivery in the rest of the body is normal. For example, a patient with severe carotid stenosis and moderate hypertension may have what appears to be adequate arterial blood pressure, but because of an inability to increase blood flow or a shift in cerebral autoregulation, cerebral perfusion is inadequate. Similarly, patients with cerebral vasospasm may require higher than normal blood pressures for adequate brain oxygen delivery. Finally, neurosurgical intervention may also compromise cerebral perfusion.

The key to a successful monitor is noninvasiveness, ease of use, relative inexpense, and portability, as well as the ability to provide useful information. At present, there are no well-accepted approaches to directly monitor the adequacy of brain oxygenation that meet all of these criteria. There are, however, emerging optical spectrophotometric technologies that may partially resolve this problem through a new monitoring modality that allows the anesthesiologist and others to track changes in brain oxygenation and, perhaps, oxygenation of other organs. Similar techniques have been used for studies of tissue oxidation-reduction reactions (for a recent review, see Chance[64]).

TISSUE OXYGEN AND PATIENT MANAGEMENT

Oxygen is crucial to organ function and preservation.[65, 66] Tissue oxygen debt is considered a determinant of organ failure.[67] Because oxygen delivery is a function of both the arterial oxygen content and cardiac output, measures of arterial oxygen are inadequate to determine the adequacy of tissue perfusion. In addition, tissue hypoxia is a function of both the oxygen supply and metabolic demand.[68] However, devices that measure tissue oxygen, a variable that changes with tissue oxygen availability, or that measure an organ function that is tissue oxygen–dependent may allow better management of many groups of patients.

TISSUE ABSORPTION OF LIGHT

Considerable work has demonstrated that light in the far red range (700–900 nm) penetrates tissue well.[69, 70] It is relatively unaffected by the presence of skin or skull,[71] and absorbance at these wavelengths is primarily related to iron-containing compounds such as hemoglobin, the cytochromes, and myoglobin. Indocyanine green provides a way of detecting the degree of light penetration. When it is injected directly into the internal carotid artery of humans during CEA, indocyanine green can be detected using a surface detector 2.7 cm away from an 803-nm transilluminating light source at a signal-to-noise ratio greater than 100:1.[72]

HEMOGLOBIN ABSORPTION OF LIGHT

Hemoglobin is a member of a group of many compounds that have strong absorption characteristics at many wavelengths (see Chapter 11). In the far red bandwidth, oxyhemoglobin has an absorption maximum at about 760 nm; both oxyhemoglobin and deoxyhemoglobin have similar absorbances at 800 nm. The 800-nm wavelength at which oxyhemoglobin and deoxyhemoglobin absorb equally is called an isosbestic point (Fig. 14–5). Because hemoglobin saturation is the ratio of oxygenated or deoxygenated hemoglobin to total hemoglobin, changes in absorbance indicate the relative abundance of oxygen and may prove to be a reasonable oxygen indicator. For example, as the oxygen concentration is changed from 100% to 0%, distinct changes occur in the relative deoxyhemoglobin absorbance at 760 nm, virtually no changes occur in light absorption at the isosbestic point (about 800 nm), and at longer wavelengths (approximately 816–925 nm), oxyhemoglobin absorption increases with increasing oxygenation. Other types of hemoglobin, such as methemoglobin and carboxyhemoglobin, also absorb light; the presence of these compounds may produce errors in saturation.[73] The technology described in the next section does not distinguish these forms of hemoglobin; however, in most clinical situations, this is not a major drawback.

MOVEMENT OF LIGHT THROUGH THE BRAIN

The movement of light through a highly absorbent medium such as brain tissue is random because of the high degree of photon scattering. It can be estimated using various probability simulation techniques,[74–76] which have recently been confirmed experimentally.[77, 78] The photon path estimated using these simulation techniques spreads out as a crescent-shaped slice from the emitter to the detector with an area of high probability in line between the emitter and detector and lower probabilities along the edge. The actual amount of brain that is seen by these probes is a function of the distance between the probes and the geometry of the skull. If the probes are too close together, no brain will be seen at all. Adequate probe separation is critical for successful interrogation of brain, though as the probe separation increases, the amount of light received decreases. In terms of the vascular beds, the greatest absorption takes place within the vascular space having the largest volume. Consequently, these transcranial techniques should be most sensitive to capillary, arteriole, and venule flow because these structures contain the largest volume of blood within the brain.

MEASUREMENT OF HEMOGLOBIN CONCENTRATION

In dilute clear solutions, the absorbance of light for many compounds is proportional to the concentration of that compound (the classic Beer-Lambert relationship):

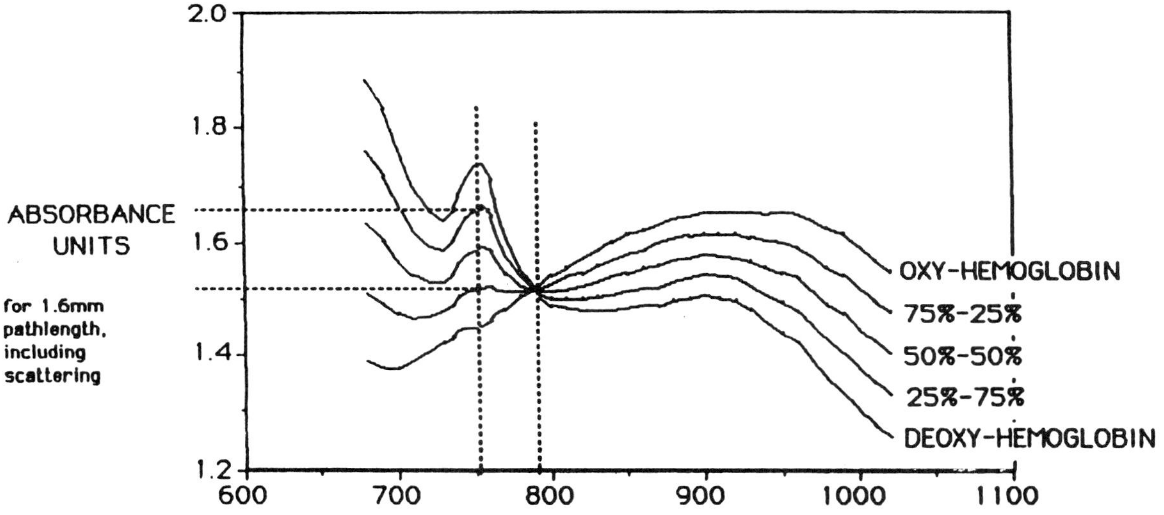

Figure 14–5. Spectrogram of hemoglobin at various degrees of saturation. A deoxyhemoglobin maximum is shown at 760 nm, the isosbestic point at roughly 800 nm, and a broader oxyhemoglobin absorbance maximum at around 900 nm. (From Chance B: Personal communication, 1992.)

$$I = I_0 10^{E \cdot C \cdot L} \qquad 14\text{–}5$$

where I = measured light, I_0 = incident light, E = molar extinction coefficient (a constant for each particular compound), C = concentration, and L = the pathlength of light through the absorbent medium. It has been demonstrated that both deoxyhemoglobin and oxyhemoglobin follow Beer's law under these conditions. This is also true in more turbid solutions, provided that the incident light is strong enough and the detectors are sensitive enough to overcome the signal losses that occur as light is scattered and subjected to greater absorption as it passes through these solutions.

ESTIMATION OF TISSUE VASCULAR HEMOGLOBIN FROM LIGHT ABSORPTION

Many investigators have explored the possibility of using the changes in oxyhemoglobin or deoxyhemoglobin as an indicator of the adequacy of organ oxygenation. Among the first was Jöbsis-Vander Vliet, who developed instrumentation that he claimed would measure both hemoglobin saturation and the redox state of cytochrome aa_3.[79] His group was particularly interested in cytochrome aa_3 because it is the oxygen acceptor of the electron transport chain, and the ability to measure cytochrome aa_3 would provide a direct indication of the redox state of the tissue. However, there are doubts as to whether or not these investigators actually separated the cytochrome aa_3 signal from the hemoglobin signal.[80] In these near red wavelengths, more than 90% of the signal is due to hemoglobin, and only a small percentage is due to cytochrome aa_3.[81] It may be irrelevant as to whether or not cytochrome aa_3 can be detected and measured in view of the fact that hemoglobin itself may be a reasonable indicator of the adequacy of tissue perfusion.[82] This is particularly true in the brain, considering its dependence on a continuing supply of oxygen and its high metabolic rate.

The first question one needs to answer is whether or not the concentration of deoxyhemoglobin or oxyhemoglobin in brain or other tissue vasculature changes in a reliable fashion with changes in inspired oxygen. A variety of studies demonstrate that this is true. One typical study was done in dogs, in which a simple two-wavelength spectrometer was placed on the dog's skull so that the incident light could be delivered through fiberoptic cables and the reflected light could be returned to a photomultiplier detector.[83] In these experiments, the dogs were caused to undergo progressive hypoxemia. Estimations of saturation using this transcranial spectrometer were compared to saturation measurements from blood obtained from sagittal sinus and femoral artery. Both the femoral artery and sagittal sinus oxygen saturations proved linear with saturation determined using the transcranial probe. However, the curves did not fit the line of identity. The saturations measured transcranially were slightly higher than those from the sagittal sinus, and the saturations measured from the artery were somewhat higher than the transcranial estimations. However, the linear fit was very good, suggesting that changes in the brain vasculature hemoglobin saturation could be measured qualitatively. Nioka and her colleagues also compared changes in brain levels of high-energy phosphates to determinations of hemoglobin saturation measured transcranially and demonstrated a break point in the saturation curve at which PCr began to decrease rapidly.[83] These findings suggest a functional linkage between brain high-energy metabolites and transcranial hemoglobin saturation.

Qualitative Approaches

Based on this work and the work of others, Chance and collaborators developed a simple portable device for measuring changes in brain vascular hemoglobin saturation.[84] This device consists of a small probe that can be strapped tightly to the skull (Fig. 14–6). There are two incandescent lamp emitters, and the diode detectors are filtered at 760 and 800 nm. The readout gives a difference spectrum (760–800 nm). This device has been used in a variety of clinical studies to be described later. Others have also developed essentially qualitative instruments of varying degrees of complexity.[79, 85, 86]

Quantitative Approaches

A problem with the measurement of deoxyhemoglobin or any other absorber in turbid media is that the photons are reflected (scattered) so that changes in optical density (OD) are related to both the concentration of absorbent and scattering (for reviews see Steinke and Shepherd[87] and Kurth et al[88]):

$$\text{OD} = \text{absorption (A)} + \text{scattering (S)} \qquad 14\text{–}6$$

where A is obtained from Equation 5. In addition, because of scattering, one cannot estimate the pathlength the light traverses using a simple linear estimator. Consequently, hemoglobin saturation can not truly be quantitated, but only the changes can be estimated, using the techniques described earlier.

A variety of approaches have been used to try to overcome the limitation of scattering and pathlength indeterminacy. One approach is to assume that scattering is constant or negligible. With this assumption, the change in optical density is proportional to the change in pathlength and the change in absorption. If one uses two wavelengths close to each other, pathlength is cancelled out, and the change in hemoglobin saturation is readily determined. In some circumstances, this approach may be appropriate, but it has yet to be proved.

Others have tried to used multiple wavelengths to solve for a change in hemoglobin saturation.[89–93] This basic approach was also taken by McCormick et al.[94] They determined absorption at several wavelengths, solved a multifactorial equation, and calibrated this value against an external source of hemoglobin. They used both tonometered hemoglobin and hemoglobin from the jugular bulb during hypoxemia as calibration standards. A reasonable fit over a narrow range, though not quite linear, was found. The degree of error in this approach depends on whether or not blood from the jugular bulb is, in fact, a good approximation of the transcranial signal. This approach also assumes that scattering is constant enough from subject to subject that an instrument calibration from one set of subjects also applies to another group and that the pathlengths of light at the frequencies used are the same. There is uncertainty as to whether these assumptions are accurate, and other approaches appear necessary. Ferrari et al used external calibration together with mathematical manipulation of the spectral signal in an attempt to reduce the effects of scattering,[90] but their approach has not yet been applied to humans.

Time of Flight

If one measures the time it takes for light to traverse a distance, one can calculate the pathlength of the light:

$$L = \frac{c \times t}{n} \qquad 14\text{–}7$$

where c = the velocity of light, t = the time from light burst to observation, and n = the average refractive index.[84] This constant behavior of the speed of light in tissue

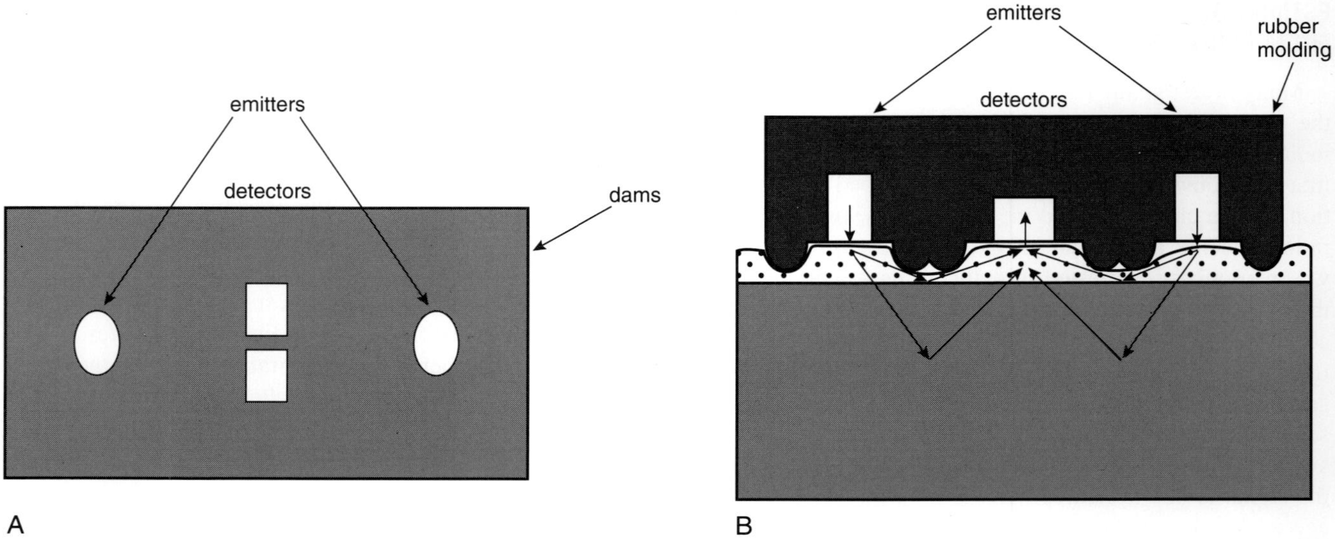

Figure 14–6. *A,* Probe for a simple, two-wavelength transcranial spectrometer. *B,* The probe is placed against a skull and the light path is delineated. (Courtesy of NIM, Inc.)

may provide an approach to the estimation of pathlength. By substituting equation 7 into equation 5, we get

$$I = I_0\, 10^{\,E \times C \times ct/n} \qquad 14\text{–}8$$

Rearranging the above equation:

$$[E \times C] = -(n/c)\log_{10}(I_0/I)\,(1/t) = \mu_a \qquad 14\text{–}9$$

If one makes these measurements at two wavelengths, then the ratio of the absorption coefficients (μ_a) at the two wavelengths is proportional to the hemoglobin saturation. This technique, "time resolved spectroscopy" (TRS), uses pulsed lasers with which the "time of flight" of the photons can be measured either through streak cameras or through pulse detection circuitry.[84, 95, 96] These lasers typically have pulse rates in the picosecond range, and the time of flight through the skull and brain is in the nanosecond range.

Phase Modulation

If instead of pulsed laser light one uses sinusoidally modulated laser light, the phase of the wave shifts relative to the phase of the incident light as light passes through the brain.[97, 98] This phase shift is also an estimator of photon pathlength.[95, 98] For example, if one places a phase modulated spectrometer (PMS) against the muscles of the arm and induces ischemia with a tourniquet, there is 1.7° of phase shift that is easily measured (Fig. 14–7).[98] If the modulation frequency is appropriate, the pathlength of light is proportional to phase shift and the information obtained from TRS and PMS is equivalent.[95] In many situations, a PMS is more convenient than TRS. The current equipment is less cumbersome, and the measurement of saturation is continuous using PMS but intermittent using TRS. The combination of PMS and TRS allows explicit determination of pathlength, scattering, and absorption.

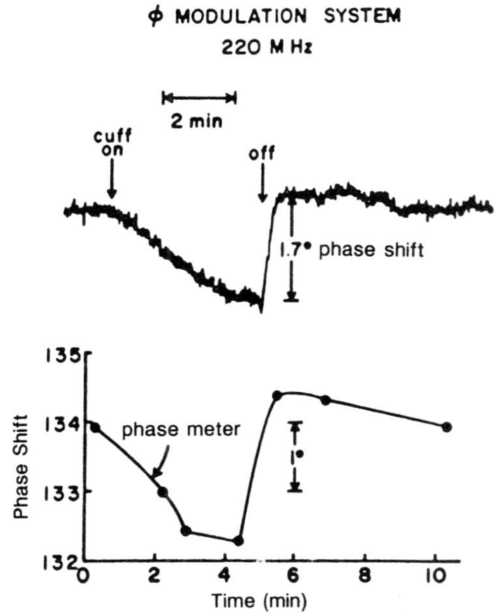

Figure 14–7. Phase shift seen in response to ischemia in an arm induced by inflation of a tourniquet (760-nm wavelength). (From Chance B, et al: A phase modulation system for dual wavelength difference spectroscopy of hemoglobin deoxygenation in tissues. Society of Photo-Optical Instrumentation Engineers 1990; 1204:481–491.)

DETERMINATION OF HEMOGLOBIN SATURATION

Hemoglobin saturation is defined as

$$\frac{HbO_2}{Hb + HbO_2} \qquad 14\text{–}10$$

and

$$\mu_a^{\lambda 1} = \epsilon_{Hb}^{\lambda 1}[Hb] + \epsilon_{HbO_2}^{\lambda 1}[HbO_2] \qquad 14\text{–}11$$

$$\mu_a^{\lambda 2} = \epsilon_{Hb}^{\lambda 2}[Hb] + \epsilon_{HbO_2}^{\lambda 2}[HbO_2] \qquad 14\text{–}12$$

where ϵ is the extinction coefficient ($cm^{-1}mM^{-1}$), λ is wavelength (nm), and μ_a (cm^{-1}) is the absorbance. Thus,

$$\frac{\mu_a^{\lambda 1}}{\mu_a^{\lambda 2}} = \frac{\epsilon_{Hb}^{\lambda 1} + S(\epsilon_{HbO_2}^{\lambda 1} - \epsilon_{Hb}^{\lambda 1})}{\epsilon_{Hb}^{\lambda 2} + S(\epsilon_{HbO_2}^{\lambda 2} - \epsilon_{Hb}^{\lambda 2})} \qquad 14\text{–}13$$

When $\lambda_1 = 754$ nm and $\lambda_2 = 816$ nm, the values of epsilon yield

$$S(\times 100\%) = \frac{38 - 18\dfrac{\mu_a^{754}}{\mu_a^{816}}}{25 + 3\,\dfrac{\mu_a^{754}}{\mu_a^{816}}} \qquad 14\text{–}14$$

The ratios of μ_a can be determined from TRS or PMS data:

$$\mu_a^{754}/\mu_a^{816} = \frac{L_0 - L_{754}}{L_0 - L_{816}} \qquad 14\text{–}15$$

where L is the pathlength and L_0 is the calculated pathlength in the absence of hemoglobin.

Newer designs of the PMS unit should simplify this calculation.

DIFFERENCES FROM CURRENT MONITORS OF OXYGENATION

It is important to recognize that these transcranial oxygen measurement techniques do not provide information similar to that gained with pulse oximetry. With pulse oximetry, only the arterial component of the hemoglobin absorption signal is measured; the pulse oximeter zeroes out the hemoglobin contribution from venous or capillary blood. With the transcranial techniques, saturation of blood in multiple vascular beds (such as arterial, venous, and capillary) are measured. One might predict that these techniques might be sensitive to relative changes in blood compartmentalization, but that has not yet been shown.

These techniques also probably do not give the same information as that given by internal jugular vein oximetry. As noted earlier, the study by Nioka et al suggests that, in dogs, transcranial saturation values are higher than those obtained from sagittal sinus blood.[83] However, one would expect a good correlation between jugular venous and transcranial values.

CLINICAL INVESTIGATIONS

Clinical instruments are as yet unavailable. Research instruments can be obtained from Somanetics Inc. (Troy, MI) and NIM Inc. (Philadelphia, PA). Many studies have been done on devices from these two companies or on devices developed by individual investigators. Data on specific instrument performance or comparisons between the various instruments are as yet not available. There is also too little experience to know for sure the sources of measurement error or patient risks. Errors can arise from inadequate sampling of brain tissue, signal contamination from extracranial tissue, regional changes in oxygenation that may not be reflected in the relatively global measures made by these devices, and errors introduced by the algorithms used to derive saturation from the measured variables. The laser-powered instruments use low-level lasers and have minimal tissue risk, though there is some potential for retinal damage if the laser is directed onto the retina for long periods. Placement over hair tends to attenuate the signal below useful levels. In our studies, the probe was placed as high on the forehead as possible but below the hair line. One might speculate that placement of the probe over a venous sinus might produce lower values than when the probe is placed over brain tissue.

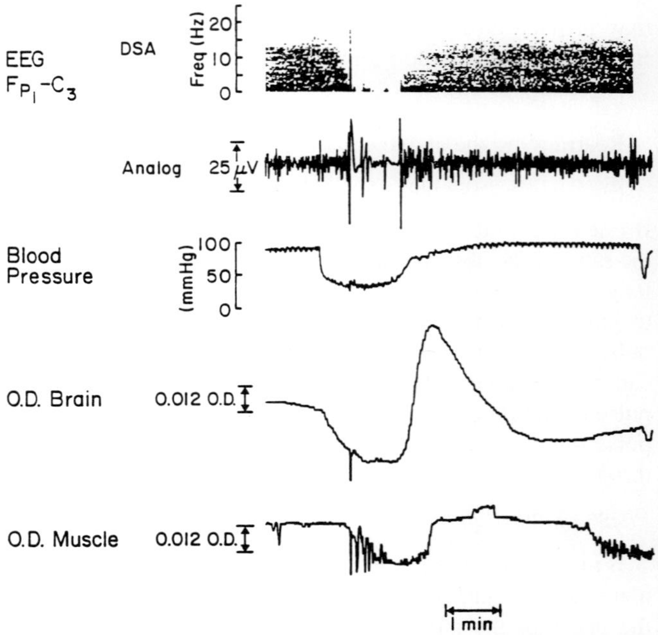

Figure 14–8. Changes in the electroencephalogram (analog and density spectral array [DSA]), blood pressure, and hemoglobin absorbance change in brain and muscle during and after an episode of cardiac arrest in patient. Downward changes in the optical density (O.D.) traces represent decreasing hemoglobin saturation. With restoration of perfusion, there is a brief overshoot of oxyhemoglobin, which may represent vasodilatation. (From Smith DS, et al: Reperfusion hyperoxia in brain after circulatory arrest in humans. Anesthesiology 1990; 73:12–19.)

The *qualitative* device developed by Chance was evaluated in patients who had survived sudden death syndrome and were undergoing implantation of automatic defibrillators into their hearts.[99] During the course of this surgery, multiple episodes of ventricular fibrillation and defibrillation occur, so that the electrodes can be placed and their sensitivities can be adjusted. Consequently, this is an excellent model of intraoperative complete ischemia, with durations of fibrillation lasting from 5 seconds to 2 minutes. In this experiment, two oxygen saturation probes were used. One was placed on the skin overlying the frontal cortex; the other was placed over the quadriceps muscle. Changes in hemoglobin saturation were recorded from these two probes simultaneously with mean arterial blood pressure and the EEG. During fibrillation and the associated decrease in blood pressure, the brain absorption of deoxyhemoglobin changed (Fig. 14–8). Blood pressure decreased slightly before the increase in brain deoxyhemoglobin. In contrast, in muscle, deoxyhemoglobin decreased much more slowly, and the onset was somewhat delayed (Fig. 14–8). There was a good time correlation between decreased brain deoxyhemoglobin and the loss of the EEG.

In another study (Fig. 14–9), a human volunteer was made progressively hypoxemic to an FIO_2 of about 0.07. In this experiment, moderate hyperventilation occurred. Pulse oximeter values decreased from 100% to roughly 55%, and there was an increase in the deoxyhemoglobin signal from the brain. The experiment was terminated at the onset of mild EEG changes.

There has been considerable interest in applying these forms of monitoring to infants. Kurth et al used qualitative instrumentation to examine the changes in oxygenated hemoglobin in neonates during cooling (target temperature was 15°C) and circulatory arrest.[100] They found an increase of brain vascular hemoglobin saturation during cooling and a progressive loss of oxygenated hemoglobin in the brain vasculature during the period of circulatory arrest, which recovered with rewarming (Fig. 14–10). This approach has also been used by several groups to demonstrate desaturation of brain vascular hemoglobin in premature infants during tracheal suctioning[101, 102] and crying.[103] This technology has progressed to allow measurement of cerebral blood volume of neonates.[103–105] With appropriate assumptions, blood volume can be obtained from qualitative systems.[105] Seeds et al applied optical probes to the heads of fetal sheep and demonstrated good correlation between fetal arterial oxygen and transcranial hemoglobin changes during cycles of ischemia and reperfusion induced by temporary occlusion of the uterine arteries.[106]

With respect to studies using *quantitative* instruments, Smith et al have used a combination of TRS and PMS to determine the variability of scattering, pathlength, and absorbance.[107] They made transcranial measurements in 36 subjects (19 men and 17 women). Thirty were Caucasian or Asian, and six were African-American. Nineteen were less than 40 years of age, 10 were between 40 and 60, and 7 were older than 60. TRS, at two different wavelengths (760 and 820 nm), was used to measure scattering and to estimate the pathlength at zero absorption. PMS was used to determine the change in pathlength. Measurements were

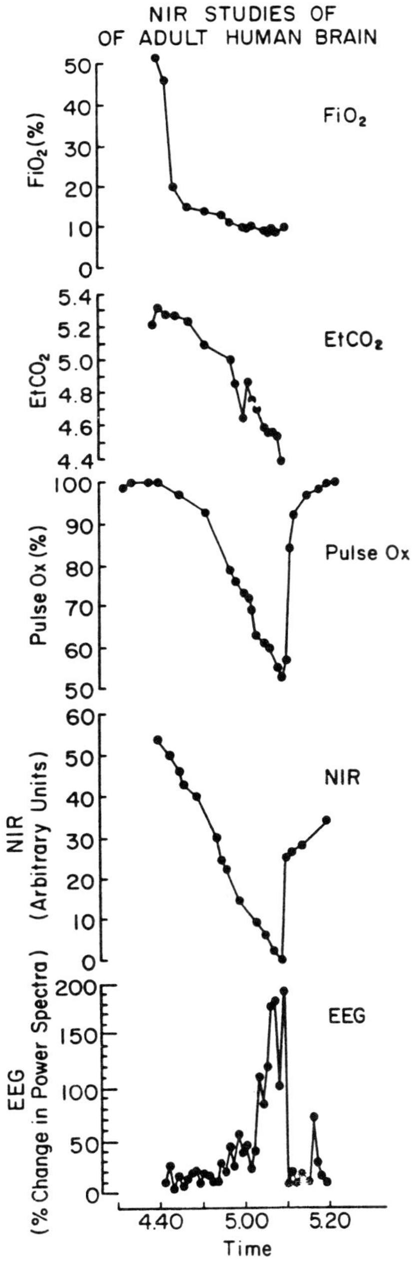

Figure 14–9. Changes in end tidal CO_2 ($Etco_2$), pulse oximetry, and brain vascular hemoglobin absorbance, as well as the electroencephalogram in a human subjected to decreasing concentrations of Fio_2. The downward changes in the NIR trace represent increasing hemoglobin desaturation. (From Chance B, et al: Comparison of time-resolved and -unresolved measurements of deoxyhemoglobin in brain. Proc Natl Acad Sci USA 1988; 85:4971–4975.)

made of the right and left frontal cortices. Results were similar for both sides of the brain and for both TRS wavelengths. Scattering (Table 14–7) was determined from the diffusion equation.[97] The hemoglobin-free photon migration pathlength was calculated from the TRS scattering data (Table 14–7). Actual photon migration pathlengths obtained at 754- and 816-nm wavelengths were measured using the PMS system (Table 14–7). As expected, they are shorter than the hemoglobin-free pathlengths because of the strong absorption of these wavelengths of light by hemoglobin. Brain vascular hemoglobin saturation was calculated using equation 10 and the hemoglobin-free and measured pathlengths (Table 14–7). Explicit calculation of scattering has not been used by others who are developing transcranial saturation instrumentation. The large intersubject variation suggests a need for explicit scattering determination.

McCormick et al studied a variety of situations with their device and reported that the normal value of saturation from the brain vasculature of adults is 64 ± 3%.[108] They noted that a reading of 50% represents an Sao_2 of less than 90% and a mixed cerebral oxygen saturation of less than 50%, if one assumes that the venous blood percentage is between 72 and 82. In a group of volunteer subjects, these researchers demonstrated the ability to track changes in brain vasculature hemoglobin saturation from an inspired oxygen of 21% (transcranial saturation, 63.9 ± 3.4%, mean ± 1 S.D.) to 7% (transcranial saturation, 35.2 ± 9.6%). They demonstrated a correlation between the onset of EEG slowing and the decrease in hemoglobin saturation as measured with their technique. McCormick et al also tracked brain vascular hemoglobin saturation changes during complete cardiac arrest, exsanguination, and profound hypothermia (15°C) for giant cerebral aneurysm repair.[109] The patterns of continued saturation during the period of complete cardiac arrest and the decreased saturation during reperfusion and rewarming are similar to those reported by Kurth et al[100] during cardiac arrest in neonates.

Transcranial oxygen measurement techniques are just emerging from the developmental stages. Few clinical studies have been done, and the role of these techniques in clinical care has not yet been determined. Ideally, they might provide a noninvasive measure of brain vascular hemoglobin saturation that could prove to be an early warning of cerebral perfusion failure that is easier to use and less

TABLE 14–7. PHOTON SCATTERING, L_0, PHOTON PATHLENGTH, AND BRAIN VASCULAR HEMOGLOBIN SATURATION FROM HUMAN BRAINS

Brain Side*	Mean	SDEV	CV (%)
Photon scattering	14.6	6	41
L_0†	77	15	19
Photon pathlength‡	22.9	4.9	22
Saturation	73	3	4

*Data were obtained from both the left and the right sides of the brain. Because the data were similar, only data from the left side are shown. Photon scattering and L_0 were measured from a calculated value of T_0 (the time of first light penetration). Time-resolved spectroscopy measurements were obtained at 670 and 820 nm; the values at both wavelengths were similar, and only the 670 data are shown. Thirty-four subjects were studied.

†L_0 is the calculated pathlength of light if hemoglobin were absent.

‡Pathlength changes were measured at two PMS wavelengths (670 and 820 nm) because the results from both were similar; only the 670 nm data are shown.

SDEV = 1 standard deviation; CV = coefficient of variation

Data from Levy et al: Personal communication, 1992.

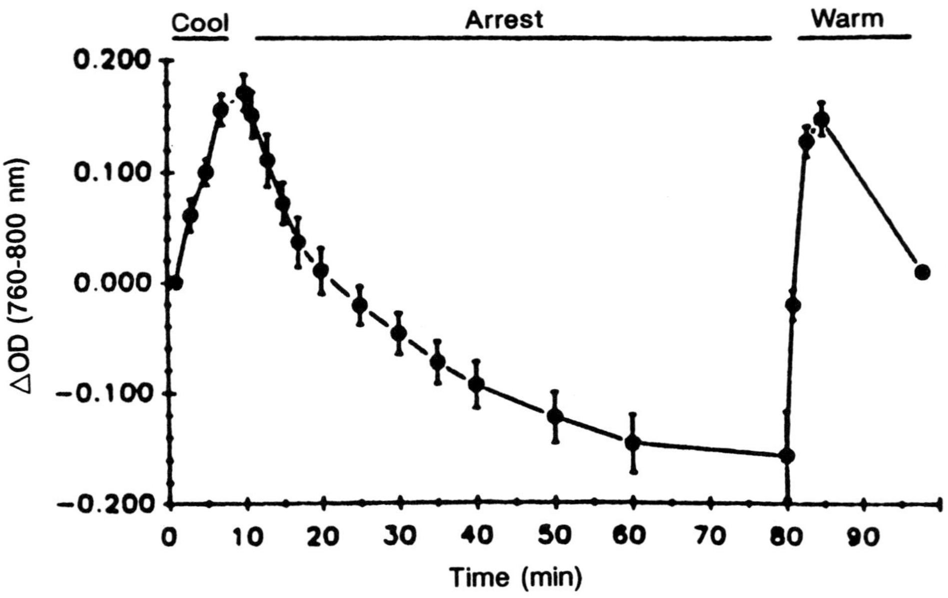

Figure 14–10. Changes in oxyhemoglobin in the brains of 15 neonates during cooling and warming on cardiopulmonary bypass and circulatory arrest. (From Kurth CD, et al: Kinetics of cerebral deoxygenation during deep hypothermic circulatory arrest in neonates. Anesthesiology 1992; 77:656–661.)

sensitive to anesthetic drugs and such factors than is the EEG or evoked potentials. Other potential roles include the monitoring of resuscitation, because improving brain vascular hemoglobin saturation might indicate improved perfusion. Noninvasive techniques might also help with early detection of intraventricular hemorrhage and cerebral ischemia in low-birthweight infants[110] and when pulse oximetry fails (as with patients with poor peripheral circulation[111]), because central circulations such as the brain will be perfused when the periphery is not.

Acknowledgments

We would like to thank Iris R. Karafin for her expert secretarial assistance and Cara Grugan for her help in assembling the bibliography. DSS would like to express his appreciation to Warren Levy and Britton Chance, his collaborators on the transcranial brain vascular hemoglobin saturation research.

REFERENCES

1. Miller JD: Transcranial Doppler instruments and accreditation for their use. Neurosurgery 1993; 33:757–761.
2. Aaslid R, Markwalder TM, Nornes H: Noninvasive transcranial Doppler ultrasound recording of flow velocity in basal cerebral arteries. J Neurosurg 1982; 57:769–774.
3. Arnolds BJ, von Reutern G-M: Transcranial Dopplersonography. Examination technique and normal reference values. Ultrasound Med Biol 1986; 12:115–123.
4. DeWitt LD, Wechsler LR: Transcranial Doppler. Stroke 1988; 19:915–921.
5. Werner C: Transcranial Doppler sonography: Trend monitor of cerebral hemodynamics? J Neurosurg Anesth 1991; 3:73–76.
6. Martin NA, Thomas KM, Caron M: Transcranial Doppler—Techniques, application, and instrumentation. Neurosurgery 1993; 33:761–763.
7. Werner C, Kochs E, Rau M, Schulte am Esch J: Transcranial doppler sonography as a supplement in the detection of cerebral circulatory arrest. J Neurosurg Anesth 1990; 2:159–165.
8. Hennerici M, Rautenberg W, Sitzer G, Schwartz A: Transcranial Doppler ultrasound for the assessment of intracranial arterial flow velocity—Part 1. Examination technique and normal values. Surg Neurol 1987; 27:439–448.
9. Schoning M, Walter J: Evaluation of the vertebrobasilar-posterior system by transcranial color duplex sonography in adults. Stroke 1992; 23:1280–1286.
10. Dahl A, Lindegaard K, Russell D, et al: A comparison of transcranial Doppler and cerebral flow studies to assess cerebral vasoreactivity. Stroke 1992; 23:15–19.
11. Seiler RW, Grolimund P, Aaslid R, et al: Cerebral vasospasm evaluated by transcranial ultrasound correlated with clinical grade and CT-visualized subarachnoid hemorrhage. J Neurosurg 1986; 64:594–600.
12. Martin NA, Doberstein C, Zane C, et al: Posttraumatic cerebral artery spasm: Transcranial Doppler ultrasound, cerebral blood flow, and angiographic findings. J Neurosurg 1992; 77:575–583.
13. Klingelhöfer J, Sander D, Holzgraefe M, et al: Cerebral vasospasm evaluated by transcranial Doppler ultrasonography at different intracranial pressures. J Neurosurg 1991; 75:752–758.
14. Brass LM, Pavlakis SG, DeVivo D, et al: Transcranial Doppler measurements of the middle cerebral artery. Effect of hematocrit. Stroke 1988; 19:1466–1469.
15. Trindle MR, Dodson BA, Rampil IJ: Effects of fentanyl and sufentanil in equianesthetic doses on middle cerebral artery blood flow velocity. Anesthesiology 1993; 78:454–460.
16. Werner C, Kochs E, Rau M, et al: Dose-dependent blood flow velocity changes in the basal cerebral arteries following low-dose ketamine. J Neurosurg Anesth 1990; 2:86–91.
17. Eng C, Lam AM, Mayberg TS, et al: The influence of propofol with and without nitrous oxide on cerebral blood flow velocity and CO_2 reactivity in humans. Anesthesiology 1992; 77:872–879.
18. Halsey JH, McDowell HA, Gelmon S, Morawetz RB: Blood velocity in the middle cerebral artery and regional cerebral blood flow during carotid endarterectomy. Stroke 1989; 20:53–58.
19. Halsey JH Jr: Risks and benefits of shunting in carotid endarterectomy. Stroke 1992; 23:1583–1587.
20. Markus H: Transcranial doppler detection of circulating cerebral emboli. A review. Stroke 1993; 24:1246–1250.
21. Padayachee TS, Parsons S, Theobald R, et al: The detection of microemboli in the middle cerebral artery during cardiopulmonary bypass: A transcranial Doppler ultrasound investigation using membrane and bubble oxygenators. Ann Thorac Surg 1987; 44:298–302.
22. Harrison MJ, Pugsley W, Newman S, et al: Detection of middle cerebral emboli during coronary artery bypass surgery using transcranial Doppler sonography [Letter]. Stroke 1990; 21:1512.
23. Spencer MP, Thomas GI, Nicholls SC, Sauvage LR: Detection of middle cerebral artery emboli during carotid endarterectomy using transcranial Doppler ultrasonography. Stroke 1990; 21:415–423.
24. Teague SM, Sharma MK: Detection of paradoxical cerebral echo contrast embolization by transcranial Doppler ultrasound. Stroke 1991; 22:740–745.

25. Siebler M, Sitzer M, Steinmetz H: Detection of intracranial emboli in patients with symptomatic extracranial carotid artery disease. Stroke 1992; 23:1652–1654.
26. Brautaset NJ: Provokable bilateral vertebral artery compression diagnosed with transcranial doppler. Stroke 1992; 23:288–291.
27. Grosset DG, Straiton J, du Trevou M, Bullock R: Prediction of symptomatic vasospasm after subarachnoid hemorrhage by rapidly increasing transcranial Doppler velocity and cerebral blood flow changes. Stroke 1992; 23:674–679.
28. Eng CC, Lam AM, Byrd S, Newell DW: The diagnosis and management of a perianesthetic cerebral aneurysmal rupture aided with transcranial Doppler ultrasonography. Anesthesiology 1993; 78:191–194.
29. Pople IK: Doppler flow velocities in children with controlled hydrocephalus: Reference values for the diagnosis of blocked cerebrospinal fluid shunts. Childs Nerv Syst 1992; 8:124–125.
30. Newell DW, Aaslid R, Stooss R, Reulen HJ: The relationship of blood flow velocity fluctuations to intracranial pressure B waves. J Neurosurg 1992; 76:415–421.
31. Myerson A, Halbran RD, Hirsch HL: Technic for obtaining blood from the internal jugular vein and internal carotid artery. Arch Neurol Psychiatry 1927; 17:807–808.
32. Gibbs EL, Lennox WG, Nims LF, Gibbs FA: Arterial and cerebral venous blood arterial-venous differences in man. J Biol Chem 1942; 144:325–332.
33. Kety SS, Schmidt CF: The nitrous oxide method for the quantitative determination of cerebral blood flow in man: Theory, procedure, and normal values. J Clin Invest 1948; 27:476–483.
34. Obrist WD, Wilkinson WE: Regional cerebral blood flow measurement in humans by xenon-133 clearance. Cerebrovasc Brain Metabol Rev 1990; 2:283–327.
35. Meyer JS, Wiederholt IC, Toyoda M, et al: A new method for continuous sampling of cerebral venous blood without extracranial contamination in man. Neurology 1969; 19:353–358.
36. Griffiths DPG, Greenbaum R: A simplified technique for cannulation of the jugular bulb. Stroke 1973; 4:955–957.
37. Goetting MG, Preston G: Jugular bulb catheterization: Experience with 123 patients. Crit Care Med 1990; 18:1220–1223.
38. Miller JD, Dearden NM, Piper IR, Chan KH: Control of intracranial pressure in patients with severe head injury. J Neurotrauma 1992; 9:S317–S326.
39. Robertson CS, Grossman RG, Goodman JC, Narayan RK: The predictive value of cerebral anaerobic metabolism with cerebral infarction after head injury. J Neurosurg 1987; 67:361–368.
40. Chan KH, Miller JD, Dearden NM, et al: The effect of changes in cerebral perfusion pressure upon middle cerebral artery blood flow velocity and jugular bulb venous oxygen saturation after severe brain injury. J Neurosurg 1992; 77:55–61.
41. Landsman MLJ, Knop N, Kwant G, Zijlstra WG: A fiberoptic reflection oximeter. Pflugers Arch 1978; 373:273–282.
42. Enson Y, Briscoe WA, Polanyi ML, Cournand A: In vivo studies with an intravascular and intracardiac reflection oximeter. J Appl Physiol 1962; 17:552–558.
43. Reinhart K, Moser N, Rudolph T, et al: Accuracy of two mixed venous saturation catheters during long-term use in critically ill patients. Anesthesiology 1988; 69:769–773.
44. Garlick R, Bihari D: The use of intermittent and continuous recordings of jugular venous bulb oxygen saturation in the unconscious patient. Scand J Clin Lab Invest 1987; 47(Suppl 188):47–52.
45. Cruz J, Gennarelli TA, Hoffstad OJ: Lack of relevance of the Bohr effect in optimally ventilated patients with acute brain trauma. J Trauma 1992; 33:304–311.
46. Sutton LN, McLaughlin AC, Dante S, et al: Cerebral venous oxygen content as a measure of brain energy metabolism with increased intracranial pressure and hyperventilation. J Neurosurg 1990; 73:927–932.
47. Meyer JS, Gotoh F, Ebihara S, Tomita M: Effects of anoxia on cerebral metabolism and electrolytes in man. Neurology 1965; 15:892–901.
48. Lennox WG, Gibbs FA, Gibbs EL: Relationship of unconsciousness to cerebral blood flow and anoxemia. Arch Neurol Psychiatry 1935; 34:1001–1013.
49. Schell RM, Kern FH, Reves JG: The role of continuous jugular venous saturation monitoring during cardiac surgery with cardiopulmonary bypass. Anesth Analg 1992; 74:627–629.
50. Gilbert J: Estimation of CBF by cerebral venous oxygen difference [Letter]. J Neurosurg 1989; 71:790.
51. Engberg M, Øberg B, Christensen KS, et al: The cerebral arteriovenous oxygen content differences ($AVDo_2$) during halothane and neurolept anaesthesia in patients subjected to craniotomy. Acta Anaesthesiol Scand 1989; 33:642–646.
52. Sanchez G, Imparato A, Ransohoff J: Internal jugular oxygen saturation and arteriovenous oxygen difference during artificial embolization of arteriovenous malformations. J Neurosurg 1969; 30:227–232.
53. Lyons C, Clark LC Jr, McDowell H, McArthur K: Cerebral venous oxygen content during carotid thrombintimectomy. Ann Surg 1964; 160:561–567.
54. Clauss RH, Hass WK, Ransohoff J: Simplified method for monitoring adequacy of brain oxygenation during carotid-artery surgery. N Engl J Med 1965; 273:1127–1131.
55. Croughwell ND, Frasco P, Blumenthal JA, et al: Warming during cardiopulmonary bypass is associated with jugular bulb desaturation. Soc Thorac Surg 1992; 53:827–832.
56. Nakajima T, Kuro M, Hayashi Y, et al: Clinical evaluation of cerebral oxygen balance during cardiopulmonary bypass: On-line continuous monitoring of jugular venous oxyhemoglobin saturation. Anesth Analg 1992; 74:630–635.
57. van der Linden J, Priddy R, Ekroth R, et al: Cerebral perfusion and metabolism during profound hypothermia in children. J Thorac Cardiovasc Surg 1991; 102:103–114.
58. Kern FH, Jonas RA, Mayer JE Jr, et al: Temperature monitoring during CPB in infants: Does it predict efficient brain cooling? Ann Thorac Surg 1992; 54:749–754.
59. Sheinberg M, Kanter MJ, Robertson CS, et al: Continuous monitoring of jugular venous oxygen saturation in head-injured patients. J Neurosurg 1992; 76:212–217.
60. Cruz J, Miner ME, Allen SJ, et al: Continuous monitoring of cerebral oxygenation in acute brain injury: Injection of mannitol during hyperventilation. J Neurosurg 1990; 73:725–730.
61. Cruz J, Miner ME, Allen SJ, et al: Continuous monitoring of cerebral oxygenation in acute brain injury: Assessment of cerebral hemodynamic reserve. Neurosurgery 1991; 29:743–749.
62. Cruz J: On-line monitoring of global cerebral hypoxia in acute brain injury. Relationship to intracranial hypertension. J Neurosurg 1993; 79:228–233.
63. Gopinath SP, Robertson CS, Contant CF, et al: Jugular venous desaturation and outcome after head injury. J Neurol Neurosurg Psychiatry 1994, in press.
64. Chance B: Optical method. Ann Rev Biophys Biophys Chem 1991; 20:1–28.
65. Siesjö BK: Pathophysiology and treatment of focal cerebral ischemia. Part I: Pathophysiology. J Neurosurg 1992; 77:169–184.
66. Schumacker PT, Cain SM: The concept of a critical oxygen delivery. Intens Care Med 1987; 13:223–229.
67. Shoemaker WC, Appel PL, Kram HB: Tissue oxygen debt as a determinant of lethal and nonlethal postoperative organ failure. Crit Care Med 1988; 16:1117–1120.
68. Connett RJ, Honig CR, Gayeski TEJ, Brooks GA: Defining hypoxia: A system view of $\dot{V}o_2$, glycolysis, energetics, and intracellular Po_2. J Appl Physiol 1990; 68:833–841.
69. Eggert HR, Blazek V: Optical properties of human brain tissue, meninges, and brain tumors in the spectral range of 200 to 900 nm. Neurosurgery 1987; 21:459–464.
70. Svaasand LO, Ellingsen R: Optical properties of human brain. Photochem Photobiol 1983; 38:293–299.
71. Wan S, Parrish JA, Anderson RR, Madden M: Transmittance of nonionizing radiation in human tissues. Photochem Photobiol 1981; 34:679–681.
72. McCormick PW, Stewart M, Lewis G, et al: Intracerebral penetration of infrared light. J Neurosurg 1992; 76:315–318.
73. Tremper KK, Barker SJ: Monitoring of oxygen. *In* Lake CL (ed): Clinical Monitoring for Anesthesia and Critical Care, 2nd Ed. Philadelphia: WB Saunders, 1994.
74. Patterson MS, Chance B, Wilson BC: Time resolved reflectance and transmittance for the non-invasive measurement of tissue optical properties. Appl Optics 1989; 28:2331–2336.
75. Bonner RF, Nossal R, Weiss GH: A random walk theory of time-resolved optical absorption spectroscopy in tissue. *In* Chance B (ed): Photon Migration in Tissues. New York: Plenum Press, 1989; 11–23.

76. Flock ST, Wilson BC, Patterson MS: Monte Carlo modeling of light propagation in highly scattering tissues—II: Comparison with measurements in phantoms. IEEE Trans Biomed Eng 1989; 36:1169–1173.
77. Flock ST, Patterson MS, Wilson BC, et al: Monte Carlo modeling of light propagation in highly scattering tissues—I: Model predications and comparison with diffusion theory. IEEE Trans Biomed Eng 1989; 36:1162–1168.
78. Cui W, Kumar C, Chance B: Experimental study of migration depth for the photons measured at sample surface. Society of Photo-Optical Instrumentation Engineers 1991; 1431:180–191.
79. Jöbsis-Vander Vliet FF: Noninvasive, infrared monitoring of cerebral and myocardial oxygen sufficiency and circulatory parameters. Science 1977; 198:1264–1267.
80. Chance B, Smith DS, Nioka S, et al: Photon migration in muscle and brain. *In* Chance B (ed): Photon Migration in Tissues. New York: Plenum Press, 1989; 121–135.
81. Wray S, Cope M, Delpy DT, et al: Characterization of the near infrared absorption spectra of cytochrome aa_3 and haemoglobin for the non-invasive monitoring of cerebral oxygenation. Biochim Biophys Acta 1988; 933:184–192.
82. Chance B: Evaluation of tissue hypoxia by optical methods. *In* Gutierrez G, Vincent JL (eds): Tissue Oxygen Utilization. Berlin, Springer-Verlag, 1991; 33–40.
83. Nioka S, Chance B, Smith DS, et al: Cerebral energy metabolism and oxygen state during hypoxia in neonate and adult dogs. Pediatr Res 1990; 28:54–62.
84. Chance B, Leigh JS, Miyake H, et al: Comparison of time-resolved and -unresolved measurements of deoxyhemoglobin in brain. Proc Natl Acad Sci USA 1988; 85:4971–4975.
85. Delpy DT, Cope MC, Cady EB, et al: Cerebral monitoring in newborn infants by magnetic resonance and near infrared spectroscopy. Scand J Clin Lab Invest 1987; 47(Suppl 188):9–17.
86. Cope M, Delpy DT: System for long-term measurement of cerebral blood and tissue oxygenation on newborn infants by near infra-red transillumination. Med Biol Eng Comput 1988; 26:289–294.
87. Steinke JM, Shepherd AP: Role of light scattering in whole blood oximetry. IEEE Trans Biomed Eng 1986; 33:294–301.
88. Kurth CD, Steven JM, Benaron D, Chance B: Near-infrared monitoring of the cerebral circulation. J Clin Monit 1993; 9:163–170.
89. Piantadosi CA, Comfort BJ: Development and validation of multiwavelength algorithms for in vivo near infrared spectroscopy. *In* Chance B (ed): Photon Migration in Tissues. New York: Plenum Press, 1989; 69–82.
90. Ferrari M, Wilson DA, Hanley DF, et al: Noninvasive determination of hemoglobin saturation in dogs by derivative near-infrared spectroscopy. Am J Physiol 1989; 25:H1493–H1499.
91. Wyatt JS, Delpy DT, Cope M, et al: Quantification of cerebral oxygenation and haemodynamics in sick newborn infants by near infrared spectrophotometry. Lancet 1986; 2:1063–1066.
92. Cope M, Delpy DT, Reynolds EOR, et al: Methods of quantitating cerebral near infrared spectroscopy data. Adv Exp Med Biol 1988; 222:183–189.
93. Delpy DT, Arridge SR, Cope M, et al: Quantitation of pathlength in optical spectroscopy. Adv Exp Med Biol 1989; 248:41–46.
94. McCormick PW, Stewart M, Goetting MG, et al: Noninvasive cerebral optical spectroscopy for monitoring cerebral oxygen delivery and hemodynamics. Crit Care Med 1991; 19:89–97.
95. Sevick EM, Chance B, Leigh J, et al: Quantitation of time- and frequency-resolved optical spectra for the determination of tissue oxygenation. Anal Biochem 1991; 195:330–351.
96. Delpy DT, Cope M, van der Zee P, et al: Estimation of optical pathlength through tissue from direct time of flight measurement. Phys Med Biol 1988; 33:1433–1442.
97. Weng J, Zhang MZ, Simons K, Chance B: Measurement of biological tissue metabolism using phase modulation spectroscopic technology. Society of Photo-Optical Instrumentation Engineers 1991; 1431:161–170.
98. Chance B, Maris M, Sorge J, Zhang MZ: A phase modulation system for dual wavelength difference spectroscopy of hemoglobin deoxygenation in tissues. Society of Photo-Optical Instrumentation Engineers 1990; 1204:481–491.
99. Smith DS, Levy W, Maris M, Chance B: Reperfusion hyperoxia in brain after circulatory arrest in humans. Anesthesiology 1990; 73:12–19.
100. Kurth CD, Steven JM, Nicolson SC, et al: Kinetics of cerebral deoxygenation during deep hypothermic circulatory arrest in neonates. Anesthesiology 1992; 77:656–661.
101. Shah AR, Kurth CD, Gwiazdowski SG, et al: Fluctuations in cerebral oxygenation and blood volume during endotracheal suctioning in premature infants. J Pediatr 1992; 126:769–774.
102. Brazy JE, Lewis V, Mitnick MH, Jöbsis-Vander Vliet FF: Noninvasive monitoring of cerebral oxygenation in preterm infants: Preliminary observations. Pediatrics 1985; 75:217–225.
103. Brazy JE: Effects of crying on cerebral blood volume and cytochrome aa_3. J Pediatr 1988; 112:457–461.
104. Ferrari M, De Marchis C, Giannini I, et al: Cerebral blood volume and hemoglobin oxygen saturation monitoring in neonatal brain by near IR spectroscopy. Adv Exp Med Biol 1986; 200:203–211.
105. Wyatt JS, Cope M, Delpy DT, et al: Quantitation of cerebral blood volume in human infants by near-infrared spectroscopy. Am J Physiol 1990; 1086–1091.
106. Seeds JW, Cefalo RC, Proctor HJ, Jöbsis-Vander Vliet FF: The relationship of intracranial infrared light absorbance to fetal oxygenation. I: Methodology. Am J Obstet Gynecol 1984; 149:679–684.
107. Smith DS, Levy WJ, Carter S, et al: Brain vascular hemoglobin saturation and light scattering in a population of normal volunteers. Anesthesiology 1992; 77:A561.
108. McCormick PW, Stewart M, Goetting MG, Balakrishnan G: Regional cerebrovascular oxygen saturation measured by optical spectroscopy in humans. Stroke 1991; 22:596–602.
109. McCormick PW, Balakrishnan G, Stewart M, et al: Cerebral oxygen metabolism measured during hypothermic circulatory arrest: A case report. J Neurosurg Anesth 1991; 3:302–307.
110. Rea PA, Crowe J, Wickramasinghe Y, Rolfe P: Non-invasive optical methods for the study of cerebral metabolism in the human newborn: A technique for the future? J Med Eng Technol 1985; 9:160–166.
111. Severinghaus JW, Spellman MJ Jr: Pulse oximeter failure thresholds in hypotension and vasoconstriction. Anesthesiology 1990; 73:532–537.

CHAPTER 15

Electroencephalography

WARREN J. LEVY, M.D.

In 1987, intraoperative electroencephalography reached a milestone—50 years had passed since the initial report[1] of the effects of various drugs on the electroencephalogram (EEG). Although the role of most monitoring techniques becomes well defined after such a time span, this has not been the case for intraoperative electroencephalography. The history of EEG monitoring can easily be divided into two periods: the early analog period, when strip-chart display of the raw signal was used, and the current, processed period, when a number of processing techniques have been used to facilitate the use of electroencephalography as a monitor.

Although this is an accurate description, historically speaking, it may give the impression that analog EEG is passé, that anesthesiologists do not need to understand or interpret it, and that the output of the next EEG processing system will provide the definitive answer to all problems of anesthetic depth, brain perfusion, and neurologic well-being. Nothing could be less accurate, for no EEG processor is better than the analog signal it receives, and no processed EEG contains information not in the original signal. Understanding the origin of the EEG is mandatory in order to record the signal, categorize its character, and interpret it for intraoperative monitoring.

ORIGINS OF THE EEG

It is generally accepted that the electrical activity ultimately recorded as the EEG originates spontaneously in the most superficial layers of the cerebral cortex.[2] In these layers, the pyramidal cells have many dendrites oriented perpendicular to the surface; the spread of the postsynaptic potentials along these structures produces electrical fields, called dipoles, which summate over adjacent neurons because of their common orientation. Ionic flow secondary to excitatory stimuli causes negativity in the extracellular space around the dendrite compared with the area near the cell body. This electrical summation process is quite complex, because the polarity, timing, and depth of different postsynaptic potentials differ. In addition, some dendrites are not perpendicularly oriented to the surface, and these also generate postsynaptic potentials and correspondingly oriented dipoles.

Studies of the time course of EEG activity have demonstrated that cortical action potentials do not play a major direct role in the generation of the EEG. Obviously, if there were no action potentials at all, there would be no synaptic transmission and thus no postsynaptic potentials to summate into the EEG. Many of the axons whose terminal synapses are responsible for cortical postsynaptic potentials originate in subcortical tissues. An alteration in the function of these subcortical neurons changes the pattern of postsynaptic activity and thus influences the EEG. However, not all subcortical structures have cortical projections, and many studies of intracerebral electrical activity have demonstrated the absence of associations of EEG with underlying subcortical structures. For this reason, it is common to utilize EEG monitoring as if the EEG were derived purely from cortical activity.

CORTICAL EEG

The EEG recorded at the cortical surface differs in many ways from that recorded on the scalp.[3] These differences arise during the passage of the electrical activity through the skull and soft tissue. The skull is fairly resistant to the transmission of electrical signals and considerably reduces their amplitude. Abrupt changes in skull thickness, such as after craniectomy, cause distortion or asymmetry of the EEG when compared with recordings made over contralateral, intact structures. In most cases, however, EEG monitoring is performed over areas of relatively uniform bone density, and transmission through the skull does not excessively distort EEG activity. The most important change in electrical activity that occurs during the transmission process is the averaging of nearby dipoles into a more uniform electrical gradient. Thus, even though areas of cortex only 1 or 2 mm apart can show different activity (recorded on the surface of the cortex), the EEG, recorded from the scalp, will only reflect a composite of nearby activity.

The process by which these signals are averaged strongly influences the distance at which a signal may be recorded, particularly in the presence of other activity originating at sites closer to the recording electrode. Studies using cortical evoked potentials suggest that the amplitude of the recording decreases dramatically when the recording electrode is more than a few centimeters from the site of the activity.[4] Thus, even though EEG activity can be recorded at a greatly reduced amplitude many centimeters away from its origin, it is likely to be masked by the presence of higher-amplitude activity generated closer to the recording electrode.

RECORDING OF THE EEG

The limited dispersion of the EEG signal has created several characteristics of the EEG recording process. First, there is the need to record from many electrodes (8–16 or more) simultaneously in order to examine different areas of the brain. Also, there is the need for careful measurement of electrode positions in order to place the electrodes in reproducible relationships to the underlying cortical structures. Third, consistent and logical electrode montages must be used, because different combinations of electrodes may make the recording appear different, even though the underlying electrical activity is unchanged.

TECHNICAL CONSIDERATIONS

Although these issues cover many of the technical considerations of EEG monitoring, issues of artifact identification and elimination and the basic electronics of biologic amplifiers must be considered as well. In fact, the technology of EEG recording is probably the single factor most responsible for the success (or failure) of efforts to monitor the EEG during anesthesia and surgery.

To appreciate the technical problems of recording the intraoperative EEG, it is only necessary to consider the characteristics of this signal in comparison to other signals recorded from the patient. The EEG is a signal of a few microvolts in amplitude (perhaps as high as 100 μV) with an irregular pattern of oscillation a few times per second (1–30 Hz). Muscle artifact generated by frontalis or extraocular muscles can be several hundred microvolts in amplitude, and the normal electrocardiogram (ECG), at 2–4 mV, is nearly 1000 times the amplitude of the desynchronized EEG recorded during some normal mental states. Finally, electrical equipment, including the ubiquitous electrocautery, can create electrical gradients of many volts across the patient. Obviously, if the EEG is to be extracted from all of this extraneous electrical noise, considerable attention to detail is required.

ELECTRODES

The recording electrode is the single most important part of the recording system, the easiest part to misuse, and the part that yields the greatest improvement in performance for the expenditure of effort. The scalp is a difficult location from which to record electrical activity, with hair impeding mechanical contact, oil and cornified skin impeding electrical contact, and a dense subcutaneous plexus of blood vessels that bleed profusely if punctured by an intradermal electrode. The type of electrode selected depends, in large measure, on which characteristics are compromised in order to optimize others.

Traditionally, anesthesiologists have opted for needle electrodes, perhaps because their biggest disadvantage, discomfort, was eliminated by the administration of anesthesia. Additionally, these electrodes can be applied much more quickly than metal and collodion systems and can be placed within a sterile field if necessary. Unfortunately, the electrical characteristics of needle electrodes are suboptimal, and their small surface area results in relatively high electrode impedances, even when properly placed. The electrodes are mechanically unstable, coming out as easily as they are inserted; and sterile technique (including needle sterilization between patients) is mandatory. Perhaps most important, when EEG monitoring is used to ensure cerebral perfusion during cerebrovascular procedures, the monitoring should begin before the induction of anesthesia, necessitating the discomfort of multiple needle insertions in an awake patient. Placement within a sterile field is probably the only situation in which needle electrodes are truly preferable.

Metal surface electrodes come in many shapes, sizes, and compositions, including gold, silver, and tin. Silver electrodes must be coated with silver-chloride in order to reduce their electrode impedance, but this can be accomplished easily by soaking them in household bleach. Although there are subtle differences among the metals, these factors do not appear to be significant for routine intraoperative monitoring. Nor does the choice of conductive agent, although the duration of some procedures allows drying of the conductive paste or jelly. This is undesirable, because it increases the electrode impedance, often in an erratic fashion. Taping over the electrode with plastic tape is often performed to reduce the drying and thus eliminate the need to refresh the conductive agent intraoperatively.

Another approach to electrode selection (and placement) is a cap, not unlike a bathing cap, which has electrodes fastened to it (Electrocap—Electrocap International, Inc., Dallas, TX). Such a system greatly simplifies proper placement of electrodes; however, for best results, a chin or chest strap is suggested to maintain the position of the cap, and this strap can interfere with access to the surgical field or airway.

Prepackaged adhesive EEG electrodes are also available, although rarely recommended by EEG technologists. In general, these electrodes cannot be placed over the scalp in close proximity to neural tissue at risk for hypoperfusion, although an occasional balding patient does permit correct placement. Such electrodes largely are recommended by manufacturers who are responding to the desires of individuals who value simplicity over precision or who are only concerned with global EEG effects, which can be assessed from frontal electrodes. For those who wish to perform multichannel recordings in hirsute individuals, prepackaged adhesive electrodes are not a satisfactory option.

The impedance—the interface between the electrode and the subject's skin—must be minimized for good EEG recordings. Recommended impedances are less than 3000–5000 Ω. Impedance reduction is achieved by meticulous skin preparation and careful electrode application.

Standard Electrode Positions

The positioning of electrodes is another area in which anesthesiologists often attempt shortcuts, usually by ''eyeballing'' positions or placing electrodes at symmetric but ill-defined locations. There are several standard systems for determining electrode placement, the International 10–20 system[6] being one of the most commonly used.

International 10–20 System. In the 10–20 system, electrode positions are defined in relation to cranial dimensions (Fig. 15–1), and the electrodes are positioned in reproducible relationships with cortical structures. Occasionally, additional nonstandard electrode positions are desirable, although these are more frequently used to optimize the amplitude of evoked potentials than to record spontaneous EEG. The advantages of anatomically reproducible electrode positions are obvious, and include both the ability to generalize and discuss the findings of one patient relative to another and the ability to correlate the EEG findings and the underlying neuropathology.

The International 10–20 system comprises 21 surface electrodes, which can be connected in many thousands of ways. Although most of these possibilities have no logical rationale, three patterns of electrode connections are commonly used that influence the appearance of the EEG. The bipolar montage is created by recording multiple channels of EEG, each of which is derived from two active electrodes placed at any of the defined electrode positions (Fig. 15–2). A third electrode is required as an electrical ground, for which the ipsilateral ear is often used. Most commonly, these electrode pairs are recorded from chains of electrodes (F_{P1}–F_3, F_3–C_3, C_3–P_3, and so on) in either parasagittal or coronal positions. Occasionally, bilateral symmetric positions are used (e.g., F_{P1}–F_{P2}, F_3–F_4), but rarely bilateral asymmetric positions.

Bipolar Montages. Bipolar chains have several important characteristics. When the EEG is recorded in a bipolar chain, the focus of unusual activity is often recognized by the increase in amplitude of the activity as the recording pairs approach the site, together with a change in the polarity of the activity as seen by channels on opposite sides of the focus. Although this is quite valuable for the encephalographer trying to identify a seizure focus, this is of little value to the anesthesiologist using processed EEG analysis techniques, because none of the techniques currently in use provides information about wave polarity or phase. A more important characteristic is the tendency for bipolar recordings to emphasize focal effects while minimizing global

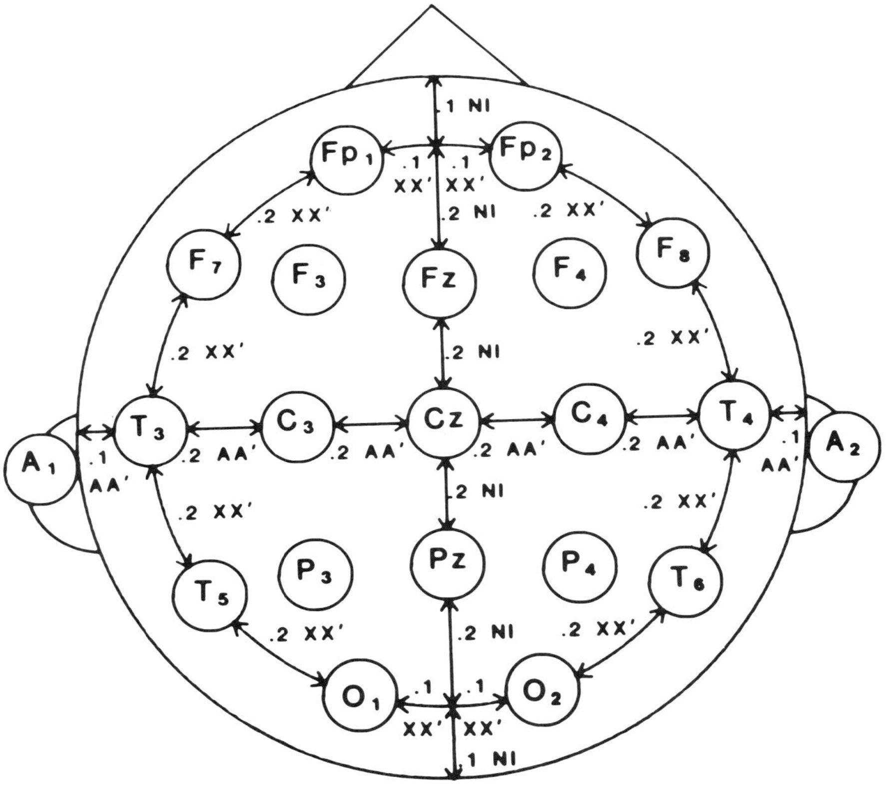

Figure 15–1. Measurements necessary to identify the 21 scalp electrodes of the International 10–20 System of electrode placement. Measurements are either 10% (.1) or 20% (.2) of a circumferential measurement. NI is the distance from the nasion to the inion, measured over the vertex of the head. The preauricular distance (AA′) is measured from tragus to tragus over the vertex.

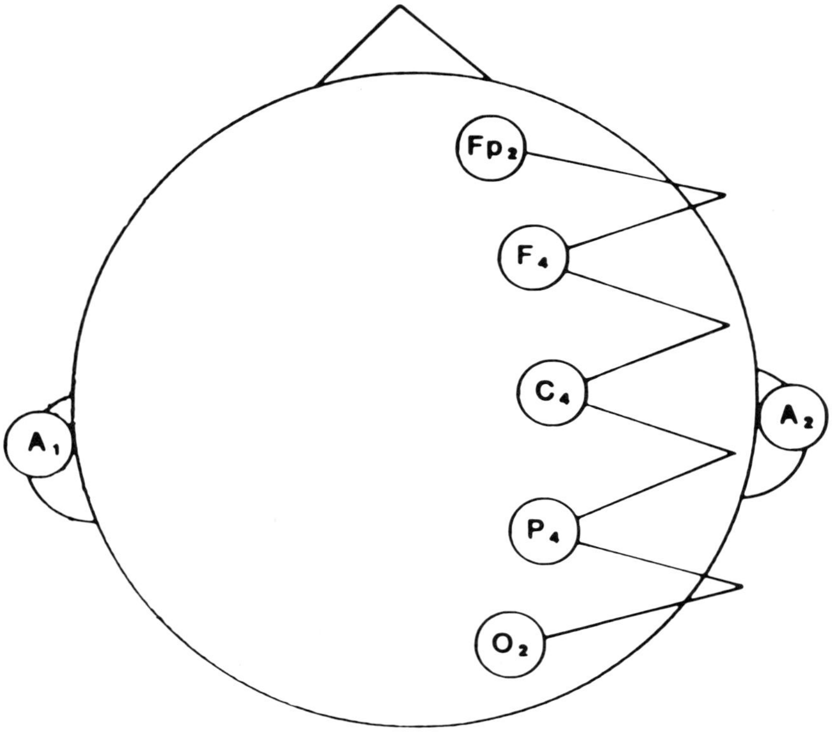

Figure 15–2. A bipolar montage is created by recording from pairs of electrodes as shown. Only the ground electrode (A_2) is common to all channels.

ones.[7] Thus, with both electrodes over an area of hypoxic slowing, the bipolar recording will show a prominent change, a highly desirable characteristic for a monitor of intraoperative ischemia. Finally, the bipolar recording is physically robust, with only one electrode (the ground electrode) common to all channels. Thus, the loss of electrical contact at any other single electrode will not preclude EEG recording, although this can happen with referential montages.

Referential Montages. Referential montages differ from bipolar montages by the existence of a reference electrode that is used in the recording of all channels of the EEG (or at least all ipsilateral channels) (Fig. 15–3). Normally, one attempts to place the common reference electrode in an area of little EEG activity, thus allowing the electrical activity directly under the other recording electrode to predominate. (This has led to the somewhat erroneous term ''unipolar recording.'') The ipsilateral ear is commonly used. Occasionally a quiescent site cannot be found, and an average reference electrode montage may be created by electrically averaging several electrodes to provide a new and more stable reference.

RECORDING PROBLEMS

Several problems are shared by both common and average reference electrode montages. First, activity occurring near the reference electrode appears on all channels. Thus, when it is used to monitor for ischemia, activity at the reference electrode can resemble adequate perfusion when areas of ischemia are present. Also, artifact derived from the reference electrode can obliterate the entire EEG recording, something that could not occur with a bipolar montage. Even worse, with an average reference electrode, artifact on any one of many channels is added into all channels of the recording, making high-quality recordings more difficult to obtain in an electrically noisy environment such as the operating room.

If the details of electrode positioning, application, and interconnection appear imposing, several approaches can be used to simplify the task, including employing the assistance of a qualified electrophysiologist technician. Although few anesthesia services can justify a full-time technician, it is often possible to utilize one of the hospital technicians to apply electrodes preoperatively, even the night before surgery, which then need only be checked or refilled with conductive jelly. Alternatively, anesthesia personnel can be trained in recording techniques in the neurology clinic by the EEG technologists. The ready availability of a reasonable patient schedule allows the rapid assimilation of the necessary experience. Such an experience will not provide all the skills of an electrophysiologist, but greatly improves the ease and quality of patient preparation for intraoperative EEG monitoring.

To use a commercial EEG monitoring system, one need not comprehend in detail the electronics involved. However, there is little doubt that a general overview of such matters not only satisfies intellectual curiosity, but also assists in understanding why certain problems occur and how best to rectify them. For example, it is not intuitively obvious how it is possible to record EEG (at an amplitude of 10–100 μV) from a patient whose ECG has an amplitude

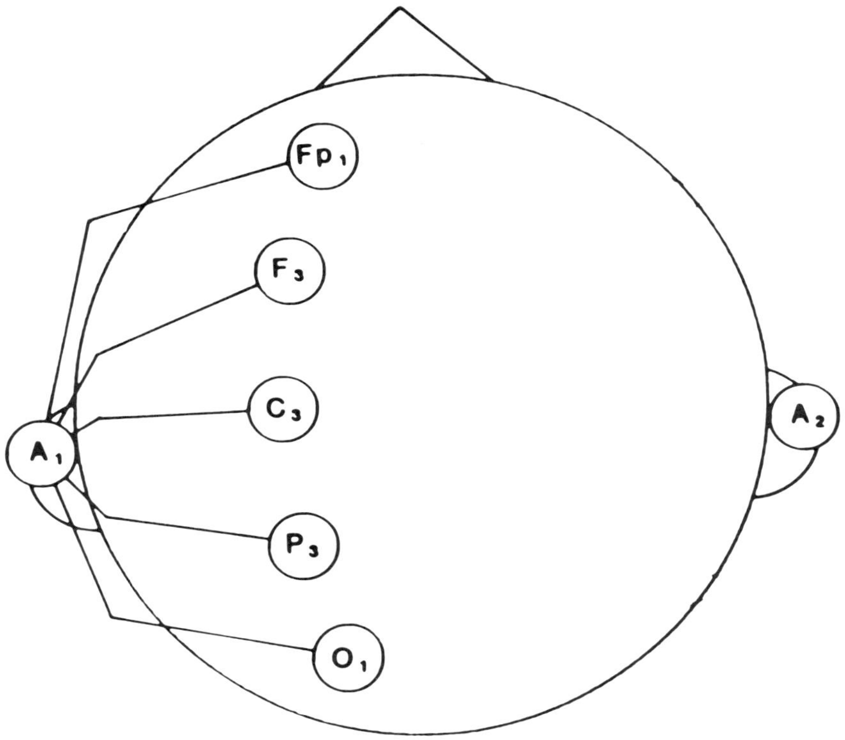

Figure 15–3. A common reference montage is created by recording each channel with one electrode in common. In this example, each of the channels has A_1, the left ear, as one of the two active electrodes. A_2, the ground electrode, also is common to all channels.

of many millivolts and who is exposed to other forms of electrical noise (especially at 60 Hz), the amplitude of which may be measured in volts. The most important step in this process occurs in the very earliest stage of amplification of the signal—the differential amplifier.

Differential Amplifiers

Although it is common to speak of a channel of EEG activity that is recorded from a pair of electrodes (e.g., E_1 and E_2), the actual amplification process requires three electrodes. The third electrode, the ground (G), is critical to the differential application of the desired signal and the rejection of artifact. The differential amplifier does not amplify a single voltage but actually amplifies only the difference in voltage between two pairs of electrodes. The pairs of electrodes are created by each single active electrode (E_1 and E_2) and the ground (G). Thus, the amplifier actually amplifies the voltage between E_1 and G minus the voltage between E_2 and G. The result is the voltage between E_1 and E_2, which is desired; even more important, any signal common to both E_1-G and E_2-G gets subtracted out (rejected) and not amplified. This process, called common mode rejection, may reduce the amplitude of a common signal such as 60-Hz artifact a million times (120 db or 99.9999% rejection), provided that the amplifiers are working optimally; this requires that the common signal be of equal amplitude on each differential channel E_1-G and E_2-G.

One of the major factors that causes common mode signal to appear to be of differing amplitude on each channel of the amplifier is a difference in the electrode characteristics, particularly unequal electrode impedances at E_1 and E_2. The amplification process is such that if the impedance at E_1 is much higher than that at E_2, a common signal (such as 60-Hz noise) will actually appear to be larger in E_1-G than in E_2-G. Because the common signal is not equal, not all of it is removed, and some common signal (noise) appears as real, amplified signal (EEG).

A similar phenomenon can be responsible for the appearance of ECG signal on the EEG, even though the electrode impedances are not unbalanced or faulty. By placing a ground electrode at a distant site (e.g., the shoulder), the amplitude of ECG signal on each side of the differential amplifier is greatly increased. In addition, volume conduction effects (which occur because of the transmission of a signal from a large volume, the chest, to a smaller one, the head) can change the amplitude of the ECG in the half-channels so that they do not completely cancel and ECG appears on the EEG. For this reason, it is usually undesirable to put the EEG ground electrode on the torso.

Filters

Another important aspect of EEG monitoring is the use of filters and the resultant potential for distortion of the EEG. Almost all EEG recording systems are equipped with filters that reduce both high-frequency and low-frequency activity. Filters are described by the frequency at which they reduce the amplitude by 70% (the 3-db point) and the rate at which they reduce activity outside of the band of interest, typically halving the voltage for a doubling of the frequency. A frequent use of high-frequency filters is reduction of 60-Hz artifact. However, a 30-Hz filter only reduces 60-Hz artifact by 50%, and a lower-frequency filter reduces the amplitude of the high-frequency EEG activity often associated with light anesthesia or barbiturates.

At the low-frequency end of the EEG, similar problems exist. Low-frequency filters at 3 Hz are capable of eliminating baseline artifact in the frequency range below 0.5 Hz, but do so at the expense of low-frequency delta activity (1.5-Hz components are 50% below 3-Hz waves of equal amplitude and 65% below 6-Hz theta activity of equal amplitude, which would be essentially unfiltered). Lower-frequency filters (e.g., 1-Hz) do far less damage to the EEG waveform but are much less effective at reducing low-frequency artifact.

CONVENTIONAL MULTICHANNEL EEG

Having amplified and filtered the electrical activity from the scalp, conventional EEG techniques do no further processing. They simply display the signal as a graph of amplitude (i.e., voltage) over time. Depending on the activity being recorded, full-scale deflection of the pen is usually 100–500 μV, and the paper speed is 15–60 mm/second. This process results in patterns of waves that can be associated with specific physiologic states, drug effects, or pathologic conditions.

EEG PATTERNS

The best known of these patterns is the alpha rhythm (Fig. 15–4), a pattern of activity containing waves of 8–12 Hz, predominating posteriorly, and masked by mental activity, particularly eye opening and attending to stimuli.[8] For any given individual, the frequency of alpha activity is quite stable, although slowing can occur with age.[9] Occasionally, this slowing is enough to cause the peak of the alpha rhythm to fall outside of the normal alpha band (8–12 Hz), and a slow alpha or 7- to 8-Hz variant alpha is seen.

Not all patients demonstrate baseline alpha rhythms. Various studies estimate the incidence of nonalpha activity to be between 15 and 35%. About half of these nonalpha patterns are low-voltage mixed patterns, with the remainder divided among pure beta (above 12 Hz), theta (4–8 Hz), and mixed and irregular variants. Pure delta activity (below 4 Hz) is not seen in healthy patients under standard recording conditions (awake with eyes closed and without psychotropic drugs).

There are other patterns of activity as well, some of which are closely associated with certain levels of mental status. For example, sleep spindles—fusiform bursts of activity at about 14 Hz—are commonly seen during certain stages of natural sleep. Spike and wave activity is classically seen during seizures at a frequency of about 3 Hz. Isolated spikes lasting 0.01–0.08 seconds can also be seen, as can slightly slower "sharp wave" activity, which is similar in shape but of slightly longer duration (0.08–0.2 seconds). Burst-suppression (Fig. 15–5) is another pattern of activity commonly observed by the anesthesiologist, who induces it with hypothermia or the administration of barbiturates, isoflurane, or other agents.

INTRAOPERATIVE EEG RECORDING

The conventional multichannel strip-chart recording is the gold standard against which all other EEG systems must be compared. However, this standard was set for diagnostic, not monitoring, purposes, and a number of problems occur in the translocation of this technique (and the equipment) to the operating room. Despite improvements due to the miniaturization of electronic components, a standard EEG machine is a large, cumbersome device without a home in the crowded operating room. It may not even be possible to put the device where the anesthetist can see both the EEG and his usual monitors and attend to the administration of an anesthetic. Another disadvantage derives from the use of electrocautery, which not only obliterates the EEG but produces wild gyrations of the pen and sprays ink over the machine and anything nearby. EEG recording at conventional rates (30 mm/second) requires prodigious amounts of paper (360 pages/hour), and simply finding a previous event for comparison may be a heroic task. Lastly, most intraoperative events of interest are not associated

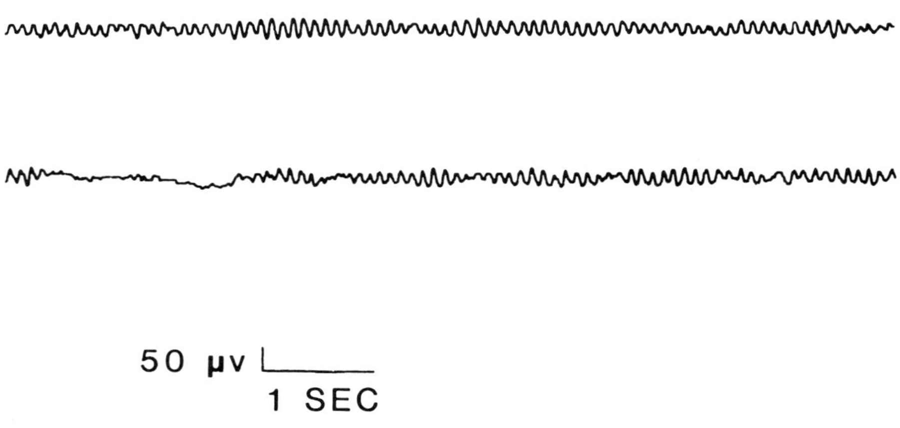

Figure 15–4. The EEG above exemplifies the rhythm and amplitude patterns characteristic of the alpha rhythm. The frequency is about 10 Hz, with an amplitude of 30–40 μV (peak to peak).

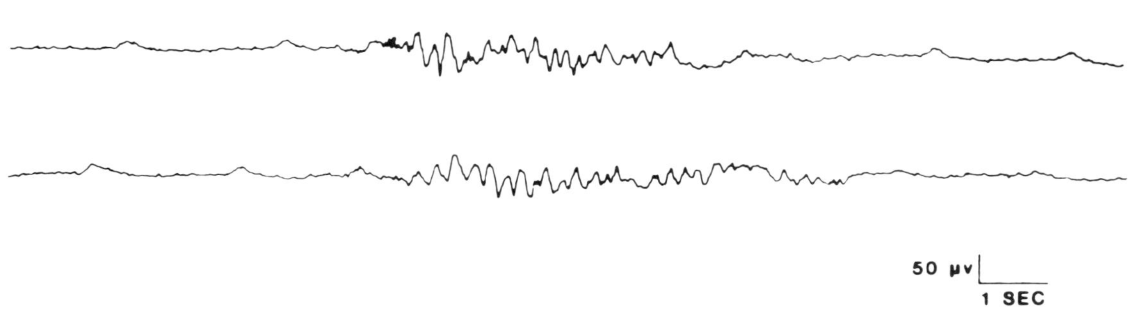

Figure 15–5. This EEG demonstrates the pattern of activity and quiescence characteristic of burst-suppression.

with specific, identifiable waveforms; thus, the ability to make such identifications does not add to the usefulness of the techniques.

Nonetheless, the ability to examine the unprocessed analog EEG, either on a strip-chart or on a video display, is most important when using processed EEG monitors. It may be necessary for EEG interpretation, when burst-suppression or seizure activity occurs. Analog display may be useful for artifact identification, including the recognition of electrocardiographic contamination of the signal. Examination of the raw signal is also helpful when trying to eliminate baseline drift and movement artifact. In short, assessment of the analog EEG is a quality-control measure to ensure that the signal being processed accurately reflects cortical electrical activity.

PROCESSED EEG MONITORS

Difficulty in using the strip chart EEG as a monitor stimulated the development of EEG processing systems for monitoring. Three distinct patterns of processing and data display emerged in the late 1960s and early 1970s: power spectrum analysis, cerebral function monitor, and aperiodic analysis. The first of these, power spectrum analysis,[10] evolved from engineering work in the 1950s and was applied to the EEG as a research tool in the 1960s.[11] Technology had not yet produced microcomputers, so the technique remained an investigational tool for many years. However, during this time, display techniques were developed and enhanced. The second analysis technique, the cerebral function monitor,[12] was developed in England in 1969 for monitoring the EEG after resuscitation, not during anesthesia. The third branch of the EEG analysis tree evolved in 1975 when Demetrescu proposed a technique he called aperiodic analysis for quantifying the EEG.[13]

Although one may discuss a monitoring technique and its implementation separately, the two are inseparably linked for the clinician who cannot (and probably should not) develop his or her own system. Unfortunately, technologic change in this area is rapid, and critiques based on specific features may suddenly become obsolete. Accordingly, the following discussion emphasizes general concerns and theoretic aspects of EEG analysis rather than the presence of specific "front panel" features on each monitor. Because many commercial systems now contain other monitors (e.g., evoked potentials), the ultimate decision to obtain a particular instrument will clearly be influenced by other factors.

THE CEREBRAL FUNCTION MONITOR AND CEREBRAL FUNCTION ANALYZING MONITOR

Although power spectrum analysis predated the cerebral function monitor (CFM), the latter was the first device specifically designed and built for monitoring the EEG in the clinical setting. It was designed for the continuous monitoring of one channel of EEG between conventional EEG recordings. The unit incorporated a continuous record of electrode impedance, which functioned to identify both movement artifact and electrode malfunction.

Unfortunately, the name of the device suggested that a quantity called "cerebral function" existed and that this device measured it. In fact, the device measured the peak voltage of a rectified, heavily filtered EEG. The filtration served to de-emphasize low-frequency activity (which tends to be higher in amplitude than high-frequency activity) and emphasize high-frequency activity. As an indicator of EEG activity in patients with decreased brain function, this is a reasonable approach. However, its appropriateness for processing the EEG during general anesthesia is questionable. Nonetheless, extensive work was done with the CFM, identifying EEG changes during carotid endarterectomy,[14] deliberate hypotension,[15] and cardiopulmonary bypass,[16–18] correlating changes with anesthetic agents,[19, 20] and even providing control of anesthetic depth in animals.[21] Despite this success, the inability to examine the behavior of different frequencies within the EEG was a major drawback of this device.

The cerebral function analyzing monitor (CFAM) evolved from the CFM to address this need.[22] The CFAM still filters the EEG before processing, and generates CFAM units as a logarithmic function of the root-mean-square (RMS) voltage generated by the filter. The output from the filter is further analyzed using a modified zero-crossing technique. This allows the computation of activity in individual frequency bands as a fraction of total activity. Like its predecessor, the CFAM analyzes only a single channel of the EEG, but improvements over CFM include the ability to display portions of unprocessed signal and to transmit digital data about the CFAM analysis to a computer for further analysis.

TECHNIQUE OF ANALYSIS

The underlying analysis technique, zero-crossing analysis, is conceptually straightforward. A signal is analyzed, as shown in Figure 15–6, by determining the amount of time (the period) that the polarity remains the same. By definition, the frequency is the inverse of the period (i.e., frequency = 1/period), so that the frequency is easily calculated. The RMS amplitude is easily computed by electronic means, and the amplitude can then be summed (integrated) into the frequency band indicated by the frequency computation for the wave.

The process of summing the EEG waves into frequency bands evolved from the classic description of wave frequency:

delta waves: $f < 4$ Hz
theta waves: $4 \leq f < 8$ Hz
alpha waves: $8 \leq f \leq 13$ Hz
beta waves: $13 \text{ Hz} < f$

The CFAM uses slightly different bandwidths, considering activity up to 13 Hz to be alpha, moving the alpha-theta transition to 7.5 Hz and the theta-delta transition to 3.5 Hz. For computer analysis, each band is further subdivided; however, the details are not relevant to this discussion. The appearance that this process imposes on the processed output is, however, most important.

When examining the behavior of the EEG during anesthesia, it is clear that there may be activity that does not fit into the classically defined bands but spreads across bands. Furthermore, as the EEG changes because of drug effects or other factors, these bands of activity shift gradually, but the use of arbitrary limits makes the transition appear abrupt (Fig. 15–7). Perhaps more importantly, the process of lumping EEG activity into bands implies that a shift within a band (e.g., from 11 to 8 Hz) is less important than a shift between bands (e.g., from 8 to 7 Hz), even though there are no data derived from the analysis of the EEG recorded during anesthesia to suggest this to be true.

APERIODIC ANALYSIS

In 1975, Demetrescu published a single abstract concerning a new EEG analysis technique[13] and began to develop a commercial application from it (patented in 1982). As a result, it was 1986 before the actual analysis technique was published.[23] In the interval, the initial machine was extensively revised and a number of important improvements were made, but the characteristic analysis technique and display format were not changed.

Unlike the CFAM, which uses polarity to identify the duration of a wave, the aperiodic analysis does so by determining the time of voltage between two voltage minima. Two different algorithms (for slow and fast activity) are used to select voltage minima (Fig. 15–8). The slow-wave algorithm operates on a signal that has been filtered by an 8.2-Hz low-pass filter and selects negative voltage minima that are separated by positive voltage EEG activity. The fast-wave algorithm operates on waveform filtered at 29.4 Hz and determines the period of the wave from successive minima regardless of polarity of the EEG activity. The minima having been identified, the largest amplitude between them is considered the peak, and the amplitude for that wave is computed as the average of the voltage differences between the peak voltage and each of the minima.

Lifescan Monitor

The Lifescan monitor displays the processed EEG (aperiodic analysis) in a unique format. Waves are displayed as vertical spikes (often called telephone poles) on an isometric three-dimensional cathode-ray tube (CRT) display. The size of the spike indicates the amplitude of the wave; its horizontal position and color are determined by the frequency; and time is displayed on the z axis by placing new data in the front and scrolling older data into a more distant-appearing position. Current versions of this device include the ability to monitor evoked potentials, computer communication protocols, and two-channel capability.

Many publications attest to the function of the device as a waveform processor. It has been used to demonstrate both

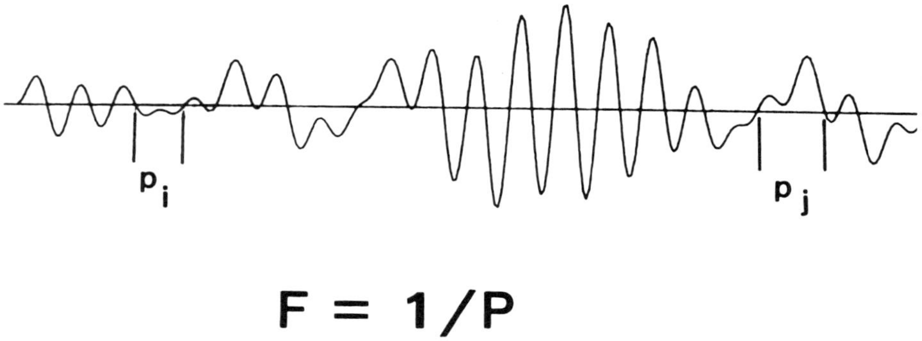

Figure 15–6. Zero-crossing analysis determines the period of a wave by measuring the time that the wave is above (or below) the isoelectric line. The frequency of the wave is the inverse of the period.

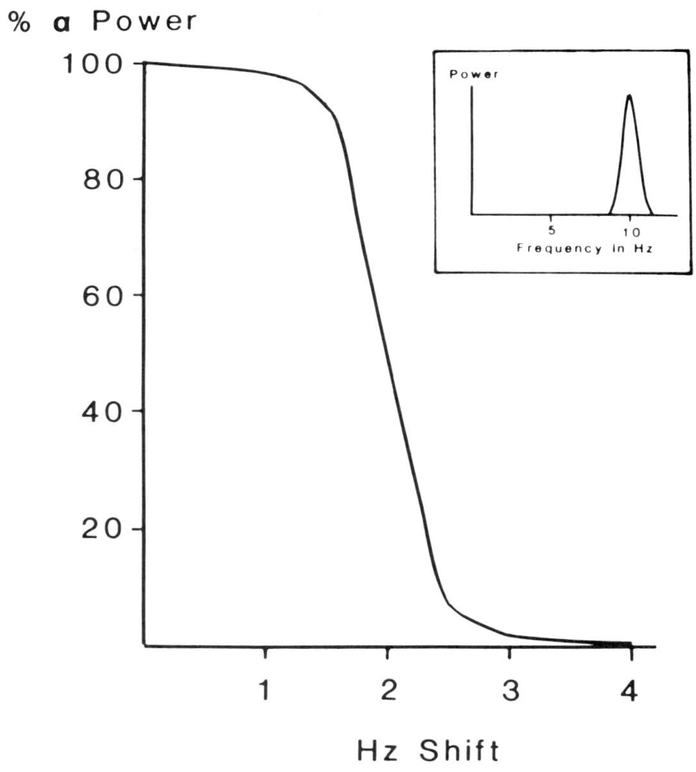

Figure 15–7. Percentage of power in the alpha band as a (hypothetic) band of activity *(inset)* is slowed. Almost no change in power is noted during the first 1 Hz of slowing, with very rapid changes in the percentage of power in the alpha band between 1.5 Hz and 2.5 Hz of slowing. Thus, the use of fixed bands makes the uniform slowing appear very sudden and nonuniform.

ischemia[24] and anesthetic effects.[25, 26] No side-by-side comparisons have been made with any other processing technique; thus, it is unclear whether aperiodic analysis truly represents an advantage over zero-crossing or power spectrum techniques. Further confusing the comparison is the unique display, which some observers enjoy and others find difficult to interpret.

POWER SPECTRUM ANALYSIS

Although Blackman and Tukey ''wrote the book'' on power spectrum analysis in 1958,[10] it was 10 years before these techniques migrated from the engineering world to anesthesia. This is hardly surprising, because a refrigerator-sized computer was required to process even a single channel of EEG data. Real-time analysis, without which monitoring is impossible, was still a gleam in the designers' eyes, realized nearly 5 years later and then only by telephone data transmission.[27] In spite of these difficulties, this period allowed for the development of two alternative display techniques.[28, 29] In addition, as computers became smaller and faster, a number of researchers developed their own systems; this research increased understanding of the technique before its clinical use became common.

Method of Analysis

Power spectrum analysis is a general-purpose technique for describing the amplitudes of component waves of a sample of EEG (or any signal that varies with time). It requires that the original signal be digitized and mathematically manipulated through a complex process known as Fourier transformation (Fig. 15–9). This transformation process defines certain characteristics of the resultant power spectra. Failure of the EEG to meet the mathematical assumptions strictly necessary for the application of this transformation has raised questions about its applicability.

To perform Fourier transformation, the analog EEG data must be sampled (digitized), a process that defines the highest frequency resolvable by the subsequent Fourier analysis. (This frequency is one half the sampling frequency.) In fact, if the data are not sampled at a sufficiently high frequency, high-frequency waves will appear at lower frequencies, an artifact known as aliasing (Fig. 15–10). (This is true of digitization for all types of analysis, not just power spectrum analysis.)

The process of Fourier transformation converts a collection of data points (an epoch) into a series of sine wave components at regularly spaced frequency intervals. For each two data points, one frequency interval can be calculated; thus, if 500 data points are transformed, there will be 250 frequency intervals ranging from zero to the highest frequency that could be resolved by the sampling rate. The relationship between the number of data points and the sampling rate defines both the length of the epoch (epoch length = number of data points/sampling rate) and the frequency resolution of the power spectra (which is simply the inverse of the epoch length in seconds).

One of the major areas of contention about power spectrum analysis is the appropriateness of the application of

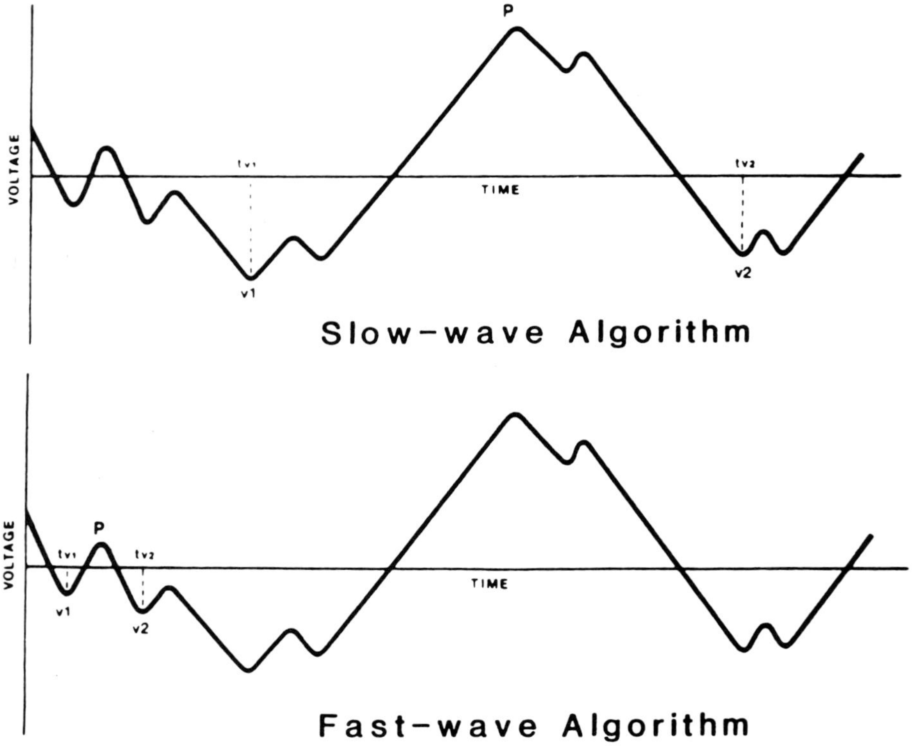

Figure 15–8. The slow- and fast-wave detection algorithms of the Lifescan monitor. The slow-wave algorithm identifies negative voltage minima separated by a positive voltage; the fast-wave algorithm identifies minima and maxima without regard to polarity.

this technique to the EEG.[30] Strictly speaking, Fourier analysis may be applied to a periodic, stationary signal. The EEG is well known to be nonstationary, although if epochs are not excessively long, stationary behavior may be reasonably well approximated. The EEG is also not, strictly speaking, periodic, because sequential epochs are not identical. These failures to meet the mathematical requirements of power spectrum analysis are often cited by those who favor other analytic approaches; however, they do not, in general, appear to be reasons for not applying power spectrum analysis to the EEG.

These issues become more problematic when the EEG demonstrates burst-suppression activity, because this is clearly nonstationary activity, and analysis with epochs shorter than a complete burst-suppression cycle can be misleading *if taken out of context.* When clinical monitoring is performed, the pattern of burst-suppression activity is easily identified in the graphic display and confirmed by examination of the unprocessed recording.[31] Investigation of the effects of epoch length (and thus spectral resolution) has supported the use of short epochs in all other monitoring situations and recommended the recognition of burst suppression by its characteristic pattern on the graphic display.[32]

Display

The graphic display of the power spectrum analysis normally takes one of two general forms: a linear graphic or a topographic picture. The linear graphic is almost always utilized for the display of a single epoch of data. Frequency is plotted on the x axis and amplitude on the y axis. Although frequency is a nearly self-explanatory concept, amplitude is not. Strictly speaking, the amplitude of the power spectrum should be plotted in units of intensity: V^2/Hz.[33] This can be converted to actual units of power (watts) if one is willing to assume that the brain behaves as a 1-Ω resistor—hardly a reasonable assumption. The normalization by spectral resolution (hertz) is necessary in order to correct for the reduction in intensity that occurs in each spectral component when the spectral resolution is increased. When all data are analyzed at the same spectral resolution, the normalization is often omitted, and occasionally the square root of this unnormalized intensity is plotted as ''volts.''

Even though a graph of intensity and frequency is relatively easy to understand, it may be difficult to describe (Fig. 15–11). Such complexity could be eliminated if the power spectrum could be reduced to one number that could summarize the behavior of the spectrum. From a mathematical standpoint, such a wish is clearly a dream. Even the gaussian distribution, or bell-shaped curve as it is commonly called, requires two numbers, the mean and the variance (which describes its width), to describe it. Such logical arguments have failed to deter clinicians, who regularly describe new combinations of spectral frequencies and powers in an attempt to derive the ideal univariate descriptor. At least 27 such descriptors have been proposed,[34] but none has proved useful in all situations.

Spectral Edge Frequency

The spectral edge frequency (SEF)[35] has been one of the most widely used of the univariate descriptors of the EEG

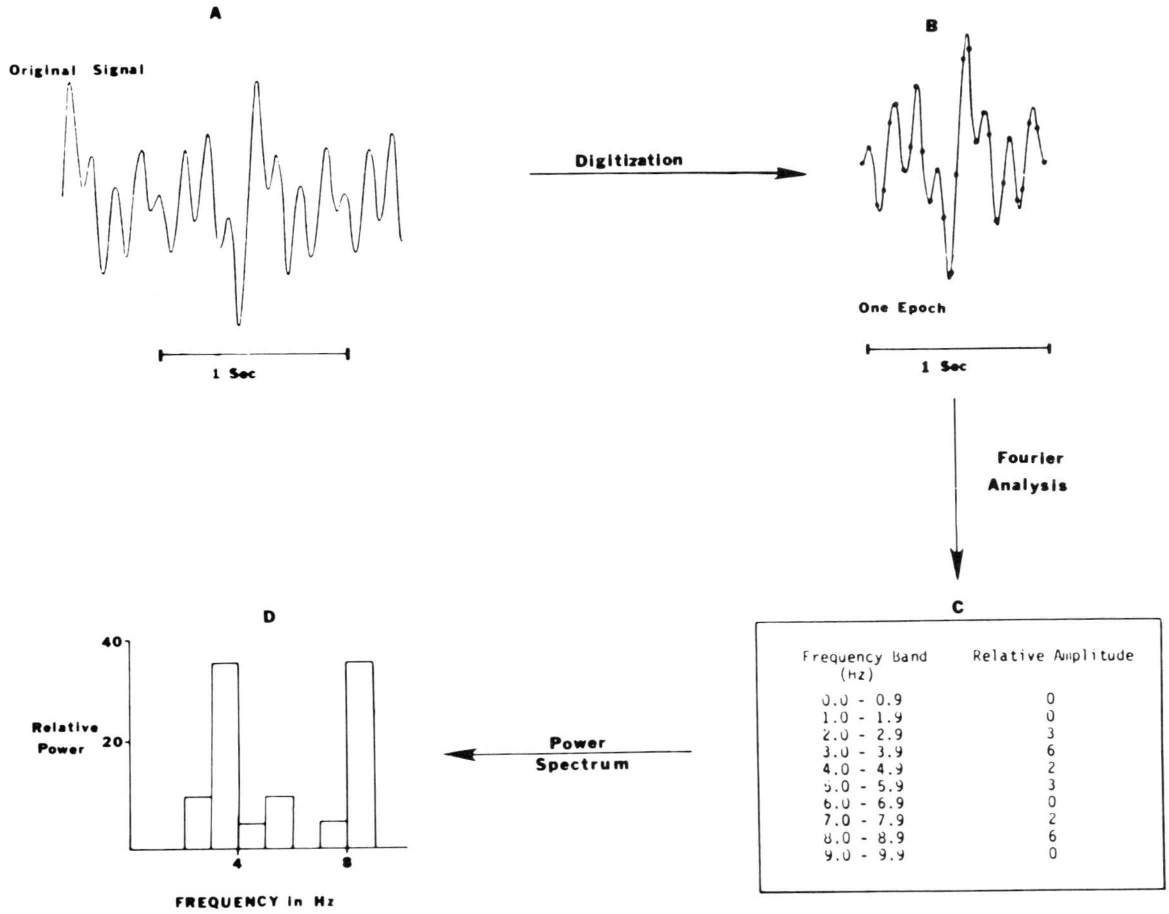

Figure 15–9. To perform power spectrum analysis, data are digitized, grouped in epochs, and transformed, and the power spectrum is computed.

power spectrum. This variable is loosely defined as the highest frequency at which there are components in the power spectrum. Many have taken this to be the frequency of the 95th percentile of the power, although this was not the original description. These differing definitions of SEF account for some of the different results obtained using it. When diffuse slowing of the EEG is a prominent component of the changes under study, the SEF is a useful adjunct for the description of the power spectrum. In this way, hypoxia during carotid endarterectomy has been monitored,[36] the pharmacodynamics of narcotic agents have been differentiated,[37] and questions of acute tolerance to thiopental have been addressed.[38] Other drugs, such as the benzodiazepines,[39] do not produce this slowing, and thus the SEF has been ineffective in analyzing the EEG effects of these agents.

The reduction of the power spectrum to a single value also simplifies the display of these data over time, because a single value is easily graphed as a trend. However, when the entire spectrum is to be displayed over time, the problem becomes more complex, because three-dimensional data must now be compressed into two dimensions. Although it is common to do so by shifting the origin both up and to the right, the initial attempts to do this for the EEG power spectrum involved only an upward displacement. The resulting display (Fig. 15–12), known as the compressed spectral array (CSA),[28] has several disadvantages for monitoring. The primary problem is difficulty in identifying reductions in EEG activity, especially in monitoring

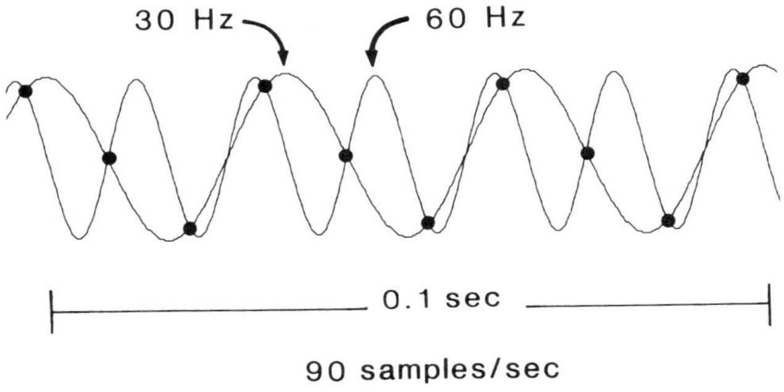

Figure 15–10. Aliasing occurs when a signal is sampled too slowly to be resolved. In this example, a 60-Hz wave is sampled at 90 samples/second; however, a 30-Hz wave also can be drawn through these points. Thus, the 60-Hz wave is made to appear to be 30 Hz, and will appear to be such in all subsequent analyses.

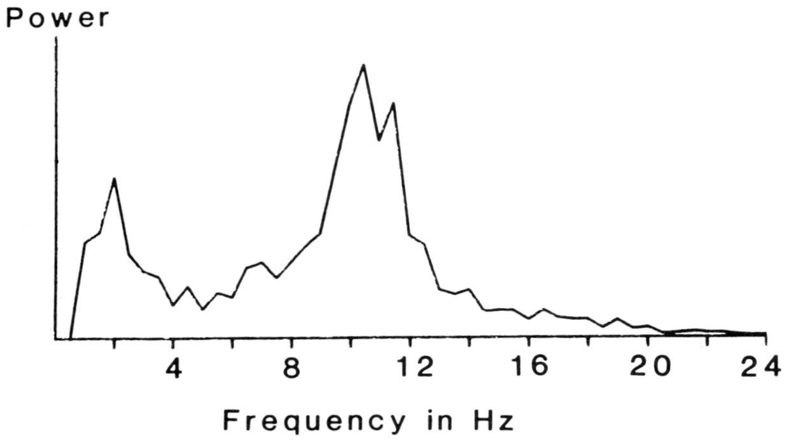

Figure 15–11. Complex power spectrum. Although it would be convenient if power spectra were narrow, bell-shaped curves, the diffuse bimodal distribution exemplified here is much more typical. Describing this spectrum as a single number must, of necessity, omit much information.

activity following artifact, because there is a tendency for low-amplitude data to be hidden by previous activity.

One solution to this problem involved modifying the time axis so that new data are placed below the old, ensuring the visibility of the most recent data (Fig. 15–13). This format improves the legibility of the data when it is displayed in this fashion and is found on commercial equipment utilizing CSA-type displays.

Density-Modulated Spectral Array

The alternative display format, known as the density-modulated spectral array (DSA),[29] utilizes a topographic compression of the three-dimensional data into two dimensions. This type of compression requires the color or grayscale encoding of amplitude information, which is then displayed on a graph of time (x axis) and frequency (y axis) (Fig. 15–14). Although it appears complex, the process of topographic compression is not only simple, but well known to grade-school children, whose maps often show mountains in various shades of brown, valleys in greens, coastlines in white, and oceans in blue—altitude data has been encoded in colors. Whether such encoding is performed by colors or by shades of gray, the result is the same. Colors, however, tend to emphasize differences more dramatically. The advantages of this display include a horizontal time axis that is easily scaled to coincide with other physiologic data and elimination of any hiding of data behind "hills."

Other Analyses Using Fourier Transformation

Power spectrum analysis is only one of the analyses that can be performed on the Fourier-transformed EEG. Coher-

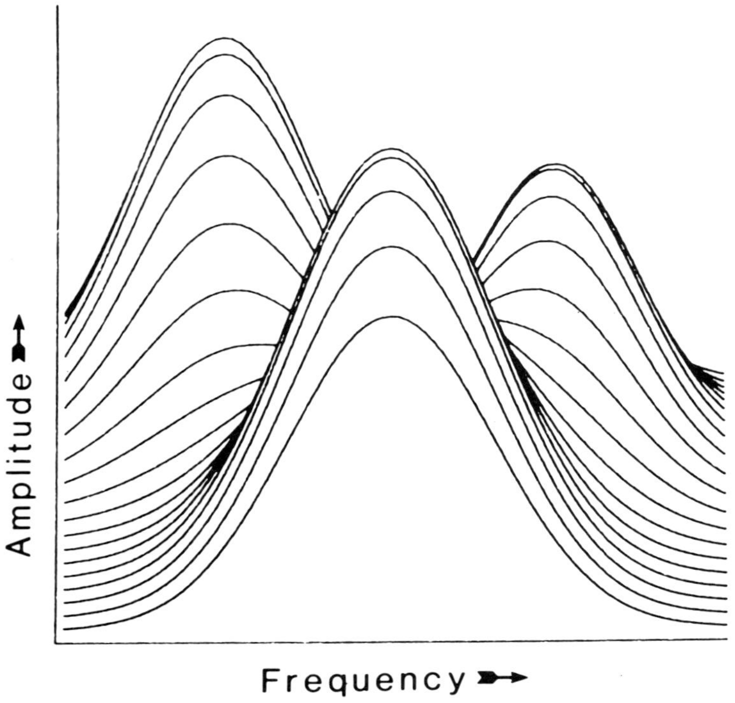

Figure 15–12. The compressed spectral array, a format for power spectral data, places time and amplitude on the same (vertical) axis. New data are placed at the back of the figure, and are easily obscured by preceding information.

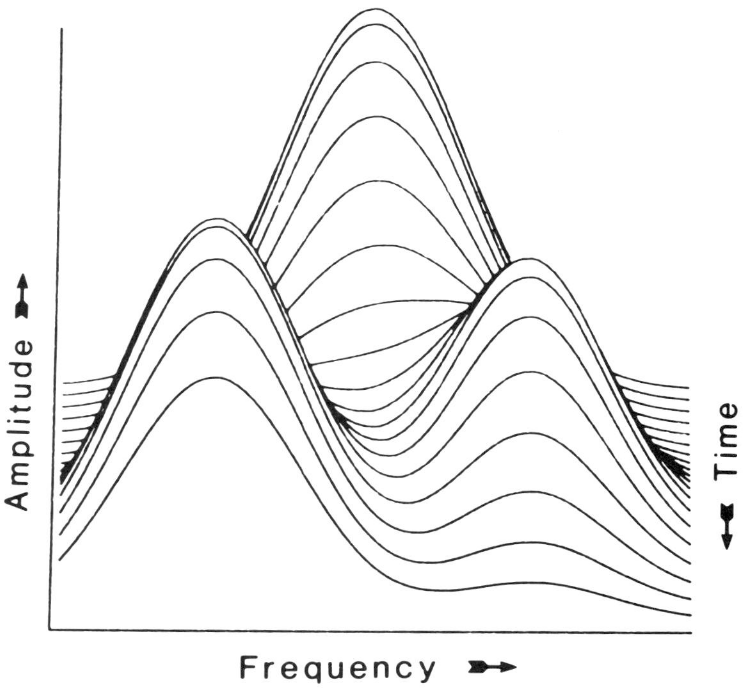

Figure 15–13. This compressed spectral array inverts the time axis (compared to Fig. 15–12). As a result, new data are placed at the front, where changes are discerned more easily.

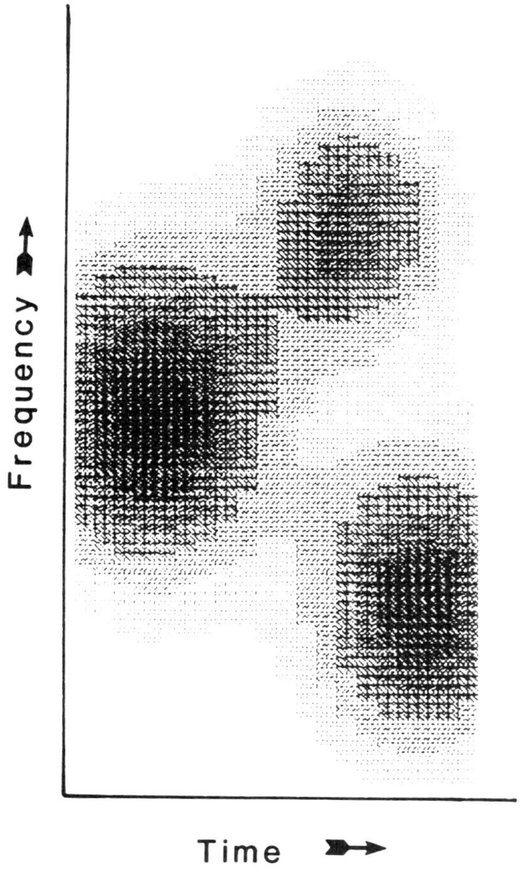

Figure 15–14. Density-modulated spectral array. The data shown in Figures 15–12 and 15–13 are replotted in the density-modulated format. Darker areas are peaks of greater intensity; new data are placed at the right margin.

ence analysis compares the phasic relationship of two channels of EEG to determine if they are synchronous.[40,41] Such synchrony suggests that the EEG generators are functionally interconnected, either by direct connections or by the presence of synchronizing input into both from a third location (e.g., thalamus). Because coherence is based on the variation in the phase angles between channels over time, the coherence must be calculated over a number of epochs. (For convenience they are usually taken sequentially, although there is no strict mathematical requirement for this.) The computation yields a dimensionless value (analogous to a correlation coefficient) that ranges between 0 and 1.0. The value of coherence that signifies a statistically significant number varies as a function of the number of epochs used in the computation.

In the unstimulated subject, the alpha rhythm is normally coherent,[42] most likely a consequence of the large number of cortical and subcortical interhemispheric connections that perform visual processing. The mu rhythm, a similar alpha-frequency rhythm derived from central somatosensory regions, is not coherent.[43] Although the coherence of the EEG during anesthesia is not thoroughly studied, it appears to increase, especially when computed from symmetric contralateral regions.[44] When anesthesia is deepened to the extent that burst suppression occurs, this activity is synchronous throughout the EEG. Whether increasing coherence is useful as a measure of anesthetic depth is unknown.

Both power and coherence comprise components of the analytic process known as bispectral analysis.[45,46] This technique also compares two channels of Fourier-processed EEG for interactions, but does so looking for harmonics rather than for individual frequencies. Because harmonics occur at frequencies that are the sum (or difference) of the interacting fundamental frequencies, bispectral analysis is capable of detecting interactions that cannot be observed with regular power or coherence analysis. Like coherence analysis, bispectral analysis must be performed over many sequential epochs. Many complexities surround the statistical interpretation of bispectral power or coherence, issues that are far beyond the extent of this review. Nonetheless, bispectral analysis has been applied to the EEG during anesthesia.[47] Its ultimate usefulness remains to be determined. Because of the limited number of studies examining these techniques, both coherence and bispectral analysis must be considered experimental.

DIFFERENCES AMONG PROCESSING TECHNIQUES

From a clinician's viewpoint, the differences among the other analysis techniques are much less significant than the characteristics of the equipment that has been designed to implement these techniques. Qualitatively, all analysis techniques show frequency changes when the EEG slows and amplitude changes when it flattens. Quantitatively, however, these techniques produce different results when applied to the same EEG, and applications that depend on quantitative analysis can be influenced by both analysis technique and the parameters that define it. This has been shown most extensively for power spectrum analysis. The variability from epoch to epoch is reduced by shortening the epoch unless burst–suppression is present.[32] The resolution of high–frequency activity is not affected by such changes, but it may be affected when other analysis techniques are used (Fig. 15–15). Most important, different frequency distributions may be observed with different analysis techniques (Fig. 15–16), thus reducing the applicability of data developed with one technique to situations in which another monitoring technique is utilized. This is most unfortunate, because it increases the importance of a particular monitoring technique, produces apparently conflicting reports of the usefulness of EEG monitoring in particular situations, and impedes research and understanding.

INDICATIONS FOR EEG MONITORING

The appropriate use of the EEG as an intraoperative monitor depends on three factors. First, the phenomenon must have identifiable EEG correlation that can be recognized by visual inspection or simple analysis of the EEG, whether in processed or analog form. Second, the phenomenon must not be associated with other, more easily identifiable signs that would eliminate the need for a more complex monitoring technique like the EEG. Third, the phenomenon should have clinically significant consequences, and therapeutic options should exist that can reduce the magnitude or the severity of these consequences.

CEREBRAL ISCHEMIA

One of the earliest uses of the EEG was in monitoring for the occurrence of cerebral ischemia during deliberate hypotension[48] and cardiopulmonary bypass.[49] Subsequently, there has been substantial interest in such monitoring for the determination of ischemia during carotid endarterectomy as well.[14, 36, 50–52] To complete the picture of ischemia/hypoxia detection, the EEG has been proposed as a way to identify hypoxia during routine anesthetics. Although each situation involves monitoring for ischemia (or hypoxia), the applicability of the EEG to each varies greatly.

Ischemia detection by electroencephalographic techniques easily fulfills the first of the criteria established earlier. Ischemia produces readily identifiable EEG changes consisting of the loss of high-frequency activity (if present) combined with an increase in low-frequency activity, particularly if such activity was not prominent before the ischemic insult. When the pre-ischemic EEG consists of high-amplitude, low-frequency activity, the early identification of ischemia may be more difficult, but continued inadequate perfusion produces the loss of low-frequency EEG activity, and the amplitude may decrease to nearly an

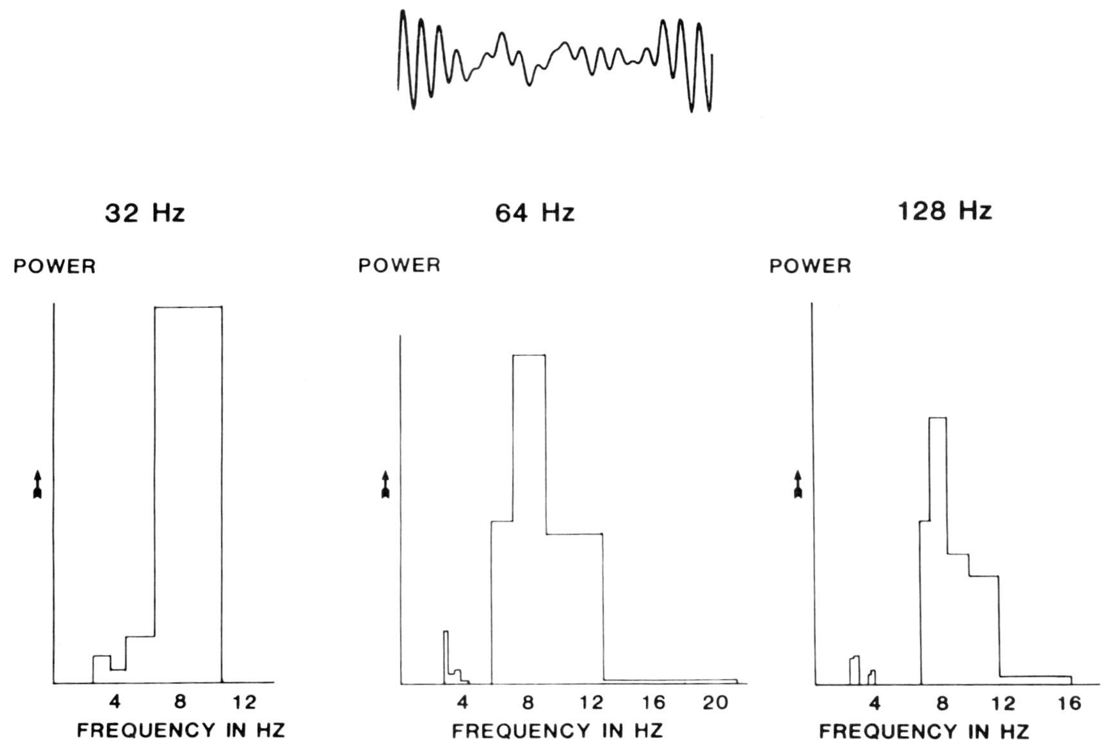

Figure 15–15. Effect of sampling frequency on zero-crossing analysis. Analysis of the 2-second waveform *(at top)* yields quantitatively different spectra when sampled at 32, 64, and 128 Hz.

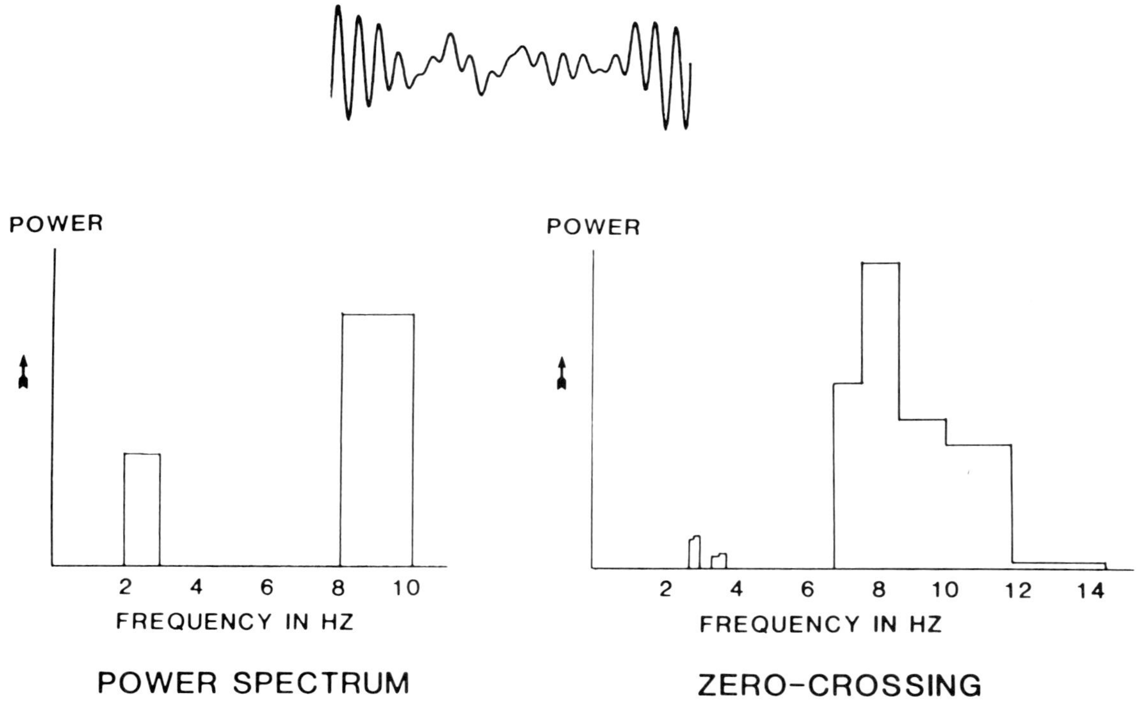

Figure 15–16. Effect of analysis technique. The spectrum on the left depicts the power spectral representation of the waveform at the top. On the right is a distribution of the waves identified by zero-crossing analysis. Although these are generally similar, there are many quantitative differences.

isoelectric level. These changes are gross and easily detected in both analog and processed EEG (Fig. 15–17).

When considering the presence of other signs of ischemia, one must distinguish end-organ ischemia (or hypoxia) from systemic hypoxia. The former is rarely accompanied by other signs and thus fulfills the second requirement for monitoring. As a general-purpose monitor of oxygenation during routine anesthesia, however, the EEG appears ineffective in comparison to the modern pulse oximeter. The pulse oximeter is a simple, robust device requiring only seconds to apply, and it yields qualitative data about systemic hypoxia at the very beginning of arterial desaturation. By comparison, the EEG takes longer to apply, is more easily obliterated by artifact, and is more difficult to interpret; it yields qualitative (not quantitative) data and is less specific (because of anesthetic influences) and less sensitive. In awake human volunteers, the EEG does not begin to change until the oxygen saturation of the blood has fallen below 60%,[53] long after the pulse oximeter has warned of the desaturation. Clearly, EEG monitoring is not indicated as a monitor of systemic hypoxia for routine anesthesia care.

The third requirement is for clinical significance and therapeutic options, and it is in this area that the indications for hypoxia monitoring begin to weaken. This is not, however, due to the lack of clinical significance of a hypoxic event. Cerebral hypoxia or ischemia severe enough to produce EEG changes is no less significant than myocardial ischemia sufficient to change the ECG. It is, by definition, a clinically significant event.

Our ability to provide therapeutic options, however, varies markedly. During deliberate hypotension, therapeutic options include increasing the blood pressure. Because many indications for deliberate hypotension are relative (e.g., reducing blood loss during orthopedic surgery), EEG monitoring may provide a margin of safety for these patients. It should be noted, however, that cerebral autoregulation begins to fail at 50–60 mmHg, and an additional 30% reduction in cerebral perfusion is required to produce EEG evidence of ischemia.[54] It is exceedingly rare for these levels of hypotension to be achieved during any procedures except neurosurgery or during cardiopulmonary bypass. Thus, for routine, modest levels of hypotension, cerebral ischemia is so rare that EEG monitoring is of marginal value.

CARDIOVASCULAR SURGERY

During cardiopulmonary bypass, neurologic complications are not rare,[55] and hypoperfusion is common. Is this

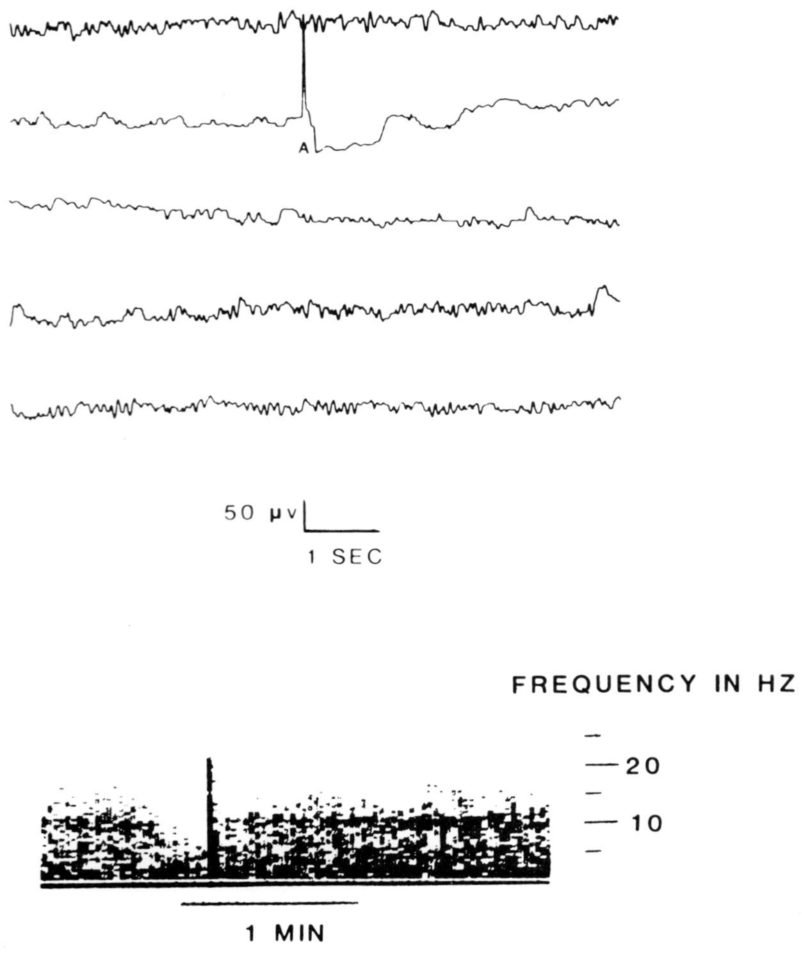

Figure 15–17. Cerebral hypoxia. Continuous EEG recorded during a severe ventricular arrhythmia (terminated at A, the artifact due to defibrillation). Diffuse slowing is evident about 4 seconds before this artifact and for about 12 seconds thereafter. The power spectral display of these data (shown below the raw signal) also depicts the ischemic slowing and recovery. The defibrillation artifact is again prominent.

an appropriate opportunity for EEG monitoring? It probably is not, because most neurologic complications during bypass are embolic,[56] and there are no specific therapies available to prevent or treat this complication. Furthermore, most cerebral ischemia during bypass occurs during hypoperfusion undertaken to facilitate specific surgical maneuvers (e.g., removing the aortic cross-clamp). Although these maneuvers may produce ischemia, there is no acceptable alternative, and these brief episodes do not appear to pose a threat to the neurologic well-being of the patient.[57] In addition, the high-dose narcotic anesthetics commonly used during cardiac anesthesia and hypothermia during bypass induce profound EEG slowing similar to changes caused by ischemia. However, the EEG can be used to titrate effects of drugs (barbiturates) during cardiac surgery.[56] Thus, routine EEG monitoring is probably unnecessary for procedures involving extracorporeal circulation.

Only in the case of cerebrovascular surgery (e.g., carotid endarterectomy) are all of the requirements for EEG monitoring met. Not only does carotid occlusion produce ischemia frequently and without systemic signs, but the placement of a vascular shunt markedly reduces the severity of ischemia or eliminates it entirely. Perhaps most importantly, shunting itself is associated with surgical morbidity due to emboli and intimal dissection; thus, shunting is undesirable except when there is evidence of ischemia. The shunt also complicates surgical access to the vessel, another reason to avoid its unnecessary use. Although this rationale strongly supports the use of EEG monitoring and selective shunting, satisfactory studies comparing selective shunting with alternative techniques have not been performed. Such comparisons may, in fact, be impossible, because the incidence of stroke is often reported to be less than 2%, and comparative studies would require thousands of subjects. Because the debate is clearly unsettled,[58] each anesthesiologist must decide the appropriateness of these monitoring techniques.

ASSESSMENT OF ANESTHETIC DEPTH

Another commonly proposed indication for EEG monitoring is the assessment of anesthetic depth. This vague term may refer either to anesthesia near the level at which recall for intraoperative events occurs or to much deeper levels of anesthesia necessary to blunt the autonomic response to painful stimulation. Others use the term to refer to EEG changes produced by anesthetic agents themselves, without surgery, in which the drug concentration represents the evidence of anesthetic depth. Although the EEG may be applicable to each of these areas, in most situations this technique seems to lack clinical utility.

If one reviews case reports and series involving intraoperative recall, EEG data is almost uniformly missing. Considering the infrequent occurrence of these events, this is not surprising—such a study would be a heroic undertaking. It does mean, however, that any usefulness of the EEG must be extrapolated from studies in unstimulated subjects using different, and largely irrelevant, stimuli.

Such extrapolation must be undertaken with caution. The onset of unresponsiveness during anesthetic induction has been shown to correlate with changes in the EEG[59]; however, these changes were specific to the drug under study. Enflurane produces high-frequency activity, whereas the addition of nitrous oxide produces similar unresponsiveness without this high-frequency activity. In other studies, analgesic doses of nitrous oxide by itself have produced high-frequency activity.[60] With isoflurane, the change in responsiveness is associated with the slowing of the alpha rhythm, if it is present. Absence of the alpha rhythm, usually the result of perioperative anxiety, precludes the use of changes in the alpha rhythm as an indication of unresponsiveness. Because attention to stimuli changes the EEG, one might also expect that attention to surgical stimuli during light anesthesia might also change the EEG. There is evidence that the EEG changes in response to surgical stimulation,[61] particularly in lightly anesthetized patients. However, there is no evidence that this would indicate awareness or cognitive function.

At greater depths of anesthesia, there is somewhat more evidence that the EEG can be used as a measure of anesthetic depth. This includes both classic studies of EEG changes with large variations in anesthetic concentration[11, 62, 63] and more recent ones that suggest that high-frequency activity in the power spectrum (spectral edge over 14 Hz) is a predictor of inadequate anesthetic depth for intubation, as evidenced by a hypertensive response.[64] Confirmation by other researchers and extension of these findings to other anesthetics and stimuli would be a valuable advance and might even justify more frequent EEG monitoring in those patients for whom a hypertensive response to intubation is particularly hazardous (e.g., patients with aneurysms and severe coronary artery disease). However, EEG monitoring only becomes valuable if there are no other signs of anesthetic depth to utilize and if the subject is sufficiently stable to allow adjustment of the anesthetic depth at will. Clearly, the clinical role for EEG monitoring of anesthetic depth remains to be defined.

In spite of the problems of applying pure pharmacologic data in the clinical setting, studies of the EEG effects of drugs continue and often demonstrate close associations between drug dosage and EEG changes.[65, 66] Thus, the EEG effects of fentanyl and alfentanil are grossly similar, but EEG studies explained differences in the clinical behavior of the drugs, which were the result of different pharmacodynamics. Similar studies have been performed with other drugs, although certain technical problems have arisen concerning the drug-specific nature of the EEG descriptors.

With the inhalational anesthetics, such pharmacologic data are extensive but older and less applicable to the mixed anesthetic techniques applied clinically. Nonetheless, the EEG changes in a dose-dependent and drug-specific fashion for all of the anesthetic agents. With light enflurane, high-frequency activity is more noticeable than with halothane or isoflurane; but at moderate concentrations, the differences are less striking. Isoflurane is the only modern inhalational agent to produce burst suppression, particularly at clinically useful doses, although this EEG pattern can also be achieved with the barbiturates. Even though each agent tends to produce a specific EEG pattern, the concept of an "anesthetic signature" that would allow identification of the anesthetic in use in any particular patient does not seem achievable, at least not at present. Perhaps this reflects the integration by the brain of many stimuli, not only the anesthetic chemicals administered. If so, each patient must be considered as an individual, not simply as a biologic mass spectrometer that converts drug input into bioelectric output.

Despite these problems and objections, physicians who are comfortable with interpreting the intraoperative EEG often identify changes in anesthetic depth using the EEG before such changes become evident by hemodynamic or somatic signs. In a given anesthetic in a particular patient, changes in anesthetic depth too small to be identified by other means can be evident in the EEG, and the presence of such change can often predict future clinical developments. The skill to detect such changes is not difficult to develop and might be worth developing for one so inclined; whether it justifies the use of a complex, albeit safe, monitoring modality like the EEG is open to question.

ELECTROENCEPHALOGRAPHY IN THE INTENSIVE CARE UNIT

There are two distinct indications for EEG recording in the ICU: for diagnosis and for monitoring. The indications for diagnostic recordings include determination of brain death and identification of seizures, both postoperatively and during status epilepticus. Such recordings are performed by technicians using standard multichannel strip-chart recorders and are interpreted by neurologists.

The applicability of processed EEG is less clear. The original CFM was developed to help confirm the diagnosis of brain death, but such monitoring has not become a criterion of brain death. Another application for EEG monitoring is to follow the progress of patients with drug overdoses.[67] Although it is interesting, there is no evidence that this monitoring improves care or modifies therapeutic choices that would be made on a purely clinical basis.

When dealing with victims of head trauma, there may be indications for continuous EEG monitoring. EEG patterns have been compared to the Glasgow coma score as a predictor of outcome, and the EEG performs comparably.[68] In such a situation, the simple clinical evaluation of patients seems preferable to something as complex as continuous EEG monitoring. On the other hand, the depth of barbiturate coma can easily be assessed from burst-suppression activity; thus, EEG monitoring may allow more rapid adjustment of this therapy than is possible with intermittent determinations of blood barbiturate concentrations. There may also be EEG evidence of "lightening" of coma, which is particularly valuable when neuromuscular blocking drugs are used to facilitate control of ventilation but patients are not heavily sedated. There is also evidence of sleep/waking patterns in monitored EEG, but it is not clear whether these findings are sufficient to indicate routine EEG monitoring in the neurologic intensive care unit.

SUMMARY

Modern technology has made intraoperative EEG monitoring reliable and practical, provided attention is given to technical detail. There are several approaches to EEG analysis. No single approach has been shown convincingly to be preferable to others. In general, clinicians select equipment based on such criteria as the number of channels of EEG processed, other monitors incorporated, flexibility, display mode, cost, user interface, length of epoch, and personal taste. The application of EEG monitoring in carotid endarterectomy procedures seems well justified, but for the identification of ischemia in other situations, the benefits are less evident. Although useful as a research tool for drug effects, the EEG cannot currently be recommended as a means of assessing anesthetic depth, although further work might change this assessment.

REFERENCES

1. Gibbs FA, Gibbs EL, Lennox WG: Effect on the electroencephalogram of certain drugs which influence nervous activity. Arch Intern Med 1937; 60:154–166.
2. Peronnet F, Sindon M, Laviron A, et al: Human cortical electrogenesis: Statigraphy and spectral analysis. *In* Petsche H, Brazier MAB (eds): Synchronization of EEG Activity in Epilepsies. New York: Springer-Verlag, 1972; 235–262.
3. Delucchi MR, Garoutte B, Aird RB: The scalp as an electroencephalographic averager. Electroencephalogr Clin Neurophysiol 1962; 14:191–196.
4. Allison T: Calculated and empirical evoked-potential distributions in human recordings. *In* Otta DA (ed): Multidisciplinary Perspectives in Event-Related Brain Potential Research. Washington, DC: US Environmental Protection Agency, 1978.
5. Blom JL, Anneveldt M: An electrode cap tested. Electroencephalogr Clin Neurophysiol 1982; 54:591–594.
6. Jasper HH: The ten-twenty electrode system of the International Federation. Electroencephalogr Clin Neurophysiol 1958; 10:371–375.
7. MacGillivray BB: Handbook of EEG and Clinical Neurophysiology, Vol 3-C. Amsterdam: Elsevier, 1974.
8. Chatrian GE, Bergamini L, Dondey M, et al: Report of the Committee on Terminology, Appendix A. Electroencephalogr Clin Neurophysiol 1974; 37:538–548.
9. Pichlmayr I, Lips U, Kunkel H: The Electroencephalogram in Anesthesia. New York: Springer-Verlag, 1984; 37.
10. Blackman RB, Tukey J: The Measurement of Power Spectra. New York: Dover, 1958.
11. Findeiss JC, Kien GA, Huse KOW, Linde HW: Power spectral density of the electroencephalogram during halothane and cyclopropane anesthesia in man. Anesth Analg 1969; 48:1018–1023.
12. Maynard D, Prior PF, Scott DF: A device for continuous monitoring of cerebral activity in resuscitated patients. Br Med J 1969; 4:545–546.
13. Demetrescu TM: The aperiodic character of the electroencephalogram (EEG): New approach to data analysis and condensation [Abstract]. Physiologist 1975; 18:189.
14. Cucchiara RF, Sharbrough FW, Messick JM, Tinker JH: An electroencephalographic filter-processor as an indicator of cerebral ischemia during carotid endarterectomy. Anesthesiology 1979; 51:77–79.

15. Patel H: Experience with the cerebral function monitor during deliberate hypotension. Br J Anaesth 1981; 53:639–644.
16. Sechzer PH, Ospina J: Cerebral function monitor: Evaluation in anesthesia/critical care. Curr Ther Res 1977; 22:335–347.
17. Kritikou PE, Branthwaite MA: Significance of changes in cerebral electrical activity at onset of cardiopulmonary bypass. Thorax 1977; 32:534–538.
18. Schwartz MS, Colvin MP, Prior PF, et al: The cerebral function monitor. Anaesthesia 1973; 28:611–618.
19. Dubois M, Savege TM, O'Carroll TM, Frank M: General anaesthesia and changes on the cerebral function. Anaesthesia 1978; 33:157–164.
20. Frank M, Savege TM, Leigh M, et al: Comparison of the cerebral function monitor and plasma concentrations of thiopentone and alphaxalone during total IV anaesthesia with repeated bolus doses of thiopentone and althesin. Br J Anaesth 1982; 54:609–616.
21. Prior PF, Maynard DE, Brierley JB: EEG monitoring for the control of anaesthesia produced by the infusion of althesin in primates. Br J Anaesth 1978; 50:993–1000.
22. Sebel PS, Maynard DE, Major E, Frank M: The cerebral function analysing monitor (CFAM). Br J Anaesth 1983; 55:1265–1270.
23. Gregory TK, Pettus DC: An electroencephalographic processing algorithm specifically intended for analysis of cerebral electrical activity. J Clin Monit 1986; 2:190–197.
24. Spackman TN, Faust RJ, Cucchiara RF, et al: A comparison of the Lifescan® EEG monitor with EEG and cerebral blood flow for detection of cerebral ischemia [Abstract]. Anesthesiology 1985; 63:A187.
25. Smith NT, Demetrescu M: The EEG during high-dose fentanyl anesthesia [Abstract]. Anesthesiology 1980; 53:S7.
26. Demetrescu M, Kavan E, Smith NT: Monitoring the brain condition by advanced EEG [Abstract]. Anesthesiology 1981; 53:A130.
27. Myers RR, Stockard JJ, Fleming NI, et al: The use of on-line telephonic computer analysis of the EEG in anaesthesia. Br J Anaesth 1973; 45:664–670.
28. Bickford RG, Fleming NI, Billinger TW: Compression of EEG data by isometric power spectral plots [Abstract]. Electroencephalogr Clin Neurophysiol 1971; 31:632.
29. Fleming RA, Smith NT: Density modulation. A technique for the display of three-variable data in patient monitoring. Anesthesiology 1979; 50:543–546.
30. Brazier MAB, Walter DO (eds): Handbook of Electroencephalography and Clinical Neurophysiology, Vol 5-A. Amsterdam: Elsevier, 1974; 33–43.
31. Levy WJ: Intraoperative EEG patterns: Implications for EEG monitoring. Anesthesiology 1984; 60:430–434.
32. Levy WJ: Effect of epoch length on power spectrum analysis of the EEG. Anesthesiology 1987; 66:489–495.
33. Walter DO: On units and dimensions for reporting spectral intensities. Electroencephalogr Clin Neurophysiol 1968; 24:486–487.
34. Matteo RS, Orenstein E, Schwartz AE, et al: Effects of low-dose sufentanil on the EEG: Elderly vs young [Abstract]. Anesthesiology 1986; 65:A553.
35. Rampil IJ, Sasse FJ, Smith NT, et al: Spectral edge frequency—A new correlate of anesthetic depth [Abstract]. Anesthesiology 1980; 53:S12.
36. Rampil IJ, Holzer JA, Quest DO, et al: Prognostic value of computerized EEG analysis during carotid endarterectomy. Anesth Analg 1983; 62:186–192.
37. Scott JC, Ponganis KV, Stanski DR: EEG quantitation of narcotic effect. The comparative pharmacodynamics of fentanyl and alfentanil. Anesthesiology 1985; 62:234–241.
38. Hudson RJ, Stanski DR, Meathe E, Saidman LJ: Does acute tolerance to thiopental exist? [Abstract] Anesthesiology 1982; 57:A501.
39. Burhrer M, Maitre PO, Ebling WF, Stanski DR: Pharmacological quantitation of midazolam's CNS drug effect in hypnotic doses [Abstract]. Anesthesiology 1987; 67:A658.
40. Benignus VA: Estimation of the coherence spectrum and its confidence interval using the fast Fourier transform. IEEE Trans Audio Electroacoustics 1969; 2:145–150.
41. Shaw JC: An introduction to the coherence function and its use in EEG signal analysis. J Med Eng Technol 1981; 6:279–288.
42. Da Silva FHL, van Lierop THMT, Schrijer CF, van Leeuwen WS: Organization of thalamic and cortical alpha rhythms: Spectra and coherences. Electroencephalogr Clin Neurophysiol 1973; 35:627–639.
43. van Leeuwen WS, Wieneke G, Spoelstra P, Versteeg H: Lack of bilateral coherence of mu rhythm. Electroencephalogr Clin Neurophysiol 1978; 44:140–146.
44. Levy WJ, Canals-Curtis E: Coherence analysis of the EEG during isoflurane anesthesia. [Abstract] Anesthesiology 1991; 75:A178.
45. Nikias CL, Raghuveer MR: Bispectrum estimation: A digital signal processing framework. Proc IEEE 1987; 75:869–891.
46. Mendel JM: Tutorial on higher-order statistics (spectra) in signal processing and system theory: Theoretical results and some applications. Proc IEEE 1991; 79:278–305.
47. Vernon J, Bowles S, Sebel PS, Chamoun N: EEG bispectrum predicts movement at incision during isoflurane or propofol anesthesia. [Abstract] Anesthesiology 1992; 77:A502.
48. Mannheimer WH, Keats AS, Chamberlin JA: Safety in hypotensive anesthesia. Surgery 1963; 54:883–890.
49. Coons RE, Keats AS, Cooley DA: Significance of electroencephalographic changes occurring during cardiopulmonary bypass. Anesthesiology 1959; 20:804–810.
50. Sharbrough FW, Messick JM Jr, Sundt TM: Correlation of continuous electroencephalograms with cerebral blood flow measurements during carotid endarterectomy. Stroke 1973; 4:674–683.
51. Sundt TM Jr: The ischemic tolerance of neural tissue and the need for monitoring and selective shunting during carotid endarterectomy. Stroke 1983; 14:93–98.
52. Chiappa KH, Burke SR, Young RR: Results of encephalographic monitoring during 367 carotid endarterectomies: Use of a dedicated minicomputer. Stroke 1979; 10:381–388.
53. Cohen PJ, Alexander SC, Smith TC, et al: Effects of hypoxia and normocarbia on cerebral blood flow and metabolism in conscious man. J Appl Physiol 1967; 23:183–189.
54. Finnerty FA Jr, Witkin L, Fazekas JF: Cerebral hemodynamics during cerebral ischemia induced by acute hypotension. J Clin Invest 1954; 33:1227–1232.
55. Slogoff S, Girgis KZ, Keats AS: Etiologic factors in neuropsychiatric complications associated with cardiopulmonary bypass. Anesth Analg 1982; 61:903–911.
56. Nussmeier NA, McDermott JP: Macroembolization. Prevention and outcome modification. *In* Hilberman M (ed): Brain Injury and Protection During Heart Surgery. Boston: Martinus Nijhoff, 1988; 85–106.
57. Levy WJ, Parcella PA: Electroencephalographic evidence of cerebral ischemia during acute extracorporeal hypoperfusion. J Cardiothorac Anesth 1987; 4:300–304.
58. Ferguson GG: Intra-operative monitoring and internal shunts: Are they necessary in carotid endarterectomy? Stroke 1983; 13:287–289.
59. Levy WJ: Power spectrum correlates of changes in consciousness during anesthetic induction with enflurane. Anesthesiology 1986; 64:688–693.
60. Yamamura T, Fukuda M, Takeya H, et al: Fast oscillatory EEG activity induced by analgesic concentrations of nitrous oxide in man. Anesth Analg 1981; 60:283–288.
61. Bimar J, Bellville J: Arousal reactions during anesthesias in man. Anesthesiology 1977; 47:449–454.
62. Martin JT, Faulconer A, Bickford RG: Electroencephalography in anesthesiology. Anesthesiology 1959; 20:359–376.
63. Clark DL, Rosner BS: Neurophysiologic effects of general anesthetics. Anesthesiology 1973; 38:564–582.
64. Rampil IJ, Matteo RS: Changes in EEG spectral edge frequency correlate with the hemodynamic response to laryngoscopy and intubation. Anesthesiology 1987; 67:139–142.
65. Sebel PS, Bovill JG, Wauquier A, Rog P: Effects of high-dose fentanyl anesthesia on the electroencephalogram. Anesthesiology 1981; 55:203–211.
66. Brandt L, Pokar H: EEG power spectrum analysis during isoflurane anesthesia in man [Abstract]. Anesthesiology 1984; 61:A340.
67. Myers RR, Stockard JJ: Neurologic and electroencephalographic correlates in glutethimide intoxication. Clin Pharmacol Ther 1975; 17:212–220.
68. Karnaze DS, Marshall LF, Bickford RG: EEG monitoring of clinical coma: The compressed spectral array. Neurology 1982; 32:289–292.

CHAPTER 16

Evoked Potentials

VEDRAN DELETIS, M.D., Ph.D.

Surgeons and anesthesiologists are becoming increasingly aware of the advantages of monitoring the functional integrity of the sensory and motor pathways during many surgical procedures that put these pathways at risk. With the wider application of standard evoked potential (EP) techniques and the advent of new EP methods, many more patients are benefiting from intraoperative monitoring. However, the use of EPs in the diagnosis of neurologic diseases will not be discussed here; for this, the interested reader is referred to Chiappa.[1]

PRINCIPLES OF MEASUREMENT

SOURCE OF EVOKED POTENTIALS

Stimulation of the nervous system initiates the transmission of neural signals along a specific pathway. These signals may be recorded as EPs from synaptic or axonal activity at various points along the pathway. The source of EPs recorded from synaptic activity is the summed activity of presynaptic and postsynaptic potentials; the source of the EPs recorded from axonal activity (traveling wave) is the summed activity produced from current propagated along the axons.

The EP is represented as a waveform of voltage over time and is described in terms of amplitude, latency, and morphology (Fig. 16–1). Amplitude is the peak-to-peak (or baseline-to-peak) voltage difference. Latency may be described as absolute or relative. Absolute latency is measured from the stimulus onset to the response onset (onset latency) or to the peak of the response (peak latency). Relative, or interpeak, latency is the interval between two peaks of interest. Morphology is the overall shape of the waveform and can be described as a series of positive and negative peaks and waves that are monophasic, biphasic, polyphasic, synchronized, or desynchronized.

RECORDING TECHNIQUES

Because resistive media impede the passage of electrical current between a neural generator and the skin, EPs should be recorded from a site as close as possible to the source of the potential. Amplification and signal averaging allow extraction of the signal from the background environmental and patient noise. Common sources of environmental noise include electrical current from the operating table, warming blanket, intravenous fluid warmers, fluorescent lights, and electrosurgical instruments. Other sources are crossed cables, improperly attached recording electrodes, poor grounding, and movement of the wires that link electrodes and preamplifier. Patient noise consists of spontaneous electrical activity of the brain as measured by the electroencephalogram (EEG), heart as measured by the electrocardiogram (ECG), and muscle as measured by the electromyogram (EMG), all of which produce activity that is many times larger than that produced by EPs.

Proper patient set-up techniques will limit the absolute amount of noise recorded. Proper preparation of electrode sites and application of the electrodes will reduce the impedance at the electrode-tissue interface. Establishing equal impedances at the electrode sites allows better noise subtraction because of common mode rejection (discussed later).

Because it is usually impossible to eliminate noise completely, techniques such as filtering, common mode rejection, and signal averaging are employed to decrease the amplitude of the noise and to increase the signal-to-noise ratio (SNR), the ratio of the amplitude of the signal of interest to the amplitude of the background noise.[2]

Filtering

To remove background noise, the frequency ranges for the noise and signal are determined, and electrical activity in the frequency range of the noise that does not overlap with the range of the signal is filtered out. EEG is composed of frequencies of 0.5–30 Hz and is considered electrical noise for EP recording. Activity in this range should be filtered out when the EP signal of interest does not include energy in this frequency range.

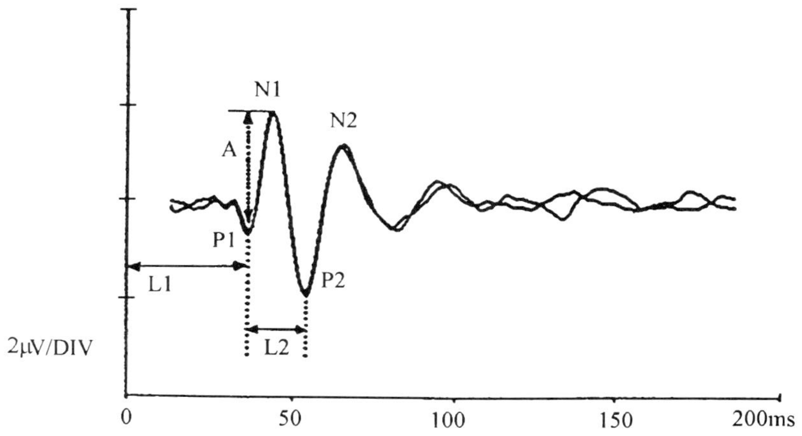

Figure 16–1. A cortical somatosensory evoked potential showing peak *P1* (first positive peak), *N1* (first negative peak), *P2* (second positive peak), and *N2* (second negative peak). Note that upward deflections are negative. *A* indicates the peak-to-peak (P1 to N1) amplitude. *L1* indicates the (absolute) latency between the onset of the stimulus and the P1. *L2* is the interpeak latency between P1 and P2.

Common Mode Rejection

Common mode rejection suppresses noise common to two recording electrodes. An active electrode is placed over the generator of interest, and a reference electrode is placed at a distance from the generator, such that it records the same noise as the active electrode but does not record the signal. A differential amplifier calculates the voltage difference between the two electrodes and extracts the signal by subtracting the noise (recorded from the reference electrode) from the signal-plus-noise (recorded from the active electrode).

Signal Averaging

Although common mode rejection and filtering greatly improve signal quality, the signal can rarely be seen in just one response (with the exception of some responses recorded directly from neural tissue). The technique of signal averaging allows one to extract a signal by averaging repeated evoked responses. The responses are averaged by summing the amplitudes at each point on the waveform and dividing each sum by the total number of recordings. Because the EP is time-locked to the stimulus, the signal will appear as a peak or wave at a fixed latency. In contrast, the background activity is not time-locked to the stimulus. Summing the EP's amplitude at each point in the waveform will therefore result in a nearly flat line.

DIRECT VERSUS NEAR-FIELD AND FAR-FIELD RECORDING

Near-field recordings are EPs recorded from locations close to the neural generator, where the current density gradients are steep and small changes in distance from the generator produce large changes in the amplitude of the response. Direct recordings are near-field recordings obtained from electrodes placed in the surgical field directly on, or very close to, the generator. Far-field recordings are those obtained from sites far from the neural generator, where the amplitude of the response is relatively constant despite changes in electrode position.[3]

Because of their proximity to the neural generator, direct recordings are of much larger amplitude than near-field or far-field recordings. They are usually obtained with higher rates of stimulation and fewer averages than is possible with the other techniques, allowing for a much shorter data acquisition time. Direct recordings are very reliable and should be monitored whenever possible in addition to near- and far-field recordings, which should be monitored before and after placement of the direct recording electrode.

PRINCIPLES OF INTRAOPERATIVE MONITORING

Intraoperative monitoring (IOM) is based on the principle that EPs reflect the moment-to-moment functional integrity of the monitored neural pathways, i.e., the ability of the pathway to conduct signals. Modalities that are at risk for injury are monitored, and significant changes in the EP responses are relayed to the surgeon. A "control" pathway (or a segment of the pathway of interest) that is not at risk is also monitored in order to assess the effects of changes due to nonsurgical factors (e.g., anesthetic regimen, temperature, blood pressure). Because many nonsurgical factors have their greatest effect on synaptic activity, the modality chosen as a control should match the at-risk modality in terms of number of synapses.

It should be noted that intraoperative EPs do not necessarily reflect the ability of the nervous system to perform complex functions, such as sensory or sensorimotor integration. Partial damage to a nerve pathway may result in destruction of some fibers or desynchronization of fibers with loss of the EP, whereas the ability to perform complex functions is preserved. Thus, preservation of EPs indicates fully intact or only slightly damaged neural function. However, loss of EPs does not necessarily indicate complete loss of function.

Accurate predictions of neural function based on EP parameters depend on the quality of the preoperative and postinduction baselines. Preoperative baseline examination, performed before the patient arrives in the operating room, establishes whether a response is present and, if so, how reliable it is. This knowledge greatly simplifies the task of establishing the postinduction (opening) EP response in the operating room. The preoperative responses may be compared to postoperative responses in order to document any effects of the surgery. Because anesthetics are known to affect EPs, only the preoperative response can be appropriately compared to the postoperative response. Postinduction responses provide a measure of EP parameters in the patient under general anesthesia. They are compared to the responses during surgical closure to determine the effects of the surgical procedure. Changes in EP parameters may occur after closing and are assessed postoperatively.

Occasionally, a patient's pathology causes an absent response or one that is too weak or desynchronized to record reliably. Anesthetics or technical difficulties may also prevent reliable recordings. These cases may be considered *unmonitorable.* The decision as to whether a case is monitorable should be based on the quality of the preoperative and postinduction responses. Poor-quality preoperative and postinduction responses are the basis for most of the reported false correlations in EP monitoring. Poor-quality signals are subject to many fluctuations during the procedure that may not correlate well with neural integrity and outcome. If each of these fluctuations is communicated to the surgeon as a cause for alarm, the information is useless and the procedure may be unnecessarily prolonged. It is better to provide no information than to misinform.[4]

SPECIFIC VERSUS NONSPECIFIC CHANGES

Intraoperative changes in EP parameters are due to surgically induced effects (specific changes) or nonsurgically induced effects (nonspecific changes). Only the specific changes are communicated to the surgeon.

Specific Changes

Specific changes are changes due to the surgeon's mechanical manipulations, such as cutting, coagulating, pulling, applying pressure on neural tissue, or clamping blood vessels supplying critical tissue. EPs show changes when cerebral blood flow decreases to 18 ml/100 gm/minute and completely disappear at 15 ml/100 gm/minute, signaling cerebral ischemia.[5] Specific changes also include changes that were indirectly caused by the procedure, such as thromboses and emboli. Changes due to surgical manipulations may manifest in the same ways as nonspecific changes (changes in amplitude, latency, and morphology) and are not uniquely described. A surgically induced change may be identified as a change occurring during or following a critical surgical manipulation that is not attributable to a nonspecific factor.

Indirect, surgically induced changes (e.g., thromboses of spinal arteries, stroke) may not occur at critical points in procedures and manifest as unexpected deleterious changes in the EP parameters that should be reported to the surgeon. Because of their timing, these changes are particularly difficult to diagnose and may be attributed to surgical manipulation only after all nonspecific factors have been eliminated.

Nonspecific Changes

Nonspecific changes may be due to anesthesia, temperature, blood pressure, oxygen and carbon dioxide tension, other changes in patient state, or noise and technical problems. Of these, general anesthesia is the most common cause of nonspecific changes in EP parameters.

Anesthesia

General anesthesia has a deleterious effect on neural transmission, and this effect is greater on synaptic activity than on nonsynaptic activity. Anesthetics influence the membranes of axons, although this influence is considered to be only slight.[6] For this reason, responses recorded from polysynaptic pathways (e.g., cortical recordings) will be affected by anesthesia to a greater extent than responses recorded from oligosynaptic pathways (e.g., recordings from the spinal cord).[7]

The effect of anesthesia on EPs is greater in neurologically impaired patients than in patients without such deficits. Almost all studies of the effects of anesthesia were performed on neurologically intact patients or healthy subjects, and the conclusions of these studies are not always valid for neurologically impaired patients.[7–9] Also, anesthetic agents have more complex effects on motor evoked potentials (MEPs) than on other EP modalities.

Inhaled Anesthetics

Volatile anesthetics such as isoflurane, halothane, enflurane, and nitrous oxide have detrimental effects on most EPs, which depend on the potency and concentration of the anesthetic as well as on concurrent administration of other drugs (additive effects). According to Peterson et al, halogenated anesthetics prolong the central sensory conduction time, with enflurane producing the greatest influence and halothane showing the weakest influence of this set of agents.[10]

The effect may vary from no effect to complete obliteration of the EP. When isoflurane is needed, concentrations of less than 0.4 minimum alveolar concentration (MAC) can usually be tolerated. The combination of N_2O and a maintenance dose of a halogenated anesthetic has an additive effect that severely depresses cortical EPs by decreasing amplitude and prolonging latency. If halogenated anesthetics cannot be avoided, N_2O should be discontinued, and the halogenated anesthetic should be increased. This regimen is not ideal and should be avoided if at all possible. However, it is preferable to the combination of the two agents.[10]

Benzodiazepines, Narcotics, and Other Intravenous Drugs

Diazepam and other benzodiazepines can increase the amount of fast EEG activity and decrease amplitude and slightly prolong latency of cortical EPs.[11] High doses of narcotics (fentanyl, sufentanil) or droperidol decrease the amplitude of the cortical EPs.[8] Because the effects of these drugs are most dramatic following bolus injections, they should be administered as a constant infusion.

Neuromuscular Blocking Drugs

Neuromuscular blocking drugs do not directly influence sensory EPs or motor EPs (MEPs) recorded epidurally or subdurally or over peripheral nerves. In some instances, neuromuscular blockade may improve the quality of EPs by eliminating muscle artifacts and increasing SNR. Neuromuscular blocking drugs can be administered to restless comatose patients to eliminate muscle artifacts and facilitate recordings of somatosensory evoked potentials (SSEPs), brainstem auditory evoked potentials (BAEPs), and EEG. Of course, neuromuscular blockers are incompatible with recordings from muscle, such as compound muscle action potentials after stimulation of the cranial nerves, the peripheral nerves, the motor roots, the bulbocavernosus reflex, and MEPs. If neuromuscular blocking drugs must be administered for airway management or other reasons, a depolarizing blocker or an intermediate-acting nondepolarizing drug should be administered, if not contraindicated.

Optimal Anesthetic Regimen

The optimal anesthetic technique for monitoring most modalities in the operating room is a combination of N_2O, O_2, and narcotics or propofol, alone or in combination with N_2O or fentanyl. In general, a regimen of total intravenous anesthesia is better than one with inhalation anesthetics. With both inhalation and intravenous anesthetics, a steady state is preferable to varying concentrations or bolus injections. Neuromuscular blocking drugs must be avoided when recording from muscle (or observing muscle contraction during cortical mapping).

Other Nonspecific Factors

Nonspecific factors such as temperature and blood pressure affect EP parameters. Core temperature and temperature of the extremities and surgical field (affected by the irrigation fluid) may affect EP amplitude and latency.[12] Very low blood pressure and hypoxia interfere with EP parameters.[13] Nonspecific changes may also be the result of technical problems, and all possible sources should be carefully examined. Changes in electrode impedance or the characteristics of environmental and patient noise may result in dramatic changes in EP parameters.

CRITERIA FOR EVALUATING SPECIFIC CHANGES IN EPs

Changes in EP parameters must first be analyzed to determine whether they are due to surgically induced or to nonspecific effects. Changes that are confidently attributed to surgically induced effects are then examined to determine whether the changes indicate damage to neural tissue—i.e., significant changes—that should be reported to the surgeon. This decision is critical; significant changes should be reported immediately so that the surgeon may alter the procedure to reverse the damage or avoid further damage, if possible. Significant EP changes may consist of changes in amplitude, latency, and/or morphology compared with control nonspecific changes and should be present for a least two consecutive traces. Criteria for determining which surgically induced changes are significant are outlined below. These criteria are based on empirical findings.[14] Although the majority of neurophysiologists performing IOM accept these criteria, they are still debated.

A decrease in *amplitude* of greater than 50% in critical peaks indicates a significant change in the integrity of a neural pathway.

An increase in *latency* of greater than 10% in the critical peak indicates a significant slowing in signal transmission (e.g., a critical peak occurring at 30 msec at baseline shifting to 33 msec).

The *morphology* of an averaged EP depends on the morphology of the individual waves. If the component waves vary greatly in amplitude and latency, the morphology of the resulting averaged responses will vary from average to average. Change in morphology may indicate strain on the underlying tissue and serves as a warning signal, rather than a definitive sign, of neural damage. Some EP systems have software programs that measure trends in amplitudes or latency of a selected wave and present the parameters as a trajectory. This display is very useful in detecting slow, usually nonspecific changes in the EPs.

METHODOLOGIES

SOMATOSENSORY PATHWAYS: ANATOMIC OUTLINE

Figure 16–2 illustrates the part of the somatosensory pathway carrying touch, pressure, vibration, and proprioception information from the trunk and lower extremities. The axons of the peripheral neurons (1) enter the spinal cord through the dorsal roots, where some branch, sending collateral axons to the anterior horn, and some continue rostrally in the dorsal column of the spinal cord. The axons of sensory neurons innervating the lower part of the body ascend in the spinal cord as the fasciculus gracilis (2), whereas the axons of sensory neurons coming from the upper part of the body ascend in the fasciculus cuneatus (3), just lateral to the fasciculus gracilis.

The fasciculi gracilis and cuneatus terminate just above the junction of the spinal cord and the medulla in the nucleus gracilis and the nucleus cuneatus (4), respectively. Second-order neurons from these nuclei immediately decussate (5) to the opposite side of the brainstem, where they regroup to form the medial lemniscus (6).

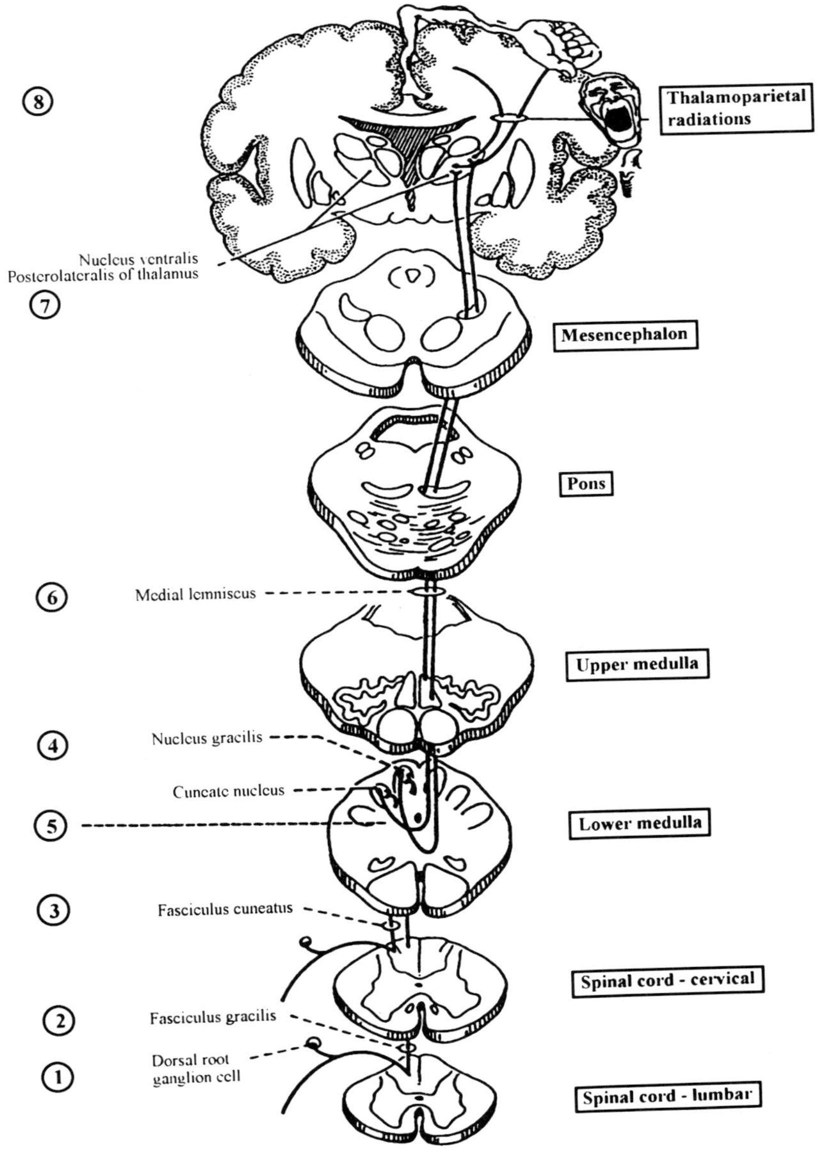

Figure 16–2. The somatosensory pathway for touch, proprioception, pressure, and vibratory stimuli. See text for details. (Modified from DeJong RN: The Neurological Examination, 5th Ed. Philadelphia: JB Lippincott, 1992.)

The neurons in the medial lemniscus continue rostrally through the midbrain and synapse in the ventral posterolateral nucleus (VPL) of the thalamus (7). Third-order neurons from the VPL leave the thalamus and travel through the posterior limb of the internal capsule to synapse in the postcentral gyrus of the parietal lobe, the primary somatosensory cortex (8). Somatotopic organization is represented according to the homunculus shown in the cortex. Note that the legs are represented deep in the superior sagittal fissure, whereas each arm is represented more laterally on the postcentral gyrus. Knowledge of this somatotopic cortical organization is critical for the placement of electrodes for recording somatosensory EPs.

Cortical Somatosensory Evoked Potentials

Somatosensory evoked potentials (SSEPs) are the electrical response of the brain or spinal cord to somatosensory stimulation and may be used to detect lesions of, or damage to, the somatosensory pathway or somatosensory cortex. SSEPs are usually elicited by transcutaneous electrical stimulation of the median nerves at the wrist (for upper extremities) and tibial nerves at the ankle or popliteal fossa (for lower extremities). The somatosensory system may be activated by stimulating peripheral nerves or the cutaneous nerves or skin (dermatomal SSEPs), or they may be activated by directly stimulating the dorsal columns of the spinal cord through an epidural electrode placed over the spinal cord.[15, 16] SSEPs may also be elicited by mechanical or laser stimulation.

SSEPs may be recorded from the cortex (cortical SSEPs-CSEP) with electrodes placed on the scalp according to the somatotopic representation of the body in the primary somatosensory cortex using the International 10–20 system of electrode placement (Fig. 16–3). To record the response to

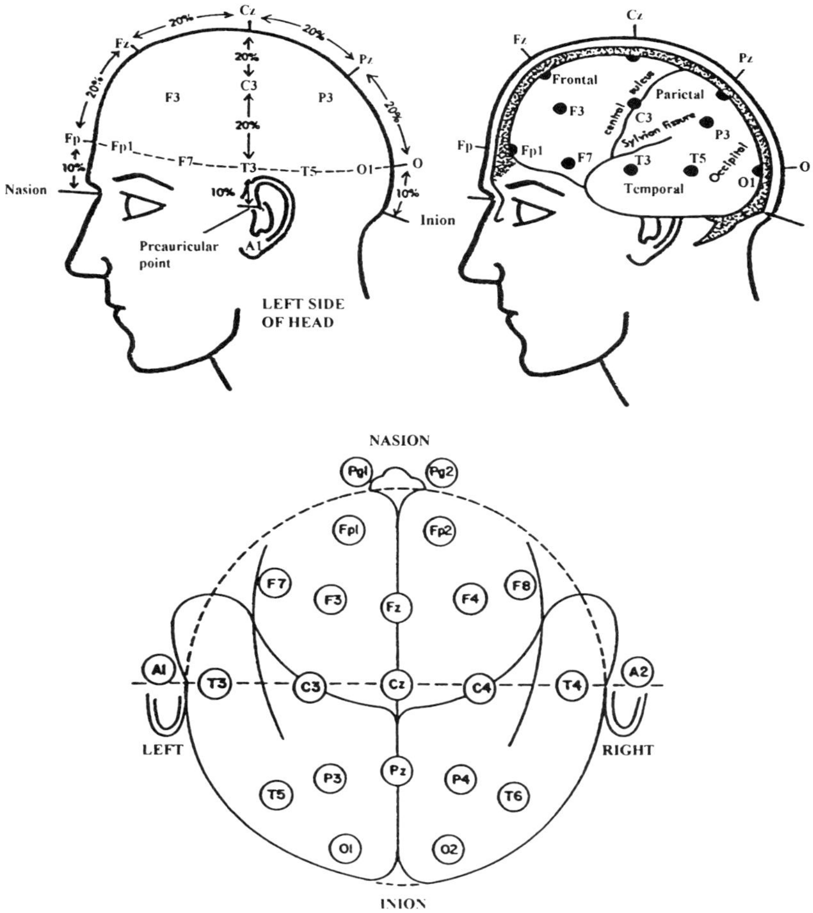

Figure 16–3. The International 10–20 system of scalp electrode positions. Electrodes are placed either 10% or 20% of the distance between landmarks on the skull. See text for details. (From Harner P, Sannit T: A Review of the International Ten-Twenty System of Electrode Placement. Grass Instruments Company, 1974; and Aminoff MJ: Electrodiagnosis in Clinical Neurology, 3rd Ed. New York: Churchill Livingstone, 1992.)

stimulation of the lower extremities, the active electrode is placed at CZ′ (2 cm posterior to CZ), and the reference electrode is placed at FPZ or FZ. For the response to stimulation of the upper extremities, the active electrode is placed at C3′ (2 cm posterior to C3) for right arm stimulation) or at C4′ (2 cm posterior to C4) for left arm stimulation) with the same reference. SSEPs may also be recorded from the brainstem or sensory cortex by placing specially designed electrodes on surgically exposed structures. SSEPs may also be recorded percutaneously from other points along the somatosensory pathway, such as Erb's point and the C2, C5, or C7 spinous processes for upper extremities and the S1, L1 (Th12), or C2 spinous processes for the lower extremities (Fig. 16–4). These recordings serve as a control for nonspecific factors and allow calculation of central conduction time, the time needed for a signal to travel from the segmental level to the cortex.

Somatosensory Evoked Potentials Recorded from the Spinal Epidural/Subdural Space

Somatosensory evoked potentials are elicited by stimulation of the peripheral nerves and are recorded from electrodes inserted into the epidural or subdural space of the spinal cord. The source of the SSEP may be axonal or synaptic. If the recording electrode is placed over the spinal cord rostral to the root entry zone (and dorsal horn synapse), the SSEP will reflect axonal activity traveling up the spinal cord. If the recording electrode is placed over the spinal cord segment where the sensory roots of the stimulated peripheral nerve synapse in the cord, the SSEP will reflect that synaptic activity.

For intraoperative monitoring, an epidural catheter-electrode is placed rostral to the spinal cord lesion to record the signal passing through the affected area of the spinal cord. Another catheter-electrode may be placed caudal to the lesion to serve as a control for nonspecific factors (Fig. 16–5). Because the SSEP from upper extremity stimulation has not yet been established as a monitoring technique, only SSEPs from lower extremity stimulation are monitored in the operating room.

The spinal SSEP has several advantages over the CSEP; it is less susceptible to nonsurgical effects and can be recorded with fast stimulation rates. This results in a shorter acquisition time and faster feedback to the surgeon. However, even when SSEPs are monitored, CSEPs should also be recorded as a ''back-up'' modality, and for monitoring before and after placement of the epidural electrode.

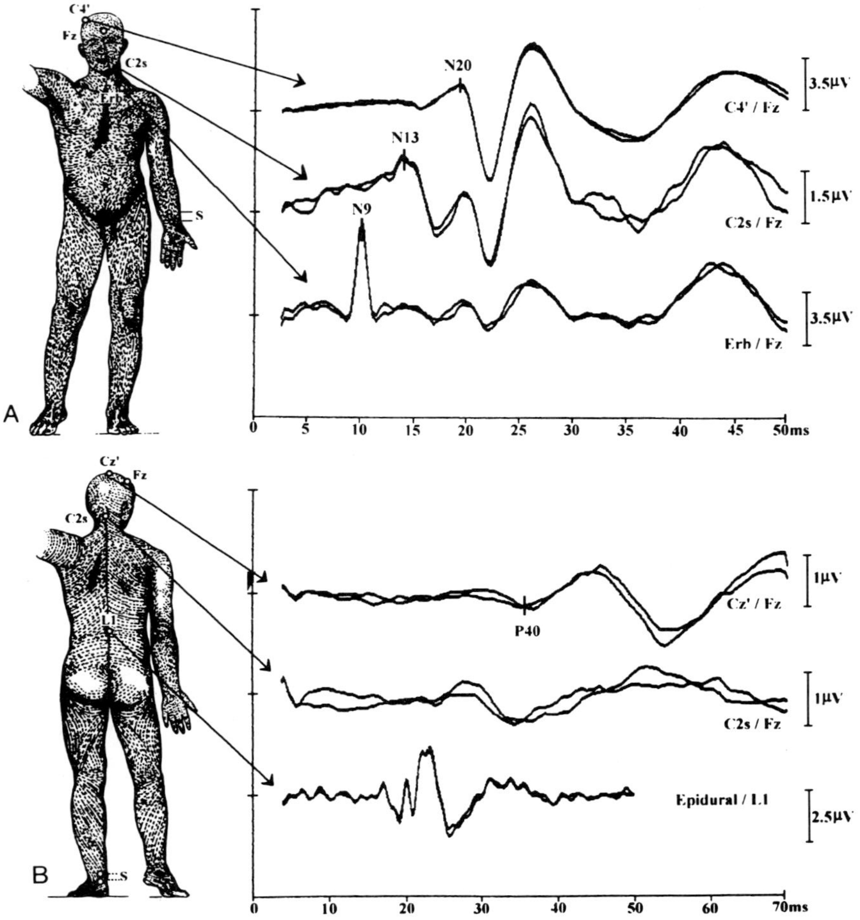

Figure 16–4. *A,* Somatosensory EPs following stimulation to the left median nerve (S), recorded transcutaneously from points along the somatosensory pathway; from Erbs point (Erb/Fz); over the C2 spinous process (C2s/Fz); and over the somatosensory cortex (C4′/Fz). The difference between N13 and N20 represents the central somatosensory conduction time. *B,* Somatosensory EPs following stimulation to the left tibial nerve (S), recorded from points along the somatosensory pathway; from the L1 epidural space (Epidural/L1); from the skin overlying the C2 spinous process (C2s/Fz); and from the scalp overlying the somatosensory cortex (CZ′/Fz).

CORTICOSPINAL TRACT: ANATOMIC OUTLINE

The corticospinal tract (CST) begins with the primary motor area of the cerebral cortex (Fig. 16–6, part 1). The motor cortex is topographically organized in the precentral gyrus, with the legs represented deep within the superior sagittal fissure and the arms represented laterally. This representation parallels that of the primary somatosensory cortex, which lies just across the central sulcus in the parietal lobe. The motor cortex contains large pyramidal cells whose axons descend ipsilaterally in the corticospinal tract through the posterior limb of the internal capsule (2) and the medial aspect of the basis pedunculi. In the ventral pons, they pass through the pontine nuclei and regroup in the medulla to form the ventrally located medullary pyramids. In the caudal medulla, near the junction of the spinal cord, 85–90% of these axons cross to the opposite side in the pyramidal decussation (3) and descend in the spinal cord as the lateral CST tract (4). The lateral CST tract controls the distal extremity muscles, and the anterior CST tract controls the proximal extremity muscles.[17]

Large diameter axons from the lateral CST tract synapse with neurons whose cell bodies lie in the anterior horn (5) of the spinal cord. The axons of these lower motor neurons, referred to as the final common pathway, then exit the spinal cord via the ventral roots and continue as peripheral nerves innervating the skeletal musculature. In its simplest configuration, the motor system can be considered a two-neuron system consisting of upper motor neurons derived from pyramidal cells and lower motor neurons originating in the anterior horn.

Motor Evoked Potentials

MEPs are the response to stimulation of the motor cortex or pyramidal tract and are recorded from different parts of the motor pathway. MEPs may be used to detect lesions or damage to the motor cortex or pyramidal tract and may be recorded from the epidural or subdural space of the spinal cord, muscle, or peripheral nerves. Ideally, MEPs should be recorded from muscle after cortical stimulation in order to assess the functional integrity of the entire pathway. However, the use of general anesthetics restricts recording from muscle and peripheral nerves. Thus, the only practical method of monitoring MEPs in the operating room is recording from the spinal epidural space.

Methods of Eliciting MEPs

MEPs may be elicited by transcranial electrical stimulation of the motor cortex, direct electrical stimulation of the

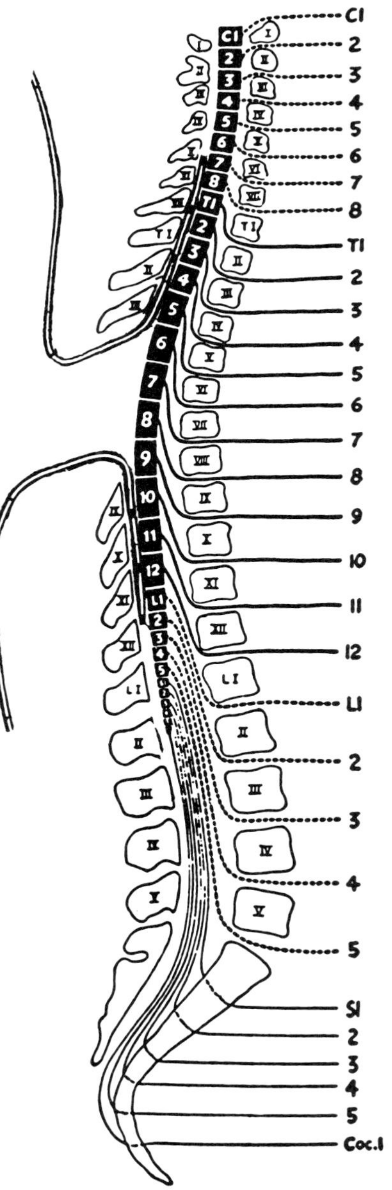

Figure 16–5. Schematic drawing of the placement of the rostral (control) and caudal catheter-electrodes in the spinal epidural space after a laminectomy. (From Deletis V: Intraoperative monitoring of the functional integrity of the motor pathways. *In* Devinski O, Beric A, Dogali M [eds]: Electrical and Magnetic Stimulation of the Brain and Spinal Cord. New York: Raven Press, 1993.)

exposed motor cortex, transcranial magnetic stimulation of the motor cortex, and stimulation of the spinal cord. Of these, transcranial and direct electrical stimulation of the motor cortex are the most practical methods of eliciting MEPs in the operating room. A more comprehensive review of methods of MEP monitoring may be found in Deletis.[12]

Transcranial Electrical Stimulation of the Motor Cortex

The introduction of a noninvasive technique of transcranial electrical stimulation of the motor cortex and spinal cord by Merton et al opened new possibilities for the direct evaluation of the functional integrity of the CST.[18] This technique uses an electrical stimulator with a low-output impedance to generate a *single* high-voltage, short-duration stimulus that can pass through the high impedance presented by the skin and bone to activate the CST neurons. The stimulus is delivered in a bipolar fashion through electrodes placed on the scalp overlying the motor cortex.

Stimulation is delivered with the Digitimer D-180 (Welwyn, Garden City, England) through electrodes placed on the scalp overlying the motor cortex. This stimulator can produce a maximum intensity of 750 V, with duration of 50 or 100 μsec and a rate of up to 0.4 Hz. For intraoperative monitoring, intensities of 50–70% of stimulator output with a duration of 100 μsec and a rate of 0.4 Hz are recommended. Another commercially available stimulator, the Digitimer D-180A, is more powerful and can produce a maximal stimulus intensity of 1200 V. This more powerful stimulator is preferred for percutaneous stimulation over the vertebral column extraoperatively, but may also be used for transcranial electrical stimulation with intensities up to 750 V.

Common Ag/AgCl$_2$ surface cup electrodes fixed to the scalp with collodion can be used for stimulation. Corkscrew-design spiral electrodes (Nicolet N-Spiral electrodes) are preferable for percutaneous electrical stimulation in the operating room, however, because of their simple, fast, and secure attachment. The same electrodes may be used for recording the cortical SSEP.

To stimulate CST tract neurons for the arm and hand, the anode is placed at C3/C4, and the cathode is placed at CZ. To stimulate the CST neurons for lower extremities, the anode is placed at CZ, and the cathode is placed either 6 cm in front of CZ or at C3/C4. The stimulating (active) electrode is the anode (in contrast to the method of stimulating peripheral nerves). Anodal stimulation is generally considered superior to cathodal stimulation in its ability to excite the motor cortex.[19] This is probably because anodal stimulation causes hyperpolarization of the apical dendrites of the CST neurons and depolarization of the initial internodal segments of the axons.

In addition to the bipolar method, a transcranial unipolar method of electrical stimulation may be used.[20, 21] With this technique, the anode is placed over the motor area of interest, and eight electrodes are positioned circumferentially above the nasion-inion line to serve as the cathode. This method allows more focused stimulation and motor cortex stimulation with the intensities available with regular neurophysiologic electrical stimulators. However, the unipolar technique has the disadvantages of requiring the additional placement of eight electrodes with matched impedances, which is often difficult to achieve in the operating room.

Direct Stimulation of the Exposed Motor Cortex

When the motor cortex is surgically exposed, it can be stimulated through electrodes placed directly on the cortex. This method of stimulation allows one to *map* some of the

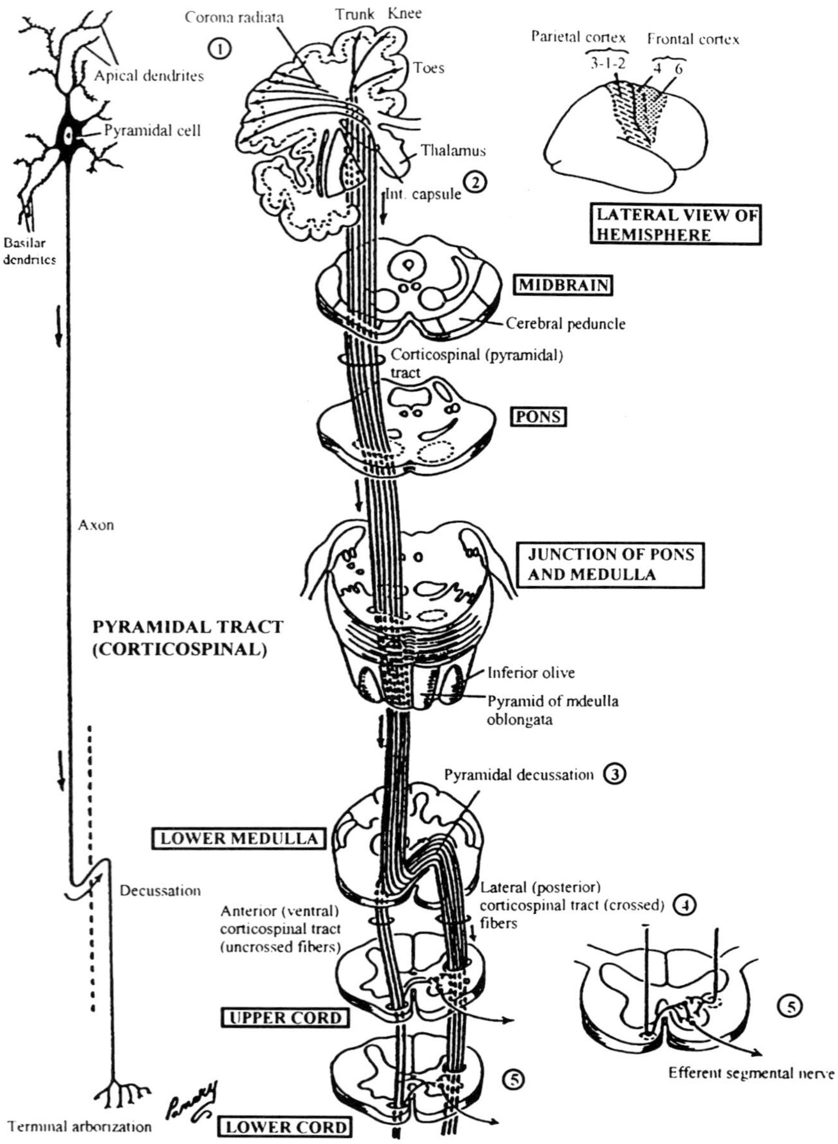

Figure 16–6. The corticospinal tract showing its path from the cerebral cortex through the brainstem to the spinal cord and efferent segmental nerves. See text for details. (From Pansky B, Allen DJ: Review of Neuroscience. New York: Macmillan, 1980.)

functional areas of the motor cortex, as well to *monitor* the functional integrity of the CST throughout the surgical procedure.

Direct Stimulation of the Motor Cortex for Mapping

Stimulation of the exposed motor cortex allows one to visually observe contractions of contralateral facial and extremity muscles and to identify areas of the motor cortex responsible for movement in different muscle groups. This information can be used by the surgeon in order to avoid damage to these areas. Stimulation of the exposed motor cortex in order to map motor areas was originally applied in awake subjects[22, 23] but is now performed in patients under general anesthesia. A few reports of intraoperative use of this technique have been published.[24–26] The mapping procedure is as follows: the exposed motor cortex is stimulated by the surgeon with a handheld monopolar ball electrode, which serves as the anode; a needle electrode inserted into the wound muscles serves as the cathode while the face, arms, and legs are observed for movement. (A bipolar method of stimulation may also be used.) A 50-Hz *train* of electrical impulses (0.2 msec duration), with intensity up to 15 mA, is delivered for 3–5 seconds while the face, arms, and legs are observed for movement. The movements appear as slow, sustained contractions of isolated muscle groups.[23] It is important to note that this technique is only successful if halogenated anesthetics and muscle relaxants are not used. An N_2O/narcotic or total intravenous anesthesia regimen should be used.

Mapping of Cortical Speech Areas

In some cases, the speech area of the motor or the parietal/temporal cortex may be at risk of damage. To identify the speech area, the surgeon may stimulate the appropriate area of the cortex while the patient speaks. The patient will undergo speech arrest when the surgeon stimulates Broca's or other areas involved in speech. This area is marked so that the surgeon may avoid damage to it during the surgical procedure. The patient must, of course, be awake (under local anesthesia) during the procedure to map speech areas. (A detailed description of the procedure to map the speech areas can be found in Luders and Lesser.[27]) Brain topography may be studied in more detail with an implanted grid of subdural electrodes on patients undergoing epilepsy surgery.[28]

Direct Stimulation of the Motor Cortex for Monitoring

It is possible to continuously monitor the CST during neurosurgical procedures in which the motor cortex is exposed. Monitoring is usually performed after the arm or the leg area has been identified with the mapping procedure described in the preceding section. For direct stimulation, a cottonoid-tipped Teflon insulated wire (anode) and a needle electrode inserted in the wound (cathode) are used. The motor cortex may also be stimulated in a bipolar fashion with a strip electrode.[29] Constant-current electrical impulses (0.2 msec duration) with an intensity of up to 15 mA are delivered with a maximal frequency of 1 Hz during the procedure. A technique of stimulation with a train of five high-frequency stimuli (300–500 Hz, 0.2–0.4 msec duration, 10–15 mA intensity) over the exposed motor cortex has been introduced.[30]

Transcranial Magnetic Stimulation of the Motor Cortex

Magnetic stimulation is an effective and painless way to stimulate the motor cortex.[31] Magnetic stimulation is delivered through a circular (or otherwise shaped) coil placed over the motor cortex. A voltage is discharged through the coil, producing a time-varying magnetic field that induces an electrical current in the brain and activates the pyramidal tract neurons. The field intensity is maximal under the edge of the coil, which is positioned over the point of the motor cortex that produces the maximal response in the target muscles (Fig. 16–7). To stimulate the leg area of the motor cortex, the coil stimulator is positioned such that the edge of the coil is over CZ; to stimulate the hand area of the motor cortex, the coil is placed such that the edge of the coil is over the C3 or C4 area.

Although transcranial magnetic stimulation is as effective as transcranial electrical stimulation in activating the CST, it is difficult to perform in the operating room. The stimulating coils are generally large and heavy. Placing and securing the coil over the vertex and keeping it in the same position throughout the surgery is difficult and often obstructive to the surgical and anesthetic teams. Almost all commercially available coils rapidly overheat and cannot sustain the repeated stimulation demanded by intraoperative monitoring. For these reasons, one cannot rely on the coil at the critical points of the surgical procedure. Magnetic stimulation is thus not well suited to intraoperative use and provides no advantages over transcranial electrical stimulation. MEPs following magnetic stimulation are recorded in preoperative and postoperative evaluations and in diagnostic studies of conscious patients, in whom electrical stimulation may cause discomfort.

A magnetic stimulator capable of delivering rapid stimulation of up to 60 Hz has been developed. Rapid-rate stimulation is painless and may be applied in awake patients in order to map areas of the cortex. This technique allows one to identify speech areas of the cortex (by identifying areas that cause speech arrest when stimulated) and hemispheric dominance, which is not possible with traditional low-frequency magnetic stimulation, and may eventually serve as a substitute for the Wada test.[32] This rapid-rate stimulator is the only magnetic stimulator that does not overheat with repeated stimulation.

Stimulation of the Spinal Cord

MEPs may also be elicited by *intraoperative* electrical stimulation of the spinal cord. Two techniques have been developed: Machida et al developed a technique in which electrical stimulation is delivered to the spinal cord by means of epidural wire electrodes,[33] and Owen et al introduced the technique of electrical stimulation of the spinal cord through electrodes inserted at the base of the spinous process.[34] These techniques are problematic because the stimulation activates the CST and the dorsal columns both orthodromically and antidromically. The anterior horn cells and peripheral motor nerves are most likely activated via the CST, and because the dorsal column is the continuation of the axons in the dorsal roots, the dorsal roots and mixed peripheral nerves are antidromically activated.

Because these techniques stimulate both the ascending and descending tracts, it is difficult to separately record sensory and motor EPs.[12] Recording from mixed peripheral nerves using Owen's method of stimulation is problematic for this reason. In principle, spinal cord stimulation could be used in conjunction with recordings over muscle, which excludes the contribution of the antidromically activated sensory part of mixed nerves. However, intraoperative recording from muscle is not reliable (see section on recording from muscle and peripheral nerves).

There are also several methods of *extraoperative* stimulation of the spinal cord or spinal roots. The descending pathways of the spinal cord may be stimulated by percutaneous application of a single electrical stimulus over the spine with a high-voltage stimulator. Although this method is not used in the operating room, it is useful in clinical examinations. In conjunction with motor cortex stimulation, it allows calculation of central motor conduction time. Central motor conduction time may be easily measured by subtracting the latency of the response from muscle following spinal stimulation from the latency of the response from muscle following cortical stimulation. The difference represents the conduction time from the motor cortex to the appropriate spinal segment.

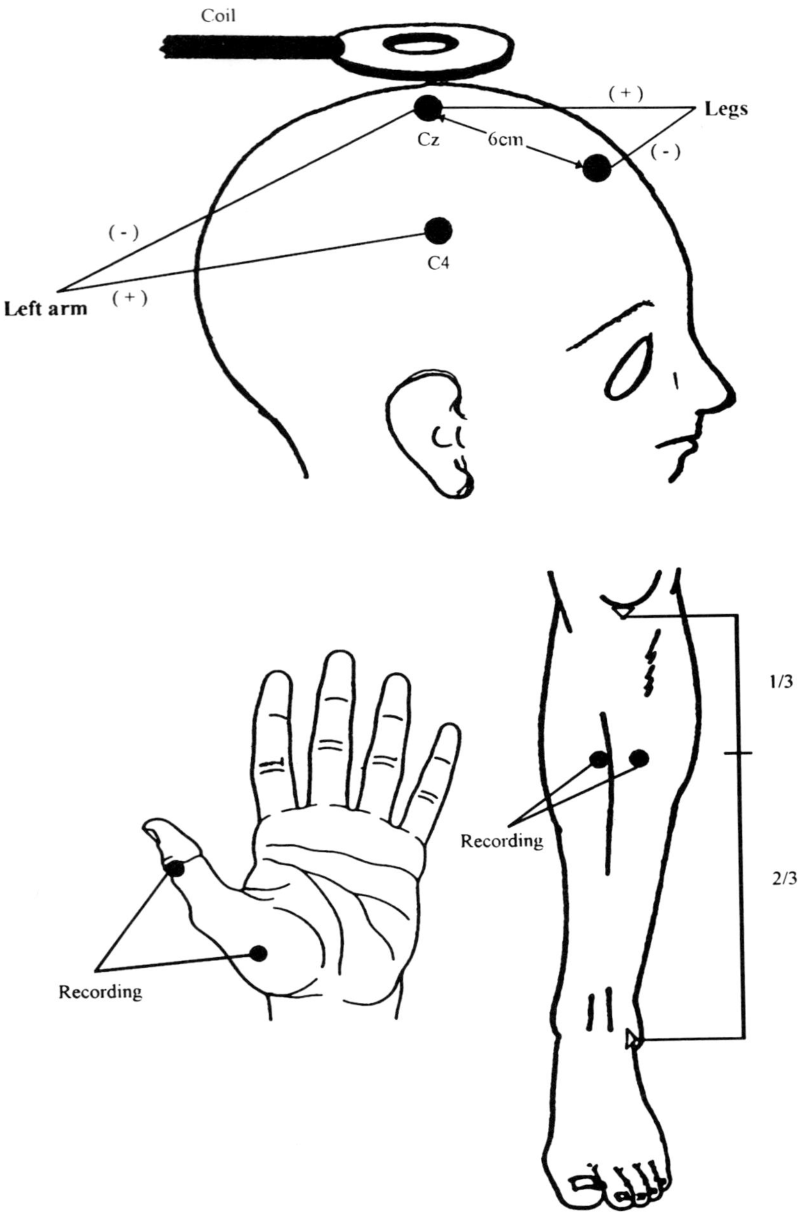

Figure 16–7. Stimulating and recording sites for magnetic and electrical transcranial stimulation of the arm (abductor pollicis brevis) and leg (anterior tibial muscle) areas of the motor cortex. See text for details.

Methods of Recording MEPs

Intraoperative MEPs may be recorded from the spinal epidural space, peripheral nerves, or muscle.

Recording from the Epidural or Subdural Space of the Spinal Cord

To record from the epidural (or subdural) space of the surgically exposed spinal cord, a catheter-electrode is inserted into the spinal epidural space (see Fig. 16–5). When the spine is not exposed, an epidural catheter-electrode is inserted percutaneously using a Tuohy needle.[29] The same electrode may be used to record SSEPs. In spine or spinal cord surgery, two catheter-electrodes are placed, one rostral to and one caudal to the lesion, if possible. Recordings from the catheter-electrode rostral to the pathology serve as a monitoring control, and recordings caudal to the lesion allow one to monitor the functional integrity of the motor pathways traversing the lesion.

Responses recorded from the epidural or subdural space of the spinal cord consist of a series of negative waves.[19, 35] The first negative wave is called a D wave because it represents the direct activation of the CST neurons. The D wave is transmitted through a pathway without intervening synapses, which makes it highly resistant to anesthetics. This wave is followed by I waves, which are generated after indirect reactivation of the same CST neurons. These waves are the result of transynaptic activation of CST neurons and thus may be affected by general anesthetics. For this reason, only D waves are monitored for surgically induced changes.[29]

Epidural recording of MEPs following transcranial electrical stimulation and direct stimulation of the exposed cortex are recommended for intraoperative monitoring, because these recordings are generally stable and of large amplitude. The signals recorded from the spinal epidural space do not traverse any synapses and are very robust even with high concentrations of anesthetics (e.g., 2% isoflurane[36]) (Fig. 16–8).

Recording from Muscle and Peripheral Nerves

In addition to recording from the epidural space of the spinal cord, MEPs can also be recorded from muscle. However, MEPs recorded from muscle are not reliable in the operating room. Neuromuscular blocking agents must be administered during most surgical procedures and greatly reduce or completely eliminate the muscular response. Halogenated anesthetics also have a detrimental effect on MEPs recorded from muscle and can completely obliterate the response in even low concentrations (0.2–0.6%).[37] The amplitude of MEPs recorded from muscle is significantly diminished by N_2O,[38] propofol (at 2 mg $\times$ kg^{-1}), midazolam (at 0.05 mg $\times$ kg^{-1}), and etomidate (at 0.3 mg $\times$ kg^{-1}).[39] However, fentanyl does not seem to have an effect on the MEP recorded from muscle.[39]

Even when anesthetics are not used, MEPs recorded from muscle are prone to a great amount of trace-to-trace variability because of changes in excitation in the anterior horn cells. Furthermore, when muscle relaxants are avoided, the muscle twitches evoked by the stimulation often interfere with the surgical procedure. For these reasons, the technique of recording MEPs from muscle is not generally employed in the operating room and will not be described. This method should be used exclusively for the neurophysiologic evaluation of comatose patients or as a method of diagnosing upper motor neuron dysfunction.

It is also possible to record responses from the peripheral motor nerves. Owen et al described a method for recording responses from the mixed peripheral nerves (neurogenic motor response) after electrical stimulation of the spinal cord.[34] However, the motor response recorded at the peripheral nerve must traverse the ventral horn synapse and is thus affected by halogenated and other anesthetics. Despite the serious limitations described here, recording from muscle and peripheral nerves is advantageous in some situations. These techniques allow one to monitor some of the roots of the cauda equina, the peripheral nerves, and the left and right descending motor tracts separately.

Identification of the Central Sulcus by Phase Reversal of Median Nerve CSEPs

It is difficult to identify the primary motor cortex in a surgically exposed brain by anatomy alone. Neurophysiologic mapping of the sensory and motor cortices is achieved by recording median nerve CSEPs directly from the exposed cortex. This allows the surgeon to identify the central sulcus, the primary somatosensory cortex, and consequently the primary motor cortex. This technique does not involve MEPs, but is included here because it indirectly identifies the motor cortex for subsequent CST monitoring.

Identification of the central sulcus is based on the interpretation of the pattern of responses recorded from a multielectrode array overlying the primary sensorimotor cortex after electrical stimulation of the contralateral median nerve. The response recorded from the hand area of exposed somatosensory cortex after contralateral median nerve stimulation is a *negative* peak with a latency of 20 ms (N_{20}), followed by a *positive* peak with a latency of 30 ms (P_{30}). The response recorded simultaneously from the exposed precentral gyrus is of opposite polarity, with a

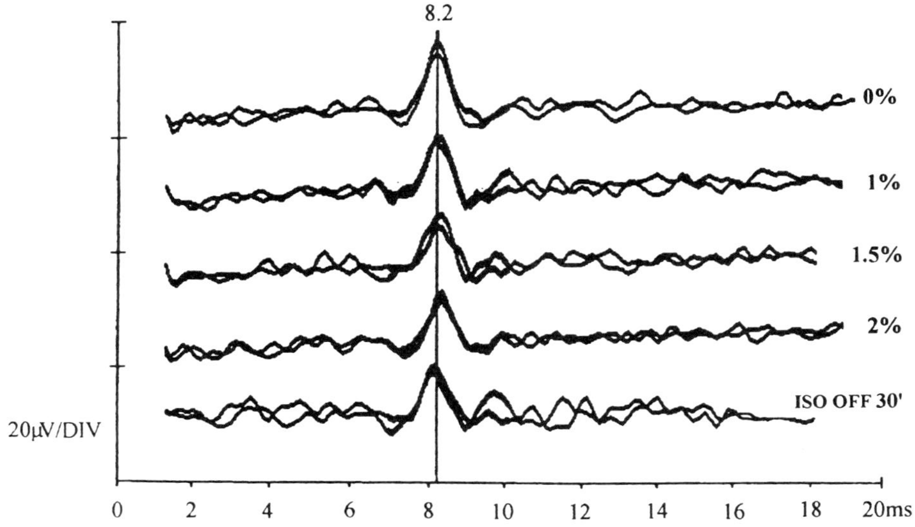

Figure 16–8. Motor EPs recorded from the epidural space of the low thoracic spinal cord after direct stimulation of the motor cortex showing the influence of different concentrations of isoflurane. (DIV = division.)

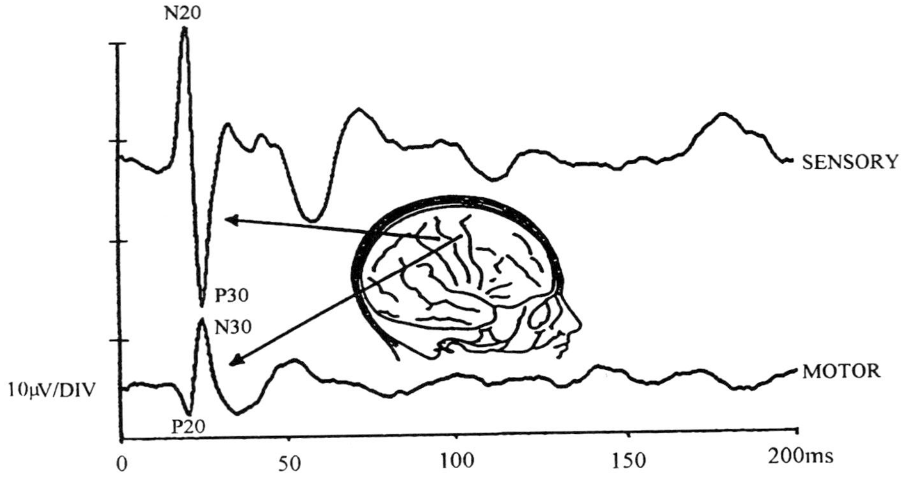

Figure 16–9. The phase-reversed response recorded over the exposed sensory-motor cortex after stimulation to the contralateral median nerve in a patient undergoing resection of an epileptic focus. The response recorded over the sensory cortex is of the same shape as the evoked potential recorded from the surface of the scalp, and the response recorded over the motor cortex shows "phase-reversed" potentials (i.e., the mirror image of the potentials recorded over the sensory cortex). Note the large amplitude of the response. (DIV = division.) (From Deletis V: The Sentinel-4 Evoked Potential/Electroencephalographic Analyzer. Anesth Rev 1991; 16(6):27–31.)

positive peak at 20 ms (P_{20}) and a *negative* peak at 30 ms (N_{30}). The response over motor cortex is the *mirror image* or *phase reversal* of the response recorded over the somatosensory cortex (Fig. 16–9). This response recorded from motor cortex is believed to be generated by the same source as the response recorded over the somatosensory cortex.[40, 41]

AUDITORY SYSTEM: ANATOMIC OUTLINE

Figure 16–10 shows the afferent auditory pathway from the eighth nerve to the auditory cortex and the neural substrates believed to be the generators of the short latency brainstem auditory evoked potentials (BAEP). The first-order neurons from the cells of the organ of Corti synapse with cells of the ventral and dorsal cochlear nuclei (CN). The axons of the second-order neurons synapse with cells in the superior olivary complex (SOC) in the caudal pons. Most of the axons of the third-order neurons branch, with some collateral axons crossing the midline. Axons from these cells then pass in the lateral lemniscus (LL) in each side of the brain as fourth-order neurons to form synapses in the inferior colliculi (IC). Fifth-order cells of the inferior colliculi branch, again partially decussate, and travel to synapse in the medial geniculate nuclei (MGN) of the thal-

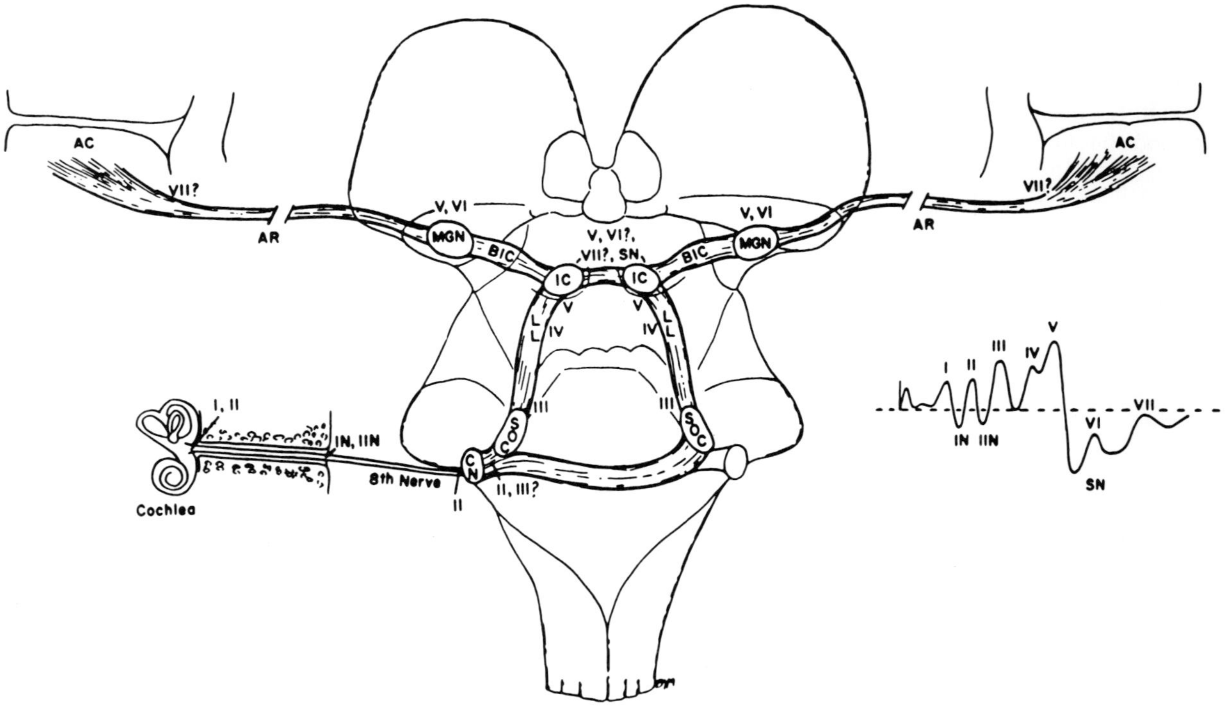

Figure 16–10. Schematic drawing of the auditory system and possible generators of different waves of the BAEP. See text for details. (From Legatt AD, Arezzo JC, Vaughan HG: Neurologic Clinics: Evoked Potentials. Philadelphia: WB Saunders, 1988.)

amus. Finally, medial geniculate cells project to the superior part of the temporal lobe (auditory radiations, or ARs) of the cerebral cortex to synapse with the cortical cells of the superior temporal gyrus (transverse gyri of Heschl), which is the primary auditory cortical area (AC).

Brainstem Auditory Evoked Potentials

The BAEP is the electrical response of the eighth nerve and various brainstem structures to auditory stimulation. BAEPs are very useful in identifying lesions and detecting surgically induced damage to the eighth nerve and the brainstem rostral to the entrance of the eighth nerve. They cannot, however, detect lesions below this level or in the ventral portion of the brainstem.

BAEPs are elicited by stimulating the ear with a series of click stimuli delivered by stimulators placed in the patient's ear. Masking noise is delivered to the contralateral ear in order to prevent the stimulation from conducting through bone to the contralateral ear.

The simplest way to record auditory EPs is to record the far-field response from the brainstem. To record BAEPs, the active electrode is placed at CZ or FPZ, and the reference electrode is placed over the ipsilateral mastoid. The response can also be recorded directly from electrodes placed on the surgically exposed floor of the fourth ventricle.[42] Direct recordings are generally of higher amplitude, and a reliable response may be acquired in only a few seconds (Fig. 16–11).

The BAEP is recorded as a series of five (and sometimes seven) peaks. The anatomic structures that are believed to generate these peaks[43] are:

Wave I:	Distal portion of the eighth nerve
Wave II:	Intracranial portion of the eighth nerve
Wave III:	Dorsal and ventral cochlear nuclei of the rostral medulla
Wave IV:	Superior olivary complex of the caudal pons
Wave V:	Lateral lemniscus in the midpons
Waves VI and VII:	Inferior colliculus of the tectum, not always recorded

The waves of primary importance for IOM are waves I–V. The wave I–wave III interpeak latency provides information concerning the integrity of the peripheral component of the auditory pathway, and wave III–wave V interpeak latency provides information about central brainstem pathways.

Direct Recording of Compound Action Potentials from the Eighth Cranial Nerve

The auditory response may also be recorded directly from the eighth nerve with an electrode placed on the surgically exposed nerve.[43] The eighth nerve compound action potential (CAP) is often preferred over the far-field BAEP because it is of much larger amplitude, and because a reliable response can be obtained with many fewer traces (Fig. 16–12). This results in a better SNR, shorter acquisition time, and faster feedback to the surgeon. However, in most cases in which eighth nerve CAPs are recorded, far-field BAEPs are also recorded as a back-up modality.

Compound Muscle Action Potentials after Stimulation of the Motor Cranial Nerves

The compound muscle action potential (CMAP) is recorded in order to identify a motor cranial nerve from the surrounding tissue and tumor as well as to monitor the functional integrity of the nerve, once identified.[43] The surgeon stimulates the nerve (or tumor) with a handheld stimulator. The CMAP from the muscles innervated by stimulated nerve is amplified and presented as auditory feedback to the surgeon. It is imperative that neuromuscular blocking agents not be administered during this type of nerve monitoring. The nerves most commonly monitored in the operating room are the facial nerve, the hypoglossal nerve, and the motor part of the trigeminal nerve. Table 16–1 lists the

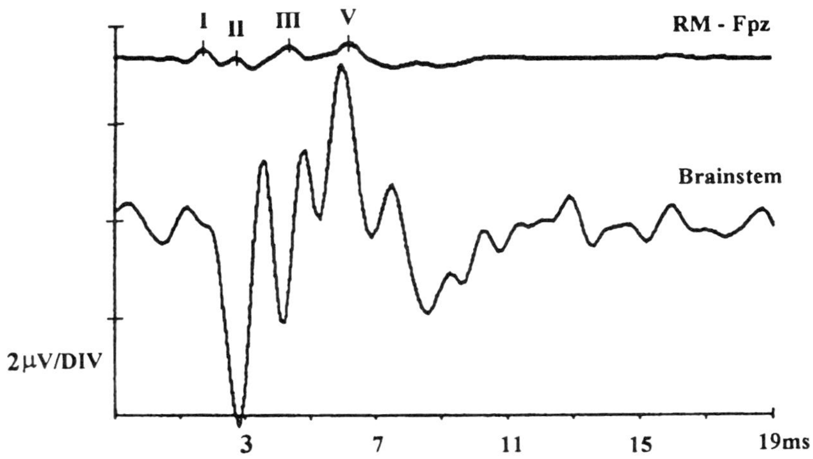

Figure 16–11. The direct BAEP recorded from the floor of the fourth ventricle (brainstem) and the far-field BAEP recorded simultaneously from the ipsilateral mastoid (RM-Fpz) after stimulation to the ipsilateral ear in a patient undergoing resection of a brain stem tumor. Note the large difference in the amplitudes of the recordings.

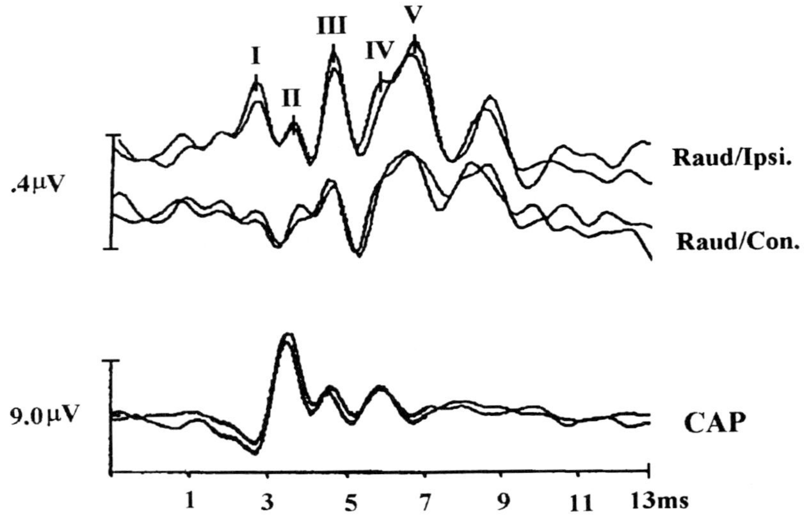

Figure 16–12. Far-field BAEPs recorded from the right (Raud/Ipsi.) and left (Raud/Con.) mastoid *(top two traces),* and the eighth nerve compound action potential (CAP) *(bottom trace)* recorded from a cottonoid electrode placed over the surgically exposed eighth nerve, after right ear stimulation. Note different scales.

cranial nerves and the appropriate muscles for recording the CMAP for each nerve.

Visual Evoked Potentials

Although visual evoked potentials (VEPs) are a very useful diagnostic tool in clinical neurophysiology, they have not been shown to be useful in the operating room. Although there is a need for visual system monitoring, current methodologies are not appropriate for use with patients under general anesthesia, and intraoperatively recorded VEPs do not correlate well with neurologic outcome.

Pattern-reversal visual stimuli cannot be used in patients under general anesthesia, for whom gaze direction cannot be controlled. Only flash stimuli or stimuli from light-emitting diodes incorporated into goggles or fiberoptic cables embodied into contact lenses are used in the operating room.[2] However, flash VEP is not correlated with visual function,[44, 45] and there is evidence that flash stimuli are processed by different neural channels than pattern-reversal stimuli.[44] The utility of VEP monitoring could be improved with the development of more effective methods of intraoperative visual stimulation.

TABLE 16–1. COMPOUND MUSCLE ACTION POTENTIAL GENERATORS

Cranial Nerve	Muscles
Oculomotor	Rectus medialis
	Rectus superior
	Rectus inferior
	Obliquus inferior
Trigeminal	Masseter
	Temporalis
Trochlear	Obliquus superior
Abducens	Rectus lateralis
Facial	Orbicularis oris
	Orbicularis oculi
	Nasal
Glossopharyngeal	Stylopharyngeus
Vagus	Laryngeal
Accessory	Sternocleidomastoid
Hypoglossal	Lateral tongue

NEW METHODOLOGIES

Pudendal Nerve Monitoring

The functional integrity of the sacral roots responsible for micturition and sexual function may be monitored by recording electrically elicited pudendal nerve activity. Sacral root function may be evaluated by recording the dorsal root action potential (DRAP), the bulbocavernous reflex (BCR), the spinal pudendal EP, or the cortical pudendal EP. All of these responses are elicited by stimulation to the penile or clitoral nerves with two silver or silver chloride cup electrodes placed on the dorsal surface of the penis (cathode proximal) or one electrode placed on the dorsal surface of the clitoris (cathode) and one on either adjacent labium (anode) (Fig. 16–13).

The DRAP is recorded by the surgeon from the surgically exposed sacral roots with a handheld bipolar hooked electrode. Recording DRAPs allows one to map the pudendal afferents in the sacral roots in order to determine which roots or rootlets are the primary carriers of pudendal activity (Fig. 16–14). This method is used primarily to preserve pudendal afferents in selective dorsal rhizotomies that produce lesions in the sacral roots in order to relieve spasticity,[46] but this method may be used to map pudendal afferents in surgery for other pathology of the conus medullaris or cauda equina.

Another method of assessing the functional integrity of the sacral roots is by monitoring the BCR, recorded from the anal sphincter with intramuscular wire electrodes (Fig. 16–15). This method allows for continuous monitoring in the operating room, which is not technically feasible with DRAP recordings. The BCR is easily obtainable with an

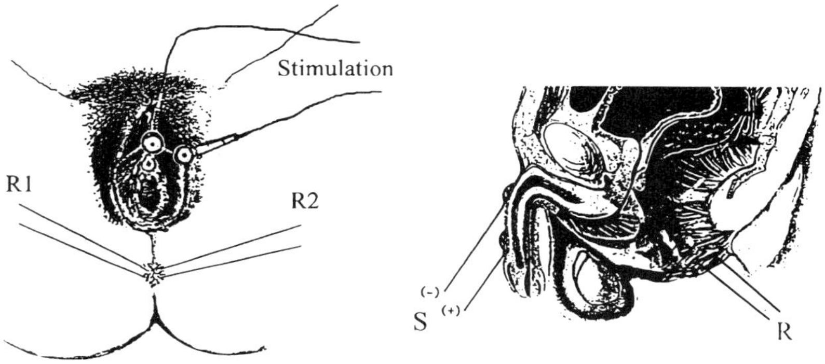

Figure 16–13. *Left,* Stimulation sites for the clitoral nerves and recording sites for anal EMG (R1, R2). *Right,* Stimulation sites for the penile nerves (S) and recording sites for anal EMG (R).

anesthesia regimen of propofol or narcotic but is not reliably recorded when neuromuscular blocking agents and volatile anesthetics are administered.[47] It is also possible to record a stationary wave over the conus with an epidural or subdural electrode after stimulation of the pudendal nerves (spinal pudendal SSEP). This response is of large amplitude and is reliably recorded (Fig. 16–16). Finally, it is possible to record pudendal nerve activity from the scalp (cortical pudendal SSEP). Unfortunately, the cortical response is seldom obtainable in patients under general anesthesia and is not commonly monitored in the operating room.

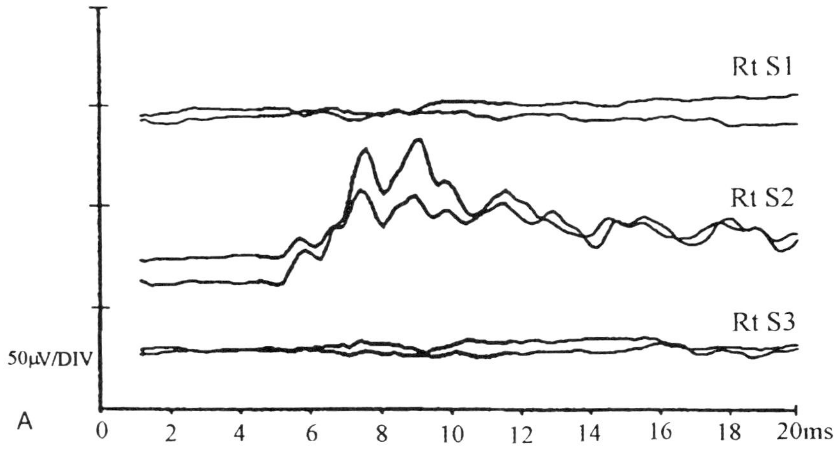

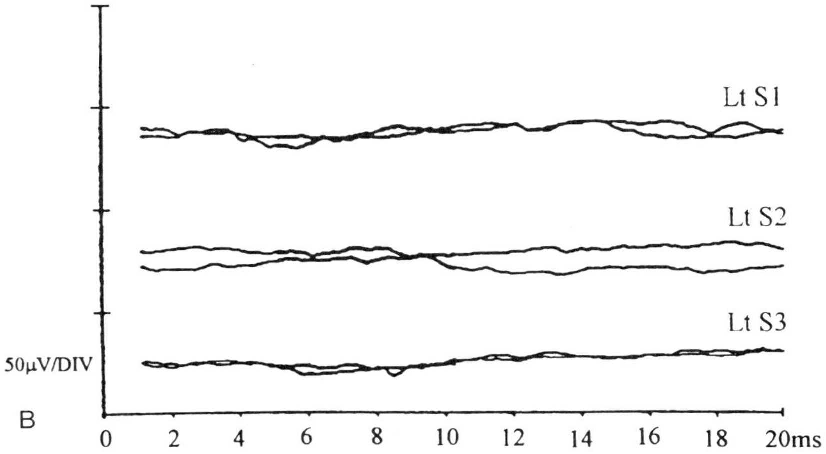

Figure 16–14. Dorsal root action potentials recorded from the surgically exposed right *(A)* and left *(B)* sacral roots in a 4-year-old boy after stimulation of the penile nerves. All afferent activity is limited to the right S2 (Rt S2) root. Two averages of 100 responses from each root are superimposed. (From Deletis V, Vodusek D, Abbott R, et al: Intraoperative monitoring of the dorsal sacral roots: minimizing the risk of iatrogenic micturition disorders. Neurosurgery 1992; 30(1):72–75.)

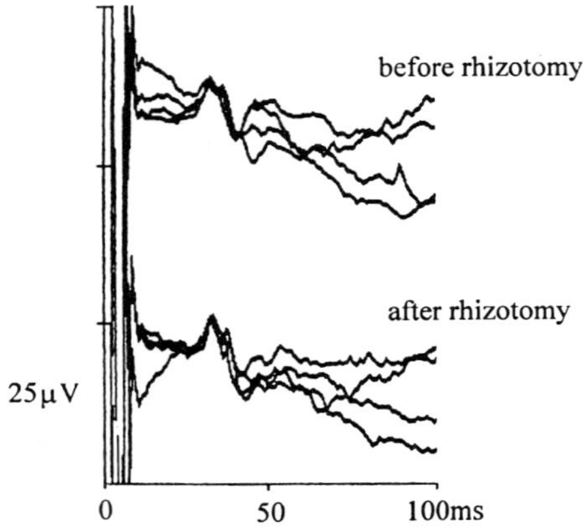

Figure 16–15. Intraoperative recording of bulbocavernosus reflex in a 4-year-old boy before and after selective dorsal rhizotomy of the lumbosacral roots, showing no surgically induced changes.

SAFETY CONSIDERATIONS

There are no known risk factors associated with recording EPs, even with electrodes placed directly on neural tissue. There are also no known risk factors associated with stimulation of the peripheral or cranial nerves. There are no reports of adverse sequelae associated with these stimulating techniques, with the rare exception of burns at the site of percutaneous stimulation of peripheral nerves. The incidence of burns is very low and is speculated to be due to a problem in the monopolar coagulator. Electrical and magnetic stimulation of the brain and spinal cord presents very little risk to the patient when used in the manner described in this chapter. However, when used with other parameters of stimulation, these methods may present some risks, which are outlined below.

LOW-FREQUENCY MOTOR CORTEX STIMULATION

At present, most methods of motor cortex stimulation employ ''single'' electrical or magnetic stimuli, i.e., a stimulation rate of less than 1 Hz. There have been no reports of complications resulting from the use of low-frequency *electrical* stimulation in awake, comatose, or anesthetized patients. There is no evidence that delivering low-frequency electrical stimulation to the motor cortex produces kindling, the phenomenon in which repeated delivery of initially subconvulsive stimuli results in seizures. It has been shown that the EEG does not change following low-frequency electrical motor cortex stimulation,[48, 49] and that there are no significant differences between serum prolactin levels before and after stimulation.[48] (Increased serum prolactin levels are a well-known correlate of seizures.[50])

Animal studies suggest that damage to the neural tissue immediately below cortical stimulating electrodes can occur when charge densities exceed 40 $\mu C/cm^2$/phase and the charge per phase exceeds 0.4 μC/phase at pulse frequencies of 50 Hz, with stimulating electrodes of surface area of 10 mm^2.[51] The charge density during the peak of the transcranial magnetic and electrical impulse is 2.4 $\mu C/cm^2$/phase, which is well below the level found to cause damage.[52]

It is possible, however, that stimulation of the cortex with low-frequency electrical stimuli changes systemic blood pressure. Approximately 10% of patients undergoing prolonged intraoperative cortical stimulation with low-frequency stimuli (at greater than 60% of stimulator output) exhibit systemic hypertension. In these cases, when the interval between sets of low-frequency stimuli is increased, the blood pressure returns to baseline. No adverse sequelae have been noted.

There is also evidence that low-frequency transcranial magnetic stimulation does not damage the human or animal

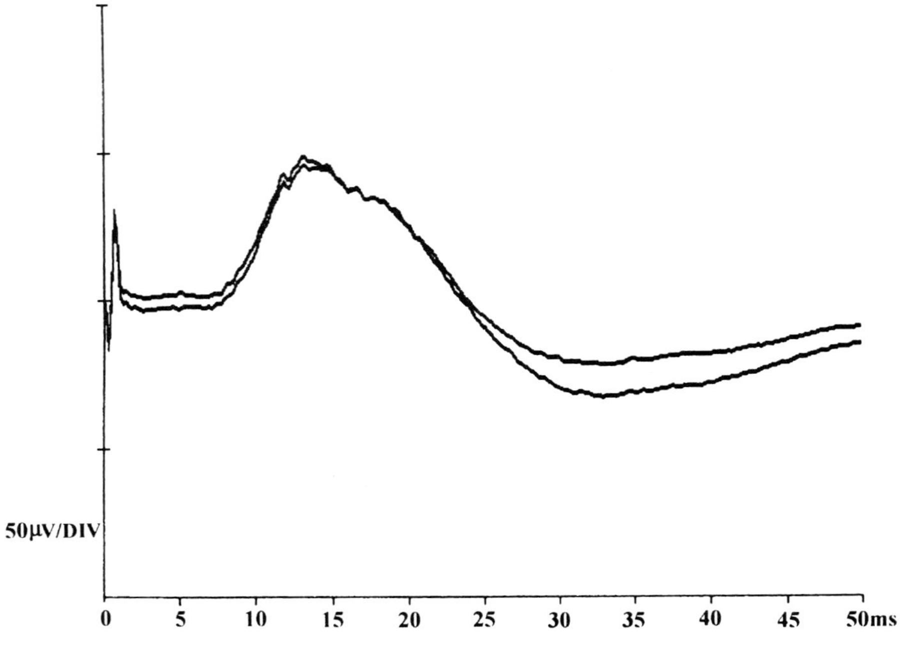

Figure 16–16. Spinal pudendal SEPs recorded subdurally over the conus with an epidural electrode in a 4-year-old patient undergoing selective dorsal rhizotomy.

brain[52, 53] or induce seizures in most patients. There is no evidence of changes of the plasma levels of pituitary hormones after transcranial magnetic stimulation with low-frequency stimuli.[54] However, there are a few cases of induced seizure in patients with neurologic disorders: epilepsy,[55] multiple sclerosis,[56] and ischemic stroke.[57, 58]

Some patients have seizures following low-frequency magnetic stimulation, although there are no reports of seizures induced by low-frequency electrical stimulation. This may be explained by the fact that many more awake patients have undergone magnetic stimulation than have undergone electrical stimulation. (Electrical stimulation is used primarily on patients under general anesthesia, which suppresses seizure activity.) Finally, there is one report of acoustic trauma in rabbits due to the acoustic artifact produced by the magnetic coil following low-frequency stimulation.[59] However, this finding was not confirmed in humans.[60]

HIGH-FREQUENCY MOTOR CORTEX STIMULATION

Repetitive stimulation with a train of electrical or magnetic stimuli has been associated with an increased risk of seizure activity. Early researchers discovered that stimulating the motor cortex with a high rate (55–65 Hz) of *electrical* stimulation produced epileptic seizures in some patients.[22] High rates of stimulation (50–60 Hz) are still employed with direct electrical stimulation of the motor cortex for mapping purposes, because low-frequency stimuli do not elicit the complex muscle movements necessary for mapping the motor cortex in the operating room. Although this procedure can elicit seizures, this risk is justified, because the procedure is extremely valuable in locating and preserving critical areas of the motor cortex.

The risk of seizures may be minimized by increasing the intensity of stimulation in small increments, starting at steps of 2 mA. The EEG should be recorded during this procedure and observed for possible after-discharges. The risk of seizure is greater in epileptic patients who are not under general anesthesia, and fast-acting antiepileptic drugs should be available for these patients. Histologic studies of human cortex after electrical stimulation of the exposed cortex with trains of stimuli performed during temporal lobectomies showed no histologic changes.[61] Although this technique may elicit seizures, it does not damage brain tissue.

Rapid-rate (up to 60 Hz) transcranial *magnetic* stimulation has also been shown to elicit seizures in a single epileptic patient[62] and even in one healthy subject.[63] Stimulating parameters that are not associated with seizures have been suggested,[63] but more research is needed to established their safety. Finally, it is possible to produce burns at the site of metal electrodes under a magnetic coil if rapid-rate magnetic stimulation is used.[64]

CLINICAL APPLICATIONS

NEUROPHYSIOLOGIC EVALUATION OF COMATOSE PATIENTS

Neurophysiologic assessment of comatose patients with EEG and multimodal EPs provides information about the functional integrity of both the reticular formation and the sensory and motor tracts. The appearance of EEG desynchronization indicates that the reticular activating system is functional,[65] and EP recordings from the somatosensory, motor, and auditory pathways determine which pathways are intact and allow calculation of central conduction time.[66] This information is not available from clinical evaluations. EEG and/or multimodal EP parameters correlate with outcome in comatose patients.[65, 67–71]

Neurophysiologic monitoring of comatose patients may be performed sequentially or continuously. Continuous evaluation is advisable because of the dynamic nature of coma, particularly in the acute stage. Twenty-four–hour recordings are relatively easy to obtain with modifications of standard EP recording techniques and use of appropriate software for prolonged serial registrations of different EP modalities. Continuous monitoring is especially important in patients with a great amount of muscle artifact. Twenty-four–hour monitoring allows one to catch rare periods of quiescence, when usable data are obtainable. Continuous monitoring also provides data that warn of acute neurologic

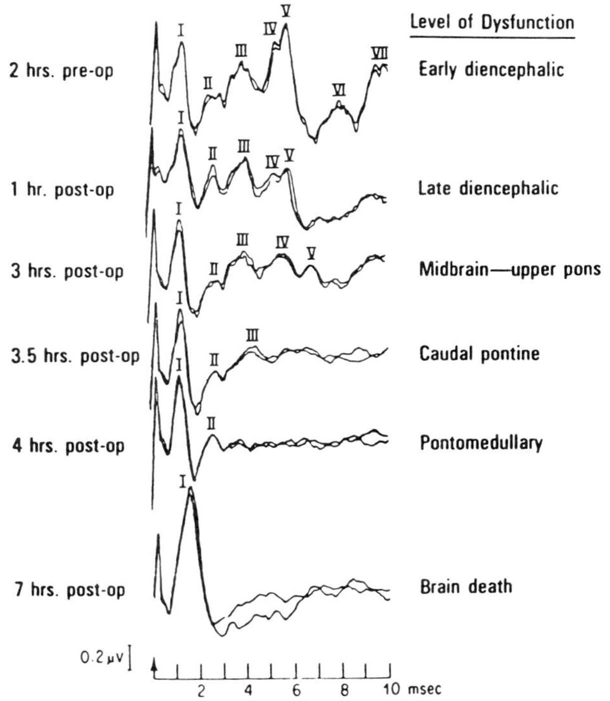

Figure 16–17. Serial recordings of BAEPs in a 37-year-old male patient with progressive central herniation syndrome. The EPs reflect the patient's progressive rostral-caudal deterioration. (From Plum F, Posner JB: The Diagnosis of Stupor and Coma, 3rd Ed. Philadelphia: FA Davis, 1980.)

deterioration (Fig. 16–17), allowing more timely treatment or identification of brain-dead patients for selection of candidates for organ donation.[72]

RESECTIONS OF INTRAMEDULLARY TUMORS AND ARTERIOVENOUS MALFORMATIONS OF THE SPINAL CORD

Surgery for the removal of intramedullary tumors and spinal arteriovenous malformations (AVMs) is associated with a great risk of damage to the spinal cord and may result in paralysis and incontinence.[73] Resection may involve damage to the CST, dorsal columns, or both. To obtain direct information concerning the functional integrity of both the sensory and motor tracts, both SSEPs and MEPs must be monitored. However, if it is not possible to monitor one of these modalities, information from the other modality will provide indirect evidence of the integrity of the other spinal tract. Patients with intramedullary tumors often exhibit poor-quality or absent SSEPs or may lose SSEPs following myelotomy (Fig. 16–18), in which case MEPs are the only means of monitoring spinal pathways.

MEPs from the epidural space following transcranial electrical stimulation and SSEPs from the epidural space following stimulation to the peripheral nerves should be monitored. Cortical SSEPs should also be monitored, especially before placement and after removal of the epidural catheter-electrode, as a back-up modality. The following surgical manipulations are particularly likely to damage neural tissue:

1. Laminectomy or laminotomy
2. Myelotomy
3. Retraction of the dorsal column
4. Manipulation and resection of the tumor
5. Resection of AVMs involving the anterior spinal artery

RESECTIONS OF TUMORS OF THE CONUS MEDULLARIS OR CAUDA EQUINA

Surgery for the removal of tumors of the conus medullaris and cauda equina can damage the spinal roots or conus medullaris, and may result in paralysis, micturition disorders, and sexual dysfunction. In cases of relatively small tumors involving only one or more roots, the sacral roots should be mapped with DRAPs in order to determine which roots carry pudendal afferents.[46] However, mapping may not be possible in patients with large tumors. Roots should therefore be monitored with spinal pudendal EPs recorded over the conus or the BCR. SSEPs after stimulation of the tibial nerves should also be monitored with an epidural electrode from the spinal epidural space. During these procedures, the following surgical manipulations may damage neural tissue:

1. Laminectomy or laminotomy
2. Manipulation and resection of the tumor
3. Manipulation of the nerve roots

RESECTION OF BRAINSTEM TUMORS

Surgery for the removal of brainstem tumors can injure the brainstem, cranial nerves, and sensory and motor tracts.[74] It is advisable to monitor all modalities that can cause damage; the specific modalities will depend on the location of the tumor. In these patients, the CMAP from muscles innervated by motor cranial nerves following direct stimulation to the nerve should be recorded with direct BAEP, far-field BAEP, and CSEPs as back-up modalities.

Resection of tumors located in the ventral aspect of the brainstem can damage the CST. MEPs following transcranial stimulation should be recorded in these cases. Although there is usually very little space available to place a recording electrode on the field, MEPs may be recorded with an electrode placed percutaneously into the epidural space of the midthoracic spine. Critical surgical manipulations include:

1. Dural opening and cerebrospinal fluid (CSF) drainage
2. Retraction of the vermis
3. Retraction of the brainstem (ventrally located tumor)
4. Manipulation of the fourth ventricle floor
5. Manipulation and resection of the tumor

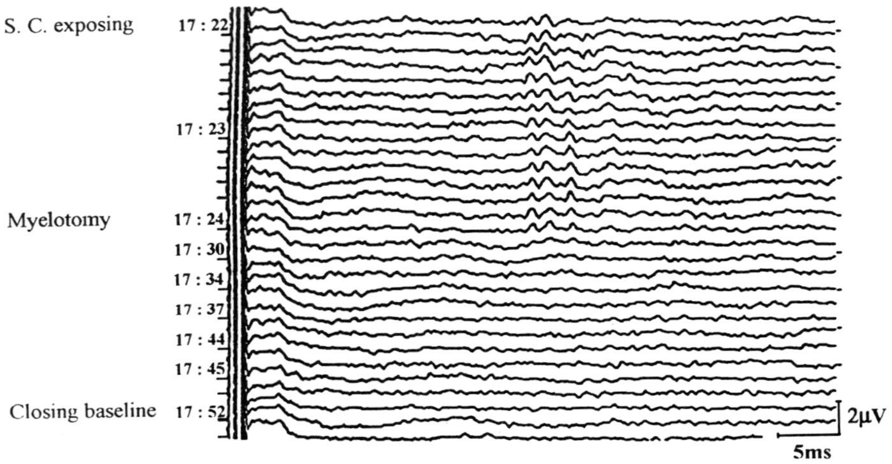

Figure 16–18. Spinal somatosensory EPs recorded from the T6 epidural space (cranial to the tumor) in a 79-year-old patient with a lower thoracic spinal cord (S.C.) tumor, following bilateral tibial nerve stimulation The EPs disappeared after the myelotomy (17:24) was performed.

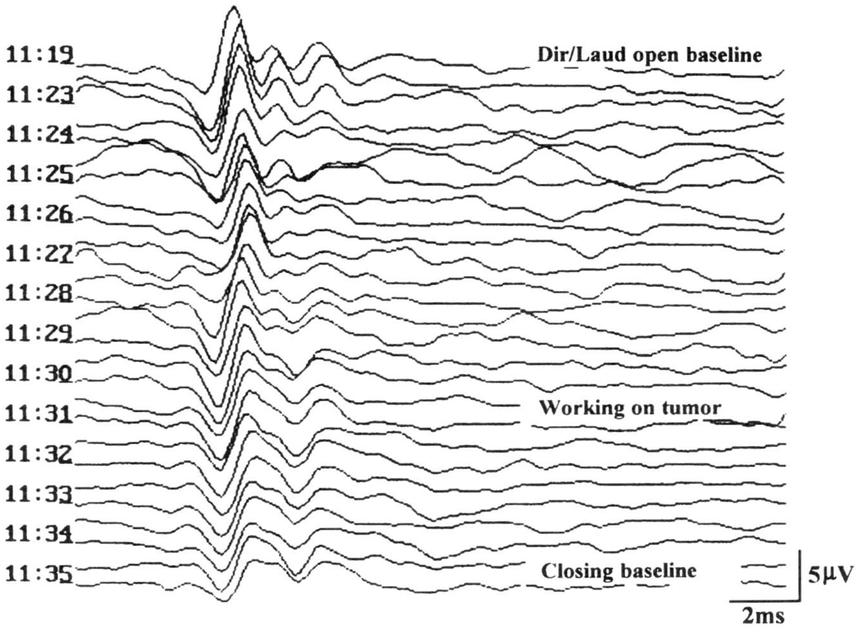

Figure 16–19. Eighth nerve compound action potential recorded in a patient undergoing removal of a small acoustic neuroma. The response was diminished but present at the end of surgery; postoperatively, the patient's hearing was preserved. (Dir/Laud = direct/left auditory.)

RESECTION OF ACOUSTIC NEUROMAS

Removal of acoustic neuromas can damage the vestibulocochlear (VIII) and facial (VII) nerves; in some cases, it can damage brainstem structures. Monitoring the CAP of the eighth cranial nerve following stimulation of the ipsilateral ear is the preferred method, when possible (Figs. 16–19 and 16–20). Large tumors sometimes obscure the eighth nerve and preclude placement of a direct electrode. The far-field BAEP is also recorded in order to allow monitoring of the eighth nerve before and after the direct recording electrode is placed. Far-field BAEPs from the unaffected ear should be recorded as a control over non–surgically induced changes. It should be noted that patients with acoustic neuromas often have abnormal BAEPs, and patients with large tumors may have significant brainstem compression, in which case no signal can be monitored from the affected side.

The tumor often grows along the facial nerve; thus, the facial nerve should be mapped with the CMAP before and during resection. Cortical SSEPs from upper extremity stimulation should be monitored throughout the procedure in order to evaluate the effect of the procedure on the brainstem lemniscal pathway. Neural damage is particularly likely during the following procedures:

1. Dural opening and CSF drainage
2. Retraction of the cerebellar hemisphere/application of pressure on the brainstem and eighth nerve
3. Drilling of the petrosal bone
4. Manipulation and resection of the tumor
5. Coagulation of critical blood vessels

RESECTION OF BRAIN TUMORS INVADING THE MOTOR CORTEX OR THE CORTICOSPINAL TRACT

The removal of tumors of the primary somatosensory and motor cortices carries the risk of damaging functionally important cortex. Damage to the motor cortex is associated with motor deficits and is usually considered more serious than damage to the somatosensory cortex. The motor cortex is usually not evident by anatomy alone (and the anatomy may be abnormal because of the pathology) and should be identified neurophysiologically so that the surgeon may avoid damage to it.

Neurophysiologic mapping of the cortices using the phase reversal procedure should be performed. After identification of the motor cortex, specific motor areas may be mapped by direct stimulation of the cortex while observing the arm, leg, and face for movements. In some cases, continuous monitoring of the arm or leg area of the motor cortex and CST may be performed in order to assess its functional integrity throughout the procedure. In these cases, MEPs may be recorded from an electrode inserted percutaneously into the spinal epidural space.[12]

REPAIR OF VASCULAR ABNORMALITIES (ANEURYSMS AND AVMs) OF THE BRAIN AND BRAINSTEM

Surgery for the clipping of cerebral aneurysms or resection of AVMs can damage the sensory and motor systems or selectively damage one of these systems. Proximal and distal clipping of the feeding arteries of the aneurysm can result in ischemia to the brain if collateral circulation is insufficient. This surgery is further complicated by individual differences in vascular anatomy.

Clipping the middle cerebral or anterior cerebral arteries may result in cerebral ischemia and damage to both the sensory and motor pathways—or it may result in compromise to the perforating arteries supplying the motor pathway of the internal capsule and leave the sensory pathways unaffected. The consequence may be "pure" motor hemi-

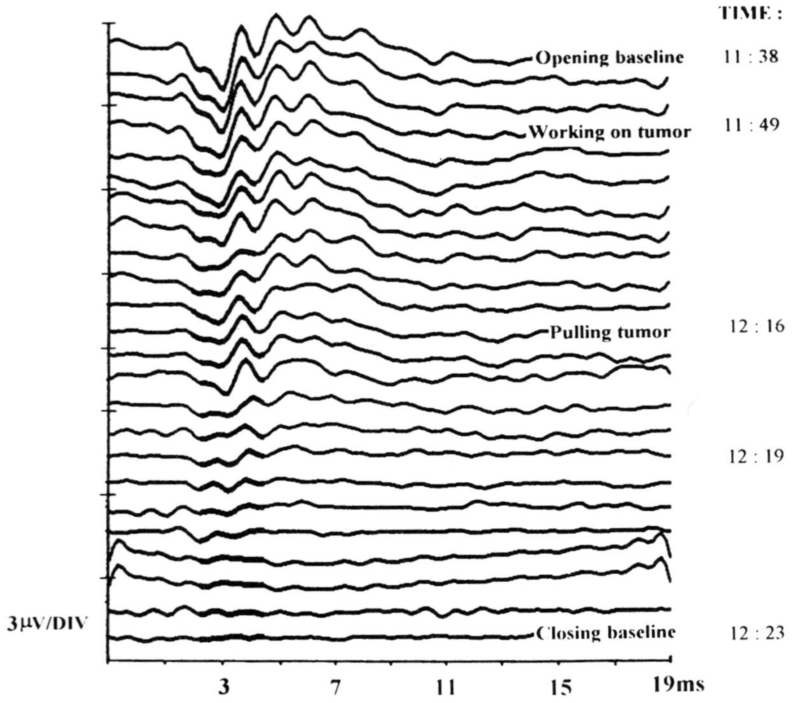

Figure 16–20. Eighth nerve compound action potential recorded in a patient undergoing resection of an acoustic neuroma. The response decreased in amplitude during resection and finally disappeared. Postoperatively, the patient had no hearing on the affected side.

plegia, the loss of motor function and MEPs, and preservation of somatosensory function and SSEPs[12] (Fig. 16–21). In the same way, occlusion of the perforating branches of the basilar artery may compromise the blood supply to the motor nuclei or motor tracts traversing the brainstem. This event may also result in postoperative motor deficits while leaving SSEPs and BAEPs unaffected.[75] Thus, MEPs should be monitored during surgery for the repair of basilar artery aneurysms to detect this occurrence.

To reduce arterial pressure or prevent blood flow in the aneurysm or AVM nidus, the surgeon may place a temporary clip on the parent artery of the aneurysm or feeding artery of the AVM. CSEPs and MEPs are recorded during the clipping to detect the occurrence of ischemia. If the EP is reduced or obliterated during the clipping, it indicates that the clipped artery is a critical blood supply to the sensory or motor cortex or tracts. Even temporary clipping of that blood vessel may result in sensory or motor deficits and should be avoided if the EPs indicate cerebral ischemia.

CAROTID ENDARTERECTOMY

Cross-clamping the carotid artery during a carotid endarterectomy may restrict the blood supply to the ipsilateral hemisphere. Collateral circulation through the anterior and posterior communicating arteries from the opposite internal carotid artery and the vertebral artery system may or may not be sufficient to support the affected side once the cross-clamping is complete. Information obtained from EP or EEG monitoring can detect whether the collateral circulation provides sufficient blood flow to the affected cerebral hemisphere. That EPs and EEG are extremely sensitive to cerebral ischemia has been demonstrated in a large group of patients.[76, 77]

The cortical SSEP should be monitored to assess the adequacy of the collateral circulation. The cortical SSEP following stimulation to the median nerve contralateral to the clamped artery will assess the degree of perfusion in the cortex at risk. The cortical SSEP following stimulation to the median nerve ipsilateral to the clamped artery will control for nonsurgical effects. Insufficient collateral flow is evidenced by dramatic changes in EP parameters, indicating a need for a shunt to bypass the clamped internal carotid artery. However, monitoring should be performed even when shunting is planned, because EPs may detect shunt malfunctioning or damage during shunt placement. Monitoring is not necessary when the procedure is performed under local anesthesia in cooperative patients.

EEG may also be used to monitor the brain perfusion; an asymmetry indicates insufficient blood supply to the affected cortex. Changes in EEG recorded during cross-clamping of the carotid artery have also been shown to indicate postoperative neuropsychologic deficits that are often undetected with routine neurologic examination.[2] It is not necessary to monitor MEPs during this procedure, because the motor tracts are not specifically at risk.

REPAIR OF SCOLIOSIS

There is a small risk of damage to the spinal cord during surgery for the repair of scoliosis. Approximately 1% of patients undergoing this procedure experience permanent paralysis of the lower extremities. Because the paralysis is such a devastating outcome and intraoperative monitoring

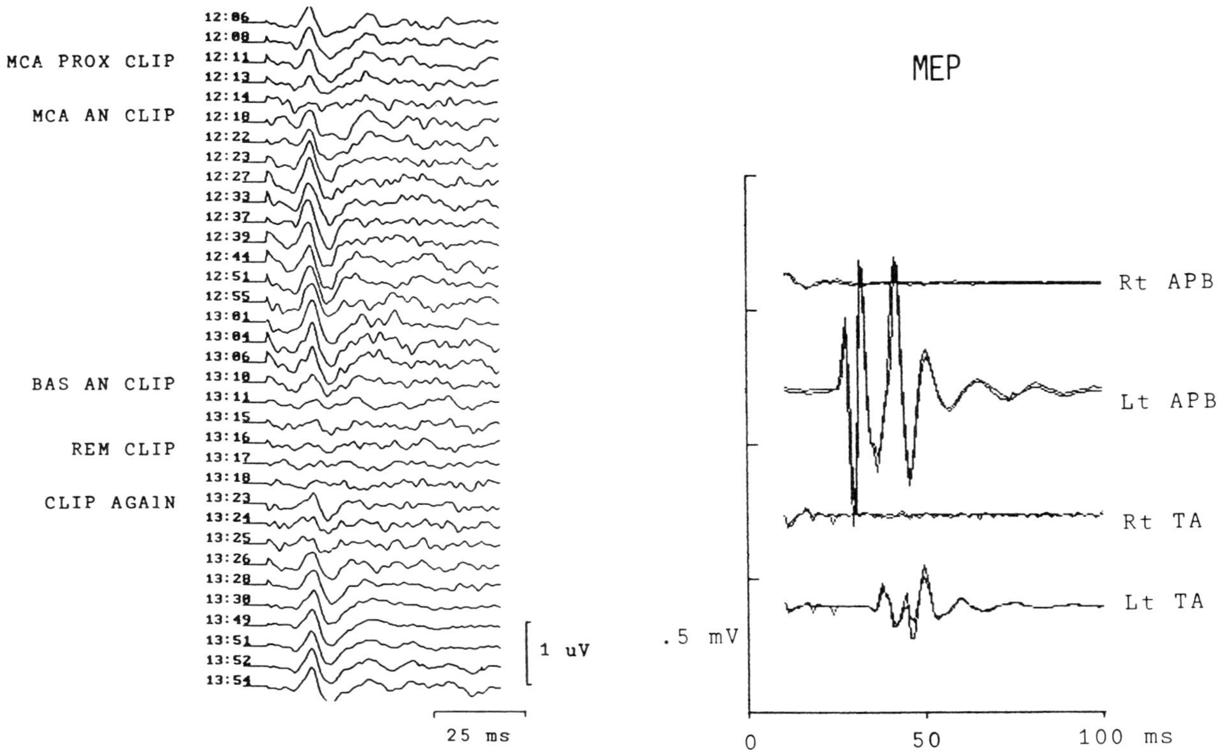

Figure 16–21. Cortical SEPs recorded from a patient undergoing surgical repair of a middle cerebral artery (MCA) aneurysm and a basilar artery aneurysm, after stimulation of the right median nerve. The SEP disappeared temporarily after clipping the proximal middle cerebral artery (MCA PROX CLIP) and basilar aneurysm (BAS AN CLIP), but recovered fully by the end of the surgery. The patient woke up with intact sensation, but with right side hemiplegia. MEPs recorded postoperatively after transcranial magnetic stimulation showed the absence of a motor response from the right extremities (abductor pollicis brevis [APB] and tibialis anterior [TA] muscles). (From Deletis V: Intraoperative monitoring of the functional integrity of the motor pathways. In Devinski O, Beric A, Dogali M [eds]: Electrical and Magnetic Stimulation of the Brain and Spinal Cord. New York: Raven Press, 1993.)

can easily detect spinal cord damage, EP monitoring is standard in surgery for the repair of scoliosis (Fig. 16–22). This procedure was one of the first procedures to use routine EP monitoring.[78] SSEPs have been used to directly evaluate the functional integrity of the ascending tracts and to indirectly assess the integrity of the motor tracts. However, because there are reports of patients who experienced loss of motor function and preserved SSEPs with this surgery,[79] it is necessary to monitor both SSEPs and MEPs.

The ideal methodology for monitoring procedures for the correction of scoliosis is a combination of SSEPs and epidurally recorded MEPs. This allows high-speed acquisition

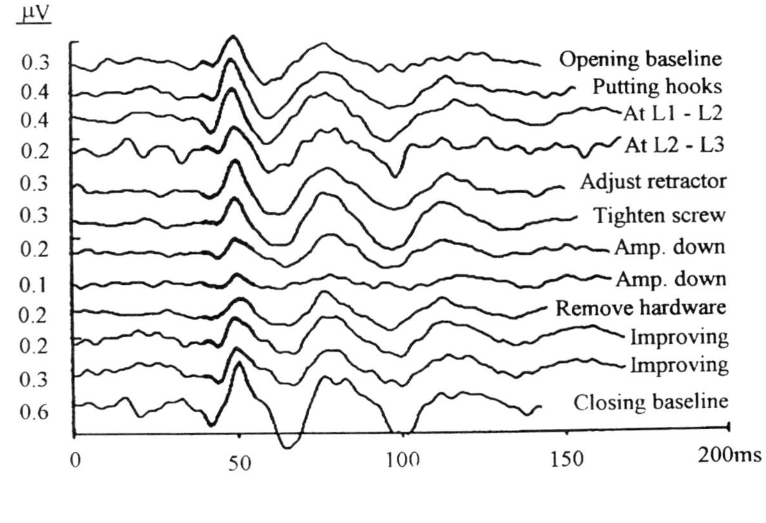

Figure 16–22. Cortical SEPs recorded in a patient with idiopathic scoliosis undergoing Cotrel-Dubousset instrumentation following bilateral tibial nerve stimulation. After spinal distraction, the CSEP amplitude decreased to 0.1 μV. The surgeon was warned of the evoked potential change, and he removed the instrumentation. The CSEPs fully recovered, and the patient had no postoperative neurologic deficits. (Numbers on left refer to the amplitude of the first negative peak.) (From Deletis V: The Sentinel-4 Evoked Potential/Electroencephalographic Analyzer. Anesth Rev 1991; 16(6):27–31.)

of data on the functional integrity of both the ascending and the descending tracts. To insert the epidural recording electrodes, the surgeon must perform a flavectomy or small laminectomy. Cortical SSEPs following lower extremity stimulation are monitored before and after the placement of the epidural electrodes and throughout the case if SSEPs and epidurally recorded MEPs are not monitored. Cortical SSEPs from upper extremity stimulation are also monitored to check for non–surgically induced changes and to detect brachial plexus traction, which can result from improper patient positioning.

The following surgical manipulations risk damage to neural tissue during scoliosis repair:

1. Securing sublaminar hooks
2. Placement of rods
3. Rotation of correcting rod or distraction of spine

SPINAL DECOMPRESSION AND FUSION

Spinal cord decompression and fusion is a procedure for surgical management of compressive spinal cord lesions. The spine is usually stabilized with instrumentation; depending on the location of the lesion, the surgeon may approach the spine from either the anterior or the posterior direction. These procedures present a risk to both the ascending and descending pathways of the spinal cord, and both SSEPs and MEPs should be monitored.

Ideally, both SSEPs and MEPs should be monitored, because these techniques allow high-speed data acquisition and yield information on the functional integrity of both the ascending and descending spinal pathways. However, these methodologies may not be applicable in procedures involving an anterior approach to the spine where it is not possible to surgically insert an epidural electrode unless the electrode is inserted percutaneously.

Cortical SSEPs should be monitored before and after placement of the catheter-electrode or throughout the procedure when it is not possible to monitor SSEPs and MEPs. Both upper and lower extremity cortical SSEPs should be monitored in all cases. If the compression is in the thoracic or lumbar spine, cortical SSEPs from upper extremities serve as a control for non–surgically induced changes and detect brachial plexus traction resulting from improper patient positioning.

EMBOLIZATION OF SPINAL CORD AVMs AND TUMORS

Neuroradiologic embolization is the occlusion of pathologic blood vessels by the injection of an occluding substance. Spinal cord AVMs may be treated by embolization of the abnormal vessels so that normal blood flow to the capillary bed is restored. Tumors may be treated by embolization of the feeding vessels. Because many of the vessels to be embolized are intermingled with the normal vascular architecture of the spinal cord, therapeutic embolization carries the risk of occluding, damaging, or rupturing normal spinal cord blood vessels. EP monitoring is critically important in identifying which blood vessels may be safely occluded. Cortical SSEPs from all four extremities should be monitored. If the lesion is in the thoracic or lumbar spinal regions, cortical SSEPs following upper extremity stimulation serve as a control for nonspecific factors.

In addition to monitoring for inadvertent damage, EPs may be used in conjunction with a technique that causes temporary blockage of nerve conduction. This technique allows one to test whether a vessel feeds critical neural tissue before it is permanently occluded. Amobarbital, a short-acting barbiturate, is injected into the vessel to be occluded while EPs are recorded. Because amobarbital blocks nerve conduction in the tissue supplied by the vessels, a loss of EPs during this test indicates that the vessel supplies critical tissue and should not be occluded (Fig. 16–23).[80] Another method of testing whether a vessel supplies critical neural tissue is the inflation of a balloon occluder while EPs are recorded.[81]

In these procedures, the critical incidents are:

1. Injection of dye during fluoroscopic imaging
2. Occlusion of vessels by balloon occluder
3. Embolization of vessels

CROSS-CLAMPING OF THE AORTA

Repair of thoracic aortic aneurysms or other aortic anomalies usually involves aortic cross-clamping and may be performed with or without aorta-to-femoral bypass. Bypass is usually considered imperative if the clamping is expected to exceed 30 minutes in order to perfuse the spinal cord.

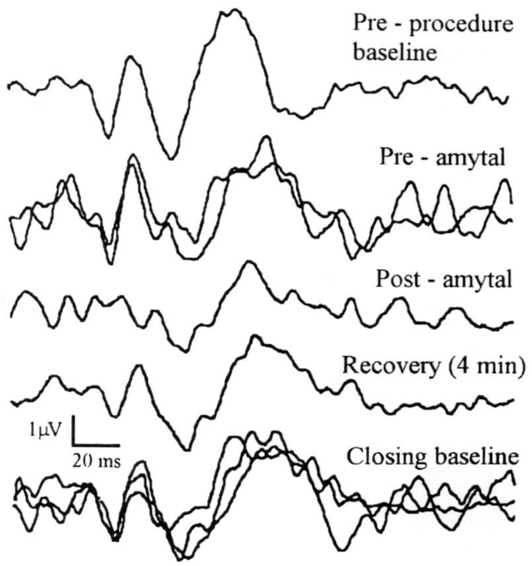

Figure 16–23. Cortical SEPs showing the effect of an injection of amobarbital (Amytal) into a high thoracic feeding vessel in a patient undergoing embolization of vessels feeding a spinal cord tumor. (From Young W, Mollin D: Intraoperative somatosensory evoked potential monitoring of spinal surgery. *In* Desmedt JE [ed]: Neuromonitoring in Surgery. Amsterdam: Elsevier, 1989;165–173.)

EP monitoring may be performed in these cases in order to detect insufficient spinal cord perfusion or ischemia (due to low distal blood pressure or a malfunction in the bypass) so that the surgeon may increase the blood supply to the spinal cord. If bypass is not performed, EPs can only document the occurrence of ischemia (Fig. 16–24).

Cortical SSEPs following tibial nerve stimulation are monitored as a measure of the functional integrity of the dorsal columns and the spinal cord as a whole. However, the dorsal and ventral columns of the spinal cord have different blood supplies and may be separately affected, as in the anterior spinal artery syndrome.[82] In fact, there are several reports of patients undergoing repair of thoracic aneurysms who experienced motor deficits despite preserved cortical SSEPs. For this reason, MEPs should be monitored in addition to cortical SSEPs to test for the functional integrity of the CST. MEPs following transcranial electrical stimulation should be recorded with an epidural electrode inserted percutaneously into the spinal epidural space.

EVOKED POTENTIALS IN EVALUATION OF PATIENTS WITH SPINAL CORD INJURIES

SSEPs are useful in predicting recovery in patients with spinal cord injuries.[83, 84] However, MEPs are not commonly employed in evaluating patients with spinal cord injuries, because motor cortex stimulation produces paraspinal muscle movements that may compromise the stability of the spine in acute patients. The value of MEPs in predicting recovery of the motor system has not yet been established.

CLASSIFICATION OF SURGICAL MANIPULATIONS BASED ON THEIR EFFECT ON NEURAL TISSUE

The surgical and neuroradiologic manipulations that have been presented may be classified according to their effect on neural tissue—whether the damage they incur is reversible or irreversible. An understanding of the relationship between particular manipulations and the resulting EP changes may clarify the role of EP monitoring in the preservation of neural tissue. This understanding will also allow the neurophysiologist to provide more meaningful feedback to, and to work more closely with, the surgeon or neuroradiologist.

Information that permanent damage has occurred may not be useful to the surgeon in a procedure. However, information that temporary, or reversible, damage has occurred is very useful. This information alerts the surgeon to the fact that critical neural tissue is being manipulated and that continuing that manipulation or performing a permanent version of that manipulation may result in permanent damage.

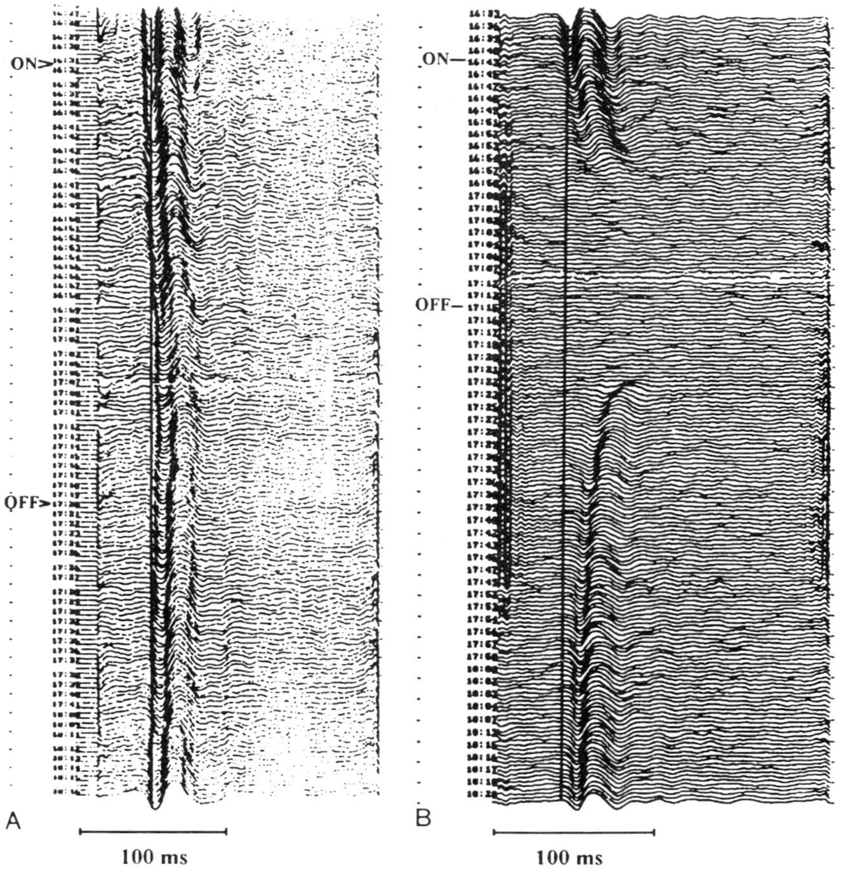

Figure 16–24. *A,* Cortical SEPs after left tibial nerve stimulation during cross clamping of the aorta, with aortal-femoral bypass. When the aorta was clamped and bypass installed at 16:31 (ON), a slow decrease in amplitude and an increase in latency were noted. The EPs showed partial recovery when the clamp was released at 17:20 (OFF). *B,* Cortical SEPs after right tibial nerve stimulation during cross clamping of the aorta without aortal-femoral bypass. Following the aortic clamping at 16:43 (ON), the EPs showed decreased amplitude and increased latency and finally disappeared because of compromised blood flow to the spinal cord. Blood flow was reestablished after the clamp was released at 17:14 (OFF), and the SEPs slowly reappeared. The closing baseline (18:20) showed delayed latency and decreased amplitude. (Vertical lines indicate the latency of peak P1 before the aortic cross clamping. Note that EP changes appear clearer when the figure is observed at an angle of 15°.)

A *provocative* surgical manipulation is one that is always reversible. By noting whether EPs are stable or changed following the manipulation, the surgeon can determine whether it is necessary to reverse the manipulation. If significant EP changes are observed, permanent EP changes may result if the procedure is not reversed. If no EP changes are observed following the manipulation, the manipulation probably was not damaging.

A provocative manipulation can be performed to test the effect of a surgical occlusion of the blood supply to a part of the nervous system. For example, clipping an intracranial artery during a procedure for the repair of cerebral aneurysm may produce reversible ischemia of the cerebral cortex. If the cortical EPs recorded after clipping are significantly depressed, there probably is insufficient collateral blood flow to the cortex, and prolonged clipping will result in neural damage. In this case, the clip would be removed or replaced (Fig. 16–25). However, if no changes are noted, the surgeon may proceed with the knowledge that the cortex is receiving enough blood.

The following procedures utilize provocative manipulations: injection of amobarbital into spinal blood vessels, cross-clamping of the carotid artery, cross-clamping of the intracranial cerebral vessels, insertion of spinal hardware, and positioning the patient with an unstable spine on the operating table.

During neuroradiologic procedures, the incidence of complications from selective spinal angiography and embolization decreased dramatically from over 20% to less than 2%, in part from the introduction of provocative testing using EP monitoring.[4]

A *nonprovocative* manipulation is one that causes permanent damage to neural tissue and irreversible loss of EPs. In these situations, intraoperative monitoring fails to prevent neural damage and does little more than document the time that the lesion occurred. In some cases, however, the surgeon may not know whether the EP changes are temporary or permanent immediately following the manipulation. In this situation, the surgeon should presume that the changes are only temporary and reverse the manipulation if possible. Specific examples of nonprovocative manipulations are cutting of nervous tissue with dissection instruments, coagulation of critical blood vessels, and tissue resection with the ultrasonic aspirator.

Feedback to the surgeon concerning EP changes due to nonprovocative manipulations does not aid the surgeon in reducing neurologic complications in that particular patient. However, the knowledge gained from documenting the time the lesion occurred may be used to correlate specific surgical manipulations with irreversible damage to nervous tissue. Identification of deleterious surgical manipulations may result in an avoidance of these manipulations whenever possible.

Finally, *neurophysiologic mapping* is a procedure in which anatomically indistinct neural structures are identified by their neurophysiologic features so that the surgeon can avoid producing lesions in critical structures during the procedure. This procedure is not a surgical manipulation, in that it is not instrumental in achieving the goals of the surgical procedure. However, the information gained from neurophysiologic mapping allows the surgeon to operate more safely.

The following procedures utilize a neurophysiologic mapping technique: mapping of the sensory motor cortex with phase reversal median nerve SSEP, mapping of the pudendal afferents (DRAP), and intracranial mapping of the motor cranial nerves. The incidence of urinary complications decreased, from 24% to zero after the introduction of

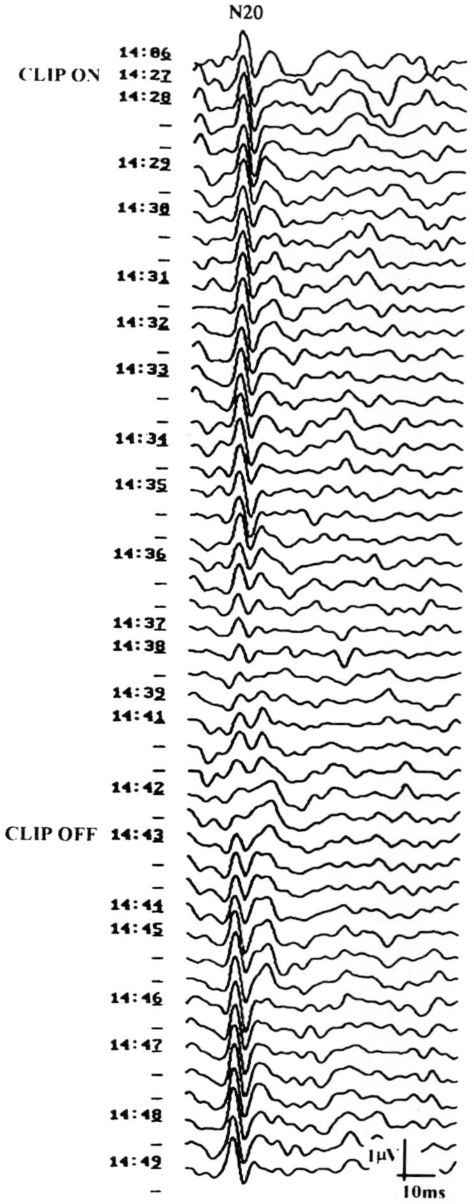

Figure 16–25. CSEPs recorded over the scalp in a 58-year-old patient undergoing surgical repair of a middle cerebral artery aneurysm after left median nerve stimulation. The artery was clipped at 14:27, but the EPs did not deteriorate until approximately 10 minutes later. When the EPs deteriorated further, the surgeon removed the clip, and the EPs recovered.

pudendal nerve mapping in selective dorsal rhizotomy cases, including production of lesions in the S2 root.[46]

Acknowledgment

I express my great appreciation and thankfulness to Miss Ann Demarais, Ph.D., for her critical readings of the text and for using her sharp mind and logic, the result of which was a significant improvement in the presented material.

REFERENCES

1. Chiappa KH: Evoked Potentials in Clinical Medicine, 2nd Ed. New York: Raven Press, 1990.
2. Nuwer M: Evoked Potential Monitoring in the Operating Room. New York: Raven Press, 1986.
3. Emerson RG, Pedley TA: Somatosensory evoked potentials. *In* Daly DD, Pedley TA (eds): Current Practice in Clinical Electroencephalography, 2nd Ed. New York: Raven Press, 1990; 679–705.
4. Young W, Mollin D: Intraoperative somatosensory evoked potentials monitoring of spinal surgery. *In* Desmedt JE (ed): Neuromonitoring in Surgery. Amsterdam: Elsevier, 1989; 165–173.
5. Branston NM, Symon L: Cortical EP, blood flow and potassium changes in experimental ischemia. *In* Barnes C (ed): Evoked Potentials. Baltimore: University Press, 1980; 527–530.
6. Richard CD: The action of general anaesthetics on synaptic transmission in the CNS. Br J Anesth 1983; 55:201–207.
7. Samra SK, Vanderzant CW, Domer PA, Sackellares JC: Differential effects of isoflurane on human median nerve somatosensory evoked potentials. Anesthesiology 1987; 66:29–35.
8. Kimovec MA, Koht A, Sloan TB: Effect of Sufentanil on median nerve somatosensory evoked potentials. Br J Anesth 1990; 65:169–172.
9. Wolfe DE, Drummond JC: Differential effect of isoflurane/nitrous oxide on posterior tibial somatosensory evoked responses of cortical and subcortical origin. Anesth Analg 1988; 67:852–895.
10. Peterson DO, Drummond JC, Todd MM: Effects of halothane, enflurane, isoflurane, and nitrous oxide on somatosensory evoked potentials in humans. Anesthesiology 1986; 65:35–40.
11. Sloan TB, Fugina ML, Toleikis JR: Effects of midazolam on median nerve somatosensory evoked potentials. Br J Anaesth 1990; 64:590–559.
12. Deletis V: Intraoperative monitoring of the functional integrity of the motor pathways. *In* Devinski O, Beric A, Dogali M (eds): Electrical and Magnetic Stimulation of the Brain and Spinal Cord. New York: Raven Press, 1993; 201–214.
13. Lesnick JE, Michele JJ, Simeone FA, et al: Alteration of somatosensory evoked potentials in response to global ischemia. J Neurosurg 1984; 60:490–494.
14. Jones SJ, Howard L, Shawkat F: Criteria for detection and pathological significance of response decrement during spinal cord monitoring. *In* Ducker TB, Brown RH (eds): Neurophysiology and Standards of Spinal Cord Monitoring. New York: Springer-Verlag, 1988; 201–206.
15. Beric A, Dimitrijevic MR, Sharkey PC, Sherwood AM: Cortical potentials evoked by epidural stimulation of the cervical and thoracic spinal cord in man. Electroencephalogr Clin Neurophysiol 1986; 65:102–110.
16. North RB, Drenger B, Beattie C, et al: Monitoring of spinal cord stimulation evoked potentials during thoracoabdominal aneurysm surgery. Neurosurgery 1991; 28:325–330.
17. Rothwell JC: Control of human voluntary movement. Rockville, MD: Aspen, 1987; 158–179.
18. Merton PA, Morton HB, Hill DK, Marsden CD: Scope of a technique for electrical stimulation of human brain, spinal cord and muscle. Lancet 1982; 2:597–600.
19. Burke D, Hicks RG, Stephen JPH: Corticospinal volleys evoked by anodal and cathodal stimulation of the human motor cortex. J Physiol 1990; 425:283–299.
20. Hassan NF, Rossini PM, Cracco RQ, Cracco JB: Unexposed motor cortex activation by low voltage stimuli. *In* Morocutti C, Rizzo PA (eds): Evoked Potentials: Neurophysiological and Clinical Aspects. Amsterdam: Elsevier, 1985; 107–113.
21. Rossini PM, Marciani MG, Caramia M, et al: Nervous propagation along "central" motor pathways in intact man: Characteristics of motor responses to "bifocal" and "unifocal" spine and scalp non-invasive stimulation. Electroencephalogr Clin Neurophysiol 1985; 61:272–286.
22. Penfield W, Boldrey E: Somatic motor and sensory representation in the cerebral cortex of man as studied by electrical stimulation. Brain 1937; 60:389–443.
23. Penfield WG, Rasmussen T: The Cerebral Cortex of Man. A Clinical Study of Localization of Function. New York: Macmillan, 1957.
24. Gregorie EM, Goldring S: Localization of function in the excision of lesions from the sensorimotor region. J Neurosurg 1984; 61:1047–1054.
25. King BR, Schell GR: Cortical localization and monitoring during cerebral operations. J Neurosurg 1987; 67:210–219.
26. Berger MS, Kincaid J, Ojemann GA, Lettich E: Brain mapping techniques to maximize resection, safety, and seizure control in children with brain tumors. Neurosurgery 1989; 25(5):786–792.
27. Luders H, Lesser RP, Dinner DS, et al: Localisation of cortical function: New information from extraoperative monitoring of patients with epilepsy. Epilepsia 1988; 29(Suppl 2):S56–S65.
28. Lesser RP, Gordon B, Fisher R, et al: Subdural grid electrodes in surgery of epilepsy. *In* Luders H (ed): Epilepsy Surgery. New York: Raven Press, 1991; 399–408.
29. Katayama Y, Tsubokawa T, Maejima S, et al: Corticospinal direct response in humans: Identification of the motor cortex during intracranial surgery under general anaesthesia. J Neurol Neurosurg Psychiatry 1988; 51:50–59.
30. Taniguichi M, Cedzich C, Shramm J: Modification of cortical stimulation for motor evoked potentials under general anesthesia: Technical description. Neurosurgery 1993; 32(2):219–226.
31. Barker AT, Freestone IL, Jarratt JA, Jalinous R: Magnetic stimulation of human nervous system: An introduction and basic principles. *In* Chokrovety S (ed): Magnetic Stimulation in Clinical Neurophysiology. Boston: Butterworths, 1990; 55–72.
32. Pascual-Leone A, Gates JR, Dhuna A: Induction of speech arrest and counting errors with rapid-rate transcranial magnetic stimulation. Neurology 1991; 41:697–702.
33. Machida M, Weinstein SL, Yamada T, Kimura J: Spinal cord monitoring—Electrophysiological measures of sensory and motor function during spinal surgery. Spine 1985; 10(5):407–413.
34. Owen JH, Laschinger J, Bridwell K, et al: Sensitivity and specificity of somatosensory and neurogenic-motor evoked potentials in animals and humans. Spine 1988; 13:1111–1118.
35. Kernell D, Wu CP: Responses of the pyramidal tract to stimulation of the baboon's motor cortex. J Physiol 1967; 191:653–672.
36. Hicks RG, Burke D, Stephen JPH: Corticospinal volleys evoked by electrical stimulation of human motor cortex after withdrawal of volatile anesthetics. J Physiol 1992; 456:393–404.
37. Kalkman CJ, Drummond JC, Ribberink AA: Low concentrations of isoflurane abolish motor evoked responses to transcranial electrical stimulation during nitrous oxide/opioid anesthesia in humans. Anesth Analg 1991; 73:410–415.
38. Zentner J, Kiss I, Ebner A: Influence of anesthetics—nitrous oxide in particular—on electromyographic response evoked by transcranial stimulation of the cortex. Neurosurgery 1989; 24:253–256.
39. Kalkman CJ, Drummond JC, Ribberink AA, et al: Effects of propofol, etomidate, midazolam, and fentanyl on motor evoked responses to transcranial electrical or magnetic stimulation in humans. Anesthesiology 1992; 76(4):502–509.
40. Wood CC, Spencer DD, Allison T, et al: Localization of human sensorimotor cortex during surgery by cortical surface recording of somatosensory evoked potentials. J Neurosurg 1988; 68:99–111.
41. Allison T, McCarthy G, Wood CC, et al: Human cortical potentials evoked by stimulation of the median nerve. I. Cytoarchitectonic areas generating short-latency activity. J Neurosurg 1989; 62:694–710.
42. Moller AR, Jannetta PJ: Simultaneous surface and direct brainstem recordings of brainstem auditory evoked potentials (BAEP) in man. *In* Cracco RQ, Bodis-Wollner I (eds): Evoked Potentials. New York: Alan R. Liss, 1986; 227–234.
43. Moller AR: Evoked Potentials in Intraoperative Monitoring. Baltimore: Williams & Wilkins, 1988.
44. Raudzens PA: Intraoperative monitoring of evoked potentials. Ann N Y Acad Sci 1982; 388:308–326.
45. Cedzich C, Schramm J, Mangedoht CF, Fahlbusch R: Factors that limit the use of flash visual evoked potentials for surgical monitoring. Electroencephalogr Clin Neurophysiol 1988; 71:142–145.
46. Deletis V, Vodusek D, Abbott R, et al: Intraoperative monitoring of

the dorsal sacral roots: Minimizing the risk of iatrogenic micturition disorders. Neurosurgery 1992; 30(1):72–75.
47. Deletis V, Vodusek D, Kiprovski K, Morota N: Intraoperative recording of the bulbocavernosus (BCR) reflex [Abstract]. American Academy of Clinical Neurophysiology, San Francisco, 1993.
48. Boyd SG, De Silva LVK: EEG and serum prolactin studies in relation to transcutaneous stimulation of central motor pathways. J Neurol 1986; 49:954–956.
49. Cohen LG, Hallett M: Non-invasive electrical stimulation of the brain does not cause short-term changes in the electroencephalogram. *In* Rossini PM, Marsden CD (eds): Non-Invasive Stimulation of Brain and Spinal Cord. New York: Alan R. Liss, 1988; 159–161.
50. Pitkanen A, Jolkkonen J, Riekkinen P: B-endorphin, somatostatin, and prolactin levels in cerebrospinal fluid of epileptic patients after generalized convulsion. J Neurol Neurosurg Psychiatry 1987; 50:1294–1297.
51. Agnew WF, McCreery DB: Considerations for safety in the use of extracranial stimulation for motor evoked potentials. Neurosurgery 1987; 20:143–147.
52. Barker AT, Freeston IL, Jalinous R, Jarratt JA: Magnetic and electric stimulation of the brain: Safety aspects. *In* Rossini PM, Marsden CD (eds): Non-Invasive Stimulation of Brain and Spinal Cord. New York: Alan R. Liss, 1988; 131–144.
53. Eyre JA, Flecknell PA, Kenyon BR, et al: Acute effect of electromagnetic stimulation of the brain on cortical activity, cortical blood flow, blood pressure and heart rate in the cat: An evaluation of safety. J Neurol Neurosurg Psychiatry 1990; 53:507–513.
54. Thomas S, Merton WL, Boyd SG: Pituitary hormones in relation to magnetic stimulation of the brain. J Neurol Neurosurg Psychiatry 1991; 54(1):89–90.
55. Hufnagel A, Elger CE: Induction of seizures by transcranial magnetic stimulation in epileptic patients. J Neurol 1991; 238:109–110.
56. Kandler R: Safety of transcranial magnetic stimulation. Lancet 1990; 335:469–470.
57. Homberg V, Netz J: Generalized seizures induced by transcranial magnetic stimulation of motor cortex. Lancet 1989; 2:1223.
58. Fauth C, Meyer B-U, Prosiegel M, et al: Seizure induction and magnetic brain stimulation after stroke. Lancet 1992; 339:362.
59. Counter SA, Borg E, Lofquist L: Acoustic trauma in extracranial magnetic brain stimulation. Electroencephalogr Clin Neurophysiol 1991; 78:173–184.
60. Pascual-Leone A, Cochen LG, Shotland LI, et al: No evidence of hearing loss in humans due to transcranial magnetic stimulation. Neurology 1992; 42(3):647–651.
61. Gordon B, Lesser R, Rance NE, et al: Parameters for direct cortical stimulation in the human: Histopathologic confirmation. Electroencephalogr Clin Neurophysiol 1990; 75:371–377.
62. Dhuna A, Gates JR, Pascual-Leone A: Transcranial magnetic stimulation in patient with epilepsy. Neurology 1991; 41:1067–1071.
63. Pascual-Leone A, Valls-Sole J, Brasil-Neto JP, et al: Seizure induction and transcranial magnetic stimulation. Lancet 1992, 339:997.
64. Pascual-Leone A, Dhuna A, Roth BJ, et al: Risk of burns during rapid-rate magnetic stimulation in presence of electrode. Lancet 1990; 336:1195–1196.
65. Bricolo A, Turazzi S, Faccioli F, et al: Clinical application of compressed spectral array in long-term EEG monitoring of comatose patients. Electroencephalogr Clin Neurophysiol 1978; 45:211–225.
66. Hume AL, Cant BR, Shaw NA: Central somatosensory conduction time in comatose patients. Ann Neurol 1979; 5:379–384.
67. Tsubokawa T, Yamamoto T, Katayama Y: Prediction of outcome of prolonged coma caused by brain damage. Brain Injury 1990; 4:329–337.
68. Greenberg RP, Mayer DJ, Becker DP: Evaluation of brain function in severe human head trauma with multimodality evoked potentials. Part 1: Evoked brain injury potentials, methods and analysis. J Neurosurg 1977; 47:150–162.
69. Greenberg RP, Becker DP, Miller JD, Mayer DJ: Evaluation of brain function in severe human head trauma with multimodality evoked potentials. Part 2: Localization of brain dysfunction and correlation with posttraumatic neurological conditions. J Neurosurg 1977; 47:163–177.
70. Ebner A, Zentner J: Prognostic value of somatosensory and motor evoked potentials in comatose patients with severe head injury. *In* Rossini P, Marsden C (eds): Noninvasive stimulation of brain and spinal cord. New York: Alan R. Liss, 1988; 313–319.
71. Facco E, Baratto F, Munari M, et al: Sensorimotor central conduction time in comatose patients. Electroencephalogr Clin Neurophysiol 1991; 80:469–476.
72. Deletis V, Simunovic V, Ransohoff J: Neurophysiologic evaluation. *In* Sandel E, Ellis DW (eds): The Coma-Emerging Patient. Philadelphia: Hanley & Belfus, 1990; 421–432.
73. Coooper PR, Epstein F: Radical resection of intramedullary spinal cord tumors in adults. J Neurosurg 1985; 63:492–499.
74. Epstein F, McCleary EL: Intrinsic brain-stem tumors of childhood: Surgical indications. J Neurosurg 1986; 64:11–15.
75. Little JR, Lesser RP, Luders H: Electrophysiological monitoring during basilar aneurysm operation. Neurosurgery 1987; 20:421–427.
76. Haupt WF, Horsch S: Evoked potential monitoring in carotid surgery: A review of 994 cases. Neurology 1992; 42:835–838.
77. Chiappa KH, Burke SR, Young RR: Results of electroencephalographic monitoring during 367 carotid endarterectomies. Stroke 1979; 10:381–388.
78. Engler GL, Spielholz NI, Bernhard WN, et al: Somatosensory evoked potentials during Harrington instrumentation for scoliosis. J Bone Joint Surg 1978; 68(4):528–532.
79. Lesser RP, Raudzens P, Luders H, et al: Postoperative neurological deficits may occur despite unchanged intraoperative somatosensory evoked potentials. Ann Neurol 1986; 19:22–25.
80. Berenstein A, Young W, Ransohoff J, et al: Somatosensory evoked potentials during spinal angiography and therapeutic transvascular embolization. J Neurosurg 1984; 60:777–785.
81. Young W, Berenstein A: Somatosensory evoked potential monitoring of intraoperative procedures. *In* Schramm J, Jones SJ (eds): Spinal Cord Monitoring. Heidelberg: Springer-Verlag, 1985; 197–212.
82. Zornov MH, Grafe MR, Tybor C, Swenson R: Preservation of evoked potentials in a case of anterior artery syndrome. Electroencephalogr Clin Neurophysiol 1990; 77:133–139.
83. Young W: Somatosensory evoked potentials (SEPs) in spinal cord injury. *In* Schramm J, Jones SJ (eds): Spinal Cord Monitoring. Heidelberg: Springer-Verlag, 1985; 127–142.
84. Young W, Mollin D: Somatosensory evoked potentials in chronic spinal cord injury: An update. *In* Ducker TB, Brown RH (eds): Neurophysiology and Standards of Spinal Cord Monitoring. New York: Springer-Verlag, 1988; 277–288.

CHAPTER

17

Monitoring Peripheral Nervous System Function

STUART C. LAW, M.D. and D. RYAN COOK, M.D.

Neuromuscular blocking drugs (NBD) are administered in nearly three quarters of general anesthetics in order to facilitate endotracheal intubation, control of mechanical ventilation, and surgery.[1] Despite their widespread use, use of these agents is not without risk.

In 1954, Beecher and Todd conducted a retrospective study of 599,548 patients and showed a six-fold increased mortality rate when an NBD had been used.[2] Even though this study has been criticized, it nonetheless pointed out the need for increased diligence when using these agents. Over 25 years have passed since Beecher and Todd's study and Churchill-Davidson and Christie's proposal to use nerve stimulators to monitor neuromuscular blockade.[3] Several studies, however, have shown that neuromuscular blockers are still administered without nerve stimulators and that many patients have significant degrees of neuromuscular block in the immediate postoperative period. Viby-Mogensen and colleagues demonstrated that patients receiving NBDs had a 42% incidence of residual neuromuscular blockade on arrival in the recovery room.[4] Other studies have shown a 21–25% incidence.[5,6]

Two general problems are encountered each time neuromuscular blockade is performed. The proper dose of drug and antagonist must be determined, and residual blockade must be evaluated in the operating room and in the recovery room. It is impossible to accurately predict the response of a given patient to an NBD based solely on pharmacokinetic data. Katz has demonstrated the marked individual variability in response to d-tubocurarine.[7] A dose of 0.1 mg/kg produced no demonstrable blockade in 6% of patients, whereas 7% of the patients developed complete blockade.[7] There may be as much as a four-fold difference in the serum concentration of an NBD required to produce a given degree of relaxation in different patients.[8]

In addition to the normal wide variability in response to relaxants, many other factors are known to influence neuromuscular blockade. Temperature, plasma pH, plasma protein concentration, age, and coexisting disease, including renal and hepatic function, affect the response to relaxants. The concomitant administration of a variety of drugs may also alter the response to relaxants. Even in a single patient, changing physiologic parameters may alter the dose-response relationship.

THE NEUROMUSCULAR JUNCTION

ANATOMY

The motor unit is composed of a motor neuron and a group of muscle fibers to which it branches. The interface between the nerves and the muscle fibers is called the neuromuscular junction (NMJ). Motor neurons are single cells that extend, uninterrupted, from the ventral horn of the spinal cord to the muscle. After entering the muscle, they branch and send unmyelinated axons to individual muscle fibers. In most muscles, there is only one NMJ. The extraoccular muscles of the eye, however, have multiple NMJs and, unlike other muscles, contract in response to depolarizing relaxants. The NMJ is required to amplify the electrical impulse in nerve fibers in order to depolarize the relatively large muscle fibers.

The NMJ consists of a nerve terminal and a specialized area of the muscle fiber known as the motor end-plate. The nerve terminal is an unmyelinated extension of the axon that has an abundance of mitochondria and 300-Å spheres, called vesicles, which contain acetylcholine (ACh), adenosine triphosphate, calcium, choline, and a variety of lipids and proteins.[9] The motor end-plate is contiguous with the muscle fiber membrane and features extensive infoldings that contain concentrated amounts of acetylcholinesterase.[10] The nerve terminal and motor end-plate are separated by a distance of 500 Å. The motor end-plate is literally paved with ACh receptors at a density of 10,000–20,000/μm (Fig. 17–1).[2,11] Electron micrographs have demonstrated specialized areas of the terminal axon membrane, called active

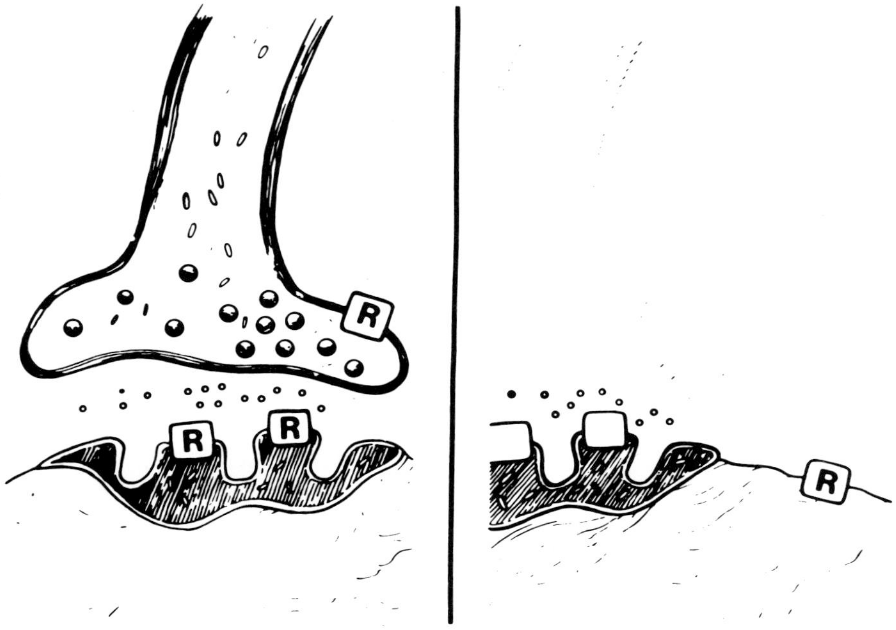

Figure 17–1. *Left,* The anatomy of the normal neuromuscular junction includes the motor nerve containing vesicles of acetylcholine, which diffuse across the junction to activate receptors (R) on the postjunctional membrane of the skeletal muscle. *Right,* The denervated muscle junction with extrajunctional receptors. (From Standaert FG: Donuts and holes: Molecules and muscle relaxants. *In* Katz RL [ed]: Muscle Relaxants. Basic and Clinical Aspects. Orlando, FL: Grune & Stratton, 1985; 2, with permission. See also Semin Anesth 1984; 3:4.)

zones, that face invaginations of postsynaptic folds on the outside and feature a twin row of 20–30 synaptic vesicles on the inside. There are 500–1000 zones per terminal (Fig. 17–2).[12]

PHYSIOLOGY

ACh, Synthesis, Storage, and Release

Synthesis and Storage

ACh is synthesized in the axon terminal of the motor nerve from acetylcoenzyme A (AcCoA) and choline by the enzyme choline-O-acetyltransferase, which is synthesized in the motor neuron cell body and transported to the nerve terminal (Fig. 17–3). AcCoA is derived from pyruvate, which in turn is a product of glycolysis. Hydrolysis of ACh and dietary intake provide choline, which is actively transported into the cell.[13] Muscle fibers are also known to produce ACh, probably through the enzyme carnitine acetyltransferase.[14] The rate of ACh synthesis and choline uptake increases with impulse activity of the axon terminal.[15] About 50% of the ACh within the neuron terminal is free in the cytosol, whereas the other 50% is in vesicles.[10] Each

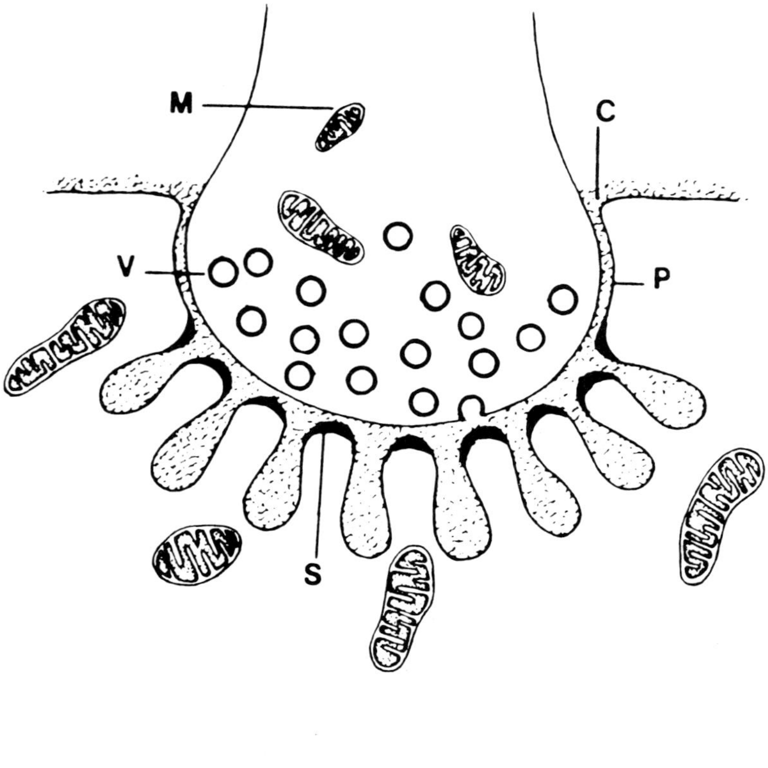

Figure 17–2. Microscopic anatomy of the neuromuscular junction showing the twin row of 20–30 synaptic vesicles on the inside of the nerve ending, which face the invaginations of the postsynaptic folds in the "active zones." (M = mitochondria, V = vesicles, P = postjunctional membrane, S = synaptic fold, C; eq synaptic cleft. (From Maclean IC: Neuromuscular function. *In* Johnson EW [ed]: Practical Electromyography. Baltimore: Williams & Wilkins, 1980; 75, with permission.)

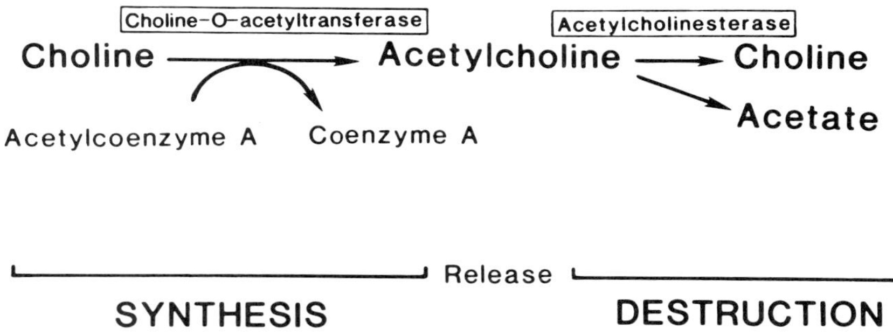

Figure 17–3. Acetycholine is synthesized in the motor nerve terminal from choline and acetyl coenzyme A by the enzyme choline-O-acetyltransferase. It is degraded by acetylcholinesterase to choline and acetate. (From Durant NN: The physiology of neuromuscular transmission. *In* Katz RL [ed]: Muscle Relaxants. Basic and Clinical Aspects. Orlando, FL: Grune & Stratton, 1985; 24, with permission. See also Semin Anesth 1984; 3:4.)

vesicle contains approximately 5000–10,000 molecules of ACh.[16]

Release of ACh

Role of Calcium. Stimulation of a motor neuron causes voltage-responsive ion channels to propagate an action potential down the axon to the nerve terminal. Nerve terminals, however, lack Na^+ channels and cannot generate an action potential.[17] Depolarization is spread through the nerve terminal by cable conduction and causes voltage-sensitive calcium channels to open. The resulting flux of calcium ions into the terminal initiates ACh release. The released ACh molecules cross the synaptic cleft and bind to ACh receptors. The ACh-bound receptors open channels that allow ionic flux to depolarize the motor end-plate and generate an end-plate potential (EPP). The EPP is conducted to the surrounding membrane where it triggers opening of voltage-sensitive channels and thereby generates a muscle fiber action potential that is transmitted through the T tubule system to initiate contraction. Calcium channels close in response to terminal repolarization induced by an outward potassium current. Thesleff suggests that these voltage-dependent calcium channels may exist exclusively at the active zones.[12]

The mechanism by which calcium promotes the release of ACh at the active zones is not known. It is known, however, that calcium is required for quantal release of ACh. Without Ca^{2+} the nerve terminal can depolarize, but no quantal ACh release occurs.[18] Agents that block potassium channels, such as 4-aminopyridine, prolong the influx of calcium and thereby increase calcium-mediated ACh release. Other mediators of ACh release have been identified. Calcium and magnesium ions have opposite actions. Magnesium has been shown to decrease the number of quanta released in response to an action potential.[19]

Quantal Theory. Quantal release implies that ACh is released from the nerve terminals in discrete packets of a uniform size called a quantum. Each quantum contains 5000–10,000 ACh molecules.[20] Spontaneous release of a quantum of ACh produces a postsynaptic voltage potential change called a miniature end-plate potential (MEPP). Neurally evoked ACh release produces an EPP that is actually a summation of many MEPPs. The vesicular hypothesis was developed to incorporate the observance of nerve terminal vesicles into the quantal theory. The central theme of this hypothesis is that ACh is stored in vesicles and is released into the synaptic cleft. Spontaneous discharge of a single vesicle produces an MEPP, whereas the neurally evoked release of many vesicles produces an EPP. The EPP after nerve terminal depolarization consists of a summation of several hundred quanta.[9] Unfortunately, the actual mechanism for ACh release appears to be more complicated than the vesicle hypothesis suggests. There now appear to be at least three different mechanisms of ACh release into the synaptic cleft (Table 17–1). There is, at present, debate regarding the validity of the vesicular hypothesis (Table 17–2).

Receptor Types

Three populations of nicotinic ACh receptors are involved with neuromuscular transmission. They are classified according to their location as prejunctional, postjunctional, or extrajunctional (see Fig. 17–1).

Prejunctional Receptors

The prejunctional receptors are located in the membrane of the nerve terminal and modulate ACh mobilization and release. They have different binding characteristics and possibly different channel characteristics than the postjunctional receptors do.[20] Antagonism of this receptor results in diminished ACh release from neurons stimulated at high frequency. These nicotinic receptors increase ACh mobilization to readily releasable stores and provide feedback control during high-frequency stimulation.

TABLE 17–1. DIFFERENT TYPES OF ACh RELEASE

Calcium-Mediated Quantal Release
- Responsible for neurally evoked transmission[9]
- Quantal release may be a summation of MEPP size discharges, which may in turn consist of smaller subunits[9]

Quantal Release That Is Not Calcium-Mediated
- Consists of events larger than MEPPS, referred to as giant MEPPS
- Unaffected by nerve terminal depolarization or by presynaptic calcium fluxes[22]

Nonquantal Leakage
- May account for 99% of the ACh in the synaptic cleft
- Does not appear to be involved with the process of neurally evoked transmission[23]

TABLE 17–2. VALIDITY OF THE VESICLE HYPOTHESIS

Factors in Favor of the Vesicular Hypothesis:
- Vesicles contain an amount of ACh that corresponds to a MEPP.
- Rapid-freeze techniques show that depolarization results in the appearance of pits in the membrane that seem to be associated with vesicles.
- The transmembrane potential does not influence the amount of ACh released as would be expected if ACh was transported through a gate mechanism.
- Osmotically induced changes in the nerve terminal volume and a corresponding decrease in cytosolic ACh concentration do not alter ACh release.

Factors Against:
- Newly synthesized ACh is released preferentially by nerve stimulation.[50] Newly synthesized ACh is found in the cytoplasm but not in the vesicles.[9]
- The number of vesicles is not altered by physiologic levels of stimulation, whereas cytoplasmic free ACh is depleted.[9]
- Vesicles contain both ACh and ATP. The ACh /ATP ratio within vesicles differs from the ratio observed within the synapse after stimulation.[9]
- Stimulation depletes cytoplasmic stores of ACh in the same amount released during depolarization, whereas the vesicular content does not change.[11]

Postjunctional Receptors

Postjunctional receptors are packed into the end-plate region at a density of 10,000–20,000/m^2.[11] The receptor consists of five subunits ranging from 40,000–65,000 daltons. There are two alpha subunits (45,000 daltons), both of which must be bound by ACh in order to initiate channel opening and the resultant flux of Na^+, K^+, and Ca^{2+} ions.[21]

Extrajunctional Receptors

The extrajunctional receptors are located in the muscle fiber membrane outside of the motor end-plate region. They respond to agonists by allowing ionic flow to occur, as do the other ACh receptors. They are not capable of producing an action potential, because their density is insufficient to allow the development of threshold EPP. A deficiency of neural stimulation (as after spinal cord injuries) may initiate the production of these extrajunctional receptors. Although the density of these receptors is low, the absolute numbers may be very high. It is postulated that the receptors bind to agonists quite avidly and allow for ionic flux, resulting in the well-described increase in potassium after administration of succinylcholine chloride.[22–24]

Impulse Formation

Neurons, muscle fibers, and most other living cells maintain ionic gradients across their membranes. Energy-requiring pump mechanisms transport Na^+ into and K^+ ions out of the cell while producing a voltage gradient of −70 to −90 mV. The K^+ ions are able to slowly leak back out along the concentration gradient and thus leave the inside of the cell negatively charged with respect to the outer membrane.[25] The membrane possesses voltage-gated channels that allow rapid ionic flux to occur if the membrane is depolarized beyond a threshold value.[26] Thus, an electric current sufficient in amplitude to depolarize a motor neuron membrane to more than −50 mV triggers a propagated wave of depolarization. When this impulse reaches the nerve terminal, it must be transmitted across the synaptic cleft to the muscle fiber that it supplies. This is accomplished by the transmitter ACh. Its effect is terminated rapidly as ACh is enzymatically degraded by acetylcholinesterase (see Fig. 17–2).

NEUROMUSCULAR BLOCKERS

Neuromuscular blockers currently in clinical use are described as either depolarizing or nondepolarizing, depending on their effect on the motor end-plate. A thorough review of the relaxant-receptor interaction has been done by Standaert.[21]

DEPOLARIZING BLOCKADE

Succinylcholine is the most common nondepolarizing relaxant. It is unusual in that it produces two different types of block: phase 1 and phase 2.

Phase 1 Block

During phase 1, succinylcholine chloride binds to ACh receptors and causes membrane ionic channels to open in the same fashion as ACh does. The molecules remain bound to the receptor for an extended period and cause the membrane to remain depolarized and unable to trigger any further muscle action potentials. Characteristics of phase 1 block include (1) muscle fasciculation prior to onset of block, (2) absence of fade with fast or slow stimulation, including train-of-four (TOF) stimulation and tetanus, (3) absence of post-tetanic facilitation, (4) antagonism by prior administration of a nondepolarizing relaxant, (5) potentiation by other depolarizing agents,[27] and (6) absence of tachyphylaxis.

Phase 2 Block

With prolonged exposures and doses of 2–5 mg/kg, a succinylcholine-induced block assumes the characteristics of a nondepolarizing block and is referred to as phase 2, desensitization, or dual block.[28–31] As phase 2 block develops, fade is seen with both tetanus and TOF stimulation. The TOF ratio decreases to 0.3–0.4.[28] Additional doses of succinylcholine chloride demonstrate tachyphylaxis and even reversal of the block (Fig. 17–4).[32] Phase 2 block may be more likely to develop in the presence of potent inhalation agents than during nitrous oxide narcotic anesthesia.[33] Characteristics of a phase 2 block include (1) fade with tetanic or TOF stimulation, (2) post-tetanic facilitation, (3) antagonism with anticholinesterase agents, and (4) diminished response after repeated doses (tachyphylaxis).

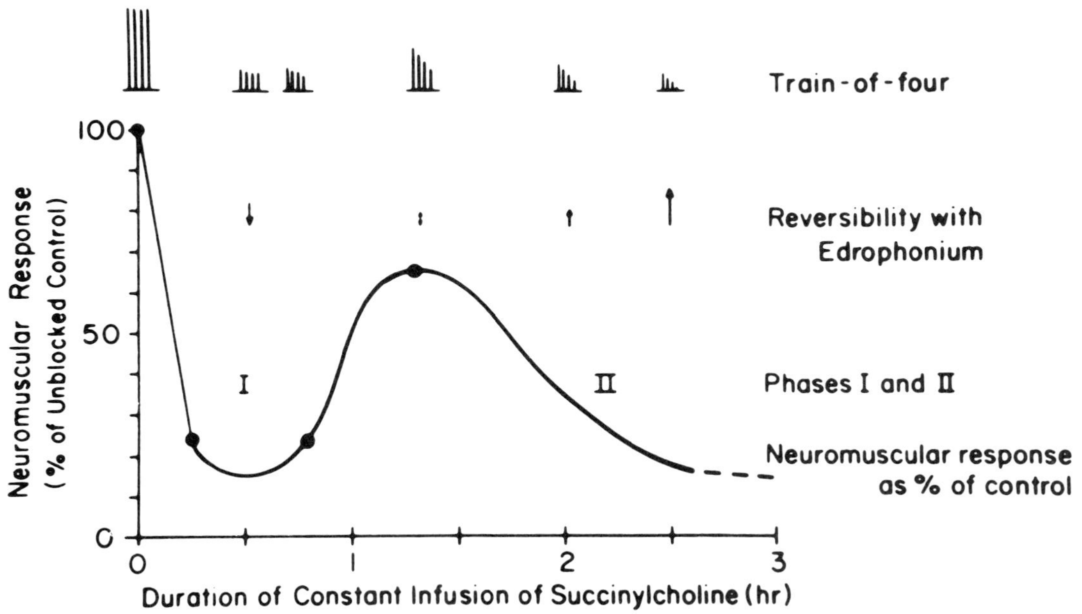

Figure 17–4. During continuous infusion of succinylcholine, a phase 1 block—characterized by reduced neuromuscular response, little fade on train-of-four, and increased blockade with edrophonium—is seen initially. During phase 2, there is fade on train-of-four, increasing reversibility of the block by edrophonium, and accumulation of the slowly recovering residual block. (From Lee C: Succinylcholine: Its past, present, and future. *In* Katz RL [ed]: Muscle Relaxants. Basic and Clinical Aspects. Orlando, FL: Grune & Stratton, 1985; 78, with permission. See also Semin Anesth 1984; 3:4.)

Reversal of Phase 2 Block

Phase 2 block, produced by 5 mg/kg succinylcholine chloride given over a period of more than 90 minutes, can be antagonized by neostigmine. The infusion must be stopped 10 minutes prior to the neostigmine in order to allow circulating succinylcholine levels to diminish and thus terminate phase 1 block.[34] Furthermore, a 90% block produced by succinylcholine chloride after development of phase 2 can be reversed with neostigmine more rapidly than a 90% pancuronium bromide–induced block.[34, 35]

NONDEPOLARIZING BLOCKADE

This type of block is produced by d-tubocurarine chloride, pancuronium bromide, metocurine iodide, atracurium besylate, gallamine triethiodide, vecuronium bromide, mivacurium chloride, pipecuronium bromide, and doxacurium chloride. All these agents bind to the alpha subunits of the ACh receptor or physically block the ion channel in the motor end-plate. Some agents cause direct physical blockade of channels. This effect is more common at high concentrations of relaxant in the synaptic cleft. Characteristics of nondepolarizing blockade include (1) absence of fasciculations, (2) fade with rapid stimulation, (3) post-tetanic facilitation, and (4) antagonism by anticholinesterase drugs.

RECEPTOR FUNCTION

Administration of nondepolarizing NBDs diminishes the peak tension developed in response to neural stimulation. Besides this diminution in tension, there is also a phenomenon called fade. When tetanic stimulation or stimulation greater than 0.1 Hz is applied to a motor neuron, the developed motor tension progressively decreases (fades). At present, it is thought that these two phenomena, diminished tension and fade, are the result of postjunctional and prejunctional receptor blockade, respectively (Table 17–3). These observations indicate that depression of twitch and peak tetanic tension differ from fade of TOF or tetanus in that they are the result of ACh receptor antagonists acting at different sites. It is thought that prejunctional receptor

TABLE 17–3. EVIDENCE SUPPORTING PREJUNCTIONAL ETIOLOGY FOR FADE

- The motor end-plate response to ACh does not change during rapid stimulation that causes fade.[24]
- d-Tubocurarine causes progressive decline in ACh release during high-frequency stimulation.[24]
- Postjunctional blockers erabutoxin or alpha-bungarotoxin decrease twitch tension without fade of TOF or tetanus.[24]
- The onset and recovery of fade and twitch depression have differing pharmacokinetics.*
- Pancuronium bromide, primarily a postjunctional blocker, may not cause much tetanic fade.†

*Powers SF, Jones RM: Relationship between single twitch depression and train-of-four fade: Influence of relaxant dose during onset and spontaneous offset of neuromuscular blockade. Anesth Analg 1987; 66:633–636; and Pearce AC, Casson WR, Jones RM: Factors affecting train-of-four fade. Br J Anaesth 1985; 57:602–606.

†Cashman JN, Jones RM, Vella LM: Fade characteristics and onset times following administration of pancuronium, tubocurarine and a mixture of both agents. Br J Anaesth 1985; 57:488–492; and Stanec A, Baker T: Prejunctional and postjunctional effects of the tubocurarine and pancuronium in man. Br J Anaesth 1984; 56:607–611.

antagonists prevent these receptors from promoting ACh synthesis and mobilization.[24] Postjunctional effects can be measured by single twitch, peak tetanic tension, or the first twitch in a TOF. Prejunctional effects are evaluated by the T-1/T-4 ratio and by tetanic fade.

EVALUATION OF NEUROMUSCULAR BLOCKADE

CLINICAL CRITERIA VERSUS EVOKED RESPONSES

Neuromuscular blockade is frequently evaluated purely on the basis of clinical impression. Doses of relaxants are selected empirically, and clinical cues such as gross movement and muscle tone are used to determine subsequent doses of NBD. Postoperatively, the evaluation of neuromuscular blockade is based on observation of various volitional motor responses of the awake patient.

Clinical criteria commonly used to indicate adequate recovery of neuromuscular function are listed in Table 17–4. These criteria represent a variety of ways in which the integrity of the NMJ can be evaluated during stress. Such methods are imprecise and nonrigorous, and they cannot be used to evaluate the anesthetized patient. They usually do not compare the response after antagonism of neuromuscular blockade to a measured preoperative control. For example, the majority of patients can perform a head lift for much longer than 5 seconds preoperatively; hence, the ability to do this for only 5 seconds postoperatively does not indicate a return to baseline. Viby-Mogensen and colleagues demonstrated that 28% of patients evaluated in the recovery room were able to sustain a 5-second head lift but still had evidence of residual blockade using TOF.[4] The head lift test was useful only as a gross indicator of residual blockade, because no patient with a TOF ratio < 0.40 was able to perform the test.[4]

More recent studies have confirmed these findings.[5, 6] Russell and Serle evaluated hand grip as an indicator of residual blockade.[36] They used a hydraulic hand dynamometer to establish a preanesthetic baseline, and they showed that patients able to sustain head lift for 5 seconds had a mean hand grip strength about 29% of preoperative baseline as compared with hand grip strength of 77% in those patients who had not received muscle relaxants. Half the patients who could perform a 5-second head lift had less than 25% of baseline hand grip strength. This study shows that the lack of sensitivity demonstrated by the usual clinical tests is primarily due to failure to obtain an accurate baseline measurement. Although it is clear that individual bedside tests of neuromuscular function are insensitive, there are no studies evaluating the ability of experienced clinicians using a variety of examinations to detect residual blockade.

TABLE 17–4. CLINICAL CRITERIA FOR ADEQUACY OF NEUROMUSCULAR TRANSMISSION

Head lift for 5 seconds[42, 113]
Sustained hand grasp[39, 113]
Absence of nystagmus/diplopia[42]
Coordinated breathing pattern
Wide opening of the eyes[113]
Normal voice
Coordinated swallowing[113]
Tongue protrusion[113]
Normal abdominal and sternocleidomastoid tone
Negative inspiratory force of at least -55 cmH_2O (adults), -32 cmH_2O (children)*
Vital capacity of 15 ml/kg[113]
Sustained leg lifting*
Sustained arm lift (45 seconds)[49]

*Mason LJ, Betts EK: Leg lift and maximum inspiratory force, clinical signs of neuromuscular blockade reversal in neonates and infants. Anesthesiology 1980; 52:441–442.

TABLE 17–5. COMMONLY UTILIZED PERIPHERAL NERVES

Nerve	Location	Movement Observed
Ulnar	Wrist or elbow	Thumb adduction Fifth digit movement
Posterior tibial	Posterior to the medial malleolus	Plantar flexion of the big toe
Peroneal	Lateral to the neck of the fibula	Foot dorsiflexion
Facial	Near the earlobe where the nerve emerges from the stylomastoid foramen	Orbicularis oculi contraction
Mandibular	At the condyle and ramus angle	Jaw closure

EVOKED RESPONSES

The most reliable method for evaluating recovery from neuromuscular blocking agents is to stimulate a peripheral motor nerve and evaluate the resultant motor response. The first step in the process is accomplished by delivering electrical impulses to a superficial motor nerve. Motor responses to electrical stimuli are determined by (1) the contractile state of the muscle (electromyogram [EMG] excluded), (2) the functional state of the NMJ, (3) the site of stimulation, (4) electrical stimuli characteristics (duration, intensity, waveform), and (5) the pattern of frequency of stimulation (single twitch, tetanus, TOF, post-tetanic).

Site of Stimulation

Although any motor nerve can be stimulated, it is best to use a nerve that is close to the skin surface (readily accessible to the anesthesiologist) and a muscle whose action is easily monitored. Common monitoring sites are listed in Table 17–5. The adductor pollicis is a deep muscle, the major portion of which is covered dorsally by the first dorsal interosseous muscle; its palmar aspect is partially covered by the flexor pollicis brevis and the first lumbrical. The ulnar nerve–adductor pollicis muscle is a particularly useful nerve-muscle unit, because stimulation over the ulnar

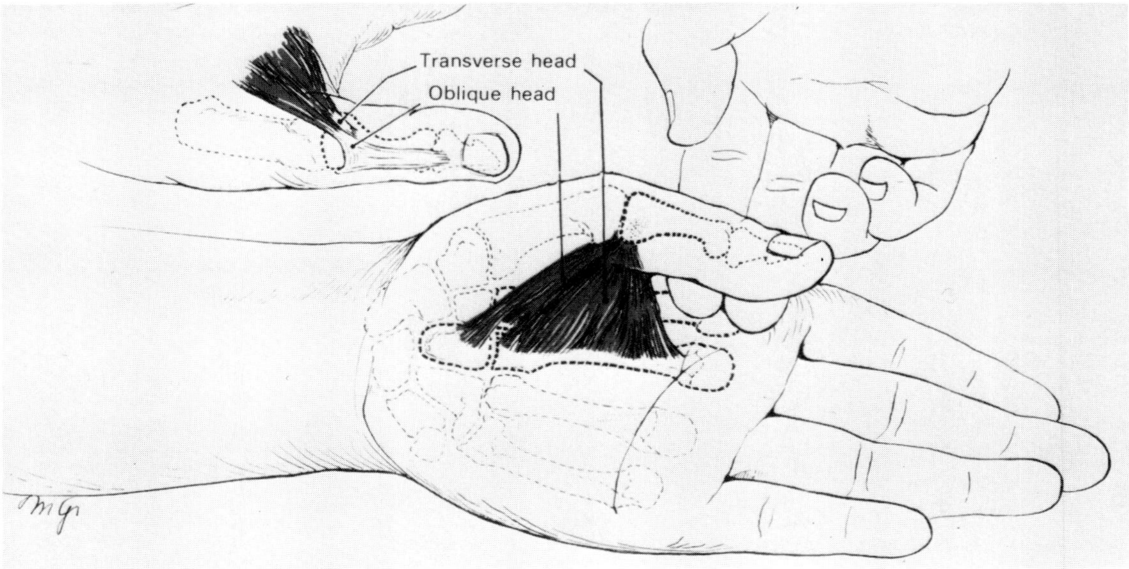

Figure 17–5. The adductor pollicis muscle of the thumb, innervated by the ulnar nerve, is a convenient site for monitoring neuromuscular blockade. (From Kendall FP, McCreary ER: Muscles Testing and Function. Baltimore: Williams & Wilkins, 1983; 61, with permission.)

nerve can cause thumb movement only by transmission through the nerve and not by direct muscle stimulation (Fig. 17–5; Table 17–6). In contrast, movement of the finger can result from either depolarization of the ulnar nerve or from direct depolarization of the forearm flexors that lie underneath the stimulating electrodes.

The response to NBDs varies somewhat with the nerve-motor unit being monitored. The facial nerve, for example, is relatively resistant to NBDs and tends to underestimate the degree of relaxation.[37] Caffrey and coworkers compared twitches in the thumb with orbicularis oculi twitch using force transducers.[38] They noted that during recovery from atracurium, four facial twitches could be present before the thumb had recovered a single twitch of the TOF! By measuring transdiaphragmatic pressures during bilateral phrenic nerve stimulation, Chauvin and coworkers showed that vecuronium bromide–induced block had more rapid onset and offset of blockade in the diaphragm than the adductor pollicis (1.6 minutes versus 2.5 minutes).[39] Despite having a shorter onset time, several studies have demonstrated that the diaphragm is only about 50% as sensitive to NBDs as is the adductor pollicis.[37, 40–42]

TABLE 17–6. HAND MUSCLES SUPPLIED BY THE ULNAR NERVE

Abductor digiti minimi
Adductor pollicis
Dorsal and palmar interossei
Flexor digiti minimi
Flexor pollicis brevis (deep head)
Lumbricales 3 and 4
Opponens digiti minimi
Palmaris brevis

Characteristics of Electrical Stimuli

Motor responses are evoked by stimulating peripheral nerves with electrical impulses. The physical characteristics of electrical stimuli will influence the motor responses that they evoke. As a result, there are standard methods of stimulating peripheral nerves.

Supramaximal

The stimulation current required to trigger an action potential varies between nerves in a given bundle. As stimulation current is increased, the number of nerves reaching the threshold increases until all the nerves are responding (Fig. 17–6). Once the threshold has been reached for a given nerve, it depolarizes and releases ACh at the motor end-plates of all the muscle fibers it supplies. In the absence of neuromuscular blockers, motor end-plate depolarization induces these muscle fibers to contract in an all-or-none fashion. In theory, a plateau is reached at which further increments in stimulating current will not increase motor response. If all the neurons are being depolarized, any subsequent changes in motor response result from effects at the NMJ or from changes in contractility. It is usual practice to stimulate at *supra*maximum currents, 25–50% greater than that required to elicit maximum response.[43] This ensures that despite alterations in electrode impedance or position, all neurons in the bundle are depolarized.

Duration and Waveform

Pulses greater than 0.2–0.3 m/second that are not square waves may exceed the nerve refractory period, thereby causing repetitive firing.[44, 45]

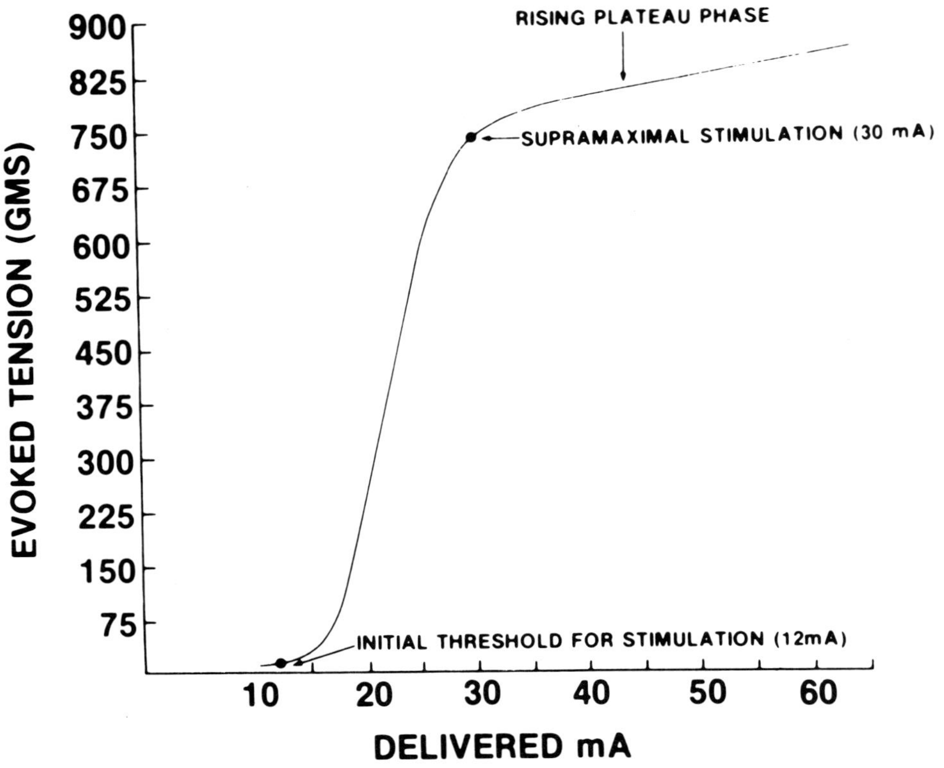

Figure 17–6. The evoked tension of the muscle varies with the stimulating current. As current increases, the number of nerves reaching threshold increases until all are responding. After all nerves have reached threshold, further increases in current fail to increase the motor response (plateau). Supramaximal currents are used to ensure depolarization of all neurons. (From Kopman EA, et al: Milliamperage requirements for supramaximal stimulation of the ulnar nerve with surface electrodes. Anesthesiology 1984; 61:84, with permission.)

Patterns of Stimulation

There are five methods in which individual, supramaximal, 0.1- to 0.2-msec square wave impulses are used clinically: single twitch, TOF, tetanic, post-tetanic single twitch, and double burst. It is important to understand the basis for their use and their individual limitations in clinical practice.

Single Twitch

The simplest pattern of stimulation is the single twitch. The degree of relaxation is determined by dividing the measured elicited response (T_1) by the control response (Tc). Recovery from relaxants is sometimes measured by the recovery index or interval between 25% and 75% recovery.

Frequency. In the presence of NBDs, high-frequency neural stimulation results in a progressive decline in the amount of ACh released from the motor neuron terminals.[46, 47] In the absence of NBDs, no decrement in response is observed below frequencies of 50 Hz because of the margin of safety afforded by the NMJ.[48, 49] When a nondepolarizing NBD is administered, prejunctional effects greatly decrease the amount of ACh released. As a result, the motor response to single stimuli exceeding 0.15 Hz (1 twitch/7–10 seconds) declines to a baseline that is less than the initial response and represents an equilibrium between ACh liberation and synthesis.[50, 51] Thus, rapid stimulation rates potentiate the NBD-induced stress of the NMJ.

Without neuromuscular block, a response that has been conditioned (conditioning means a stimulation occurring in the 10-second interval preceding the measured response) by a preceding response less than 10 seconds earlier has an increased amplitude. In the presence of a nondepolarizing relaxant, however, the second response is reduced.[51] Ali and Savarese demonstrated that as stimulation frequency is increased, the apparent dose-response curve to d-tubocurarine is shifted to the left.[50] The dose of d-tubocurarine required to produce 50% and 95% depression of the response height (ED_{50} and ED_{95}, respectively) was greater at 0.1 Hz than at 1.0 Hz. A key point is that the dose of d-tubocurarine producing 95% twitch depression at 0.1–0.15 Hz was associated with excellent intubating conditions, whereas at 1.0 Hz there was inadequate relaxation (Fig. 17–7). Single twitch frequency of 0.1–0.15 Hz, therefore, provides a means of monitoring neuromuscular blockade over a clinically significant range of muscle relaxation.

There are two drawbacks to the single twitch method of stimulation: (1) a baseline prior to administration of relaxants must be established; hence, the technique is not helpful in patients who have already received NBDs, and (2) it is insensitive for the detection of residual blockade.

Train of Four

The use of TOF stimuli to monitor neuromuscular block during anesthesia was first introduced by Ali and colleagues in 1970.[52] Conventionally, TOF stimulation consists of four supramaximal, 0.1- to 0.2-msec, square wave impulses delivered at a rate of two/second (2 Hz) (see Fig. 17–8 for TOF). The TOF method is based on the principle that

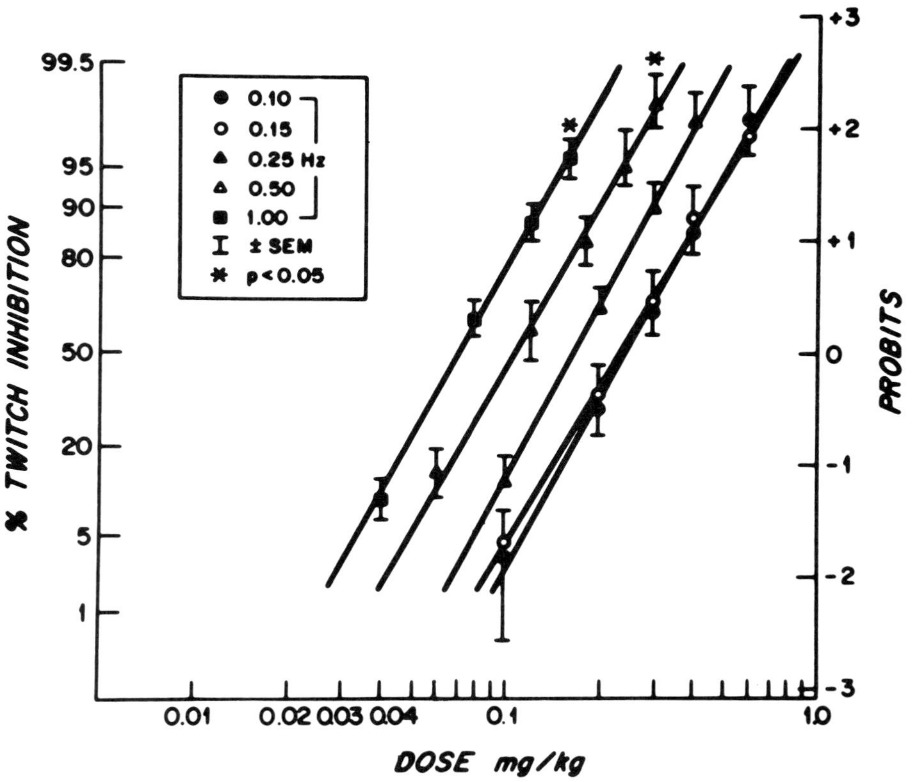

Figure 17–7. Cumulative dose (mg/kg)–response (% twitch inhibition) curves for a d-tubocurarine at different stimulation frequencies (symbols in box). Increases in stimulation frequency shift the dose-response curve to the left. The dose of curve required to produce 50% or 95% twitch inhibition is increased by stimulation at 1 Hz compared to 0.1 Hz. (From Ali HH, et al: Stimulation frequency and dose response to d-tubocurarine in man. Anesthesiology 1980; 52:37, with permission.)

stimulation at frequencies greater than 0.1–0.15 Hz in the presence of nondepolarizing NBDs causes a rapid decline in the evoked response until a new baseline is reached, usually after the third stimulus. The degree of relaxation determines the response height of the second, third, and fourth stimuli. Blockade can thus be evaluated by comparing the ratio of the fourth response with that of the first response. Because this method uses the first response as the reference point, no preblock baseline needs to be established. There must be at least a 10-second quiescent interval between each TOF, so that the first twitch of each is unconditioned. In each TOF, the three twitches after the first are conditioned. Failure to wait 10 seconds until the next TOF conditions the first response in the train and thus decreases the difference between the first and the last response. As a result, the degree of blockade is underestimated. Stimulation with fewer trains or slower frequencies sacrifices sensitivity, whereas higher-frequency stimulation causes fusion of individual mechanical responses.[52]

The TOF method can be used to monitor both mild and intense relaxation. For monitoring residual blockade, a TOF ratio of 0.7 has been used as a benchmark to indicate a level of relaxation that does not compromise respiration. Surgical degrees of relaxation are monitored by counting the number of twitches present in a TOF. Adequate surgical relaxation is usually indicated by the presence of only one or two twitches in a TOF. Lee compared the first and last twitches in a TOF after administration of d-tubocurarine using a force transducer to measure thumb abduction.[53] He found that there was no change in the single twitch until the TOF ratio was decreased by 20–25%. He also demonstrated the relationship between fade of TOF and the depression of single response at varying levels of block (Table 17–7). Intense neuromuscular block is evaluated by counting the number of twitches after tetanic stimulation.

The advantages of the TOF method include greater sensitivity than single twitch for evaluation of residual blockade, lack of need to establish a baseline response, and performance in awake patients with minimum discomfort. It has also been shown to be useful in monitoring high degrees of blockade and avoids the distortion of neuromuscular transmission that may result from tetanic stimulation.

A problem with the method is that the TOF ratio can only be determined by quantitative methods such as EMG or mechanomyography (MMG). It has also been clearly

TABLE 17–7. COMPARISON OF TRAIN-OF-FOUR AND SINGLE STIMULATION TECHNIQUES

Twitch Disappearance	T_1 Depression
Fourth	75%
Third	80%
Second	90%
First	100%

The relationship between the depression of the first mechanical thumb twitch (T_1) of a train-of-four and the last twitch in the train during dTC relaxation.

(Data from Lee CM: Train-of-4 quantitation of competitive neuromuscular block. Anesth Analg 1975; 54:649–653.)

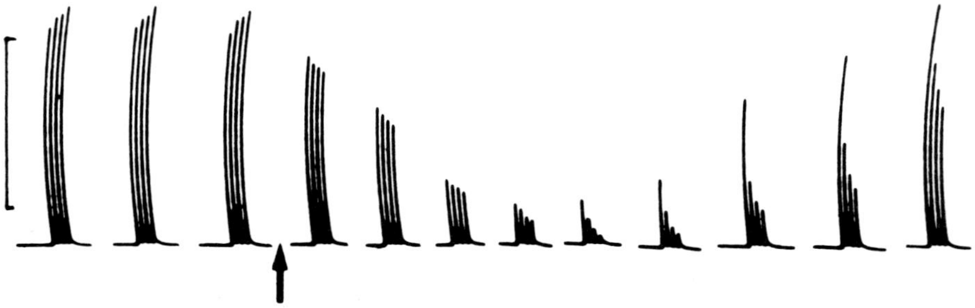

Figure 17–8. The train-of-four varies during onset and offset of nondepolarizing block. Vecuronium was given (*arrow*) to a cat nerve–tibialis muscle preparation. Fade of the train-of-four is more marked during recovery of neuromuscular function than with initial twitch depression. (From Bowman WC: Prejunctional and postjunctional cholino-receptors at the neuromuscular junction. Anesth Analg 1980; 59:940, with permission.)

demonstrated that the TOF ratio varies with onset and offset of block as well as with relaxant dose, duration of relaxation, and different reversal agents. There is usually significantly more fade during offset of block than during onset. This probably reflects differing pharmacokinetic properties at prejunctional and postjunctional receptors (Fig. 17–8).

Tetanus

Tetanic stimulation consists of single, supramaximum, 0.1- to 0.2-msec square waves delivered at rates of 20 or more per second. Tetanic stimulation, therefore, is rapid single twitch stimulation taken to the extreme. At stimulation rates greater than 5 Hz, the mechanical response begins to fuse and fails to return to its original position. Complete fusion occurs at 20–30 Hz.[54] By using EMG techniques, it is possible to observe the individual muscle responses to each stimulation within a tetanic burst. As previously mentioned, rapid stimulation stresses the mechanisms responsible for ACh release. Although there is a margin of safety, sustained rapid stimulation produces fade even in the absence of NBDs (Table 17–8).[55] The range of frequencies used clinically has been 30–200 Hz. Most investigators now feel that 50-Hz tetanic stimulation for 5 seconds should be used. This conclusion is based on the findings by Merton in 1954, demonstrating that with 50-Hz stimulation, the force of contraction is the same as that produced by a maximum effort of an awake patient (Fig. 17–9).[56] Other investigators demonstrated that tetanic pulses of 80 Hz applied during maximum voluntary contraction do not produce an increase in contractile force or in compound action potential.[57] Waud and Waud showed that with d-tubocurarine, tetanic stimulation is more sensitive than single twitch stimulation for detecting residual blockade. They showed that the sustained response to single twitches required 25% of receptors to be free, whereas sustained 100-Hz tetanus response required 50% receptor availability.[48]

TABLE 17–8. TETANIC STIMULATION WITHOUT FADE

Tetanus (Hz)	Duration (seconds)
300	1
150–200	2
80–100	3
70	5
50	10

The maximum duration of tetanic stimulation at various frequencies that can be delivered in the absence of relaxants without developing fade.

(Data from Stanec A, Heyduk J, Stanec G, Orkin LR: Tetanic fade and post tetanic tension in the absence of neuromuscular blocking agents in anesthetized man. Anesth Analg 1978; 57:102–107.)

A significant limitation of this technique is that tetanus of 50 Hz causes considerable discomfort and therefore is not well suited for use in conscious patients. Conditioning of responses following tetanic stimulation is probably not a significant problem, because TOF returns to normal within about 2 minutes following tetanic stimulation.

The typical practice of simply observing the tetanic response against no resistance is not acceptable, because patients can sustain this type of contraction preoperatively for extended periods without much effort. Counterforce to thumb movement should be provided in order to compare the force with the estimated baseline force (Fig. 17–10). It is imperative to note that if supramaximum stimulating current is used with 50-Hz tetanus, the resultant contraction is identical to the patient's maximum voluntary response.

Post-Tetanic Potentiation

Tetanic stimulation enhances the response of a twitch that immediately follows it. This is called post-tetanic potentiation and may be due to both augmentation of contraction and facilitation of transmission.[58] Augmentation of contraction occurs as a result of increased calcium release within the muscle fiber and is detected in the absence of NBDs by all methods of measurement except EMG.[59] Facilitation of transmission occurs only in the presence of nondepolarizing NBDs and is the result of increased ACh synthesis/mobilization that persists after tetanic stimulation. Facilitation is not observed in the absence of neuromuscular blockade, because an excess of ACh is normally released.[60] The number of responses to a single twitch following 50-Hz tetanic stimulation for 5 seconds is the post-tetanic count.[61]

The technique of post-tetanic stimulation may be used to demonstrate either nondepolarizing or phase 2 block or the intensity of neuromuscular blockade.[61–63] Ridley and Hatch used tetanic stimulation of 50 Hz for 5 seconds followed by a single twitch at 1 Hz to evaluate depth of block, a modification of the post-tetanic count method. They have noted that a post-tetanic count less than 10 ensured adequate surgical relaxation, whereas a count greater than 15 indicated easy reversibility.[64]

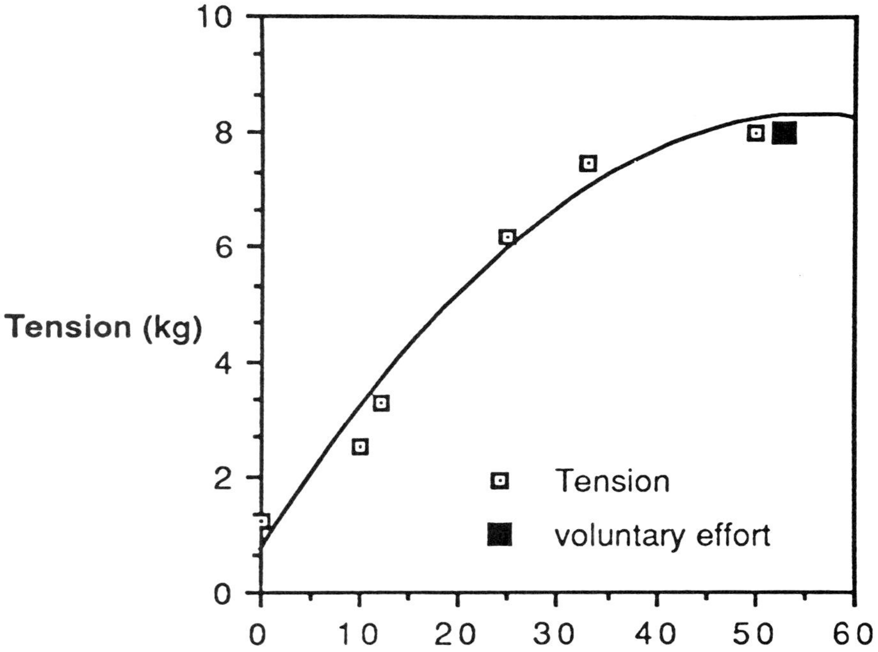

Figure 17–9. This relationship between the force of a maximal voluntary effort of the adductor pollicis and its response to tetanic stimulation at different frequencies demonstrates that at 50 Hz, the tension (force) is identical. (Adapted from Merton PA: Voluntary strength and fatigue. J Physiol 1954; 123:553–564.)

Double-Burst Stimulation

Double-burst stimulation (DBS) is a relatively new technique that was developed by Engbaek and colleagues to improve the detection of residual neuromuscular blockade using visual or tactile evaluation of motor responses.[65] DBS consists of two 50-Hz bursts of square wave stimuli with a 0.75-second pause separating the bursts. Subscripts are used to denote the number of pulses in each burst. $DBS_{3,3}$, for example, consists of three square wave impulses followed by a 0.75-second pause and a second burst of three impulses (Fig. 17–11).[65] This stimulation pattern elicits two distinct motor responses, which are evaluated using visual or tactile methods. Although the responses are more forceful than those elicited by TOF stimulation, a study by Gill and colleagues showed that the ratio of last response to first response is identical for both DBS and TOF methods.[66] A number of studies have convincingly demonstrated that clinicians using visual or tactile methods to evaluate motor responses are more likely to detect residual neuromuscular blockade by using double-burst rather than TOF stimulation.[67–71]

Despite this advantage over TOF stimulation $DBS_{3,3}$ can reliably detect fade only when the TOF ratio is <0.6.[72] $DBS_{3,2}$ is more sensitive than $DBS_{3,3}$ at detecting residual neuromuscular blockade (defined as TOF ratio < 0.7) but tends to demonstrate fade when the actual TOF ratio is > 0.9.[72–74] Evaluation of awake patients may be limited somewhat, because DBS is more painful than TOF stimulation.[75] A potential solution to this problem has been developed by Brull and colleagues, who showed that submaximum stimulating currents may actually provide better results than supramaximum stimulation.[73, 74]

Nerve Stimulators

Requirements

Because current density causes nerve depolarization, peripheral nerve stimulators (PNSs) should deliver a constant current over a range of impedances. Constant-voltage stimulators have been shown to provide inadequate stimulation with high impedances that are typical of surface electrodes.[75] The amount of current required to produce supra-

Figure 17–10. Developed twitch tension varies with the load or counterforce on the muscle (thumb). Function of the neuromuscular junction should always be evaluated against a resistance and at baseline conditions before administration of a neuromuscular blocking drug. *, $p < 0.001$ from 100, 200, 300 g. †, $p < 0.05$ from 200, 300 g. (From Donlon JV, et al: Cumulative dose response curves for gallamine. Effect of altered resting thumb tension and mode of stimulation. Anesth Analg 1979; 58:379, with permission.)

Resting thumb tension	Developed twitch tension
g	*g* ± *SE*
50	312.8 ± 34.8*
100	371.3 ± 39.0†
200	399.8 ± 37.7
300	410.0 ± 35.6

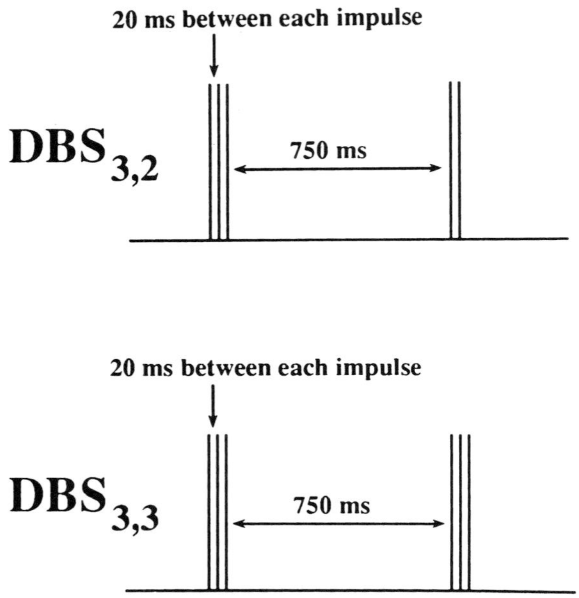

Figure 17–11. Double-burst stimulation. (See text for details.) (From Brull SJ, et al: Correlation of train-of-four and double burst stimulation ratios at varying amperages. Anesth Analg 1990; 71:489, with permission of International Anesthesia Research Society.)

maximum stimulation varies between patients and is a function of electrode type and position, skin resistance, edema, obesity, and wrist diameter. Pollmaecher and associates demonstrated that, with surface electrodes, maximum stimulation required 38 ± 23 mA, but 6% of patients required greater than 80 mA.[54] Kopman and Lawson showed that 30 mA was adequate to produce supramaximum stimulation using surface electrodes with wrist circumference ≤ 16 cm. They concluded that battery-operated PNSs should deliver no less than 50–60 mA.[76] The requirements for needle electrodes are considerably less. Gravenstein and Paulus reported supramaximum stimulation with 5–8 mA using needle electrodes.[77] A test of six commercially available PNSs showed that none was able to produce either constant current or constant voltage over the range of clinically relevant impedances. The output current in all of the tested PNSs decreased at resistances > 1 kΩ.[78]

Electrode Placement and Nerve Depolarization

Electrode placement affects the ability to deliver supramaximum stimuli using clinically available PNSs. As electrodes are moved further apart, the interelectrode impedance increases, and eventually, stimulating current is inadequate. Care must be taken when applying the surface electrodes to seal the outer edges before applying pressure to the central portion; otherwise, gel can be extruded beyond the electrode, creating a large contact area or possibly forming a direct contact with the other electrode (cathode-anode bridge). This bridging effect can be observed on the ohmmeter as very low impedance (< 1–2 kΩ).

An electrode placed over a nerve is called the active electrode and concentrates the current on the nerve. The effect is greatest on the nerve wall closest to the electrode. Nerve depolarization resulting from electrical current takes place under the cathode (black, −), whereas hyperpolarization occurs under the anode (red, +).[43, 79–81]

Needles versus Surface Electrodes for Stimulation

Electrodes can be either needles that are inserted through the skin or surface electrodes that are placed on the skin. Needle electrodes have lower impedance than surface electrodes do, but they are more invasive and can cause infection and tissue trauma. Normally, surface electrodes are satisfactory to provide supramaximum stimulation, and in the case of the EMG, they provide accurate recording of evoked potentials. Pierce and coworkers showed that reliable supramaximum stimulation could be achieved using either surface or needle electrodes as long as adequate current was provided.[82]

The adequacy of surface or needle electrodes can be checked by a variable output stimulator. By incrementally increasing the applied current, one should be able to achieve a maximum response followed by a plateau. The stimulator can then be set at 25–50% above the maximum response (*supra*maximum stimulation). If no plateau is reached, inadequate current is being delivered to the nerve, and the electrodes should be changed or a more powerful stimulator should be used. Another approach is to set the delivered current at 2.75 times the current required to produce a barely visible twitch.[76] In some cases, however, surface electrodes produce *sub*maximum stimulation, resulting in overestimation of neuromuscular block. In a study of 50 awake volunteers, surface electrodes resulted in 6% incidence of submaximum stimulation despite the use of a stimulator capable of 80-mA output.[54]

Preparation of the skin prior to placement of surface electrodes markedly decreases the measured impedance. An effective method is to lightly abrade the skin with an abrasive pad (ECG preparation pad, Marquette Electronics, Milwaukee, WI), which removes the high-resistance superficial layers of skin. This technique reduces impedance about 50%, whereas wiping with alcohol or lightly rubbing with gauze have minimal effect (Fig. 17–12). It is also imperative to use fresh electrodes, because extended storage can lead to drying of the electrolyte gel.

Complications of Monitoring

There are very few reported complications related to monitoring neuromuscular transmission. Burn injuries have been reported secondary to interaction with an electrocautery and by intermittent stimulation using spherical metal electrodes.[83, 84] A case of ulnar nerve palsy resulting from pressure over the ulnar groove by a surface electrode connector and improper arm positioning has been described, as has a thumb paresthesia lasting 4–14 days following the use of a particular type of thumb twitch force transducer.[85, 86] Interference with pacemaker function has been described as a result of stimulation of evoked potential testing.[87] Although there are no reports to date, it is also

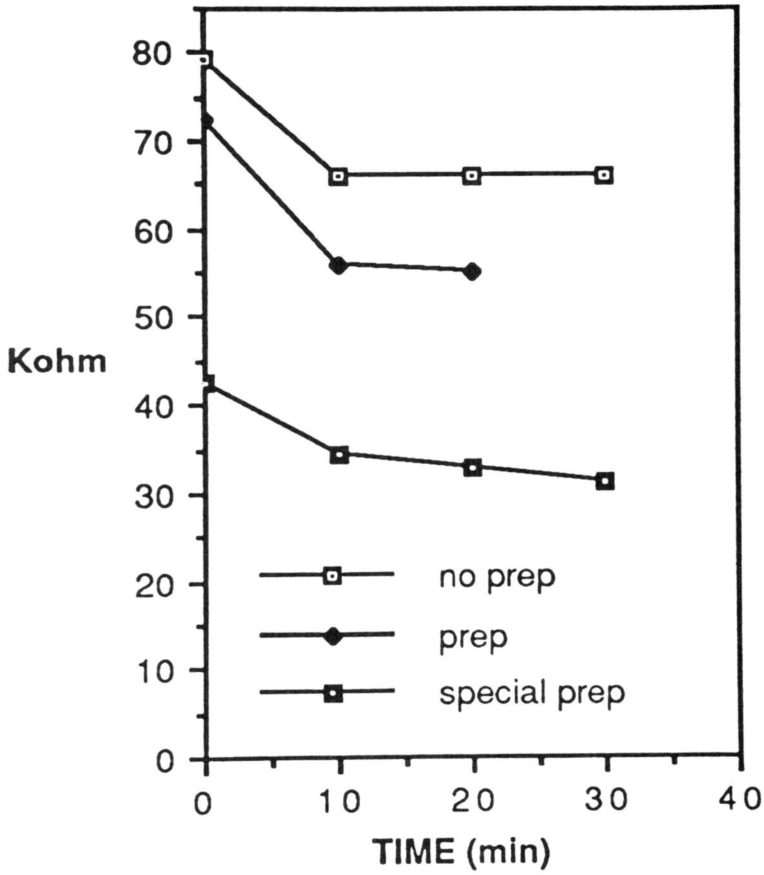

Figure 17–12. A comparison of the impedances of surface electrodes after no skin preparation, skin preparation with alcohol, and skin preparation with alcohol/abrasion/electrolyte gel, as described in text.

possible that a PNS could be inadvertently attached to the leads from a temporary pacemaker.

PNS Testing

Actual testing of stimulator output is rarely done. One can set the stimulator on a low setting and feel the electrodes for a shock. An alternative is to attach the leads to a neon lamp (type NE-2) available from most electronic parts suppliers.[88]

Quantifying Evoked Responses

The simplest method of evaluating mechanical responses is by visual or tactile estimation. Although these methods are suitable for monitoring relatively intense neuromuscular blockade, they are unreliable for the detection of residual blockade. It has been consistently demonstrated that the diagnosis of residual paralysis cannot be excluded by the lack of palpable or observable fade with TOF, double-burst, or tetanic stimulation. TOF ratios, for example, must be less than 0.4 for experienced observers to reliably identify fade.[66, 72, 89, 90] In a study by Brull et al, some observers did not detect fade even when actual TOF ratios were as low as 0.1.[74] Reliable detection of residual neuromuscular blockade using TOF or DBS requires precise quantitative methods. Three methods currently are available to quantify the motor response to nerve stimulation. The graphic depiction of developed tension is MMG. The second method, EMG, measures the compound action potential generated by the summation of the individual action potentials of contracting muscle fibers. The third method, accelerometry, measures the acceleration of the thumb.

Mechanomyography

Measurement of the adductor pollicis contraction tension in response to ulnar nerve stimulation is generally considered the gold standard of quantitative methods. A force transducer is used to convert the contractile force into electrical current that can be quantified. The motor response lasts longer than the EMG; therefore, the response can be recorded on a strip chart (Fig. 17–13). Accurate measurement requires maintenance of a constant thumb angle and resting tension. A 200- to 800-gm preload on the muscle is necessary to provide maximum tension development.[49, 60] Movement during the use of MMG that reduces resting tension from 200 to 50 gm may decrease twitch tension by 20–25%.[91] The transducer should be capable of responding to tensions in the 0- to 15-kg range, because the maximum force generated by thumb abduction is about 8 kg (see Fig. 17–10).[56] The Grass transducer that is most commonly used is the FT-10, which accurately responds to a maximum force of 10 kg. The FT-03 overloads with tensions greater than 2.2 kg and, therefore, is unsuitable for abductor pollicis monitoring in the adult.[6]

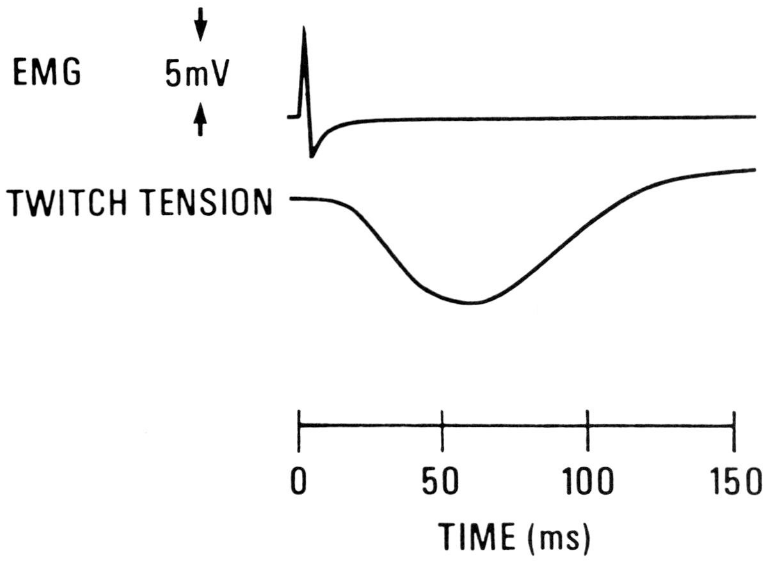

Figure 17–13. The motor response (twitch tension) is longer in duration than the EMG and can be recorded on a strip chart. (From Donati F, et al: Neuromuscular blocking drugs in anesthesia. Can Anaesth Soc J 1984; 31:326, with permission.)

Electromyography

This technique measures a summation of biphasic action potentials called the compound muscle action potential. The compound action potential is a brief, low-voltage event that must be amplified. This response is a biphasic wave that can be quantified either by amplitude or by integration of the area under the curve. Both techniques produce similar results.[92] An example of a commercially available EMG monitor is the Datex Relaxograph (Datex Medical Instrumentation, Inc., Tewksbury, MA) (Fig. 17–14). This device produces TOF stimuli and then measures the integrated compound action potential of the muscle being monitored. The supramaximum stimulation current level is determined after start-up by giving single twitches at 5-mA increments until no further increase in EMG is produced. The current is then increased by 20% to produce supramaximum stimulation. The maximum stimulation current is 70 mA. The compound action potential resulting from each stimulation is amplified, rectified, and then electronically integrated. A stimulation artifact is produced with each twitch that occurs before and is independent of the resultant muscle response. The amplitude of this artifact after each TOF is compared with the initial artifact; a decrease of 30% or more is presumed to be secondary to an increase in electrode impedance, and "ELEC OFF" is noted in the display. The first twitch of the TOF is compared with the prerelaxation baseline and is displayed as a ratio (first twitch/reference). If four twitches are present, the ratio of last twitch to first twitch is displayed. The monitor can be moved with the patient from operating room to postanesthesia recovery area, because the calibration values are retained for 15 minutes after power disconnect. An RS-232 port is provided for computerized data acquisition (see Chapter 21).

EMG Electrodes. The key to successful EMG monitoring is skin preparation and placement of the surface electrodes. A pair of electrodes, called the reference and the active electrodes, monitors the compound action potential. These electrodes convert varying ion currents generated by nerve and muscle activity into varying electric currents in wires that are connected to the amplifier. The optimum location for the active (−) electrode of the pair is over the innervation zone of the muscle, usually midway between origin and insertion. Some authors suggest using a strip electrode oriented perpendicular to the muscle belly and positioned over the innervation zone.[93] The reference (+) electrode is positioned away from muscles that are innervated by the nerve being stimulated. Some investigators position the reference electrode over the insertion of the muscle, because this ensures that no contracting muscle is under the electrode and, at the same time, places the electrodes parallel to the axis of depolarization, thus maximizing the signal. Kalli compared several electrode placements and demonstrated that positioning the active electrode over the adductor pollicis innervation zone and the reference electrode on the index finger produced the least drift and variation in response.[94]

Pregelled silver–silver chloride surface electrodes work well with adequate skin preparation. Surface electrodes that connect to the EMG leads through a hinged flap work best. This design allows lead movement without transmission to the skin-electrode interface. A ground electrode should be positioned between the stimulating and the recording electrodes in order to decrease stimulation artifact. The ground electrode should be large in order to decrease skin-electrode impedance.[95] The EMG also depends on the location of the stimulating electrodes. The positioning of the stimulating electrodes affects the ability to achieve supramaximum stimulation and alters the shape of the compound action potential. As the stimulating electrodes, specifically the

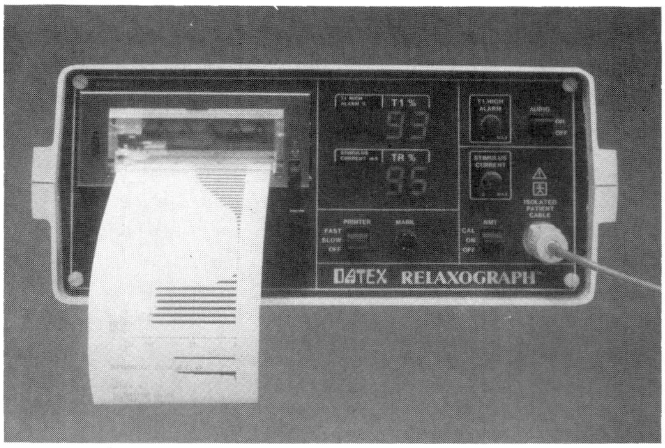

Figure 17–14. A clinical EMG monitor is the Datex NMT-100 Relaxograph. It measures the compound action potential resulting from train-of-four stimulation. The first twitch is compared to that prior to neuromuscular blockade as well as to the fourth twitch (if present). (From Datex Medical Instrumentation, Inc., Tewksbury, MA, with permission.)

cathode, are moved to a more proximal position, the EMG response demonstrates diminished amplitude and longer duration. This occurs because differential conduction velocity along the motor neuron is magnified by increased distance. This disperses motor unit activation over a larger time span.[95]

Actual use of an EMG is somewhat more complicated than simply attaching five surface electrodes to the patient. The skin must be adequately prepared, the wrist must be secured in a splint, and a system must be devised to maintain core and surface temperature. Electrodes should be attached 15 minutes ahead of time in order to minimize surface electrode-skin impedance. It may be useful to check the electrode impedance with an ohmmeter designed for this purpose.

EMG versus MMG. Both EMG and MMG are ways to quantitate the number of muscle fibers that contract with a given stimulus. Because supramaximum stimuli are used, the motor response depends on the number of motor endplates that are depolarized beyond threshold. In the case of MMG, the measured response also depends on the contractile state of the muscle fibers. For example, a patient given dantrolene sodium has a diminished force tension but an unchanged EMG response. Post-tetanic potentiation in the absence of NBDs is observed on MMG, whereas post-tetanic potentiation during EMG indicates phase 2 depolarizing block or of nondepolarizing blockade.[59, 60]

Many studies have correlated the EMG and the MMG. For nondepolarizing agents, the EMG method tends to show less blockade than does MMG.[6, 96] Depolarizing agents produce the opposite results, with EMG overestimating the degree of block.[92] Thus, EMG underestimates nondepolarizing blockade and overestimates depolarizing blockade when compared with the gold standard, MMG. The results produced by either of these techniques depend largely on the nerve-muscle unit being monitored. Muscles vary in their response to NBDs. The reasons for this are not clear but may be related to differences in temperature, perfusion, and content of slow- and fast-twitch fibers. An example is the difference observed between the thenar MMG and the hypothenar EMG. Kopman has shown that the single thumb twitch MMG was depressed 15% more than was hypothenar EMG.[97] Epstein and Epstein also demonstrated 14% greater depression of the thenar MMG than the hypothenar EMG.[60] These studies indicate that the relationship between thenar and hypothenar EMG is MMG thenar + 0.14% = EMG hypothenar. It may be appropriate to use different criteria for onset and reversal of nondepolarizing blockade based on the type of monitoring used.

Advantages and Disadvantages of EMG. The advantages of EMG over MMG are listed in Table 17–9. Common recording sites are the abductor pollicis (thenar), the abductor digiti minimi (hypothenar), and the first dorsal interosseous muscles of the hand. The hand and electrode leads should be well secured, because movement can produce artifacts resembling action potentials. The EMG is a brief event and, therefore, cannot be recorded on a polygraph. The response can be photographed from an oscilloscope or stored in memory and then displayed on paper. This method avoids some of the problems that are inherent with MMG, including extremity fixation, transducer overload, preload requirement, and twitch angle. Unfortunately, the EMG method has its own assortment of problems. The available EMG monitors are somewhat unreliable, requiring readjustment by the manufacturer. Furthermore, the methodology is not well established, especially in regard to electrode types and placement. The output from two EMG monitors on the same patient may not be identical.

Accelerometry

In 1988, Viby-Mogensen and associates described a new method of monitoring neuromuscular blockade called accelerometry.[98] The basis of this technique is a very small piezoelectric transducer that generates an electrical signal proportional to acceleration. A commercial unit called Accelograph (Biometer) is available that has a built-in nerve stimulator and that graphically records TOF responses.[5] The set-up for this technique is simple compared with EMG and MMG. The only equipment besides standard peripheral nerve stimulating electrodes is the transducer, which must be taped to the thumb. As a result, this is the only quantifiable method that is practical for routine monitoring.[98–102] This technique produces results that compare favorably with EMG and MMG,[98–101] although, for unclear reasons, TOF ratios greater than 100% are sometimes recorded.[98] One obvious limitation is that the thumb must be free to move.

TABLE 17–9. ADVANTAGES OF EMG OVER MMG

- Less immobilization required
- Greater flexibility in muscles monitored
- Easier to perform on infants
- Individual responses to tetanic train measurable
- Measure of neuromuscular refractory period
- Enhanced portability

CLINICAL CORRELATIONS

Applications of the phenomenon of neuromuscular transmission and monitoring methods to clinical management is difficult, because anesthetic depth, type of anesthetic agent used, monitoring site, technique, and patient-determined variables are interrelated and together determine the response to NBDs.

INTUBATION

When NBDs are utilized to facilitate tracheal intubation, the goal is to produce a relaxed glottis and a motionless patient. In essence, this amounts to relaxation of laryngeal, jaw, abdominal, and intercostal muscles. Diaphragmatic relaxation is of less concern during intubation, because the diaphragm contracts during inspiration rather than during the forceful expiration that is characteristic of ''bucking.''

Several groups have studied the response of the laryngeal adductors to relaxants by positioning a tracheal tube cuff between the vocal cords and measuring the pressure developed during recurrent laryngeal nerve stimulation.[103–106] It has been demonstrated that the laryngeal adductors are less sensitive than the adductor pollicis to nondepolarizing relaxants and that the response is similar in intensity and time course to the orbicularis oculi.[103] This means that thumb twitch may cease prior to complete relaxation of the vocal cords.[104] The opposite is true for succinylcholine, which may explain why excellent intubating conditions are achieved so rapidly with this drug.[105]

In the majority of patients, disappearance of an adductor pollicis response to single twitch, post-tetanic, or double-burst stimulation produces good to excellent intubating conditions in over 75% of patients.[72] Another approach is to monitor the orbicularis oculi, because this muscle is relatively resistant to neuromuscular blockade and should thereby signal that relaxation has been achieved in other muscle groups.[103] Abolition of twitch responses can be monitored with a peripheral nerve stimulator combined with visual or tactile evaluation of the elicited responses. It is imperative to note that total suppression of the peripheral twitch response does not guarantee lack of response to noxious stimuli when anesthesia is inadequate.[104]

SURGICAL RELAXATION

The degree of blockade required during a procedure depends on the type of surgery being performed and the risk associated with spontaneous movement. The most common surgical requirement for muscle relaxation is during intra-abdominal surgery. Several studies have compared the effect of muscle relaxants on abdominal muscles and the adductor pollicis. Katz used abdominal EMG and noted that the spontaneous abdominal EMG correlated with degree of thumb twitch, anesthetic depth, and mechanical hyperventilation.[107] He noted that 90–95% depression of the single twitch was sufficient to produce adequate abdominal relaxation in most patients. This is probably an overestimation, because he used stimulation rates of 0.3 Hz, which would indicate more profound block than is actually present.[50] He also demonstrated an increase in spontaneous abdominal EMG activity during skin incision that could have been prevented by prior infiltration with local anesthetic. This degree of relaxation corresponds to the presence of one twitch in TOF.[53] Another study using EMG-derived TOF ratios demonstrated that recovery from relaxants took about 30% longer in the hand than in the rectus abdominis.[106] This may partially explain the common situation in which the surgeon complains of increased abdominal tone despite thumb twitch evidence of adequate relaxation.

During surgical procedures in which patient movement constitutes a hazard, it is imperative to use supramaximum stimulation. When a PNS is used, the utilization of needle electrodes in patients with large wrist diameters increases the likelihood of delivering adequate stimulation current. With EMG, it is possible to continuously check electrode contact by evaluation of the stimulus artifact. It is also necessary to use intense degrees of muscle relaxation that will eliminate all responses to TOF stimulation. This degree of neuromuscular blockade is best evaluated by the post-tetanic count method.[61, 63, 108] By maintaining at least one post-tetanic twitch, the degree of block can be assessed, the recovery time can be predicted, and the stimulator's function can be evaluated.

ASSESSMENT OF RECOVERY FROM RELAXANTS

In an ideal world, no patient would have residual blockade after surgery. Because this is not the case, it is necessary to determine what degree of recovery is adequate for a given patient to support and clear the airway and to ventilate the lungs without assistance.

Respiratory Function and Residual Blockade

A margin of safety separates the minimum degree of relaxation that can be detected from the level of relaxation that causes ventilatory failure. Several factors contribute to this margin of safety. In their classic study of receptor occupancy, Waud and Waud demonstrated that patients may have normal inspiratory force and vital capacity even when 75–80% of the ACh receptors are blocked.[48] Another contribution comes from the relative sensitivities of respiratory and nonrespiratory muscle groups to NBDs. Investigators have repeatedly shown that the diaphragm is less sensitive to muscle relaxants than are peripheral muscles.[39, 41, 42, 109] The other muscles involved in respiration—abdominal, intercostal, scalene, and laryngeal muscles—are more sensitive to these agents than is the diaphragm.[110] As a result, neuromuscular blockade has an effect on respiratory function tests that depends on the muscle group being tested.

In unanesthetized subjects, Foldes and coworkers demonstrated the effect of "inspiratory sparing" by showing that 77% depression of grip strength induced by d-tubocurarine was associated with only a 12% decrease in vital capacity.[41] Gal and Goldberg administered d-tubocurarine to healthy subjects and noted no change in tidal volume even though head lift and hand grip were completely abolished.[42] They attributed this phenomena to the fact that tidal volume breathing is almost entirely due to diaphragmatic function. Of the other muscles involved with ventilation and airway protection, those required for swallowing appear to be the most sensitive to NBDs.[111] Unfortunately, monitoring of these muscles in the clinical setting is nearly impossible. Demonstrating the variable response of different muscles to NBDs has been relatively simple. The more difficult task has been to develop criteria to indicate when patients can be safely extubated.

Several investigators compared the response to TOF stimulation with respiratory parameters in order to develop criteria to be applied to anesthetized or uncooperative patients. In 1973, Ali and Kitz noted that after neostigmine reversal, patients with an MMG TOF ratio to thumb adduction of 74 ± 5% had clinical evidence of full recovery.[112] Subsequent studies in awake volunteers and in American Society of Anesthesiologists class 3 and 4 patients demonstrated that recovery to a TOF ratio of 0.70 (thumb twitch) is associated with clinical signs of complete recovery and a return to baseline respiratory parameters, including vital capacity at 96.5% of control, control peak inspiratory force, and vital capacity of 17 ml/kg.[113–115] The conclusion from these studies is that patients with recovery to a TOF ratio of 0.70 have cough and ventilatory capabilities comparable with their baseline values. These ratios were determined using MMG evaluation of the adductor pollicis. As a result of the relative insensitivity of the hypothenar EMG, Kopman suggested using a TOF ratio of ≥ 0.9 to indicate adequate reversal when monitoring this particular muscle group.[97]

It is useful for the clinician to realize that this gold standard of TOF ratio > 0.7 may be misleading in some situations. Any TOF ratio of < 100% is evidence of residual relaxant effect. In a patient compromised by surgically induced upper airway dysfunction, pulmonary disease, obesity, or metabolic acidosis, it is difficult to prove that that any degree of blockade is unimportant. An area that has not received much attention is the potential for mild degrees of residual blockade to cause patient discomfort and anxiety. Given these considerations, it is probably best to strive for complete antagonism of relaxation whenever possible.

Evaluation of Antagonism

Accurate evaluation of the TOF ratio requires quantitative methods such as EMG or MMG.[51, 92, 116] As previously discussed, visual and tactile evaluation of the TOF ratio or fade with tetanus and DBS is not adequately sensitive to reliably detect patients with a TOF ratio < 0.7.[66–72] Of these stimulation patterns, however, DBS appears to be the most sensitive. Accurate evaluation of TOF ratios requires quantitative methods such as MMG, EMG, and accelerometry. The TOF and tetanic methods of stimulation are more sensitive than single twitch, because the TOF may show significant fade when the single twitch has returned to baseline.[117, 118]

Because most clinicians do not have access to quantitative equipment, bedside tests of recovery can be employed and evoked responses can be assessed using visual and tactile methods. There should be no detectable fade with either tetanus, TOF, or DBS as measured by tactile or visual means. If tetanus is used, the response should be of the same magnitude as a maximum volitional contraction. As mentioned previously, DBS appears to offer the greatest sensitivity in detecting significant residual relaxant effect. The potential for nerve stimulation to cause discomfort in the awake or near awake patient has been addressed by Brull and coworkers. They have demonstrated that TOF or double-burst ratios can be successfully determined by using just enough current to elicit the appropriate responses.[73, 74] Regardless of the stimulation pattern utilized, tactile and visual evaluation will not rule out the possibility of significant residual neuromuscular blockade. In this situation, the clinician must use bedside tests to assess recovery.

The ability to raise the head for 5 seconds has been shown to indicate adequate strength to swallow, perform a Valsalva maneuver, and approximate the teeth.[119] Although the ability to perform these maneuvers suggests return of adequate strength for safe extubation, the ability to perform a 5-second head lift should not be interpreted as complete recovery. Numerous studies have demonstrated that patients who are able to do a 5-second head lift may have TOF ratios < 0.7 and may have muscle strength well below their baseline values.[120]

SUMMARY

The most rational approach to the issue of residual neuromuscular blockade is the use of precise relaxant doses directed by intraoperative monitoring in order to avoid intense relaxation at the conclusion of surgery. It is well known that reversal of intense blockade is unpredictable. The presence of three or four adductor pollicis responses to TOF stimulation *prior* to administration of antagonists is probably the best approach, because rapid recovery to a TOF ratio > 0.7 is virtually guaranteed.[128] It is clear that most practitioners do not have access to the quantifiable techniques available with either MMG or EMG. Even if these monitors were widely available, the additional time and attention they require render them unsuitable for use in all cases. Indeed, the margin of safety present in most patients allows for competent administration and reversal of NBDs using only a nerve stimulator and bedside tests.

REFERENCES

1. Lunn JN, Mushin WW: Mortality associated with anaesthesia. Nuffield Provincial Hospital Trust 1982; 48.
2. Beecher HK, Todd DP: A study of the deaths associated with anesthesia and surgery based on a study of 599,548 anesthesias in ten institutions 1948–1952 inclusive. Ann Surg 1954; 140:2–34.
3. Churchill-Davidson HC, Christie TH: The diagnoses of neuromuscular block in man. Br J Anaesth 1959; 31:390–395.
4. Viby-Mogensen J, Jorgenson BC, Ording H: Residual curarization in the recovery room. Anesthesiology 1979; 50:539–541.
5. Beemer GH, Rozental P: Postoperative neuromuscular function. Anaesth Intens Care 1986; 14:41–45.
6. Lenmarken C, Lofstrom JB: Partial curarisation in the postoperative period. Acta Anesthesiol Scand 1984; 28:260–262.
7. Katz RL: Neuromuscular effects of d-tubocurarine, edrophonium and neostigmine in man. Anesthesiology 1967; 28:327–336.
8. Matteo RS, Spector S, Horowitz PE: Relation of serum d-tubocurarine concentration to neuromuscular blockade in man. Anesthesiology 1974; 41:440–443.
9. Dunant Y: On the mechanism of acetylcholine release. *In* Smythies JR, Bradley RJ (eds): International Review of Neurobiology. Orlando: Academic Press, 1985; 27:55–92.
10. Durant NN: The physiology of neuromuscular transmission. *In* Katz RL (ed): Muscle relaxants. Basic and Clinical Aspects. Orlando: Grune & Stratton, 1985; 13–38.
11. Heuser JE, Salpeter SR: Organization of acetylcholine receptors in quick frozen, deep etched and rotary-replicated *Torpedo* post synaptic membrane. J Cell Biol 1979; 82:150–174.
12. Thesleff S: Different kinds of ACh release from the motor nerve. *In* Smythies JR, Bradley RJ (eds): International Review of Neurobiology. Orlando: Academic Press, 1986; 59–88.
13. Collier B, Katz HS: Acetylcholine synthesis from recaptured choline by a sympathetic ganglion. J Physiol (Lond) 1970; 206:145–166.
14. Tucek S: The synthesis of acetylcholine in skeletal muscles of the rat. J Physiol (Lond) 1982; 322:53–69.
15. Thesleff S: The mode of neuromuscular block caused by acetylcholine, nicotine, decamethonium and succinylcholine. Acta Physiol Scand 1955; 34:218–224.
16. Kuffler SW, Yoshikami D: The number of transmitter molecules in a quantum: An estimate from ionophoretic application of acetylcholine at the neuromuscular synapse. J Physiol (Lond) 1975; 251:465–482.
17. Brigent JL, Mallant A: Presynaptic currents in mouse motor endings. J Physiol (Lond) 1982; 333:619–636.
18. Katz B: Nerve, Muscles and Synapse. New York: McGraw Hill, 1966.
19. Hubbard JI, Jones SF, Landau EM: On the mechanisms by which calcium and magnesium affect the release of neurotransmitter by nerve impulses. J Physiol (Lond) 1968; 196:75–86.
20. Standaert FG: Donut and holes: Molecules and muscle relaxants *In* Katz RL (ed): Muscle Relaxants. Basic and Clinical Aspects. Orlando: Grune & Stratton, 1985; 1–18.
21. Standaert FG: Basic physiology and pharmacology of the neuromuscular junction. In Miller RD (ed): Anesthesia, 3rd Ed. New York: Churchill Livingstone, 1990; 659–684.
22. Tobey RE, Jacobsen PM, Cahil CT, et al: The serum potassium response to muscle relaxants in neural injury. Anesthesiology 1972; 37:332–337.
23. Pepper K, Bradley RJ, Dreger K: The ACh receptor at the neuromuscular junction. Physiol Rev 1982; 62:1271–1340.
24. Bowman WC: Prejunctional and postjunctional cholinoreceptors at the neuromuscular junction. Anesth Analg 1980; 59:935–943.
25. Vassalle M: Contribution of the Na^+/K^+ pump to the membrane potential. Experientia 1987; 43:1135–1140.
26. Brown WF: The Physiological and Technical Basis of Electromyography. Boston: Butterworths, 1984; 12–13.
27. Ali HH, Savarese JJ: Monitoring neuromuscular function. Anesthesiology 1976; 45:216–249.
28. Lee C: Dose relationships of phase II, tachyphylaxis and train-of-four fade in suxamethonium-induced dual neuromuscular block in man. Br J Anaesth 1975; 47:841–845.
29. Bevan JC, Donati F, Bevan DR: Prolonged infusion of suxamethonium in infants and children. Br J Anaesth 1986; 58:839–843.
30. Sutherland GA, Bevan JC, Bevan DR: Neuromuscular blockade in infants following intramuscular succinylcholine in two or five percent solution. Can Anaesth Soc J 1980; 30:342–346.
31. Goudsouzian NG, Liu LM: The neuromuscular response of infants to a continuous infusion of succinylcholine. Anesthesiology 1984; 60:97–101.
32. Lee C: Self antagonism: A possible mechanism of tachyphylaxis in suxamethonium induced-neuromuscular block in man. Br J Anaesth 1976; 48:1097–1101.
33. Donati F, Bevan DR: Long term succinylcholine infusion during isoflurane. Anesthesiology 1983; 58:6–10.
34. Donati F, Bevan DR: Antagonism of phase II succinylcholine block by neostigmine. Anesth Analg 1985; 64:773–776.
35. Futter ME, Donati F, Sadikot AS, Bevan DR: Neostigmine antagonism of succinylcholine phase II block: A comparison with pancuronium. Can Anaesth Soc J 1983; 30:575–580.
36. Russell WJ, Serle DG: Hand grip force as an assessment of recovery from neuromuscular block. J Clin Monit 1987; 3:87–89.
37. Stiffel P, Hammeroff SP, Blitt C, Cork RC: Variability in assessment of neuromuscular blockade. Anesthesiology 1980; 52:436–437.
38. Caffrey RR, Warren ML, Becker KE: Neuromuscular blockade monitoring comparing the orbicularis oculi and adductor pollicis muscles. Anesthesiology 1986; 65:95–97.
39. Chauvin M, Lebrault C, Duvaldestin P: The neuromuscular blocking effect of vecuronium on the human diaphragm. Anesth Analg 1987; 66:117–122.
40. Wymore ML, Eisele JH: Differential effects of d-tubocurarine on inspiratory muscles and two peripheral muscle groups in anesthetized man. Anesthesiology 1978; 48:360–362.
41. Foldes FF, Monte AP, Brunn HM, Wolfson B: Studies with muscle relaxants in unanesthetized subjects. Anesthesiology 1961; 22:230–236.
42. Gal TJ, Goldberg SK: Relationship between respiratory muscle strength and vital capacity during partial curarization in awake subjects. Anesthesiology 1981; 54:141–147.
43. Swett JE, Bourassa CM: Electrical stimulation of peripheral nerve. *In* Patterson M, Kesner RP (eds): Electrical stimulation research techniques. New York: Academic Press, 1981; 244–298.
44. Epstein RA, Jackson SH: Repetitive muscle depolarization from a single indirect stimulation in man. J Appl Physiol 1970; 28:407–410.
45. Epstein RA, Wyte SR, Jackson SH, Sitter S: The electrical response to stimulation by the Block-Aid monitor. Anesthesiology 1969; 30:43–47.
46. Brooks VB, Theis RD: Reduction of quantum content during neuromuscular transmission. J Physiol (Lond) 1962; 162:298–310.
47. Liley AW, North AK: An electrical investigation of the effects of repetitive stimulation on mammalian neuromuscular junction. J Neurophysiol 1953; 16:509–527.
48. Waud BE, Waud DR: The relation between tetanic fade and receptor occlusion in the presence of competitive neuromuscular block. Anesthesiology 1971; 35:456–464.
49. Stanec A, Heyduk J, Stanec G, Orkin LR: Tetanic fade and post tetanic tension in the absence of neuromuscular blocking agents in anesthetized man. Anesth Analg 1978; 57:102–107.
50. Ali HH, Savarese JJ: Stimulation frequency and dose response to d-tubocurarine in man. Anesthesiology 1980; 52:36–39.
51. Lee C, Katz RL: Neuromuscular pharmacology. A clinical update and commentary. Br J Anaesth 1980; 52:173–188.
52. Ali HH, Uting JE, Gray C: Stimulus frequency in the detection of neuromuscular block in humans. Br J Anaesth 1970; 42:967–977.
53. Lee CM: Train-of-4 quantitation of competitive neuromuscular block. Anesth Analg 1975; 54:649–653.
54. Pollmaecher JT, Steirt H, Buzello W: A constant current peripheral nerve stimulator (neurostim T_4). Br J Anaesth 1986; 58:1443–1446.
55. Katz RL: Clinical neuromuscular pharmacology of pancuronium. Anesthesiology 1971; 34:500–506.
56. Merton PA: Voluntary strength and fatigue. J Physiol (Lond) 1954; 123:553–565.
57. Moritani T, Muro M, Kijima A, et al: Electromechanical changes during electrically induced and maximal voluntary contractions: Surface and intramuscular EMG responses during sustained maximal voluntary contraction. Exp Neurol 1985; 88:484–489.
58. Calvey TN: Assessment of neuromuscular blockade by electromyography: A review. J R Soc Med 1984; 77:56–59.
59. Katz RL: Electromyographic and mechanical effects of suxamethonium and tubocurarine on twitch, tetanic and post-tetanic responses. Br J Anaesth 1973; 45:849–859.

60. Epstein RA, Epstein RM: The electromyogram and the mechanical response of indirectly stimulated muscle in anesthetized man following curarization. Anesthesiology 1973; 38:212–223.
61. Viby-Mogensen J, Howardy-Hansen P, Chraemmer-Jorgensen B, et al: Posttetanic count (PTC). A new method of evaluating an intense nondepolarizing neuromuscular blockade. Anesthesiology 1981; 55:458–461.
62. Muchhal KK, Viby-Mogensen J: Evaluation of intense neuromuscular blockade caused by single bolus vecuronium using posttetanic count (PTC). Anesthesiology 1987; 66:846–849.
63. Bonsu AK, Viby-Mogensen J, Fernando PU, et al: Relationship of post-tetanic count and train-of-four response during intense neuromuscular blockade caused by atracurium. Br J Anaesth 1987; 59:1089–1092.
64. Ridley SA, Hatch DJ: Post-tetanic count and profound neuromuscular blockade with atracurium infusion in paediatric patients. Br J Anaesth 1988; 60:31–35.
65. Engbaek J, Ostergaard D, Viby-Mogensen J: Double burst stimulation (DBS): A new pattern of nerve stimulation to identify residual neuromuscular block. Br J Anaesth 1989; 70:578–581.
66. Gill SS, Donati F, Bevan DR: Clinical evaluation of double-burst stimulation. Its relationship to train-of-four stimulation. Anaesthesia; 1990; 45:543–548.
67. Ueda N, Viby-Mogensen J, Olsen NV, et al: The best choice of double burst stimulation pattern for manual evaluation of neuromuscular transmission. J Anesth 1989; 3:94–99.
68. Drenck NE, Ueda N, Olsen NV, et al: Manual evaluation of residual curarization using double burst stimulation: A comparison with train-of-four stimulation to assess neuromuscular blockade in children. Anesthesiology 1990; 70:578–581.
69. Saddler JM, Bevan JC, Donati F, et al: Comparison of double-burst and train-of-four stimulation to assess neuromuscular blockade in children. Anesthesiology 1990; 73:401–403.
70. Ueda N, Muteki T, Tsuda H, et al: Is the diagnosis of significant residual neuromuscular blockade improved by using double-burst stimulation? Eur J Anaesth 1991; 8:213–218.
71. Brull SJ, Silverman DG: Visual assessment of train-of-four and double burst–induced fade at submaximal stimulating currents. Anesth Analg 1991; 73:627–632.
72. Drenck NE, Ueda N, Olsen NV, et al: Manual evaluation of residual curarization using double burst stimulation: A comparison with train-of-four. Anesthesiology 1989; 70:578–581.
73. Brull SJ, Ehrenwerth J, Silverman DG: Stimulation with submaximal current for train-of-four monitoring. Anesthesiology 1990; 72:629–632.
74. Brull SJ, Ehrenwerth J, Connelly NR, Silverman DG: Assessment of residual curarization using low-current stimulation. Can J Anaesth 1991; 38:164–168.
75. Connelly NR, Silverman DG, O'Connor TZ, Brull SJ: Subjective responses to train-of-four and double-burst stimulation in awake patients. Anesth Analg 1990; 70:650–653.
76. Kopman AF, Lawson D: Milliamperage requirements for supramaximal stimulation of the ulnar nerve with surface electrodes. Anesthesiology 1984; 61:83–85.
77. Gravenstein J, Paulus D: Monitoring practice in clinical anesthesia. Philadelphia: JB Lippincott, 1982; 178.
78. Mylrea KC, Hameroff SR, Calkins JM, et al: Evaluation of peripheral nerve stimulators and relationship to possible errors in assessing neuromuscular blockade. Anesthesiology 1984; 60:464–466.
79. Rosenberg H, Greenhow DE: Peripheral nerve stimulator performance: The influence of output polarity and electrode placement. Can Anaesth Soc J 1978; 25:424–426.
80. de Weerd JPC: Instrumentation, electrodes, electrical interference and safety. *In* Notermans SLH (ed): Current Practice of Electromyography. New York: Elsevier, 1984; 29–56.
81. Ranck JB: Extracellular stimulation: *In* Patterson M, Kesner RP (eds): Electrical Stimulation Research Techniques. New York: Academic Press, 1981; 2–36.
82. Pierce PA, Mylrea KC, Watt RC, et al: Effects of pulse duration on neuromuscular blockade monitoring: Implications for supramaximal stimulation. J Clin Monit 1986; 2:169–173.
83. Lippman M, Fields WA: Burns of the skin caused by a peripheral nerve stimulator. Anesthesiology 1974; 40:82–84.
84. Brock-Utne JG, Downing JW: Rectal burn after the use of an anal stainless steel electrode/transducer system for monitoring myoneural junction. Anesth Analg 1984; 63:1139–1144.
85. Gertel M, Shapira SC: Ulnar nerve palsy of unusual etiology. Anesth Analg 1987; 66:1337.
86. Sia RL, Straatman NJ: Thumb paresthesia after neuromuscular twitch monitoring. Anaesthesia 1985; 40:167–169.
87. Merritt WT, Brinker JA, Beattie C: Pacemaker-mediated tachycardia induced by intraoperative somatosensory evoked potential stimuli. Anesthesiology 1988; 69:766–768.
88. Sarnat JA: A simple device for testing peripheral nerve stimulators. Anesthesiology 1984; 61:624–625.
89. Donati F, Bevan DR, Bevan JC: Neuromuscular blocking drugs in anesthesia. Can Anaesth Soc J 1984; 31:324–336.
90. Viby-Mogensen J, Jensen NH, Engbaek J, et al: Tactile and visual evaluation of the response to train-of-four nerve stimulation. Anesthesiology 1985; 63:440–443.
91. Donlon JV, Savarese JJ, Ali HH: Cumulative dose response curves for gallamine: Effect of altered resting thumb tension and mode of stimulation. Anesth Analg 1979; 58:379–381.
92. Weber S, Muravchick S: Monitoring technique affects measurement of recovery from succinylcholine. J Clin Monit 1987; 3:1–5.
93. McComas AJ: Neuromuscular Function and Disorders. Woburn, MA: Butterworths, 1977.
94. Kalli I: Effect of surface electrode positioning on the compound action potential evoked by ulnar nerve stimulation in anesthetized infants and children. Br J Anaesth 1989; 62:188–193.
95. Jabre JF, Hackett ER: EMG Manual. Springfield, IL: Charles C Thomas, 1983.
96. Weber S, Muravchick S: Electrical and mechanical train of four responses during depolarizing and nondepolarizing neuromuscular blockade. Anesth Analg 1986; 65:771–776.
97. Kopman KF: The relationship of evoked electromyographic and mechanical responses following atracurium in humans. Anesthesiology 1985; 63:208–211.
98. Viby-Mogensen J, Jensen E, Werner M, Nielsen HK: Measurement of acceleration: A new method of monitoring neuromuscular function. Acta Anaesthesiol Scand 1988; 32:45–48.
99. May O, Kirkegaard Nielsen H, Werner MU: The acceleration transducer—An assessment of its precision in comparison with a force displacement transducer. Acta Anaesth Scand 1988; 32:239–243.
100. Meretoja OA, Wirtavuori K: Two-dose technique to create an individual dose-response curve for atracurium. Anesthesiology 1989; 70:732–736.
101. Meretoja OA, Brown WA, Cass NM: Simultaneous monitoring of force, acceleration and electromyogram during computer-controlled infusion of atracurium in sheep. Anaesth Intens Care 1990; 18:486–489.
102. Jensen E, Viby-Mogensen J, Bang U: The accelerograph: A new neuromuscular transmission monitor. Acta Anaesthesiol Scand 1988; 32:49–52.
103. Ungurcanu D, Meistelman C, Frossard J, Donati F: The obicularis oculi and the adductor pollicus muscles as monitors of atracurium block of laryngeal muscles. Anesth Analg 1993; 77:775–779.
104. Meistelman C, Plaud B, Donati F: Rocuronium (Org 9426) neuromuscular blockade at the adductor muscles of the larynx and adductor pollicis in humans. Can J Anaesth 1992; 39:665–669.
105. Meistelman C, Plaud B, Donati F: Neuromuscular effects of succinylcholine on the vocal cords and adductor pollicis muscles. Anesth Analg 1991; 73:278–282.
106. Donati F, Meistleman C, Plaud B: Vecuronium neuromuscular block at the adductor muscles of the larynx and adductor pollicis. Anesthesiology 1991; 74:833–837.
107. Katz RL: Comparison of electrical and mechanical recording of spontaneous and evoked muscle activity. Anesthesiology 1965; 26:204–211.
108. Howardy-Hansen P, Viby-Mogensen, Gottschau A, et al: Tactile evaluation of the posttetanic count (PTC). Anesthesiology 1984; 60:372–374.
109. Gal TJ, Goldberg SK: Diaphragmatic function in healthy subjects during partial curarization. J Appl Physiol 1980; 48:921–926.
110. DeTroyer A, Bastenier J, Delhez L: Function of respiratory muscles during partial curarization in humans. J Appl Physiol 1980; 49:1049–1056.
111. Isono S, Ide T, Kochi T, et al: Effects of partial paralysis on the

swallowing reflex on conscious humans. Anesthesiology 1991; 75:980–984.

112. Ali HH, Kitz RJ: Evaluation of recovery from nondepolarizing neuromuscular block using a digital neuromuscular transmission analyzer: Preliminary report. Anesth Analg 1973; 52:740–745.
113. Brand JB, Cullen DJ, Wilson NE, Ali HH: Spontaneous recovery from nondepolarizing neuromuscular blockade: Correlation between clinical and evoked responses. Anesth Analg 1977; 56:55–58.
114. Jones RM, Pearce AC, Williams JP: Recovery characteristics following antagonism of atracurium with neostigmine or edrophonium. Br J Anaesth 1984; 56:453–457.
115. Ali HH, Wilson RS, Savarese JJ, Kitz RJ: The effect of tubocurarine on indirectly elicited train-of-four muscle response and respiratory measurements in humans. Br J Anaesth 1975; 47:570–574.
116. Pedersen T, Viby-Mogensen J, Bang U, et al: Does perioperative tactile evaluation of the train-of-four response influence the frequency of postoperative residual neuromuscular blockade? Anesthesiology 1990; 73:835–839.
117. Ali HH, Savarese JJ, Lebowitz PN, Ramsey FM: Twitch, tetanus and train-of-four as indices of recovery from nondepolarizing neuromuscular blockade. Anesthesiology 1981; 54:294–297.
118. Gissen AJ, Katz RL: Twitch tetanus and posttetanic potentiation as indices of nerve-muscle block in man. Anesthesiology 1969; 30:481–487.
119. Pavlin EG, Holle RH, Schoene RB: Recovery of airway protection compared with ventilation in humans after paralysis with curare. Anesthesiology 1989; 70:381–385.
120. Jones KA, Lennon RL, Hosking MP: Method of intraoperative monitoring of neuromuscular function and residual blockade in the recovery room. Minn Med 1992; 75:23–26.

SECTION FIVE

Monitoring in Special Situations

CHAPTER 18

Maternal and Fetal Monitoring

ANDREW M. WOODS, M.D.

Obstetric monitoring frequently begins with a very inexpensive device, an oral thermometer. By monitoring body temperature for the specific pattern associated with ovulation, a woman is able to identify the narrow time frame when conception may be possible. Once conception has occurred, obstetric monitoring takes on a unique duality because there are at least two patients with separate, but interdependent, physiologic systems to be assessed. The ideal of maternal-fetal monitoring is the early detection of physiologic abnormalities that, in the absence of intervention, might progress to serious organ injury.

MATERNAL MONITORING

MATERNAL PHYSIOLOGY IN NORMAL PREGNANCY

Pregnancy is associated with a number of physiologic changes; some subserve the increased metabolic burden imposed by the fetus, whereas others alter the maternal physiognomy to accommodate the mechanical burden of the fetus during pregnancy and delivery. One objective of antepartum maternal monitoring is to determine whether the alterations fall within expected norms and to document the normal progression in these changes.

Cardiovascular Physiology in Normal Pregnancy

Cardiac Output and Vascular Resistance

Normal pregnancy is characterized by a 30–50% increase in cardiac output (Figs. 18–1*A* and 18–2) that results from a 30% increase in stroke volume and a 15% increase in heart rate. The increase in cardiac output appears to plateau at the end of the second trimester. Thereafter, there is considerable variability in cardiac output; in some women it continues to increase, but in most, it decreases after the 32nd week of gestation because of a decreasing stroke volume.[1]

Easterling and colleagues found no correlation between body surface area and cardiac output in normal pregnancies, and therefore recommend reporting cardiac output rather than cardiac index (cardiac output divided by body surface area).[2] The purpose of normalization of cardiac output for body surface area is to reduce intersubject variability based on differences in body size. However, to do so in pregnant patients results in the inclusion of tissues such as amniotic fluid, edema fluid, the fetal mass, and the increased maternal blood volume. Because these are not maternal oxygen-consuming tissues, normalization based on a weight-derived body surface area only serves to obscure changes in cardiovascular parameters during pregnancy.

The increase in maternal cardiac output during normal pregnancy parallels a modest decrease in mean arterial blood pressure (Fig. 18–1*B*). The direction and magnitude of these physiologic changes necessitate a commensurate decrease in peripheral vascular resistance (Fig. 18–1*C*). Of these three variables, cardiac output and blood pressure are measured directly, either invasively or noninvasively, and vascular resistance is calculated as follows:

$$\text{Resistance} = (\text{pressure/cardiac output}) \times 80 \qquad 18\text{–}1$$

When invasive techniques are used, the value for pressure is mean arterial pressure minus central venous pressure, and resistance is referred to as systemic vascular resistance (SVR). When, as is increasingly frequent in obstetrics, noninvasive techniques are used to measure cardiac output, central venous pressures are not measured, and the value for pressure refers solely to mean arterial pressure; in this case, resistance is reported as total peripheral resistance. In most circumstances, central venous pressures are inconsequentially small compared to mean arterial pressures, and the two measures of resistance are interchangeable.

A major component of the decrease in vascular resistance during pregnancy is the low-resistance uteroplacental circulation, which receives a large proportion of the increase in cardiac output. Abnormalities of vascular resistance can

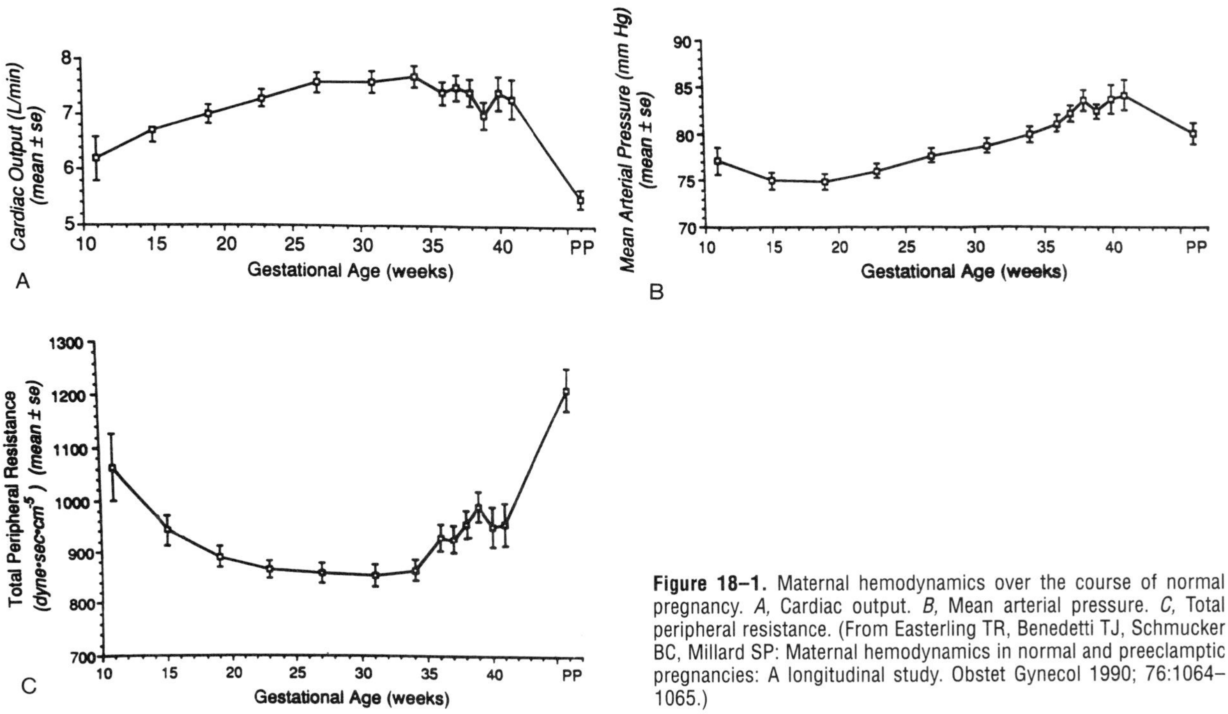

Figure 18–1. Maternal hemodynamics over the course of normal pregnancy. *A*, Cardiac output. *B*, Mean arterial pressure. *C*, Total peripheral resistance. (From Easterling TR, Benedetti TJ, Schmucker BC, Millard SP: Maternal hemodynamics in normal and preeclamptic pregnancies: A longitudinal study. Obstet Gynecol 1990; 76:1064–1065.)

involve primarily the placental circulation, the maternal peripheral vasculature, or both.

Almost all pregnant women develop a grade 2/4 systolic murmur that is best heard along either the left or the right upper sternal border. Such murmurs are almost always related to increased flow, either across the pulmonic or aortic outflow tracts or through the mammary vessels. Murmurs that are diastolic, pansystolic, late systolic, or associated with an abnormal electrocardiogram (ECG) cannot be classified as benign and warrant echocardiographic assessment.[3]

Cardiac Size and Function

In normal pregnancy, the left ventricle enlarges without changing wall thickness (eccentric enlargement).[4] Thus, the radius-to-wall thickness ratio is increased. This physiologic change places the heart at a structural disadvantage for dealing with acutely increased arterial pressure because an increase in ventricular size without a change in wall thickness results in an increase in wall tension. The force generated by heart muscle can be approximated by ventricular wall tension (force per unit area). LaPlace's law states that wall tension is directly proportional to both the intracavitary (ventricular) pressure and the ventricular radius and inversely proportional to wall thickness. Concomitant increases in intracavitary pressure, as occurs with increases in arterial blood pressure, produce additive increases in wall tension that may precipitate heart failure.

Multiple gestations (e.g., twins, triplets) are associated with even greater increases in cardiac output than normal pregnancies.[5] The increase in output appears to be related to increases in contractility and heart rate rather than further increases in chamber size above that in single gestation pregnancies. Thus, cardiac reserve is reduced in multiple gestations, which may have implications for patients with pre-existing cardiac disease.

Uterine Vascular Changes

The blood supply to the placenta travels through the uterine musculature (myometrium) via an arterial network that includes the spiral arteries. In normal pregnancy, the

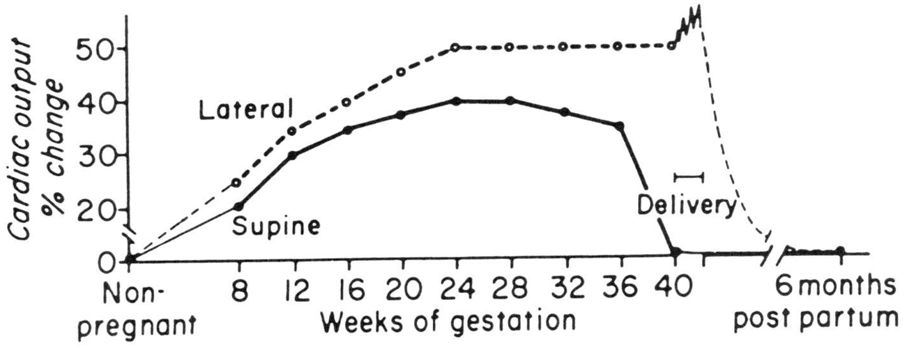

Figure 18–2. Change in cardiac output over the course of normal pregnancy in the supine and lateral positions. (From Bonica JJ: Obstetric Analgesia and Anesthesia, 2nd Ed. Amsterdam: World Federation of Societies of Anesthesiologists, 1980, 5.)

trophoblast, which is derived from the fertilized ovum and is thus of fetal origin, invades the wall of the spiral arteries and obliterates the encircling vascular smooth muscle and the internal elastic lamina, leaving the external elastic lamina. The resultant large-lumen vessels lose the ability to vasoconstrict. Thus, in normal pregnancy, the uterus becomes a very low-resistance vascular bed with minimal ability to vasoconstrict and autoregulate blood flow in response to changes in maternal blood pressure. Uterine flow thus becomes pressure-dependent; thus, even modest hypotension during anesthesia for the pregnant patient should be controlled.

Arterial Pressure

There is an approximate 5-mmHg decrease in mean arterial pressure during the first half of normal pregnancy. The pressure nadir is reached at midgestation (around 20 weeks); from that point on, mean pressure increases (Fig. 18–1*B*).[1, 6] By term, the mean pressure is slightly higher than in the nonpregnant state and returns to normal in the early postpartum period. The change in mean blood pressure is primarily because of changes in the diastolic pressure.

Effects of Patient Position on Arterial Blood Pressure. Blood pressure in the left lateral decubitus position is consistently less (about 15 mmHg) than it is in the supine position, in both the nonpregnant and the pregnant states, when the cuff is placed on the right (up) arm. However, this difference is not found when central pressures are measured, indicating that it is due to the elevated position of the right brachial artery relative to the heart. The magnitude of the effect is approximately 0.77 mmHg/cm of the vertical distance above the heart. This positional difference should be considered when evaluating blood pressure in a recumbent patient, as after epidural block. Conversely, if the cuff is placed on the dependent arm, pressures will be slightly higher than central pressures.

During pregnancy, there appear to be no differences between blood pressures measured in the sitting and in the standing position, in contrast to the nonpregnant state, in which systolic pressures are higher in sitting than in standing subjects.[7] The hemodynamic explanation for this is unclear and would require knowledge of cardiac output and regional vascular resistances, which may be quite different for the same blood pressure recorded in different positions.

In evaluating the effect of patient position on hemodynamic variables, Clark and colleagues found no significant changes in blood pressure when comparing the recumbent position to the standing position.[8] However, there were major differences in cardiac output and vascular resistance in pregnant patients at term as compared to the same patients 3 months postpartum, depending on position. Pregnant patients maintained their blood pressure on standing primarily by maintaining cardiac output, whereas the same patients in the postpartum period had a large decrease in cardiac output on standing that was offset by a large increase in vascular resistance (42%). Thus, it would appear that the hypervolemic and vasodilated state of pregnancy provides some protection against gravitational changes in the distribution of blood volume and impairment of venous return to the heart.

The supine position may have profound effects on cardiovascular function as the parturient approaches term and the gravid uterus impairs blood return to the right side of the heart from the lower body (Fig. 18–2). Although the resultant decrease in cardiac output may be modest in some patients (10%), others will develop symptoms of shock (dizziness, nausea, vomiting, pallor, sweating, decreased level of consciousness) if the obstruction is not relieved. This obstruction to vena cava flow by the gravid uterus is referred to as the supine hypotensive syndrome. Pirhonen and Erkkola reported an increase in maternal blood pressure of 11 mmHg and an increase in heart rate of 23 beats/minute when the supine position was assumed by parturients with a history of supine position dizziness (Fig. 18–3).[9] However, the change in blood pressure is partially artifactual and reflects a lower position of the cuffed right arm relative to the heart in the supine position as opposed to the left lateral semirecumbent position. After 5 minutes, a decrease in blood pressure (an average of 20 mmHg) coincided with maternal symptoms in some patients and impairment of the uterine circulation in others; two fetuses demonstrated heart rate decelerations during this period.

Although the blood pressure at which symptoms are present is only about 20 mmHg below normal, it is clearly associated with a marked decrease in cardiac output to both the maternal cerebral and the uterine circulations. Modest changes in blood pressure in this situation may give little indication of the marked changes in the underlying components of blood pressure—cardiac output and vascular resistance. Both maternal symptoms and the uterine hemodynamic disturbances are usually effectively relieved when the pregnant woman shifts from the supine to the lateral recumbent or semirecumbent position.

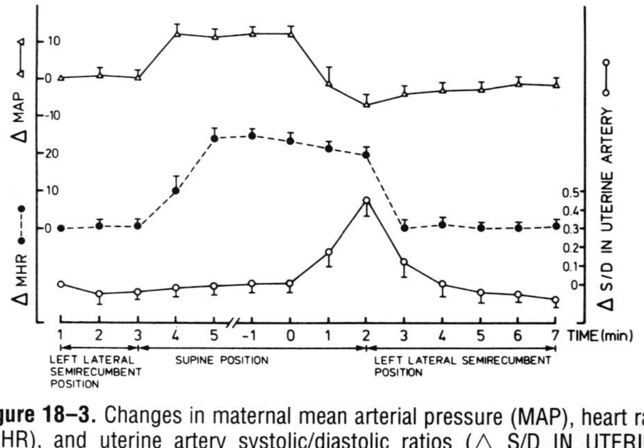

Figure 18–3. Changes in maternal mean arterial pressure (MAP), heart rate (MHR), and uterine artery systolic/diastolic ratios (Δ S/D IN UTERINE ARTERY) in 10 patients experiencing the supine hypotensive syndrome. Time zero is the point at which blood pressure begins to decrease after a period of stability. The increase in the S/D ratio is indicative of increased uterine impedance to blood flow. (From Pirhonen JP, Erkkola RU: Uterine and umbilical flow velocity waveforms in the supine hypotensive syndrome. Obstet Gynecol 1990; 76: 177.)

Altered Sensitivity to Vasoactive Compounds. Normal pregnancy is characterized by decreased sensitivity to endogenous vasopressors such as norepinephrine and angiotensin II.[10] Figure 18–4 depicts the dose of angiotensin II required to increase diastolic blood pressure by 20 mmHg at various intervals over the course of normal pregnancy. At the end of the second trimester, approximately twice the dose of angiotensin II is required compared with nonpregnant controls. The decrease in vasopressor sensitivity parallels an increase in plasma renin activity (PRA)[7] and is important in preventing a hypertensive response to a state of increased vascular volume plus increased PRA, because both of these factors tend to increase blood pressure in the absence of changes in resistance. These findings have important implications for obstetric patients. Patients with uncontrollable uterine bleeding requiring hysterectomy demonstrate no response to a number of vasoconstrictors,[11] whereas patients with hypertensive pregnancies have increased vasopressor sensitivity.

Venous Pressure

Venous pressures are unchanged in pregnancy as long as the measurements are not performed in the leg or in a supine patient. Venous pressures in the lower extremities increase sharply after the first trimester, reflecting in part the increased hydrostatic load imposed by the expanded blood volume and the obstruction to venous return caused by the enlarging uterus (Fig. 18–5).[12] To the degree that these conditions promote venous stasis, they place the mother at risk for embolic complications; pulmonary embolism now ranks as a leading cause of maternal mortality.[13]

Blood Volume and Oxygen Transport

Maternal blood volume increases by 30–40% over the course of normal pregnancy (Fig. 18–6). Red cell volume increases 15%, and plasma volume increases 40–50%, resulting in a dilutional decrease in the hematocrit level from a nonpregnant value of 39–41% to 34–35% during pregnancy.[14–17] Despite the reduced oxygen-carrying capacity associated with a lower hemoglobin concentration, oxygen transport during pregnancy is actually increased, particularly to vital organs such as the kidneys and the uterus. Oxygen transport and delivery is facilitated by an increase in maternal cardiac output and an increase in 2,3-diphosphoglycerate. The latter causes a rightward shift in the maternal oxyhemoglobin dissociation curve, with P_{50} increasing from 26.7 mmHg to 30.4 mmHg; this increases the availability of oxygen at the tissue level by decreasing the affinity of hemoglobin for oxygen.[18]

Fluid Balance

Total body water increases by 7.5 L during pregnancy in a distribution described in Table 18–1.[19] Sodium plays a key role in body water balance, and an increase in total body sodium of almost 1000 mmol brought about by increased renal reabsorption of sodium drives the expansion in body water. A balanced increase in both salt and water leaves plasma sodium concentration unchanged.

Colloid osmotic pressure (COP) decreases from a range of 25–28 mmHg in the nonpregnant patient to 21–23 mmHg in the pregnant patient at term.[20] COP decreases still further to 13–18 mmHg following delivery. Pulmonary capillary wedge pressure (PCWP) is unchanged during normal pregnancy.[21] The net result is a modest decrease in the

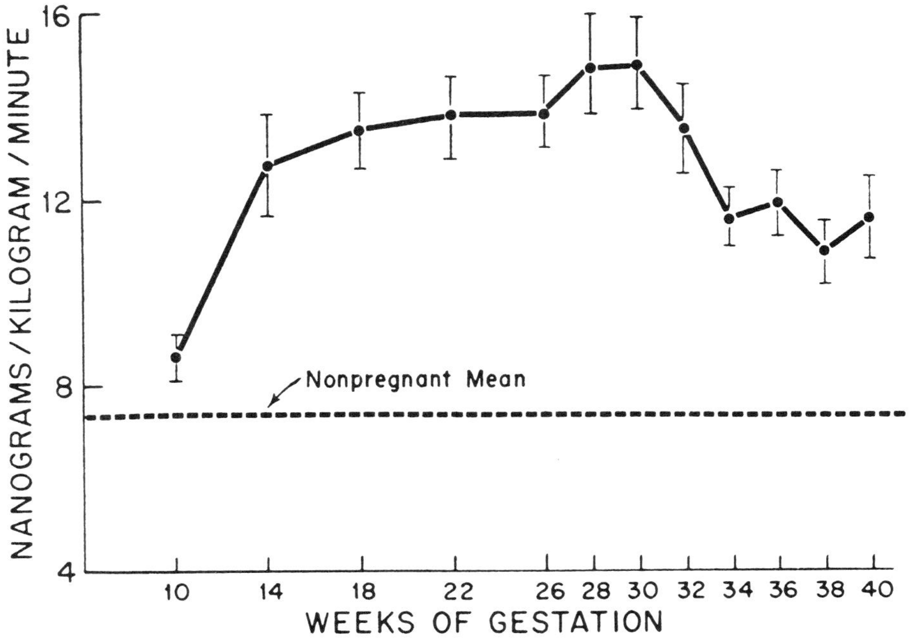

Figure 18–4. Decreased angiotensin II sensitivity over the course of normal pregnancy. The closed circles represent the mean dose of angiotensin II (± standard error of the mean) required to elicit a pressor response of 20 mmHg in diastolic blood pressure in normotensive pregnant patients. The broken line represents the mean for nonpregnant patients. (From Gant NF, Daley GL, Chand S, et al: A study of angiotensin II pressor response throughout primigravid pregnancy. J Clin Invest 1973; 52:2682–2689, by copyright permission of the American Society for Clinical Investigation.)

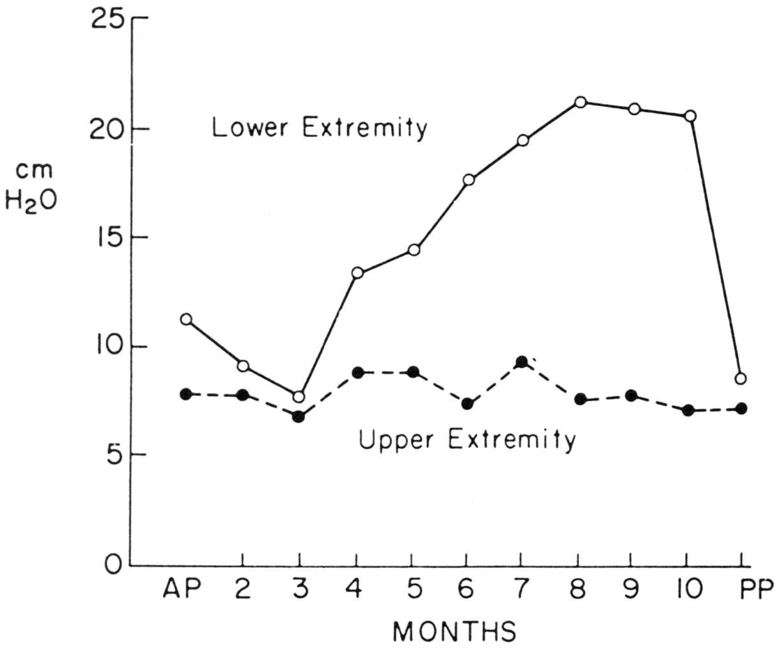

Figure 18–5. Comparison of venous pressures in the upper and lower extremities before (AP), during, and after (PP) pregnancy. (From Brinkman CR: Biologic adaptations to pregnancy. *In* Creasy R, Resnik R [eds]: Maternal-Fetal Medicine, 2nd Ed. Philadelphia: WB Saunders, 1989; 741.)

COP-PCWP gradient and a potential narrowing of the margin of safety against the development of pulmonary edema.

Fluid balance between the capillaries and the interstitium is maintained by opposing forces; capillary and interstitial hydrostatic pressure oppose each other, as do capillary and interstitial COP. Although the capillary hydrostatic pressure cannot be measured directly, it can be calculated from measured COP in plasma and interstitial fluid and from the hydrostatic pressure of the interstitial fluid.

Capillary hydrostatic pressure increases approximately 30% from the first to the third trimester of pregnancy.[22] Increased capillary hydrostatic pressure, coupled with the decrease in plasma COP, favors the movement of fluid across the capillary membrane, yet normal pregnancy is not associated with generalized tissue edema. The distribution of fluid between the vascular space and the interstitium is unchanged[23] because interstitial COP decreases markedly over the course of pregnancy, presumably because of increases in local lymphatic flow (Table 18–2). The dependent edema seen in the feet of ambulatory women in the late stages of normal pregnancy is associated with capillary hydrostatic pressures in the ankle region that are 35% higher than capillary pressures in the upper part of the body. The resultant edema reflects an inability of the distri-

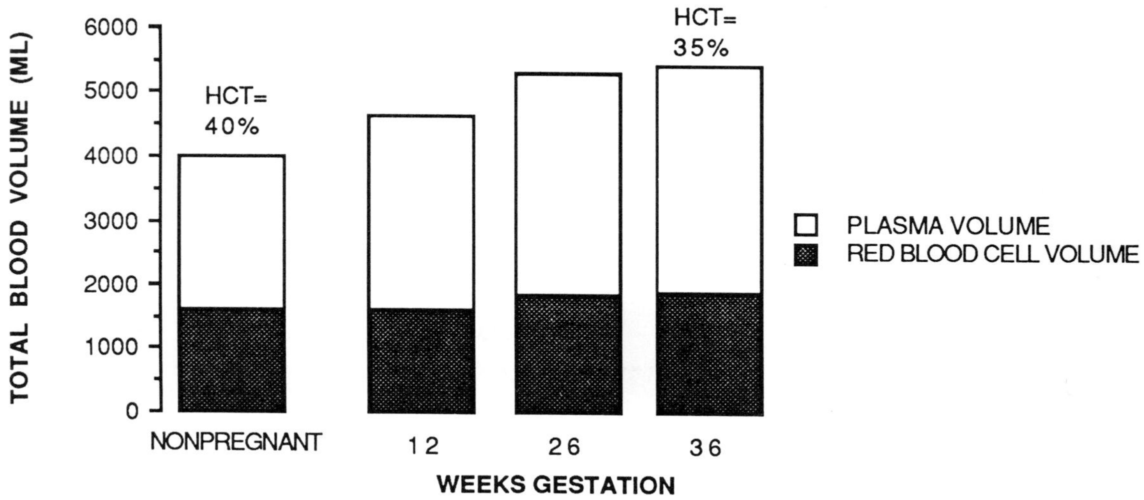

Figure 18–6. Blood volume, plasma volume, and red cell volume over the course of normal pregnancy. Most of the increase in blood volume is accounted for by an increase in plasma volume, producing a modest dilutional "anemia of pregnancy." (HCT = hematocrit.) (Compiled from Blekta, Hlavatý, Trnková, et al: Am J Obstet Gynecol, 1970; Davidson: Scand J Clin Lab Invest [Suppl], 1984; Goodlin, Quaife, Dirksen: Semin Perinatol, 1981; Hayes, Cruikshank, Dunn: Am J Obstet Gynecol, 1985; Gallery: Clin Exp Hypertens, 1982.)

TABLE 18–1. DISTRIBUTION OF INCREASED TOTAL BODY WATER IN PREGNANCY

Tissue	Volume (Liters)
Interstitial fluid	1.7
Plasma	1.2
Fetus	2.0
Amniotic fluid	1.2
Uterus, placenta, and breasts	1.4

Modified from Davison JM: Renal hemodynamics and volume homeostasis in pregnancy. Scand J Clin Lab Invest Suppl 1984; 169:15–27, with permission of Blackwell Scientific Publications.

bution of plasma and interstitial proteins to counterbalance the increase in hydrostatic pressure in the capillaries, and there is a net movement of water across the capillary membrane into the interstitium.

Cardiovascular Changes During Labor and Delivery

During active labor, cardiac output increases over prelabor values as a result of catecholamine-mediated increases in heart rate and stroke volume, as long as the patient is not in the supine position. The increase correlates with the degree of cervical dilatation (Fig. 18–7).[24] Both stroke volume and heart rate increase with each contraction. The increase in stroke volume is caused by an autotransfusion effect that accompanies each contraction as uterine blood (500 ml) is forced into the central circulation. The peak increase in cardiac output occurs immediately after delivery, as uterine involution relieves the obstruction to venous return and also displaces a large volume of uterine blood into the maternal circulation. Because the uterus is now removed as a parallel circuit in the maternal vascular bed, additional maternal vasodilatation is necessary to maintain low peripheral vascular resistance and to avoid hypertension. Potent vasoconstrictors such as phenylephrine and ergonovine maleate, an oxytocic, can produce severe systemic and pulmonary hypertension if administered in the immediate postpartum period. Endogenous catecholamines, as often accompany tracheal suctioning and extubation, can produce similar results. Such hypertension places the patient at risk for both pulmonary edema and cerebral vascular injury, particularly in the presence of underlying disease.

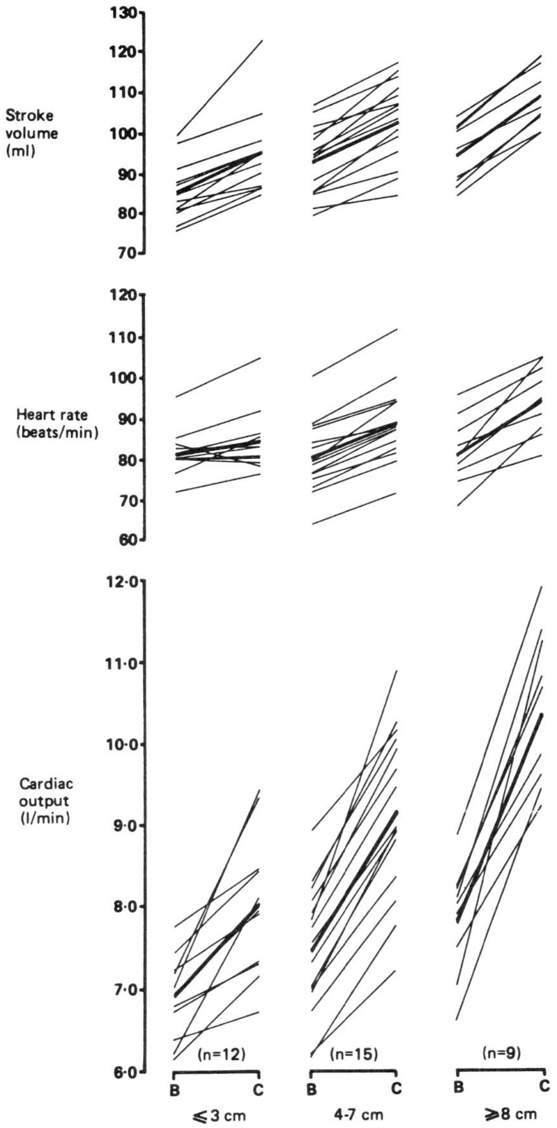

Figure 18–7. Changes in stroke volume, heart rate, and cardiac output during uterine contractions at progressive stages of cervical dilatation. Darker lines represent the mean values. (From Robson SC, Dunlop W, Boys RJ, Hunter S: Cardiac output during labor. Br Med J 1987; 295:1170.)

TABLE 18–2. COLLOID OSMOTIC PRESSURES AND HYDROSTATIC PRESSURES IN THE CAPILLARIES AND INTERSTITIUM OVER THE COURSE OF PREGNANCY

	First Trimester (mmHg)	Third Trimester (mmHg)
Colloid osmotic pressure—capillary	23.2 ± 0.8	21.1 ± 1.2
Colloid osmotic pressure—interstitium (thorax)	13.1 + 1.2	8.4 + 0.8
Colloid osmotic pressure—interstitium (ankle)	9.6 + 5.5	5.5 + 1.4
Hydrostatic pressure—interstitium (thorax)	−1.6 + 0.7	−1.2 + 0.9
Hydrostatic pressure—interstitium (ankle)	−0.9 ± 0.5	−0.1 ± 0.4
Hydrostatic pressure—capillary (thorax)	8.3 ± 1.9	11.5 ± 2.3
Hydrostatic pressure—capillary (ankle)	12.7 ± 2.1	15.5 ± 2.3

Modified from Oian P, Maltau JM: Calculated capillary hydrostatic pressure in normal pregnancy and preeclampsia. Am J Obstet Gynecol 1987; 157:104, with permission.

Respiratory Physiology in Normal Pregnancy

Minute ventilation increases 50% during pregnancy to accommodate increased maternal-fetal oxygen consumption and carbon dioxide production. The increase in minute ventilation is due almost entirely to increased tidal volume; respiratory rate is unchanged.[25] Carbon dioxide tension in the blood decreases to 30–32 mmHg; the mechanism for this hyperventilation is thought to be related to the effects of increased progesterone on the respiratory centers in the central nervous system. Serum bicarbonate decreases to about 22 mEq/L, such that arterial pH remains normal.

Both oxygen consumption and carbon dioxide production increase significantly during the third trimester (Fig. 18–8). The change is proportional, and there is minimal change in the respiratory exchange ratio.

During labor, hyperventilation accompanying painful contractions may result in pronounced hypocarbia ($Pa{CO_2}$ less than 20 mmHg) and respiratory alkalemia. Although such acid-base abnormalities have not been shown to directly affect uterine blood flow or fetal oxygenation, the hypoventilation that may occur between contractions when the mother is extremely alkalotic can cause maternal and fetal hypoxemia.[26] These ventilatory abnormalities are not seen if effective epidural analgesia is employed during parturition.

Lung volumes and lung capacities show little change with pregnancy except for a 15–20% decrease in functional residual capacity that results from the cephalad displacement of the diaphragm by the enlarging uterus (Fig. 18–9). Although the 45° sitting position has been shown to improve the functional residual capacity of nonpregnant subjects and to prolong the time to desaturation during apnea, this position change is of no benefit to the parturient.[27]

Expiratory reserve volume decreases as a result of the expanded tidal volume. There is a decrease in total pulmonary resistance during pregnancy that is felt to be mediated by progesterone, a known smooth muscle relaxant. Forced expiratory volume in 1 second and peak expiratory flow rate are unaffected.[28] Pregnancy does not protect against the deleterious effects of cigarette smoking on lung function, and smokers have a 25% impairment of flow in small airways.[29]

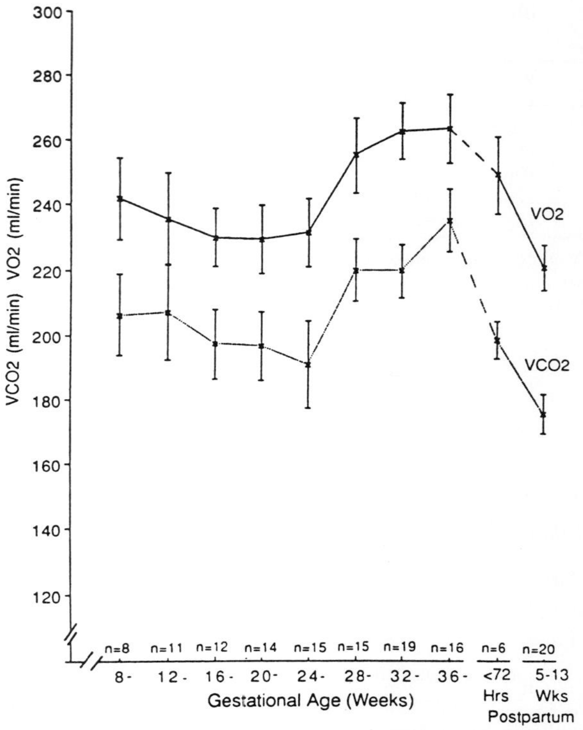

Figure 18–8. Variation in oxygen consumption (V_{O_2}) and carbon dioxide production (V_{CO_2}) over the course of normal pregnancy. The number (n) of subjects studied at each stage of gestation is shown. (From Rees GB, Pipkin FB, Symonds EM, Patrick JM: A longitudinal study of respiratory changes in normal human pregnancy with cross-sectional data on subjects with pregnancy-induced hypertension. Am J Obstet Gynecol 1990; 162:827.)

Closing volume refers to the lung volume at which airway closure begins to occur in dependent zones of the lungs, resulting in areas that are perfused but not ventilated. If the lung volume at end-expiration is less than the closing volume, closure occurs and favors an increased oxygen

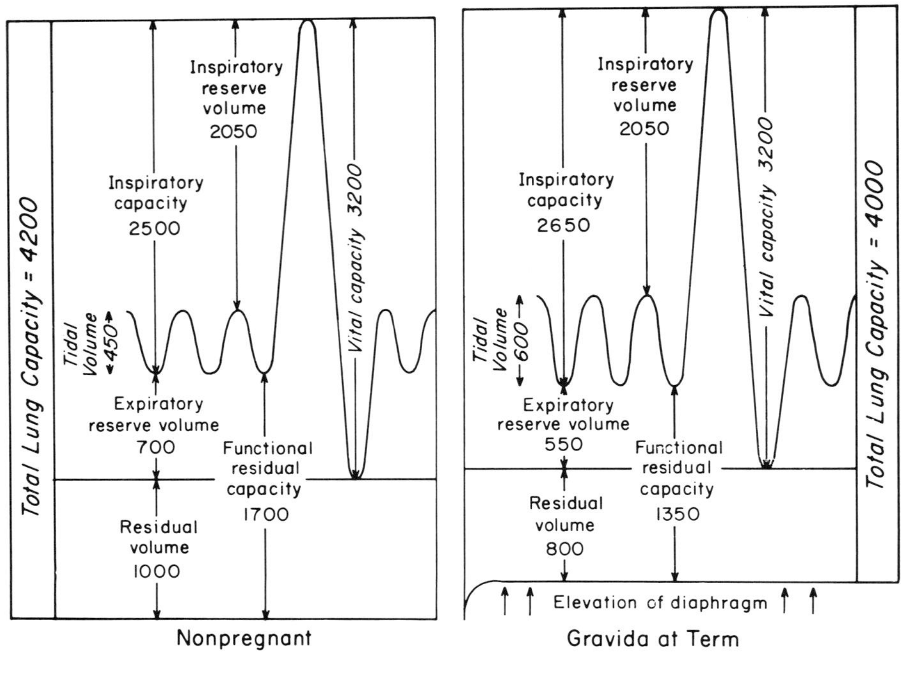

Figure 18–9. Pulmonary volumes and capacities at term compared to the nonpregnant state. (From Bonica JJ: Principles and Practice of Obstetric Analgesia and Anesthesia. Philadelphia: FA Davis, 1967; 24.)

alveolar-arterial (A-aO_2) gradient. Although there is some controversy in this area, it appears that as many as one half of all pregnant women develop airway closure in the supine position.[30]

The decreased functional residual capacity and the tendency toward airway closure in the supine position have particular significance for the gravida during anesthesia. Both conditions effectively decrease the time to hypoxia in the event of an interruption of oxygen delivery to the alveoli, as might result from airway obstruction associated with induction of general anesthesia. Thus, adequate preoxygenation prior to induction is mandatory. Also, the decrease in functional residual capacity and the increase in minute ventilation accelerate induction of anesthesia with inhalation agents, particularly in the supine position with the resultant decrease in cardiac output.

Capillary engorgement during pregnancy affects both the nasal and the laryngeal mucosa. This increases the likelihood of bleeding if the nasal route is used for the passage of tubes. Also, the narrowed upper airway may not be able to accommodate standard-size endotracheal tubes; a tube one size smaller than normal is recommended for the pregnant patient.

Renal Physiology in Normal Pregnancy

Renal plasma flow and glomerular filtration rate are 50% above normal by the end of the second trimester, resulting in lower values for blood urea nitrogen (8 mg/dl) and creatinine (0.46 mg/dl). However, during the third trimester, renal plasma flow and glomerular filtration rate tend to return toward nonpregnant levels, in part as a result of aortic compression by the gravid uterus. Both mild glucosuria and moderate proteinuria (< 300 mg/day) are very common during pregnancy. Neither condition necessarily indicates underlying disease.

Gastrointestinal Physiology in Normal Pregnancy

Pregnancy is associated with a loss of competency of the gastroesophageal junction, leading to reports of "heartburn" and esophagitis in roughly half of all pregnant patients. This effect occurs early in pregnancy and is caused in part by increased levels of progesterone, a smooth muscle relaxant. Gastric acidity and volume are elevated in late pregnancy as a result of increased gastrin levels. Gastric emptying is not affected by pregnancy.[31] However, the onset of labor has a profound retardant effect on gastric emptying. Ultrasound examination of parturients in active labor has shown that two thirds of patients have solid food in the stomach independent of the time between the last intake of food and the examination.[32] Although the risk associated with pulmonary aspiration of nonparticulate gastric fluid, irrespective of the pH, is controversial and undefined, a high morbidity rate is associated with the aspiration of partially digested food; this is an event that continues to contribute to maternal morbidity and mortality in association with general anesthesia in the pregnant patient, particularly in the setting of emergency cesarean delivery for fetal distress during labor.

Nervous System Physiology in Normal Pregnancy

Anesthetic requirement, or minimal alveolar concentration (MAC), is decreased approximately 40% during pregnancy. This is most likely due to increased maternal endorphins, because the decreased MAC is reversible with naloxone hydrochloride. Also, a smaller amount of local anesthetic drug is required for epidural and subarachnoid blockades in pregnancy. Although a number of factors have been implicated, including engorgement of the epidural veins and acid-base changes in the spinal fluid, the onset of the decrease in local anesthetic requirement during early pregnancy adds credence to another explanation: progesterone and possibly other pregnancy-related compounds potentiate the effects of both endogenous and exogenous opiates[33] and alter the nerve membrane to make it more easily penetrated by local anesthetic molecules.[34]

Hemostasis in Normal Pregnancy

The blood of pregnant patients becomes slightly hypercoagulable as gestation progresses, a useful adaptation to decrease blood loss at delivery. Factor I (fibrinogen) levels and factor VIII (antihemophilic factor) activity are increased 50–100%. Other coagulation factors increase slightly or not at all. Platelet reactivity to adrenaline and arachidonic acid increases during the third trimester, which further contributes to the hypercoagulable state and increases the risk of thromboembolic complications.[35] Although the platelet count decreases 20% in pregnancy, no clinically significant change in bleeding occurs.

MATERNAL MONITORING IN LOW-RISK PREGNANCY

Antepartum Monitoring

Routine antepartum monitoring in low-risk pregnancies consists of periodic examinations with particular attention to blood pressure, weight, uterine size, hematocrit, blood glucose, urinalysis (particularly for protein), and cultures and blood serology for sexually transmitted diseases. Increasingly, ultrasonography is included in routine antepartum monitoring, although the maternal indications are rather limited. The image produced by ultrasound can identify a gestational sac as early as 3 weeks following conception (Fig. 18–10). This can help in the diagnosis of an ectopic pregnancy. Placental problems such as placenta previa and abruption can be diagnosed using ultrasound. There is some evidence that placental position (laterally vs. centrally located within the uterus) may be a risk factor for the development of fetal growth retardation and maternal hypertensive disorders during pregnancy.[36] A centrally lo-

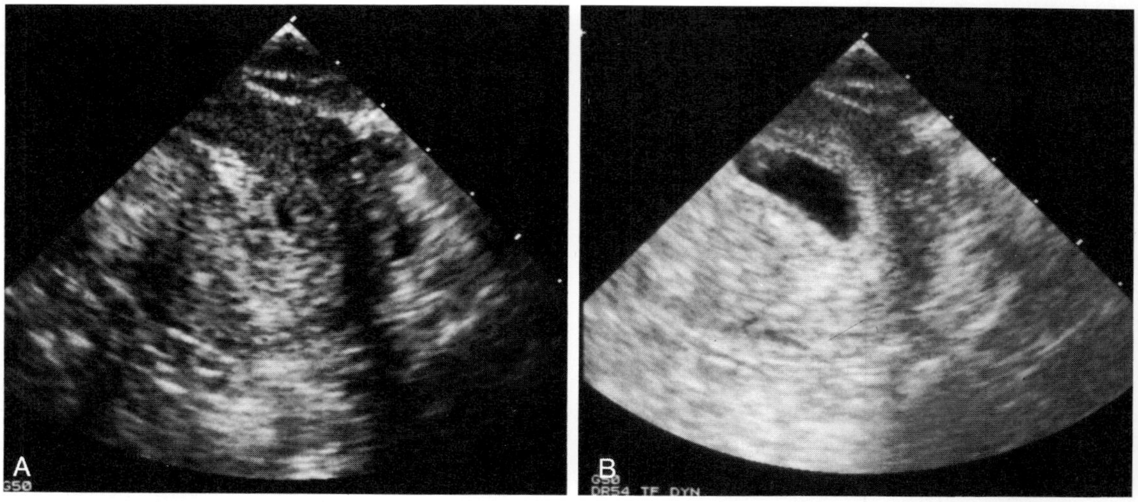

Figure 18–10. *A,* Ultrasound scan allowing visualization of an intrauterine gestational sac 3 weeks following conception. The sac is the small black spot in the center of the scan. The dark shadows on both sides of the sac outline the uterus. *B,* Same patient, 12 days later. The gestational sac is much larger, and a tiny fetus is visible. Real time ultrasonography is able to record the pumping of the fetal heart at this early stage.

cated placenta receives an equal blood supply from both uterine arteries, whereas laterally situated placentas have a decreased blood supply from the contralateral uterine artery in the absence of collateral circulation through major vascular anastomoses.

The significance of routine monitoring (e.g., vital signs, weight, blood glucose) during low-risk pregnancy is that abnormalities, if detected, often result in reclassification of the pregnancy into one of high risk.

Blood Pressure

Blood pressure monitoring is important, because maternal hypertension in pregnancy is a major risk factor affecting fetal outcome. In a large study involving almost 15,000 patients, Page and Christianson reported that each 5-mmHg increase in mean arterial pressure (MAP) recorded during the fifth and sixth months of gestation was associated with an increase in perinatal mortality, with the largest increase in mortality occurring when the MAP was 90 mmHg or higher.[37]

Unfortunately, this extremely important vital sign is subject to considerable error in measurement.[38] Interobserver variability arises from observer bias (expecting certain pressures), lack of standard technique (fourth vs. fifth Korotkoff sound as the diastolic value), observer terminal digit preference (values ending in zero occurring at a frequency many times higher than values ending in a digit other than zero), and improper technique (letting the mercury column fall too fast). Interobserver variability increases with gestation and is greater for diastolic pressures than for systolic pressures.

Some of the problems with observer bias can be corrected by use of a random-zero sphygmomanometer. This device masks the true zero level of the mercury, and the correct pressure is determined by adding or subtracting the baseline value from the measured value.

Use of an automated device such as the Dinamap can also eliminate much of the bias of manually measured blood pressure (see Chapter 5). The MAP is the most reliable of the pressures reported by the Dinamap. Both the systolic and particularly the diastolic pressures are less accurate. Unfortunately, studies that utilize automated devices based on oscillometry often calculate the mean pressure from the systolic and diastolic pressures rather than simply using the directly measured value. For example, a major study by Easterling and colleagues [1] used an automated blood pressure device yet derived MAP from the following formula:

$$\text{MAP} = \text{diastolic blood pressure} \times 2 + \text{systolic blood pressure}/3 \qquad 18\text{–}2$$

Use of such formulas, in which the diastolic pressure is doubled relative to the systolic pressure for calculation purposes, tends to further magnify the variation in the derived mean pressure because of the inherent variability in diastolic measurements using oscillometry as well as manual sphygmomanometry.

The importance of accurate and precise blood pressure measurements is illustrated by studies that, early in gestation, find abnormally increased blood pressures in women who are destined to become preeclamptic (Fig. 18–11, 18–12, and 18–13).[1, 6, 39] However, in part because of the degree of variability in blood pressure measurements, there is too much overlap between normal persons and patients destined to become preeclamptic to accurately and precisely predict the outcome of any individual patient. To the degree that accuracy in blood pressure determinations can be maximized and variability minimized, zones of overlap can be minimized and distinctions between normals and those destined to become preeclamptic can be optimized.

Routine use of *automated devices* to record *mean blood pressures* in a *standard position* would allow for more reliable data with less variability, and would also facilitate

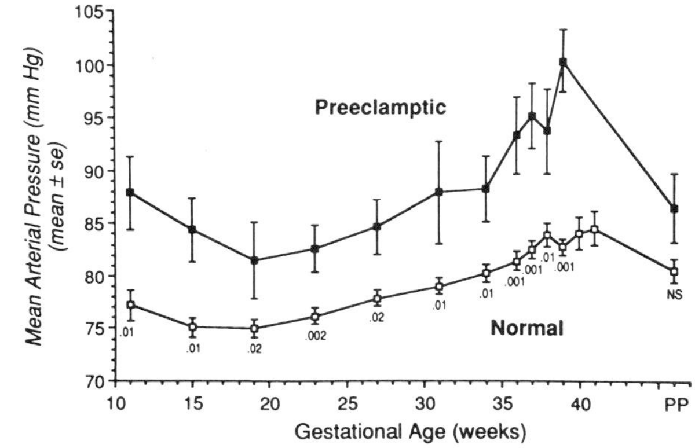

Figure 18–11. Mean arterial pressure (± standard error) over the course of pregnancy in normotensive and preeclamptic nulliparous pregnancies as measured by an automated oscillometric device. Measurements were made with subjects in the left lateral recumbent position with the cuff on the left arm. Differences are significant at all gestational ages but not in the postpartum period. (From Easterling TR, Benedetti TJ, Schmucker BC, Millard SP: Maternal hemodynamics in normal and preeclamptic pregnancies: A longitudinal study. Obstet Gynecol 1990; 76:1064.)

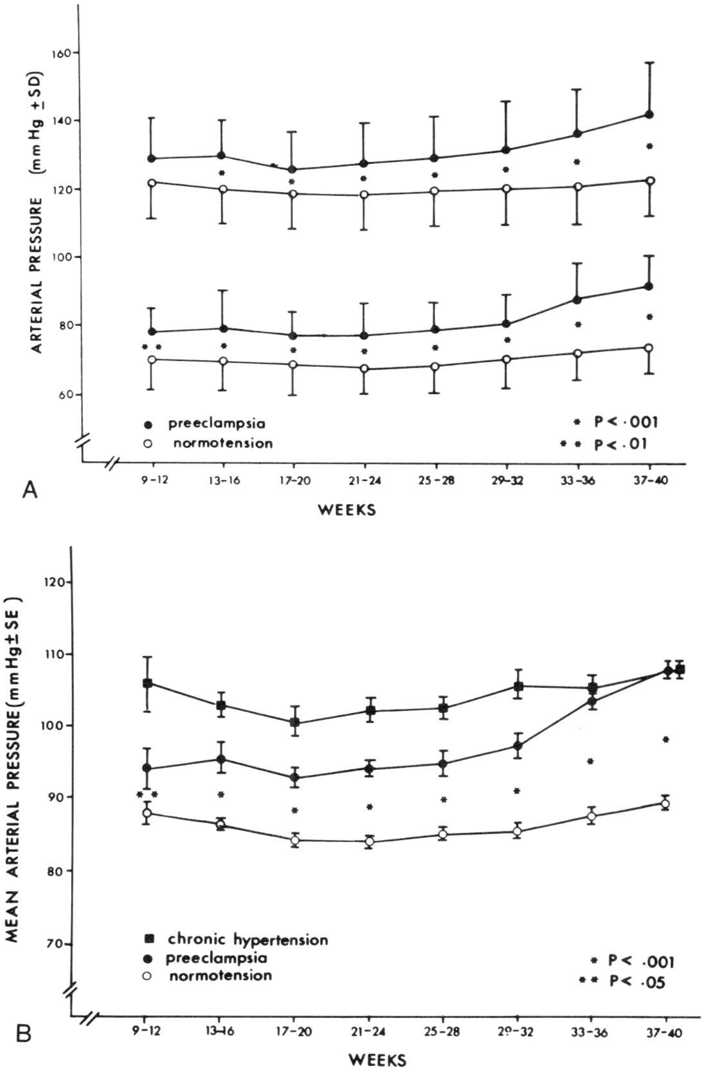

Figure 18–12. Systolic and diastolic *(A)* and mean *(B)* blood pressures over the course of normal and preeclamptic nulliparous pregnancies. Mean pressure measurements also are given for pregnant patients with chronic hypertension. Measurements were made with patients in the sitting position, using a cuff on the right arm and an automatic oscillometric device. (From Moutquin JM, Rainville C, Giroux L, et al: A prospective study of blood pressure in pregnancy: Prediction of preeclampsia. Am J Obstet Gynecol 1985; 151:192.)

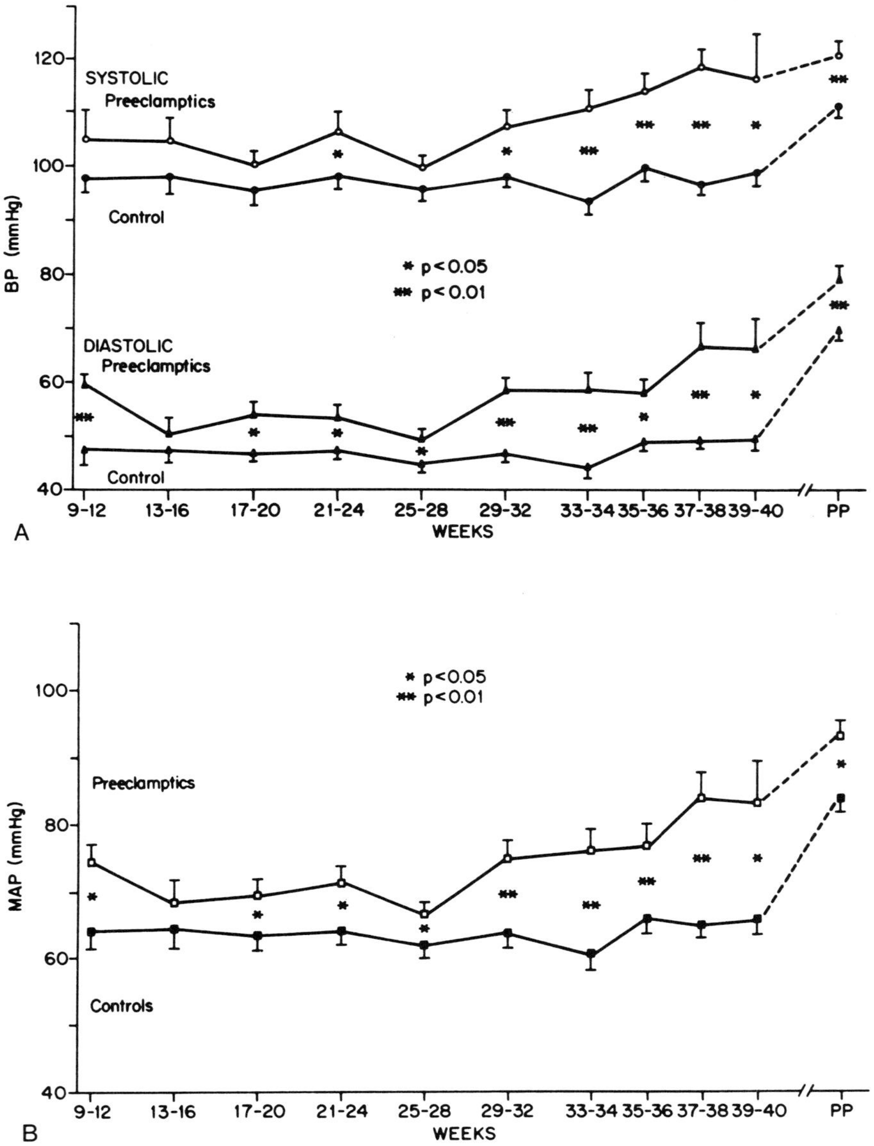

Figure 18–13. Systolic and diastolic *(A)* and mean *(B)* blood pressures over the course of normal and preeclamptic pregnancies. Measurements were made with patients in the left lateral recumbent position with the cuff on the right arm, using a manual sphygmomanometer. (From Reiss RE, O'Shaughnessy RW, Quilligan TJ, Zuspan FP: Retrospective comparison of blood pressure course during preeclamptic and matched control pregnancies. Am J Obstet Gynecol 1987; 156:895.)

cross-study comparisons. When one study uses the fourth Korotkoff sound for determining diastolic pressure and another uses the fifth Korotkoff sound, and diastolic pressures are used to calculate mean arterial pressures, comparisons are meaningless.

The lack of uniformity in blood pressure measurement leads to confusing results. The discrepant data in Figure 18–11 were obtained with the patients in the left lateral recumbent position and with the cuff on the left (down) arm, whereas the data in Figure 18–13 were obtained from the right (up) arm in patients in the left lateral recumbent position. Use of the cuff on the dependent arm more closely corresponds to results obtained in the sitting and standing positions.

On the basis of the combined results from the studies by Easterling et al,[1] Moutquin et al,[6] and Reiss et al,[39] a mean blood pressure in excess of 90 mmHg prior to the 36th week of gestation measured in the standing, seated, or left recumbent position with the cuff on the left arm should raise the suspicion of pregnancy-induced hypertension. Between 36 weeks and term, but prior to the onset of labor, a mean blood pressure greater than 95 mmHg is clearly two standard deviations above normal, and patients with mean pressures in this range should be considered at risk for preeclampsia.

Heart Rate

Maternal heart rate is monitored to detect abnormalities that may affect the mother and/or the fetus. Extremes of heart rate may be associated with maternal thyroid disease, for example. An increase in maternal heart rate in the supine position is associated with the supine hypotensive syndrome.[9]

Temperature

Temperature monitoring detects the timing of ovulation. The major significance of maternal body temperature variations once pregnancy is established is to detect an infectious process. During the first trimester particularly, maternal infection carries a risk of fetal morbidity, particularly with such agents as cytomegalic virus, toxoplasmosis, rubella, herpes, and syphilis. Later in pregnancy, and particularly once there has been rupture of the membranes, increases in maternal body temperature may be a sign of chorioamnionitis, an intrauterine infection that affects both the mother and the fetus.

Uterine Activity

The pain usually associated with uterine contractions allows the mother to be a very good monitor of uterine activity. When such activity occurs prior to term, it is an ominous sign. Premature labor and subsequent delivery of immature infants is still the leading cause of perinatal morbidity and mortality. Once detected, the uterine activity of premature labor may be closely monitored to assess the efficacy of tocolytic therapy, if initiated.

In addition to maternal reporting, uterine activity can be monitored by manual palpation of the lower abdomen and by external and internal devices. External monitors can document the frequency and duration of contractions, but not the intensity. Internal monitors are able to quantify the intensity of contractions but require that the membranes be ruptured in order to place a catheter in the uterus. Thus, internal monitors are not appropriate for antepartum monitoring.

Intrapartum Monitoring

Because low-risk pregnancies can abruptly attain high-risk status without prior identifiable factors, the following guidelines apply to all healthy parturients. The most important maternal monitor is continuous observation and frequent assessment by an experienced obstetric nurse. For example, a patient complaint of chest pain or shortness of breath must be recognized as suggestive of a pulmonary embolus from a thrombus arising in either a deep vein or amniotic fluid. Such complaints may seem less obvious in a patient having painful uterine contractions during labor. Unusual abdominal or shoulder pain must be distinguished from normal labor pains, because the former may herald uterine rupture. Frequent visual inspection and occasional digital examination of the vaginal canal are necessary to detect prolapse of the umbilical cord.

The purpose of routine monitoring is to detect abnormal events or trends early enough to allow intervention; because many obstetric events can happen with great rapidity, frequent monitoring is essential. Blood pressure should be monitored at least every hour in all patients in labor. Heart rate and respiratory rate should be monitored along with blood pressure. Temperature is measured every 4 hours. Once maternal membranes are ruptured, the frequency of temperature measurement is increased to every 2 hours for detection of chorioamnionitis. Urine should be examined initially for protein, glucose, and cellular elements.

During labor, Marx and colleagues reported discrepancies between systolic and diastolic blood pressures obtained by auscultation as opposed to automatic oscillometric devices, with individual differences as high as 20 mmHg.[40] Mean pressure measurements were not significantly different; thus, these authors recommend that the diagnosis of hypertension and hypotension during labor be based on the mean rather than on the systolic or diastolic pressure. Unfortunately, they identified a mean pressure of 105 mmHg in a previously normotensive patient as diagnostic of pregnancy-induced hypertension. The work of other investigators suggests that this figure is too high.[1,6] A mean pressure of 95 mmHg during labor in the presence of adequate analgesia should be considered abnormal.

Hypertension is usually asymptomatic and can be detected only by measurement. Low blood pressure due to vena caval obstruction is usually accompanied by clinical signs of lightheadedness or nausea.

The frequency of uterine contractions can be monitored noninvasively by manual palpation of the abdomen or use of an external tocodynamometer. However, internal monitoring of the uterine cavity is necessary to accurately assess the quality of contractions (Fig. 18–14). The cessation of uterine activity in a patient previously having regular contractions, particularly in the setting of a previous cesarean section, could signal uterine rupture.

Monitoring During Lumbar Epidural Analgesia

Monitoring during lumbar epidural analgesia is focused on detection of the possible complications of the technique: hypotension, intravascular injection, and subarachnoid injection. The risk of all these events is increased in the pregnant patient.

Hypotension. Maternal hypotension is infrequent in patients who are adequately prehydrated (at least 1000 ml of crystalloid), maintained in the lateral recumbent position, and given limited amounts of local anesthetic (8 ml of 0.25% bupivacaine). However, blood pressure should be monitored once every 5 minutes after initiation of lumbar epidural analgesia for at least 15 minutes, and then once every 15 minutes for the duration of the block.

In the absence of regional anesthesia, hypotension may still occur because of vena caval obstruction or maternal hemorrhage. However, these conditions usually present with other symptoms of maternal compromise.

Intravascular Injection. The incidence of blood vessel cannulation is much higher in pregnant than in nonpregnant patients, presumably because of engorgement of the veins in the epidural plexus. Intravascular injection of large amounts of local anesthetic can result in loss of consciousness, seizures, arrhythmias, and cardiovascular collapse.

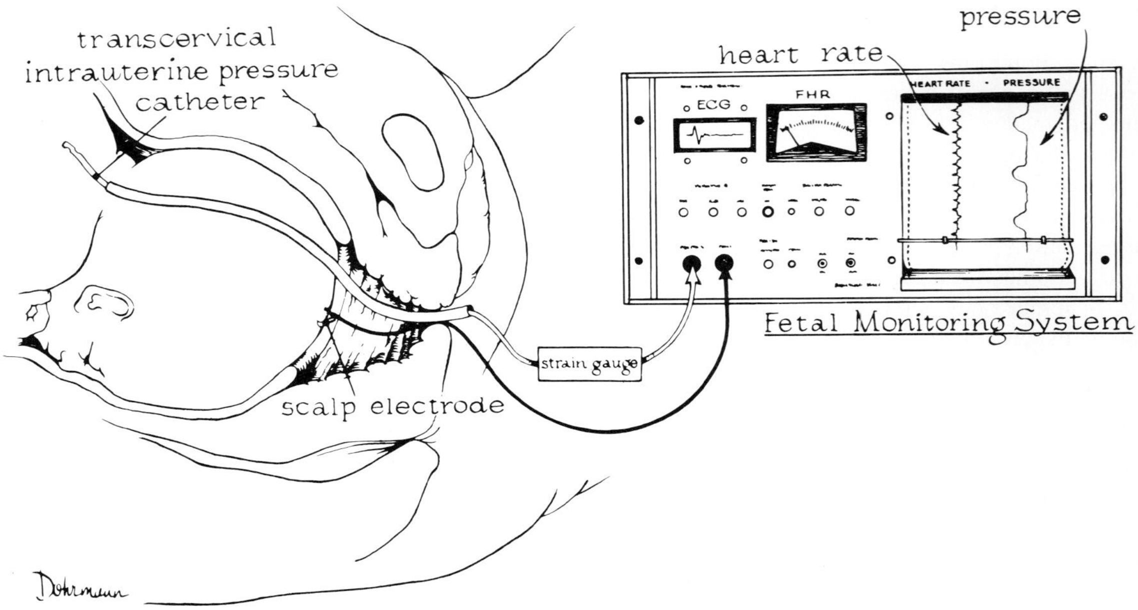

Figure 18–14. Fetal heart rate and intrauterine pressure are recorded from a fetal scalp electrode and a transcervical pressure catheter in the uterus. (From Parer JT: Biophysical evaluation of fetal status: Fetal heart rate. *In* Creasy R, Resnik R [eds]: Maternal-Fetal Medicine. Philadelphia: WB Saunders, 1984; 292.)

This risk is avoided by the incremental injection of doses of local anesthetic that, even if given intravenously, are below the toxic threshold. Incremental doses (2–3 ml) of 0.25% bupivacaine will produce blood levels well below the seizure threshold if accidentally injected intravascularly during performance of an epidural block. An aspiration test should be performed before every injection of local anesthetic, including repeat doses through an indwelling catheter. It is possible for a catheter to migrate into an epidural vein at any time. Total failure of an apparently correctly placed epidural catheter also suggests an intravascular location, as do patient complaints of tinnitis, perioral tingling, and mental confusion.

The use of epinephrine in an epidural test dose in order to detect an intravascular injection has proponents as well as detractors. Particularly in a laboring patient, any increase in heart rate caused by epinephrine may be difficult to distinguish from increases due to the pain of uterine contraction.[41] There is also the concern that the use of low doses of epinephrine (40–50 μg) in the epidural space may contribute to systemic hypotension through its $beta_2$ agonist properties. Epinephrine may also decrease uterine blood flow; in one study, 2 of 10 healthy laboring patients who receiving 15 μg of epinephrine, a standard test dose, developed new ominous fetal heart rate changes lasting 10–12 minutes.[41] Isoproterenol has also been evaluated for detection of intravascular injections; however, neurotoxic studies have yet to document the safety of this drug within the neuraxis.

The most sensitive technique available for the safe detection of an intravascular catheter during attempted epidural analgesia or anesthesia is injection of 1–2 ml of vigorously shaken saline.[42] The microbubbles created by shaking just prior to injection through the epidural catheter will cause an obvious audible change in Doppler heart sounds detected over the sternum. A Doppler ultrasound device should always be readily available in an obstetric suite.

Because of the unreliability of changes in heart rate as a marker for intravascular injection, many obstetric anesthesiologists who do not use chronotropic agents in their test dose solutions see no need for continuous electronic maternal heart rate monitoring during lumbar epidural analgesia.

Subarachnoid Injection. Unsuspected subarachnoid injection of a volume of drug sufficient for epidural blockade can produce a total spinal anesthetic with loss of diaphragmatic function and protective airway reflexes in a patient who is likely to have partially digested food in her stomach. This possibility can be greatly reduced by the incremental administration of small doses of local anesthetic and testing for evidence of subarachnoid block between each injection.

Monitoring During Continuous Epidural Infusions. When epidural analgesia is administered by continuous infusion, the lack of need for frequent redosing does not eliminate the requirement for periodic reassessment by the anesthesiologist. The fact that the patient has no pain is not a sufficient level of assessment. Development of significant lower extremity weakness or sensory loss above the T-8 level warrants slowing of the rate of infusion. Loss of previous analgesia despite an adequate rate of infusion requires aspirating the catheter for blood before administering a supplemental bolus injection, because the catheter may have migrated to an intravascular location. Rapid increases in the level of block may be due to subarachnoid catheter penetration. Infusion pumps must be frequently checked to make sure the correct infusion rate is set and that the correct volume of drug is being delivered. The safety of continuous infusion techniques is increased by the use of the lowest effective concentration of local anesthetic, often supplemented with small concentrations of epidural narcotics.

Monitoring During Routine Cesarean Section

Many cesarean sections are performed on an elective basis, usually because of a prior cesarean delivery. Healthy parturients with presumably healthy fetuses who require cesarean delivery can be considered low-risk patients.

Regional Anesthesia. Anesthesia for cesarean delivery requires a much higher level of sensory blockade than analgesia for vaginal delivery does. Even though the incision is made in the lowest thoracic dermatomal region (T-12) when a low transverse (Pfannenstiel) incision is employed for cesarean section, peritoneal retraction involves nerve fibers that originate at much higher thoracic levels. Adequate epidural anesthesia for cesarean delivery, particularly if the surgeon exteriorizes the uterus for closure, requires a sensory blockade above the level of T-4. This degree of blockade is associated with a much higher incidence of systemic hypotension due to vasodilatation of all vascular beds below the level of the block, particularly the splanchnic circulation.

Maternal heart rate monitoring is essential during regional anesthesia, regardless of whether or not a chronotropic test dose is employed. Epinephrine is more reliable as a marker for intravascular injection in nonlaboring patients undergoing cesarean delivery, because there is much less heart rate variability compared to a patient in labor. If a drug such as epinephrine is used, the patient should be asked if she has symptoms of adrenergic stimulation (sudden pounding heart and anxiety) in order to detect intravascular injection. This marker is more reliable than asking about sensations related to local anesthetic effects, because the 50–60 mg of lidocaine in a test dose may not be readily detectable to some patients.

Abrupt decreases in maternal heart rate shortly after regional blockade (epidural or spinal) usually immediately precede patient complaints of nausea; the next recorded blood pressure is almost invariably in the hypotensive range. The heart rate decrease is due to the "right atrial reflex."[43] Because the right side of the heart is a passive filling system, the only way it can accommodate a sudden decrease in venous return is by slowing its rate. If bradycardia fails to allow adequate filling for the maintenance of cardiac output, the various receptor systems in the systemic circulation initiate the compensatory responses of adrenergically mediated vasoconstriction and tachycardia. As soon as the heart rate decreases, corrective measures should be instituted, including left uterine displacement and elevation of both legs (not the Trendelenburg position). The head-down position is of no benefit to patients with an intravascular volume deficit, presumably because there is already redistribution of blood flow to the brain.[44, 45]

Because larger volumes and higher concentrations of local anesthetic are required for surgical anesthesia as opposed to analgesia for labor, the risk of toxicity from intravascular injection is greater, particularly with long-acting, highly lipid-soluble amide anesthetics. As with epidural analgesia, safe epidural anesthesia requires frequent patient contact, eliciting symptoms of intravascular or subarachnoid injection, as well as frequent monitoring of blood pressure and heart rate. Pulse oximetry should be available in all delivery suites and should be used during regional anesthesia.

ECG monitoring during cesarean section frequently detects changes in the ST segments. This phenomenon has been evaluated in healthy parturients using transthoracic 2D echocardiography and myocardial specific creatine kinase levels.[46] Although the incidence of ST segment changes is greater when using epidural anesthesia than when using spinal anesthesia, the difference may relate to the presence of epinephrine in the epidural solution. No evidence of myocardial ischemia has been found, and the phenomenon is presumed to be benign and enigmatic.

General Anesthesia. In the healthy parturient receiving general anesthesia for cesarean delivery, the special monitoring considerations include the likelihood of a "full stomach" in all patients, regardless of the timing of the last oral intake; the shorter time to hypoxia if gas exchange is interrupted; potential difficulties in intubation due to obesity, breast engorgement, and airway mucosal swelling; the decreased anesthetic requirement; and the possibility of amniotic fluid embolism. Because it is difficult to monitor gastric contents, gastric acid prophylaxis is recommended in all patients undergoing general anesthesia. Such prophylaxis, however, offers no protection against regurgitation and pulmonary aspiration of partially digested food fragments. Essential operating room monitoring includes ECG, blood pressure measurement, pulse oximetry, and capnography for the detection of unsuspected esophageal intubation as well as for assessment of cardiac output. The unconscious, anesthetized patient is still at risk for pulmonary embolism from venous thrombi or amniotic fluid but is unable to communicate the usual symptoms of extreme shortness of breath and chest pain. A sudden decrease in expired carbon dioxide, particularly in association with other signs such as hypotension, oxygen desaturation, and abnormal breath sounds, suggests a pulmonary embolus. As in all operating rooms where general anesthesia is administered, the capability for temperature monitoring and assessment of neuromuscular blockade must be available. The decrease in plasma cholinesterase associated with pregnancy is not clinically significant; however, for the occasional patient with a plasma cholinesterase deficiency, a nerve stimulator will be necessary to explain the inability to resume spontaneous respirations following a dose of succinylcholine for a rapid intubation sequence.

MATERNAL MONITORING IN HIGH-RISK PREGNANCIES

Preeclampsia

Perhaps no other disorder of pregnancy involves such extensive maternal physiologic derangement as that associated with preeclampsia. Most invasive hemodynamic monitoring in obstetric units takes place in patients with severe preeclampsia.

Definition of Preeclampsia

The American College of Obstetricians and Gynecologists classification of hypertensive disorders of pregnancy is listed in Table 18–3. Hypertension is defined as an increase in blood pressure of 30 mmHg systolic or 15 mmHg diastolic over baseline or a blood pressure greater than 140/90 if the baseline blood pressure is unknown. Hypertension occurring before the 20th week of gestation is classified as chronic hypertension. Preeclampsia is defined as hypertension plus proteinuria, edema, or both occurring after the 20th week of gestation. Eclampsia refers to the new onset of seizures during a hypertensive pregnancy in the absence of other central nervous system pathology. The degree of hypertension in preeclampsia does not necessarily correlate with the severity of the disease, and 20% of patients who become eclamptic do not have preeclampsia by the above definition. This may reflect that the values chosen for the definition of hypertension are too high or that blood pressure per se is not the best indicator for the presence of preeclampsia. On the other hand, some patients will be extremely hypertensive, with blood pressure in the range of 250/150 mm Hg.

Preeclampsia is further categorized into mild and severe forms. Criteria for the severe form include blood pressure > 160 mmHg systolic or > 110 mmHg diastolic while at bed rest, proteinuria > 5 gm in 24 hours (3+ or 4+ on qualitative examination), oliguria (< 500 ml urine in 24 hours), cerebral or visual disturbances, epigastric pain, pulmonary edema, and cyanosis. Epigastric pain can signal impending rupture of the liver and is an ominous finding irrespective of other signs and symptoms.

It is now clear that patients destined to develop preeclampsia have measurable hemodynamic abnormalities as early as the tenth week of gestation and that changes in cardiac output and vascular resistance are much more significant to the disease process than is the blood pressure.[1] It also appears that if preeclampsia is a single disease, it has a spectrum of severity. Subclassifications based on differences in hemodynamic profiles, plasma volumes, and fetal size may be more relevant to clinical management and pregnancy outcome than the present categories based primarily on the degree of hypertension and proteinuria.

TABLE 18–3. CLASSIFICATION OF HYPERTENSIVE DISORDERS OF PREGNANCY

Chronic hypertension
Preeclampsia/eclampsia
Preeclampsia superimposed on chronic hypertension
Transient hypertension
Unclassified

Cardiovascular Physiology in Preeclampsia

Noninvasive assessment of cardiac output has provided dramatic new insights into the cardiovascular abnormalities associated with preeclampsia. Pulsed Doppler ultrasound measurements of cardiac output have been validated in both nonpregnant and pregnant subjects and have consistently demonstrated high degrees of correlation with thermodilution techniques using pulmonary artery catheters.[2, 47]

Cardiac Output and Vascular Resistance. Cardiac output and vascular resistance may by extraordinarily high or extraordinarily low in patients with preeclampsia. However, patients with vastly different hemodynamic profiles in terms of cardiac output and vascular resistance may be indistinguishable based solely on blood pressure and clinical appearance. Until recently, preeclampsia was considered a disease characterized by major increases in vascular resistance, somewhat lesser increases in blood pressure, and hence, decreased cardiac output. If vascular resistance increases proportionally more than mean blood pressure, cardiac output must decrease. Hemodynamic data to support this view were primarily obtained from parturients with preeclampsia requiring pulmonary artery catheterization. Most such patients had been treated with fluids and medications affecting hemodynamics (e.g., crystalloid, colloid, magnesium sulfate, hydralazine), so there was uncertainty as to the baseline hemodynamic state. Another problem with most of the studies on which we have based our understanding of hemodynamics is that they are cross-sectional and not longitudinal, and they evaluate patients at a point in time rather than over the course of pregnancy.

One cross-sectional study during the past decade was a landmark paper by Groenendijk and associates that was unique in that 10 patients with moderate to severe preeclampsia underwent pulmonary artery catheterization for hemodynamic measurements upon admission to the hospital *before* volume or antihypertensive therapy was instituted.[48] Mean blood pressure ranged between 110 and 135 mmHg (Fig. 18–15). Cardiac output was uniformly abnormally decreased, and SVR was abnormally increased. After initial measurements, the patients were given an infusion of a synthetic colloid solution until the PCWP increased to 8 mmHg. Volume therapy alone insignificantly changed blood pressure but increased cardiac output and decreased SVR. At this point, vasodilator therapy using dihydralazine was instituted, and SVR decreased further into the normal range for pregnant patients; blood pressure decreased as well. A marked improvement in cardiac output with no change in PCWP occurred primarily because of decreased afterload. This study has been one of the cornerstones of current management principles for the patient with severe preeclampsia and has reinforced the view of preeclampsia

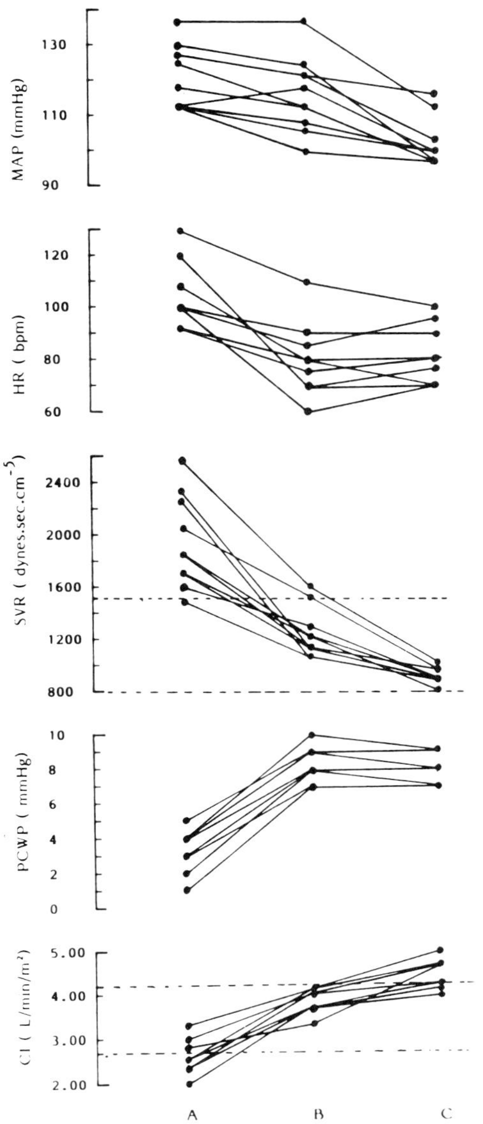

Figure 18–15. Hemodynamic responses in patients with severe preeclampsia prior to treatment *(A)*, following volume expansion *(B)*, and after vasodilatation *(C)*. (MAP = mean arterial pressure, HR = heart rate, SVR = systemic vascular resistance, PCWP = pulmonary capillary wedge pressure, CI = cardiac index.) (From Groenendijk R, Trimbos JBMJ, Wallenburg HCS: Hemodynamic measurements in preeclampsia: Preliminary observations. Am J Obstet Gynecol 1984; 150:234.)

as a disease of an intensely vasoconstricted vascular bed clamped down around a reduced intravascular volume.

The patients in Groenendijk et al's study all exhibited increased vascular resistance and decreased cardiac output. Thus, it seemed reasonable to assume that the hemodynamic findings in severe preeclampsia represented a progression in severity from the hemodynamic state found in milder forms of the disease. However, other studies involving patients who were not as ill showed hemodynamic findings that were more heterogeneous, with cardiac outputs ranging from 4 to 13 L/minute. Figure 18–16*A* compares the hemodynamic profile of 36 untreated preeclamptic patients monitored noninvasively with similarly obtained parameters from patients in the third trimester of normal pregnancies. Figure 18–16*B* provides similar hemodynamic data in preeclamptic patients monitored with pulmonary artery catheters. Note the similarity of the ranges of cardiac output

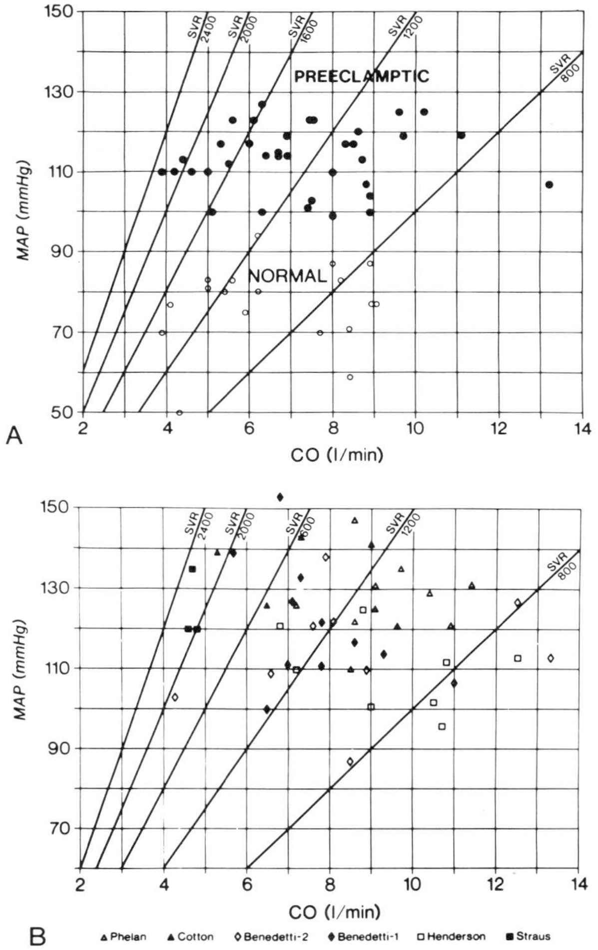

Figure 18–16. *A,* Cardiac output (CO), mean arterial pressure (MAP), and peripheral vascular resistance (SVR) in normal (open circles) and untreated preeclamptic (black circles) pregnancies. The cardiac output was measured noninvasively using Doppler ultrasonography. Although the variation in mean blood pressure among preeclamptic patients is limited (range 95–125 mmHg), there is a tremendous variation in cardiac output and vascular resistance, with over a threefold increase from the lowest to the highest values. *B,* Cardiac output, mean arterial pressure, and systemic vascular resistance in 46 preeclamptic patients monitored with pulmonary artery catheters. (Data is from six different studies that are differentiated by the various symbols: Phelan JP, Yurth DA: Severe preeclampsia. I. Peripartum hemodynamic observations. Am J Obstet Gynecol 1982; 144:17; Cotton DB, Gonik G, Dorman KF: Cardiovascular alterations in severe pregnancy-induced hypertension: Acute effects of intravenous magnesium sulfate. Am J Obstet Gynecol 1984; 148:162; Benedetti TJ, Cotton DB, Read JC, et al: Hemodynamic observations in severe pre-eclampsia with a flow-directed pulmonary artery catheter. Am J Obstet Gynecol 1980; 136:465; Benedetti TJ, Kates R, Williams V: Hemodynamic observations in severe preeclampsia complicated by pulmonary edema. Am J Obstet Gynecol 1984; 150:232; Henderson DW, Vilos GA, Milne KJ, et al: The role of Swan-Ganz catheterization in severe pregnancy-induced hypertension. Am J Obstet Gynecol 1984; 148:570; and Strauss RG, Keefer JR, Burke T, et al: Hemodynamic monitoring of cardiogenic pulmonary edema complicating toxemia of pregnancy. Obstet Gynecol 1980; 55:170, as reproduced in Easterling TR, Watts DH, Schmucker BC, Benedetti TJ: Measurement of cardiac output during pregnancy: Validation of Doppler technique and clinical observations in preeclampsia. Obstet Gynecol 1987; 69:848–849.)

and vascular resistance obtained by different methods in different patients and by multiple investigators. Unfortunately, in many of the studies utilizing pulmonary artery catheters, the patients were treated either with volume or with vasodilators before hemodynamic measurements were made, and thus the true hemodynamic picture could not be known, and the clinical significance of this widely disparate information was not fully appreciated.

Further studies have offered new insights into the pathophysiology of preeclampsia and indicate that mild to moderate preeclampsia may be a disease of high cardiac output and low peripheral resistance, which is just the opposite of our current thinking. Easterling and colleagues, in a blinded longitudinal study of women in their first pregnancy, have challenged our current models of preeclampsia as a disease of systemic hypoperfusion.[1] These researchers measured a number of hemodynamic variables beginning at the first clinic visit, usually around the 10th week of conception. As in several previous studies of blood pressure changes over the course of pregnancy, they found that the patients destined to develop preeclampsia had a significant increase in mean arterial pressure detectable in the first trimester that

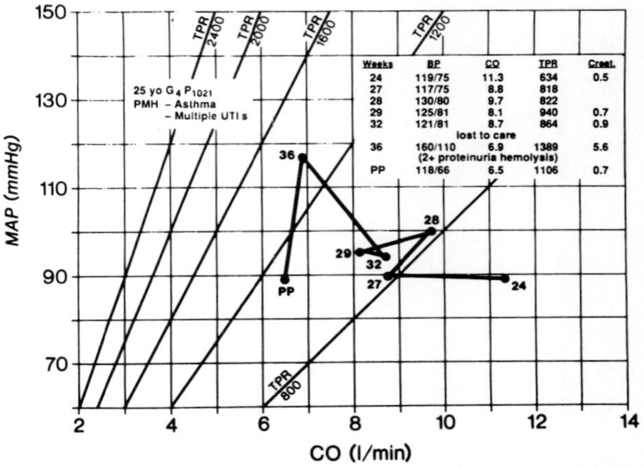

Figure 18–18. Serial hemodynamic data from a single patient who presented initially with a high cardiac output (CO) and a low vascular resistance (TPR) profile, and who subsequently crossed over to a category of low cardiac output and high vascular resistance. Numbers adjacent to each point indicate gestational age in weeks. PP = postpartum, MAP = mean arterial pressure, BP = blood pressure, Creat. = creatinine in mg/dl. (From Easterling TR, Benedetti TJ, Schmucker BC, Millard SP: Maternal hemodynamics in normal and preeclamptic pregnancies: A longitudinal study. Obstet Gynecol 1990; 76:1067.)

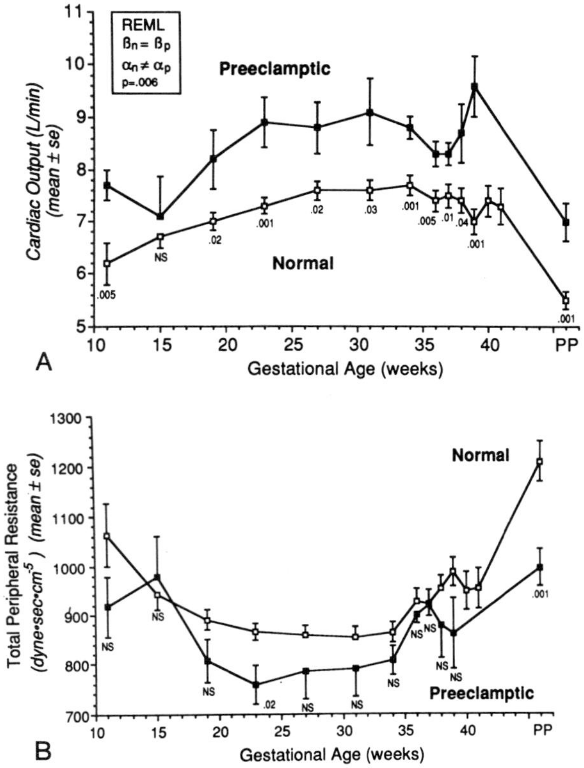

Figure 18–17. Cardiac output *(A)* and total peripheral resistance *(B)* over the course of normal and preeclamptic pregnancies. Levels of statistical significance are given for each gestational age. To control for the effects of multiple comparisons, the curves for the normotensive (n) and the preeclamptic (p) group were analyzed by the technique of restricted maximal likelihood (REML), where β indicates the slope and α indicates the intercept of the line. The hypothesis that the slopes are equal ($\beta_n = \beta_p$) but the intercepts are different ($\alpha_n \neq \alpha_p$) was significant at the p = .006 level. (From Easterling TR, Benedetti TJ, Schmucker BC, Millard SP: Maternal hemodynamics in normal and preeclamptic pregnancies: A longitudinal study. Obstet Gynecol 1990; 76:1065.)

continued throughout the pregnancy, with the differences becoming even greater at term (see Fig. 18–11).[7, 9] However, unlike researchers in most previous longitudinal studies, they also measured cardiac output and calculated peripheral vascular resistance (Fig. 18–17). Patients who eventually developed preeclampsia had higher cardiac outputs compared to normotensive pregnant controls at almost every measuring interval (monthly) over the course of gestation; cardiac output was on the average about 2 L/minute greater in preeclamptic patients than in normal patients. Peripheral resistance was actually lower in preeclamptics than in normal patients. Thus, in the patients with higher blood pressures, the pathophysiology was an increase in cardiac output rather than an increase in vascular resistance! In the postpartum period, even though there was no significant difference in blood pressure between preeclamptic patients and controls, there was still a very significant difference in both cardiac output and total peripheral resistance.

All women in the study were delivered once they became overtly preeclamptic (developed hypertension and proteinuria). The authors raised the question as to whether or not some of these patients may, without prompt delivery, have subsequently crossed over from a high output/low resistance condition to one of low output/high resistance. As an example of this condition, they reported one patient (Fig. 18–18) with a slightly increased mean blood pressure of 90 mmHg (77 mmHg was the normal value at 24 weeks of gestation) who initially presented with a high output/low resistance picture (cardiac output 11.3 L/minute). At 27, 28, 29, and 32 weeks, her cardiac output measured between 8 and 10 L/minute with normal resistance for pregnancy. Her mean blood pressure remained above normal for pregnancy. She was lost to care for approximately 1 month, then presented with an elevation in blood pressure to 160/110, 2+ proteinuria and hemolysis. Her cardiac output at that time had decreased to slightly less than 6.9 L/minute, and she had a marked increase in peripheral vascular resistance. Her creatinine was 5.6 mg/dl, a markedly abnormal value for pregnancy. Post partum, her blood pressure and creatinine returned to normal.

In considering a pregnant patient with a diagnosis of preeclampsia, it is essential to recognize that a mean blood pressure of 100 mmHg can be associated with an extremely wide range of cardiac outputs and vascular resistances. Equation 18–1 may be rewritten and substituted for as follows:

$$\text{Mean arterial pressure} = \frac{\text{vascular resistance} \times \text{cardiac output}}{80} \qquad 18\text{–}3$$

$$100 = \frac{4000 \times 2}{80}$$

for the case in which there is very high vascular resistance (4000 dynes-cm-sec^{-5}) and very low cardiac output (2 L/minute), and

$$100 = \frac{500 \times 16}{80}$$

for the case in which there is very low vascular resistance (500 dynes-cm-sec^{-5}) and very high cardiac output (16 L/minute). In preeclampsia, these hemodynamic extremes still present with an identical mean blood pressure of 100 mmHg.

It is still unclear whether all patients with preeclampsia go through a hyperdynamic phase (high cardiac output/low resistance), with some eventually progressing to a low output/high resistance state, or whether this latter group represents a different disease process. Evidence that the difference is important, at least to the fetus, was suggested in a study of preeclamptic patients that compared the hemodynamic parameters of mothers of infants whose birth weights were appropriate for gestational age (AGA) to those whose infants were small for gestational age (SGA).[49] The mean birth weight of the AGA babies was 3576 gm, which was more than 1 kg greater than the 2478-gm mean birth weight of the SGA infants (Table 18–4). The mothers of the AGA babies had higher mean blood pressures than the mothers of the smaller babies, which would suggest that the mothers of the AGA babies had more severe preeclampsia. However, when maternal cardiac output was measured, it was found to be significantly higher in the mothers of AGA babies (8.2 L/minute) compared to those with SGA infants (5.8 L/minute). The lower cardiac outputs in the mothers of the small infants was associated with much higher measurements of vascular resistance. This paper suggests that preeclamptic patients with low cardiac output/high peripheral resistance are more likely to have SGA babies than preeclamptic mothers who, despite their hypertension, have a normal or supranormal cardiac output.

Cardiac Size and Function. Left ventricular performance is usually well maintained in patients with pregnancy-induced hypertension. For example, Kuzniar and colleagues found that of 42 patients with preeclampsia, all but three had normal indices of left ventricular performance; of the three who had depressed ventricular function, only one had clinically apparent heart failure.[50] The maintenance of normal ventricular function in preeclampsia may be partially explained by the absence of gestational cardiac enlargement in most patients.[4] Thus, although wall tension is increased by increases in ventricular pressure, this is not usually compounded by increases in the ratio of radius to wall thickness as occurs in normotensive pregnancies.

Factors that acutely increase ventricular pressure and/or the ratio of radius to wall thickness may precipitate heart failure in preeclamptic patients. The usual scenario is either (1) a hypertensive response to tracheal intubation or extubation in association with general anesthesia or (2) massive fluid overload, often due to fluid management based on low central venous pressures when there is poor correlation between right-sided and left-sided pressures in the heart.[51]

Uterine Vascular Changes. In normal pregnancy, a dramatic increase in the cross-sectional area of the uterine arterial tree results from obliteration of vascular smooth muscle in the spiral arteries. The autonomic innervation of these vessels is also interrupted. In preeclampsia, the normal invasion of the spiral arteries by the trophoblast is impaired, and the vessels maintain much of their encircling smooth muscle and autonomic innervation and, hence, the

TABLE 18–4. MATERNAL HEMODYNAMIC VARIABLES AND NEONATAL BIRTH WEIGHTS IN PREGNANCY-INDUCED HYPERTENSION

Variable	AGA n = 16	SGA n = 5	p
Mean arterial pressure (mmHg)	115 ± 3	102 ± 3	<.05
Cardiac output (L/minute)	8.2 ± 0.3	5.8 ± 0.2	<0.01
Stroke volume (ml)	100 ± 5	76 ± 7	<0.01
Heart rate (beats/minute)	82 ± 2	79 ± 5	NS
Systemic vascular resistance (dynes-cm-sec^{-5})	1450 ± 80	1770 ± 80	NS
Birth weight (gm)	3576 ± 76	2478 ± 220	<0.01

AGA = appropriate for gestational age; SGA = small for gestational age.

Modified from Nisell H, Lunell N, Linde B: Maternal hemodynamics and impaired fetal growth in pregnancy-induced hypertension. Obstet Gynecol 1988; 71:164–165, with permission.

ability to vasoconstrict. Thus, in preeclampsia, uterine perfusion is primarily a function of uterine vascular resistance rather than maternal blood pressure. Blood pressure may be markedly elevated, but if resistance is elevated to an even greater extent, uterine flow will be decreased.

Altered Sensitivity to Vasoactive Compounds. Preeclampsia is associated with increased responses to vasopressors such as epinephrine, norepinephrine, and angiotensin II, whereas in normal pregnancy, vasopressor responsiveness decreases. In Figure 18–19, the response of patients with pregnancy-induced hypertension to angiotensin II is compared to the normal response, which was presented in Figure 18–4. This differential sensitivity has been utilized to identify women with preeclampsia prior to the onset of clinical symptoms.[52] However, because of the complexity of infusing angiotensin II and uncertain safety in pregnant patients, this test is not routinely used. Platelet angiotensin II binding has been reported to be increased as early as the 12th week of gestation in patients who develop preeclampsia, a fact that may permit a less invasive screening test.[53]

The enhanced responsiveness requires careful titration of all vasopressor drugs. Similarly, preeclamptic parturients are five times more sensitive to the chronotropic effects of isoproterenol than are normal parturients.[54]

Although the maternal circulatory response to vasoactive agents is altered in preeclampsia, *in vitro* the placental arteries (of fetal origin) display no increased sensitivity to either vasodilator or vasoconstrictor compounds.[55] *In vivo*, flow studies demonstrate a vasoconstrictive response to angiotensin II in the uterine vessels (maternal) but no change in flow in the umbilical vessels (fetal) in normal pregnancies.[56] These findings suggest that, even though it is the presence of fetal tissue (trophoblast) that is necessary to initiate the disease of preeclampsia, the vascular pathology in terms of altered vasoactivity is limited to the mother.

Fluid Balance. In preeclampsia, the expected increase in plasma volume seen in normal pregnancy is impaired, and the degree of impairment is related to the severity of the disease.[14, 17] Two studies using different techniques found plasma volume increases of 10–15% in patients with preeclampsia compared with increases of 45–50% in normal pregnancies.[14, 17] The normal increase in red cell mass is also impaired in preeclampsia, but parallels the modest increase in plasma volume, so the hematocrit is often unchanged. Preeclamptic patients have the same increase in total body water as is seen in normal pregnancies.[16] However, because less of this volume is distributed to the intravascular space, it must be accounted for by abnormal increases in interstitial and/or intracellular water. Increases in both interstitial and intracellular water contribute to the edematous, puffy appearance of some patients. The edema is generalized, as opposed to the dependent edema that is typical of normal pregnancy. This generalized edema is one of the main reasons for mismanagement of patients with severe preeclampsia. The usual treatment of edema is fluid restriction and diuretics, which is inappropriate treatment in severe preeclampsia. Although these patients are edematous, their intravascular volume is decreased.

Capillary permeability is increased in patients with preeclampsia, regardless of whether or not proteinuria is present. This suggests that the mechanism for glomerular leak may be different from that for capillary leak.[22]

Although capillary hydrostatic pressure is increased in normal pregnancy (see Table 18–2), it is significantly lower in preeclampsia, despite increased blood pressure (Fig. 18–20), because arteriolar vasoconstriction decreases capillary flow. To some extent, this helps to defend against further

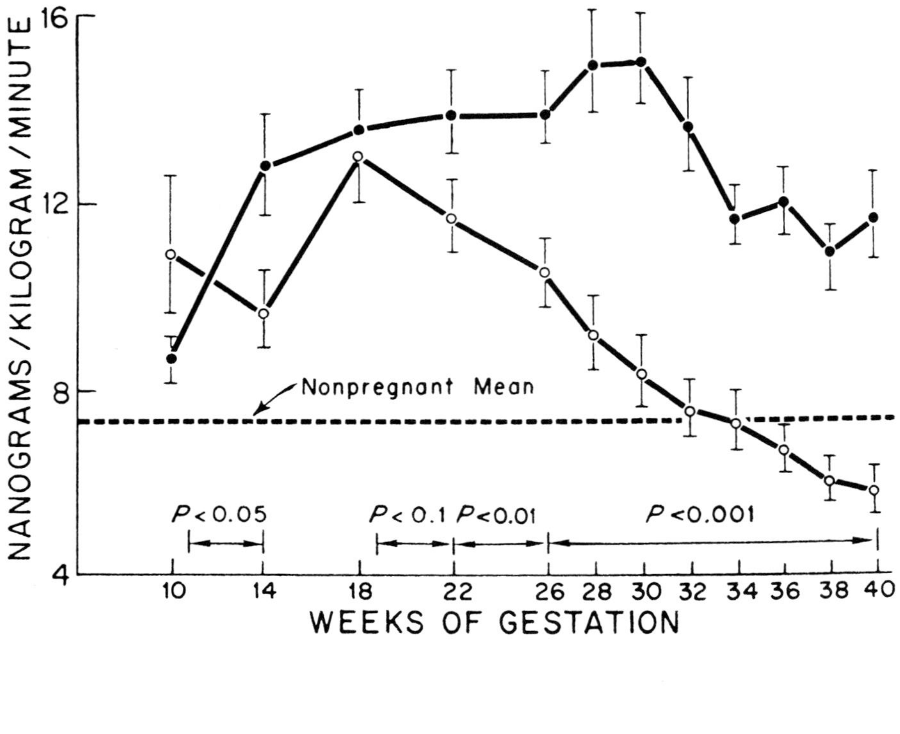

Figure 18–19. Increased angiotensin II sensitivity in patients with preeclampsia. Although normal pregnancy (closed circles) is associated with a decreased sensitivity to vasopressors such as angiotensin II, patients with preeclampsia have an increased sensitivity, such that small doses produced a marked pressor response. (From Gant NF, Daley GL, Chand S, et al: A study of angiotensin II pressor response throughout primigravid pregnancy. J Clin Invest 1973; 52:2682–2689.)

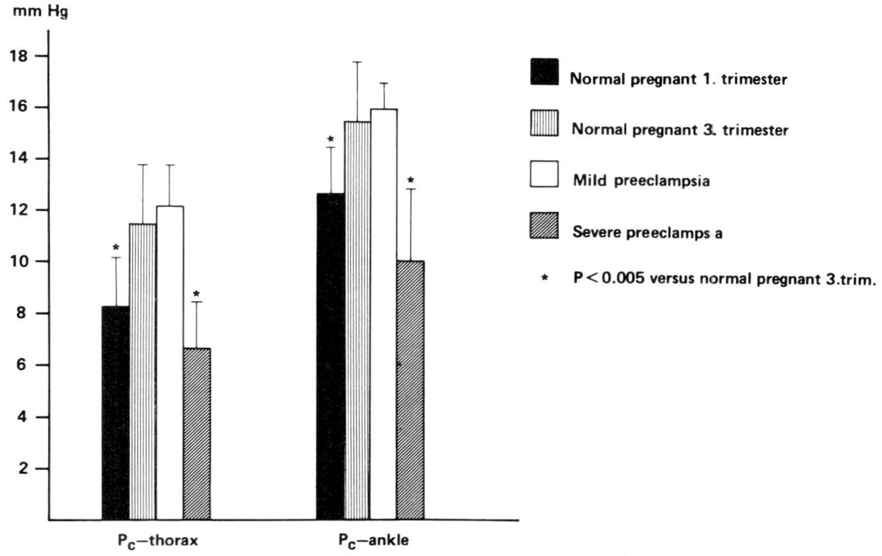

Figure 18–20. Capillary hydrostatic pressure (P_c) at the thorax and ankle in normal pregnancies, mild preeclampsia, and severe preeclampsia. (From Oian P, Maltau JM: Calculated capillary hydrostatic pressure in normal pregnancy and preeclampsia. Am J Obstet Gynecol 1987; 157:105.)

fluid losses to the interstitium, because higher capillary pressures coupled with the decreased osmotic pressures associated with preeclampsia would favor fluid movement out of the capillaries. However, very high precapillary resistance, although resulting in lower capillary hydrostatic pressure and potentially less edema, may in fact be more detrimental to the fetus and maternal organ systems. Brown and colleagues found a mean fetal birth weight of 3180 gm in 10 infants born to preeclamptic mothers with edema; in a corresponding group of preeclamptic parturients with similar arterial pressures and plasma volumes but without edema, the mean birth weight was 715 gm lower.[23]

The significance of the decreased maternal plasma volume in preeclampsia is that it correlates strongly with fetal size, the single most important determinant of outcome.[15, 23] Hays and colleagues (Fig. 18–21) found that normotensive mothers had an increase in plasma volume from approximately 1600 ml/m^2 to over 2300 ml/m^2, whereas parturients with preeclampsia and AGA babies had an increase to only 1900 ml/m^2. Preeclamptic parturients with SGA babies actually had a slight contraction in plasma volume.[14] Clearly, plasma volume abnormalities are much more central to the pathophysiology and fetal morbidity of preeclampsia than increased blood pressure is, which bears no predictable relation to fetal outcome.

The decrease in colloid osmotic pressure seen in normal pregnancy is even more pronounced in preeclampsia.[57] This decrease results in a greater likelihood of pulmonary edema should PCWP increase. Such increases are very common following endotracheal intubation and extubation, and the development of acute pulmonary edema is not uncommon at such times. The COP continues to decline in the immediate postpartum period when there is an increase in central blood volume due to involution of the uterus. Overly zealous volume administration in this period can increase PCWP and result in pulmonary edema.[51]

Volume Therapy in Severe Preeclampsia. The hemodynamic responses of individual patients with severe untreated preeclampsia to intravascular volume expansion using a colloid solution are increased cardiac index and decreased SVR (Fig. 18–15).[48] Vasodilator therapy with dihydralazine after volume expansion further decreased mean blood pressure and increased cardiac index, but did not increase PCWP. Data from such studies confirm the physiologic rational for using volume and vasodilator therapy in the management of patients with severe preeclampsia. Volume expansion is essential prior to treatment of severe hypertension, because acute vasodilatation in a hemoconcentrated, hypovolemic, hypertensive patient may result in cardiovascular collapse.[58]

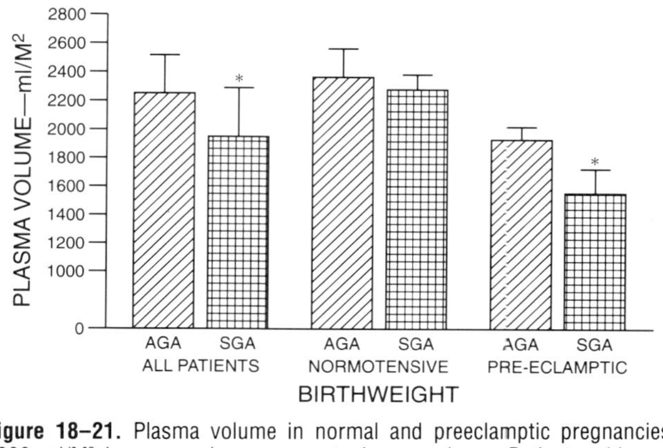

Figure 18–21. Plasma volume in normal and preeclamptic pregnancies. 1600 ml/M^2 is a normal nonpregnant plasma volume. Patients with preeclampsia and AGA babies had a lesser expansion in plasma volume than normotensive patients, regardless of the size of the baby. Severe preeclampsia was associated with a contraction in plasma volume and SGA babies. (* = $p < 0.05$, AGA = appropriate for gestational age, SGA = small for gestational age.) (From Hays PM, Cruikshank DP, Dunn LJ: Plasma volume determination in normal and preeclamptic pregnancies. Am J Obstet Gynecol 1985; 151:962.)

Oliguric Preeclamptic Patients: Hemodynamic Subsets. Clark and coworkers have further characterized the range of hemodynamic abnormalities found in severe preeclampsia and the role of fluid therapy in the oliguric patient.[59] Studies were made in patients who were oliguric (< 30 ml of urine/hour for 3 consecutive hours) in spite of maintenance fluid therapy of 100–125 ml/hour and a fluid bolus of 300–500 ml of crystalloid. One subset of patients (category I, Table 18–5) had a cardiac index of 3.8 L/minute/m^2, a PCWP of 4 mmHg, and an SVR of 1330 dynes-second-cm^{-5}. A diagnosis of hypovolemia was made, and following an additional volume of crystalloid, the oliguria resolved in these patients. After additional volume therapy, the cardiac index was 4.5 L/minute/m^2; PCWP, 10 mmHg; and SVR, 1150 dynes-second-cm^{-5}. These results are similar to the findings of Groenendijk et al in severe preeclamptics following fluid therapy alone.[48]

However, there were two other subsets of patients identified in the Clark study, both of which had persistent oliguria following a fluid challenge with crystalloid. Because one subset (category II) had normal or elevated PCWPs and low SVRs, it was postulated that selective renal artery vasoconstriction maintained the oliguric state of these patients. The administration of hydralazine and additional fluid was followed by resolution of the oliguria in the patients with normal PCWP. The observation that dopamine is efficacious in preeclamptic oliguria suggests dopaminergic receptor–mediated decreases in renal vascular resistance.[60]

One patient in the Clark study had a PCWP of 18 mmHg and a cardiac index of 6.1 L/minute/m^2. The diagnosis of volume overload was established, and the patient was given an infusion of nitroglycerin to decrease both preload and afterload. Nitroglycerin therapy resulted in a decrease in blood pressure and resolution of the oliguria. It should be stressed that nitroglycerin is usually an inappropriate vasodilator for patients with preeclampsia. Nitroglycerin acts on the venous side of the circulatory bed to a greater degree than it acts on the arterial side. The vasoconstriction of preeclampsia is primarily arteriolar. Thus, one could predict that giving nitroglycerin would result in venous dilatation with pooling of blood and decreased return to the heart. Although this may be desirable in a patient with volume overload, it is poorly tolerated by patients with intravascular volume depletion, such as those with severe preeclampsia. Venodilatation in such patients may result in fetal distress, presumably owing to impaired placental perfusion and fetal hypoxemia.[61]

The third subset in the Clark study included only one patient, but one who helps to illustrate an important aspect of preeclampsia. This oliguric patient had a mean arterial pressure of 140 mmHg, a cardiac index of only 2.6 L/minute/m^2, a PCWP of 18 mmHg, and an SVR of 2790 dynes-second-cm^{-5}. This patient demonstrated left ventricular dysfunction and was managed with fluid restriction and aggressive afterload reduction with hydralazine.

Cardiovascular Physiology During Epidural Analgesia and Anesthesia in Patients with Preeclampsia. Epidural blockade can produce profound hypotension in patients with severe preeclampsia, as it does in any patient with a severe intravascular volume deficit. This concern has led to the blanket condemnation of epidural blockade by some,[62] whereas others have demonstrated that the risk of serious hypotension can be greatly reduced by intravascular volume repletion prior to performance of the block. This is true for both lumbar epidural analgesia for labor[63] with a segmental block to T-10 and epidural anesthesia for cesarean section[64–66] with a T-4 level.

Lumbar epidural analgesia has the unique potential to increase uterine blood flow while decreasing maternal blood pressure. Most vasodilators affect both the maternal systemic and uterine circulations fairly equally, so that the flow relationships remain constant. Lumbar epidural analgesia (maximum height T-8) selectively blocks the sympathetic innervation of the uterus without blocking sympathetic innervation of other vascular beds, particularly the splanchnic bed. This preferentially reduces uterine vascular resistance relative to maternal peripheral resistance, thereby increasing the fraction of flow through the low-resistance bed. In one study of severe preeclamptics in labor, lumbar epidural analgesia resulted in a 77% increase in intervillous blood flow over controls when maternal blood pressure was maintained at prelumbar epidural analgesia levels.[63] The modest decrease in blood pressure that is usually seen following lumbar epidural analgesia in adequately hydrated severe preeclamptics is due to uterine vasodilatation as well as to lower levels of endogenous catecholamines as maternal pain is relieved.

The same beneficial effect on maternal blood pressure seen with epidural analgesia has also been documented for epidural anesthesia in severe preeclamptic patients (Fig. 18–22).[65] In adequately hydrated patients, there is a modest decrease in mean arterial pressure, with no change in PCWP. Cardiac output is well maintained following epidural anesthesia in spite of the decrease in blood pressure (Fig. 18–23).[64] It must be stressed that uterine displacement is essential if cardiac output is to be maintained in the supine position, regardless of whether or not maternal preeclampsia is present.

Our knowledge of the wide range of underlying hemodynamic patterns that may be present in preeclamptic patients clearly has implications for management of epidural analgesia and anesthesia in such patients. For example, in patients with a high cardiac output/low peripheral vascular resistance profile, modest volume supplementation (~500 ml) is adequate to attenuate the vasodilatory effects of epidural analgesia, and 1000–1500 ml is adequate for epidural anesthesia for cesarean section. These patients have moderately decreased intravascular volumes relative to normal pregnant patients, despite the presence of high cardiac outputs. In patients with low cardiac output/high peripheral vascular resistance profiles, much more careful attention to volume replacement is required, because this pattern may reflect either a severe intravascular volume deficit or cardiac dysfunction. In either case, a more careful program of

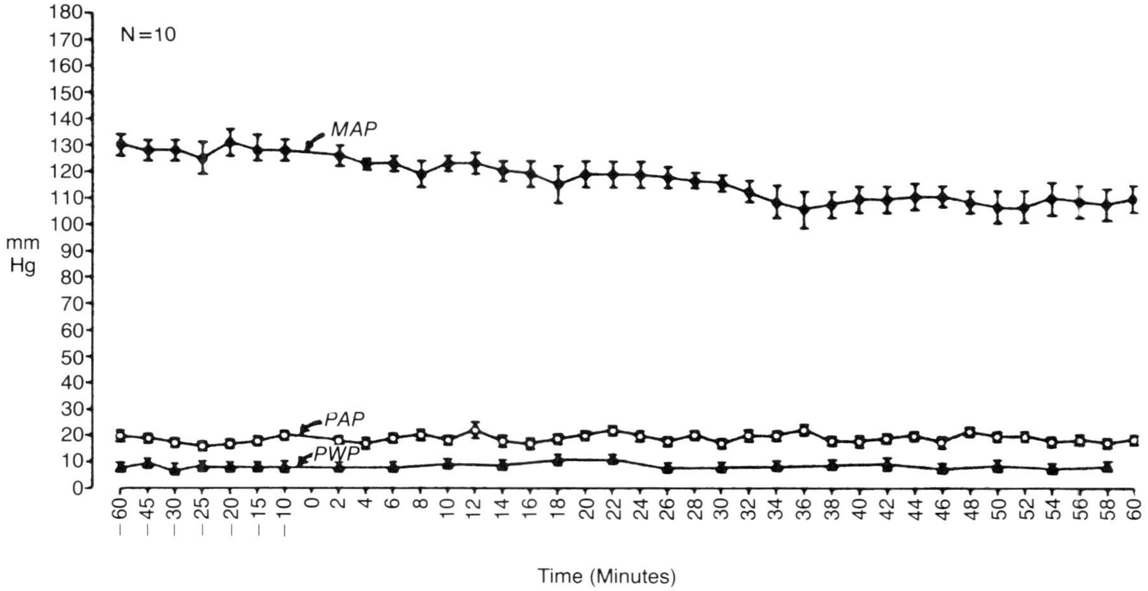

Figure 18–22. Hemodynamic response to lumbar epidural anesthesia for cesarean section in patients with severe preeclampsia. Injection of epidural anesthetic was at time zero. MAP = mean arterial pressure, PAP = pulmonary artery pressure, PWP = pulmonary wedge pressure. (From Hodgkinson R, Husain FJ, Hayashi RH: Systemic and pulmonary blood pressure during cesarean section in parturients with gestational hypertension. Can Anaesth Soc J 1980; 27:392.)

volume and vasodilator therapy is required for optimum patient management.

Cardiovascular Physiology During General Anesthesia in Patients with Preeclampsia. General anesthesia is associated with potentially dangerous increases in maternal blood pressure and cardiac filling pressures. The most extreme elevations are related to tracheal intubation and extubation, an absolute requirement in anesthetized pregnant women. Hodgkinson and coworkers documented a 45-mmHg increase in mean arterial pressure and a 20-mmHg increase in PCWP during both intubation and extubation of the trachea in patients with severe preeclampsia (Fig. 18–24).[65] These changes reflect the increased sensitivity to vasopressors, including endogenous catecholamines, seen in preeclamptic patients. Severe and abrupt pulmonary and systemic hypertension of the magnitude documented by Hodgkinson et al has been associated with acute heart failure, pulmonary edema, and cerebral hemorrhage in patients with preeclampsia. Optimum patient management requires continuous monitoring of cardiovascular changes and carefully titrated drug therapy to prevent adverse changes. James has demonstrated that a combination of magnesium sulfate (30 mg/kg) and alfentanil (7.5 μg/kg) is superior to larger doses of either drug alone as well as to lidocaine

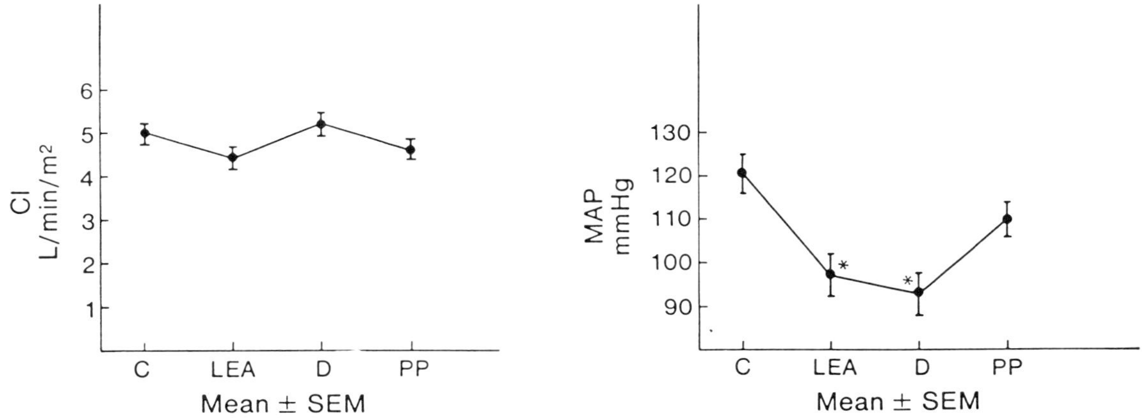

Figure 18–23. Cardiac index and mean arterial pressure in patients with severe preeclampsia at control (C), following lumbar epidural anesthesia (LEA), at delivery (D), and 2 hours postpartum (PP). *indicates statistical significance, $p < 0.05$. SEM = standard error of the mean. (From Newsome LR, Bramwell RS, Curling PE: Severe preeclampsia: Hemodynamic effects of lumbar epidural anesthesia. Anesth Analg 1986; 65:32. Reprinted with permission from the International Anesthesia Research Society.)

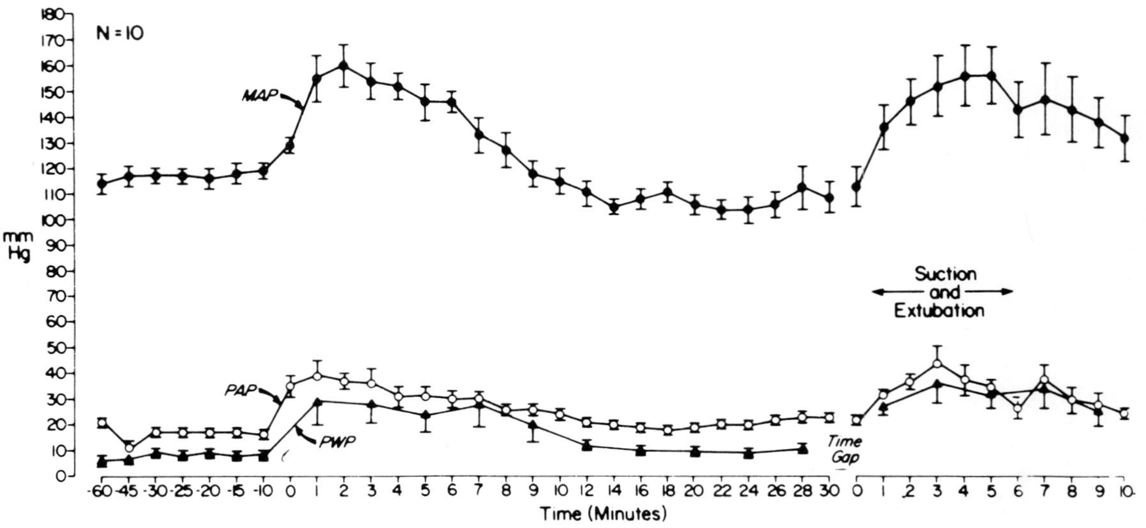

Figure 18–24. Hemodynamic responses in patients with severe preeclampsia undergoing cesarean section under general anesthesia. The first zero indicates induction, the second suctioning and extubation. MAP = mean arterial pressure, PAP = pulmonary artery pressure, PWP = pulmonary wedge pressure. (From Hodgkinson R, Husain FJ, Hayashi RH: Systemic and pulmonary blood pressure during cesarean section in parturients with gestational hypertension. Can Anaesth Soc J 1980; 27:392.)

(1.5 mg/kg) in controlling the hypertensive response to tracheal intubation in patients with preeclampsia.[67] Bolus doses of sodium nitroprusside (100–200 μg) in adequately hydrated patients are also effective in blunting the hypertensive response, whereas nitroglycerin is somewhat less efficacious.[68]

Renal Alterations in Preeclampsia

Renal function in preeclampsia is affected adversely by numerous factors. Decreased cardiac output in severe preeclampsia decreases renal blood flow and glomerular filtration rate. There may also be selective renal artery vasoconstriction that further impairs renal perfusion.[59] Preeclampsia is associated with varying degrees of endothelial injury, and injury to the glomeruli and renal tubules may be so severe as to require dialysis. Renal tubular injury can be estimated by following levels of uric acid, a substance handled by the tubule.[69] The injury to the glomerulus is reflected by significant proteinuria, which is defined as 0.1 gm/L of protein in a random sample or 0.3 gm/L in a 24-hour specimen. Severe preeclampsia is diagnosed in the presence of proteinuria of 5 gm or more in a 24-hour period. Fetal mortality is directly related to the amount of proteinuria and to the uric acid levels, which suggests a common etiology of injury to both the kidney and the placenta. However, the presence and severity of proteinuria do not correlate with the occurrence of seizures (eclampsia), suggesting a different mechanism for central nervous system injury.

Decreased urine output is a usual feature of severe preeclampsia and correlates with the severity of the disease. In most patients, volume and vasodilator therapy, guided by sophisticated cardiovascular monitoring when required, will correct the prerenal causes of oliguria. If not, the diagnosis of acute renal failure must be considered. This diagnosis may be difficult to establish, because urinary diagnostic indices, such as the fractional excretion of sodium and urinary sodium concentration, may not correlate with measurements of effective intravascular volume as determined by the PCWP.[70] Management of a preeclamptic patient in renal failure is very challenging and usually demands immediate delivery of the infant and, possibly, renal dialysis.

It appears likely that many patients with preeclampsia have pre-existing subclinical renal disease that possibly predisposes them to the development of preeclampsia. One study, using phase contrast microscopy to examine urine for dysmorphic erythrocytes (which has a high specificity for glomerulonephritis), found that two thirds of preeclamptic patients presenting before 37 weeks of gestation had underlying renal disease, with mesangial IgA nephropathy being the most common finding.[71] Another study found a high incidence of preeclampsia (33%) in women with a history of asymptomatic bacteriuria in childhood but with renal scarring demonstrated by an intravenous pyelogram. Women with a history of childhood bacteriuria but a normal subsequent pyelogram had a preeclampsia incidence of $< 5\%$ (1 in 22 patients), not significantly different from a control group of women without a history of bacteriuria (1 in 36 developed preeclampsia).[72] Leduc and colleagues reported that the urine sediment of 30 patients with severe preeclampsia uniformly contained granular, hyaline, red-cell, and tubular casts, indicative of both glomerular and tubular injury.[73] No casts were found in the urine of parturients having normal pregnancies. It is possible that preeclampsia is a high cardiac output disease that is relatively benign in 80% of patients, but in those with underlying renal insufficiency, however modest and subclinical, it progresses to severe preeclampsia.

Central Nervous System in Preeclampsia

Generalized central nervous system irritability is a common feature in preeclampsia. Mild degrees of irritability are manifested by the presence of hyperreflexia or clonus on physical examination; extreme irritability results in convulsions, a condition referred to as eclampsia. Routine management of preeclampsia involves minimizing stimulation of the patient in order to decrease the risk of convulsions. Seizures may occur in patients with seemingly mild disease in terms of blood pressure, proteinuria, and edema.

Patients with preeclampsia are at risk for cerebral edema; at our institution, a patient with minimal symptoms who was at bed rest for preeclampsia suffered brain herniation secondary to acute cerebral edema. However, cerebral edema is not the etiology of eclamptic convulsions. One report of seven eclamptic patients with repetitive seizures while receiving intravenous magnesium sulfate found only one with cerebral edema, two with venous thrombosis, two with low-density white matter, and two with normal computerized axial tomographic findings.[74] Autopsy findings usually show only petechial hemorrhages and other nondiagnostic changes and not brain swelling. It is possible that seizures are due to platelet microthrombi blocking tiny capillaries in the brain and increasing CNS irritability on an ischemic basis; alternatively, cerebral vasculitis due to diffuse endothelial injury may be the cause. It has been suggested that magnesium sulfate is effective as an anticonvulsant in preeclampsia not because of any inherent anticonvulsant properties, but because it is a cerebral vasodilator.[67]

One large series of hypertensive pregnant patients was managed during labor with lumbar epidural analgesia and without specific anticonvulsant medications.[75] In 1106 patients, there were no convulsions in any patient treated with effective lumbar epidural analgesia. Two patients experienced seizures after catheter placement but before onset of analgesia. Four patients had seizures in the postpartum period, hours after termination of the local anesthetic effect. The most likely explanation is that, at the low systemic blood levels that result following epidural analgesia, local anesthetics tend to be mild central nervous system depressants and thus exert anticonvulsant effects. It is only at toxic doses that local anesthetics cause seizures. Also, effective lumbar analgesia decreases endogenous catecholamines; epinephrine is known to enhance platelet aggregation.

Should a seizure occur, it can be terminated with a small dose of barbiturate or benzodiazepine. Oxygen by mask should be given, and cricoid pressure should be maintained to protect the airway. This is one instance of an unconscious patient with a potentially full stomach in which succinylcholine and prompt tracheal intubation may not be indicated. The extreme hypertensive response associated with tracheal intubation in an unanesthetized patient may pose a greater hazard to the mother than the risk of aspiration, and the seizure can usually be terminated rapidly using intravenous drugs.

Hemostasis in Preeclampsia

The gamut of coagulation abnormalities in preeclampsia ranges from the hypercoagulable state of normal pregnancy to the opposite extreme of disseminated intravascular coagulation. Fortunately, clinical bleeding is rarely the basis for patient morbidity or mortality.

Standard tests of coagulation (prothrombin time, partial thromboplastin time) usually yield normal results, even in severe preeclampsia.[76] A decreased platelet count is the most frequent hematologic abnormality found. Katz and associates reported platelet counts below 150,000 mm^3 in approximately 50% of 237 patients with preeclampsia, and counts below 100,000 mm^3 were seen in 25% of patients.[77] In 100 patients with severe preeclampsia, Leduc and colleagues found 36 with platelet counts below 100,000 mm^3 and 14 with platelet counts below 50,000 mm^3.[76] Bone marrow analysis in preeclamptic patients demonstrates a hypercellular marrow with a proliferation of megakaryocytes and increased platelet production, which occurs in response to increased platelet consumption. A decreasing platelet count indicates worsening disease as platelet consumption exceeds replacement.

Platelet activation, which results in aggregation and consumption, is favored by the imbalance between thromboxane and prostacyclin and by increased sympathetic nervous tone associated with elevated plasma catecholamines. Platelet consumption is accelerated by endothelial damage with subsequent platelet adherence, and endothelial injury is probably central to the pathophysiology of preeclampsia.[78] In some cases, platelet destruction may involve immunologic mechanisms.[79] There may also be a qualitative platelet defect, because patients may have prolonged bleeding times in spite of adequate numbers of platelets.[80, 81]

Thrombocytopenia in pregnancy, with or without hypertension, may also be associated with diseases other than preeclampsia, such as hemolytic uremic syndrome, thrombotic thrombocytopenic purpura, immune thrombocytopenic purpura, and systemic lupus erythematosus. The HELLP syndrome (*he*molysis, *l*iver enzyme abnormalities, and *l*ow *p*latelets) is a manifestation of severe preeclampsia.

Plasma epinephrine levels are increased during labor in both normal and preeclamptic patients, and epinephrine is a potent platelet activator. Epidural analgesia during labor has been shown to decrease maternal epinephrine levels, which may have a favorable effect on platelet aggregation.[82]

Impaired platelet function increases the risk of an epidural or subarachnoid hematoma, as do other coagulation defects. There are insufficient data to even suggest the risk associated with epidural analgesia and anesthesia in preeclamptic patients with clotting abnormalities. One case report describes epidural bleeding (but no hematoma) in a patient with the HELLP syndrome and a bleeding time in excess of 15 minutes in association with an epidural catheter.[83] No treatment was required. It is important to know that epidural hematomas may occur spontaneously in patients with impaired clotting mechanisms, and that the avoidance of an epidural needle neither prevents this complication nor removes the need for vigilance. It is critical that the symptoms of back pain in association with neurologic deficits in the legs and/or urogenital region not be ignored, because prompt evacuation of an intraspinal hematoma is crucial to avoid permanent injury. Long-term neurologic sequelae are unlikely when high-risk patients are properly observed and evaluated.

There is no consensus on the minimum acceptable platelet count prior to performing regional anesthesia, in part because platelet function depends on both quantity and quality. Although it would seem that a bleeding time might be a more meaningful test than a simple platelet count, because it is an *in vivo* test of platelet function, it has been demonstrated that there is no correlation between skin bleeding, as measured by the bleeding time test, and organ bleeding during surgery.[84] Thus, even though some institutions use bleeding times as an absolute criterion in determining the suitability of preeclamptic patients for regional anesthesia,[81] it must be stressed that there are no scientific or clinical data to support the validity of this practice.

A study by Ramanathan found that 2% of normal pregnant patients had abnormal bleeding times in spite of normal numbers of platelets; 20% of patients with preeclampsia had abnormal bleeding times. Because the true incidence of preeclampsia in this country is in the 2–3% range, there are, if the Ramanathan data is valid, many more normal pregnant patients with prolonged bleeding times (2% of 97%, or 19 in 1000) than there are preeclamptic patients with prolonged bleeding times (20% of 3%, or 6 in 1000). Data from the same study (Fig. 18–25) show that, in preeclampsia, when 100,000 platelets/mm^3 is used as a cutoff, more patients with platelet counts above this value will have bleeding times in excess of 15 minutes than will patients with platelet counts below 100,000 platelets/mm^3. This indicates that many preeclamptic patients with platelet counts that are deemed adequate nonetheless have abnormal bleeding times. There is no clinical evidence that

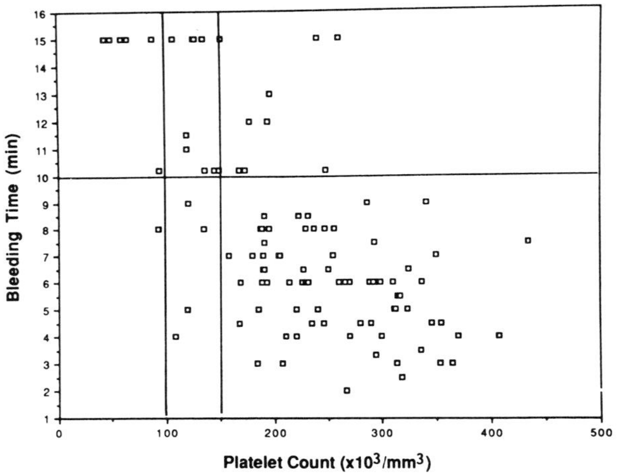

Figure 18–25. Bleeding times plotted against platelet counts in parturients with preeclampsia. (From Ramanathan J, Sibai BM, Vu T, Chauhan D: Correlation between bleeding times and platelet counts in women with preeclampsia undergoing cesarean section. Anesthesiology 1989; 71:190.)

regional anesthesia in these patients has been associated with increased bleeding complications.

The fact that regional anesthesia is the preferred anesthetic technique for operative delivery in preeclamptic pregnancies as well as in normal pregnancies and the fact that bleeding complications are so rare confirm the clinical irrelevance of bleeding time tests. Thus, it appears that there is no rational basis for using this test as a factor in clinical decision making in the patient with preeclampsia.

A more rational policy is to base the decision regarding regional anesthesia in the preeclamptic patient on a number of factors, with the most significant being not the platelet count but the clinical status of the patient. For example, is there bruising around intravenous catheter sites? Is there bleeding of the gums when the patient brushes her teeth? Patients with clinical evidence of abnormal bleeding would be considered at higher risk for regional anesthesia, regardless of the absolute platelet count or the results of a bleeding time test. Patients with such symptoms may receive platelet transfusions prior to cesarean section based on surgical considerations; if so, regional anesthesia can be performed after the platelet transfusion with a presumably increased margin of safety, assuming that the clinical bleeding is corrected by the platelet transfusion.

It must be stressed that the bleeding risks associated with regional anesthesia in severe preeclampsia must be viewed as relative risks. Ramanathan and colleagues reported a maternal death due to an inability to secure an airway following induction of general anesthesia in a patient in whom regional anesthesia was felt to be contraindicated because of thrombocytopenia (platelet count 55,000/mm^3) and an abnormal bleeding time ($>$ 15 minutes).[85] The authors felt that laryngeal edema contributed to the failure to ventilate/intubate. Thus, the decision to avoid regional anesthesia must be weighed against the potential risks associated with general anesthesia in patients with preeclampsia, which include pulmonary edema, heart failure, and cerebral hemorrhage, as well as the ever-present risk of pulmonary aspiration of gastric contents in patients who may present challenges to tracheal intubation because of edema of the head and neck, including the larynx. Cerebral hemorrhage still ranks as a leading cause of maternal mortality in preeclampsia and is a much more serious bleeding complication than an epidural hematoma. Thus, potential bleeding complications are associated with both regional and general anesthesia, and choices in anesthetic management should reflect these risks.

The placenta in normal pregnancy produces roughly equal amounts of thromboxane A_2 and prostacyclin. With preeclampsia, placental prostacyclin production is decreased, and thromboxane A_2 production is increased.[86] This imbalance favors platelet aggregation, vasoconstriction, decreased uteroplacental blood flow, and increased uterine activity, factors detrimental to both the fetus and the mother. However, the imbalance may be reversible with drugs affecting prostaglandin synthesis. Low-dose aspirin (60 mg/day) appears to decrease both the incidence and the severity of preeclampsia when therapy is begun at 24 weeks of gestation.[87] At this aspirin dose, there is no clinically significant impairment of hemostatic mechanisms in either the mother or the fetus. The beneficial effects of aspirin appear to derive from the fact that, at low doses, aspirin inhibits thromboxane biosynthesis without altering prostacyclin production. However, despite the initial promise that attended clinical trials of aspirin therapy, there are still patients who develop severe preeclampsia in the face of documented blood salicylate levels. At this stage, treatment of all pregnancies with aspirin does not appear warranted, and at present there are no tests sensitive enough to identify high-risk patients for selective prophylaxis.[88]

Treatment of Maternal Hypertension

A lack of understanding of the relationship between maternal blood pressure and uterine flow may lead to suboptimal management in patients with preeclampsia. The standard of practice on many obstetric services is that maternal hypertension is not treated until the diastolic pressure exceeds 110 mmHg; hypertension is maintained in order to "ensure adequate uterine perfusion."[89] However, in preeclampsia, hypertension does not equal adequate uterine perfusion. Despite elevated blood pressure, uterine blood flow is reduced 50%, and, in severe cases, reduced 70%; the highest blood pressures are often associated with the lowest uterine blood flows.[90] Decreasing maternal blood pressure by decreasing peripheral vascular resistance, using vasodilating agents such as hydralazine, vasodilates the uterine vessels such that placental flow is not impaired as long as maternal hypotension is avoided.[91]

Allowing the maternal blood pressure to remain elevated has consequences for the mother as well as for the fetus. The upper limit of cerebral blood flow autoregulation occurs at a mean perfusion pressure of 150 mmHg; above this, the blood-brain barrier begins to break down, and cerebral injury results. Many patients with severe preeclampsia will have mean pressures close to this limit and exceed it during painful labor. Also, untreated hypertension increases the work load on the left ventricle. It is not uncommon for preeclamptic patients to develop acute left-sided heart failure during the stress of labor or in association with endotracheal intubation and surgery.

Sodium nitroprusside is the drug of choice for acute control of severe hypertension in preeclampsia. This drug has seen limited use in obstetrics, in part because of misinterpretation of animal studies in which supraclinical doses were given to pregnant ewes in order to produce acidosis in the fetuses.[92] However, sodium nitroprusside has been shown to have no detectable adverse effects on the human fetus when used in usual clinical doses.[93, 94]

Other drugs for the treatment of hypertension in patients with preeclampsia include labetalol[95] and hydralazine,[96] which decrease maternal blood pressure without altering uterine blood flow. However, fetal blood flow is affected; hydralazine tends to decrease the pulsatility index of the umbilical artery, whereas labetalol causes an increase,[96] indicating that hydralazine decreases vascular resistance in the fetoplacental circulation. The increase in resistance in the fetal circulation seen with labetalol appears to be due to transplacental passage of the drug and beta-adrenoceptor–mediated vasoconstriction. Labetalol should be used cautiously when the infant is stressed, because it may interfere with the normal cardiovascular responses to stress.

Hydralazine is not readily available because of problems in the manufacturing process. Nifedipine appears to be the drug most likely to replace hydralazine in patients with preeclampsia and from a hemodynamic standpoint may, in fact, be a superior agent. In a comparative study of the treatment of maternal hypertension in severe preeclampsia, nifedipine was a more efficacious antihypertensive drug and was associated with a much lower incidence of fetal distress.[97] Infants of nifedipine-treated mothers spent an average of 11 days in intensive care as opposed to 33 days for the hydralazine group. The overall maternal-infant cost in the nifedipine group was 31% lower than in the hydralazine group. Other investigators, using Doppler technology, showed that nifedipine has no adverse fetal or uteroplacental hemodynamic side effects when used in the treatment of preeclampsia.[98] In the postpartum period, nifedipine lowers maternal mean arterial pressure while enhancing urine output.[99]

Sophisticated noninvasive monitoring techniques, such as Doppler ultrasonography, are necessary to accurately define the hemodynamic state of patients with preeclampsia. Volume therapy and antihypertensive therapy can then be tailored to the specific hemodynamic pattern.[100] For example, patients with high output and low resistance would be better candidates for treatment with drugs to lower cardiac output, such as beta-adrenergic blockers, and do not require volume resuscitation, whereas patients with low output and high resistance would be better treated with volume expansion and peripheral vasodilatation using such drugs as nifedipine.

Invasive Cardiovascular Monitoring in Patients with Preeclampsia

The risk/benefit ratio of invasive cardiovascular monitoring in patients with preeclampsia, as well as with other cardiovascular disorders, must incorporate the skill and experience of the physicians and nursing staff as well as the severity of the patient's disease. Placement of intra-arterial and pulmonary artery catheters in patients with preeclampsia is not warranted, regardless of maternal status, if the obstetric and anesthetic decision makers are either unable or unwilling to incorporate the information to be obtained into the medical and anesthetic management of the patient. Recognition of the significance of various pulmonary artery waveforms, such as a continuously wedged position, requires specially trained individuals; pulmonary artery catheters should not be used without the continuous presence of personnel experienced in their use.

In patients with coagulation problems, as may occur in preeclampsia, introduction of central venous and pulmonary arterial catheters through the median basilic vein in the antecubital fossa or an external jugular vein is preferable to an internal jugular vein approach in order to minimize the risk of a neck hematoma in the event of carotid artery cannulation. The blood of preeclamptic patients may be hypocoagulable or hypercoagulable; in the latter case, the risk of axillary vein thrombosis is increased with prolonged use of brachial venous catheters long enough to reach the central circulation.

Arterial Pressure. In severe preeclampsia, an in-dwelling arterial catheter is warranted for beat-to-beat assessment of maternal blood pressure during either regional or general anesthesia. Both tracheal intubation and extubation may cause extreme systemic and pulmonary hypertension (see Fig. 18–24); direct arterial monitoring is necessary in order to guide antihypertensive therapy with rapid-acting agents. During epidural or spinal anesthesia, direct arterial monitoring permits earlier correction of hypotension. Such prompt therapy is mandated in the setting of a compromised fetus with minimal cardiovascular reserve, as is the usual case in severe preeclampsia.

Central Venous Pressure. A central venous catheter may be useful in cases of moderate to severe preeclampsia in which there is reduced urine output. If the initial central venous pressure (CVP) is low (0–3 mmHg) and the patient has a normal chest examination and normal arterial oxygen saturation on room air, it is appropriate to assume that the oliguric patient has persistent intravascular volume depletion and to continue with fluid and, possibly, arteriolar vasodilator therapy. However, it must be recognized that in patients with preeclampsia, central venous pressures may not reliably predict left-sided cardiac filling pressures, either in absolute values or in trends.[101] Figure 18–26 indicates that for any level of CVP, the PCWP may be equal to or 2–3 times greater than the measured CVP. Thus, although a very low CVP will usually indicate a low PCWP, there will be an occasional patient in whom a very low CVP is associated with a PCWP high enough to pose a risk for pulmonary edema. If the CVP is increased (6–12 mmHg) in a patient with preeclampsia, one must assume that the PCWP is of similar magnitude and probably much higher. Such a patient will have much less tolerance for aggressive volume therapy.

Disparities between right-sided and left-sided heart filling pressures may occur in the absence of any underlying cardiac abnormality and are primarily due to differences in afterload. For example, the left ventricle in severe preeclampsia is required to pump against an abnormally high peripheral resistance, whereas the right heart sees a normal afterload. Pulmonary vascular resistance is not increased in preeclampsia, even in the face of precipitous increases in SVR.[102] Thus, intercavitary pressure differences between the right and the left heart are to be expected, with the differences being more pronounced with greater differences in pulmonary and systemic afterload.

The limitations of CVP measurements in preeclampsia do not require that every patient have a pulmonary catheter

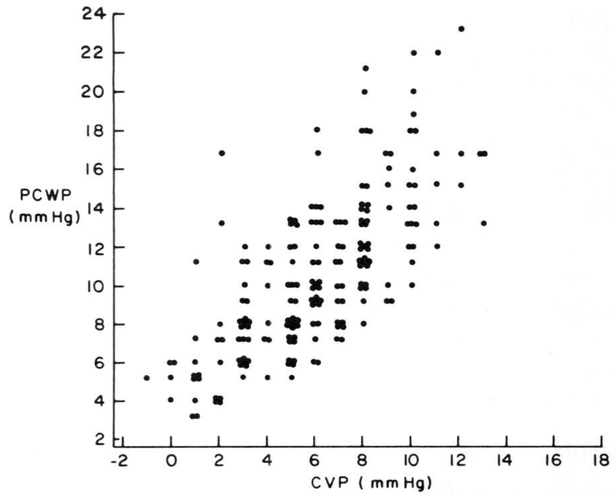

Figure 18–26. Relationship of central venous pressure (CVP) to pulmonary capillary wedge pressure (PCWP) in patients with severe preeclampsia. (From Cotton DB, Gonik B, Dorman K, Harrist R: Cardiovascular alterations in severe pregnancy-induced hypertension: Relationship of central venous pressure to pulmonary capillary wedge pressure. Am J Obstet Gynecol 1985; 151:763.)

to guide volume therapy. However, one should not rely entirely on a CVP measurement, particularly in the face of persistent oliguria. If fluid and vasodilator therapy are ineffective in establishing adequate urine output and the CVP is above 6–8 mmHg, a measurement other than CVP is required to assess cardiac filling. The two available options are pulmonary artery catheterization (PAC) and echocardiography.

Pulmonary Artery Pressure. The most frequent indication for monitoring pulmonary artery pressures in patients with preeclampsia is persistent oliguria in the face of presumably adequate fluid therapy. Although most oliguria patients will have low to normal PCWP, indicative of a persistent intravascular volume deficit, a minority will have markedly increased wedge pressures.[59] Increased wedge pressures in the absence of aggressive fluid therapy usually indicate left ventricular dysfunction. PAC allows for measurement of cardiac output and calculation of SVR, and preeclampsia is associated with widely disparate values for these variables, as seen in Figure 18–16 and Table 18–5. Knowledge of these parameters in a particular patient allows optimal hemodynamic management in cases of severe preeclampsia.

Another indication for PAC is when a central venous catheter is placed and the initial CVP is > 15 mmHg. Such pressures indicate either massive volume overload or heart failure; additional hemodynamic data are necessary for further assessment and management.

A pulmonary artery catheter is recommended for management of preeclamptic patients with pulmonary edema to accurately determine the cause of the pulmonary edema and the underlying hemodynamic state. COP is decreased in pregnancy and further decreased in preeclampsia. Thus, pulmonary edema can occur at "normal" levels of PCWP in such patients. Even when the PCWP is much lower than

TABLE 18–5. HEMODYNAMIC DATA FROM NINE PREECLAMPTIC PATIENTS WITH PERSISTENT OLIGURIA

	Patient No.—Category I					Patient No.—Category II			Patient No.—Category III
	1	*2*	*3*	*4*	*5*	*6*	*7*	*8*	*9*
Following Unsuccessful Fluid Challenge									
Mean arterial pressure (mmHg)	120	110	101	118	107	117	129	130	140
PCWP (mmHg)	7	3	4	5	1	9	10	18	18
CVP (mmHg)	6	1	0	2	2	5	9	9	3
Cardiac index (L/minute/m²)	3.5	4.2	3.5	4.1	4.0	4.8	5.1	6.4	2.6
SVR (dynes-cm-sec^{-5})	1378	1245	1393	1497	1135	1093	1043	921	2790
Left ventricular stroke work index	54	90	54	66	59	88	94	89	33
Therapy	Fluid	Fluid	Fluid	Fluid	Fluid	Fluid/ hydralazine	Fluid/ hydralazine	Nitroglycerin	Hydralazine
Following Therapy and Resolution of Oliguria									
Mean arterial pressure (mmHg)	117	123	120	107	107	110	107	105	104
PCWP (mmHg)	11	7	11	9	11	9	15	2	8
CVP (mmHg)	11	5	4	—	—	8	10	—	—
Cardiac index (L/minute/m²)	4.6	4.5	4.1	5.0	4.4	5.4	5.1	5.6	4.0
SVR (dynes-cm-sec^{-5})	961	1237	1367	1138	1049	884	843	910	1867
Left ventricular stroke work index	66	111	65	59	50	65	60	65	51

From Clark SL, Greenspoon JS, Aldahl D, Phelan JP: Severe preeclampsia with persistent oliguria: Management of hemodynamic subsets. Am J Obstet Gynecol 1986; 154:490–494, with permission.

COP, pulmonary edema may be present on the basis of altered capillary permeability.[51] Increased PCWP and cardiac output with decreased to normal SVR, particularly in the immediate postpartum period and with a history of aggressive fluid therapy, suggest volume overload as the etiology of pulmonary edema. Increased PCWP and SVR with decreased cardiac output are consistent with pulmonary edema due to acute left heart failure.

Volume loading prior to epidural or spinal anesthesia can be guided by CVP if oliguria is not present. However, if there is no increase in the CVP following 1500 ml of crystalloid or 500 ml of colloid, and the catheter position is confirmed, it is likely that there is poor correlation between the CVP and the PCWP. Further fluid management should be based on careful clinical assessment or a PAC.

In a preeclamptic patient who experiences decreased oxygen saturation immediately after tracheal intubation or extubation, acute heart failure must be considered in the differential diagnosis. After problems with oxygen delivery have been ruled out, a PAC is useful for diagnosis and treatment of the cardiac dysfunction.

Noninvasive Cardiovascular Monitoring in Patients with Preeclampsia

Noninvasive cardiovascular monitoring is increasingly used in patients with preeclampsia, obviating the need in many cases for PAC. This approach offers desirable benefits in terms of patient safety, particularly in patients with coagulation defects. Noninvasive Doppler echocardiography can readily differentiate patients with high cardiac output and low vascular resistance from those with low cardiac output and high resistance. However, in preeclamptic patients with persistent oliguria, Doppler echocardiography may not be able to reliably differentiate the patient with low cardiac output and extremely high vascular resistance due to severe intravascular hypovolemia from the patient with myocardial dysfunction and similar indices. Transesophageal echocardiography (TEE) allows for better imaging of cardiac function than transthoracic echocardiography. TEE may identify wall motion abnormalities that will permit better assessment and management of the wide range of hemodynamic profiles occurring in preeclamptic patients. In addition, Doppler echocardiographic techniques are now being used to study the flow characteristics of the uterine arteries.

Maternal Heart Disease

The normal hemodynamic changes associated with pregnancy may have severe adverse consequences for patients with cardiac disease, even those with previously asymptomatic lesions. Increases in blood volume (40–50%) and cardiac output (40–50% during pregnancy and 80% during labor and delivery) may precipitate pulmonary edema and heart failure in patients with mitral valve disease, whereas patients with aortic stenosis or right-to-left shunt are most imperiled by systemic hypotension such as might occur during episodes of the supine hypotensive syndrome or following regional anesthesia. Obstetric anesthetic management of patients with cardiac disease is lesion-specific; thus, it is essential that the exact nature of the heart lesion be known. Inappropriate intrapartum management can result in cardiac decompensation in a patient who has tolerated pregnancy quite well. The underlying pathophysiology of various cardiac lesions, the expected physiologic effects during pregnancy, labor, and delivery of such lesions, and the likely hemodynamic consequences of anesthetic interventions must be carefully considered.

Indications for Invasive Cardiovascular Monitoring in Parturients with Heart Disease

Because most of the increase in cardiac output occurs before the 24th week of gestation, the parturient presenting with a viable fetus has already undergone a prolonged and quite strenuous cardiac stress test. The response of the mother to the stress of pregnancy can usually be ascertained by a careful history and physical examination. In many cases, this information alone is sufficient to determine the need for invasive cardiovascular monitoring. Asymptomatic patients who have had an uneventful pregnancy without worsening of their cardiopulmonary status can be expected to tolerate the additional stress of labor and delivery *as long as obstetric and anesthetic management is appropriate for the specific cardiac lesion.* In such cases, invasive hemodynamic monitoring is usually not required. Some suggested exceptions to this rule include any parturient with a right-to-left shunt, primary pulmonary hypertension, severe coarctation of the aorta, or severe aortic stenosis.

Use of data obtained from a PAC requires an understanding of the limitations inherent in measurements made in patients with structural or functional cardiac abnormalities. In many patients, trends provide more reliable information than any one absolute value, underscoring the importance of frequent observation and early recognition of ominous trends.

Mitral Stenosis

Pathophysiology. In mitral stenosis, there is an impediment to filling of the left ventricle due to narrowing of the mitral valve orifice (Fig. 18–27). The normal gradient of 3–5 mmHg across the valve is increased several times, and gradients in excess of 25 mmHg are present in patients with severe mitral stenosis. The obstruction to left atrial outflow increases pressures in the left atrium, pulmonary veins, and pulmonary capillaries.

Pulmonary congestion accounts for the symptoms of dyspnea and orthopnea that occur as the disease progresses in severity. Chronic volume overload usually presents as right ventricular failure with hepatic congestion. Thus, the presence of right ventricular hypertrophy on ECG carries a significant risk of cardiac failure. Acute volume overload in pregnant patients with mild to moderate mitral stenosis is more likely to overstress the left ventricle.[103]

Atrial contraction contributes 33% of left ventricular filling in mitral stenosis, compared to 20% in the normal heart. Hence, sinus rhythm is important for maintaining cardiac output in patients with mitral stenosis. The distention of the left atrium in mitral stenosis predisposes patients to atrial fibrillation, which can rapidly result in pulmonary edema and cardiac insufficiency for two reasons: the loss of atrial contraction and decreased diastolic filling time if the heart rate increases during atrial fibrillation. The sluggish flow of blood through the distended left atrium in patients with mitral stenosis favors thrombus formation. The risk of systemic embolization is further enhanced by the presence of atrial fibrillation.

Patients with mitral stenosis may not tolerate the normal physiologic changes of pregnancy, particularly the increase in pulmonary blood volume. Labor, delivery, and the immediate puerperium are considered the times of maximum risk. Each uterine contraction increases central blood volume by 15–25%, worsening any pulmonary congestion. The further distention of the left atrium by this increased blood volume increases the probability of atrial fibrillation. The greatest increase in central blood volume occurs immediately after delivery as a result of uterine involution and relief of vena caval obstruction. Clark and colleagues doc-

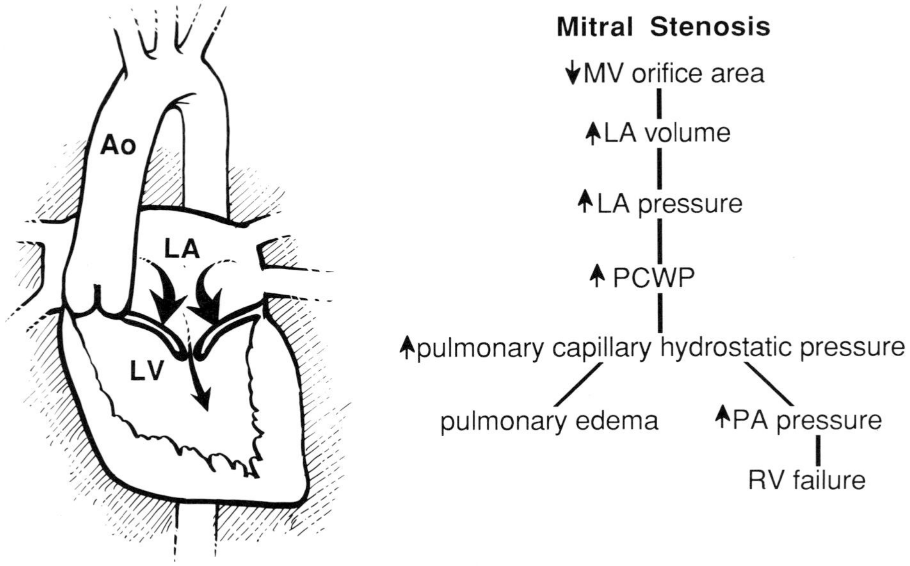

Figure 18–27. Mitral stenosis (diastole). Restricted flow through the narrowed mitral valve orifice results in elevated blood volumes in the cardiopulmonary circuit proximal to the mitral valve. (MV = mitral valve, LA = left atrium, PCWP = pulmonary capillary wedge pressure, PA = pulmonary artery, RV = right ventricle, LV = left ventricle, Ao = aorta.)

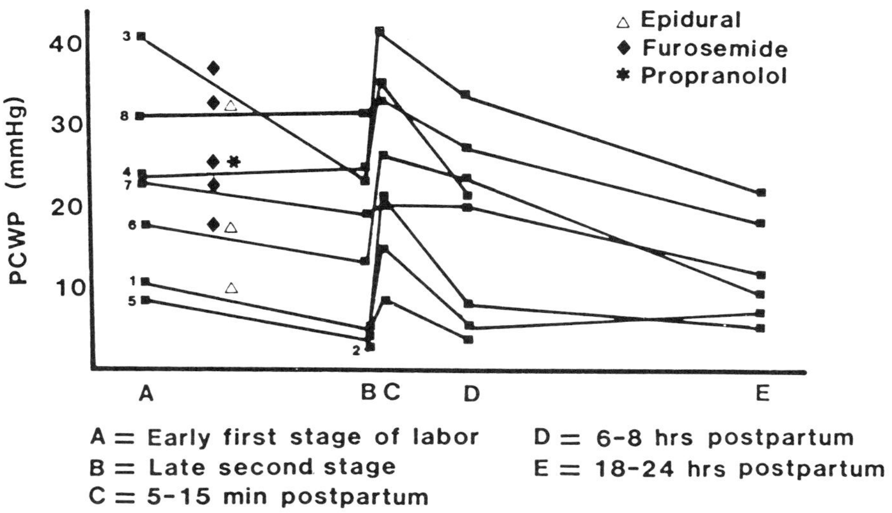

Figure 18–28. Intrapartum changes in pulmonary capillary wedge pressure (PCWP) in eight patients with mitral stenosis. Delivery is consistently associated with an abrupt increase in PCWP and the risk of pulmonary edema. (From Clark SL, Phelan JP, Greenspoon J, et al: Labor and delivery in the presence of mitral stenosis: central hemodynamic observations. Am J Obstet Gynecol 1985; 152:984–8; as reproduced in Mangano DT: Anesthesia for the pregnant cardiac patient. *In* Shnider SM, Levinson G [eds]: Anesthesia for Obstetrics, 2nd Ed. Baltimore: Williams & Wilkins, 1987.)

umented a 10-mmHg (± 6 mmHg) increase in PCWP after vaginal delivery in a series of patients with severe mitral stenosis (Fig. 18–28).[103] However, the range (0–18 mmHg) was wide, and the greatest increases occurred in patients beginning labor with the highest wedge pressures. Cunningham and coworkers reported four patients with mitral stenosis in a series of patients with unsuspected and asymptomatic cardiac disease who developed peripartum congestive heart failure. All four patients became symptomatic *after* delivery (within 48 hours).[104] Thus, careful monitoring of patients with mitral stenosis should continue for several days post partum.

The risk of cardiac decompensation during delivery is also increased by tachycardia, as can be expected with painful uterine contractions. The rapid rate allows less time for ventricular filling through the stenotic mitral orifice; as forward flow decreases, pulmonary congestion increases.

A number of reports have confirmed the efficacy of balloon valvotomy during pregnancy in women with severe mitral stenosis with pliable mitral valves.[105–108] In all the studies, the average cross-sectional area of the mitral orifice was less than 1.0 cm^2 before balloon dilatation; afterwards, the cross-sectional area increased to approximately 2.0 cm^2 in most patients. Almost every patient exhibited functional improvement following valvotomy, moving from New York Heart Association class III or IV to class I or II. Given the efficacy of this procedure during pregnancy, it is likely that the incidence of pregnant patients with symptomatic mitral stenosis presenting for delivery will be mainly confined to those parturients lacking sophisticated prenatal care. Also, this procedure should reduce the frequency of emergent delivery of premature infants necessitated because of worsening maternal condition associated with mitral stenosis.

Monitoring. Parturients with mild mitral stenosis without episodes of pulmonary edema or atrial fibrillation do not require invasive monitoring during labor and delivery. However, the ECG should be monitored continually during this period, and equipment for cardioversion must be available. Volume status must be carefully assessed in the postpartum period. All patients with mitral stenosis should be considered at risk for development of pulmonary edema, regardless of the severity of their lesions. Pulse oximetry is useful for early detection of worsening pulmonary congestion in such patients.

Symptomatic patients should be monitored with both a peripheral arterial and a pulmonary artery catheter; CVP monitoring is not sufficiently reliable in this situation. In patients with mitral stenosis, there is very poor correlation between CVPs and PCWPs, with differences of 10 mmHg or greater in 85% of patients in one study.[103] Clark recommends maintaining the PCWP in the 14-mmHg range.[109] This value is based on the expected increase in PCWP following delivery being somewhat less than 18 mmHg in most patients and the observation that clinically significant pulmonary edema does not usually occur with wedge pressures below 28–30 mmHg. Attaining a PCWP of 14 mmHg may require diuresis in some patients; this must be done with extreme caution, because the PCWP does not accurately reflect left ventricular filling volumes in the presence of mitral stenosis.[110] Treating increased PCWP when in fact the left ventricular end-diastolic volume is decreased may severely impair cardiac output; many patients with mitral stenosis require elevated left atrial pressures for adequate ventricular filling. Therapeutic alterations in intravascular volume should be guided by additional information, such as blood pressure, urine output, weight change, and preferentially, noninvasive measurement of stroke volume and cardiac output.

Anesthetic Considerations. Because of the severity of the consequences of atrial fibrillation, pregnant patients with mitral stenosis usually receive prophylactic digitalis. Drugs causing tachycardia, such as atropine, ketamine, and pancuronium, should be avoided. If tachycardia occurs, it may be treated with adenosine, verapamil, or beta-blocking drugs such as propanolol or esmolol.

Epidural analgesia helps to prevent increases in heart rate associated with painful uterine contractions. Perineal analgesia blocks the urge to push, a beneficial effect because Valsalva maneuvers are detrimental; the increased intrathoracic pressure impedes venous return and markedly reduces cardiac output.[111] The venodilatation resulting from epidural anesthesia is likewise helpful in reducing central blood volume.[112] Hypotension should be treated with a pure $alpha_1$ agonist such as phenylephrine rather than ephedrine, a mixed agent that produces tachycardia by virtue of its $beta_1$ properties. The addition of epinephrine to solutions of local anesthetics for epidural injection also increases the risk of tachycardia.

One report described the use of the Trendelenburg position to adjust PCWP during epidural anesthesia in patients with severe mitral stensois.[113] The initial PCWP of 37 mmHg decreased to 15 mmHg following epidural blockade; associated with this decrease in preload was a decrease in cardiac index, from 2.4 to 1.8 L/minute/m^2. By selecting the appropriate angle of the Trendelenburg position, the authors were able to optimize cardiac output; at a PCWP of 25 mmHg, the mean cardiac index was 3.1 L/minute/m^2. As previously discussed, the Trendelenburg position does not improve cardiac output in patients with severe hypovolemia; patients with severe mitral stenosis undergoing epidural anesthesia occupy the opposite end of the hemodynamic spectrum compared with patients in hypovolemic shock.[44, 45]

General anesthesia utilizing a standard rapid intubation sequence and a potent inhalational agent is acceptable only for patients with mild disease. This regimen may precipitate rapid cardiac decompensation as a result of tachycardia. Increased pulmonary artery pressures associated with tracheal intubation worsen pre-existing right ventricular dysfunction. Patients with severe stenosis and cardiac compromise requiring general anesthesia are more safely managed with regional blockade of the glossopharyngeal and superior laryngeal nerves and topical anesthesia of the trachea,[114, 115] followed by a narcotic induction and then tracheal intubation. Alfentanil, a short-acting narcotic, has been used successfully in patients with severe mitral stenosis with pulmonary hypertension to avoid myocardial depression and permit extubation at the end of the surgical procedure.[116] Anesthetic inductions using primarily high-dose narcotics may be associated with a slightly increased risk of pulmonary aspiration of gastric contents, because the cough reflex and the glottic closure reflex are greatly obtunded by opiates.[117] The best assurance against this possibility is the maintenance of effective cricoid pressure until the airway is secure. Antagonism of narcosis in the neonate may be required. If so, it should be done with very small, incremental doses of naloxone (1 μg/kg) rather than the larger doses suggested in standard pediatric texts.[118]

Pulse oximetry is particularly important if general endotracheal anesthesia is utilized, because of the potential for rapid worsening of pulmonary function. Pulse oximetry is also useful to assess the adequacy of oxygenation prior to extubation of the trachea.

Mitral Regurgitation

Pathophysiology. Incompetence of the mitral value permits regurgitant flow from the left ventricle into the left atrium (Fig. 18–29). The compliant atrial walls readily distend to accommodate the increased blood volume, and, until late in the course of the disease, there is no significant increase in pulmonary vascular pressures. Forward flow through the aortic valve depends on the resistance across this valve compared to the resistance across the incompetent mitral valve. Factors that lower peripheral vascular resistance tend to favor forward flow and improve cardiac output. For this reason, normal pregnancy is usually well tolerated by individuals with isolated mitral regurgitation. However, parturients with longstanding mitral regurgitation may have increased left atrial pressures and left ventricular

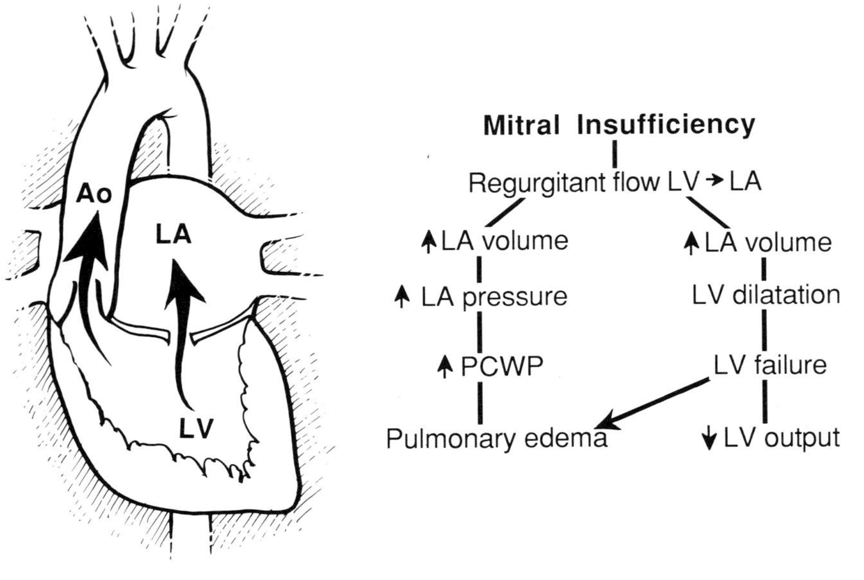

Figure 18–29. Mitral regurgitation (systole). A portion of the left ventricular output is ejected in a retrograde manner into the left atrium, resulting in increased blood volume in the pulmonary venous circuit. During diastole, this extra volume overloads the left ventricle, resulting in chamber enlargement. (LV = left ventricle, LA = left atrium, PCWP = pulmonary capillary wedge pressure, Ao = aorta.)

dysfunction based on chronic volume overload. The elevated left atrial pressures are transmitted to the pulmonary circulation, predisposing the patient to pulmonary congestion. In such patients, labor can be quite hazardous, because enhanced sympathetic nervous system activity increases vascular resistance and worsens the regurgitant flow, and further pulmonary blood volume overload occurs with the autotransfusion associated with each uterine contraction. This combination of factors may precipitate acute left-sided heart failure and pulmonary edema.

Atrial fibrillation may occur, but is less likely to adversely affect cardiac output than it is in patients with mitral stenosis. Mild degrees of tachycardia may be beneficial by decreasing the regurgitant volume. Bradycardia often decreases cardiac output, because stroke volume tends to be relatively fixed.

Monitoring. Monitoring concerns are similar to those for mitral stenosis. The amount of regurgitant flow parallels the intensity of the insufficiency murmur as well as the size of the V wave on the PCWP tracing. These findings may be a better guide to hemodynamic management than PCWP, because there may be little correlation between left atrial pressure and left atrial volume in a chronically dilated atrium. Such lack of correlation precludes any valid estimate of left ventricular end-diastolic volume.

Anesthetic Considerations. Epidural anesthesia is beneficial in decreasing peripheral resistance, which is very desirable in patients with mitral regurgitation. One potential concern with epidural anesthesia is the bradycardia that usually accompanies the sharp decrease in blood pressure resulting from extensive venodilatation and decreased cardiac return. Contrary to what one might expect, the initial response of the right heart and the sinoatrial node to *acute* hypovolemia is bradycardia.[43] Only in this manner can the right ventricle fill enough to maintain an adequate fiber length in order to permit contraction. If the hypovolemia persists, sympathetically mediated responses will dominate, and tachycardia eventually ensues.

The abrupt decrease in cardiac filling volume following venodilatation induced by epidural anesthesia, coupled with reflex slowing of the heart rate, severely decreases cardiac output. This hemodynamic impairment occurs in normal patients and frequently results in nausea. When the patient has mitral regurgitation, the combination of hypotension and bradycardia is of particular concern, because it may cause myocardial ischemia and heart failure. This can be minimized by judicious volume administration as the epidural anesthetic is being administered, maintaining the patient in the left lateral decubitus position until the block reaches the upper thoracic dermatomes, and by steeply elevating the patient's legs (while maintaining uterine displacement) at the first sign of hypotension (nausea, slowing of heart rate). Small doses of ephedrine are also useful, providing both inotropic and chronotropic support without an excessive increase in afterload. It is likely that a portion of the hypotension associated with epidural anesthesia results from the use of epinephrine in the epidural solution, either as a test dose or to decrease systemic absorption of the local anesthetic. Low doses of systemic epinephrine produce predominantly $beta_2$ effects, and adrenergically mediated venodilatation may occur even with epidural blockade below the levels that innervate the splanchnic circulation. The same concerns for hypertension with tracheal intubation apply as discussed for mitral stenosis. The capability for careful titration of a rapid-acting vasodilator such as sodium nitroprusside must be present. Potent agents may cause excessive myocardial depression in already compromised patients.

Mitral Valve Prolapse

Pathologic mitral valve prolapse is a connective tissue abnormality of the leaflets, annulus, and chordae tendineae of the mitral valve. It must be distinguished from the normal superior displacement of the mitral valve leaflets, a very common condition occurring in 5–15% of healthy patients examined using 2D echocardiography.[119] Table 18–6 lists diagnostic criteria for identifying patients with pathologic mitral valve prolapse. One or more major criteria are necessary and sufficient to establish the diagnosis. Patients with one or more minor criteria do not warrant this diag-

TABLE 18–6. CRITERIA RELATED TO THE DIAGNOSIS OF MITRAL VALVE PROLAPSE

Major criteria that establish the diagnosis of mitral valve prolapse
Auscultation
Mid to late systolic clicks and a late systolic murmur at the cardiac apex
Mobile mid to late systolic clicks at the cardiac apex
Late systolic murmur at the cardiac apex in the young patient
Auscultation plus Echocardiography
Apical holosystolic murmur of mitral regurgitation plus echocardiographic criteria
Two-Dimensional/Doppler Echocardiography
Marked systolic displacement of mitral leaflets with coaptation point at or on the left atrial side of the annulus
Moderate systolic displacement of the leaflets with at least moderate mitral regurgitation, chordal rupture, and annular dilatation
Two-Dimensionally Targeted M-mode Echocardiography
Marked (≥ 3 mm) late systolic buckling posterior to the C-D line (annular plane)
Minor criteria that arouse suspicion but do not establish the diagnosis of mitral valve prolapse
History
Focal neurologic attacks or amaurosis fugax in the young patient
First-degree relatives with major criteria
Recurrent supraventricular tachycardia (documented)
Auscultation
Soft, inconstant, or equivocal mid to late systolic sounds at the cardiac apex
Other Physical Signs
Low body weight, asthenic habitus
Low blood pressure
Thoracic bony abnormalities
Two-Dimensional/Doppler/Color Flow Echocardiography
Moderate superior systolic displacement of mitral leaflets with Doppler mitral regurgitation
Two-Dimensionally Targeted M-mode Echocardiography
Moderate (2 mm) late systolic buckling posterior to the C-D line (annular plane)
Holosystolic displacement (3 mm) posterior to the C-D line (annular plane)

From Perloff JK, Child JS: Clinical and epidemiologic issues in mitral valve prolapse. Am Heart J 1987; 113:1324, with permission.

nosis, but they may still have cardiac abnormalities, particularly in the presence of a holosystolic murmur.

Fortunately, mitral valve prolapse remains asymptomatic in most patients, and pregnancy, labor, and delivery are well tolerated.[120, 121] Pregnancy may present complications for the small percentage of patients who present with significant mitral regurgitation.

Pathophysiology. In mitral valve prolapse, the chordae tendineae are elongated, allowing the mitral valve leaflets to prolapse into the left atrium when the ventricular volume decreases during systole. This accounts for the mid- to late-systolic click and murmur of mitral regurgitation that are characteristic of mitral valve prolapse. The volume status of the left ventricle affects the degree of regurgitant flow. Conditions that augment left ventricular volume (hypervolemia, increased afterload, bradycardia, and decreased myocardial contractility) decrease regurgitant flow. Regurgitant flow increases when left ventricular volume decreases (hypovolemia, sustained increases in intrathoracic pressure, and tachycardia with resultant decreased filling time). Thus, patients with mitral valve prolapse and severe preeclampsia may be at increased risk for cardiac compromise due to the hypovolemia and tachycardia seen in these conditions.

Monitoring. Invasive cardiovascular monitoring is rarely necessary in patients with isolated mitral valve prolapse. Dysrhythmias are common, particularly supraventricular tachyarrhythmias, and continuous ECG monitoring during labor facilitates their prompt treatment.

Anesthetic Considerations. Preload should be maintained in patients with mitral valve prolapse. Epidural anesthesia is appropriate as long as sympathetic blockade (decreased SVR) is induced slowly, and intravascular volume is carefully evaluated. Ephedrine is not advisable for treating hypotension, because its inotropic and chronotropic properties are undesirable in the setting of mitral valve prolapse. Antibiotic prophylaxis against subacute bacterial endocarditis is recommended for all patients with *pathologic* mitral valve prolapse. Antiarrhythmic medications should be continued, regardless of anesthetic technique. The hyperdynamic cardiac response to tracheal intubation can worsen the degree of prolapse, and control of tachycardia and hypertension is important for optimum management.

Aortic Stenosis

Pathophysiology. Aortic stenosis is rarely symptomatic during the childbearing years. However, in symptomatic patients, pregnancy causes severe hemodynamic derangements. As the aortic valve narrows from a normal cross-sectional area of 2.6–3.5 cm^2 to less than 1 cm^2, increasing left ventricular pressures are required to maintain cardiac output (Fig. 18–30), leading to concentric hypertrophy of the left ventricle. The elevation in end-diastolic pressure combined with a thickened left ventricular wall impairs subendocardial blood flow, resulting in myocardial ischemia.

The outflow tract obstruction results in a relatively fixed stroke volume, so that increases in cardiac output are determined primarily by increases in heart rate. However, decreased diastolic compliance may be the major pathophysiologic abnormality in many patients with aortic stenosis, and tachycardia with resultant decreased ventricular filling times worsens cardiac output.[122]

Monitoring. Invasive hemodynamic monitoring is required in patients with severe stenosis (gradient $>$ 50 mmHg), symptoms of congestive failure, angina, or a history of syncopal episodes. However, because of decreased left ventricular compliance, left ventricular end-diastolic pressure may be increased although actual chamber volume is low. Higher than normal PCWP may be necessary to maintain cardiac output, but such increases in pressure increase the likelihood of pulmonary edema. ECG monitoring is recommended in order to detect myocardial ischemia.

Anesthetic Considerations. Pregnant patients with aortic stenosis may not tolerate large decreases in preload (filling volumes), afterload (peripheral vascular resistance), or heart rate. Thus, epidural anesthesia, which can cause all three of these undesirable responses, must be administered

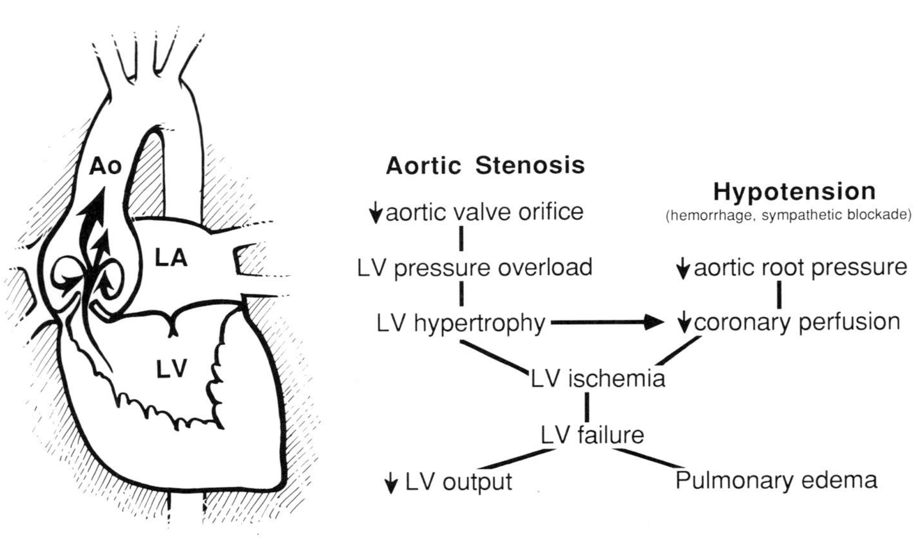

Figure 18–30. Aortic stenosis (systole). The narrow aortic valve orifice requires elevated left ventricular pressures to overcome the resistance to ejection. There is turbulent flow just distal to the valve, resulting in dilatation of the aortic root. (LV = left ventricle, LA = left atrium, Ao = aorta.)

carefully, with attention given to adequate fluid pretreatment and prompt correction of hypotension. The recommended treatment for hypotension is administration of a predominantly $alpha_1$ agent, such as phenylephrine, to elevate aortic root pressures as a consequence of arteriolar vasoconstriction.

Light general anesthesia such as that typically used for cesarean section is usually tolerated quite well, because both blood pressure and heart rate are well maintained. The hemodynamic response to laryngoscopy and tracheal intubation can precipitate left ventricular dysfunction, and alfentanil (35 μg/kg) has been recommended for use in blocking this response.[123] The expected side effects of alfentanil at this dose include maternal hypotension and neonatal respiratory depression. Regional and topical anesthesia of the airway prior to induction, as described for patients with mitral stenosis, coupled with reduced dosages of intravenous induction agents offer another option for minimizing hemodynamic alterations. In patients with evidence of left ventricular failure, potent inhalational agents should be avoided owing to their propensity for myocardial depression.

Aortic Regurgitation

Pathophysiology. In aortic regurgitation, the incompetent valve allows blood in the aorta to flow back into the left ventricle (Fig. 18–31). This "runoff" lesion decreases diastolic pressure and widens pulse pressure. Regurgitant blood causes volume overload of the left ventricle and, if chronic, dilatation of the left ventricle. Thus, left ventricular end-diastolic pressure may remain normal despite an increased left ventricular end-diastolic volume. With progressive distention, the left ventricle eventually fails, and left ventricular end-diastolic pressure increases. Bradycardia allows more time for regurgitant flow during diastole and should be avoided. Increased SVR enhances regurgitant flow and may precipitate congestive heart failure.

Pregnancy is well tolerated in patients with mild to moderate aortic regurgitation, because pregnancy-induced decreases in peripheral resistance decrease the ratio of regurgitant volume to total stroke volume. However, in patients with myocardial dysfunction, increased blood volume worsens pulmonary congestion, and the increase in SVR associated with labor in such a patient can lead to acute decompensation.

In severe aortic regurgitation, there are abnormalities of coronary flow, with phasic coronary flow occurring mainly during systole rather than during diastole,[124] reversal of flow during part of diastole, and redistribution of coronary flow from the endocardium to the epicardium.[125] Systemic hypotension may additionally impair coronary flow, precipitating myocardial ischemia and cardiac failure.[126]

Monitoring. Isolated aortic regurgitation is usually asymptomatic in patients of childbearing age. In patients with left ventricular dysfunction or echocardiographic evidence of a significantly dilated left ventricle, invasive hemodynamic monitoring is warranted to guide titration of vasodilator and inotropic therapy. The dilated ventricle accommodates a large end-diastolic volume without an increase in pressure, and thus PCWP fails to accurately assess left ventricle volume. However, any increase in PCWP must be investigated and promptly treated, if necessary, because such a change may herald a rapid deterioration in cardiac function.

Anesthetic Considerations. The anesthetic considerations in aortic regurgitation are similar to those for mitral regurgitation: avoid increased peripheral resistance, bradycardia, and myocardial depression. Carefully administered epidural anesthesia is usually hemodynamically beneficial in patients with aortic regurgitation.

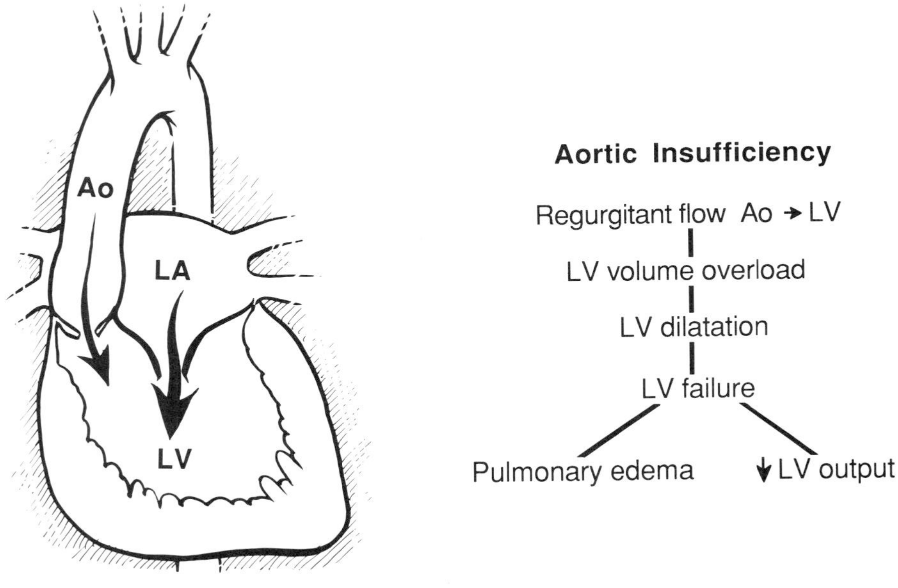

Figure 18–31. Aortic regurgitation (diastole). The incompetent aortic valve allows ejected blood to flow back into the left ventricle during diastole at the same time that the ventricle is being filled from the left atrium. This volume overload causes the left ventricle to enlarge and possibly fail. (Ao = aorta, LV = left ventricle, LA = left atrium.)

Intracardiac and Extracardiac Shunts

Left-to-Right Shunts

Pathophysiology. Atrial septal defect, ventricular septal defect, and patent ductus arteriosus differ in the location of the shunt site, yet they have in common an increase in pulmonary blood flow due to a left-to-right shunt. Small defects produce small shunts and minimal symptoms, whereas large defects, in which pulmonary blood flow may be four to five times systemic flow, eventually overload the pulmonary circuit, leading to pulmonary hypertension and right ventricular failure. Increases in SVR normally worsen the shunt.

The increased blood volume associated with pregnancy adds to the already excessive pulmonary blood flow, but this effect is offset somewhat by the decrease in SVR occurring in normal pregnancy. Maternal and fetal outcomes are usually satisfactory.[127]

Monitoring. Invasive hemodynamic monitoring is not required in patients with small defects and no symptoms. However, patients with pulmonary hypertension and right ventricular dysfunction warrant pulmonary and peripheral arterial monitoring and, in the case of an atrial septal defect, right atrial pressure monitoring. Cardiac output determined by thermodilution methods will be unreliable in situations in which pulmonary flow is much greater than systemic flow.[128] Doppler ECG may be preferable if cardiac output must be measured.

Anesthetic Considerations. Patients with shunts are always at risk for systemic embolization of any air introduced into a blood vessel, regardless of the normal direction of the shunt. For example, in patients with an atrial septal defect with a left-to-right shunt, air bubbles introduced into the right atrium may nonetheless traverse the septal defect in a right-to-left direction and gain access to the systemic circulation, notably the cerebral vessels and the coronary arteries. This phenomenon is referred to as ''paradoxical'' shunting.

Epidural and spinal anesthesia result in peripheral vasodilatation and decreased peripheral resistance, conditions that generally benefit patients with left-to-right shunts. Extreme arterial hypotension, however, can cause shunt reversal and hypoxemia. Conversely, general anesthesia and the necessity for tracheal intubation carry the risk of increasing peripheral resistance and worsening the left-to-right shunt.

Right-to-Left Shunts

Pathophysiology. In right-to-left shunts, deoxygenated blood bypasses the pulmonary capillary bed, resulting in systemic arterial desaturation and cyanosis. The shunt can occur at any level in the cardiopulmonary circuit—atrial, ventricular, aortopulmonary, or intrapulmonary. Right-to-left shunts also develop as a consequence of pulmonary hypertension in lesions normally resulting in left-to-right shunting. This reversal of shunt flow is known as Eisenmenger's syndrome. Cyanosis and reversed shunt flow carry a high risk for both maternal and fetal morbidity and mortality.

There are a number of congenital cardiac lesions that produce cyanosis, including transposition of the great vessels, pulmonary atresia, tricuspid atresia, and tetralogy of Fallot. In tetralogy of Fallot, the pulmonic stenosis can be either fixed or dynamic, the latter involving infundibular hypertrophy. In cases of fixed obstruction, increased right ventricular contractility is necessary to maintain adequate pulmonary blood flow. On the other hand, if there is dynamic infundibular obstruction, increases in right ventricular contractility tend to worsen the outflow obstruction, as does hypovolemia and tachycardia.

Pregnancy can be very deleterious for patients with right-to-left shunts, and even more so in the presence of pulmonary hypertension. One study noted deterioration of cardiac status in all pregnant patients with pulmonary artery pressures greater than 50 mmHg.[129] The thickened pulmonary vessels in patients with pulmonary hypertension are minimally responsive to the factors producing peripheral vasodilatation in pregnancy, and pulmonary vascular resistance does not decrease. The imbalance between pulmonary and systemic vascular resistance in pregnancy worsens the right-to-left shunt, producing severe cyanosis, a detriment to both the mother and the fetus. In patients with tetralogy of Fallot and right ventricular infundibular hypertrophy, the sympathetic nervous system response to labor increases right ventricular contractility and increased pulmonary vascular resistance, conditions that worsen the amount of right-to-left shunt.

Monitoring. Pulse oximetry is the most useful monitor in patients with right-to-left shunts. These patients tend to be on the steep portion of the oxygen-hemoglobin dissociation curve, and thus they are very sensitive to any of the factors adversely affecting oxygen saturation (Sa_{O_2}): (1) decreased inspired fraction of oxygen, (2) increased right-to-left shunting, (3) increased oxygen consumption, (4) decreased cardiac output, and (5) decreased mixed venous oxygen tension.[130] Pulse oximetry correlates well with *in vitro* Sa_{O_2} determined by co-oximetry in children with cyanotic congenital heart disease over an oxygen saturation range of 35–95%.[131] Measurement of CVP is helpful in patients with tetralogy of Fallot and infundibular hypertrophy, because it is important to maintain an adequate central volume.

Anesthetic Considerations. Epidural and spinal anesthesia carry the risk of decreased peripheral resistance with consequent worsening of right-to-left shunting. Resistance can be adjusted with careful volume and appropriate vasopressor therapy. Ephedrine, with its $beta_1$ enhancement of cardiac contractility and inotropy, should not be used to correct venodilatation in patients with tetralogy of Fallot and infundibular hypertrophy. Rather, a more selective $alpha_1$ agent is preferable.

Light general anesthesia for cesarean section tends to maintain peripheral resistance, a desirable goal in patients with a right-to-left shunt. Halothane is particularly efficacious in reducing right ventricular contractility in patients with tetralogy of Fallot and dynamic outflow tract obstruction, but may be deleterious in patients with tetralogy and a fixed obstruction. Factors increasing pulmonary vascular resistance, such as hypercarbia, hypoxia, and extremes of lung volume,[132] must be assiduously avoided in patients with right-to-left shunts. For example, prolonged coughing on an endotracheal tube empties the lung to residual volume and causes hypoxia and tachycardia, conditions adversely affecting pulmonary flow in patients with right-to-left shunts.

MONITORING OF PATIENTS RECEIVING SPINAL NARCOTICS

Epidural and intraspinal narcotics are extensively used in obstetrics, primarily for postoperative analgesia following cesarean section and, usually in combination with local anesthetics, labor analgesia and anesthesia for cesarean section. The advantages of neuraxial opiates include good pain relief without motor blockade, prolonged duration of action compared to other routes of administration, and negligible narcotic blood levels in the fetus when used in appropriate doses. The disadvantages include pruritus, nausea, dizziness, urinary retention, and the potential for respiratory depression. These side effects are reversible with naloxone at dosages that do not reverse the analgesic effects, because naloxone does not antagonize the analgesic activity of mu agonists in the spinal cord as it does in the brain, and the mechanism of action of neuraxial (epidural and intraspinal) opiates appears to predominantly involve mu receptors in the dorsal horn of the spinal cord.

One approach to the problems inherent in mu agonists such as morphine and fentanyl is the use of mixed agents such as butorphanol, a kappa agonist with partial mu antagonism. However, this drug has been shown to cause irreversible neurologic injury in sheep when administered intrathecally.[133] Because unsuspected intrathecal injection is always a possibility during epidural drug administration, use of butorphanol in the neuraxis in humans would appear to involve an as yet unspecified risk.

After injection of an epidural opiate, there is some systemic absorption through the epidural vessels that is related to the lipophilicity of the particular opiate and is roughly equivalent to an intramuscular injection of the same dose of drug. There is also the potential for an unsuspected intravascular or intrathecal injection when administering epidural opiates. Thus, patients should be continuously observed following each injection for the possibility of immediate respiratory depression in the same manner that patients should be monitored after parenteral narcotic administration.

However, it is the potential for delayed respiratory depression that has been the greatest concern in the use of neuraxial narcotics.[134] This effect is thought to be caused by the interaction of the narcotic with respiratory centers in the fourth ventricle of the brain. The narcotic reaches this area of the central nervous system through the cerebrospinal fluid rather than the systemic circulation, and the flow characteristics of spinal fluid are such that it takes several hours for usual doses of lumbar epidural morphine to achieve significant brain levels.[135] Because pruritus and nausea are also centrally mediated, these side effects exhibit the same delay. The peak period for delayed respiratory depression is from 4 to 8 hours after epidural morphine administration, although Abboud and coworkers have demonstrated a 30–50% depression of ventilatory response to CO_2 beginning 1.5 hours after administration of 5 mg of epidural morphine and lasting 24 hours.[136]

Other narcotics that are more lipid-soluble than morphine, such as fentanyl, sufentanil, and meperidine, are more extensively absorbed by lipid tissues near the site of injection; consequently, a smaller proportion of the drug is available for rostral migration to the brain compared to morphine. However, sufficient quantities of highly lipid-soluble agents do reach the brain via the cerebrospinal fluid to cause depression of the CO_2 response in a dose-dependent manner.[137] The onset (15 minutes) of respiratory depression is much more rapid than that seen after epidural administration of morphine, and the duration of action is shorter. One case report described apnea and hypoxemia 100 minutes after epidural administration of 100 μg of fentanyl to a healthy 27-year-old woman undergoing cesarean section.[138]

Use of the more lipid-soluble agents does reduce the likelihood of delayed respiratory depression occurring after the patient has left the operating room and postanesthesia recovery area. Unfortunately, it also reduces the duration of analgesia. For example, epidural fentanyl (75 μg) has an analgesic action of approximately 6 hours, whereas epidural morphine (5 mg) has a duration of 18–24 hours.

One solution to the problem of delayed respiratory depression is a naloxone infusion. Rawal and Wattwil demonstrated that a naloxone infusion (5 μg/kg/hour) reversed the ventilatory depression produced by 10 mg of epidural morphine in healthy volunteers, a dose twice that used clinically.[139] Addition of 1 or 2 ampules (0.4–0.8 mg) of naloxone to postoperative intravenous fluids at a maintenance rate (125 ml/hour) provides 50–100 μg/hour of naloxone. If continued for 16 hours, the risk of delayed respiratory depression in patients receiving epidural morphine (3–5 mg) is extremely low. An additional benefit of the naloxone infusion is that it lessens the severity of nausea and pruritus if initiated shortly after the administration of epidural morphine.

Naloxone infusions are not standard practice at many leading obstetric centers; this in part reflects a cost/benefit ratio that imposes an expense on every patient receiving epidural morphine in order to prevent the rare (probably less than 1 in 1000) case of significant respiratory depression. Postpartum patients receiving epidural morphine are presumably at even less risk for delayed respiratory depression than other patients because of the respiratory stimulant effects of elevated progesterone levels that accompany pregnancy. Also, obstetric patients tend to be young and free of concurrent lung disease, factors that affect the likelihood of delayed respiratory depression.

All cases of clinically significant respiratory depression attributable to epidural narcotic administration have been accompanied by somnolence on the part of the patient. Thus, monitoring of patients receiving epidural opiates should include an assessment of their state of arousal. Excessive sedation should be a cause for concern. Likewise, sedating drugs such as systemic opiates, antihistamines, and benzodiazepines should be used with caution, because their use may mask an early indication of excessive respiratory depression, and certain of these drugs potentiate respiratory depression when the patients already have a depressed response to increases in carbon dioxide. It is essential to note that merely documenting respiratory rate does not ensure a lack of respiratory depression in patients receiving epidural opiates. In contrast to systemic opiates, which decrease minute ventilation primarily by decreasing respiratory rate, *epidural opiates decrease tidal volumes.* Thus, minute ventilation may be markedly impaired in sleeping patients who appear to be breathing at a normal rate.

Even though all patients receiving neuraxial opiates have a depressed response to CO_2, very few will have any significant changes in respiratory parameters such as minute ventilation. Only those patients who are asleep or very sedate are at risk, and in the healthy parturient, that risk is still very low. There are as yet no studies that compare either the efficacy or the cost of dealing with this low risk through the use of naloxone infusions as opposed to electronic monitors (capnography, pulse oximetry, impedance respiratory monitors) or frequent nursing assessment.

FETAL MONITORING

Fetal monitoring consists of assessments of fetal well-being and developmental progress. This process begins in early pregnancy and continues until delivery.

FETAL CARDIOVASCULAR PHYSIOLOGY

An understanding of fetal cardiovascular physiology is important in the interpretation and evaluation of fetal heart rate patterns, the cornerstone of the assessment of fetal well-being.

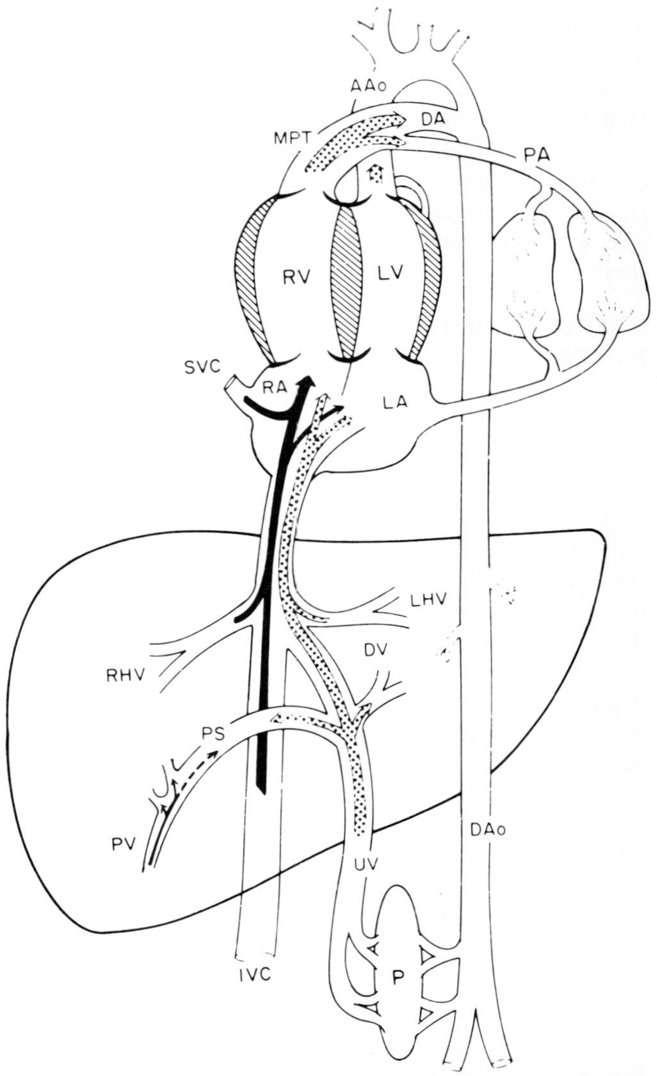

Figure 18–32. The fetal circulation. Dark arrows indicate deoxygenated blood; stippled arrows, deoxygenated blood. P = placenta, UV = umbilical vein, IVC = inferior vena cava, DV = ductus venosus, RHV = right hepatic vein, LHV = left hepatic vein, PV = portal vein, PS = portal sinus, RA = right atrium, LA = left atrium, SVC = superior vena cava, RV = right ventricle, LV = left ventricle, MPT = main pulmonary trunk, DA = ductus arteriosus, AAo = ascending aorta, PA = pulmonary artery, DAo = descending aorta. (From Heymann MA: Biophysical evaluation of fetal status. *In* Creasy R, Resnik R [eds]: Maternal-Fetal Medicine. Philadelphia: WB Saunders, 1984; 260.)

Fetal Circulation

Oxygenated blood from the placenta has a normal oxygen tension of about 30 mmHg. However, owing to the presence of fetal hemoglobin, this represents a saturation of 80%. The saturated blood is carried by the umbilical vein (Fig. 18–32). A portion goes to the liver, but the majority bypasses the liver by traversing the ductus venosus and empties into the inferior vena cava. Streaming occurs, so that much of the oxygenated blood from the placenta is directed across the foramen ovale into the left atrium and, subsequently, the left ventricle. This oxygenated blood is then preferentially supplied to the brain and myocardium. Desaturated blood from the head and upper body returns via the superior vena cava and is directed into the right ventricle, where it mixes with saturated blood from the placenta. Because of the high pulmonary vascular resistance, most of the right ventricular output crosses the ductus arteriosus and enters the descending aorta. A portion of this blood then goes to the placenta via the umbilical arteries to be reoxygenated. The normal oxygen tension of this desaturated umbilical artery blood is 20 mmHg, with a saturation of approximately 55%.

Fetal Hypoxic Response

The response of the fetus to hypoxia consists of a redistribution of blood flow to essential organs, decreased oxygen consumption, and anaerobic glycolysis. The favored organs are the brain, heart, placenta, and adrenal glands. Blood flow to the adrenal gland increases markedly during periods of asphyxia, a response necessary to sustain the tenfold increase in plasma norepinephrine that occurs during periods of hypoxia. The redistribution of blood flow is accomplished by vasoconstriction of certain vascular beds and alterations in downstream impedance. Increased impedance in the descending aorta favors blood flow to the cerebral and coronary circulation (Fig. 18–32).

With hypoxia, heart rate decreases because of increased vagal stimulation, and overall oxygen consumption decreases. Fetal pH decreases owing to a metabolic acidosis caused by lactic acid production in vascular beds receiving inadequate oxygen for aerobic metabolism. Asphyxia with a marked decrease in placental flow impairs carbon dioxide exchange and contributes a respiratory component to the acidosis.

The assessment of fetal well-being, both before and during birth, consists primarily of methods to infer the absence of asphyxia by documenting the absence of features of the fetal hypoxic response—heart rate slowing, acidosis, and alterations in patterns of fetal blood flow.

ANTENATAL MONITORING

Antenatal monitoring consists of efforts to assess fetal well-being and developmental progress. There are simple as well as highly complex technologies associated with such monitoring. For example, manual estimation of uterine size (fundal height) is performed sequentially to infer fetal growth and development. However, ultrasonography is the most sophisticated modality for the assessment of fetal development. During the third trimester, the most important aspect of fetal development becomes the maturation of the lungs, because lung immaturity is the primary determinant of infant morbidity and mortality following premature delivery. In preterm fetuses, pulmonary maturity is inferred by the evidence of sufficient lung surfactant production.

Fetal well-being is inferred primarily by documenting the absence of changes that suggest a hypoxic response. The technologies associated with this documentation range from simple auscultation of fetal heart tones to measurement of blood flow velocity in the middle cerebral artery of the fetus using pulsed Doppler ultrasonography.

Fetal well-being and fetal maturity are not the same thing. A fetus can be mature and not well or very immature and quite well as long as it continues an intrauterine existence. Certain high-risk fetuses warrant assessment of well-being before the onset of labor. The most frequent pregnancies so monitored are those complicated by hypertension, diabetes, or a growth-retarded fetus. How early in pregnancy monitoring should be initiated depends on how soon one is willing to intervene if a distressed fetus is detected. The 26th week of gestation is usually the earliest time for this type of assessment.

Ultrasound in Fetal Assessment

Technical Terminology

Ultrasound refers to sound waves whose frequency exceeds 20,000 Hz. Diagnostic ultrasound involves the application of electrical current to a crystal in order to produce vibrations, thus emitting ultrasonic waves that are reflected off target tissues and returned to the crystal to be converted back to electrical energy. The timing and the intensity of the returning echo allow the electrical signals to be displayed on a 2D cathode ray tube, with time (distance) on one axis and intensity on the other. In modern obstetric ultrasonography, the electrical signal is converted to a spot on the oscilloscope, and the brightness of the spot varies with the intensity of the signal. This display is referred to as B-mode or brightness-mode. Real-time imaging displays the echoes so rapidly that it is possible to visualize target motion. Thus, real-time B-mode ultrasound imaging allows a dynamic view of the fetus, permitting both structural and functional evaluations.

In addition to structural imaging, Doppler ultrasound technology is also employed to evaluate the hemodynamics of various vascular regions in the fetus and the uteroplacental circulation. Both pulsed-wave and continuous-wave Doppler ultrasound have been used and produce similar results for most of the clinically useful parameters.[140] Continuous-wave Doppler is less expensive and uses a lower energy output. Color Doppler imaging easily identifies reversal of blood flow. Duplex systems that combine B-mode and pulsed-wave Doppler may provide the greatest degree of sensitivity, because this technology allows precise and specific vessel imaging prior to measurement of flow. The importance of this is that different results may be obtained from different sites in the same vascular structure. For example, assessment of vascular resistance in the umbilical arteries was higher at a site near the abdominal wall of the fetus than it was at a site near the placental insertion.[141] At this time, the cost/benefit ratio associated with the use of more sophisticated imaging technology to improve specificity and thus avoid the identification of fetal distress when in fact none exists remains to be established.

Uses of Ultrasound: Imaging

Ultrasonic imaging can document an intrauterine pregnancy as early as 3 weeks after impregnation (see Fig. 18–10). It is also valuable for estimating gestational age by measuring such features as gestational sac volume as early as 4 weeks, crown-rump length at 5 weeks, and biparietal diameter at 12 weeks.[142] Accurate estimation of gestational age is important in determining fetal maturity and reducing the incidence of respiratory distress syndrome of prematurity following elective cesarean section. Fetal growth can be documented using ultrasound, and the finding of intrauterine growth retardation may, in cases in which the cause is uteroplacental insufficiency, require an early delivery. Ultrasound imaging is used to determine fetal position, such as breech presentation.

Ultrasonographic measurement of amniotic fluid volume allows the identification of pregnancies with disorders of either too much fluid (polyhydramnios) or too little fluid (oligohydramnios). Volume replacement in cases of oligohydramnios decreases the risk of umbilical cord compromise during labor and delivery.

Ultrasound permits detection of a wide range of congenital disorders, both structural and functional, with a high degree of precision (Fig. 18–33). In some cases, early detection permits beneficial therapy. Fetal supraventricular tachycardia can be treated with maternal beta blockade, possibly avoiding fetal heart failure. A new area of fetal medicine emerged after the performance by Harrison and associates of bilateral ureterostomies in a 21-week-old fetus.[143] Subsequently, numerous surgical procedures have been performed on fetuses to correct lesions that, if left untreated, would cause further damage to the newborn.[144] An example is hydrocephalus due to aqueductal stenosis. Insertion of a ventriculoamniotic shunt *in utero* prevents the development of hydrocephalus in some fetuses. In other cases, ultrasound reveals lethal anomalies, such as anencephaly, and prevents unnecessary maternal surgery and morbidity.

Elevated maternal alpha-fetoprotein levels suggest neural tube or abdominal wall defects in the fetus and placental abnormalities in the mother. High maternal levels can result either from very high fetal levels or normal fetal levels with mixing of maternal and fetal blood. The latter can result from placental hemorrhage and infarctions, as well as abnormally adherent placentas (accreta, percreta, and increta).[145] Ultrasonography is essential in the evaluation of abnormally high maternal alpha-fetoprotein; correct diagnosis allows for appropriate peripartum management of both mother and infant.

Ultrasonography is routinely used to determine the sex of the fetus as early as 16–22 weeks of gestation. It is also used to document fetal death.

Uses of Ultrasound: Doppler Flow Velocimetry

Combination real-time and Doppler ultrasonography has recently enabled noninvasive hemodynamic studies of the fetus and its supporting circulation. Doppler flow velocimetry is now used to evaluate blood velocity waveforms in the pulsatile fetal and uteroplacental vessels and appears to be a powerful new tool in the identification of fetal distress in pregnancy.[146]

One specific application of Doppler velocimetry involves computation of the ratio of systolic to diastolic (S/D) flows in specific vessels. As downstream resistance to flow increases, diastolic flow is disproportionally impeded, and the S/D ratio increases. This ratio is an indirect but reproducible estimate of vascular resistance. These techniques are less reliable prior to 26 weeks of gestation and display a wide standard deviation.[147]

Use of ratios rather than values for absolute flow permits assessments that are independent of the angle of incidence of the ultrasound beam. The S/D ratio is also identified as

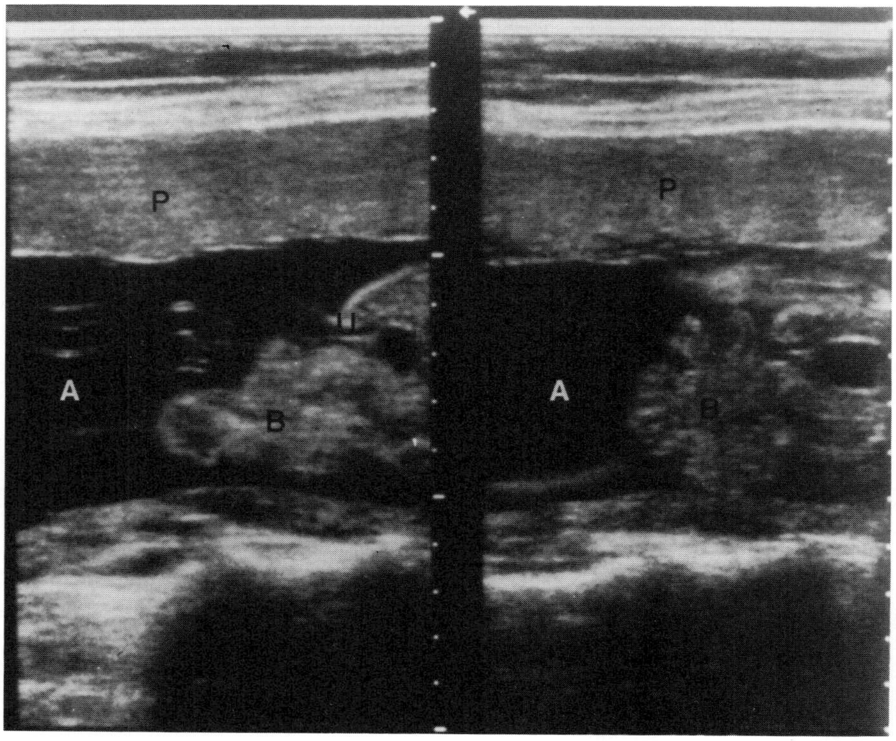

Figure 18–33. Ultrasonographic visualization of a fetus with gastroschisis, two views. The lesion is distinguished from omphalocele by the fact that the bowel (B) can be seen extruding from the abdomen along the umbilical cord (UC) in the view on the left. This distinction is significant, because omphalocele is associated with a high rate of associated anomalies, whereas gastroschisis tends to be an isolated lesion. A = amniotic cavity, P = placenta.

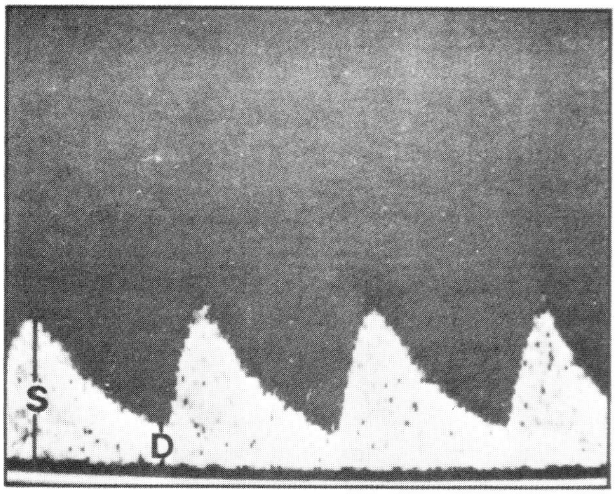

Figure 18–34. Flow velocity waveform from the fetal umbilical artery. The A/B ratio compares the peak systolic (S) flow velocity to the end-diastolic (D) velocity. (From Fleischer A, Anyaegbunam AA, Schulman H, et al: Uterine and umbilical artery velocimetry during normal labor. Am J Obstet Gynecol 1987; 157:41.)

the A/B ratio and compares the peak systolic flow to the end-diastolic flow (Fig. 18–34). The resistance index (RI) is computed as the peak systolic minus the end-diastolic frequencies divided by the peak systolic frequency. The pulsatility index (PI) is computed by subtracting the nadir, or the negative peak, of the diastolic frequencies from the peak systolic frequencies and dividing this value by the mean maximum frequency over one cardiac cycle (Fig. 18–35).

Uterine Artery Doppler Velocimetry. After the 26th week of gestation, a uterine artery S/D ratio > 2.6 is highly suggestive of increased resistance to uterine artery blood flow and correlates with increased maternal and fetal morbidity (Figs. 18–36 and 18–37). Fleischer and coworkers have documented the power of uterine S/D ratios to identify the at-risk fetus in hypertensive pregnancies; infants born

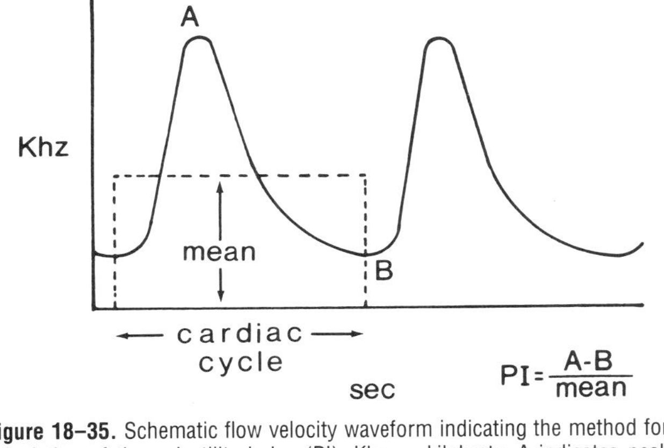

Figure 18–35. Schematic flow velocity waveform indicating the method for calculation of the pulsatility index (PI). Khz = kilohertz, A indicates peak systolic frequency, B indicates lowest diastolic frequency. (From McCowan LM, Mullen MB, Ritchie K: Umbilical artery flow velocity waveforms and the placental vascular bed. Am J Obstet Gynecol 1987; 157:901.)

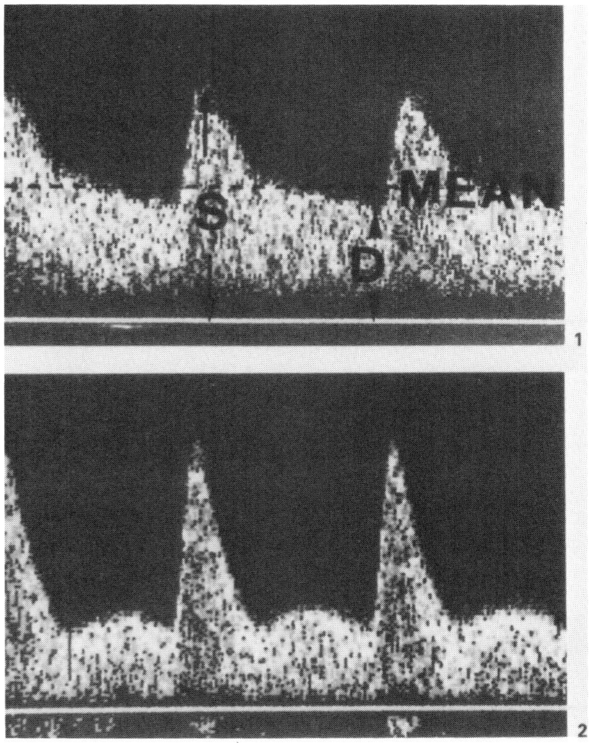

Figure 18–36. *1,* Normal uteroplacental flow velocity waveform, with peak systolic (S) and end-diastolic (D) frequencies marked. *2,* Abnormal uteroplacental flow velocity waveform characterized by decreased end-diastolic velocity as well as diastolic notching at the beginning of diastolic flow. (From Grab D, Hutter W, Sterzik K, Terinde R: Reference values for resistance index and pulsatility index of uteroplacental Doppler flow velocity waveforms based on 612 uneventful pregnancies. Gynecol Obstet Invest 1992; 34:83. With permission from S. Karger AG, Basel.)

to hypertensive mothers with S/D ratios > 2.6 were delivered 5 weeks earlier and weighed 1125 gm less than infants born to hypertensive mothers with S/D ratios < 2.6.[148] The 17 stillbirths in the study all occurred in mothers with abnormal uterine S/D ratios. In spite of the dramatic differences in fetal outcomes, the difference in mean blood pressure between the two groups (mothers with high vs. mothers with normal S/D ratios) was 5 mmHg and not statistically or clinically significant. Because Doppler flow velocimetry estimates vascular resistance, it has been shown to be a more powerful tool for predicting the outcome of pregnancy than is blood pressure.[149, 150]

Not only is the S/D ratio significant, but, as it reflects the mean of both uterine arteries, divergent ratios between the two sides are also significant. A difference of greater than one between the left and right uterine artery S/D ratios is associated with an increased risk for growth retardation, preeclampsia, and premature delivery. This divergence most likely reflects placental laterality, a factor shown to have an adverse outcome on pregnancy.[36]

Umbilical Doppler Velocimetry. In the umbilical circulation, both the arterial and the venous flow can be studied. The umbilical arteries carry desaturated blood from the fetal descending aorta to the placenta. Umbilical artery S/D ra-

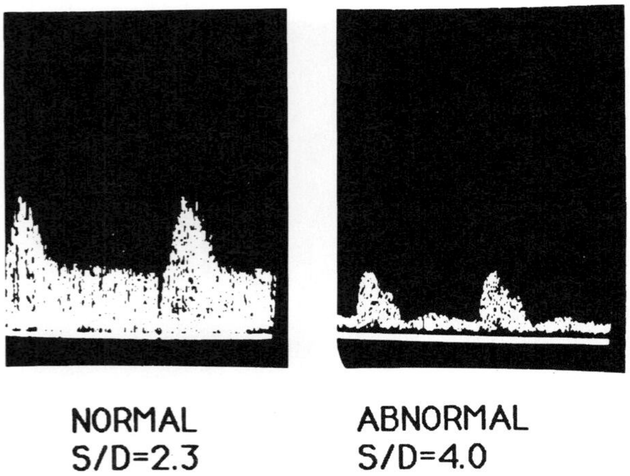

Figure 18–37. *Left,* Normal uterine artery flow velocity waveform with systolic/diastolic (S/D) ratio < 2.6. *Right,* Abnormal uterine artery flow velocity waveform with systolic/diastolic (S/D) ratio = 4.0. There is markedly decreased velocity (notching) at the beginning of diastole as well as at end-diastole. (From Ducey J, Schulman H, Farmakides G, et al: A classification of hypertension in pregnancy based on Doppler velocimetry. Am J Obstet Gynecol 1987; 157:682.)

tios are calculated as for the uterine circulation; however, the cutoff value for term infants is a ratio of 3, whereas for preterm infants 3.5 is a more appropriate value (Fig. 18–38).

Systolic/Diastolic Ratio Patterns. Because the uterine and umbilical vasculatures develop independently, there are four different patterns of umbilical and uterine S/D ratios that may arise: uterine > 2.6 and umbilical > 3 (both abnormal); uterine > 2.6 and umbilical normal; uterine normal and umbilical > 3; and uterine and umbilical both normal.

In the surveillance of *hypertensive* pregnancies, those with normal S/D ratios in uterine and umbilical circulations (50% of patients) have pregnancy outcomes that are similar to outcomes for normotensive patients. Thus, once this pattern is documented at the beginning of the third trimester, additional monitoring need only be maternal blood pressure and routine assessment of fetal well-being, as in normal pregnancy, with velocimetry repeated once at 32–34 weeks.[142]

When the fetal umbilical circulation is abnormal and the maternal uterine circulation is normal, the usual consequence is fetal growth retardation. Even if the mother is normotensive, 70% of infants will be SGA if the umbilical S/D ratio is abnormally high. Conversely, despite the presence of maternal hypertension, if the umbilical flow velocity waveforms are normal, only 3% of infants will be SGA. The circumstance of an abnormal umbilical circulation coupled with a normal uterine circulation is usually caused by a decrease in the number of small muscular arteries in the placenta and probably represents a failure of angiogenesis.

The value of Doppler velocimetry in evaluation of the SGA fetus is illustrated in a study by Hitschold and colleagues.[151] The placentas from SGA fetuses with umbilical S/D ratios < 3 had no evidence of placental insufficiency; perfusion and diffusion capacities and placental/fetal weight ratios were not different from those in AGA babies. However, SGA babies with S/D ratios > 3 were markedly smaller than SGA fetuses with normal flow velocimetry, and there was a reduction in vascularization in the terminal villi and impaired diffusion conditions in the placentas of these infants. Thus, Doppler flow velocimetry is able to distinguish fetuses who are genetically small from those who are small because of placental insufficiency. This distinction is important, because, in the Hitschold et al study, all SGA infants with abnormal S/D ratios required cesarean delivery because of additional evidence of fetal distress, whereas the SGA fetuses with S/D ratios < 3 were all delivered vaginally following spontaneous labor.

The pattern of abnormal uterine S/D ratios and a normal umbilical flow pattern occurs in only 10% of hypertensive patients and is not associated with severe fetal growth retardation or an increased risk of fetal distress during labor. However, the mothers may be symptomatic with headaches, hypertension, and decreased urine output, which often prompts premature delivery of the baby.

The 20% of hypertensive pregnancies with both abnormal uterine and umbilical circulations are associated with the highest degrees of maternal and fetal morbidity and warrant the most intense surveillance. Fetal growth retardation is the most severe for this group (50% of normal), because the increased resistance to uterine blood flow is compounded by increased resistance to fetal blood flow through the placenta and represents true uteroplacental insufficiency. Fetuses under such conditions will most likely display signs of distress (late heart rate decelerations, absent Doppler end-diastolic flow, and umbilical venous pulsations) during the intrapartum period.[152] Appearance of these distress patterns during the antepartum period is particularly ominous.

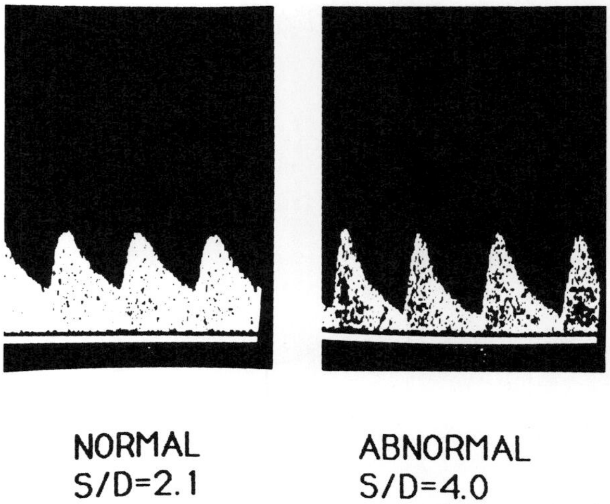

Figure 18–38. *Left,* Normal umbilical artery flow velocity waveform with systolic/diastolic (S/D) ratio < 3.0. *Right,* Abnormal umbilical artery flow velocity waveform with systolic/diastolic (S/D) ratio = 4.0. (From Ducey J, Schulman H, Farmakides G, et al: A classification of hypertension in pregnancy based on Doppler velocimetry. Am J Obstet Gynecol 1987; 157:682.)

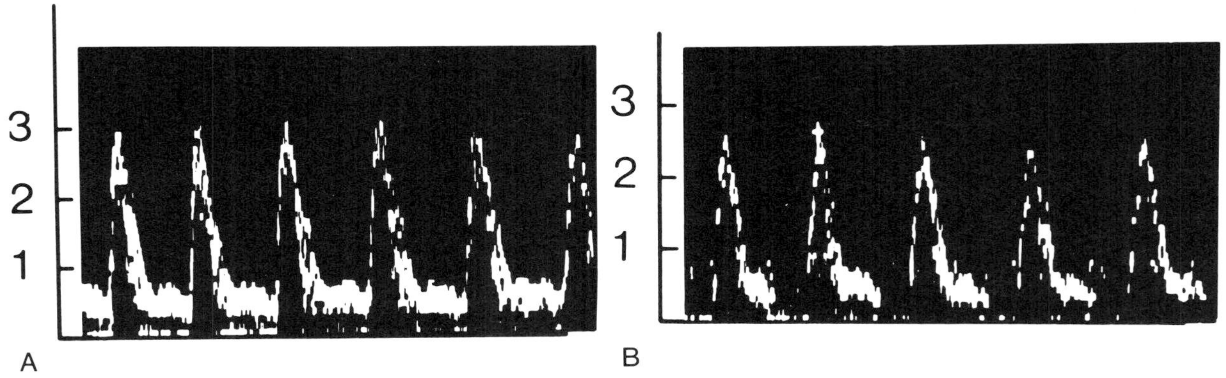

Figure 18–39. *A,* Normal flow velocity waveform from the descending aorta of a fetus at 39 weeks' gestation. Scale is in kilohertz. *B,* Flow velocity waveform from the descending aorta of a fetus in distress with absent end-diastolic frequencies. (From Jouppila P, Kirkinen P: Blood velocity waveforms of the fetal aorta in normal and hypertensive pregnancies. Obstet Gynecol 1986; 67:857–858.)

Absent or Reversed Umbilical Artery Diastolic Flow. Absent or reversed diastolic flow in the fetal aorta or umbilical artery is a velocimetry pattern that is highly suggestive of fetal asphyxia, particularly with a high-risk pregnancy (Fig. 18–39). In a study of 37 pregnancies in which there was no end-diastolic flow in the umbilical arteries, the fetal death rate was 38%.[153] Fairlie and colleagues, in a study of patients with pregnancy-induced hypertension, reported that absent end-diastolic frequencies in the fetal umbilical artery that presented *before* 30 weeks of gestation were associated with a perinatal death rate of 62%, whereas the same pattern presenting *after* 30 weeks had a mortality of only 14%.[149] The difference reflects the increased severity of preeclampsia presenting early in gestation.

The explanation for the loss of the diastolic waveform is very high placental resistance, impaired fetal myocardial function, or both. The phenomenon of absent flow usually precedes the onset of abnormal fetal heart rate patterns in cases of asphyxia; the interval from the occurrence of absent diastolic flow to the occurrence of abnormal fetal heart rate ranges from 1 day to several weeks. Thus, this ominous finding requires intensive monitoring.

Umbilical Vein Pulsations. The normal Doppler flow pattern obtained from the umbilical vein is seen in Figure 18–40, along with umbilical arterial and venous waveforms. Pulsations in the umbilical vein are often associated with absent end-diastolic velocities in the umbilical arteries. In one study of 21 fetuses with absent end-diastolic velocities, 11 had venous pulsations, and 10 did not[154]; 6 of the 11 with pulsations died (55% mortality rate), whereas all but 1 of the 10 without pulsations survived (10% mortality rate). In another study of fetuses with absent end-diastolic velocities in the umbilical arteries, 10 of 16 (62.5%) with pulsations in the umbilical vein died, compared with 4 deaths in a group of 21 fetuses (19%) without venous pulsations.[153] It thus appears that pregnancies complicated by absent end-diastolic velocities can be further subdivided on the basis of the presence or absence of venous pulsations in the

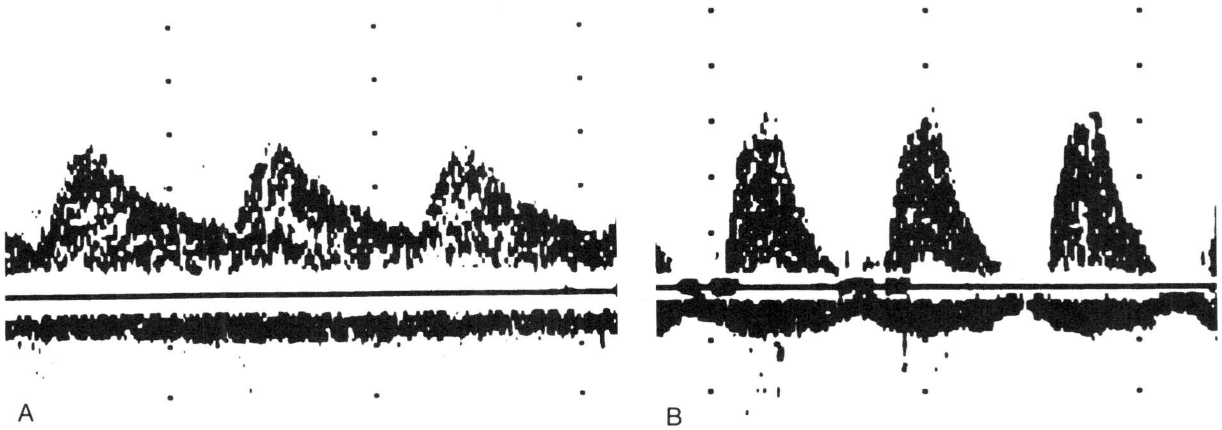

Figure 18–40. *A,* Umbilical arterial and venous Doppler flow velocity waveform in a normal fetus. The venous velocities have no variation with the cardiac cycle. *B,* Abnormal flow velocity waveform from the umbilical artery and vein of a fetus with absent diastolic umbilical arterial blood flow and pulsations in the umbilical venous flow tracing. (From Reed KL, Anderson CF, Shenker L: Changes in intracardiac Doppler blood flow velocities in fetuses with absent umbilical artery diastolic flow. Am J Obstet Gynecol 1987; 157:775.)

umbilical vein, with the presence of pulsations carrying an ominous prognosis.

The venous pulsations are due to large increases in the amount of reverse blood flow from the right atrium into the inferior vena cava, with the waveform being reflected back into the umbilical vein. Venous pulsations are invariably present when there are extremes of fetal heart rate. Rates > 180 beats/minute increase end-diastolic pressure in the ventricles because of either insufficient ejection time or inadequate time during diastole for coronary perfusion with resultant ischemia and decreased compliance. When the right atrium contracts and the ventricular pressure is increased, a portion of the blood will be pumped into the vena cava as it follows the path of least resistance. Venous pulsations also occur with heart rates < 120 beats/minute, and the end-diastolic timing is the same as during tachycardia except in cases of complete heart block (Fig. 18–41). The explanation for venous pulsations with slow heart rates is that maximal ventricular filling occurs during the lengthened diastole, and the atrial contraction ejects a portion of blood in a retrograde direction rather than forward into the already full ventricle. During complete heart block, atrial contractions occur independently of ventricular volume changes, and those occurring during ventricular systole will tend to eject blood in a retrograde direction or across the foramen ovale. In the study by Indik and colleagues, all infants with venous pulsations due to extremes of heart rate survived.[154]

In the presence of a normal heart rate and in the absence of fetal breathing movements, which affect intrathoracic pressures, reversal of flow is primarily due to decreased ventricular compliance secondary to ischemia. The vena cava becomes a lower-resistance circuit than the path of forward flow through the ventricle. Retrograde flow decreases the volume of potentially oxygenated blood reaching the coronary arteries, further compromising myocardial blood flow and exacerbating the ischemia and decreased

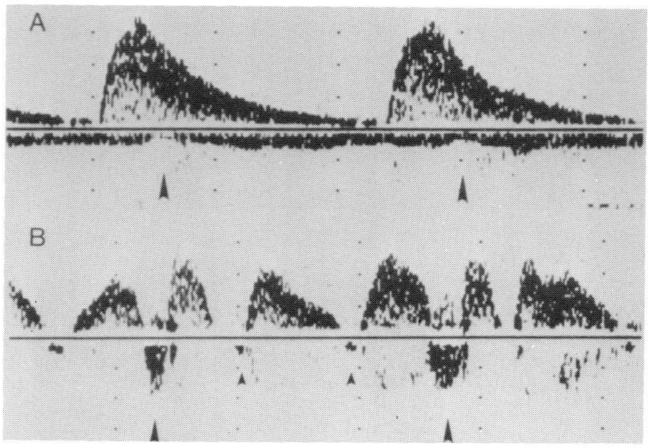

Figure 18–41. *A*, Umbilical arterial and venous flow velocity waveform from a fetus with complete heart block. Atrial contractions (arrowheads) result in venous pulsations when they occur in midsystole. *B*, Inferior vena cava flow velocity waveform in the same fetus. Venous pulsations are associated with reversal of flow in the inferior vena cava. (From Indik JH, Chen V, Reed KL: Association of umbilical venous with inferior vena cava blood flow velocities. Obstet Gynecol 1991; 77:554.)

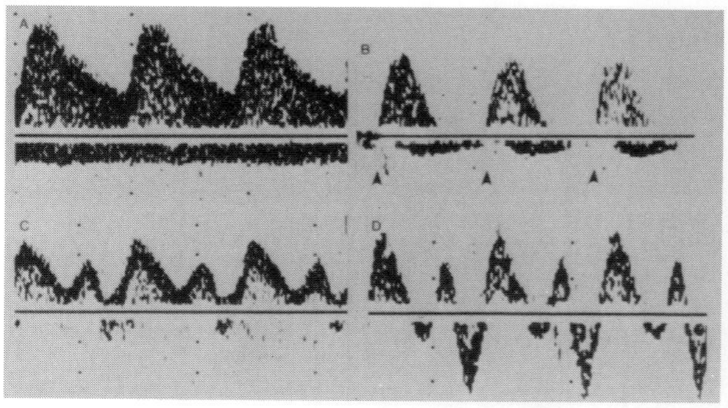

Figure 18–42. *A*, Umbilical arterial and venous flow velocity waveform in a normal 38-week fetus. *B*, Umbilical arterial and venous flow velocity waveform in a 34-week fetus with absent diastolic velocities and venous pulsations. *C*, Inferior vena cava flow velocity waveform from the normal fetus in *A*. *D*, Inferior vena cava flow velocity waveform from the fetus in *B*. There is reversal of flow during atrial contraction (arrowheads in *B*). (From Indik JH, Chen V, Reed KL: Association of umbilical venous with inferior vena cava blood flow velocities. Obstet Gynecol 1991; 77:552.)

compliance. Thus, it appears that the pattern of absent end-diastolic velocities in the umbilical arteries coupled with venous pulsations in the umbilical vein that are not due to irregularities of heart rate or fetal breathing movements carry an extremely high mortality rate. Once detected, such a pattern demands intense efforts to improve fetal oxygenation or deliver the fetus, if it is at a viable gestational age.

Inferior Vena Cava Waveforms. Pulsed Doppler studies of inferior vena cava flow in the fetus may provide even more sensitive information regarding myocardial function than umbilical artery studies. The ratio of systolic and diastolic peak flow velocities for vena caval flow can be measured just as for other vascular beds, and reverse flow can also be estimated (Fig. 18–42). Rizzo and associates found evidence of decreased cardiac function (increased S/D ratios, increased percentage of reverse flow) on the basis of vena cava waveforms in fetuses in which there were no significant abnormalities seen in umbilical artery waveforms, and the subsequent clinical course was consistent with uteroplacental insufficiency.[155] Likewise, Indik and colleagues found a high association between venous pulsations in the fetal umbilical vein and abnormal flow velocities in the inferior vena cava, a result that is not surprising, because the two vascular beds are closely linked in series.[154]

Cerebral Waveforms. The PI of the cerebral waveforms has been found to be a strong predictor of subsequent neonatal neurologic abnormalities.[156] Such information may have great relevance in cases of cerebral palsy, in which intrapartum events are often blamed for neurologic injury in spite of evidence that intrauterine events are much more significant.[157, 158] When the ratio of PIs in the umbilical artery relative to the middle cerebral artery in the fetus is abnormally high, it indicates a "brain sparing" state in which the vascular resistance in the umbilical vessels is increased while the vascular resistance in the brain is decreased. This is the opposite of the findings in other vascular beds during periods of hypoxemia (Fig. 18–43). Such findings may be present at the end of the second trimester and warrant Doppler monitoring several times per week to detect evidence of further deterioration in fetal well-being.

Cerebral blood flow increases linearly with decreases in the arterial oxygen tension of umbilical venous blood. Fetal hypoxia is associated with a decreased PI in the internal carotid artery (due to cerebral vasodilatation or loss of cerebral autoregulation); simultaneous increases in the PIs in the umbilical arteries and the descending aorta are caused by increases in vascular resistance in these circulations.[159–161] Thus, evaluation of cerebral vascular resistance appears to provide additional information to answer the question: is this fetus at risk for asphyxia? A decreased PI results when cerebral oxygenation is impaired, and this finding places the fetus at increased risk.[162] In the face of continuing and severe hypoxemia, the cerebral PI may subsequently increase because of cerebral edema.[163]

Amniocentesis

Amniocentesis performed early in the second trimester allows the antenatal determination of the cytogenetic constitution of the fetus, the diagnosis of inborn errors of metabolism, and the detection of neural tube and abdominal wall defects (identified by elevated alpha-fetoprotein levels in the amniotic fluid). In late pregnancy, amniocentesis is used to assess the severity of Rh-isoimmunization, estimate fetal lung maturity, and decompress polyhydramnios.

If amniocentesis is necessary, ultrasound is required to locate fluid for aspiration and to avoid the placenta, the umbilical cord, and the fetus. Fetal death from exsanguination has occurred following undetected injury to the umbilical vessels during amniocentesis. Nevertheless, the role of fetal heart rate monitoring following amniocentesis to detect evidence of fetal distress is controversial.

Antepartum Fetal Heart Rate Monitoring

The fetal heart rate may be monitored as early as 4–5 weeks following conception using ultrasound. Subsequently, auscultation over the maternal abdomen may detect gross abnormalities of rate, such as tachycardia and bradycardia. However, electronic monitoring is necessary to detect the presence or absence of more subtle rate changes that may indicate the state of fetal well-being. For this purpose, electronic ECG from the abdominal wall is more accurate than Doppler ultrasound devices.

Nonstress Test

The nonstress test (NST) monitors fetal heart rate variability and accelerations with fetal movement over a 20-minute period. The fetal heart rate is monitored using ultrasound. If the long-term baseline variability (irregular sine waves with cycles of 3–6/minute) is at least 10 beats/minutes and the heart rate acceleration is at least 15 beats/minute with fetal movement, and there are at least two episodes of fetal movement, the test result is considered *reactive.* A reactive test result correlates highly with fetal well-being. If there is no fetal movement or no acceleration of fetal heart rate with movement over the 20-minute test period, the result is classified as *nonreactive.* Long-term variability is usually minimal or absent. A nonreactive test result is associated with a poor neonatal outcome or a depressed newborn in approximately 20% of cases. The result is classified as *uncertain reactivity* when there are less than two fetal movements in the test period, accelerations with movement are less than 15 beats/minute, or long-term variability amplitude is less than 10 beats/minute. In the area of fetal monitoring, ''reactive'' thus indicates both normal variability and accelerations with movement, whereas ''nonreactivity'' indicates the absence of these

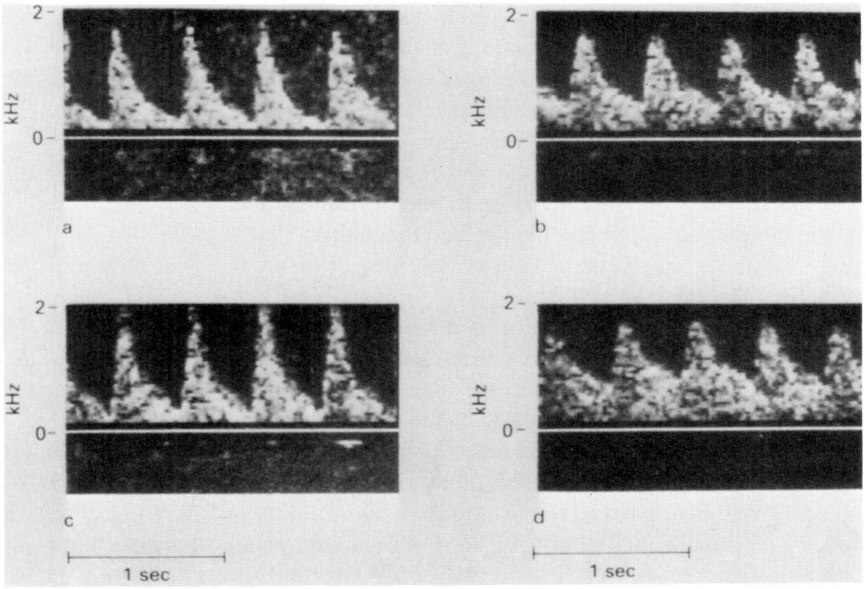

Figure 18–43. Internal carotid artery blood flow velocity waveforms. *a* and *c* are from a normal fetus at 27 and 37 weeks' gestation; *b* is from a growth-retarded fetus at 27 weeks, and *d* is from the same fetus at 37 weeks. The increase in diastolic flow is abnormal, and is due to decreased cerebral vascular resistance and possible loss of autoregulation. (From Wladimiroff JW, Tonge HM, Stewart PA: Doppler ultrasound assessment of cerebral blood flow in the human fetus. Br J Obstet Gynecol 1986; 93:471–475.)

changes. A nonreactive result does not necessarily indicate a depressed fetus but does require further evaluation, which most commonly takes the form of an oxytocin challenge test.

Oxytocin Challenge Test

An oxytocin challenge test (OCT) evaluates the fetal heart rate pattern in response to uterine contractions induced by oxytocin. Ultrasonography is used to record the heart rate. The appearance of abnormal heart rate slowing (late decelerations) with contractions indicates a ''positive'' result. A nonreactive (absent variability and accelerations), positive (late decelerations) contraction stress test result indicates a distressed fetus and demands immediate intervention to either reverse the maternal condition causing the distress or to deliver the fetus if the gestational age is greater than 30 weeks.[164]

Accuracy of Antepartum Heart Rate Observations

Tests such as the nonstress test that rely on human observation and ultrasound detection of the fetal heart rate have been shown to be notoriously inaccurate.[165, 166] There is poor interobserver and intraobserver agreement in the detection of heart rate accelerations and decelerations as well as in the determination of the clinical significance of patterns. One study of five expert observers found that 92% of fetal heart rate decelerations went undetected when compared to computer analysis of the same tracings.[167] The new generation of antenatal fetal monitors that incorporate wide-range ultrasound transducers and autocorrelation, while greatly reducing signal loss, detect a considerable incidence of erroneous decelerations and accelerations. Autocorrelation is a method of processing ultrasound signals from the fetal heart rate to derive the best estimate of pulse interval. Dawes and associates found a 20% incidence of erroneous decelerations in fetuses of less than 30 weeks of gestational age; the frequency of erroneous accelerations was 11%.[168] The errors typically involved abrupt changes in the heart rate and were felt to be due to fetal events (movement, hiccups) that inject impulses at frequencies close to those generated by the fetal heart. Other errors may arise when there is transient detection of the maternal rather than the fetal pulse. The faults did not depend on the manufacturer of the monitor and were readily detected by computer analysis of the tracings. Once so identified, most errors were visually identifiable by skilled readers.

Computerized analysis eliminates reader variability and monitor artifact in antepartum heart rate analysis and facilitates longitudinal comparisons in the same fetus. It remains to be proven whether computer-facilitated heart rate analysis will improve perinatal outcomes. Current methodology is associated with a degree of intraobserver and interobserver variability that calls into question the validity of specific test results as well as the results of outcome studies based on such data.

Assessment of Fetal Maturity

Prematurity is still the most significant cause of perinatal morbidity and mortality. Fetal maturity in present perinatal practice is synonymous with pulmonary maturity, the rate-limiting step in the process that allows the fetus to become independent of the placenta. Because of variability in the timing of lung maturation relative to gestational age, specific markers for lung maturity have been sought. The most reliable tests at present assess surfactant production in the fetal lung.

A major limitation of all tests of fetal lung maturity is that although they are quite sensitive in identifying fetuses who will develop respiratory distress syndrome of prematurity (RDS), they are much less specific in identifying fetuses who will not, if delivered at the time of the test, develop RDS. Thus, in a high-risk pregnancy in which it is deemed necessary to deliver the fetus as soon as the lungs are mature, tests of lower specificity will unnecessarily delay some cases.

Lecithin/Sphingomyelin Ratio

Until recently, the standard method for assessing lung maturity was the lecithin/sphingomyelin ratio. This test compares the concentrations of two phospholipids, lecithin and sphingomyelin, in amniotic fluid obtained by amniocentesis. Before 34 weeks of gestation, both substances are present in approximately equal amounts. After 34 weeks, the amount of lecithin increases, and the amount of sphingomyelin decreases (Fig. 18–44). A lecithin/sphingomyelin ratio of 2:1 indicates lung maturity. However, a recent study found that 20% of infants developed RDS in spite of a ratio > 2.[169]

Phosphatidylglycerol

One possible reason that a significant number of fetuses with lecithin/sphingomyelin ratios greater than 2:1 develop RDS if delivered at that point is a lack of phosphatidylglycerol. This compound appears to stabilize lecithin in surfactant. Phosphatidylglycerol measurements of 3% or greater in the amniotic fluid indicate functional lung maturity. Phosphatidylglycerol is not present in blood, vaginal secretions, or meconium, so these contaminants do not confuse the interpretation as they do in all surfactant tests.

Foam Stability Index

This semiquantitative test, a commercial modification of the ''shake'' test, is based on the ability of pulmonary surfactant to generate stable foam in the presence of ethanol, an inhibitor of foaming. Serial tube dilutions of amniotic fluid and ethanol are shaken for 15 seconds and then, after 15 minutes, observed for the presence of stable foam. A complete ring of bubbles in the meniscus constitutes a positive result. Results are reported in terms of the volume fraction of ethanol, and the foam stability index value is the highest ethanol volume fraction (volume of ethanol/volume of ethanol + volume of amniotic fluid) that

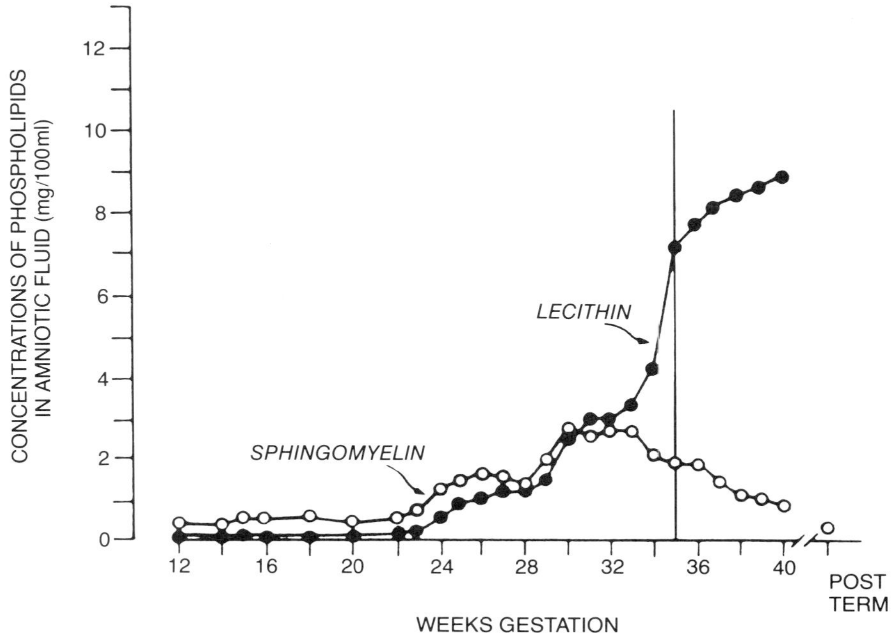

Figure 18–44. Changes in concentrations of lecithin and sphingomyelin in amniotic fluid over the course of normal pregnancy. (From Gluck L, Kulovich MV: Lecithin/sphingomyelin ratios in normal and abnormal pregnancy. Am J Obstet Gynecol 1973; 115:541.)

will allow foam to persist. Thus, a foam stability index of 47 indicates that when 0.45 ml of ethanol was added to 0.5 ml of centrifuged amniotic fluid and shaken, there was a continuous ring of bubbles around the meniscus, but when 0.46 ml of ethanol was added, the meniscal ring was discontinuous.

Fluorescent Polarization Techniques

Two current tests utilize fluorescent dyes, synthetic derivatives of lecithin, which have binding and solubility characteristics similar to those of surfactant-associated phospholipids. One such dye is NBD-phosphatidylcholine (NBD-PC), and the other is PC16; the latter is used in an automated kit marketed as the TDx Fetal Lung Maturity (FLM) assay (Abbott Laboratories, Abbott Park, IL). The fluorescent dye distinguishes between albumin and phospholipid in amniotic fluid samples, and the degree of partitioning can be measured using a standard TDx fluorescent polarimeter, available in virtually all laboratories. The polarization measured by the analyzer reflects the ratio of surfactant to albumin in the amniotic fluid sample, and this value correlates with lung maturity.

There is still no accepted value for the surfactant/albumin ratio determined by fluorescence polarization. In one large study in which the cutoff was 50 mg/gm (milligrams of surfactant per gram of albumin), the sensitivity was 96% and the specificity was 88%; 24 of 312 newborns developed RDS with surfactant/albumin ratios of 50 mg/gm or greater.[170] If a higher cutoff is used, such as the 70 mg/gm recommended by the manufacturer of the TDx FLM assay, the sensitivity remains at 96%, but the specificity decreases to 81%.[171] This means that the lung studies will demonstrate maturity (surfactant/albumin ratio of > 70 mg/gm), and the infant will not develop RDS in 81% of cases, whereas in 19% of cases, the lung studies will indicate immaturity and yet the infant will not develop RDS. Some institutions use a higher value (120 mg/gm) as an absolute cutoff, assuring a very high sensitivity. For values between 70 and 120 mg/gm, an additional test such as the lecithin/sphingomyelin ratio is performed. Other investigators have found that sequential testing of this nature, when the first test indicates maturity, offers very little additional predictive ability.[169] Although such cascade testing increases the specificity of some combinations of tests, much more experience will be necessary to determine sensitivity and specificity ranges for various combinations of lung maturity tests.[172]

Lamellar Body Count

Pulmonary surfactant is packaged into structures known as lamellar bodies within type II pneumocytes in the lung, and these lamellar bodies are released by exocytosis into the alveolus. A count of these lamellar bodies in amniotic fluid, which can be performed quickly using standard automated counters, has been proposed as a rapid technique for estimating fetal lung maturity.[173]

Evaluation of the Fetal Lung Maturity Tests

A major advantage of fluorescence polarization, foam stability, and lamellar body count analyses is speed; results can be available in less than 30 minutes. This is much faster than the lecithin/sphingomyelin assay, which takes several hours. The latter test also suffers from poor precision (at best $\pm$ 15%) and very poor interlaboratory agreement.[174] This is because lecithin/sphingomyelin assays, as well as phosphatidylglycerol assays, require 2D thin-layer chromatography; this technology is very dependent on the technical skill of the person performing the test. The assignment of quantitative values to a smear on a gel plate is inherently imprecise. In contrast, fluorescence polarization, whether PC16 or NBD-PC is used, is very precise (less than 2% variation).[175]

The foam stability index test also has excellent interlaboratory and intralaboratory agreement. Because the fluorescence polarization results are reported as the ratio of surfactant to albumin, fetal conditions that result in decreased levels of albumin in the amniotic fluid, such as urinary tract obstruction, can give a normal ratio, when in fact surfactant production is in a below normal range. The foam stability index test is one third as expensive as fluorescence polarization or lecithin/sphingomyelin assays, and the rapid lamellar count should be even less expensive than foam stability tests that use a commercial kit. Because a positive test, indicating lung maturity, has a very high predictive rate (> 96%) regardless of the test used, performing a second test following a positive result contributes very little to improving predictive ability. However, because of the weakness of all tests in correctly predicting RDS when the test indicates immaturity, cascade testing does improve predictive ability.

Cascade, or sequential, testing requires more than one test indicating immaturity before that determination is made. For all cascade testing, starting with a low-cost test such as the foam stability index test is most cost-efficient.[176] As medical costs are subjected to greater and greater scrutiny, it is likely that simple and inexpensive tests, such as the ''shake'' test and its modifications, will enjoy a revival at the expense of more costly and technologically intensive tests that provide no greater predictive value.

Another consideration that has greatly altered the assessment of fetal lung maturity is the success of exogenously administered surfactant. This therapy has reduced the incidence of hyaline membrane disease in newborns who would have previously developed the disease. It will be very difficult to evaluate the predictive valve of lung maturity tests in the future because of the absence of a control group in which surfactant therapy is not used immediately after delivery of an infant with immature lungs.

INTRAPARTUM FETAL MONITORING

Intrapartum Fetal Heart Rate Monitoring

Evaluation of fetal heart rate patterns remains the cornerstone of monitoring for the purpose of assessing fetal well-being during labor. Auscultation of the fetal heart rate using a stethoscope provides very limited information other than extremes of heart rate and arrhythmias. Owing to the intermittent nature of this technique, significant pathology may be present but not detected. Maximum information from fetal heart rate monitoring is obtained with continuous beat-to-beat monitoring for an extended period using electronic monitoring equipment.

Fetal Heart Rate Changes

Fetal heart rate changes consist of baseline changes and periodic changes. Baseline changes include beat-to-beat variability, tachycardia, and bradycardia. Periodic changes refer to deceleration patterns: early, late, and variable.

Baseline Fetal Heart Rate Changes

Beat-to-Beat Variability. The baseline fetal heart rate is normally 120–160 beats/minute. In the healthy fetus, there is a slight difference in the interval between successive heart beats. This is referred to as beat-to-beat variability or short-term variability. Beat-to-beat variability produces the irregular baseline seen in normal fetal heart rate tracings (Fig. 18–45). The physiologic origins and significance of this variability are uncertain, but clinical evidence suggests that its presence confirms an intact pathway from the cerebral cortex to the midbrain to the vagus nerve to the cardiac conduction system.[177, 178] Sporadic input from various areas in the cerebral cortex is transmitted to the cardiac centers in the medulla oblongata. This results in continuously vary-

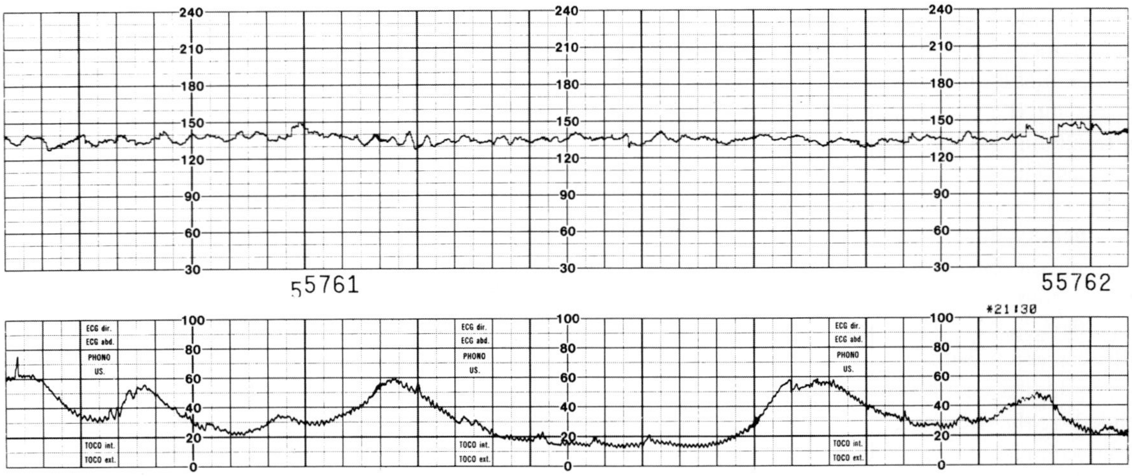

Figure 18–45. Normal fetal heart rate tracing (upper trace) showing good beat-to-beat variability, a baseline rate of 135 beats per minute, and no heart rate changes with uterine contractions (lower trace).

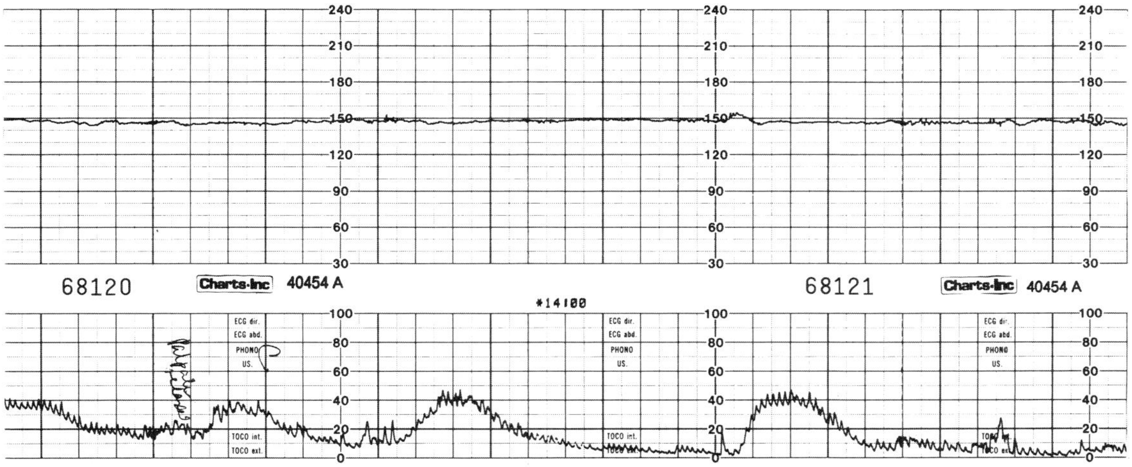

Figure 18–46. Decreased beat-to-beat variability. Compare the fetal heart rate pattern (upper trace) with the tracing in Figure 18–45.

ing levels of vagal stimulation, and the heart rate reflects this uneven input. Cerebral asphyxia decreases heart rate variability (Fig. 18–46), possibly because of decreased cerebral input to the midbrain. Absent beat-to-beat variability is seen in anencephalic infants, in whom there is an absence of cerebral cortex. It may also be caused by drugs, such as narcotics and sedatives, that depress higher brain centers. Anticholinergic drugs in high doses decrease variability. Defects in the fetal cardiac conduction system also cause loss of variability.

During labor, one should rarely, if ever, base the diagnosis of fetal asphyxia solely on a lack of heart rate variability. However, in the presence of other indicators of fetal distress, the presence or absence of heart rate variability is highly significant.

Fetal Tachycardia. Fetal tachycardia is defined as a heart rate greater than 160 beats/minute. If normal variability is present, tachycardia does not indicate asphyxia (Fig. 18–47). However, tachycardia may be seen in the recovery phase following a period of asphyxia and the resultant catecholamine release. Other causes of tachycardia are maternal or fetal infection, especially chorioamnionitis, drugs such as $beta_2$ agonists or parasympathetic blockers, tachydysrhythmias, and thyrotoxicosis.

Fetal Bradycardia. Bradycardia is the initial response of a normal fetus to acute hypoxia. Deceleration refers to a slowing of the heart rate to less than 120 beats/minute lasting for less than 2 minutes, whereas moderate bradycardia is defined as a heart rate between 100 and 120 beats/minute lasting longer than 2 minutes. If variability is normal, the fetus is able to tolerate mild hypoxic states by the compensatory mechanisms already discussed, namely, redistribution of blood flow, decreased oxygen consumption, and anaerobic glycolysis. In some patients, moderate bradycardia is idiopathic and benign and does not represent hypoxia. For example, moderate bradycardia may result from prolonged head compression and is vagally mediated.

Other causes of bradycardia are less common. Complete

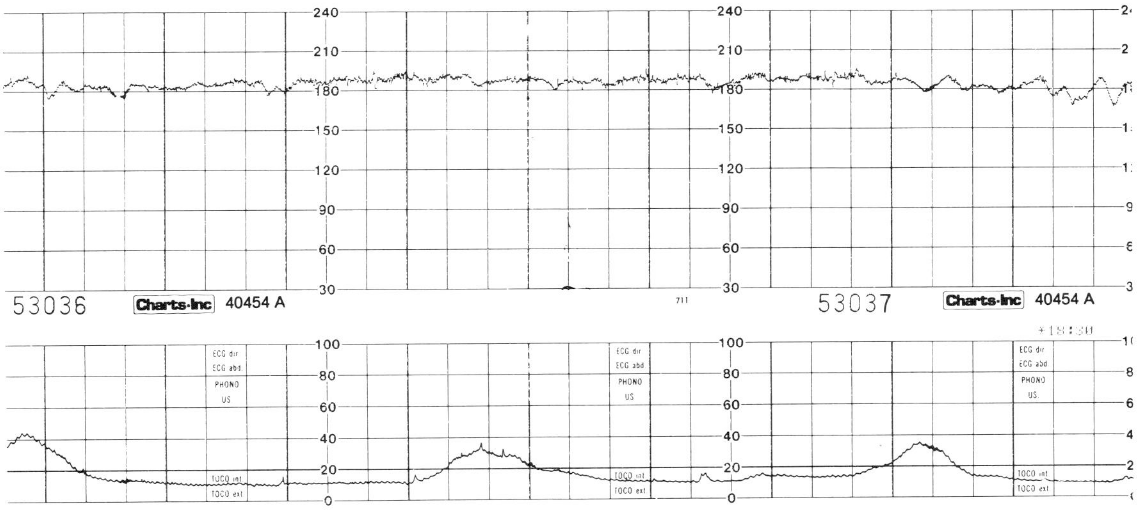

Figure 18–47. Fetal tachycardia. The baseline fetal heart rate is 190 beats/minute, but there is good beat-to-beat variability, and there are no deceleration patterns.

heart block, a condition associated with a significant incidence of structural heart disease, may be present. Congenital heart block may also be seen in the offspring of mothers with systemic lupus erythematosus. Bradycardia can be caused by maternal medications, such as beta blockers or local anesthetics. Of particular note is the high incidence of fetal bradycardia following paracervical block.

Bradycardia due to complete heart block, in the absence of structural heart disease, is better tolerated than sinus bradycardia at the same rate (e.g., 50 beats/minute). This is because the atrial rate tends to be twice as fast in complete heart block than in sinus bradycardia (see Fig. 18–41), in which the sinus rate is as slow as the ventricular rate. The slow atrial rate is associated with greater abnormalities of blood flow streaming, so that there is greater mixing of oxygenated and deoxygenated blood in the right atrium and, therefore, a lower oxygen saturation associated with blood leaving the left ventricle for the brain and myocardium. Also, there is a greater amount of reversed flow in the vena cava during sinus bradycardia than during comparable episodes of bradycardia due to complete heart block.[179]

Severe bradycardia, with heart rates below 60 beats/minute, eventually results in cardiac decompensation and must be managed urgently. In the fetus, cardiac output is primarily determined by heart rate, and a decrease in heart rate signifies a decrease in cardiac output. The decreased cardiac output causes less blood to circulate through the placenta, causing progressively lower oxygen tension in circulating blood and the accumulation of tissue acids. Unless this process is reversed, severe bradycardia will eventually result in insufficient oxygen delivery to support myocardial demand, and the fetus will die.

Periodic Fetal Heart Rate Changes. Periodic changes are those patterns that occur in association with uterine contractions. There are three specific periodic patterns: early decelerations, late decelerations, and variable decelerations. It should be emphasized that heart rate slowing with contractions is not normal. Thus, as shown in Figure 18–45, a normal fetal heart rate pattern has a baseline rate between 120 and 160 beats/minute with good beat-to-beat variability and no periodic changes (i.e., no heart rate decelerations with contractions).

Early Decelerations. Early decelerations occur concomitantly with the uterine contraction. They start at the same time, are smooth, and are a mirror image of the uterine contraction (Fig. 18–48). Early decelerations are mild (less than 20 beats/minute below baseline). The etiology is unknown, although the usual explanation is fetal head compression.

Late Decelerations. Late decelerations are also smooth and associated with contractions, but the onset and recovery are delayed 10–30 seconds (Fig. 18–49). The onset usually coincides with the peak of the uterine contraction, and the fetal heart rate is slowest at the end of the contraction. This pattern indicates uteroplacental insufficiency. Uterine blood flow decreases during the contraction, and fetal blood returning from the placenta is not adequately oxygenated. Chemoreceptors sense the low oxygen tension and trigger a

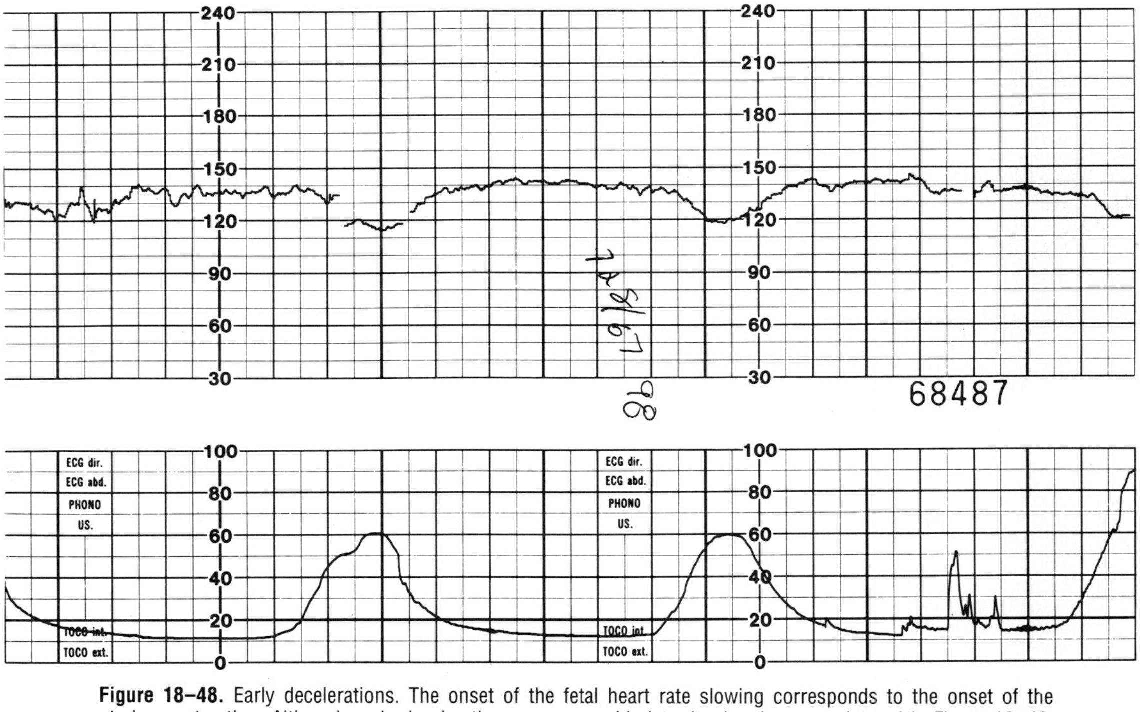

Figure 18–48. Early decelerations. The onset of the fetal heart rate slowing corresponds to the onset of the uterine contraction. Although early decelerations may resemble late decelerations, as pictured in Figure 18–49, this pattern is not associated with fetal distress but is attributed to vagal discharge, possibly in response to fetal head compression. This infant was subsequently delivered by cesarean section for prolonged bradycardia. At delivery, the infant had a tight nuchal cord, but Apgar scores of 9 and 9 at 1 and 5 minutes.

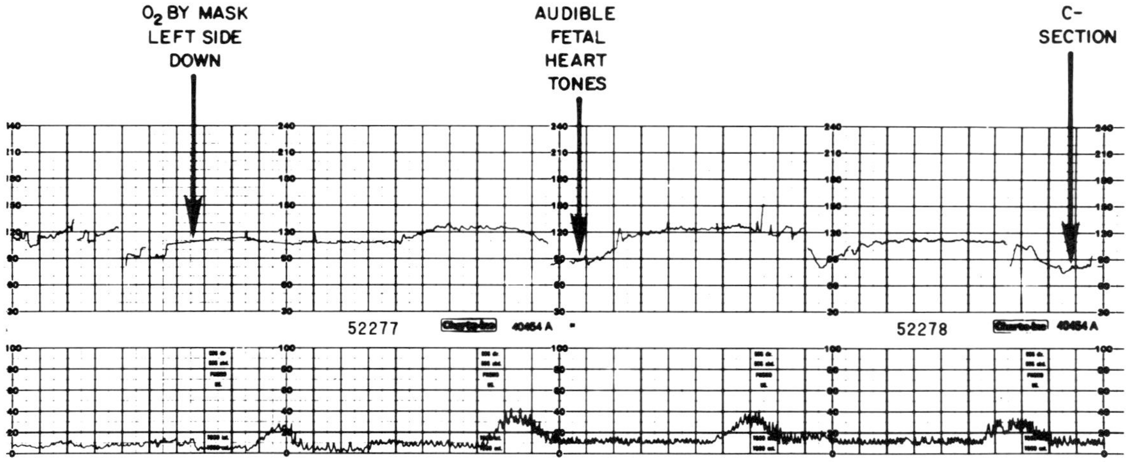

Figure 18–49. Late decelerations. The slowing of the fetal heart rate coincides with the peak of the uterine contraction. The absence of beat-to-beat variability indicates a decompensated fetus. The persistence of late decelerations and a low baseline heart rate compared to an earlier rate of 145 beats per minute prompted an emergency cesarean section. The infant was severely depressed; Apgar scores were 1 (1 minute), 2 (5 minutes), and 6 (10 minutes).

vagal discharge. As long as cerebral oxygenation is maintained, fetal heart rate variability should also remain normal, in spite of the late decelerations. However, if the deoxygenation is severe enough, it may affect the central nervous system. Cerebral hypoxia will cause decreased or absent beat-to-beat variability, as seen in Figure 18–49.

Late decelerations often occur in the setting of an already impaired placental reserve, such as preeclampsia or intrauterine growth retardation. The key to assessing the severity of the pattern is the degree of variability. The combination of late decelerations with absent variability is an ominous pattern, because it indicates that each contraction stresses the fetus beyond its compensatory capacity.

The treatment of the maternal-fetal unit when late decelerations occur consists of efforts to optimize placental blood flow and oxygenation. Maternal position should be changed, particularly if the mother is lying supine, in order to eliminate the mechanical effects of the uterus on the aorta or vena cava. In Figure 18–49, note that the response to the fetal heart rate of 110 beats/minute but with absent variability was to administer oxygen, place the patient on her left side, and notify the obstetrician. If the mother is hypotensive after correct positioning, then volume and blood pressure support with ephedrine is indicated. In patients with significant mouth breathing, as is often taught in prepared childbirth courses, oxygen should be delivered to the mother by a sealed face mask rather than by nasal prongs. Uterine activity can be reduced by stopping oxytocin if it is being infused, or with tocolytic agents. Uterine hypertonus can be most rapidly treated by the intravenous administration of small-bolus doses (100 μg) of nitroglycerin.

Measures to increase uterine perfusion and oxygenation will often correct late decelerations in which beat-to-beat variability is still good; the presence of variability indicates a margin of fetal reserve. In a decompensated fetus, these measures, though still important, are less likely to improve the status of the fetus, and immediate delivery is required.

Variable Decelerations. Variable decelerations differ in duration, depth, and shape from contraction to contraction. The onset and the termination of the deceleration are usually very abrupt. There is no definite relationship to uterine contractions (Figs. 18–50 and 18–51). Severe variable decelerations are defined as those that decrease 60 beats/minute below baseline, decrease below 60 beats/minute, or last longer than 60 seconds. Variable decelerations are felt to represent vagal firing in response to cord compression or sustained head compression, as when the mother is pushing during the second stage of labor. These postulated mechanisms have been given additional credence by studies in humans by Weiss and colleagues.[180] Temporary mechanical occlusion of the umbilical vein causes increased resistance to fetal umbilical arterial flow. If the pressure in the umbilical vein, and hence in the placenta vessels, is higher than the diastolic pressure in the umbilical artery, flow will reverse during part of the cardiac cycle, resulting in a to-and-fro movement of the blood column that is readily recorded using Doppler flow velocimetry. This decrease in arterial perfusion causes a prompt and often dramatic heart rate deceleration. However, in other cases the decrease in perfusion appears to be the result and not the cause of the deceleration of the fetal heart rate. Weiss et al postulate that this is the result of a parasympathetic reaction in the central nervous system caused by either systemic or local hypoxemia; the latter might occur when the head is compressed. Fetal head compression pressures in the range of 38–390 mmHg (mean 158 mmHg) have been measured during the second stage of labor.[180]

The presence or absence of baseline variability correlates with oxygenation of central tissues and indicates the sever-

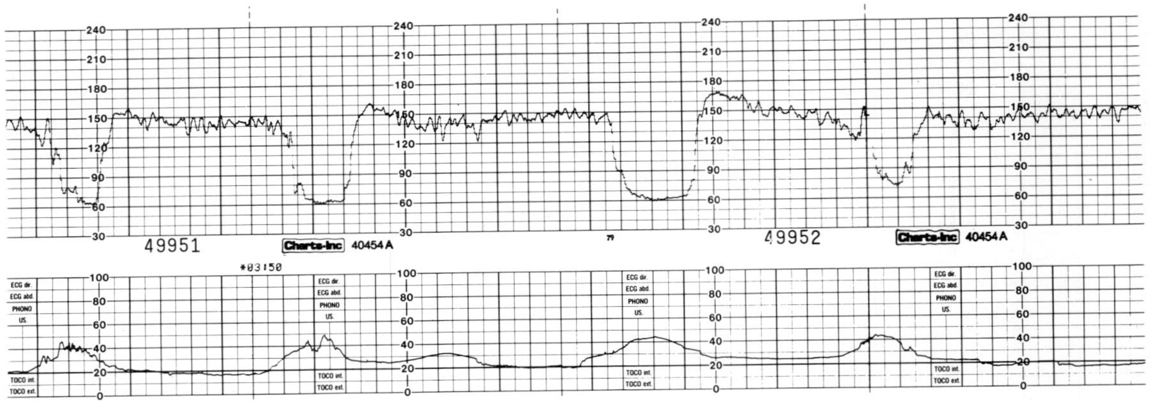

Figure 18–50. Severe variable decelerations. The deceleration tends to mirror the uterine contraction. Fetal heart rate often overshoots the baseline at the termination of the deceleration. Note the variable appearance of each deceleration tracing relative to the preceding tracing. Despite the dramatic appearance of this "severe" pattern, there is still good beat-to-beat variability, and this infant was delivered vaginally with Apgar scores of 7 (1 minute) and 9 (5 minutes).

ity of the stress producing the decelerations. The same techniques used to treat late decelerations—namely, measures to improve uterine perfusion and oxygenation—are applicable in patients with variable decelerations.

Techniques of Fetal Heart Rate Monitoring

Meaningful fetal heart rate monitoring requires both the fetal heart rate pattern and the pattern of uterine contractions in order to assess the relationship between the two. There are four methods for obtaining fetal heart rate. Intermittent stethoscopic auscultation remains the main form of surveillance during labor in low-risk pregnancies and continues to be used in high-risk pregnancies despite the fact that there is no auscultatory pattern of early fetal distress. Auscultation can identify only the extreme condition. The patterns of variable and late decelerations were only described in 1967 with the advent of electronic monitoring techniques.[182] They were never recognized through the stethoscope by generations of skilled clinicians.

Phonocardiography and Doppler ultrasound both are noninvasive and detect sounds produced by the fetal heart valves. Neither technique is adequate for assessing beat-to-beat variability but can be used to detect deceleration patterns.

ECG can be either indirect from the maternal abdomen or direct from stainless steel spiral electrodes placed in the infant's scalp (see Fig. 18–14). This latter technique is invasive and cannot be performed if the maternal membranes are intact. It carries the risk of fetal scalp infection, facial injury (specifically the eye), and bleeding. However, this technique provides the most precise data on beat-to-beat variability for clinical decision making.

Predictive Value of Fetal Heart Rate Patterns

A normal fetal heart rate pattern (120–160 beats/minute with good beat-to-beat variability and no late or variable decelerations) during the last 30 minutes of labor predicts a vigorous infant at birth more than 98% of the time, even in high risk pregnancies, assuming that the delivery is atrau-

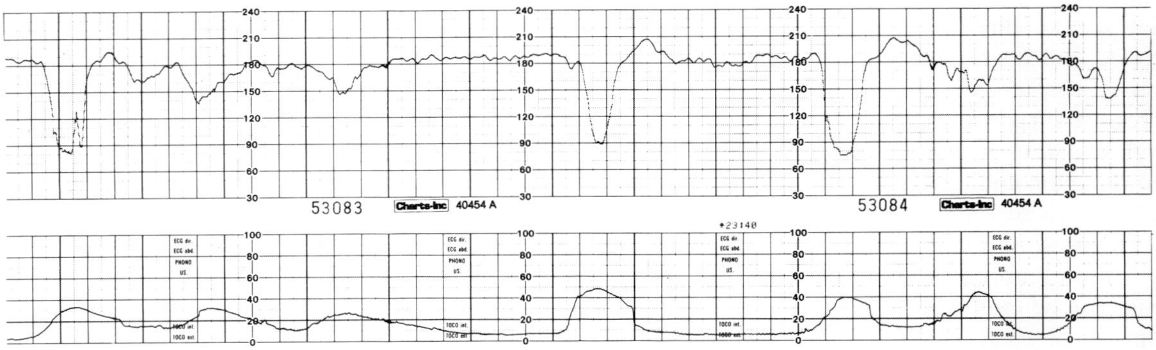

Figure 18–51. Variable decelerations. Compared to Figure 18–50, there is less beat-to-beat variability. Also note the lack of uniformity of the deceleration tracings. This heart rate tracing is from the same infant as in Figure 18–47, but 5 hours later. The baseline tachycardia is still present, but now there is decreased beat-to-beat variability and persistent variable decelerations. The mother was an insulin-dependent diabetic. She was allowed to deliver vaginally. The infant weighed 3680 gm, and had a 1-minute Apgar score of 3 and a 5-minute score of 8.

matic and the infant has no congenital malformation inconsistent with extrauterine life, such as tracheal atresia or aplastic lungs.[183] However, the converse is not true. Heart rate patterns of variable or late decelerations do not guarantee a depressed newborn. Earlier studies of late and variable decelerations showed very little correlation between these patterns and depressed newborns. One reason for this is that these studies failed to subdivide the patient population based on heart rate variability.[184] Patients with decelerations and adequate variability often have a low 1-minute Apgar score but usually have a 5-minute Apgar score of 8 or above. Decelerations and decreased variability increase the risk for significant neonatal depression. Severe deceleration patterns with the absence of variability are almost always associated with an asphyxiated fetus who will likely require active resuscitation.

The vast majority of fetuses with major congenital anomalies will have normal fetal heart rate patterns. Exceptions are anencephaly and congenital heart disease with complete heart block.

Controversies in Fetal Heart Rate Monitoring

The optimal monitoring technique for the intrapartum period is unclear; one side advocates intermittent auscultation, and the other insists on electronic fetal monitoring. The reason that stethoscopic surveillance is acceptable, even though it cannot identify early fetal distress, is that the true incidence of fetal distress is so low—about 2%. Thus, 98% of low-risk mothers monitored in this fashion, or any other manner, can be expected to deliver vigorous infants. Advocates of auscultation point to studies such as one that found fewer cases of cerebral palsy in infants monitored by auscultation than by electronic means.[185] However, as previously discussed, cerebral palsy is probably not primarily a condition resulting from intrapartum hypoxia.[157, 158, 186] On the basis of a number of studies in which there has been no demonstrable benefit associated with electronic monitoring compared to a strict protocol of intermittent auscultation, the American College of Obstetricians and Gynecologists has indicated that either technique is adequate. However, the protocols on which their decision was based require that the fetal heart rate be auscultated within 15 minutes of arrival in the delivery suite, every 15 minutes for a full minute during the first stage of labor, and every 5 minutes during the second stage of labor, again for a full minute.

The data must also be recorded at the time they are measured. This requires a 1:1 nurse-patient ratio and consumes a considerable amount of nursing time. When this protocol was applied in a busy university setting, over half the patients had to be initially excluded, because 1:1 nursing care was not available. In 19 of 442 patients in whom intermittent auscultation was attempted, auscultation was impossible because of maternal obesity. In the remaining 423 patients, auscultation as the mode of monitoring was discontinued in 392, because the stringent frequency of auscultation and recording could not be maintained.[187] Acceptance of intermittent monitoring without provision of staffing requirements would appear to raise concerns regarding standard of care, and failure to meet the stringent frequency requirement may involve an unacceptable liability exposure.

No major randomized controlled trial has clearly established the benefits of fetal monitoring. Because of the small numbers of affected fetuses, it takes very large numbers to generate meaningful studies. Such numbers (> 100,000 births) have been obtained from nonrandomized surveys, generating the following information. The interpartum stillbirth rate decreased from 2.4 to 0.5 per 1000 with monitoring ($p < .0001$), and the neonatal death rate decreased from 8.1 to 3.6 per 1000 with monitoring ($p < .0001$).[188] The data suggest, but do not conclude, that routine fetal monitoring improves neonatal outcomes. On the basis of these data, Parer (in 1984) predicted that future studies should expect to show a benefit of 5 saved lives per 1000 high-risk births through the proper use of electronic monitoring and 1 saved life per 1000 low-risk births.[188]

A randomized study, although including only 1428 patients, reported that patients monitored electronically had a greater incidence of nonreassuring fetal heart rate patterns compared with those monitored by intermittent auscultation (23.4% vs. 10.7%) and a higher rate of cesarean delivery for suspected fetal distress (5.3% vs. 2.3%).[189] There were no differences in 1- and 5-minute Apgar scores, fetal acidosis at birth, need for neonatal resuscitation, neonatal intensive care unit admission, use of assisted ventilation, neonatal hospital stay, or any other neonatal complications between the two groups. This would tend to support the position that electronic monitoring leads to increased rates of operative delivery without altering outcomes.

However, there was one major difference between the two groups in this study. The perinatal death rate related to fetal hypoxia was significantly less in the electronically monitored group (0 of 746 vs. 6 of 682; $p = .03$). This randomized, prospective study confirms that in the vast majority of cases, the nature of intrapartum fetal surveillance is of little consequence. However, it also provides evidence that in a small number of cases, possibly less than 1%, electronic monitoring detects early fetal hypoxia and allows accelerated delivery, likely by cesarean section, and thus decreases neonatal mortality when compared to intermittent auscultation, which does not detect fetal distress early. The results of this study in 1993 are thus in line with the predictions of Parer.[178, 188] Electronic monitoring provides information that may be lifesaving in a small number of cases and carries a very low risk of fetal or maternal injury. Thus, my position is at odds with that of the American College of Obstetricians and Gynecologists, and electronic monitoring and intermittent auscultation are not considered equivalent, particularly in the high-risk patient.

It is unclear whether electronic monitoring has increased the rate of cesarean sections. The number has increased, but it reflects factors other than monitoring, such as changed management for genital herpes and breach presentation, as well as the decline of midforceps interventions. It is likely that part of this increase has resulted from inadequate interpretation of fetal heart rate patterns. Another consideration is the likelihood that in a number of cases in which vigorous infants were delivered by emergent cesarean section for suspected fetal distress based on fetal heart tracings, the fetal condition would have deteriorated over time if labor had been allowed to continue. Higher rates of cesarean delivery do not necessarily equal unnecessary surgery. For example, even though the cesarean rate for fetal distress was twice as high (5.3% vs. 2.3%) in patients monitored electronically as opposed to those monitored by auscultation in the study by Vintzileos, there was a significantly lower incidence of fetal deaths due to intrapartum hypoxia in the electronically monitored group.[189]

Intrapartum Doppler Velocimetry

Increasingly, physicians are seeking information in addition to heart rate data to assess the status of the fetus in order to decrease the rate of cesarean delivery of vigorous infants with a diagnosis of suspected fetal distress. A study of 300 high-risk infants using umbilical artery Doppler flow velocimetry showed a cesarean rate of 13% in the group with Doppler flow monitoring as compared to a rate of 23% in control patients.[190] The neonatal outcomes in terms of length of stay in the intensive care nursery were also better for the monitored group. As discussed earlier, other Doppler findings such as umbilical venous pulsations may be even more sensitive than umbilical artery flow parameters in the detection of fetal decompensation. Clearly, monitoring should be both highly sensitive and highly specific. Properly interpreted fetal heart tracings are quite sensitive but not highly specific. Computer-assisted analysis may improve the specificity. However, better clinical management may result from Doppler flow analysis of fetuses with distress-type heart rate patterns. Thus, it is likely that sophisticated monitoring will live up to its initial promise and actually result in a lower rate of emergent cesarean delivery, especially of vigorous infants.

Fetal Scalp pH Sampling

When a fetal heart rate pattern suggests fetal compromise, fetal scalp pH is often recommended in order to confirm the suspected acidosis. This requires that the amniotic membranes be ruptured. The normal range for fetal capillary blood pH is 7.25–7.35; below 7.15, the fetus is definitely acidotic. Between 7.15 and 7.25, a clinical interpretation is required. What is the maternal pH? Acidotic babies born to acidotic mothers are usually vigorous. Before a fetus is diagnosed as acidotic on the basis of a scalp sample, the maternal pH should be measured, and the maternal-fetal pH difference should be evaluated. This approach resulted in a 33% reduction in the rate of false-positive scalp samples (vigorous infant with ''acidotic'' scalp pH before delivery).[191] Also, what is the type of acidosis? Metabolic acidosis suggests that anaerobic glycolysis is present, possibly as a result of tissue asphyxia due to placental failure. Respiratory acidosis is more likely to reflect umbilical cord compression.[192] Was there any preceding maternal event, such as a seizure or anesthetic-induced maternal hypotension, to account for the fetal acidosis? Also important is the timing of the fetal scalp sampling in relation to maternal contractions. The best information regarding the well-being of the fetus is obtained by sampling just before a contraction.

The predictive value of pH measurements is limited. A normal pH (above 7.25) reliably predicts a vigorous fetus in 90% of cases, whereas a very low pH (below 7.15) correctly predicts a depressed fetus with a reliability of only 80%. Thus, 20% of infants with a scalp pH below 1.5 will be vigorous. Additional clinical data is necessary in order to assess the significance of any single pH value.

The presence of normal fetal heart rate variability reliably predicts a vigorous fetus in almost 100% of cases; consequently, mild to moderate decelerations in the presence of good variability do not correlate with fetal acidosis.[193] Thus, there is little point in performing fetal scalp sampling when heart rate variability is good. Severe decelerations with decreased baseline variability predict an acidotic fetus, and there is little benefit to be gained in scalp sampling when the heart rate pattern is ominous and persistent or when ominous patterns (umbilical venous pulsations) are present on Doppler flow velocity waveforms.

Fetal blood sampling should not be done when there is any known or suspected bleeding disorder such as hemophilia or von Willebrand's disease. Sampling in such cases has resulted in fetal death.

Indications for sampling include (1) moderate to severe decelerations with somewhat decreased heart rate variability that do not respond to standard treatment, (2) the need to monitor a fetus during labor when maternal drug therapy affecting fetal heart rate variability is required, and (3) the absence of variability without obvious cause on initial measurement of the fetal heart rate. However, improvements in noninvasive pulse oximetry may obviate the need for fetal scalp sampling.

Intrapartum Pulse Oximetry

Standard pulse oximeters have not been routinely applicable to the fetus during a late stage of labor, because the light has to pass through a tissue bed. Because only one surface, the scalp, usually presents itself, placement of a transmission sensor is not feasible.

Reflectance, as opposed to transmission, pulse oximetry has recently been reported for *in utero* assessment of oxygen saturation. The amniochorionic membranes do not absorb light at either 660 or 940 nm, which are used by the oximeter, and thus reflectance oximetry can be used in the presence of intact membranes, a distinct advantage compared to fetal scalp blood sampling.[194] However, reflectance oximetry, like scalp samples, can provide erroneously low oxygen saturation data in the presence of scalp congestion or caput succedaneum.[195] Meconium interferes with light transmission at the crucial wavelengths used by the oximeter and can result in artificially low saturation readings.[196] Reflectance oximetry has been used to document improvement in fetal oxygen saturation during maternal oxygen administration.[197]

The standard algorithms used in transmission pulse oximeters were clinically derived for use over a range from 70 to 100% saturation. Pulse oximetry readings at low oxygen saturations have been extrapolated. In fetal sheep, and presumably in humans, recalibration is necessary for saturations in the range of 0–70%.[198] The presence of fetal versus adult hemoglobin is of no consequence for pulse oximetry at the standard light wavelengths.

Amniotic Fluid Volume

Real-time ultrasonography is used to estimate amniotic fluid volume, and an abnormally low amniotic fluid volume increases the risk of fetal distress during labor.[199] Once the fetal membranes are ruptured, oligohydramnios increases the likelihood of umbilical cord compression. Patients so identified may benefit from infusion of fluid into the amniotic cavity. Doppler velocimetry has been used in this setting and has been reported to be a good predictor of adverse outcome. Lombardi and coworkers found that in parturients with oligohydramnios, normal umbilical artery waveforms were associated with a normal perinatal outcome in 12 of 13 patients, whereas abnormal waveforms resulted in perinatal morbidity 100% of the time.[200]

NEONATAL ASSESSMENT

With severance of the umbilical cord at delivery, the infant must rapidly make the transition from intrauterine dependency to extrauterine independence. Careful monitoring of the fetus during this period is essential if one is to intervene promptly in the event of failure of transition, the consequences of which are devastating and lifelong.

The standard method for assessing the immediate well-being of a newborn is the Apgar score. Although many think that this is a mnemonic for appearance, pulse, grimace, activity, and respiration, it is actually named for Virginia Apgar, the anesthesiologist who first proposed the scoring system.[201] The Apgar scoring system assigns a score of 0, 1, or 2 in the categories listed in Table 18–7. For example, an absent heart rate results in a score of 0, any heart rate below 100 beats/minute gets a score of 1, and a heart rate over 100 gets a score of 2. The Apgar score is measured at 1 and 5 minutes and occasionally at 10 minutes. A 1-minute score of 0–2 indicates a severely depressed neonate who needs active resuscitation. In a newborn with this severity of depression, active resuscitation efforts should be underway before waiting for a 1-minute Apgar score. A score of 3–7 indicates a moderately depressed infant who will probably respond to oxygen administration by mask, possibly with positive pressure ventilation. Infants with scores higher than 8 rarely need respiratory assistance. The Apgar score is not a good predictor of long-term neurologic outcome. For any individual infant, a very low score at 5 minutes is of little value in predicting either the likelihood of survival or the neurologic outcome.

In addition to the Apgar scoring system, newborn assessment in the delivery room requires the same clinical observations used in other critical care settings. It is essential to recall the ABCs of basic life support: airway, breathing, circulation. Is the airway patent? Are bilateral breath sounds present? What is the quality of respiratory effort? Are there sternal retractions or nasal flaring? Is the abdomen distended? Is capillary refill adequate?

Recently, pulse oximetry has been introduced into the delivery room as a monitor of newborn oxygen saturation (SpO_2). This allows an immediate assessment of the infant's initial oxygen saturation as well as documentation of the normal transition from the low saturation state found *in utero* to the much higher saturations associated with pulmonary gas exchange (Figs. 18–52 and 18–53). Pulse oximetry has been shown to be unreliable at low saturations (< 60%) in sick neonates, and it should not replace direct arterial blood gas sampling in such infants.[202]

One major benefit is that oxygen saturation by oximetry immediately after birth correlates with umbilical vein oxygen tension.[203] This can document the absence of birth asphyxia at the time of delivery, knowledge with significant medicolegal value.

TABLE 18–7. APGAR NEONATAL SCORING SYSTEM*

Sign	Score: *0*	Score: *1*	Score: *2*
Heart rate	Absent	Under 100 beats/minute	Over 100 beats/minute
Respiratory effort	Absent	Slow, irregular	Good, crying
Color	Blue, pale	Acrocyanosis (pink body, blue extremities)	Completely pink
Reflex irritability (response to nasal catheter)	Absent	Grimace	Cough, sneeze
Muscle tone	Limp	Some flexion of extremities	Active motion

*Each sign is evaluated and scored from 0 to 2 at 1 and 5 minutes after birth. The sum of each individual score is the Apgar score for that period.

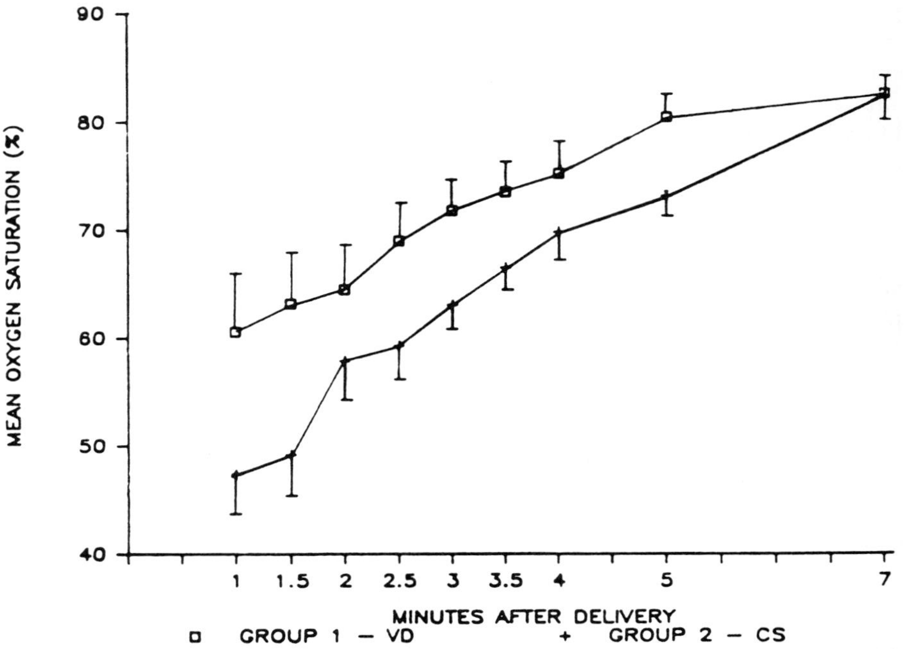

Figure 18–52. Oxygen saturation in the lower extremity in the immediate newborn period as measured by pulse oximetry. Open squares represent newborns delivered vaginally (VD); crosses indicate cesarean delivery (CS). The lower oxygen saturation in infants delivered by cesarean section, presumably accounted for by increased lung fluid, also is seen in Figure 18–53, but there the differences are much smaller. (From Harris AP, Sendak MJ, Donham RT: Changes in arterial oxygen saturation immediately after birth in the human neonate. J Pediatr 1986; 109:117–119.)

Because of the presence of right-to-left shunting through the ductus arteriosus in the transition period immediately after birth, Spo_2 will be higher in the right hand than in the left hand or lower extremities (Fig. 18–53).[204] At 1 minute after delivery, Spo_2 recorded from the right hand was higher than that recorded from the lower extremities (72% vs. 63%). By 5 minutes, Spo_2 increased to 83% in the right hand, compared with 76% in the foot. At 10 minutes, these differences diminished, and they almost completely disappeared after 24 hours. It is noteworthy that this study found much less difference in oxygen saturations based on mode of delivery (vaginal vs. cesarean section) than that in Figure 18–52. There is no obvious explanation for this. Also, because the saturations reported in the latter study are all postductal, their clinical significance is marginal. The brain and myocardium derive their blood supply from preductal flow.

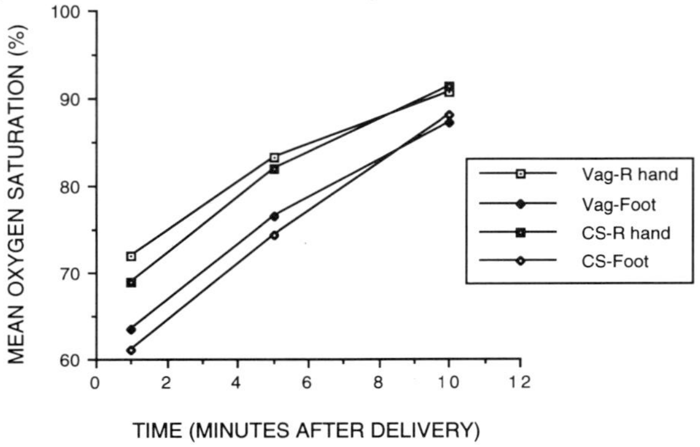

Figure 18–53. Oxygen saturation in the right hand (preductal) and lower extremity (postductal) in the immediate newborn period as measured by pulse oximetry. Note that the readings from the lower extremity are lower at all points compared to those taken from the right hand, regardless of the mode of delivery. (Vag = vaginal delivery, CS = cesarean delivery, R hand = right hand.) (From Dimich I, Singh PP, Adell A, et al: Evaluation of oxygen saturation monitoring by pulse oximetry in neonates in the delivery system. Can J Anaesth 1991; 38:985–988.)

When utilizing pulse oximetry in the delivery room, it is important to be aware that an oxygen saturation of 80% in the hand, or 75% in the foot, at 5 minutes after delivery is normal and does not warrant aggressive respiratory intervention in the absence of clinical signs of respiratory distress.

Capnography is also useful of assessing neonatal status in cases of severe asphyxia requiring cardiopulmonary resuscitation.[205] A capnogram provides information concerning both systemic and pulmonary blood flow. Capnography is not useful for the confirmation of tracheal intubation in the setting of cardiac arrest in an asphyxiated neonate; extremely high pulmonary artery pressures favor shunting of blood through the ductus arteriosus, and in the absence of pulmonary blood flow, there will be no carbon dioxide flux in the trachea to be detected by capnography.

REFERENCES

1. Easterling TR, Benedetti TJ, Schmucker BC, Millard SP: Maternal hemodynamics in normal and preeclamptic pregnancies: A longitudinal study. Obstet Gynecol 1990; 76:1061–1069.

2. Easterling TR, Watts DH, Schmucker BC, Benedetti TJ: Measurement of cardiac output during pregnancy: Validation of Doppler technique and clinical observations in preeclampsia. Obstet Gynecol 1987; 69:845–850.
3. Mishra M, Chambers JB, Jackson G: Murmurs in pregnancy: An audit of echocardiography. Br Med J 1993; 304:1413–1414.
4. Veille JC, Hosenpud JD, Morton MJ, Welch JE: Cardiac size and function in pregnancy-induced hypertension. Am J Obstet Gynecol 1984; 150:443–449.
5. Veille JC, Morton MJ, Burry KJ: Maternal cardiovascular adaptations to twin pregnancy. Am J Obstet Gynecol 1985; 153:261–263.
6. Moutquin JM, Rainville C, Giroux L, et al: A prospective study of blood pressure in pregnancy: Prediction of preeclampsia. Am J Obstet Gynecol 1985; 151:191–196.
7. Wilson M, Morganti AA, Zervoudakis I, et al: Blood pressure, the renin-aldosterone system and sex steroids throughout normal pregnancy. Am J Med 1980; 68:97–104.
8. Clark SL, Cotton DB, Pivarnik JM, et al: Position changes and central hemodynamic profile during normal third-trimester pregnancy and postpartum. Am J Obstet Gynecol 1991; 164:883–887.
9. Pirhonen JP, Erkkola RU: Uterine and umbilical flow velocity waveforms in the supine hypotensive syndrome. Obstet Gynecol 1990; 76:176–179.
10. Gant NF, Daley GL, Chand S, et al: A study of angiotensin II pressor response throughout primigravid pregnancy. J Clin Invest 1973; 52:2682–2689.
11. Nelson SH, Suresh MS: Lack of reactivity of uterine arteries from patients with obstetric hemorrhage. Am J Obstet Gynecol 1992; 166:1436–1443.
12. Brinkman CR: Biologic adaptations to pregnancy. *In* Creasy R, Resnik R, (eds): Maternal-Fetal Medicine, 2nd Ed. Philadelphia: WB Saunders, 1989; 741.
13. Sachs BP, Brown DA, Driscoll SG, et al: Maternal mortality in Massachusetts. Trends and prevention. N Engl J Med 1987; 316:667–672.
14. Hays PM, Cruikshank DP, Dunn LJ: Plasma volume determination in normal and preeclamptic pregnancies. Am J Obstet Gynecol 1985; 151:958–966.
15. Gallery EDM: Pregnancy-associated hypertension: Interrelationships of volume and blood pressure changes. Clin Exp Hypertens [B] 1982; 1:39–47.
16. Bletka M, Hlavaty V, Trnkova M, et al: Volume of whole blood and absolute amount of serum proteins in the early stages of late toxemia of pregnancy. Am J Obstet Gynecol 1970; 106:10–13.
17. Goodlin RC, Quaife MA, Dirksen JW: The significance, diagnosis, and treatment of maternal hypovolemia as associated with fetal/maternal illness. Semin Perinatol 1981; 5:163–174.
18. Kambam JR, Handte RE, Brown WU, Smith BE: Effect of normal and preeclamptic pregnancies on the oxyhemoglobin dissociation curve. Anesthesiology 1986; 65:426–427.
19. Davison JM: Renal hemodynamics and volume homeostasis in pregnancy. Scand J Clin Lab Invest 1984; 169(Suppl):15–27.
20. Cotton DB, Gonik B, Spillman T, Dorman KF: Intrapartum to postpartum changes in colloid osmotic pressure. Am J Obstet Gynecol 1984; 149:174–177.
21. Mashini IS, Albazzaz SJ, Fadel HE, et al: Serial evaluation of cardiovascular hemodynamics during pregnancy. Am J Obstet Gynecol 1987; 156:1208–1213.
22. Oian P, Maltau JM: Calculated capillary hydrostatic pressure in normal pregnancy and preeclampsia. Am J Obstet Gynecol 1987; 157:102–106.
23. Brown MA, Zammit VC, Lowe SA: Capillary permeability and extracellular fluid volumes in pregnancy-induced hypertension. Clin Sci 1989; 77:599–604.
24. Robson SC, Dunlop W, Boys RJ, Hunter S: Cardiac output during labor. Br Med J 1987; 295:1169–1172.
25. Rees GB, Pipkin FB, Symonds EM, Patrick JM: A longitudinal study of respiratory changes in normal human pregnancy with cross-sectional data on subjects with pregnancy-induced hypertension. Am J Obstet Gynecol 1990; 162:826–830.
26. Huch A, Huch R, Schneider H, Rooth G: Continuous transcutaneous monitoring of fetal oxygen tension during labor. Br J Obstet Gynaecol 1987; 84:1–39.
27. Baraka AS, Hanna MT, Jabbour SI, et al: Preoxygenation of pregnant and nonpregnant women in the head-up versus the supine position. Anesth Analg 1992; 75:757–759.
28. Baldwin GR, Moorthi DS, Whelton JA, MacDonnell KF: New lung functions and pregnancy. Am J Obstet Gynecol 1977; 127:235–239.
29. Das TK, Moutquin J, Parent J: Effect of cigarette smoking on maternal airway function during pregnancy. Am J Obstet Gynecol 1991; 165:675–679.
30. Russell IF, Chambers WA: Closing volume in normal pregnancy. Br J Anaesth 1981; 53:1043–1046.
31. Sandhar BK, Elliot RH, Windram I, Rowbotham DJ: Peripartum changes in gastric emptying. Anesthesiology 1992; 77:196–198.
32. Carp H, Jayaram A, Stoll M: Ultrasound examination of the stomach contents of parturients. Anesth Analg 1992; 74:683–687.
33. Jayaram A, Carp H: Progesterone-mediates potentiation of spinal sufentanil in rats. Anesth Analg 1993; 76:745–750.
34. Datta S, Lambert DH, Gregus J, et al: Differential sensitivities of mammalian nerve fibers during pregnancy. Anesth Analg 1983; 62:1070–1072.
35. Louden KA, Pipkin FB, Heptinstall S, et al: A longitudinal study of platelet behavior and thromboxane production in whole blood in normal pregnancy and the puerperium. Br J Obstet Gynaecol 1990; 97:1108–1114.
36. Kofinas AD, Penry M, Swain M, Hattjis CG: Effect of placental laterality on uterine artery resistance and development of preeclampsia and intrauterine growth retardation. Am J Obstet Gynecol 1989; 161:1536–1539.
37. Page EW, Christianson R: The impact of mean arterial blood pressure in the middle trimester upon the outcome of pregnancy. Am J Obstet Gynecol 1976; 125:740–744.
38. Villar J, Repke J, Markush L, et al: The measuring of blood pressure during pregnancy. Am J Obstet Gynecol 1989; 161:1019–1024.
39. Reiss RE, O'Shaughnessy RW, Quilligan TJ, Zuspan FP: Retrospective comparison of blood pressure course during preeclamptic and matched control pregnancies. Am J Obstet Gynecol 1987; 156:894–898.
40. Marx GF, Schwalbe SS, Cho E, et al: Automated blood pressure measurements in laboring women: Are they reliable? Am J Obstet Gynecol 1993; 168:796–798.
41. Leighton BL, Norris MC, Sosis M, et al: Limitations of epinephrine as a marker of intravascular injection in laboring woman. Anesthesiology 1987; 66:688–691.
42. Leighton BL, Gross JB: Air: An effective marker of intravenously located catheters. Anesthesiology 1989; 71:848–851.
43. Baron JF, Decaux-Jacolot A, Edouard A, et al: Influence of venous return on baroreflex control of heart rate during lumbar epidural anesthesia in humans. Anesthesiology 1986; 64:188–193.
44. Taylor J, Weil MH: Failure of the Trendelenburg position to improve circulation during clinical shock. Surg Gynecol Obstet 1967; 124:1005–1010.
45. Sibbald WJ, Paterson AM, Holliday RL, Baskerville J: The Trendelenburg position: Hemodynamic effects in hypotensive and normotensive patients. Crit Care Med 1979; 7:218–224.
46. Zakowski MI, Ramanathan S, Baratta JB, et al: Electrocardiographic changes during cesarean section: A cause for concern? Anesth Analg 1993; 76:162–167.
47. Lee W, Rokey R, Cotton DB: Noninvasive maternal stroke volume and cardiac output determinations by pulsed Doppler echocardiography. Am J Obstet Gynecol 1988; 158:505–510.
48. Groenendijk R, Trimbos JBMJ, Wallenburg HCS: Hemodynamic measurements in preeclampsia: Preliminary observations. Am J Obstet Gynecol 1984; 150:232–236.
49. Nisell H, Lunell NO, Linde B: Maternal hemodynamics and impaired fetal growth in pregnancy-induced hypertension. Obstet Gynecol 1988; 71:163–166.
50. Kuzniar J, Piela A, Skret A: Left ventricular function in preeclamptic patients: An echocardiographic study. Am J Obstet Gynecol 1983; 146:400–405.
51. Benedetti TJ, Kates R, Williams V: Hemodynamic observations in severe preeclampsia complicated by pulmonary edema. Am J Obstet Gynecol 1980; 152:330–334.
52. Oney T, Kaulhausen H: The value of the angiotensin sensitivity test in the diagnosis of hypertensive disorders in pregnancy. Am J Obstet Gynecol 1982; 142:17–20.
53. Baker PN, Broughton PF: Serial measurements of platelet angiotensin II binding in two patients with hypertension in pregnancy: Case reports. Am J Obstet Gynecol 1992; 167:487–488.
54. Leighton BL, Norris MC, DiSimone CA, et al: Pre-eclamptic and

healthy term pregnant patients have different chronotropic responses to isoproterenol. Anesthesiology 1990; 72:392–393.
55. Inayatulla A, Chemtob S, Nuwayhid B, Varma DR: Response of placental arteries from normotensive and preeclamptic women to endogenous agents. Am J Obstet Gynecol 1993; 168:869–874.
56. Erkkola RU, Pirhonen JP: Flow velocity waveforms in uterine and umbilical arteries during the angiotensin II sensitivity test. Am J Obstet Gynecol 1990; 162:1193–1197.
57. Benedetti TJ, Carlson RW: Studies of colloid osmotic pressure in pregnancy-induced hypertension. Am J Obstet Gynecol 1979; 135:308–311.
58. Wasserstrum N, Cotton DB: Hemodynamic monitoring in severe pregnancy-induced hypertension. Clin Perinatol 1986; 13:781–799.
59. Clark SL, Greenspoon JS, Aldahl D, Phelan JP: Severe preeclampsia with persistent oliguria: Management of hemodynamic subsets. Am J Obstet Gynecol 1986; 154:490–494.
60. Kirshon B, Lee W, Maurer MB, Cotton DB: Effects of low-dose dopamine therapy in the oliguric patient with preeclampsia. Am J Obstet Gynecol 1988; 159:604–607.
61. Cotton DB, Longmire S, Jones MM, et al: Cardiovascular alterations in severe pregnancy-induced hypertension: Effects of intravenous nitroglycerin coupled with blood volume expansion. Am J Obstet Gynecol 1986; 154:1053–1059.
62. Lindheimer MD, Katz AI: Hypertension in pregnancy. N Engl J Med 1985; 313:675–680.
63. Jouppila P, Jouppila R, Hollmen A, Koivula A: Lumbar epidural analgesia to improve intervillous blood flow during labor in severe preeclampsia. Obstet Gynecol 1982; 59:158–161.
64. Newsome LR, Bramwell RS, Curling PE: Severe preeclampsia: Hemodynamic effects of lumbar epidural anesthesia. Anesth Analg 1986; 65:31–36.
65. Hodgkinson R, Husain FJ, Hayashi RH: Systemic and pulmonary blood pressure during cesarean section in parturients with gestational hypertension. Can Anaesth Soc J 1980; 27:389–393.
66. Ramanathan J, Bottorff M, Jeter JN, et al: The pharmacokinetics and maternal and neonatal effects of epidural lidocaine in preeclampsia. Anesth Analg 1986; 65:120–126.
67. James MFM: Clinical use of magnesium infusions in anesthesia. Anesth Analg 1992; 74:129–136.
68. Longmire S, Leduc L, Jones MM, et al: The hemodynamic effects of intubation during nitroglycerin infusion in severe preeclampsia. Am J Obstet Gynecol 1991; 164:551–556.
69. Shuster E, Weppleman B: Plasma urate measurements and fetal outcome in preeclampsia. Gynecol Obstet Invest 1981; 12:162–167.
70. Lee W, Gonik B, Cotton DB: Urinary diagnostic indices in preeclampsia-associated oliguria: Correlation with invasive hemodynamic monitoring. Am J Obstet Gynecol 1987; 156:100–103.
71. Ihle BU, Long P, Oats J: Early onset pre-eclampsia: Recognition of underlying renal disease. Br Med J 1987; 294:79–81.
72. Sacks SH, Roberts R, Jones KV, et al: Effect of symptomless bacteriuria in childhood on subsequent pregnancy. Lancet 1987; 2:991–994.
73. Leduc L, Lederer E, Lee W, Cotton DB: Urinary sediment changes in severe preeclampsia. Obstet Gynecol 1991; 77:186–189.
74. Dunn R, Lee W, Cotton DB: Evaluation by computerized axial tomography of eclamptic women with seizures refractory to magnesium sulfate therapy. Am J Obstet Gynecol 1986; 155:267–268.
75. Merrell DA, Koch MA: Epidural anesthesia as an anticonvulsant in the management of hypertensive and eclamptic patients in labor. S Afr Med J 1980; 58:875–877.
76. Leduc L, Wheeler JM, Kirshon B, et al: Coagulation profile in severe preeclampsia. Obstet Gynecol 1992; 79:14–18.
77. Katz VL, Thorp JM, Rozas L, Bowes WA: The natural history of thrombocytopenia associated with preeclampsia. Am J Obstet Gynecol 1990; 163:1142–1143.
78. Roberts JM, Taylor RN, Musci TJ, et al: Preeclampsia: An endothelial cell disorder. Am J Obstet Gynecol 1989; 161:1200–1204.
79. Borrows RF, Hunter DJ, Andrew M, Kelton JG: A prospective study investigating the mechanism of thrombocytopenia in preeclampsia. Obstet Gynecol 1987; 70:334–338.
80. Kelton JG, Hunter DJ, Neame PB: A platelet function defect in preeclampsia. Obstet Gynecol 1985; 65:107–109.
81. Ramanathan J, Sibai BM, Vu T, Chauhan D: Correlation between bleeding times and platelet counts in women with preeclampsia undergoing cesarean section. Anesthesiology 1989; 71:188–191.
82. Abboud T, Artal R, Sarkis F, et al: Sympathoadrenal activity, maternal, fetal, and neonatal responses after epidural anesthesia in the preeclamptic patient. Am J Obstet Gynecol 1982; 144:915–918.
83. Sibai BH, Taslimi MM, El-Nazer A, et al: Maternal-perinatal outcome associated with the syndrome of hemolysis, elevated liver enzymes, and low platelets in severe preeclampsia-eclampsia. Am J Obstet Gynecol 1986; 155:501–509.
84. Lind SE: The bleeding time does not predict surgical bleeding. Blood 1991; 77:2547–2552.
85. Ramanathan J, Khalil M, Sibai BM, Chauhan D: Anesthetic management of the syndrome of hemolysis, elevated liver enzymes, and low platelet count (HELLP) in severe preeclampsia: A retrospective study. Reg Anesth 1988; 13:20–24.
86. Walsh SW: Preeclampsia: An imbalance in placental prostacyclin and thromboxane production. Am J Obstet Gynecol 1985; 152:335–340.
87. Hauth JC, Goldenberg RL, Parker R, et al: Low-dose aspirin therapy to prevent preeclampsia. Am J Obstet Gynecol 1993; 168:1083–1093.
88. Dekker GA, Sibai BM: Low-dose aspirin in the prevention of preeclampsia and fetal growth retardation: Rationale, mechanisms, and clinical trials. Am J Obstet Gynecol 1993; 168:214–227.
89. Roberts JM: Pregnancy-related hypertension. *In* Creasy R, Resnik R (eds): Maternal-Fetal Medicine. Philadelphia: WB Saunders, 1984; 739.
90. Lunell NO, Lewander R, Mamoun I, et al: Uteroplacental blood flow in pregnancy induced hypertension. Scand J Clin Lab Invest 1984; 169(Suppl):28–35.
91. Jouppila P, Kirkinen P, Koivula A, Ylikorkala O: Effects of dihydralazine infusion on the fetoplacental blood flow and maternal prostanoids. Obstet Gynecol 1985; 65:115–118.
92. Naulty J, Cefalo RC, Lewis PE: Fetal toxicity of nitroprusside in the pregnant ewe. Am J Obstet Gynecol 1981; 139:708–711.
93. Shoemaker CT, Meyers M: Sodium nitroprusside for control of severe hypertensive disease of pregnancy: A case report and discussion of potential toxicity. Am J Obstet Gynecol 1984; 149:171–173.
94. Stemple JE, O'Grady JP, Morton MJ, Johnson KA: Use of sodium nitroprusside in complications of gestational hypertension. Obstet Gynecol 1982; 60:533–538.
95. Jouppila P, Kirkinen P, Koivula A, Ylikorkala O: Labetalol does not alter the placental or fetal blood flow or maternal prostanoids in preeclampsia. Br J Obstet Gynaecol 1986; 93:543–547.
96. Harper A, Murnaghan GA: Maternal and fetal hemodynamics in hypertensive pregnancies during treatment with intravenous hydralazine or labetalol. Br J Obstet Gynaecol 1991; 98:453–459.
97. Fenakel K, Fenakel G, Appelman Z, et al: Nifedipine in the treatment of severe preeclampsia. Obstet Gynecol 1991; 77:331–337.
98. Moretti MM, Fairlie FM, Akl S, et al: The effect of nifedipine therapy on fetal and placental Doppler waveforms. Am J Obstet Gynecol 1990; 163:1844–1848.
99. Barton JR, Hiett AK, Conover WB: The use of nifedipine during the postpartum period in patients with severe preeclampsia. Am J Obstet Gynecol 1990; 162:788–792.
100. Easterling TR, Benedetti TJ, Schumaker BC, Carlson KL: Antihypertensive therapy in pregnancy directed by noninvasive hemodynamic monitoring. Am J Perinatol 1989; 6:86–89.
101. Cotton DB, Gonik B, Dorman K, Harrist R: Cardiovascular alterations in severe pregnancy-induced hypertension: Relationship of central venous pressure to pulmonary capillary wedge pressure. Am J Obstet Gynecol 1985; 151:762–764.
102. Cotton DB, Lee W, Huhta JC, Dorman KF: Hemodynamic profile of severe pregnancy-induced hypertension. Am J Obstet Gynecol 1988; 158:523–529.
103. Clark SL, Phelan JP, Greenspoon J, et al: Labor and delivery in the presence of mitral stenosis: Central hemodynamic observations. Am J Obstet Gynecol 1985; 152:984–988.
104. Cunningham FG, Pritchard JA, Hankins GD, et al: Peripartum heart failure: Idiopathic cardiomyopathy or compounding cardiovascular events? Obstet Gynecol 1986; 67:157–168.
105. Patel JJ, Mitha AS, Hassen F, et al: Percutaneous balloon mitral valvotomy in pregnant patients with tight pliable mitral stenosis. Am Heart J 1993; 125:1106–1109.
106. Ben Farhat M, Maatouk F, Betbout F, et al: Percutaneous balloon mitral valvuloplasty in eight pregnant women with severe mitral stenosis. Eur Heart J 1992; 13:1658–1664.
107. Ribeiro PA, Fawzy ME, Awad M, et al: Balloon valvotomy for pregnant patients with severe pliable mitral stenosis using the Inoue

technique with total abdominal and pelvic shielding. Am Heart J 1992; 124:1558–1562.
108. Esteves CA, Ramos AI, Braga SL, et al: Effectiveness of percutaneous balloon mitral valvotomy during pregnancy. Am J Cardiol 1991; 68:930–934.
109. Clark SL: Labor and delivery in the patient with structural cardiac disease. Clin Perinatol 1986; 13:695–703.
110. Nadeau S, Noble WH: Misinterpretation of pressure measurements from the pulmonary artery catheter. Can Anaesth Soc J 1986; 33:352–363.
111. Woods AM, Queen JS, Lawson D: Valsalva maneuver in obstetrics: The influence of peripheral circulatory changes on the function of the pulse oximeter. Anesth Analg 1991; 73:765–771.
112. Hemmings GT, Whalley DG, O'Connor PJ: Invasive monitoring and anaesthetic management of a parturient with mitral stenosis. Can J Anaesth 1987; 34:182–185.
113. Ziskind Z, Etchin A, Frenkel Y, et al: Epidural anesthesia with the Trendelenburg position for cesarean section with or without a cardiac surgical procedure in patients with severe mitral stenosis: A hemodynamic study. J Cardiothoracic Anesth 1990; 4:354–359.
114. Woods AM, Longnecker DE: Endoscopy. *In* Marshall BE, Longnecker DE, Fairley HB (eds): Anesthesia for Thoracic Procedures. Boston: Blackwell Scientific, 1988; 338–341.
115. Stone DJ, Gal TJ: Airway management. *In* Miller RD (ed): Anesthesia, 3rd Ed. New York: Churchill Livingstone, 1990.
116. Batson MA, Longmire S, Csontos E: Alfentanil for urgent caesarean section in a patient with severe mitral stenosis and pulmonary hypertension. Can J Anaesth 1990; 37:685–688.
117. Kopriva CJ, Eltringham RJ, Siebert PE: A comparison of the effects of intravenous Innovar and topical spray on the laryngeal closure reflex. Anesthesiology 1974; 40:596–598.
118. Behrman RE, Vaughan VC, (eds): Nelson Textbook of Pediatrics, 13th Ed. Philadelphia: WB Saunders, 1987; 1529.
119. Perloff JK, Child JS, Edwards JE: New guidelines for the clinical diagnosis of mitral valve prolapse. Am J Cardiol 1986; 57:1124–1129.
120. Alcantara LG, Marx GF: Cesarean section under epidural analgesia in a parturient with mitral valve prolapse. Anesth Analg 1987; 66:902–903.
121. Shapiro EP, Trimble EL, Robinson JC, et al: Safety of labor and delivery in women with mitral valve prolapse. Am J Cardiol 1985; 56:806–807.
122. Dineen E, Brent BN: Aortic valve stenosis: Comparison of patients with to those without chronic congestive heart failure. Am J Cardiol 1986; 57:419–422.
123. Redfern N, Bower S, Bullock RE, Hull CJ: Alfentanil for caesarean section complicated by severe aortic stenosis. Br J Anaesth 1987; 59:1309–1312.
124. Karp RB, Roe BB: Effects of aortic insufficiency on phasic flow patterns in the coronary artery. Ann Surg 1966; 164:959–966.
125. Buckberg GD, Kattus AA: Factors determining the distribution and adequacy of left ventricular myocardial blood flow. *In* Bloor CM, Olsson RA (eds): Current Topics in Coronary Research. New York: Plenum, 1975; 95.
126. Alderson JD: Cardiovascular collapse following epidural anaesthesia for caesarean section in a patient with aortic incompetence. Anaesthesia 1987; 42:643–645.
127. Shime J, Mocarski EJM, Hastings D, et al: Congenital heart disease in pregnancy: Short- and long-term implications. Am J Obstet Gynecol 1987; 156:313–322.
128. Pearl RG, Siegel LC: Thermodilution cardiac output measurement with a large left-to-right shunt. J Clin Monit 1991; 7:146–153.
129. Sugishita Y, Ito I, Kubo T: Pregnancy in cardiac patients: Possible influence of volume overload by pregnancy on pulmonary circulation. Jpn Circ J 1986; 50:376–383.
130. Laishley RS, Burrows FA, Lerman J, Roy WL: Effect of anesthetic induction regimens on oxygen saturation in cyanotic congenital heart disease. Anesthesiology 1986; 65:673–677.
131. Boxer RA, Gottesfeld I, Sharanjeet S, et al: Noninvasive pulse oximetry in children with cyanotic congenital heart disease. Crit Care Med 1987; 15:1062–1064.
132. Simmons DH, Linde LM, Miller JH, O'Reilly RJ: Relationship between lung volume and pulmonary vascular resistance. Circ Res 1961; 9:465–471.
133. Rawal N, Nuutinen L, Paj PP, et al: Behavioral and histopathologic effects following intrathecal administration of butorphanol, sufentanil, and nalbuphine in sheep. Anesthesiology 1991; 75:1025–1034.
134. Gustafsson LL, Schildt B, Jacobsen K: Adverse effects of epidural and intrathecal opiates: Report of a nationwide survey in Sweden. Br J Anaesth 1982; 54:479–485.
135. Bromage PR, Camporesi EM, Durant PAC, Nielsen CH: Rostral spread of epidural morphine. Anesthesiology 1982; 56:431–436.
136. Abboud TK, Moore M, Zhu j, et al: Epidural butorphanol or morphine for the relief of post-cesarean section pain: Ventilatory responses to carbon dioxide. Anesth Analg 1987; 66:887–893.
137. Cohen SE, Labaille T, Benhamou D, Levron J-C: Respiratory effects of epidural sufentanil after cesarean section. Anesth Analg 1992; 74:677–682.
138. Brockway MS, Noble DW, Sharwood-Smith GH, McClure JH: Profound respiratory depression after extradural fentanyl. Br J Anaesth 1990; 64:243–245.
139. Rawal N, Wattwil M: Respiratory depression after epidural morphine—An experimental and clinical study. Anesth Analg 1984; 63:8–14.
140. Chan FY, Pun TC, Lee CP, et al: A comparative study of continuous- and pulsed-wave Doppler velocimetry in fetal and uteroplacental circulation. J Ultrasound Med 1991; 10:277–280.
141. Forouzan I, Cohen AW, Arger P: Measurement of systolic-diastolic ratio in the umbilical artery by continuous-wave and pulsed-wave Doppler ultrasound: Comparison at different sites. Obstet Gynecol 1991; 77:209–212.
142. Manning FA: General principles and application of ultrasound. *In* Creasy R, Resnik R (eds): Maternal-Fetal Medicine, 2nd Ed. Philadelphia: WB Saunders, 1989; 203.
143. Harrison MR, Golbus MS, Filly RA, et al: Fetal hydronephrosis: Selection and surgical repair. J Pediatr Surg 1987; 22:556–558.
144. Touloukian RJ: What's new in pediatric surgery. Pediatrics 1988; 81:692–696.
145. Zelop C, Nadel A, Frigoletto FD, et al: Placenta accreta/percreta/increta: A cause of elevated maternal serum alpha-fetoprotein. Obstet Gynecol 1992; 80:693–694.
146. Jouppila P, Kirkinen P: Blood velocity waveforms of the fetal aorta in normal and hypertensive pregnancies. Obstet Gynecol 1986; 67:857–858.
147. Farmakides G, Schulman H, Schneider E: Surveillance of the pregnant hypertensive patient with Doppler flow velocimetry. Clin Obstet Gynecol 1992; 35:387–396.
148. Fleischer A, Schulman H, Farmakides G, et al: Uterine artery Doppler velocimetry in pregnant women with hypertension. Am J Obstet Gynecol 1986; 154:806–813.
149. Fairlie FM, Moretti M, Walker JJ, et al: Determinants of perinatal outcome in pregnancy-induced hypertension with absence of umbilical artery end-diastolic frequencies. Am J Obstet Gynecol 1991; 164:1084–1089.
150. Bekedam DJ, Visser GHA, Van der Zee AGJ, et al: Abnormal umbilical artery waveform patterns in growth retarded fetuses: Relationship to antepartum late heart rate decelerations and outcome. Early Hum Dev 1990; 24:79–90.
151. Hitschold T, Weiss E, Beck T, et al: Low target birth weight or growth retardation: Umbilical Doppler flow velocity waveforms and histometric analysis of fetoplacental vascular tree. Am J Obstet Gynecol 1993; 168:1260–1264.
152. Ducey J, Schulman H, Farmakides G, et al: A classification of hypertension in pregnancy based on Doppler velocimetry. Am J Obstet Gynecol 1987; 157:680–685.
153. Arduini D, Rizzo G, Romanini C: The development of abnormal heart rate patterns after absent end-diastolic velocity in umbilical artery: Analysis of risk factors. Am J Obstet Gynecol 1993; 168:43–50.
154. Indik JH, Chen V, Reed KL: Association of umbilical venous with inferior vena cava blood flow velocities. Obstet Gynecol 1991; 77:551–557.
155. Rizzo G, Arduini D, Romanini C: Inferior vena cava flow velocity waveforms in appropriate- and small-for-gestational-age fetuses. Am J Obstet Gynecol 1992; 166:1271–1280.
156. Rizzo G, Arduini D, Luciano R, et al: Prenatal cerebral Doppler ultrasonography and neonatal neurologic outcome. J Ultrasound Med 1989; 8:238–240.
157. Paneth N: Birth and the origins of cerebral palsy. N Engl J Med 1986; 315:124–126.

158. Nelson KB, Ellenberg JH: Antecedents of cerebral palsy. Multivariate analysis of risk. N Engl J Med 1986; 315:81–86.
159. Arduini D, Rizzo G, Romanini C, Mancuso S: Are blood velocity waveforms related to umbilical cord acid-base status in the human fetus? Gynecol Obstet Invest 1989; 27:183–187.
160. van den Wijngaard JA, Groenenberg IA, Wladimiroff JW, Hop WC: Cerebral Doppler ultrasound of the human fetus. Br J Obstet Gynaecol 1989; 96:845–849.
161. Veille JC, Cohen I: Middle cerebral artery blood flow in normal and growth-retarded fetuses. Am J Obstet Gynecol 1990; 162:391–396.
162. Mari G, Deter RL: Middle cerebral artery flow velocity waveforms in normal and small-for-gestational-age fetuses. Am J Obstet Gynecol 1992; 166:1262–1270.
163. Vyas S, Nicolaides KH, Bower S, Campbell S: Middle cerebral artery flow velocity waveforms in fetal hypoxaemia. Br J Obstet Gynaecol 1990; 97:797–803.
164. Freeman RK: Contraction stress testing for primary fetal surveillance in patients at high risk for uteroplacental insufficiency. Clin Perinatol 1982; 9:265–270.
165. Nielsen PV, Stigsby B, Nickelson C, Nin J: Intra- and inter-observer variability in the assessment of intrapartum cardiotocograms. Acta Obstet Gynaecol Scand 1987; 66:421–424.
166. Borgata L, Shrout PE, Divon MY: Reliability and reproducibility of nonstress test readings. Am J Obstet Gynecol 1988; 159:554–558.
167. Gagnon R, Campbell MK, Hunse C: A comparison between visual and computer analysis of antepartum fetal heart rate tracings. Am J Obstet Gynecol 1993; 168:842–847.
168. Dawes GS, Moulden M, Redman CW: Limitations of antenatal fetal heart rate monitors. Am J Obstet Gynecol 1990; 162:170–173.
169. Chen C, Roby PV, Weiss NS, et al: Clinical evaluation of the NBD-PC fluorescence polarization assay for prediction of fetal lung maturity. Obstet Gynecol 1992; 80:688–692.
170. Russell JC, Cooper CM, Ketchum CH, et al: Multicenter evaluation of TDx test for assessing fetal lung maturity. Clin Chem 1989; 35:1005–1010.
171. Talt JF, Foerder CA, Ashwood ER, Benedetti TJ: Prospective clinical evaluation of an improved fluorescence polarization assay for predicting fetal lung maturity. Clin Chem 1987; 33:554–558.
172. Herbert WNP, Chapman JF, Schnoor MM: Role of the TDx FLM assay in fetal lung maturity. Am J Obstet Gynecol 1993; 168:808–812.
173. Pearlman ES, Baiocchi JM, Lease JA, et al: Utility of a rapid lamellar body count in the assessment of fetal maturity. Am J Clin Pathol 1991; 95:778–780.
174. Statland BE, Sher G: Reliability of amniotic fluid surfactant measurements. Am J Clin Pathol 1985; 83:1629–1641.
175. Ashwood ER, Palmer SE, Lenke RR: Rapid fetal lung maturity testing: Commercial versus NBD-phosphatidylcholine assay. Obstet Gynecol 1992; 80:1048–1053.
176. Herbert WNP, Chapman JF: Clinical and economic considerations associated with testing for fetal lung maturity. Am J Obstet Gynecol 1986; 155:820–823.
177. Martin CB: Physiologic and clinical use of fetal heart rate variability. Clin Perinatol 1982; 9:339–351.
178. Parer JT, Livingston EG: What is fetal distress? Am J Obstet Gynecol 1990; 162:1421–1427.
179. Reed KL, Appleton CP, Anderson CF, et al: Doppler studies of vena cava flows in human fetuses. Insights into normal and abnormal cardiac physiology. Circulation 1990; 81:498–505.
180. Weiss E, Hitschold T, Berle P: Umbilical artery blood flow velocity waveforms during variable deceleration of the fetal heart rate. Am J Obstet Gynecol 1991; 164:534–540.
181. Svenningsen L, Lindemann R, Eidal K: Measurements of fetal head compression pressure during bearing down and their relationship to the condition of the newborn. Acta Obstet Gynaecol Scand 1988; 67:129–133.
182. Hon EH: Instrumentation of fetal heart rate and fetal electrocardiography. Obstet Gynecol 1967; 30:281–286.
183. Krebs HB, Petres RE, Dunn LJ, et al: Intrapartum fetal heart rate monitoring: Classification and prognosis of fetal heart rate patterns. Am J Obstet Gynecol 1975; 133:762–772.
184. Paul RH, Suidan AK, Yeh SY, et al: Clinical fetal monitoring. VII. The evaluation and significance of intrapartum baseline FHR variability. Am J Obstet Gynecol 1975; 123:206–210.
185. Shy KK, Luthy DA, Bennett FC, et al: Effects of electronic fetal-heart-rate monitoring, as compared with periodic auscultation, on the neurologic development of premature infants. N Engl J Med 1990; 322:588–593.
186. Rosen MG, Dickinson JC: The paradox of electronic fetal monitoring: More data may not enable us to predict or prevent infant neurologic morbidity. Am J Obstet Gynecol 1993; 168:745–751.
187. Morrison JC, Chez BF, Davis ID: Intrapartum fetal heart rate assessment: Monitoring by auscultation or electronic means. Am J Obstet Gynecol 1993; 168:63–66.
188. Parer JT: Fetal heart rate. *In* Creasy R, Resnik R (eds): Maternal-Fetal Medicine. Philadelphia: WB Saunders, 1984; 314.
189. Vintzileos AM, Antsaklis A, Varvarigos I, et al: A randomized trial of intrapartum electronic fetal heart rate monitoring versus intermittent auscultation. Obstet Gynecol 1993; 81:899–907.
190. Trudinger BJ, Cook CM, Giles WB, et al: Umbilical artery flow velocity waveforms in high-risk pregnancy. Randomized controlled trial. Lancet 1987; 1(8526):188–190.
191. Bowen LW, Kochenour NK, Rehm NE, Woolley FR: Maternal-fetal pH difference and fetal scalp pH as predictors of neonatal outcome. Obstet Gynecol 1986; 67:487–495.
192. Wible JL, Petrie RH, Koons A, Perez A: The clinical use of umbilical cord acid-base determinations in perinatal surveillance and management. Clin Perinatol 1982; 9:387–397.
193. Miller FC: Prediction of acid-base values from intrapartum fetal heart rate data and their correlation with scalp and fundic values. Clin Perinatol 1982; 9:353–361.
194. Johnson N, Johnson VA, Fisher J, et al: Fetal monitoring with pulse oximetry. Br J Obstet Gynaecol 1991; 98:36–41.
195. Johnson N, Johnson VA, Bannister J, Lilford RJ: The effect of caput succedaneum on oxygen saturation measurement. Br J Obstet Gynaecol 1990; 97:493–498.
196. Johnson N, Johnson VA, Bannister J, McNamara H: The effect of meconium on neonatal and fetal reflectance pulse oximetry. J Perinat Med 1990; 18:351–355.
197. McNamara H, Johnson N, Lilford R: The effect on fetal arteriolar oxygen saturation resulting from giving oxygen to the mother measured by pulse oximetry. Br J Obstet Gynaecol 1993; 100:446–449.
198. Harris AP, Sendak MJ, Chung DC, et al: Validation of arterial oxygen saturation measurements in utero using pulse oximetry. Am J Perinatol 1993; 10:250–254.
199. Sarno AP, Ahn MO, Brar HS, et al: Intrapartum Doppler velocimetry, amniotic fluid volume, and fetal heart rate as predictors of subsequent fetal distress. Am J Obstet Gynecol 1989; 161:1508–1514.
200. Lombardi SJ, Rosemond R, Ball R, et al: Umbilical artery velocimetry as a predictor of adverse outcome in pregnancies complicated by oligohydramnios. Obstet Gynecol 1989; 74:338–341.
201. Apgar V: A proposal for a new method of evaluation of the newborn infant. Anesth Analg 1953; 32:260–267.
202. Fanconi S: Reliability of pulse oximetry in hypoxic infants. J Pediatr 1988; 112:424–427.
203. McNamara H, Chung DC, Lilford R, Johnson N: Do fetal pulse oximetry readings at delivery correlate with cord blood oxygenation and acidaemia? Br J Obstet Gynecol 1992; 99:735–738.
204. Dimich I, Singh PP, Adell A, et al: Evaluation of oxygen saturation monitoring by pulse oximetry in neonates in the delivery system. Can J Anaesth 1991; 38:985–988.
205. Woods AM: Cardiopulmonary resuscitation. *In* Berry FA, Steward DJ (eds): Pediatrics for the Anesthesiologist. New York: Churchill Livingstone, 1993; 322–323.

CHAPTER 19

Monitoring in Radiology

STEVEN C. HALL, M.D.

Monitoring for radiologic procedures incorporates multiple equipment, space, and patient considerations. Anesthesiologists are usually involved in patient care during radiologic procedures for one of two reasons. The first and most common reason is that the patient is not cooperative enough to allow the radiologic procedure to be performed in an efficient and effective manner. As a practical matter, pediatric patients are much more likely to be uncooperative. Even when the radiologic procedure involves some discomfort, such as embolization procedures, adults usually tolerate the process without the need for significant sedation or anesthesia. Therefore, planning for monitoring during radiologic procedures usually is oriented to the needs of the pediatric patient. The basic principles of monitoring and safe administration of sedatives or anesthetics are similar for adult and pediatric patient populations. Most of this chapter, however, will be oriented to the pediatric patient.

The second reason that monitoring may be indicated is that the patient is medically unstable. Patients with cardiopulmonary, metabolic, or central nervous system (CNS) instability may need intensive continuous monitoring related to the underlying medical condition. The intubated, ventilated victim of a motor vehicle accident may undergo a variety of radiologic examinations as part of initial evaluation. This patient may have injuries to a number of systems that may complicate monitoring and medical management. Increased intracranial pressure and hypovolemia from blood loss, for instance, are two sources of instability during the radiologic procedure, potentially requiring both increased monitoring and therapeutic intervention. The anesthesiologist's role in this situation is primarily to monitor the patient's abnormal and, possibly changing, medical status. The degree of monitoring, then, is largely determined by the patient's status, not the radiologic procedure.

Monitoring during radiologic procedures is determined by the needs of the patient and the limitations of the radiologic suite. When general anesthesia is administered, monitoring is based on the usual standards for intraoperative monitoring practiced in that institution. These standards usually are adapted from the recommendations of the American Society of Anesthesiologists for basic intraoperative monitoring.[1] When sedation is used instead of general anesthesia, many anesthesiologists apply general anesthesia guidelines for monitoring. However, these rigorous guidelines are not often used during sedation in the radiologic suite when nonanesthesiologists are providing the care.[2] The appropriate level of care in these situations is a source of controversy. Although there are no formal guidelines from the radiologic professional societies on the need for monitoring during procedures, the American Academy of Pediatrics has revised guidelines to be applied whenever sedation is used in children.[3]

RADIATION SAFETY

Ionizing radiation, whether x-rays, gamma rays, or other accelerated particles, can cause tissue damage and chromosomal changes. The opportunity for exposure to ionizing radiation varies with the procedure and equipment. X-rays are generated and emitted from a single source, pass through the tissue to be imaged, and then are detected by either a film or an image intensifier. The closer the tissue is to the source of the x-ray, the higher the level of radiation exposure. With fluoroscopy, there is a greater amount of radiation emitted, as well as a longer exposure. Computed tomography (CT) is based on emission of x-rays in a narrow beam that is detected by an image intensifier after passing through the body. Although the slice of exposed tissue is narrow (1–13 mm), the exposure in that area is high. The technique requires multiple exposures to build a useful image.[4] Radioisotope techniques are based on a tracer that is labeled with a gamma ray–emitting isotope. The tracer that is used is picked for its ability to identify and be concentrated in a particular organ or tissue. Also, the amount of isotope is selected to provide an adequate view of the target tissue.[5] Anesthesiologists rarely are significantly exposed to radioisotopes.

When the anesthesiologist or anesthetist is caring for a patient in the presence of ionizing radiation, it is the responsibility of the radiologist to provide the minimum amount of radiation to the patient. However, it is the responsibility of the anesthesiologist to take adequate safety precautions to prevent personal radiation exposure.

The objectives of radiation safety are twofold. The first objective is to eliminate, as far as possible, any exposure to ionizing radiation. The lowest amount of radiation that can induce subtle or significant damage or changes in a human is not known. The second goal is to minimize exposure to radiation when exposure is unavoidable. Although it is unusual for an anesthesiologist to be placed directly in the beam of radiation, this can happen by accident. The more common and pervasive source of radiation exposure is scatter radiation.

RADIATION SOURCES

Radiation scattered from the field is the primary source of exposure for both anesthesia and radiology personnel. The anesthesiologist should understand the nature of scatter as a basis for limiting exposure. The amount of scatter increases in a more than linear fashion when either the power output of the beam or the size of the imaged field increases. Therefore, the scatter for a film of the entire abdomen is greater than the scatter for a film of the hand. Fluoroscopy uses a high-power beam for prolonged periods, increasing scatter. Thus, fluoroscopy of the heart during a cardiac catheterization produces a high level of scatter, whereas a chest film of a neonate produces very little scatter. Another example is the CT scanner. Although the beams of a CT scanner are relatively powerful, they are tightly focused, reducing the amount of scatter.

The exposure to scatter radiation falls off at a rate equal to the inverse square of the distance from the field. The farther from the field, the greater the reduction in exposure. Because this is not a linear relationship, the greater distance results in significant protection; at 1 meter from the field, the exposure is usually less than 1/1000 the exposure at the field. Radiation is commonly expressed in the United States as rad (*r*adiation *a*bsorbed *d*ose) and rem (*r*oentgen *e*quivalent *m*an) units. However, the rest of the world uses the metric system of measurements, with the *sievert,* equivalent to 1 joule/kg, as the measurement of dose. One sievert (Sv) is equivalent to 100 rad or rem. The various nomenclatures can be confusing, with recommendations for exposure limits in multiple terms.

Quantifying exposure depends on the size of the target, the size of the patient, and the length of exposure. For instance, a 10-year-old patient is exposed to about 25 mrem for a chest radiograph, but fluoroscopy for 4 minutes delivers 6800 mrem to the skin and 200 mrem to the whole body.[6] These are single exposures. In comparison, background radiation provides exposure, over the course of a year, that varies from 40 to 200 mrem in the United States, depending on location. Thus, occupational exposure may be less than normal exposure from the environment. However, when monitoring radiologic procedures, there is the risk of additional exposure.

RADIATION RISKS

Two of the major risks of occupational exposure to ionizing radiation for anesthesiologists are the risk of genetic damage and the risk of cancer. The National Council on Radiation Protection and Measurements (NCRP) has published guidelines for acceptable radiation exposure. A single whole-body dose of 0.1 Sv produces an excess lifetime probability risk of 0.04 for fatal cancer and a risk of 0.008 for severe genetic effect or nonfatal cancer. Because of this, the NCRP recommended an annual occupational exposure maximum of 50 mSv (0.05 Sv). The annual limit for nonoccupational exposure is 5 mSv (5 rem). The risk of genetic damage has been based primarily on studies of civilians exposed to atomic bomb blasts during the Second World War. This risk appears to be less than previously thought, although the risk of cancer is higher.[6]

The risk of cancer is of greatest concern to those exposed to radiation repeatedly. It is well known that large doses of radiation cause cancer in humans.[7] The primary cancer risks after excessive exposure include leukemia and thyroid cancer. However, individuals rarely are exposed to excessive doses of radiation. It appears that the cancer risk to a patient from diagnostic radiologic procedures is low.[8] At lower doses, there are two important factors: first, the total amount of radiation exposure; second, the rate of exposure. A large total dose received over a long period is less likely to produce adverse effects than is the same dose in a single exposure. A single individual exposure greater than 50 rad (0.5 Sv) is considered a significant risk factor for development of cancer.[9]

Is there specific epidemiologic evidence that exposure during radiologic diagnostic procedures is safe or harmful? A retrospective study of children undergoing cardiac catheterization under fluoroscopy looked at the incidence of subsequent cancer. The study of 4891 patients followed the children for an average of 13 years after catheterization.[10] There were no cases of breast or thyroid carcinoma detected, and the incidence of leukemia and other solid tumors was normal. It is certainly possible that 13 years is not long enough to get a true picture of the potential risk of cancer development. However, these data are encouraging about the safety of exposure for diagnostic purposes.

Localized exposure to radiation can cause circumscribed damage. This potential is especially problematic for radiology personnel, whose hands are at risk for repeated exposure from holding young pediatric patients still for films. The lens of the eye is extraordinarily susceptible to damage and cataract formation. This is a complication that is related to the cumulative effect of multiple exposures, not to a single exposure. Consequently, there are NCRP recommendations for maximum annual exposures for specific areas of the body. The annual limit is 150 mSv for the lens of the eye and 500 mSv for localized skin or extremity exposure.

Exposure of high doses of radiation to the fetus can result in noticeable damage, specifically in the CNS. Mental retardation and small head size were the only abnormalities reported above statistical norms for newborns after *in utero* exposure to high levels of radiation.[11] The NCRP recommends a monthly dose limit of 0.5 mSv to the fetus once pregnancy is detected.

PREVENTION OF EXPOSURE

Anesthesiologists must observe the same safety precautions as full-time radiology department personnel. Lead aprons should be worn whenever there is a chance of exposure. If the anesthesiologist will be turning away from the radiation beam, the apron must cover his or her front, back, and sides. It is also considered prudent to wear a thyroid collar if exposure is going to be prolonged. Especially in the cardiac catheterization laboratory, there is a risk of long, repeated exposures during fluoroscopy. In this situation, the risk of cataracts from eye lens exposure should be considered. Leaded glass screens are available that allow observation of the patient and equipment without direct exposure to the radiation. Treated glasses and goggles are also available but tend to be cumbersome.

It should be stressed that protection from radiation should be a prospective aspect of delivering care and monitoring in at-risk sites. The anesthesiologist must minimize the potential for exposure, as well as wear protective attire. Personnel should only be exposed to the potential of scatter radiation when presence in the exposure area is necessary for patient welfare. Radiologists are often not accustomed to having anesthesia personnel present during their procedures, and anesthesiologists are often not aware of the protocols, procedures, and customs of the radiology suite. Radiologists must also ensure that anesthesia personnel are properly protected and situated to minimize exposure to scatter. The anesthesiologist should also be told when radiation is about to be emitted. At this point, the anesthesiologist should not only recheck protective attire and shielding but also should move as far from the beam as possible without interfering with patient monitoring. Moving 2 meters from the beam decreases scatter exposure to the same level as does having 2.5 mm of lead (the equivalent of five lead aprons) or 9 inches of concrete between the beam and the anesthesiologist.[12]

If anesthesia personnel repeatedly are exposed to radiation, it may be useful to wear the same radiation measuring devices used by the radiology department. However, an anesthesiologist rarely will be exposed enough to activate safety measures based on overexposure. More importantly, the monitoring of exposure provides positive information only after the exposure has already occurred. The two keys to minimizing the risk of radiation exposure continue to be increased distance from the beam and field and protective shielding.

COMPUTED TOMOGRAPHY

CT has significantly advanced cross-sectional visualization of areas of the body. The patient is placed in the core of an instrument that has image intensifier detectors arranged in a circle around the core. The x-ray source then rotates in the circle, emitting a narrow beam. The multiple images are compiled and displayed on a monitor and on film.[6] The computer reconstruction of sectional views allows a great deal of flexibility in the presentation of the data. The narrow beam allows visualization of cross-sectional areas that are only 1–13 mm thick; however, multiple exposures of the area are needed to build a useful image.[4] For this reason, there is significant radiation exposure with CT imaging, although in a narrow "window."

INDICATIONS

Elective or emergency CT imaging is particularly useful to evaluate the brain and spinal cord, facial bone structure, thoracic masses, abdominal masses, and potential knee injuries. CT imaging of the brain has been found useful in detecting generalized cerebral edema,[13] neonatal hypoxic/ischemic brain damage,[14] and intracerebral and subarachnoid bleeding.[15] These images provide information not only for diagnosis, but also as a practical guide to surgical intervention.

Emergency CT imaging is usually of the CNS and the abdomen.[6] CNS evaluations are important in evaluation of the patient with potential head injury or altered state of consciousness. The examination is useful for identifying increased intracranial pressure, such as ventriculoperitoneal shunt malfunction, or presence of space-occupying lesions, such as a subdural hematoma. These evaluations are often used as the basis of determining the need for surgical versus medical interventions.

The other area commonly scanned in an emergency is the abdomen. Combined with abdominal ultrasound, CT scanning has revolutionized the evaluation and treatment of the patient with blunt abdominal trauma. In the past, the traumatized patient with signs of an "acute abdomen" underwent exploratory laparotomy,[16] which was associated with significant morbidity and mortality. However, with the availability of ultrasound and CT scanning on an emergency basis, liver, spleen, or kidney injuries can be identified without laparotomy. Traumatized patients can then often be medically managed with blood and fluid replacement and close observation instead of surgical intervention, reducing morbidity and mortality.[17]

ANESTHESIA MANAGEMENT

All commonly available monitors work in the presence of the CT scanner without need for modification. The CT room is often small, requiring resourceful spacing of equipment and personnel. The patient is moved in and out of the scanner, potentially kinking or dislodging leads and cables.

As with angiography and magnetic resonance imaging (MRI), intravenous contrast media are occasionally used in the CT evaluation, with the potential risk of adverse reactions. These reactions have included transient increase in neurologic signs in children with sickle cell disease and seizures in patients with CNS tumors.[15]

The need for patient monitoring depends on the status of the patient. Unstable patients, such as a trauma victim, deserve the same monitoring in the CT scanner that they would receive in the emergency room or intensive care unit. Often, critically ill patients being treated in an intensive care setting are brought to the CT scanner for reassessment of their CNS status. These patients may require significant cardiopulmonary support and monitoring, which can be provided with portable equipment brought with the patient. Monitors, ventilators, and infusion pumps work normally in the presence of the CT scanner.

Sedation Versus General Anesthesia

For CT imaging and other radiologic procedures, patient immobility is crucial. Patient motion during the examination degrades the images.[18, 19] Although the periods of radiation exposure and imaging are short, the patient must be relatively motionless during the entire period of the scan. The time of each scan is usually only 2–3 minutes, and the total time in the newest scanners has dropped from an hour to less than half an hour. Nevertheless, some children, anxious adults, or patients with altered levels of consciousness will not cooperate. In these situations, a decision must be made about the need for the study and the means by which to complete it. Sedation and general anesthesia are two techniques that can be used to provide patient immobility. When these techniques are employed, the need for patient monitoring increases.

MONITORING

Monitoring during general anesthesia is straightforward. The same standards and guidelines used in the operating room can and should be used in the CT scanner.[1] These monitors can be arranged such that the anesthesiologist can be outside the scanning room during the brief periods of radiation and continue to watch both the monitors and the patient through a leaded glass window or open doorway.

However, for three reasons, the sedated patient is a practical problem in the CT scanner. First, sedation in this setting is often given by radiologists or other nonanesthesia practitioners. Their expertise in giving sedation to patients of different ages and medical conditions varies from individual to individual. Second, the primary attention of the radiologist is often on the scan, with less attention paid to the patient. The responsibility for monitoring the patient may or may not be the primary responsibility of another individual. Third, the intensity of monitoring of the sedated patient has been minimal in many circumstances. An understanding of the risks of the sedated patient is necessary for safe monitoring of these patients.

The most common complications related specifically to sedation are airway obstruction and hypoventilation.[18, 20–25] In a prospective study of children sedated for CT, respiratory depression was the leading cause of serious risk to the patient, and the depression from sedative medications lasted for a prolonged period after the scan was over.[26] Monitoring for adequacy of ventilation, such as capnography, chest plethysmography, and direct observation, address the primary complications of sedation, whereas pulse oximetry, blood pressure, and heart rate and rhythm monitoring identify secondary signs of hypoxemia and cardiac decompensation.

Monitoring is relatively easy for sedated patients in the CT scanner. However, recent evidence has demonstrated that monitoring is not widely used for sedated patients, at least for sedated pediatric patients. A questionnaire was sent in 1988 to 834 hospitals to survey their sedation and monitoring practices. The institutions ranged from small community hospitals to large teaching hospitals.[2] Several interesting findings came from the study. First, the radiologist was responsible for ordering the sedation in 47% of the cases; a primary care physician was responsible for 37% of the cases. Anesthesiologists were responsible in only 3% of the cases. Second, the institutions characterized the sedation prescribed as being ''light'' or ''conscious'' sedation in the vast majority of cases. Third, the radiologist was often not in attendance during the procedure, being present in about 55% of the cases. The person most likely to be present was the CT technician performing the study. A registered nurse was present in 27% (light sedation) or 47% (deep sedation) of the cases.

However, the most disturbing part of this study was the degree of monitoring employed. The common monitoring technique was visual inspection from the control room. When the child received light sedation, blood pressure measurement was used in 25% of the institutions and an electrocardiogram (ECG), respiratory monitor, pulse oximeter, or automated blood pressure machine were used in 5% or less of the reporting institutions. When the child received deep sedation, ECG was used in 45% of the institutions, respiratory monitoring in 25%, pulse oximetry in 20%, and automated blood pressure in 15%. This lack of monitors is undesirable, especially when the most commonly present person—the CT technician—is occupied with responsibilities other than the direct observation of the patient.

The question of monitoring the sedated patient is important. One review discussed an article on the safety of chloral hydrate during CT scanning. The author noted vomiting in 4% of patients, hyperactivity in 1%, and respiratory complications in 1%.[20] A close look at the data gives a different interpretation, however. Although chloral hydrate causes less ventilatory depression than do barbiturates or narcotics, respiratory complications can occur. There were four episodes of respiratory complications in this study. One patient developed wheezing; one had copious secretions; but two patients developed upper airway obstruction that required intubation! This and other articles demonstrate that significant airway obstruction can occur, even with light sedation. Monitoring is needed to detect this obstruction.

When deeper levels of sedation are used, monitoring becomes even more important. Radiologists are increasingly aggressive in using intravenous medications in relatively high doses to sedate patients.[22, 27] An example of this is an article demonstrating the use of intravenous pentobarbital and propofol during imaging procedures.[28] At the beginning of the study, anesthesiologists were present with the radiologists during the propofol infusions. However, as the study progressed, the radiologists became the only physicians present. An accompanying editorial by anesthesiologists question the safety of administration of anesthetic agents by radiologists or other nonanesthesiologists.[29] Monitoring and safety issues, as well as liability issues, are involved.

Each institution should have guidelines covering the monitoring of sedated patients, as well as the qualifications of those administering the sedation. The Joint Commission on Accreditation of Healthcare Organizations (JCAHO) has published rules for the development of guidelines for accredited institutions. Their rules state that when medications are given that can result in loss of consciousness, there should be mechanisms or processes specified for evaluating and monitoring these activities, as well as guidelines for safe administration.[30] The anesthesia department has a responsibility, through its director, to participate with services that administer these drugs to develop and establish guidelines. A recent letter from the JCAHO and the chairman of the American Society of Anesthesiologist's (ASA) Committee on Standards has clarified the responsibility of the anesthesia director to participate in, though not necessarily control, development of guidelines.[31] It remains the responsibility of the service providing the sedation to provide safe conditions.

There are no published standards for monitoring during CT or other radiologic procedures by a national organization. Suggestions about appropriate monitoring have been made by individual authors.[32, 33] However, standards and guidelines have been published by several national nonradiologic organizations for safe monitoring and care in sedated patients,[3, 34, 35] such as the guidelines published by the American Academy of Pediatrics (AAP).[3]

The AAP guidelines are specifically aimed at children but can be used for any patient. In terms of monitoring the sedated patients, there are four points of interest. First, conscious sedation is defined as a state of depressed consciousness in which the patient retains a patent airway and protective reflexes, as well as being arousable by verbal command or physical stimulation. Deep sedation is defined as a state from which the patient is not easily aroused or does not maintain an adequate airway. This distinction is made to determine the level of monitoring but is probably artificial, because patients can move from one level of depression to another. Second, there should be documentation of vital signs during the sedation and in the recovery period. Third, monitoring during conscious sedation should include continuous pulse oximetry or other measurement of oxygen saturation and heart rate in addition to intermittent respiratory rate and blood pressure measurements. For the patient receiving deep sedation, ECG monitoring is added. The fourth requirement of interest is for monitoring personnel. Conscious sedation requires a person in addition to the practitioner performing the procedure to monitor the child. Deep sedation requires that monitoring personnel be concerned solely with monitoring.

These guidelines from the AAP suggest standards for monitoring patients undergoing sedation, on which each institution can develop its own standards. However, it should be recognized that sedatives often are administered by radiologists or others with limited training in the use of these drugs. Physicians who administer sedatives are responsible for providing adequate and timely monitoring. Such care requires guidelines developed in conjunction with the director of anesthesia services. If the radiology department can not provide adequate conditions safely, the anesthesia department should help out.

THE RADIOLOGY SUITE—ANGIOGRAPHY AND EMBOLIZATION

INDICATIONS

Angiography usually is performed because of vascular disease or malignancy. In the CNS, angiography is useful in diagnosing and delineating tumors, aneurysms, and arteriovenous malformations. Peripheral vascular angiography is commonly performed for clarification of arterial and venous lesions, especially those associated with arteriosclerosis. Anesthesiologists may be requested to help monitor and provide sedation or anesthesia for a variety of reasons.

First, angiography can be painful. Large-bore catheters are inserted, often via the femoral vessels. Patients may find the discomfort of these manipulations and injection of media painful, and they may find the prolonged period of immobility on the examining table distressing. A feeling of doom has been described with some angiographic injections. Second, some patients may not stay still enough, especially children. If the patient moves during the injection of dye, the subsequent image may not be adequate. Lastly, the patient may require direct attention. The comatose patient may require controlled ventilation and monitoring of intracranial pressure, the trauma patient may have evolving CNS or cardiopulmonary instability, and the patient with significant arteriosclerotic disease may suffer cardiovascular compromise with the stress of the angiography.

MONITORING

Monitoring for the patient undergoing angiography is based on both the patient's medical condition and the anticipated stress of the angiography. The patient's anticipated medical status is the primary factor in determining the monitoring to be used. For instance, if the patient may have increased intracranial pressure from cerebral edema or a mass lesion, the monitoring (and anesthetic technique) used will be equivalent to that used during a surgical procedure.

Blood Pressure

Blood pressure monitoring is an important tool for modifying therapy. Hypertension during laryngoscopy or other maneuvers must be treated quickly, because there is a danger of hemorrhage in patients with an aneurysm or vascular malformation[36, 37] and a danger of increased cerebral blood flow and volume in patients who have lost autoregulation, such as in the presence of global ischemia. Although blood pressure can be measured using any of the standard methods, intra-arterial monitoring is considered if the patient is critically ill to allow beat-to-beat evaluation of the blood pressure.

Ventilation

The patient with intracranial pathology may also benefit from alteration in cerebral blood flow by controlling and monitoring ventilation.[38, 39] Hyperventilation decreases elevated intracranial pressure by decreasing cerebral blood volume. On the other hand, spontaneous ventilation during administration of anesthetic volatile agents increases cerebral blood flow and volume, an undesirable result if intracranial pressure is already increased.[40] Mild hyperventilation and cerebral vasoconstriction have the additional benefit of a slower transit of dye through the brain, enhancing the quality of the films.[6] On the other hand, sedation without control of the airway can increase carbon dioxide tensions[41] and depress arterial oxygen tensions,[22] both of which can be detrimental in patients with increased intracranial pressure.

Electrocardiogram

Electrocardiographic monitoring is standard in patients undergoing anesthesia.[1] It can also be important in the sedated patient if the patient is at risk for cardiac disease. If the patient has significant coronary artery disease, there may be a risk of dysrhythmias or ischemia during the stress of angiography. ECG monitoring in this situation is evaluated for both rhythm and ST-T wave configuration. The same leads and analysis should be used in the angiographic suite as in the operating room (see Chapters 4 and 5).

General Monitors

The only limits on the type of monitoring that can be used in the angiography suite are those of mobility and space. The angiography suite is often crowded with multiple machines and personnel. Access to the patient often is restricted because of other fixed equipment. Also, lighting is often not of the same bright caliber one is used to in the operating room. The anesthesiologist must be able to see and access both the patient and the monitors. There must also be enough electrical outlets for both monitors and other anesthesia-related equipment. There should be an understanding with the radiology staff about provision of adequate conditions before committing to assisting with the procedure instead of scrambling to make adjustments at the last minute. If additional personnel are needed to help with the monitoring or to assist in tasks such as blood gas analysis, this should be arranged before the procedure begins. As the radiographic intervention proceeds, close communication between the radiologist and anesthesiologist is essential to ensure successful and expeditious care.

A special adjunct to angiography used for lesions such as arteriovenous malformations is embolization. The malformations can be located peripherally or in internal organs such as the liver.[42] These patients may require aggressive monitoring because of the additional cardiovascular stress of the lesion. For instance, newborns and infants with large arteriovenous malformations can suffer high-output cardiac failure.[43] The heart failure should be treated and the patient should be stabilized as much as possible before proceeding with sedation or anesthesia.[44] The patient may also be relatively hypovolemic secondary to persistent bleeding from the lesion. After angiography to delineate the lesion, materials such as Gelfoam pledgets, wire coils, or cyanoacrylates are used as emboli. Toxic chemicals can cause local and systemic reactions. However, the more common problems of bleeding or migration of the embolic material to a distal site may require surgical intervention. This may require transporting the patient to an operating room to gain wider exposure to the area at risk.

Special mention should be made of cerebral angiography and embolization. Rarely, embolization of a cerebral arteriovenous malformation is done on an awake patient. The purpose is to use the patient's level of consciousness and other signs as a monitor of effectiveness of the procedure. If this is done, the anesthesiologist must be able to provide sedation, but not anesthesia, to allow patient cooperation.[45]

Monitoring for Complications

Media contrast reactions are of particular concern during angiography. Contrast media are associated with cardiovascular, CNS, and renal complications. There are two types of media contrast agents, the older high-osmolality agents (1400–1500 mOsm/L) and the newer low-osmolality agents (600–700 mOsm/L).[46] The incidence of reactions is higher with the older agents.[47] These agents have direct myocardial depressant, arrhythmogenic, and vasodilating properties; after injection, there is often transient hypertension followed by hypotension. Seizures and cerebral edema can also result. There is diuresis from the dye that can become hemodynamically significant. Monitoring of output with a urinary catheter may be necessary to guide intravenous fluid replacement. Because the media are nephrotoxic in large doses,[48] a running total of the amount of dye used should be kept, with a limit, usually 4–6 ml/kg, established with the angiographer.[15]

There can also be systemic chemotoxic responses, such as release of histamine and complement activation.[6, 49] Although some reactions are mild, bronchospasm, angioneurotic edema, and anaphylaxis can be immediately life-threatening. Treatment includes diphenhydramine, steroids, oxygen, fluids, and, if necessary, epinephrine.[50] If the patient had a previous reaction, prophylactic steroids and antihistamines may be useful.[51, 52]

MYELOGRAPHY

Anesthesiologists are not often involved in the monitoring of patients undergoing myelography. However, the medically unstable patient may require monitoring or, if uncooperative, general anesthesia. In visual evaluation and monitoring, attention must be paid to patient position and padding. The patient is positioned prone initially. Proper padding, diaphragmatic freedom, a clear airway, and avoidance of stretch on the brachial plexus require attention. A subarachnoid puncture and injection of dye are done in the prone position. The patient is then repositioned in the lateral and/or supine positions. There may be several position changes in an effort to allow the dye to flow to different areas of the subarachnoid space up and down the neuraxis. During these changes, the patient must be reevaluated for padding, securing of the airway, and lack of stretch on nerves. Care is taken to prevent the dye from rising above the supratentorium; dye above the supratentorium can induce seizures.

A particularly troublesome radiologic technique, pneumoencephalography, is rarely performed. This injection of air into the ventricular system has been followed by turning the patient into extreme positions to facilitate movement of air into cerebral ventricles. Patients often have significant headache, nausea, and vomiting during and after the procedure.[15]

A CT scan after the myelogram is becoming increasingly popular. If the patient is sedated or anesthetized, transport of the patient to the CT scanner may involve significant logistic difficulties and preparation. The need for the additional procedure should be discussed with the radiologist before the intervention begins.

RADIATION ONCOLOGY THERAPY

Radiation therapy is becoming increasingly common, especially with the success of bone marrow transplantation. As part of the bone marrow transplantation therapy, total body irradiation or total lymphoid tissue irradiation may be used. The therapy usually involves multiple treatments, every day or so, for several weeks.[53] Radiation therapy can also be used to treat radiation-sensitive tumors, such as retinoblastoma and medulloblastoma.[54–56] The treatments are usually short, lasting only a few minutes, though some treatments have taken up to an hour.[57] This therapy provides several monitoring challenges. A linear accelerator provides a high-energy beam in a specially shielded room. The particle beam does not interfere with the action of commonly available monitors. However, the radiation levels in the target room are too high to allow observers. Therefore, monitoring must be adequate to provide safe conditions without an observer in the room. Not only is the observer away from the patient, but reentering the room is delayed. The heavily shielded door is sealed during the therapy; usually, several minutes are required to reopen the door and to regain access to the room and patient.

Because of the high energy of the beam, the patient must rest on the table with only minimal movement during the treatment. Adults usually have no difficulty with this, but children often require sedation or general anesthesia.[58] Nonsedated patients are observed by closed-circuit television, but sedated and anesthetized patients are monitored more intensively.[59–61] Patients being sedated or anesthetized usually have been given medication before entering the treatment room; monitoring should start before the medication is administered and should continue until recovery.

It is possible to use standard ECG, pulse oximetry, automated blood pressure, and capnography monitors in the treatment room.[57, 62] Although some units have the monitoring displays transmitted into the outside control room, most radiation therapy facilities have free-standing monitors without distal displays. It has been common to focus a remote-controlled television camera on the monitor display and watch the television monitor when in the control room.[53, 57, 63] This technique requires easily readable displays.

General endotracheal anesthesia can be used for patients undergoing radiotherapy.[64, 65] However, it is common to manage these patients with either sedation or anesthesia without an artificial airway. No matter what agent or combination of agents is used for this purpose, these techniques can cause upper airway obstruction and hypoventilation. Monitoring of the patient should include efforts to evaluate adequacy of the airway and ventilation. The pulse oximeter certainly can act as a hypoxemia alarm, but it is best to detect obstruction or hypoventilation before low oxygen saturations develop.

Capnography has been used during radiotherapy. For the intubated patient, this is a common modality. In the unintubated patient, efforts have been made to use nasal prongs attached to a capnograph as an indicator of continued ventilation and patency of the airway.[54] Although this technique has worked well in some cases, it has not been uniformly successful.[62] Another alternative is chest plethysmography, if available.

Observation of the patient by television camera is the most common method of monitoring both patient movement and adequacy of ventilation. A camera other than the one focused on monitors must be used. After the patient is sedated or anesthetized, the head, neck, and shoulders are positioned to provide an open airway. Padding and support (i.e., sandbags) are placed to maintain the position. The television camera is then oriented to give a clear view of the patient's head, neck, and chest, and the image is checked to ensure an adequate view of the patient. During treatment, the patient's airway and ventilatory pattern are observed via the television image. If there is evidence of airway obstruction or hypoventilation, the treatment is stopped until the observer can enter the room and verify airway and ventilation adequacy.

GAMMA KNIFE

The "gamma knife" has many characteristics of conventional radiotherapy. The radiation beams come from a ^{60}cobalt source.[66] By using stereotactic localization of the cranial tumor or vascular malformation, it is possible to target a small area deep within other tissue for specific radiation. Like conventional radiotherapy, the treatment takes little time, but multiple treatments on succeeding days are not required. Also, because of the high-energy beam, observers cannot be in the treatment room. Both the monitors and the patient can be observed by a solid-state television camera. However, there are significant differences in the time involved for the entire process and in the sites of treatment.[67]

Initially, a stereotactic head frame is applied to the cranium, followed by a CT examination. If this is done under local anesthesia, no specific monitoring is indicated. However, if sedation or general anesthesia is used, the same monitoring as is used for other CT scans is appropriate. Based on the CT images, extensive computations are made to determine the orientation of the radiation beams; these computations take several hours. Some patients undergo angiography during this period. At the end of the computing period, the patient is taken into the radiation therapy room for treatment similar to conventional radiotherapy.[68, 69]

Monitoring during CT and radiation therapy are the same as with other patients in these situations. The two unique challenges are monitoring during multiple transports and during a prolonged waiting period. The patient is often sedated or anesthetized between application of the stereotactic head frame and the final radiotherapy. The frame is applied to the patient's head for transport between the CT scanner, the angiography suite, a waiting area, and the gamma knife room.

TRANSPORT

Transport of a patient who is anesthetized or sedated requires planning and attention to details. Although it is theoretically desirable to maintain the same monitoring that is used during the radiologic procedure, this is often not practical. It is necessary to determine what is needed to safely transport the patient before starting the procedure.

If the patient is being transported to the recovery area after sedation or anesthesia for a radiologic procedure, the need for monitoring depends on the state of the patient. An awake, healthy patient, responding appropriately to commands with a clear airway and adequate ventilation, is often monitored only with visual observation. Especially in children, however, undetected hypoxemia can occur during transport to the postanesthesia care unit, even with the shorter distances of the operating room setting.[70] Whether all healthy patients have oxygen saturation continuously monitored whenever they are being transported is unclear. Until more data demonstrate that hypoxemia is a clinical problem during transport of healthy patients, visual observation will probably continue to be the dominant monitor. However, continuous pulse oximetry is probably desirable.

The patient who is significantly sedated or who is not medically stable is in a different category. These patients are at increased risk for airway obstruction, hypoventilation, and/or cardiovascular instability during transport.[71] The longer the transport, the greater the risk. Although it is rare to experience elevator malfunction during transport, it can happen. (I was once delayed for 15 minutes in a stuck elevator.) Visual and tactile observation of the patient are important components of effective monitoring. For observation to be effective, the anesthesiologist must be able to examine the airway, chest movement, skin color and perfusion, and a palpable pulse. If the patient is not anesthetized, checking on the level of consciousness or arousability is useful.

Of all the mechanical and electronic monitors available to assist in effective monitoring during transport, the pulse oximeter is probably used the most often. Many models of pulse oximeter have adequate battery capacity to work during transports of short to moderate length. Light-emitting diode (LED) displays are bright enough to be read during the changing light conditions of transport. If the pulse oximeter can visually represent the pulse signal, this simulation can be compared to a palpable pulse for confirmation that the machine is adequately capturing the patient's pulse for accurate determination of the oxygen saturation. The rhythm is depicted to the extent of the timing of the beats, though the sources of the beats (atrial, junctional, ventricular) are not delineated. The presence of a strong peripheral pulse, coupled with an adequate oxygen saturation and regular heart rate, is often viewed by practitioners as evidence of acceptable cardiopulmonary status during short transports.

For long transports or medically unstable patients, more extensive monitoring may be indicated. Portable ECG monitors can provide heart rate and rhythm, ST-T wave representation, and arterial and central venous pressure wave displays. Many available models run on battery power and have easily read displays and the same alarm functions found on other standard machines. Although automated sphygmomanometry for determination of blood pressure is not usually used for transport, a simple cuff and manometer can easily be used. Likewise, the humble stethoscope can be useful during transport for evaluation of breath and heart sounds. Although it is not routinely used, there is a lightweight CO_2 detector that can be used to confirm presence of CO_2 in exhaled gas.[72] This device can be used in a variety of situations, such as during transport or in a resuscitation situation, if there is a question about endotracheal tube placement.

If extensive monitoring is desired during transport, it is useful to have the equipment on a free-standing cart, instead of on the patient's stretcher. At Children's Memorial Hospital, there are small, lightweight carts that are used for transport of anesthetized, intubated, or medically unstable patients. These ''arks'' (named after their designer, Zehavah Noah) contain air and oxygen 3AA cylinders connected to a blender and flowmeter, a pulse oximeter, and an ECG machine with one pressure channel. The cart also contains a variety of ventilating bags (including a self-inflating system), masks, and oral airways. These carts allow positive pressure ventilation during transport and monitoring of oxygen saturation, ECG, and arterial or venous blood pressure. For transporting anesthetized patients between sites, a vaporizer can be added to a gas source, but scavenging of waste gases is a concern. A reasonable alternative is the use of intravenous agents, such as a benzodiazepine/narcotic combination or a propofol infusion, to maintain the anesthetized state during transport.

In the specific case of gamma knife therapy, adequacy of the airway and of ventilation are major concerns, because the head frame impairs easy access to the airway. Both the bulk and the weight of the head frame are a concern because of the risk of neck torsion if the frame is not adequately supported and immobilized. If the patient is sedated, pulse oximetry, palpation of the pulse, and visual observation are commonly used monitors that reasonably assess the status of most patients. If the patient is anesthetized, the addition of blood pressure monitoring allows assessment of cardiovascular instability.

WAITING PERIOD

The time between the beginning of application of the frame and the end of the therapy can exceed 7–8 hours. For most of this time, the patient is waiting, in the head frame, without other stimulation. Many adults and older children can actually be sent to a floor bed and wait without significant sedation. However, sedation or anesthesia is often administered for this period. The patients tend to be remarkably stable with little need for ''deep'' levels of sedation or anesthesia. The challenge for this period is managing the resources necessary to provide adequate monitoring. General anesthesia or sedation can be administered with an anesthesiologist in attendance, using all the monitors used in the operating room.[69] Another alternative is to provide continuous sedation in an area such as the postanesthesia recovery area or intensive care area. If the nursing personnel are adequately trained and willing to provide continuous monitoring, the patient could be monitored in this setting during the hours of waiting for completion of the computations. An anesthesiologist must ensure that the patient is stable and be readily available if there is a change in patient status.

Monitoring after the radiotherapy is equivalent to that after other procedures under anesthesia or sedation. It is useful to note that the two most common complications related to the procedure are vomiting and seizures. Seizures occur in less than 5% of cases; prophylactic seizure medication and steroids have been used to reduce the risk.[66] Nausea and vomiting occur in less than 10% of patients and are usually self-limited.

MAGNETIC RESONANCE IMAGING

MRI has revolutionized imaging of several areas of the body, especially the CNS.[73, 74] Unlike CT or other x-ray imaging, MRI bases the image on alterations in orientation of nuclei in response to a magnetic field and radiofrequency energy instead of ionizing radiation. This technique, originally called nuclear magnetic resonance (NMR), is based on the principle that atomic nuclei possess a charge because of the presence of protons. The rotation or spin, of these protons and any accompanying neutrons produces a local magnetic field. This weak magnetic field, then, is oriented in a specific direction. By surrounding these nuclei with a strong magnetic field, it is possible to bring the orientation of the nuclei in parallel with the external field. Hydrogen ions are the most sensitive nuclei for this technique in currently used machines; MRI uses these nuclei in water as the basis of their images.[75] With commonly used MRI machines, there is a net orientation of nuclei along the axis of the external field. The patient is usually placed such that this axis is also the longitudinal axis of the patient.

The external magnetic field is very powerful, using a supercooled electromagnetic coil. This coil is oriented to maintain a fixed field in a tunnel that runs through the center of the coil; the patient is placed in this tunnel. The strength of the field varies, from 0.5 to 1.5 tesla. (Most clinically used machines are now 1.5 tesla.) Tesla units are used to measure the magnetic field. One tesla is the same as 10,000 gauss.[76] The earth's magnetic force is often thought of as 1 gauss, but may actually vary between 0.5 and 1 gauss. Thus, the magnetic force exerted in the core of the magnetic field is 10–15,000 times greater than the earth's magnetic force.

Once a patient is placed in the core of the electromagnet, there is a net orientation of hydrogen nuclei along the field of the magnet. Oscillating magnetic pulses are then induced, using radiofrequency energy. These pulses change the orientation of the nuclei. When the pulse energy ends, the nuclei return to their original orientation, releasing an electrical signal. This weak electrical signal is detected by a receiver coil.[6] Three pulse sequences are commonly used; using different sequences, different information can be gathered.

The MRI picture is based on averaging data from multiple signals. The components that affect the image are the density of water in the area imaged, the time between excitation and collection of the signal, and the time between repeated signals. The manipulation of the radiofrequency pulses produces different relaxation constants known as T_1 and T_2. This manipulation allows differentiation of tissues not obtainable with other imaging devices.[75, 77] By altering the field gradients, it is possible to gather data for sections in axial, sagittal, and coronal planes simultaneously at multiple anatomic levels without moving the patient. The images generated can be visualized in tomographic sections that are 7 mm thick, allowing fine differentiation of structures.

MRI can differentiate white and gray matter in the CNS, for instance, allowing identification of acute ischemia of the brain and discrimination of acute and resolving phases of intracerebral hemorrhage.[6] Bone, with a minimum of hydrogen nuclei, is easily identified, eliminating the problem of artifact seen with CT scans. This delineation of bone from soft tissue and blood is especially important in identifying subdural and subarachnoid hemorrhages as well as delineating posterior fossa abnormalities. Outside of the CNS, MRI is useful in evaluating the thoracic and abdominal regions, as well as joints.

MRI can also be used to identify nuclei other than water. This spectroscopic activity has exciting potential for identification of tumors and metabolic defects. Significant work is proceeding on the use of MRI for evaluation of the cardiovascular system. Blood flow in vessels of the heart generates very little MRI signal. Consequently, there is a large contrast between the blood filling the chambers of the heart and blood vessels and the surrounding tissue. MRI differentiates tissues without the use of contrast, making it appropriate for delineating cardiac anatomy. Wall motion of the heart or blood vessel decreases the effective signal. Consequently, it is common to use gating of the ECG to measure signal decay when movement is minimized.[78, 79] The R wave of the ECG synchronizes the cardiac cycle, allowing beat-to-beat evaluation of signals. It is possible to detect thrombi, aneurysms, valve abnormalities, and thinning of the ventricular wall, as after a myocardial infarction.[78] Some centers use repetitive images to develop a cine evaluation not only of static anatomy, but also of wall motion. This angiographic capability may dramatically alter the evaluation of vascular and cardiac problems in the future.

Because the signals from relaxation of the nuclei are very transient, patient movement can produce an artifact, because the emitted signal comes from a different point in space for that short period. Therefore, patient movement must be minimized. Because the signals are weak, any external radiofrequency signals, such as radio waves or induced signals from electronic equipment, will distort the signal. For this reason, the scanner is housed in a room that is placed as far from potential sources of electronic signal as possible. The scanning room is built to minimize external signal entry. The inside of the inner wall is covered with copper sheeting. This produces a "Faraday cage" that drains off external electromagnetic radiation, such as radio and television signals. Any added monitoring equipment can defeat the purpose of this environment by producing an electronic signal that interferes with the normal working of the MR.

MONITORING

Monitoring equipment not only can interfere with the imaging, but the monitor itself can be affected in two ways. First, the powerful magnetic field extends beyond the 6-foot cylindrical core of the magnet. Ferromagnetic objects can be drawn into the core with considerable force, damaging the patient or anything else in the path of the object.[75, 80, 81] The magnetic force drops off quickly the farther from the core one gets. The extent of the field into the rest of the scanning room depends on both the strength of the magnetic field and the amount of active shielding built into the unit.[38, 82] The strength of the fields are measured in gauss, with the 5-gauss and the 50-gauss limits most commonly used. Ferromagnetic items are drawn into a 50-gauss field easily; there may be dysfunction of pacemakers in fields as low as 5 gauss and degradation of cathode ray images in fields as low as 1–2 gauss.[75, 79]

As a practical matter, ferromagnetic items should be kept at least 5 meters away from the magnet, and, if at all possible, outside the scanning room. Not only can hemostats, keys, ferromagnetic gas tanks, pens, and scissors be drawn into the magnet, but the magnetic field can demagnetize watches and destroy the magnetic information included on credit cards and magnetic tapes.[81, 83] Because of the potential danger of ferromagnetic objects, it is important to determine the ferromagnetic content of items brought into the scanning room. A simple method of doing this is to place a pacemaker magnet next to the object and determine if there is noticeable attractive force. When the object in question is brought into the scanning room for the first time, the anesthesiologist should carefully observe the object to monitor any attraction.

The magnetic field can also affect ferromagnetic devices inside a patient. Cardiac pacemakers are of special concern, because the magnetic field can convert the pacemaker to the asynchronous mode, inactivate the pacemaker, create a microshock, or pull on the unit enough to cause discomfort.[80, 84–86] This is not just a theoretic problem; pacemakers have clinically failed during MRI.[86] Patients with pacemakers have been restricted from MRI in all except the weakest field units. The presence of other ferromagnetic objects should also be ascertained before allowing a patient to undergo MRI. Metallic clips used for hemostasis on cerebral vessel can be detached by the magnetic field, with subsequent hemorrhage.[80, 87] Hemostatic clips in other parts of the body are not at the same risk because of the normal development of fibrotic scar around the clip.[88] When MRI was first used, there was concern about prosthetic heart valves containing metal, but this has not been a problem with modern valves.[89–91] Some dental implants are also significantly ferromagnetic.[92] Objects made of stainless steel (high grades only), tantalum, aluminum, nickel, and most alloys are not attracted by the magnet.[90, 93]

The trauma patient presents a unique challenge in relation to possible metallic material. The patient is often comatose and may not be able to communicate about the presence of clips, pacemakers, or other metallic objects. The presence of healed surgical scars can alert the anesthesiologist and radiologist to the possible presence of metallic objects. Also, some pellets and bullets are ferromagnetic.[94] If these are the cause of the trauma, they may be dislodged by the magnet, changing the patient's clinical status. If there is a question about potential metallic objects, an initial radiograph or CT scan can at least tell if a radiolucent object is present that could be ferromagnetic. This is especially important not only for metallic objects that may be close to vital thoracoabdominal structures, but also for intraocular foreign bodies.[95–97] The clinician must then decide if the potential risk of dislodgement is greater than the anticipated benefit of the study.[90] It is unlikely that a surface hand magnet would demonstrate enough noticeable attraction to allow ruling out the possibility of a bullet being ferromagnetic.

The patient can be affected not only by the magnetic field, but also by the radiofrequency energy used to induce a signal. This energy can produce core body heating. The energy used is now calculated to not exceed basal metabolic rate.[80, 98] This may be more troublesome if field strengths above 2.0 tesla are used. Although concern has been expressed about heating of implanted metallic prosthesis, this has not been a practical problem.[99]

The second problem with monitoring in this environment is that the monitor itself may not work properly in the presence of the strong magnetic field. There may be a degradation of the signal, the internal processing of the signal, or the display. Modern electronic monitors specifically designed for use in MRI combine shielding and filters to minimize the interference of the magnetic field.

Monitors for a New MRI Unit

Although the radiologists in charge of the new unit may not feel that sedation or anesthesia will be used in their area, practical experience has shown otherwise. Because of the isolation of the patient for prolonged periods, sedation or anesthesia is increasingly recognized as a useful adjunct, especially in children. Therefore, it is reasonable for anesthesiologists to consult about potential needs for anesthesia services and monitoring when a new MRI unit is being planned and built.[82] Discussions before the unit is actually built provide for monitoring equipment in both the design and budget of the scanner. The manufacturers of MRI units and their engineers are especially helpful in educating both the radiology and anesthesia staff about the capabilities and limitations of monitoring for the installation. They also often can provide advice based on other installations.

The type and amount of monitoring that is initially provided with the installation is controversial. ECG capability is provided by most manufacturers to allow gating of signals, as mentioned earlier. However, these ECG waveforms may not be diagnostic for clinical monitoring. Additional monitoring can be provided as either a complete system or a collection of individual devices. It is possible to purchase a system from a single company that includes a variety of functions, such as ECG, automated blood pressure, pulse oximetry, capnometry, and chest plethysmography. The alternative is to purchase individual MRI-compatible monitors. A decision should also be made about where the output of the monitors should be directed. If the monitors are free-standing and remain in the scanning room, they must either be observed by a knowledgeable person inside the scanning room or be easily visible from the control room.

If adequate monitors are not supplied with the scanning room, it is the responsibility of the practitioner supplying anesthetic or sedative services to provide appropriate monitors. If the monitors to be used are not known to be MRI-compatible, they should be evaluated before starting the sedation or anesthetic. The two factors that should be evaluated are the presence of magnetic attraction (by using a magnet) and their effect on the image. The specific problems seen with individual monitors are discussed in the next section.

Monitoring Equipment

There are multiple problems with specific monitors in the MRI environment. The magnetic field can distort the electron beam that produces a cathode ray display, making the display inaccurate or unreadable. The monitors may not function at all because of interference with the electrical connections and activity within the monitor. One of the recurring and serious problems with monitors involves external wires and leads. The wires, which are ferromagnetic, can act as an antenna if they form a loop. A current may be induced in this antenna by the outside energy. The current produces a signal that can interfere with the MRI signal. Also, the current in the loop can cause the wire to heat up and eventually burn the patient.[100] Lastly, leakage of radiofrequency energy from the electrical activity within the monitor can degrade the scanner's signal and distort the accumulated image.

In general, several principles apply to monitor use in the MRI scanner. First, it is desirable to use monitors with a low amount of ferromagnetic material. Second, monitors designed with a low ferromagnetic content, extensive shielding, and in-line filters can often be used in the scanning room without modification. Third, placing the monitor as far from the magnetic field as possible decreases interaction.[101] Lastly, if a monitoring system or combination of monitors that contains all the expected needs for the scanner is introduced at once, the radiology staff and the manufacturer (or representative) can adequately test both the monitors and the scanner for function and interaction. It is possible to establish the distance that each monitor must be kept from the magnet to both adequately function and not interfere with the image.

Electrocardiography. Both patient monitoring and the need for cardiac gating necessitate use of an ECG. However, there are several problems with ECG monitoring. As with other electronic monitors, the ECG can cause both patient injury (burn) and signal degradation, as well as function inaccurately without proper shielding. For this reason, some practitioners have expressed concern about routinely using ECG monitoring in the scanner.[36] The basis of the reluctance to use the ECG is based on the ferromagnetic lead wires that attach the electrodes to the monitor cable.[102] Both monitor and patient safety issues are involved.

First, the ferromagnetic wires can distort the signal, because the strong magnetic field alters flow through the wires. It is possible to minimize this by using telemetric leads and a base station[84] or fiberoptic cables.[103] However, these are not widely available or used. Second, there is a risk of burns from wires that become virtual antennae, as discussed earlier. Third, the current generated in a loop induces a magnetic field of its own, potentially degrading the signal of the MRI.

There are several ways to minimize both patient injury and signal degradation.[104, 105] Filters can minimize artifact formation[104] and are incorporated on some machines.[106] Nonferromagnetic components are used as much as possible. Electrodes are usually not a problem because of the lack of ferromagnetic material. Recommendations to prevent both patient injury and degradation of the image are listed in Table 19–1.

The ECG signal may demonstrate ST-T wave changes in the MRI environment.[80, 107, 108] These changes have been seen in even low-tesla machines. The alterations are seen most commonly in leads I, II, V_1, and V_2.[105] However, these changes do not appear to represent true myocardial ischemia but are caused by changes in the signal from regional blood flow.[107] There is a change in the orientation of magnetic forces in the charged elements of flowing blood and not a change in actual perfusion of the myocardium.[109] The changes in T waves disappear as soon as the patient is not in the magnetic field, with no evidence of damage.[110] There is also a theoretic risk of induction of currents in the heart because of the rapid changing of magnetic fields.[111] However, the currently used field strengths are thought to pose an insignificant risk.[78, 102]

However, the presence of T wave abnormalities as artifact may be of concern, especially in patients with suspected coronary artery disease. Some authors have suggested using a monitor other than the ECG to monitor cardiac function, such as standard pulse plethysmography.[112] A more sophisticated system is a fiberoptic light system for detection of capillary blood flow. A laser Doppler probe placed on either the earlobe or the lip measures capillary blood flow. The cardiac cycle is monitored by measuring fluctuations in the capillary blood volume. The signal is transmitted by fiberoptic cable, eliminating the risk of interference by the magnetic field.[78]

The AAP guidelines for the sedation of children suggest that ECG monitoring is unnecessary for monitoring children, primarily because of the danger of burns.[3] No currently available studies address the incidence or demographics of burns with ECG wires in the MRI scanner. Cardiovascular monitoring should be provided for patients in the MRI scanner who are sedated, anesthetized, or medically unstable. If ECG monitoring is not used, the practitioner should be confident that the other modalities used adequately evaluate the cardiovascular status.

Pulse Oximetry. Pulse oximetry has been adopted by anesthesiologists as a standard of care[113, 114] and is used for both sedated and anesthetized patients. Most of the early models were both susceptible to interference from the magnetic field and a source of interference with the MRI signal. In low-tesla scanners, many models were acceptable but became unreliable when placed in the newer, higher-tesla units.[27]

With advances in circuitry and shielding and the economic incentive of providing monitors in the MRI suites, manufacturers have produced pulse oximeters that give accurate, continuous readings in the scanning room.[115] Some of the manufacturers that have demonstrated their models to be reliable include Nonen (Plymouth, MN),[36] Ohmeda (Madison, WI),[79] Criticare (Pewaukee, WI),[93] Biochem (Milwaukee, WI),[106] and Nellcor (Heyward, CA).[82]

Heavy insulation and shielding help to isolate the monitor signal. A low ferromagnetic content of the components, including the probe, is also useful, as is minimizing the number of electrical connections and computer chips within the monitor. The machines all have filters in the machine circuitry, and some models have filters in the cable itself to help eliminate extraneous signals. These filters appear to be very important in separating signal from background noise. The probe is usually placed as far from the center of the

TABLE 19–1. ECG USE IN MRI

1. Remove any wires or leads (already on the patient) that are not in use.
2. Add a second ground wire lead (i.e., use a four-lead system instead of a three-lead system). Two ground leads eliminate ECG artifacts on the images.
3. Make sure that all four leads are close together and over the center of the trunk of the patient.
4. Check all wires before each patient use for evidence of fraying or breaks in the insulation.
5. With the leads close together on the trunk, braid the wires together as soon as they can reach each other. This braiding prevents the formation of a loop, with subsequent induction of current.
6. Once the wires are connected to the leads, place a folded cloth sheet between the wires and the patient's skin. This prevents the lead wires from contacting the skin. Even if the lead wires become heated, the cloth will prevent heat transfer.
7. Whenever the patient is moved into or out of the scanner, wires may coil and form a loop anywhere along the course of the wires. It is necessary to visually check all wires each time the patient is moved. The wires also can realign if the patient moves spontaneously. Wires need to be checked before proceeding.

magnet as possible to minimize interference. In adults, this allows much greater separation from the magnet than in children. There has been some experimentation with trying to isolate the probe by placing aluminum foil over it.[116] Placing the monitor box as far from the magnet as possible also decreases both the interference of the monitor with the image and the interference of the monitor with the image and the interference of the magnet with the oximeter. With some units, the cable goes through initial filters, but the main monitor box is kept outside the scanning room. As with ECG wires, a loop in the cable can act as an antenna, leading to a buildup of heat and subsequent burning.[117] Burns have been reported in both adult and pediatric patients at either the probe site or along the course of the probe cable.[117, 118] The loop can also produce a radiofrequency signal that degrades the image.[112]

As with the CT scanner, more patients are sedated in MRI scanners with monitoring by radiology staff than with monitoring by anesthesiologists. When the patient is in the bore of the magnet, direct observation is difficult, especially in the dim light of the scanning room. Pulse oximetry acts as a hypoxemia alarm that can be very useful in ensuring safe conditions for patients.[119] The oximeter should be a model that gives accurate readings both in the presence of the magnetic field and during routine data collection. As a practical matter, oximeters that have a display easily seen from both the scanning room and the control room allow evaluation by personnel in either location. LED displays are usually much easier to read from a distance than the gray tones of liquid crystal displays. If necessary, a camera can be focused on the monitor to allow visualization from a distal site. The working pulse oximeter is an important safety device for all patients, and the anesthesia department should strongly encourage its use, even when an anesthesiologist is not participating in patient care for MRI.

Arterial Pressure. Blood pressure measurements in MRI are easy using standard cuffs and manometers.[76] If the manometer has a high ferromagnetic content, extra-long plastic tubing must be used with the cuff to place the manometer 7–10 meters from the magnet's center. A plastic stethoscope can be used to monitor Korotkoff sounds. However, if the stethoscope tubing is long, it becomes increasingly difficult to hear the sounds. In these situations, it is possible to use the first bounce of needle on deflation of the cuff as an indication of systolic pressure.

Of interest, automated cuffs of several different manufacturers, such as Critikon (Tampa, FL),[79] Invivo Research (Broken Arrow, OK),[120] and Datascope (Paramus, NJ),[81] can be used without modification in the scanning room without inducing MRI artifact. Extra-long plastic tubing is attached to the cuffs, and any ferromagnetic couplings on the tubing are removed.[112] The length of tubing is limited when used on infants because of the dampening of transduced signal. However, on children and adults, the use of long tubing allows the monitor unit to be placed close to the console room window for direct observation. This also keeps the monitor unit as far from the magnet as possible. Some systems are designed to transmit the data to a monitor in the control room.

For critically ill patients, intra-arterial pressure can be measured. If the ferromagnetic content of the transducer is not known, low-compliance arterial line tubing is extended to place the transducer as far as possible from the magnet, decreasing the chance of artifact.[121] With the longer tubing, dampening of the tracing may give more of a mean value than with shorter tubing. For this reason, the opposite advice—keeping the transducer as close to the patient as possible—has also been given.[122] It is also possible to monitor intracranial pressure in this setting by using a nonferromagnetic subdural bolt or plastic intraventricular catheter.[122]

Capnography. Side-stream, withdrawal-type capnographs can be used for both anesthetized and sedated patients in the MRI scanner. In sedated patients, nasal prongs can be used to detect both the presence of carbon dioxide and the rhythm of breathing.[123] The presence of carbon dioxide is important because of the risk of airway obstruction in the sedated patient. The rhythm and rate of breaths may give some indication of the degree of sedation to the experienced observer. A decrease in the rate of breaths may indicate significant respiratory depression, whereas an increase in rate may indicate increased agitation and the need for more sedation. In anesthetized patients, the capnograph can be used to alter controlled ventilation parameters as well as warn of airway obstruction or hypoventilation.

Most capnographs are placed as far from the magnet as possible. Plastic tubing is extended from the sampling port to the base unit.[79, 124] This long tubing delays the gas sample in reaching the base unit, though this delay can be minimized by using low-compliance tubing with a small diameter. Although there is a delay in detecting apnea or changes in carbon dioxide sampling, it is usually not extensive. The capnograph tracing is dampened, giving more of a mean value instead of the normal pattern seen with shorter tubing. However, the mean value can still be used as a trend monitor to guide adjustment of ventilation and anesthetic depth. Also, it is usually possible to notice irregular breathing efforts by a change in the configuration of the trace, such as a ventilated patient beginning to breath spontaneously. Both the change in pattern and amount of exhaled carbon dioxide are specific enough to guide ventilatory management.

At Children's Memorial Hospital, an unmodified capnograph is placed outside the scanning room. A copper conduit, 2 inches in diameter, penetrates the wall and is normally capped with copper caps, keeping the Faraday cage intact and preventing intrusion of outside radiofrequency interference. A brass conduit can also be used.[79] (The conduit can be used not only for monitoring functions, but also for introducing ventilator tubing from a machine outside the scanning room.) The monitor, a Nellcor 1000, is placed in the control room, and microbore tubing extends the 25 feet through the conduit to the patient. With this system, apnea is detected within 30 seconds.

Because of the delay in detecting apnea or a circuit

disconnection with the capnograph, other monitors may be of use during general anesthesia in an intubated patient. If the patient is breathing spontaneously, collapse of the ventilating bag indicates circuit disconnection. If the patient's ventilation is mechanically driven, the ventilator's disconnect alarm should detect the disconnection as quickly as it would with shorter tubing, because the monitored air column is interrupted. Lastly, in ventilators (such as the Siemens 900 series) that monitor returned minute ventilation, partial disconnection can be detected as well as complete disconnection.

Stethoscopes. Either precordial or esophageal stethoscopes made of plastic can be used in the scanning room.[93] However, during scanning, the production of the radiofrequency pulses vibrates wires in the scanner, producing a loud ''thumping'' noise. This noise can be very distressing, especially to a child or claustrophobic adult.[125, 126] Although these noises are below regulated noise pollution levels, they can reach 95 decibels.[80, 102] Because of the extended plastic tubing usually used with the stethoscope head and the loud background noise during scanning, stethoscopes are most useful for intermittent evaluation of breath and heart sounds, especially if there is question about the endotracheal tube placement or difficulty with the other monitoring equipment.

Alternative designs of the standard stethoscope have been used. For instance, one design used an amplified microphone connected to a stethoscope to increase definition of sound.[127] Another design used a wireless, infrared transmission of data from the sensor to the distal receiver.[128] However, neither of these stethoscopes has been widely used.

Temperature. During short MRI examinations, patient temperature is not usually monitored. Although temperature probes with filtered cables are available,[79, 101] they carry the same risks of signal interference and burns as do other electronic monitors. Patient burns have occurred even with probes specially designed for MRI use. This complication was probably caused by inadvertent formation of a cable loop during patient movement. Inspection of the probe and cable after the incident did not reveal any defects.[100] Alternatives to electronic measurement of temperature include intermittent use of a mercury thermometer or liquid crystal temperature strips.

Gas Analysis. Inspired oxygen monitors for the anesthesia machine are required to ensure appropriate gas concentrations.[106] Infrared capnographs often now also have the capability of measuring anesthetic agent concentration. As with carbon dioxide, there will be a small delay in detecting changes in concentration, but this is less important with volatile agents because of their long time constants. Both oxygen and volatile agents should be analyzed during general anesthesia, even during MRI. Vaporizers are available that have demonstrated accuracy, even when used in the scanning room.[106]

Many anesthesiologists are unaware of one important gas monitor in use in the MRI scanner. The basis of the strong electromagnet is supercooling the coil, allowing exceptional current to flow. If the liquid helium or nitrogen that is used to cool the coil heats up and evaporates, there can be a sudden quench that fills the scanning room with helium or nitrogen gas, reducing oxygen concentrations in the room to dangerous levels if not vented quickly enough. Luckily, this has not been a problem. However, most modern scanners have an oxygen alarm that sounds in the room if there is a fall in ambient oxygen levels.[102]

Monitoring Personnel. Traditionally, it is taught that the most important monitor during anesthetic or monitored care has been the trained observer. Anesthesiologists are accustomed to close contact with their patient. A ''finger on the pulse'' is an accepted practice in our profession. However, the sedated or anesthetized patient in the MRI scanner is placed in a 6-foot tunnel where direct observation of the patient is extremely difficult. Because of this, the need for an observer to be in direct contact or proximity of the patient inside the scanning room itself is controversial.

The dangers to the patient are the same as with any sedated or anesthetized patient. Because of the isolation of the patient in the bore of the magnet, there is particular concern about airway obstruction, breathing circuit disconnection, hypoventilation, and patient movement.[93] There are no reports, to my knowledge, that document an adverse patient outcome that would have been prevented or altered by having an observer in the scanning room. The difficulty of an observer in the room detecting problems, however, is well known.[129] Although there are reports of a dedicated anesthesia staff member in both the scanning room and the control room,[130] a single staff member has also been used for both monitoring and anesthesia.[121]

The lighting in the scanning room is dim because of the potential interference of fluorescent lighting. Fluorescent lighting emits radiofrequency energy that interferes with the image. Therefore, incandescent lighting at a low wattage is used. The dim light is thought to provide a quieting atmosphere for the sedated patient. However, dim lighting makes it difficult to see the patient well. Many units have a solid-state television camera to monitor the patient, but the image with these cameras is not particularly better than visual observation from the control window.

When considering the use of personnel in the scanning room, it is important to consider the concomitant dangers to those monitoring the patient. One of the great advantages of MRI is the lack of ionizing radiation. However, there has been some question about the safety of exposure to an electromagnetic field.[36, 131] Some of this concern about MRI is based on work outside of the medical environment. Reports of increased demographic risk of malignancy in people living close to high-tension electrical wires has led to investigation into MRI exposure.[131] The current evidence does not support an adverse effect from exposure to MRI fields.[132] Both *in vitro* and *in vivo* studies of the carcinogenic and teratogenic potential of MRI did not show any changes.[133, 134] Epidemiologic studies of 792 human workers has not shown evidence of increased disease in 19 potential categories.[135] The federal government, under the authority of the Food and Drug Administration, has not issued safety recommendations for either single or year-long total magnetic resonance exposure. Although there is no evidence of specific hazards, Ganagarosa has advised caution for extended exposure during the first trimester of pregnancy.[80]

The data do not support an identifiable danger from exposure to MRI fields. Also, there are no government standards limiting health care workers or others, such as parents of patients, from being in the scanning room during data collection. On the other hand, however, there is controversy about the benefit from an observer being in the room. The underlying medical condition of the patient, the duration of the scan, the adequacy and extent of monitoring, the demonstrated stability of the patient's airway and cardiopulmonary status, and the experience of the monitoring personnel are important factors in determining the need for a dedicated observer in the scanning room. Ultimately, it should be the judgment of the personnel responsible for the patient that determines if an observer needs to be present or if electronic and mechanical monitors are adequate for patient safety.

SUMMARY

Monitoring the patient undergoing radiologic procedures is an important component of modern care. The equipment, space, and personnel aspects of this monitoring should be considered. This is best done prospectively; the monitoring needs of patients should be considered when a radiologic suite is designed. The monitoring provided must be tailored to the radiologic equipment and the specific needs of the patient. Increasingly, critically ill patients are submitted to invasive and diagnostic radiologic procedures. The equipment and space must be both suitable and convenient to ensure maximum effectiveness. Most importantly, the personnel involved must be properly trained and oriented to provide the best care for these patients.

REFERENCES

1. American Society of Anesthesiologists: Standards For Basic Intra-Operative Monitoring. Park Ridge, IL: American Society of Anesthesiologists, 1992.
2. Keeter S, Benator RM, Weinberg SM, Hartenberg MA: Sedation in pediatric CT: National survey of current practice. Radiology 1990; 175:745–752.
3. Committee on Drugs, American Academy of Pediatrics: Guidelines for monitoring and management of pediatric patients during and after sedation for diagnostic and therapeutic procedures. Pediatrics 1992; 89:1110–1115.
4. Wall BF, Green DAC, Veerappan R: The radiation dose to patients from brain and body scanners. Br J Radiol 1979; 52:189–196.
5. Roedler HD: Internal dosimetry of TC 99m labeled radiopharmaceuticals used in clinical nuclear medicine. J Belge Radiol 1977; 60:23–32.
6. Gordon I: Diagnostic Imaging in Paediatrics. London: Chapman & Hall, 1987; 11–15.
7. Division of Medical Sciences, National Academy of Sciences, National Research Council, BEIR III: Report of the Advisory Committee on the Biological Effects of Ionizing Radiations: The Effects on Populations of Exposure to Low Levels of Ionizing Radiation. Washington, DC: National Academy Press, 1980.
8. Webster EW: On the question of cancer induction by small doses of X-rays. AJR 1981; 137:647–666.
9. Brent RL: Cancer risks following diagnostic radiation exposures. Paediatrics 1983; 77:288–289.
10. Sprengler RF, Cook DH, Clarke EA, et al: Cancer mortality following cardiac catheterization. A preliminary follow-up study on 4891 irradiated children. Paediatrics 1983; 71:235–239.
11. National Council on Radiation Protection and Measurements: Limitation of Exposure to Ionizing Radiation. NCRP Report No. 116. Bethesda, MD: National Council on Radiation Protection and Measurements, 1993.
12. Barker D: Protection and safety in the x-ray department. Radiography 1978; 44:45.
13. Flodmark O, Becker LE, Harwood-Nash DC, et al: Correlation between computed tomography and autopsy in premature and full-term neonates that have suffered perinatal asphyxia. Radiology 1980; 137:93–103.
14. Fitzhardinge PM, Flodmark O, Fitz CR, et al: The prognostic value of computed tomography as an adjunct to assessment of the term infant with postasphyxial encephalopathy. J Pediatr 1981; 99:777–781.
15. Kassner EG: Iatrogenic Disorders of the Fetus, Infant, and Child, Vol 1. New York: Springer-Verlag, 1985.
16. Snyder CL, Jain VN, Saltzman DA, et al: Blunt trauma in adults and children: A comparative analysis. J Trauma 1990; 30:1239–1245.
17. Cosentino CM, Luck SR, Barthel MJ, et al: Transfusion requirements in conservative nonoperative management of blunt splenic and hepatic injuries during childhood. J Pediatr Surg 1990; 25:950–954.
18. Boyer RS: Sedation in pediatric neuroimaging: The science and the art. AJNR 1992; 13:777–783.
19. Spear RM, Waldman JY, Canada ED, et al: Intravenous thiopentone for CT and MRI in children. Paediatr Anaesth 1993; 3:29–32.
20. Greenberg SB, Faerber EN, Aspinall CL: High dose chloral hydrate sedation for children undergoing CT. Comput Assist Tomogr 1991; 15:467–469.
21. Cook BA, Bass JW, Nomizu S, Alexander ME: Sedation of children for technical procedures: Current standard of practice. Clin Pediatr 1992; 31:137–142.
22. Allan MW, Laurence AS, Gunawardena WJ: A comparison of two sedation techniques for neuroradiology. Eur J Anaesthesiol 1989; 6:379–384.
23. Alexander CM, Gross JB: Sedative doses of midazolam depress hypoxic ventilatory responses in humans. Anesth Analg 1988; 67:377–382.
24. Yaster M, Nichols DG, Deshpande JK, Wetzel RC: Midazolam-fentanyl intravenous sedation in children: Case report of respiratory arrest. Pediatrics 1990; 86:463–467.
25. Snodgrass WR, Dodge WF: Lytic "DPT" cocktail: Time for rational and safe alternatives. Pediatr Clin North Am 1989; 36:1285–1291.
26. Mitchell AA, Louik C, Lacouture P, et al: Risks to children from computed tomographic scan premedication. JAMA 1982; 247:2385–2388.
27. Shepherd JK, Hall-Craggs MA, Finn JP, Bingham RM: Sedation in children scanned with high-field magnetic resonance: The experience at The Hospital for Sick Children, Great Ormond Street. Br J Radiol 1990; 63:794–797.
28. Bloomfield EL, Masaryk TJ, Caplin A, et al: Intravenous sedation for MR imaging of the brain and spine in children: Pentobarbital versus propofol. Pediatr Radiol 1993; 186:93–97.
29. Cauldwell CB, Fisher DM: Sedating patients: Is propofol a panacea? Radiology 1993; 186:9–10.
30. Joint Commission on Accreditation of Healthcare Organizations. Joint Commission Accreditation Manual for Hospitals, Vol 3. Oak Brook Terrace, IL: Joint Commission on Accreditation of Healthcare Organizations, 1992.
31. Epstein BS, Schyve PM: Anesthesiologist's interaction with other medical departments outside the operating room [Letter]. Anesth Analg 1992; 75:633.
32. Cohen MD: Pediatric sedation. Radiology 1990; 175:611–612.
33. Schecter NL, Berde CB, Yaster M: Pain in Infants, Children, and Adolescents. Baltimore: Williams & Wilkins, 1993; 145–171.
34. Feldscot AF: The new regulations on conscious sedation. N Y State Dent J 1989; 55:8–10.
35. Fleischer D: Monitoring the patient receiving conscious sedation for

gastrointestinal endoscopy: Issues and guidelines. Gastrointest Endosc 1989; 35:262–266.
36. Cote CJ: Anesthesia outside the operating room. In Coté CJ, Ryan JF, Todres ID, Goudsouzian NG (eds): A Practice of Anesthesia for Infants and Children, 2nd Ed. Philadelphia: WB Saunders, 1993; 401–415.
37. Hood JB, Wallace CT, Mahaffey JE: Anesthetic management of an intracranial arteriovenous malformation in infancy. Anesth Analg 1977; 56:236–241.
38. Brown TCK, Fisk GC: Anaesthesia for Children, 2nd Ed. London: Blackwell Scientific, 1992; 291–300.
39. Dallas SH, Moxon CP: Controlled ventilation for cerebral angiography. Br J Anaesth 1969; 41:597–602.
40. Drummond JC, Shapiro HM: Cerebral physiology. *In* Miller RD (ed): Anesthesia, 3rd Ed. New York: Churchill Livingstone, 1990; 621–658.
41. Spargo PM, Howard WV, Saunders DA: Sedation and cerebral angiography. The effect of pentazocine and midazolam on arterial carbon dioxide tension. Anaesthesia 1985; 40:901–903.
42. Allison DJ, Hordan H, Hennessy O: Therapeutic embolization of the hepatic artery: A review of 75 procedures. Lancet 1985; 1:595–598.
43. Holden AM, Fyler DC, Shillito J, et al: Congestive heart failure from intracranial arteriovenous fistula in infancy: Clinical and physiologic considerations in eight patients. Pediatrics 1972; 49:30–39.
44. Ishak B, Gutierrez F, Seleny F: Anesthetic management of arteriovenous malformations of the brain in infants and children. Anesthesiol Rev 1978; 5:23–27.
45. O'Mahoney BJ, Bolsin SNC: Anaesthesia for closed embolisation of cerebral arteriovenous malformations. Anaesth Intens Care 1988; 16:318–323.
46. King BF, Harmtan GW, Williamson B, et al: Low-osmolality contrast media. A current perspective. Mayo Clin Proc 1989; 64:976–985.
47. Cohan RH, Dunnick NR: Intravenous contrast media: Adverse reactions. AJR 1987; 149:665–670.
48. Brezis M, Epstein FH: A closer look at radiocontrast-induced nephropathy. N Engl J Med 1989; 320:179–181.
49. Goldberg M: Systemic reactions to intravascular contrast media. Anesthesiology 1984; 60:46–56.
50. Cohan RH, Dunnick NR, Bashore TM: Treatment of reactions to radiographic contrast material. AJR 1988; 151:263–270.
51. Lasser EC: Pretreatment with corticosteroids to prevent reactions to IV contrast material: Overview and implications. AJR 1988; 150:257–259.
52. Greenberger PA, Patterson R, Tapio CM: Prophylaxis against repeated radiocontrast media reactions in 857 cases. Arch Intern Med 1985; 145:2197–2200.
53. Foesel TEH, Schrimer U, Wick C: Repeated rectal methohexitone as the sole anaesthetic agent for radiotherapy. Paediatr Anaesth 1992; 2:329–331.
54. Griswold JD, Vacanti FX, Goudsouzian NG: Twenty-three sequential out-of-hospital halothane anesthetics in an infant. Anesth Analg 1988; 67:779–781.
55. Maltby JR, Watkins DMB: Repeat ketamine anaesthesia of a child for radiotherapy in the prone position. Can Anaesth Soc J 1983; 30:526–530.
56. Cronin MM, Bousfield JD, Hewett EB, et al: Ketamine anaesthesia for radiotherapy in small children. Anaesthesia 1972; 27:135–142.
57. Lo JN, Buckley JJ, Kim TH, et al: Anesthesia for high-dose total body irradiation in children. Anesthesiology 1984; 61:101–103.
58. Bennett JA, Bullimore JA: The use of ketamine hydrochloride anaesthesia for radiotherapy in young children. Br J Anaesth 1973; 45:197–201.
59. Glauber DT, Audenaert SM: Anesthesia for children undergoing craniospinal radiotherapy. Anesthesiology 1987; 67:801–803.
60. Fisher DM, Robinson S, Brett CM, et al: Comparison of enflurane, halothane, and isoflurane for diagnostic and therapeutic procedures in children with malignancies. Anesthesiology 1985; 63:647–650.
61. Martin LD, Pasternak LR, Pudimat MA: Total intravenous anesthesia with propofol in pediatric patients outside the operating room. Anesth Analg 1992; 74:609–612.
62. Aldridge LM, Gordon NH: Propofol infusions for radiotherapy. Paediatr Anaesth 1992; 2:133–137.
63. Brett CM, Wara WM, Hamilton WK: Anesthesia for infants during radiotherapy: An insufflation technique. Anesthesiology 1986; 64:402–405.
64. Whitwam JG, Morgan M, Owen JR, et al: General anesthesia for high-dose total-body irradiation. Lancet 1978; 1:128–129.
65. Bashein G, Russell AH, Momii ST: Anesthesia and remote monitoring for intraoperative radiation therapy. Anesthesiology 1986; 64:804–807.
66. Lunsford LD, Kondziolka D, Bissonette DJ, et al: Stereotactic radiosurgery of brain vascular malformations. Neurosurg Clin North Am 1992; 3:79–98.
67. Steiner L, Lindquist C: Radiosurgery with focused gamma-beam irradiation in children. *In* Edward MSB, Hoffman HJ (eds): Cerebral Vascular Disease in Children and Adolescents. Baltimore: Williams & Wilkins, 1989.
68. Kimovec M, Monma D, Meyer R, Helenowski T: Anesthesia for gamma knife radiotherapy [Abstract]. Anesthesiology 1992; 77:A1179.
69. Harris MM: Pediatric neuroanesthesia. *In* Berry FA (ed): Anesthetic Management of Difficult and Routine Pediatric Patients, 2nd Ed. New York: Churchill Livingstone, 1990; 341–362.
70. Chripko D, Bevan JC, Archer DP, Bherer N: Decreases in arterial oxygen saturation in paediatric outpatients during transfer to the postanaesthetic recovery room. Can J Anaesth 1989; 36:128–132.
71. Besag FMC, Singh MP, Whitelaw AGL: Surgery of the ill, extremely low birthweight infant: Should transfer to the operating theatre be avoided? Acta Paediatr Scand 1984; 73:594–595.
72. Ping STS, Mehta MP, Symreng T: Accuracy of the FEF CO_2 detector in the assessment of endotracheal tube placement. Anesth Analg 1992; 74:415–419.
73. Council on Scientific Affairs: Fundamentals of magnetic resonance imaging. JAMA 1987; 258:3417–3423.
74. Body AS, Gooding CA: Magnetic resonance imaging. Pediatr Rev 1986; 8:87–92.
75. Menon DK, Peden CJ, Hall AS, et al: Magnetic resonance for the anaesthetist. Part 1: Physical principles, application, safety aspects. Anaesthesia 1992; 47:240–255.
76. Nixon C, Hirsch NP, Ormerod IEC, Johnson G: Nuclear magnetic resonance imaging. Anesthesiology 1985; 62:80–83.
77. Villafana T: Fundamental physics of magnetic resonance imaging. Radiol Clin North Am 1988; 26:701–715.
78. Higgins CB, Lanzer P, Stark D, et al: Imaging by nuclear magnetic resonance in patients with chronic ischemic heart disease. Circulation 1984; 69:523–531.
79. Karlik SJ, Heatherley T, Pavan F, et al: Patient anesthesia and monitoring at a 1.5-T MRI installation. Magn Reson Med 1988; 7:210–221.
80. Gangarosa RE, Minnis JE, Nobbe J, et al: Operational safety issues in MRI. Magn Reson Imaging 1987; 5:287–292.
81. Smith DS, Askey P, Young ML, et al: Anesthetic management of acutely ill patients during magnetic resonance imaging. Anesthesiology 1986; 65:710–711.
82. Peden CJ, Menon DK, Hall AS, et al: Magnetic resonance for the anaesthetist. Part II: Anaesthesia and monitoring in MR units. Anaesthesia 1992; 47:508–517.
83. Fowler JR, TerPenning B, Syverud SA, et al: Magnetic field hazards. N Engl J Med 1986; 314:1517.
84. Roth JL, Nugent M, Gray JE, et al: Patient monitoring during magnetic resonance imaging. Anesthesiology 1985; 62:80–83.
85. Pavlicek W, Geisinger M, Castle L, et al: The effects of nuclear magnetic resonance on patients with cardiac pacemakers. Radiology 1983; 147:149–153.
86. Erlebacher JA, Cahill PT, Pannizzo F, et al: Effect of magnetic resonance imaging on DDD pacemakers. Am J Cardiol 1986; 57:437–440.
87. Dujovny M, Kossovsky N, Kossowsky R, et al: Aneurysm clip motion during magnetic resonance imaging: In vivo experimental study with metallurgical factor analysis. Neurosurgery 1985; 17:543–548.
88. Gold JP, Pulsinelli W, Winchester P, et al: Safety of metallic surgical clips in patients undergoing high-field-strength magnetic resonance imaging. Ann Thorac Surg 1989; 48:643–645.
89. Soulen RL, Budinger TF, Higgins CB: Magnetic resonance imaging of prosthetic heart valves. Radiology 1985; 154:705–707.
90. Shellock FG, Curtis JS: MR imaging and biomedical implants, materials, and devices: An updated review. Radiology 1991; 180:541–550.
91. Hassler M, LeBas JF, Wolf JE, et al: Effects of magnetic fields used in MRI on 15 prosthetic heart valves. J Radiol 1986; 67:661–666.

92. New PFJ, Rosen BR, Brady TJ, et al: Potential hazards and artifacts of ferromagnetic and nonferromagnetic surgical and dental materials and devices in nuclear magnetic resonance imaging. Radiology 1983; 147:139–148.
93. Patteson SK, Chesney JT: Anesthetic management for magnetic resonance imaging: Problems and solutions. Anesth Analg 1992; 74: 121–128.
94. Teitelbaum GP, Yee CA, Van-Horn DD, et al: Metallic ballistic fragments: MR imaging safety and artifacts. Radiology 1990; 175:855–859.
95. Mani RL: In search of an effective screening system for intraocular metallic foreign bodies prior to MR: An important issue of patient safety. Am J Neuroradiol 1988; 9:1032.
96. Williams S, Char DH, Dillon WP, et al: Ferrous intraocular foreign bodies and magnetic resonance imaging. Am J Ophthalmol 1988; 105:398–401.
97. Kelly WM, Paglen PG, Pearson JA, et al: Ferromagnetism of intraocular foreign body causes unilateral blindness after MR study. Am J Neuroradiol 1986; 7:243–245.
98. Shellock FG, Crues JV: Temperature, heart rate, and blood pressure changes associated with clinical MR imaging at 1.5 T. Radiology 1987; 163:259–262.
99. Davis PL, Crooks L, Arakawa M, et al: Potential hazards in NMR imaging: Heating effects of changing magnetic fields and RF fields on small implants. AJR 1981; 137:857–860.
100. Hall SC, Stevenson GW, Suresh S: Burn associated with temperature monitoring during magnetic resonance imaging [Letter]. Anesthesiology 1992; 76:152.
101. McArdle CB, Nicholas DA, Richardson CJ, Amparo EG: Monitoring of the neonate undergoing MR imaging: Technical considerations. Radiology 1986; 159:223–226.
102. Kanal E, Shellock FG, Talagala L: Safety considerations in MR imaging. Radiology 1990; 176:593–606.
103. Legendre JP, Misner R, Forester GV, Geoffrion Y: A simple fiber optic monitor of cardiac and respiratory activity for biomedical magnetic resonance applications. Magn Reson Med 1986; 3:953–957.
104. Wendt RE, Rokey R, Vick GW, et al: Electrocardiographic gating and monitoring in NMR imaging. Magn Reson Imaging 1988; 6:89–95.
105. Dimick RN, Hedlund LW, Herfkens RJ, et al: Optimizing electrocardiographic electrode placement for cardiac-gated magnetic resonance imaging. Invest Radiol 1987; 22:17–22.
106. Rao CC, Krishna G, Emhardt J: Anesthesia machine for use during magnetic resonance imaging. Anesthesiology 1990; 73:1054–1055.
107. Nixon C, Hirsch NP, Ormerod IEC, Johnson G: Nuclear magnetic resonance. Its implications for the anaesthetist. Anaesthesia 1986; 41:131–137.
108. Mezrich R, Reicheck N, Kressel HY: ECG effects in high-field MR imaging. Radiology 1985; 157:219.
109. Budinger TF: Nuclear magnetic resonance (NMR) in vivo studies: Known thresholds for health effects. J Comput Assist Tomogr 1981; 5:800–811.
110. Tenforde TS, Gaffey CT, Mayer BR, Budinger TF: Cardiovascular alterations in Macaca monkeys exposed to stationary magnetic fields, experimental observations and theoretical analysis. Bioelectromagnetics 1983; 4:1–9.
111. Saunders RD, Smith H: Safety aspects of NMR clinical imaging. Br Med Bull 1984; 40:148–154.
112. Sellden H, De Chateau P, Ekman G, et al: Circulatory monitoring of children during anaesthesia in low-field magnetic resonance imaging. Acta Anaesthesiol Scand 1990; 34:41–43.
113. Cote CJ, Rolf N, Liu LMP, et al: A single-blind study of combined pulse oximetry and capnography in children. Anesthesiology 1991; 74:980–987.
114. Eichhorn JH (ed): Pulse oximetry as a standard of practice in anesthesia. Anesthesiology 1993; 78:423–426.
115. Boesch C, Martin E: Combined application of MR imaging and spectroscopy in neonates and children, installation and operation of 2.35T system in a clinical setting. Radiology 1988; 168:481–488.
116. Wagle WA: Technique for RF isolation of a pulse oximeter in a 1.5 T MR unit. Am J Neuroradiol 1989; 10:208.
117. Bashein G, Syrovy G: Burns associated with pulse oximetry during magnetic resonance imaging. Anesthesiology 1991; 75:382–383.
118. Fisher DM: Sedation of pediatric patients: An anesthesiologist's perspective. Radiology 1990; 175:613–615.
119. Shellock FG: Monitoring during MRI. An evaluation of the effect of high-field MRI on various patient monitors. Med Electronics 1986; 17:93–97.
120. Tobin JR, Spurrier EA, Wetzel RC: Anaesthesia for critically ill children during magnetic resonance imaging. Br J Anaesth 1992; 69:482–486.
121. Barnett GH, Ropper AH, Johnson KA: Physiological support and monitoring of critically ill patients during magnetic resonance imaging. J Neurosurg 1988; 68:246–250.
122. Bonsu AK, Tamilarasan A, Bromage PR: A nasal catheter for monitoring tidal carbon dioxide in spontaneously breathing patients. Anesthesiology 1989; 71:318.
123. Shellock FG: Monitoring sedated pediatric patients during MR imaging. Radiology 1990; 177:586–587.
124. Flaherty JA, Hoskinson K: Emotional distress during magnetic resonance imaging. N Engl J Med 1989; 320:467–468.
125. Brummett RE, Talbot JM, Charuhas P: Potential hearing loss resulting from MR imaging. Radiology 1988; 169:539–540.
126. Henneberg S, Hok B, Wiklund L, Sjodin G: Remote auscultatory patient monitoring during magnetic resonance imaging. J Clin Monit 1992; 8:37–43.
127. Henneberg S, Hok B, Wiklund L, Sjodin G: Remote auscultatory patient monitoring during magnetic resonance imaging. J Clin Monit 1992; 8:37–43.
128. Shellock FG, Crues JV: MRI: Safety consideration in magnetic resonance imaging. Magn Reson Imaging Decisions 1988; 2:25–30.
129. Davis PJ, Gillen C, Kretchman E, et al: Experience with anesthesia for children requiring nuclear magnetic resonance imaging. Anesth Rev 1990; 17:35–40.
130. Beers GJ: Biological effects of weak electromagnetic fields from 0 Hz to 200 MHz: A survey of the literature with specific emphasis on possible magnetic resonance effects. Magn Reson Imaging 1989; 7:309–331.
131. Shellock FG: Biological effects of MRI: A clean safety record so far. Diagn Imaging 1987; 9:96–101.
132. Geard CR, Osmak RS, Hall EJ, et al: Magnetic resonance and ionizing radiation: A comparative evaluation in vitro of oncogenic and genotoxic potential. Radiology 1984; 152:199–202.
133. Osbakken M, Griffith J, Taczanowsky P: A gross, morphologic, hematologic, and blood chemistry study of adult and neonatal mice chronically exposed to high magnetic fields. Magn Reson Medicine 1986; 3:502–517.
134. Budinger TF, Bristol KS, Yen CK: Biologic Effects of Static Magnetic Fields [Abstract]. New York: Society of Magnetic Resonance in Medicine, 1984; 118.

CHAPTER

20

Metabolic Monitoring

HOWARD R. BROMLEY, M.D.,
PATRICIA M. GRAMLING-BABB, M.D.,
ROBERT W. COOK, B.A., R.R.T., R.C.P., and
THERESA PIURKOWSKY, M.Ed., R.R.T., C.P.F.T., R.C.P.

Over the past three decades, nutritional support of the hospitalized patient has improved quite dramatically. The introduction of hyperalimentation has aided in focusing extrinsic and intrinsic nutritional support on both inpatients and, more recently, outpatients. Improved nutritional maintenance has helped to decrease the incidence of morbidity and mortality.[1] One can plan these complicated alimentations using estimates of energy expenditure (EE) based on nomograms or standard formulae, which are acceptable predictors for the calculation of nutritional support in normal subjects.[2–4] However, many acute and chronic diseases cause significant alterations in energy expenditure, thereby calling into question the accuracy of these nomograms and formulae.[5, 6] Complications may be associated with excessive caloric support, including respiratory failure, hepatic insufficiency, and possible impairment of host defenses.[7–10] These complications and the desire to more closely tailor an individual patient's daily caloric balance are the reason for technical measurement of resting energy expenditure (REE) using bedside indirect calorimetry, commonly referred to as metabolic monitoring.[8]

Indirect calorimetry is frequently used to describe the technique that measures oxygen consumption ($\dot{V}O_2$) and carbon dioxide production ($\dot{V}CO_2$). Sophisticated electronic monitors can now directly measure oxygen consumption and carbon dioxide production, and they can calculate indirect caloric requirements (metabolic expenditure) on a minute-by-minute basis. From these measurements, clinicians can calculate the energy production that is associated with the patient's current activity state (e.g., basal metabolic rate, resting energy expenditure, maximum aerobic capacity). Extensive literature attests to the effectiveness of this instrument in accessing both the preoperative and postoperative metabolic condition of the patient.[6–8, 11–13] However, there is little information about the intraoperative aspects of metabolic activity.

The proliferation of commercial portable metabolic carts has aided the frequent bedside determination of a patient's REE. Previous researchers speculated that such measurements would decrease hospital stay by improving nutritional support.[1] The number of measurements needed in intensive care patients remains questionable, and many practitioners continue to use standard nomograms or formulae. Studies have shown that values for REE and estimated EE can differ significantly.

HISTORICAL PERSPECTIVE

The first reported studies that measured oxygen consumption were conducted by Antoine Lavoisier in 1777.[15] Lavoisier proved that respiratory gas exchange was a type of combustion not unlike that of a burning candle.[16] He used an ice calorimeter to measure the heat and carbon dioxide production of a guinea pig.

In 1856, Adolf Fick published his book on such topics as the mixing of air in the lungs, measurement of carbon dioxide output in humans, and the heat economy of the body. Fourteen years later, Fick published the work that yielded what has come to be known as the Fick equation for determination of total body blood flow (cardiac output) from the oxygen consumption and arterial-venous oxygen content differences.[16]

In 1849, the first closed-circuit chamber was constructed by Regnault and Rieset to measure oxygen utilization and carbon dioxide production. Pettenkofer is credited with developing the first open-circuit respirometer in 1862.[17]

Atwater and Rosa constructed a combined live-in direct and indirect calorimeter based on Pettenkofer's designs in 1899. They assumed that all dietary carbohydrate was oxidized, noting that the remaining carbon originated from fat. Their data were highly accurate.[18]

In animal studies using his respiration calorimeter, Rubner demonstrated the technique in which nitrogen balance and carbon could be used to define energy output in relation to food input by measuring the exhaled carbon dioxide and the energy and nitrogen contents of body waste.[18] Rubner was the first to use the term *indirect calorimetry*, which measures the difference between oxidation rate and heat loss.[16]

Harris and Benedict described the relationship between oxygen consumption and energy expenditure.[2] These studies were instrumental in describing the basal metabolic requirements for adults and children. Since that time, a considerable amount of research has evaluated basal and resting metabolic conditions and verified the Harris-Benedict equation.

APPARATUS: METABOLIC CARTS

The use of the metabolic cart in indirect calorimetry allows the practitioner to accurately measure $\dot{V}O_2$ and $\dot{V}CO_2$. The resulting data aid in the assessment of the patient's caloric energy needs and help in predicting the nutritional requirements for adequate metabolic functioning.[19]

Historically, the Tissot spirometer or the Douglas bag has been used to obtain $\dot{V}O_2$ and $\dot{V}CO_2$ values. However, these devices have proven to be unsatisfactory because they are large, bulky, and, in the case of the Tissot spirometer, difficult to calibrate.[20]

The metabolic cart is small, portable, and generally user-friendly. It is noninvasive, autocalibrates on a predetermined schedule, and is equipped to run self-diagnostic tests. These features, coupled with a relatively low cost, make the metabolic cart the instrument of choice for bedside measurement of REE.

INSTRUMENT COMPONENTS

Volume Measurement

All metabolic carts are equipped to measure volume in some manner. For optimal results, one of the following three devices is recommended:

Pneumotachograph. This tool converts a mechanical measurement to an electronic signal by means of a pressure transducer. The volume is obtained when the signal is amplified and integrated over a set period.[21] The pneumotachograph operates on the principle that as a fluid flows through a screen, the decrease in pressure is directly proportional to the flow.[22]

Ultrasonic Vortex-Shedding Transducer. In this method of measurement, Karmen vortices are created by a precisely sized strut within a flow tube. The tube/strut combination creates vortices, or waves, of approximately 1 ml in volume as a gas passes the strut. The resulting vortex formation (Karmen vortex) is then sensed by an ultrasonic beam directed across the tube. The vortex frequency is a function of the gaseous velocity and the strut size; the density and the temperature of the gas do not affect the readings. Consequently, the obtained vortex rate is a direct, linear measure of the gas velocity and, thus, the flow volume.[20]

Mass Flow Sensor (Wheatstone Bridge Circuitry). Two stainless steel wires heated to different temperatures (180°C and 240°C) are positioned in a laminar flow tube. The circuit, which is driven by a servo-loop bridge output, is sensed by a differential amplifier (i.e., the Wheatstone bridge). The number of gas molecules passing by the wires is measured by the mass-flow sensor. The two hot wires enable the measurement to be independent of the temperature, humidity, and viscosity of the flowing gas.[23]

Mixing Chamber

The mixing chamber is needed to completely mix the expired gases. The mixing chamber is extremely important, because the mixed expired gases are ultimately analyzed from this chamber.

A variable-volume chamber is most desirable because of the inherent differences in the exhaled minute volumes in different patients. Using a smaller mixing chamber with smaller minute volumes improves response time.[24]

Oxygen Analyzers

Zirconium Oxide. The standard oxygen analyzer is the zirconium oxide type. It consists of a zirconium oxide ceramic tube that is plated inside and out with a thin layer of platinum.

At approximately 900°C, oxygen is ionized in the presence of platinum; the zirconium oxide ceramic tube is permeable to this ionized oxygen. The oxygen generates a potential between the two platinum surfaces of the tube. This potential is directly and linearly related to the oxygen concentration[22] (see also Chapter 11).

Paramagnetic Sensor. This device functions on the principle of an oxygen molecule's attraction in a magnetic field. Two nitrogen-filled spheres are hung in a magnetic field, where they can rotate. As oxygen enters the center of the field, the spheres are displaced and rotate on their wire in relation to the number of oxygen molecules present. The displacement of the wire is then reflected onto a screen and interpreted into the percentage of oxygen[25] (see also Chapter 11).

Carbon Dioxide Analyzer

The infrared absorption analyzer is the most widely used method to measure expired carbon dioxide. It employs a beam of infrared light that passes through a sample of gas containing carbon dioxide.

Carbon dioxide, as well as other gases, absorbs specific wavelengths of infrared light. Carbon dioxide is composed of three atoms (one carbon, two oxygens). As the infrared beam passes through the gas, a portion of the infrared radiation is absorbed; this portion is compared to a reference sample with a known concentration of carbon dioxide. The resultant carbon dioxide concentration is calculated.[22, 23]

Microprocessor

The microprocessor with its associated electronics is responsible for controlling the total test routine and general operation. It collects and calculates data and is responsible for the smooth operation of the valves and solenoid switches. The microprocessor also monitors and displays inspired and expired gases, volumes, and nutritional status in either a breath-by-breath or an averaging mode.

THEORY OF OPERATION

Gas exchange, as measured by most metabolic monitors, is calculated using the following equations (with modifications for each machine)[26, 27]:

Oxygen consumption is calculated as follows:

$$\dot{V}O_2 = \frac{\dot{V}E\ (FIO_2 - FEO_2 - [FIO_2 - FECO_2])}{(1 - FIO_2)}$$

where: $\dot{V}E$ = minute volume of expired ventilation
FI = inspired fraction of gas (in decimal equivalents)
FE = expired fraction of gas (in decimal equivalents)

Carbon dioxide production is calculated as follows:

$$\dot{V}CO_2 = \dot{V}E \times FECO_2$$

Metabolic functions are computed using the technique of Bursztein[27]:

Energy metabolism (calories/minute) = 5.083 ($\dot{V}O_2$) − 0.138 ($\dot{V}CO_2$) − 0.128 (NU)

Carbohydrate metabolism (g/minute) = 4.06 ($\dot{V}CO_2$) − 2.854 ($\dot{V}O_2$) + 2.468 (NU)

Protein metabolism (g/minute) = 6.25 (NU)

Fat metabolism (g/minute) = 1.805 ($\dot{V}O_2 - \dot{V}CO_2$) − 1.681 (NU)

where: NU = urinary nitrogen (in g/minute)

$\dot{V}O_2$ and $\dot{V}CO_2$ are measured in ml/minute. Urinary nitrogen is obtained from a 24-hour urine collection; the obtained value is entered directly into the metabolic monitor.

The above formulae can be converted mathematically to be expressed in kilocalories/day or in g/day:

Energy metabolism (kcal/day) = 7.32 ($\dot{V}O_2$) − 0.198 ($\dot{V}CO_2$) − 0.184 (NU)

Carbohydrate metabolism (g/day) = 5.85 ($\dot{V}CO_2$) − 4.11 ($\dot{V}O_2$) + 3.554 (NU)

Protein metabolism (g/day) = 6.25 (NU)

Fat metabolism (g/day) = 2.6 ($\dot{V}O_2 - \dot{V}CO_2$) − 2.421 (NU)

Many techniques have been described for measuring the above parameters. The two most frequently used are the closed- and open-circuit techniques.

CLOSED-CIRCUIT TECHNIQUE

The closed-circuit technique involves the rebreathing of inspired gases from an oxygen-enriched reservoir.[28] As oxygen is consumed by the patient, the oxygen supply in the volumetric reservoir is depleted. Oxygen consumption is therefore the quotient of oxygen extraction or loss, divided by time.

Carbon dioxide production is the product of exhaled carbon dioxide concentration multiplied by the volume of exhaled gas. The exhaled carbon dioxide is removed from the closed-circuit system by chemical scrubbing to prevent hypercarbia. This closed-circuit system is essentially identical to the technique described by Lavoisier and by Harris and Benedict and is considered the gold standard for measurement of oxygen consumption.

The closed-circuit technique is primarily affected by changes in lung volume or leaks in the spirometer circuit. Acute changes in lung volume will be reflected as a decrease in $\dot{V}O_2$ if the lung volume is displaced into the spirometer. Because oxygen consumption is determined by the volume loss per unit of time, any leak will be interpreted as a change in $\dot{V}O_2$.

OPEN-CIRCUIT TECHNIQUE

The open-circuit technique involves either the timed collection of expired gases or continuous analysis of those expired gases.[28] Oxygen consumption and carbon dioxide production are the products of the difference between inspired and expired gas concentrations for oxygen and carbon dioxide multiplied by the exhaled volume. This technique has been frequently employed to determine maximum aerobic capacity during exercise performance tests.

The open-circuit technique may be affected by water vapor, gas compression, fluctuations in inspired and expired gas concentration, positive pressure, and system leaks. The assumptions underlying the open-circuit technique and the factors that may affect its accuracy make this technique questionable for use in critically ill, mechanically ventilated patients.

SYSTEM DESCRIPTIONS AND PATIENT CONNECTIONS

The bedside measurement of $\dot{V}O_2$ and $\dot{V}CO_2$ in the critically ill patient can be accomplished in several ways, depending on the type of respiratory support required by the patient. Proper connection to the patient is necessary to achieve a steady state, in which the inspiratory and expiratory gases represent the patient's true metabolic status. In all situations, it is imperative to monitor the patient closely to ensure that the system has no leaks and that expired gases are directed to the metabolic computer.

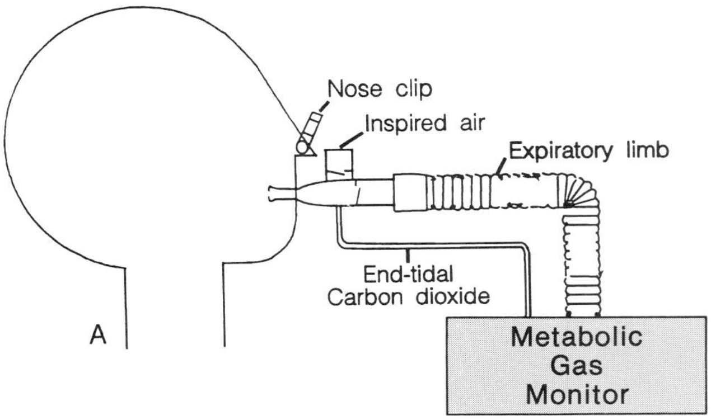

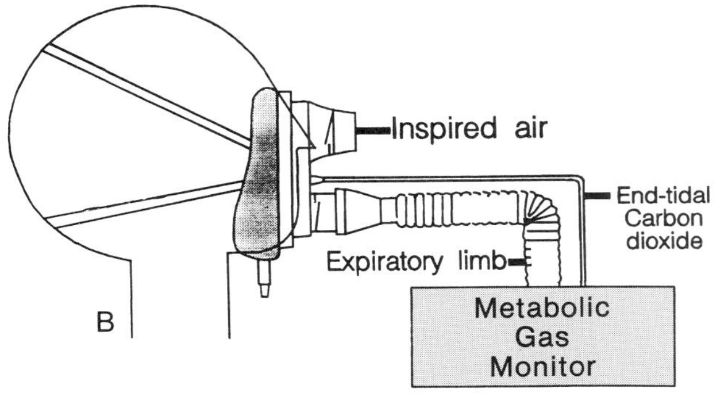

Figure 20–1. *A*, Metabolic gas monitoring in a spontaneously breathing patient using a noseclip and mouthpiece. *B*, Metabolic gas monitoring in a spontaneously breathing patient using a tight-fitting face mask.

Indirect calorimetry of the spontaneously breathing patient can be accomplished with a mouthpiece that has a nonrebreathing valve and nose clip or with a tight-fitting face mask that has inspiratory and expiratory valves (Fig. 20–1).

When a spontaneously breathing patient is receiving supplemental oxygen, the supplied supplemental oxygen must be stable and monitored by the microprocessor. Therefore, an external blender is used to provide a stable FIO_2 for the patient. The gas mixture is supplied at a flow rate high enough to meet the patient's inspiratory demand. Expired gas is directed to the metabolic computer via the nonrebreathing valve (Fig. 20–2). It is critical that the flow rate of the mixed inspired gas not be too high, because if it is, it will combine with and dilute the patient's expired gas, thereby affecting accuracy.

For a mechanically ventilated patient, a sample of inspired gas is directed to the computer; the expiratory gases flow from the expiratory valve on the ventilator to the monitor (Fig. 20–3).

During this process, the patient should be observed closely for proper exhalation. The patient and ventilator should be checked routinely to assess ventilator function and patient compatibility. Some variances in the basic procedure may be necessary because of differences in ventilator design and/or ventilator mode.

MEASUREMENT METHODS AND DEVICES

The accuracy in the Harris-Benedict formula is 80% or 90% in the normal healthy subject.[14, 29] The most accurate means of assessing EE is the metabolic cart, which requires a cooperative, stable patient. If the patient can tolerate an oral diet, food and drink should be withheld for 12 hours. If the patient is on enteral tube feeding or parenteral therapy, it should be continued at a steady state for at least 12 hours. Thirty minutes of rest prior to initiation of measurements are required for optimal results.[19]

Patients are connected directly to the calorimeter via an endotracheal tube, are placed in a ventilated hood or tent, or use a mouthpiece and nose clip.[30] If a patient must use a mouthpiece or mask, a training period is needed for the patient to become relaxed and comfortable with the procedure. It is important that the mask fit correctly, because misplacement in cachectic or edentulous patients is common. Poor mask fit results in a volume leak and incorrect measurements.[19] Tolerance for the equipment may be a problem in patients with facial fractures or bruising. Artificial airways (endotracheal or tracheostomy tubes) must be free of air leaks. Humidification should be discontinued during the period of testing.[19] Although there are differences in metabolic monitoring systems, most have similar measuring devices. Within each system, there is a method for dehumidification of the air sample by special tubing, water traps, or anhydrous materials.

The process by which the calculations are made differs according to the type of device used. Errors in measurement of $\dot{V}O_2$ can exceed 5% if FIO_2 exceeds 0.6. Theoretically, as FIO_2 approaches 1.0, it becomes difficult to detect the difference between the FIO_2 and the FEO_2.[31]

The monitors currently available include the Deltatrac Metabolic Monitor (SensorMedics, Anaheim, CA), the Engstrom Metabolic Computer (Gambro Engstrom AB, Broma, Sweden), the Hartman and Braun Metabolator (Hartman and Braun, Frankfurt, Germany), the Oxylog (PK Morgan, Kent, U.K.), and the SensorMedics MMC Horizon (SensorMedics, Anaheim, CA).

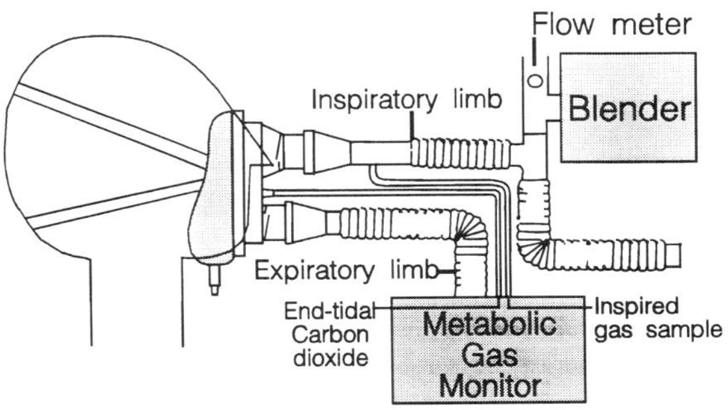

Figure 20–2. Metabolic gas monitoring in a spontaneously breathing patient receiving a continuous flow of premixed gases.

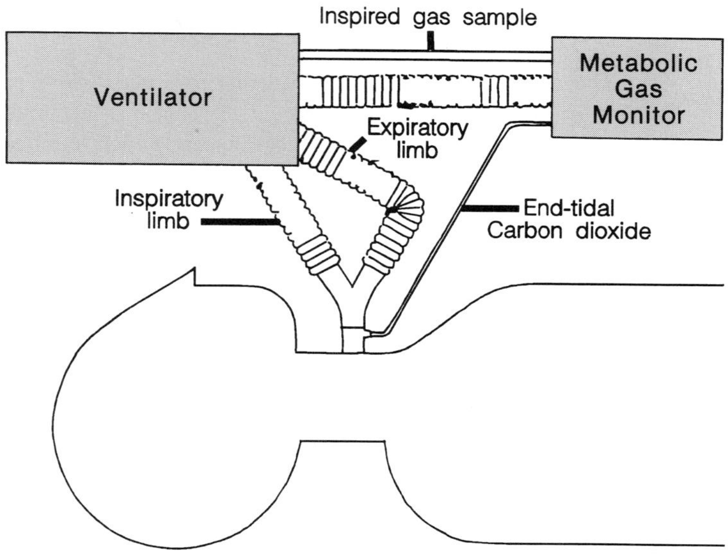

Figure 20–3. Metabolic gas monitoring of a patient on a ventilator.

DELTATRAC METABOLIC MONITOR

Oxygen is measured from a differential signal between inspired and expired gases. Actual flow is not measured directly but is calculated via an air dilution method. Because oxygen consumption is calculated, this monitor performs better, with less error, at a higher FIO_2. Calculations used by this monitor include the following:

$$\dot{V}O_2 = Q \times FECO_2 \times \frac{[(FIO_2 - FEO_2) \div FECO_2] - FIO_2}{(1 - FIO_2)}$$

where Q = a known constant generated air flow. In this calculation, $FECO_2$ = the average CO_2 concentration in expired gas after dilution with a known constant generated in airflow.[31] A mixing chamber is utilized to add the exhaled gas sample to a fixed flow of 45 L/minute. The CO_2 concentration in the effluent gas is multiplied by 45 L/minute to determine the $\dot{V}CO_2$.

$$RQ = (1 - FIO_2) \div [(FIO_2 - FEO_2) \div FECO_2] - FIO_2$$

$$\dot{V}O_2 = \dot{V}CO_2 \div RQ$$

$$REE\ (kcal/day) = 5.68\ (\dot{V}O_2) + 1.59\ (\dot{V}CO_2) - 2.17\ (NU)$$

where RQ = respiratory quotient and NU = urinary nitrogen excretion in g/day.

ENGSTROM METABOLIC COMPUTER

This metabolic monitor can be used to evaluate a ventilated patient. The unit possesses a microprocessor and utilizes an oximeter that measures inspired and expired volumes ($\dot{V}I$ and $\dot{V}E$). A reversed Haldane Transformation Factor (i.e., FI nitrogen / FE nitrogen) is used from derived FIO_2, FEO_2, and $FECO_2$, as noted below. Equations used by the microprocessor include the following:

$$\dot{V}O_2 = \dot{V}I\ (FIO_2 - K \times FEO_2)$$

$$\dot{V}CO_2 = \dot{V}I\ (K \times FECO_2 - 0.0003)$$

$$RQ = (K \times FECO_2 - 0.0003) \div (FIO_2 - K \times FEO_2)$$

where $K = (1 - FIO_2 - 0.0003) \div (1 - FEO_2 - FECO_2)$, the reversed Haldane Transformation Factor, and 0.0003 is the concentration of carbon dioxide in room air.[32]

$$EE\ (kcal/day) = 1.32\ (\dot{V}O_2) \times (1.23[RQ] + 3.81)$$

SENSORMEDICS MMC HORIZON

This is a multipurpose instrument that can be used for mechanically ventilated patients, patients in hoods or tents (canopy mode) or patients undergoing exercise testing.[32] It contains a polarographic oxygen analyzer, an infrared carbon dioxide analyzer, a turbine volume transducer, and a 3-L mixing chamber. Expired gases pass into the mixing chamber and out through the turbine volume transducer. Sample sizes of 500 ml/minute are dried and then passed through the carbon dioxide and oxygen analyzers. Eight-hour or one-hour assessment programs are available. The information is then sent to a microprocessor. Fat, carbohydrate, and protein oxidation rates can also be calculated if urinary nitrogen is obtained. The following equations are utilized by this machine[32]:

$$\dot{V}O_2 = \dot{V}E\ \{FIO_2\ (1 - FEO_2 - FECO_2) \div (1 - FIO_2 - FICO_2) - FEO_2\}$$

$$\dot{V}CO_2 = \dot{V}E\ (FECO_2 - FICO_2)$$

$$RQ = \dot{V}CO_2/\dot{V}O_2$$

$$REE\ (kcal/day) = 1.44\ (3.796[\dot{V}O_2] + 1.214[\dot{V}CO_2])$$

OXYLOG

This is a portable device for the measurement of oxygen consumption, designed for flow rates of less than 80 L/minute.[33] Expired air is directly conducted to the instrument. A small sample (about 1.5 ml/breath) is taken from both expired air and atmospheric air. The samples are dried, and oxygen is analyzed by a polygraphic oxygen analyzer. Oxygen consumption is determined by the differences among expired oxygen, atmospheric oxygen, and the volume of inspired air.[30] Equations used include:

$$EE\ (\text{kcal/day}) = \dot{V}O_2 \times 7200$$

where $\dot{V}O_2$ is in L/minute, the caloric volume of 1 L of oxygen is assumed to be 5 kcal, $\dot{V}I = \dot{V}E$, and $RQ = 1.0$.

HARTMAN AND BRAUN METABOLATOR

This monitor uses a mouthpiece and nose clip.[34] A mixing chamber collects the expired air, and a sample is drawn off and divided into two 1-ml streams. One stream is dried; the other passes through soda lime and anhydrous calcium chloride, where it is dried and voided of carbon dioxide. A Wheatstone bridge circuit containing heated measuring wires analyzes the samples. Oxygen and carbon dioxide concentrations are expressed as a percentage of the difference from atmospheric air by measuring resistance. The following equation is utilized[30]:

EE (kcal/day) = 2.58 × [barometric pressure in mmHg × volume of inspired air in 10 minutes in liters ÷ (273 + room temperature in °C)] × the corrected mean value of percentage of O_2 deficit × 79.1 ÷ [79.1 + (percentage of O_2 deficit) − the corrected mean value of percentage of CO_2 consumption]

These devices are relatively user-friendly and are usually self-calibrating. Of concern are devices that may be inaccurate when FIO_2 is high, when patients have noncompliant airways (with or without infections), and when the patient is unable to take adequate breaths.

CLINICAL APPLICATIONS

The recovery of debilitated patients with multiple organ system involvement depends on appropriate, well calculated, nutritional parameters.[8, 35, 36] Underfed, critically ill patients can be at increased risk for infection with impaired immune function,[10, 37–39] and weaning from a ventilator may be difficult because of depressed ventilatory drive and inadequate nutritional support.[35, 40]

Overfeeding has its own inherent problems when related to nutritional support.[41] As carbohydrates are metabolized, carbon dioxide production increases, causing respiratory acidosis if minute ventilation is not also proportionately increased.[42] Excess calories lead to hyperglycemia and possible liver dysfunction due to fatty infiltrates.[9, 43] Lipogenesis can increase energy expenditure by approximately 25%.[44, 45] Metabolism of proteins can cause diet-induced thermogenesis, with an increase in energy expenditure of 7–10%.[44, 46]

In general, intensivists are aware of the metabolic needs of the critically ill patient. However, the actual determination of caloric requirements differs according to which of the more than 190 available formulae are used or if determination of caloric needs is made by one of the numerous commercially available metabolic carts.[4, 47, 48] Makk et al studied 26 patients whose daily energy requirements and nutritional repletion were based on the Harris-Benedict equation.[19] Using a SensorMedics MMC Horizon metabolic cart, the researchers verified that only 32% of the patients were appropriately fed, 41% were being underfed, and 27% were being overfed. In this study, 58% of the patients were overweight, but their weight was not equated with adipose tissue or adequate nutrition. The noted weight gain could have been from volume expansion or edema. In the face of these supposedly well-fed patients, kwashiorkor patterns (three abnormal visceral proteins or two severely depressed visceral proteins) and marasma patterns (body weight of less than 90% with visceral and somatic protein depletion) of malnutrition were demonstrated.

The Harris-Benedict resting energy expenditure (HBREE), along with a metabolic activity factor, can underestimate (when using actual body weight) or overestimate (when using ideal body weight) nutritional needs in these patients. The inaccuracy of the Harris-Benedict equation is due in part to the impact of disease on energy expenditure, which can result in an approximate 30% increase. For example, major burns can cause a 100% increase, or cancer can lower requirements by 30% because of the body's response to starvation.[19]

Many factors influence true resting energy expenditure. In actuality, true REE is equal to measured REE only in a fasting, afebrile patient.[19] When formulae are being applied, the question of using ideal or actual body weight arises. Is the patient febrile, active, or paralyzed on a ventilator? Is the patient receiving inotropic support or medications such as aspirin, thyroid, caffeine, narcotics, benzodiazepines, or alpha or beta blockers?[19] Is the patient comfortable or in pain? Even the patient's circadian rhythm will make a difference in energy expenditure.[5, 49–54] An ambulatory patient can increase REE by 15%.[44]

There is also a difference in males and females of the same body weight. Men have a greater lean muscle mass and less body fat than women do. As one ages, lean muscle mass decreases and adipose tissue increases,[19] thereby lowering the body's resting energy expenditure. Bartlett et al studied critically ill surgical patients and found a correlation between cumulative caloric balance and mortality rate.[8] For obvious reasons, a controlled, prospective study on the effects of overfeeding and underfeeding on morbidity and mortality cannot be pursued without great difficulty.

PARAMETERS TO BE MONITORED

The clinical application of gas-exchange determinations has become an area of growing research. It is now well understood that fuel sources selected for nutritional support, because of their respective RQs, play a vital role in the treatment of critically ill patients, especially the ventilator-dependent patient.[40] The RQ is defined as the ratio of carbon dioxide produced to oxygen consumed ($\dot{V}CO_2/\dot{V}O_2$).

When oxidized for energy, carbohydrates, proteins, and fats result in RQs of 1.0, 0.8, and 0.71, respectively. Thus, carbohydrates generate the greatest amount of carbon dioxide, whereas fats generate the least. Increased carbon dioxide production, often indicated by an RQ greater than 1.0, will exacerbate respiratory dysfunction and possibly delay weaning (Fig. 20–4).[13, 35, 40, 55]

The nonprotein energy of parenteral nutrition is generally supplied as glucose. With nutritional depletion, the major energy source shifts from endogenous fat (RQ = 0.7) to administered glucose (RQ = 1.0), and carbon dioxide production rises concurrently with the increased RQ. Furthermore, the characteristic response to a glucose load in excess of energy needs is to convert excess glucose to fat, which is associated with an RQ of approximately 8.0. This response results in increased carbon dioxide production, with minute ventilation consequently increasing as much as 30%.[11, 12, 45] Only a small energy expenditure is associated with fat synthesis; therefore, oxygen consumption increases only minimally.[19, 56]

Ideally, every patient requiring nutritional support should be evaluated by one of the many metabolic carts available on the market today.[47, 48] Sometimes this evaluation is impractical, such as when there are air leaks around artificial airways, FIO_2 is greater than 0.6 (not an absolute contraindication), and patients are actively bleeding, are on dialysis, or have thoracic drains.[43] Accuracy of the calorimetry devices can be of concern with increased inspiratory pressures, low minute volume ventilation, and infected lung parenchyma.[20, 57, 58]

Metabolic monitoring should take place at rest during a time of stability, ranging from 30 minutes to 4 hours. A patient who is awake and alert can increase EE by approximately 10%.[5, 50, 59] Chest physiotherapy can increase EE by as much as 36%, and even an electrocardiogram can increase EE by 15%.[5, 44, 50] However, these changes do not significantly affect energy requirements. The multitude of procedures and treatments a patient must deal with in a 24-hour period in an intensive care unit only increases EE an average of about 8–10% above resting EE (Fig. 20–5).[19]

How often is metabolic testing needed? The general trend appears to be once or twice a week with extrapolation of the collected data to the other nontesting days. The day-to-day variability of true energy expenditure can exceed 31%, assuming that one day's measurements are applied to the next.[43, 54] If body temperature correction is added into the calculations, the error can be reduced to 25%.[43] Vermeij et al cited an optimal correction factor of 6% per degree Celsius,[43] whereas Dubois cited a correction factor of 13%.[60] One criticism of Dubois' study was that the patients were hyperthermic. Although Quebbeman and Ausman state that a 20% error in determination of caloric supply is acceptable,[61] the issue remains questionable. It is probably advisable to monitor REE, $\dot{V}O_2$, $\dot{V}CO_2$, and RQ on a daily basis when delivering nutritional support to a critically ill patient.

The metabolic cart accurately assesses the patient's needs and the effects of current nutritional regimens. The typical Western diet consists of 15% protein, 30% fat, and 55% carbohydrates, corresponding to an RQ of 0.82–0.83. Metabolism of alcohol or ketones (as in starvation) can decrease the RQ to 0.67, whereas the development of lipogenesis (as in overfeeding) can increase RQ to 1.2 or higher.[14, 62] An RQ of 1 or slightly less should be demonstrated when a patient is receiving total parenteral nutrition, which will represent a proper feeding combination.

SUMMARY

Researchers have determined the beneficial effects of nutritional support in critically ill patients. However, considerable debate remains as to an individual patient's caloric needs and the best method for determining those needs. Technologic advances in estimating REE have redefined the way in which nutritional support is provided.[8] In addition, further emphasis has been placed on the clinician's role of closely providing an individual's caloric needs to avoid the complications of hypocaloric or hypercaloric support.[8–10, 41, 45, 47, 48, 63]

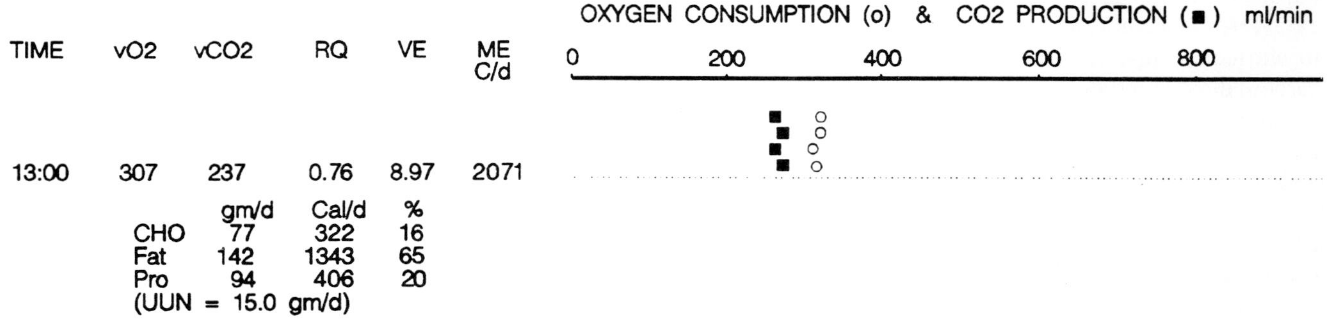

Figure 20–4. Typical printout of a simple metabolic cart monitoring record demonstrating a patient's oxygen consumption (open circles), carbon dioxide production (closed squares), respiratory quotient (RQ), and calculated mean energy expenditure (ME) in kcals/day. The record also separates the energy expenditure into carbohydrate, fat, and protein energy as g/day, kcals/day, and percentage of total energy expenditure. The protein energy portion is calculated from the urine urea nitrogen (UUN).

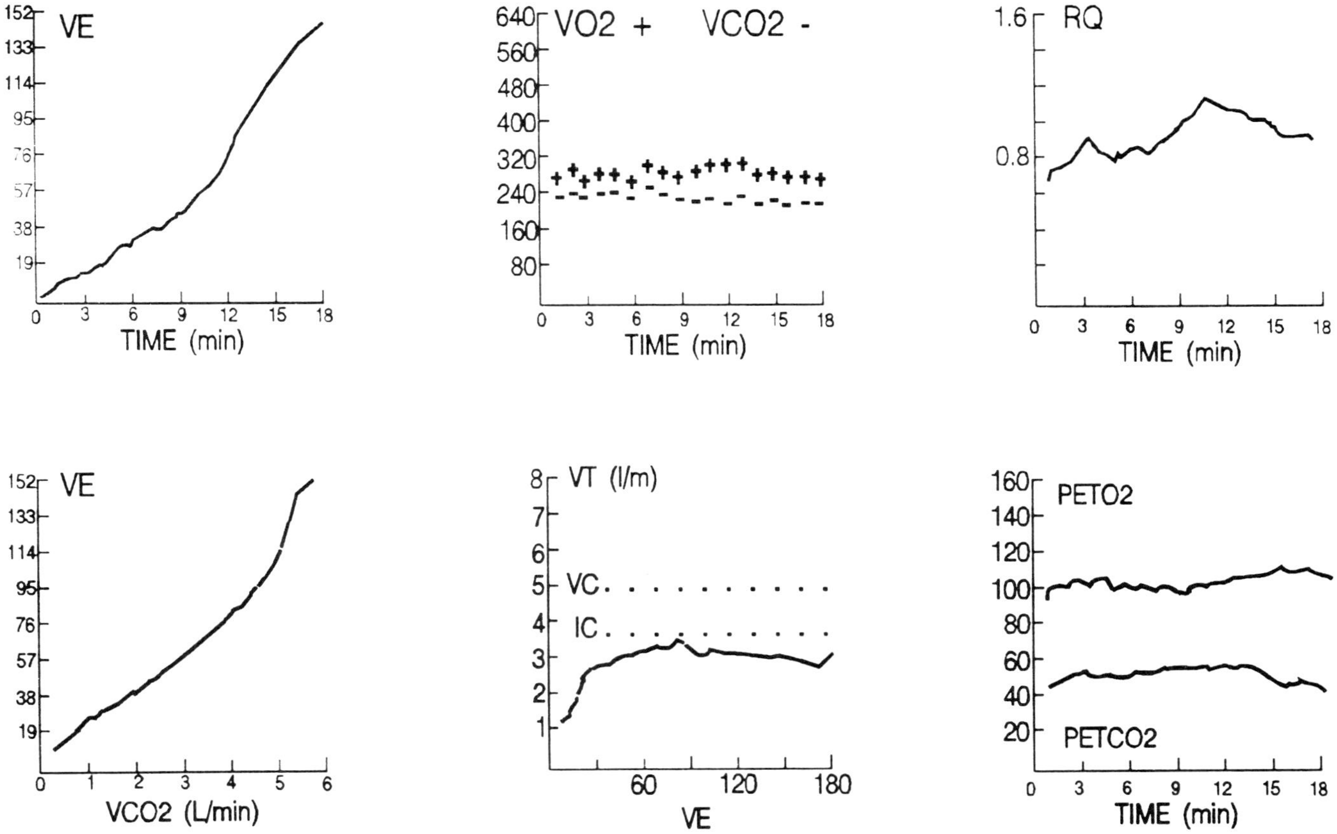

Figure 20–5. Typical graphic plot printout of a more sophisticated metabolic monitoring machine than that seen in Figure 20–4 that is capable of demonstrating pulmonary functions. (VE = expired volume, VT = tidal volume, VC = vital capacity, IC = inspiratory capacity, Vo_2 = oxygen consumption, Vco_2 = carbon dioxide production, RQ = respiratory quotient, $PETO_2$ = end-tidal partial oxygen pressure, $PETco_2$ = end-tidal partial carbon dioxide pressure.)

Caloric support in excess of expenditure (positive daily balance) will result in weight gain and an increase in body mass. However, excessive caloric support has also been associated with respiratory failure,[41, 55] hepatic encephalopathy,[9] and possible impairment of host defenses.[10] In contrast, inadequate nutritional support has been associated with weight loss, fatigue, immunodeficiency, and death. Therefore, a more precise balance of caloric intake and expenditure should improve hospital course and decrease morbidity and mortality if all other factors are equal.[1, 41] Measurement of REE with indirect calorimetry allows for a more exact determination of daily caloric balance.

Respiratory failure is one of the largest contributors to the high morbidity and mortality rates in the intensive care unit; it is exacerbated when accompanied by malnutrition.[35, 37–40] Early nutritional intervention is the primary way to prevent medical complications associated with nutritional depletion.[48] Simple techniques for nutritional assessment are available, as are the means to provide adequate calories and micronutrients.[4, 12, 47] The current recommendation is to accurately calculate both energy and protein needs to prevent overfeeding, thereby decreasing carbon dioxide production, norepinephrine excretion, and oxygen consumption.

The assessment of malnutrition and its treatment is improving. Nutritional issues will probably remain in the forefront of critical care during the remainder of this decade. Ongoing research may evolve new concepts of nutritional support, which may modify or completely replace current modes of thinking. Indeed, the prevention and management of nutritional failure appears to be the next intensive care frontier.

Acknowledgments

The authors wish to thank the following people for their assistance with this chapter: Connie Pettway, who typed the majority of the manuscript; and Victoria Kirschner, M.Ed., and Richard Stork, M.D., for their review and editorial comments.

REFERENCES

1. Kresowik TF, Dechert RE, Mault JR, et al: Does nutritional support affect survival in critically ill patients? Surg Forum 1984; 25:108–110.
2. Harris JA, Benedict FG: Biometric Studies of Basal Metabolism in Man. Washington, DC: Carnegie Institute of Washington, 1919, publication 279.
3. Swinamer DL, Grace MG, Hamilton SM, et al: Predictive equation for assessing energy expenditure in mechanically ventilated critically ill patients. Crit Care Med 1990; 18(6):657–661.

4. Wilmore DW: The Metabolic Management of the Critically Ill. New York: Plenum, 1977.
5. Weissman C, Kemper M, Elwyn DH, et al: The energy expenditure of the mechanically ventilated critically ill patient. An analysis. Chest 1986; 89(2):254–259.
6. Mann S, Westenskow DR, Houtchens BA: Measured and predicted caloric expenditure in the acutely ill. Crit Care Med 1985; 13(3):173–177.
7. Long CL, Spencer JL, Kinney JM, Geiger JW: Carbohydrate metabolism in man: Effect of elective operations and major injury. J Appl Physiol 1971; 31(1):110–116.
8. Bartlett RH, Dechert RE, Mault JR, et al: Measurement of metabolism in multiple organ failure. Surgery 1982; 92(4):771–779.
9. Fischer JF: The etiology of hepatic encephalopathy—Nutritional implications. Acta Clin Scand Suppl 1981; 507:50–68.
10. Chandra RK: Immunodeficiency in undernutrition and overnutrition. Nutr Rev 1981; 39(6):225–231.
11. Bevan DR: Metabolic response to anesthesia, surgery and trauma. *In* Cecil-Gray T, Nunn JF, and Utting JE (eds): General Anesthesia, 4th Ed. London: Butterworths, 1980; 1017–1036.
12. Negro F, Cerra FB: Nutritional monitoring in the ICU: Rational and practical application. Crit Care Clin 1988; 4(3):559–572.
13. Askanazi J, Nordenstrom J, Rosenbaum SH, et al: Nutrition for the patient with respiratory failure: Glucose vs. fat. Anesthesiology 1981; 54(5):373–377.
14. Weissman C, Kemper M, Askanazi J, et al: Resting metabolic rate of the critically ill patient: Measured versus predicted. Anesthesiology 1986; 64(6):673–679.
15. Lavoisier AL: Experiences sur la respiration des animaux et sur les changements qui arrivant a lair en passant par leur poumon. *In* Oeuvres, Tome II. Memoires de chimie et de physique. Paris: Imprimerie Imperiale, 1862; 174–179.
16. Fick A: Ueber die messung des bluntquantums in den herzventrikeln. S.B. phys-med. Ges. Wurzburg, July 9, 1870.
17. Webb P: Symposium: History of research in human energy metabolism. The measurement of energy expenditure. Am Inst Nutr 1991; 1897–1901.
18. Swyer PR: Symposium: History of research in human energy metabolism. Assumptions used in measurements of energy metabolism. Am Inst Nutr 1991; 1891–1896.
19. Makk LJ, McClave SA, Creech PW, et al: Clinical application of the metabolic cart to the delivery of total parenteral nutrition. Crit Care Med 1990; 18(12):1320–1327.
20. Westenskow DR, Cutler CA, Wallace WD: Instrumentation for monitoring gas exchange and metabolic rate in critically ill patients. Crit Care Med 1984; 12(3):183–187.
21. Sullivan WJ, Peters GM, Enright PL: Pneumotachographs: Theory and clinical application. Respir Care 1984; 29:736–749.
22. Bursztein S, Elwyn D, Askanazi J, Kinney J: Energy Metabolism, Indirect Calorimetry and Nutrition. Baltimore: Williams & Wilkins, 1989; 173–228.
23. Teirlinck H: Sensormedics 2900 Metabolic Measurement Cart: Technical and fundamental considerations in gas exchange measurements. Cardiopulmonary Review: Current Applications and Economics. Sensormedics Continuing Medical Education Group, 1991; 1–6.
24. Steinhorn DM, Rozenberg AL, Boyle MJ, et al: Modular indirect calorimeter suitable for long-term measurements in multipatient intensive care units. Crit Care Med 1991; 19(7):963–972.
25. Orkin FK: Anesthesia systems. *In* Miller RD (ed): Anesthesia. New York: Churchill Livingstone, 1986; 149.
26. Shimada Y, Hirata T, Taenaka N, et al: Evaluation of a system of breath-by-breath analysis of $\dot{V}O_2$ and $\dot{V}CO_2$ in anesthesia and intensive care. Anesthesiology 1982; 57:A487.
27. Bursztein S, Glaser P, Trichet B, et al: Utilization of protein, carbohydrate, and fat in fasting and postabsorptive subjects. Am J Clin Nutr 1980; 33(5):998–1001.
28. Johnson RE: Techniques for measuring gas exchange. *In* Kenney JM (ed): Assessment of energy metabolism in health and disease. First Ross Conference on Medical Research, Columbus: Ross Laboratories, 1980; 32–36.
29. Feurer ID, Crosby LO, Mullen JL: Measured and predicted resting energy expenditure in clinically stable patients. Clin Nutr 1984; 3:27–34.
30. Soares MJ, Sheela ML, Kurpad AV, et al: The influence of different methods on basal metabolic rate measurements in human subjects. Am J Clin Nutr 1989; 50(4):731–736.
31. Phang PT, Rich T, Ronco J: A validation and comparison study of two metabolic monitors. J Parenter Enteral Nutr 1990; 14(3):259–261.
32. Makita K, Nunn JF, Royston B: Evaluation of metabolic measuring instruments for use in critically ill patients. Crit Care Med 1990; 18(6):638–644.
33. Anonymous: The Oxylog instruction manual. Kent, UK: PK Morgan, 1983.
34. Anonymous: Basal metabolic rate indicator. Operating manual. Frankfurt: Hartman and Braun AG, 1964.
35. Bassili HR, Deitel M: Nutritional support in long term intensive care with special reference to ventilator patients: A review. Can Anaesth Soc J 1981; 28(1):17–21.
36. Gump FE, Kinney JM: Nutrition and metabolism. *In* Bartlett RH (ed): Life Support Systems in Intensive Care. Chicago: Year Book, 1984; 145–167.
37. Pingleton SK: Nutritional support in the mechanically ventilated patient. Clin Chest Med 1988; 9(1):101–112.
38. Mlynarek M, Zarowitz BJ: Individualizing nutrition in patients with acute respiratory failure requiring mechanical ventilation. Drug Intell Clin Pharm 1987; 21(11):865–870.
39. Martin TR: The relationship between malnutrition and lung infections. Clin Chest Med 1987; 8(3):359–372.
40. Deitel M, Williams VP, Rice TW: Nutrition and the patient requiring mechanical ventilatory support. J Am Coll Nutr 1983; 2(1):25–32.
41. Askanazi J, Rosenbaum SH, Hyman AI, et al: Respiratory changes induced by the large glucose loads of total parenteral nutrition. JAMA 1980; 243(14):1444–1447.
42. Askanazi J, Rosenbaum SH, Hyman AI, et al: Does nutritional support affect survival in critically ill patients? Surg Forum 1984; 35:108–110.
43. Vermeij CG, Feenstra BW, van Lanschot JJ, Bruining HA: Day-to-day variability of energy expenditure in critically ill surgical patients. Crit Care Med 1989; 17(7):623–626.
44. Swinamer DL, Phang PT, Jones RL, et al: Twenty-four hour energy expenditure in critically ill patients. Crit Care Med 1987; 15(7):637–643.
45. Askanazi J, Carpentier YA, Elwyn DH, et al: Influence of total parenteral nutrition of fuel utilization in injury and sepsis. Ann Surg 1980; 191(1):40–46.
46. Gray DS: Energetics. *In* Kaminski MV (ed): Hyperalimentation—A Guide for Clinicians. New York: Marcel Dekker, 1985; 17–20.
47. Rutten P, Blackburn GL, Flatt JP, et al: Determination of optimal hyperalimentation infusion rate. J Surg Res 1975; 18(5):477–483.
48. Mullen JL: Consequences of malnutrition in the surgical patient. Surg Clin North Am 1981; 61(3):465–489.
49. Damask MC, Askanazi J, Weissman C, et al: Artifacts in measurement of resting energy expenditure. Crit Care Med 1983; 11(9):750–752.
50. Weissman C, Kemper M, Damask MC, et al: Effect of routine intensive care interactions on metabolic rate. Chest 1984; 86(6):815–818.
51. Kirkpatrick JR, Dahn M, Lewis L: Selective versus standard hyperalimentation. A randomized prospective study. Am J Surg 1981; 141(1):116–121.
52. Mondejar EF, Duro LM, Perez de la Cruz AJ, et al: Variations in oxygen consumption and carbon dioxide production during parenteral nutrition. Intens Care Med 1982; 8(4):169–172.
53. Goldman RF: Effect of environment on metabolism. *In* Kinney JM (ed): Assessment of Energy Metabolism in Health and Disease. Columbus: Ross Laboratories, 1980; 117–121.
54. Swinamer DL, Jones RL, Grace MG, et al: Daytime variations in energy expenditure in critically ill patients. Am J Crit Care 1988; 3:190–194.
55. Askanazi J, Weissman C, Rosenbaum SH, et al: Nutrition and the respiratory system. Crit Care Med 1982; 10(3):163–172.
56. Alpers DH, Clouse RE, Stenson WF: Manual of Nutritional Therapeutics. Boston: Little Brown, 1985; 131–160.
57. Braun U, Zundel J, Freiboth K, et al: Evaluation of methods for indirect calorimetry with a ventilated lung model. Intens Care Med 1989; 15(3):196–202.
58. Damask MC, Weissman C, Askanazi J, et al: A systematic method for validation of gas exchange measurements. Anesthesiology 1982; 57(3):213–218.
59. DeVault GA: Nutritional support of the critically ill: Writing the TPN prescription. J Crit Illness 1989; 4:54–56.
60. Dubois EF: Fever and Regulation of Body Temperature. Springfield, IL: Charles C Thomas, 1948.

61. Quebbeman EJ, Ausman RK: Estimating energy requirements in patients receiving parenteral nutrition. Arch Surg 1982; 117:1281–1284.
62. Feurer ID, Mullen JL: Bedside measurement of resting energy expenditure and respiratory quotient via indirect calorimetry. Nutr Clin Pract 1986; 1:43–49.
63. Stein TP, Buzby GP, Rosato EF, Mullen JL: Effects of parenteral nutrition on protein synthesis in adult cancer patients. Am J Clin Nutr 1981; 34(8):1484–1488.
64. Criddle RS, Fontana AJ, Rank DR, et al: Simultaneous measurement of metabolic heat rate, CO_2 production, and O_2 consumption by microcalorimetry. Anal Biochem 1991; 194(2):413–417.
65. Eccles RC, Swinamer DL, Jones RL, King EG: Validation of a compact system for measuring gas exchange. Crit Care Med 1986; 14(9):807–811.
66. Farhi LE: Gas stores of the body. *In* Handbook of Physiology: Respiration. Baltimore: Waverly Press, 1976; 873–885.
67. McPherson S, Spearman C: Respiratory Therapy Equipment. St. Louis: CV Mosby, 1985; 215–216.
68. Nelson LD, Anderson HB, Garcia H: Clinical validation of a new metabolic monitor suitable for use in critically ill patients. Crit Care Med 1987; 15(10):951–957.
69. Nunn JF, Makita K, Royston B: Validation of oxygen consumption measurements during artificial ventilation. J Appl Physiol 1989; 67(5):2129–2134.
70. Weissman C, Ajoy S, Kemper M: In vitro evaluation of a compact metabolic measurement instrument. J Parenter Enteral Nutr 1990; 14(2):216–221.

SECTION SIX

Computerized Monitoring

CHAPTER 21

Computers in Monitoring

ALAN W. MURRAY, M.B., Ch.B., FRCA, and
GAVIN N. C. KENNY, B.Sc. (Hons.), M.B.Ch.B., M.D., FRCA

The computer, now a well-established tool in medicine, is used for a wide variety of functions ranging from simple clerical tasks, such as word processing, to complex clinical simulations for undergraduate and postgraduate teaching.[1] The ability to perform data acquisition; signal processing, storage, and analysis; and number manipulation is especially appropriate in anesthesia. Interpretive calculations can be performed in real time as the data are acquired; derived information can be displayed almost instantaneously with its collection. Detection of detrimental changes in physiologic functions and production of appropriate warnings distinguish computerized monitoring from simple data capture. Modern sophisticated monitors frequently contain on-board microprocessors to perform calculations of this type. Microprocessor-based drug- and anesthesia-delivery systems permit collection of physiologic data and adjustment of drug administration based on hemodynamic parameters.[2] Computerized monitors also provide storage for many hours of data and thus produce graphic displays of trends. Although humans are adept at pattern recognition (interpretation of electrocardiogram or electroencephalogram), our limited short-term memory reduces our data management capability.

Development of computerized monitoring systems requires considerable skill in engineering and programming because of the need for capturing and analyzing data in real time and for producing a system that is simple for relatively untrained operators to use. Many different groups have described monitoring and records systems, and most have approached the problems involved in different ways.

TYPES OF COMPUTERS

Before computer applications in anesthesia are discussed, the basics of computing must be considered. Two distinct types of computers are used in anesthesia: analog and digital. Their structures and functions are completely different.

ANALOG COMPUTERS

These machines are based on a unit known as an operational amplifier. Operational amplifiers cannot handle alphanumeric data (letters and numbers) but can process fixed or variable waveforms almost instantaneously when these are presented as voltages. Connecting different circuits to an operational amplifier alters the characteristics of the system and allows data manipulations such as summation, subtraction, division, multiplication, integration, and differentiation. The output from the analog computer is a voltage proportional to that of the input, and display of the calculated result occurs virtually instantaneously with the input signal.[3]

The most frequent use of analog computers in anesthesia is to calculate cardiac output from a bolus injection of dye or cold dextrose solution (thermodilution) into the circulation with blood sampling downstream from the injection site. When the concentration of the indicator is measured and plotted against time, a curve is produced. Cardiac output can then be obtained by calculating the area under the curve. Manual calculation of this area is tedious and time-consuming. Application of a computer to the problem results in almost instantaneous calculation of the result by integration of the curve in real time (see Chapter 10).

One major drawback of analog computers is the inability to use alphanumeric data. A second major disadvantage is the difficulty of changing the function of the computer. This can only be achieved by rewiring or changing the input circuit, which may require a high degree of technical skill. Analog computers have almost completely been replaced by digital computers, and most modern cardiac output computers now use digital techniques for collection of the temperature waveform and calculation of the final result.

DIGITAL COMPUTERS

The components of a digital computer system—keyboard, central processor unit, memory circuits, visual display unit, and output devices—are collectively known as computer hardware. Software is the term applied to data and programs used by the machine that determine the functions performed by the computer. Programs usually are stored on some form of magnetic medium such as a floppy disk and must be loaded into the computer before use. Firmware is an arrangement in which programs are stored permanently on a reprogrammable integrated circuit and are therefore available for immediate use.

Method of Operation

Digital computers deal directly with numbers, and all information used is coded and stored in numeric form. The computer then applies a program to process the data. A program is a series of instructions that tells the computer precisely how to perform the required tasks. Thus a finite time is required to perform a calculation or to process data. The program may consist of several thousand individual steps, each of which must be correct for the system to function appropriately. Correction, or "debugging," and maintenance of programs can require considerable time, and errors may not appear until some unusual combination of circumstances arises.

Until a digital computer is provided with a program, it cannot perform any useful operation. With a change in the program, the computer can be used for a completely different task. This provides a unique degree of flexibility, so that the same machine can be used for a wide variety of functions simply by changing the program it executes.

Binary System

The binary system is used to encode information. Thus only two "states" are required to represent information. These states represent the digits 1 and 0. The digits can be represented as arbitrarily defined voltages, the open or closed positions of a switch, the presence or absence of an electrical impulse, or the change of north-south orientation of a magnetic field. Each individual 1 or 0 is known as a *bit* of information. A group of eight bits is known as a *byte*. One byte can represent decimal numbers between 0 and 256. Values in this range are used to represent letters and control codes for activating special functions and output devices. Numbers are represented in scientific notation by a combination of two or more bytes that contain information related to the sign of the number and the exponent.

Forms of Digital Computers

Digital computers are produced in three main forms: mainframe computers, minicomputers, and microcomputers. The principles of operation, however, remain similar. Classification of computers is based on the complexity and capacity of the system.

Mainframe Computers

Mainframe computers are the largest systems. They can support several dozen users simultaneously by sharing processor time between active terminals. Each terminal consists of a keyboard with which the operator enters information and controls the functions performed by the computer and a visual display unit, which displays the results on a screen. Switching between terminals occurs so rapidly that there is usually no noticeable delay during use of any one terminal. However, if many users each require considerable processor time or frequent disk access, the response time can increase to an unacceptable level.

The advantage of mainframe computing is that it allows sharing of data, and expensive output and peripheral devices such as printers and plotters can be used efficiently. These systems are thus centralized systems and their use is controlled by a professional computing staff. Combined with the high purchase and maintenance costs, this results in a highly expensive system. Attempts have been made to link all departments within a hospital to a centralized computer, but these have had limited success (see Chapter 22).[4]

Minicomputers

Minicomputers are also capable of serving several users simultaneously, and their architecture and operation are similar to that of the mainframe. Running costs of the minicomputer are also significant but much lower than the mainframe, and response time of the processor can be unacceptably long with these systems. However, when many users must have access to a large central store of information, minicomputers can be satisfactory.

Microcomputers

Microcomputers were designed initially for single users. They are relatively simple devices with smaller memory capacity and slower processing speed than either minicomputers or mainframe computers. However, microcomputers are sufficiently powerful to handle applications when few simultaneous demands are made on the system. Their simplicity allows nonexperts to write their own programs if necessary. Microelectronic developments have resulted in microcomputers whose performance approaches that of minicomputer systems at a fraction of the cost.

Networking of microcomputers allows communication between autonomous units over short distances (local area network), thus sharing information, output, and storage devices. In contrast to minicomputers and mainframe systems, if one microcomputer within a network fails, the remainder of the network continues to function normally.

Sections of Digital Computers

Functionally, the digital computer can be divided into four sections: the central processing unit, memory system, input devices, and output devices.

Central Processing Unit

The central processing unit (CPU), or microprocessor, provides the arithmetic and decision-making capabilities of the computer. The CPU executes the programs and is responsible for the correct transfer of information between the input, output, and memory devices.

The CPU and other integrated circuits are usually connected together in such a way that data can be passed among them one byte at a time. The connection consists of many parallel tracks; one carries a timing signal that synchronizes the actions of the integrated circuits, and others carry the byte of data, one bit per track. Data are passed rapidly via this system, which is known as a data bus. More recent processors handle 16- and 32-bit data, which allows much more rapid computation than the original 8-bit data bus.

When the power supply is switched on at the start of a computing session, the CPU initiates a routine that checks the functions of the system and prepares the computer for use. This is known as *booting* the system.

Memory Systems

Memory systems are required to hold the computer operating systems, the programs, and the data to be acted on by the programs. Memory within the computer is arranged on several types of specialized integrated circuits.

Random access memory (RAM) is a form of memory that allows retrieval or storage of data one byte at a time as required. Data are transferred to a specific area of RAM by an address bus (a parallel collection of wires of high or low voltage corresponding to binary number bits). Data movement from RAM is very rapid. Modern microcomputers now have memory capacities of up to 128 megabytes. The disadvantage of RAM is that it requires a constant power supply to maintain its integrity. However, battery-backed RAM is available and can last for up to 10 years, depending on battery type.

Read-only memory (ROM) is a type of memory device that contains the operating system and the start-up instructions of the computer. ROM is not usually available to the user to store information, and its contents cannot be altered by the program. Its contents are unaffected by interruptions of the power supply.

More permanent storage is available using magnetic media to make a record of information that can be reloaded into the computer when required. Magnetic tape storage is possible, but because storage of data is sequential, retrieval is slow.

Disks coated with magnetic material are available for information storage. The data are stored on concentric tracks; when retrieval is required, any part of the disk can be accessed within one rotation of the disk. Floppy disks are relatively inexpensive and can store 1.44 megabytes of data (one–two million characters per disk). Hard disks are more expensive, but can hold up to 340–540 megabytes and are capable of much faster data storage and retrieval. A character is a letter, digit, or other special symbol. Magnetic media can be reused many times but are sensitive to damage by magnetic fields generated by electrical equipment of all kinds.

Laser disks can store billions of characters per disk. They are available in a form known as WORM technology (*w*rite *o*nce, *r*ead *m*any times) and in a rewritable form. This type of data storage is developing rapidly and should greatly ease the problems of storing information, especially for archiving.

INPUT DEVICES

Input devices can be divided into two groups: off-line and on-line. Off-line devices allow data entry after all the information has been collected, whereas on-line collection of data obtains the information directly from a source such as a blood pressure monitor. Off-line entry of data involves an operator transcribing from a print-out or graph; thus, human error is possible. The most appropriate type of input device must be selected to make the program simple and convenient to use.

Off-Line Devices

Keyboard

A keyboard is present on most computer systems and is therefore an inexpensive, readily available route for data entry. It requires no special software to support its use, although some skill is required to enter data accurately and at an acceptable speed. However, in a study comparing data entry by keyboard, light pen, and voice recognition in a group of nurses, it was found that keyboard data entry was quickest.[5] Data accuracy was good with the keyboard and comparable to that of the light pen. Voice recognition was three times slower than keyboard entry because of the high number of errors. In a separate study, medical students also expressed a preference for keyboard use when asked to compare keyboard and light pen control of teaching programs.[5] This acceptability may be the result of the increased use of computers in schools and homes and the greater familiarity with a standard keyboard: Even a decade ago 53% of the medical students had previous computer experience.[6]

Keypad

The keypad is similar to a keyboard but is restricted to fewer keys, which may be labeled with predefined functions or numbers according to the application involved. Each key may be labeled either permanently or with a changeable overlay that can be changed for the entry of different types of data, such as fluids, drugs, or anesthetic procedures. The keypad allows rapid selection of any desired item but is essentially less flexible than a standard keyboard. However, the keypad's simplicity of use allows persons unfamiliar with a typewriter keyboard to operate the computer with minimal training.

Monitor Screen

Data selection from lists or ''menus'' *directly displayed on a monitor screen* has become popular, especially with nontypists. Whereas a standard keyboard or keypad can be used to select from a list of possible items displayed on the screen by using only the numeral keys, three devices are available—the light pen, the mouse, or the touch screen—that allow the required item to be selected by simply touching the screen display directly.

Light Pen. A light pen can be interfaced with the computer. When specific blocks of light are touched on the screen, selection of the appropriate item from the screen menu is made.[7]

Mouse. A mouse is a small box housing a moveable rubber ball that is available on most microcomputers. It is moved across a work surface by the operator. As the mouse is moved, the ball on the under surface transmits the x and y coordinates via two optical sensors to the computer. Using this information, the computer's operating system moves a pointer (cursor) on the monitor screen in an equivalent direction and distance. When the pointer tip is over the required item, a button on the mouse is pressed, and the selection is made.[8] Other similar input devices are trackballs and joysticks.

This is known as the WIMP environment and refers to the combination of *w*indows (areas of the monitor screen that can show parts of a document that is larger than the whole screen could display), *i*cons (pictures representing items such as disk drives), *m*ouse, and *p*ointer. This user interface enables very rapid and easy use of a program with minimum computer knowledge. This environment has now been extended to include most types of microcomputers, and many clinical computer systems that are produced commercially use this interface.

Touch screen. The touch screen is the third method of selecting information. This system involves use of a special monitor screen that contains horizontal and vertical arrays of light sources and detectors. When the operator touches a specific item on the screen, the x and y coordinates are detected by interruption of the appropriate light beams and thus are recognized by the computer's operating system.

Touch screens allow rapid and accurate selection from screen lists but are relatively restricted by the number of items which can be displayed on the screen at any one time. The touch screen is also relatively expensive.

Bit Pad

A bit pad allows entry of x-y coordinates into the computer by touching the pad with a stylus connected to the pad. The pad can then be covered with a printed sheet containing diagrams. Touching the appropriate part of the diagram then enters information into the computer. One system permits calculation of fluid balance using the bit pad.[9]

Bar Codes

Bar codes are used increasingly to enter data into computer systems in areas such as supermarkets and have been employed to collect anesthetic information. Bar codes indicating the items available for selection may be printed on sheets of paper or attached directly to a syringe. Passing the bar code reader over the parallel bars of the code enters the selected item into the computer.

Voice Recognition

Voice recognition at present tends to be inaccurate, especially in areas with high background noise.[10] However, development of voice input is progressing rapidly, and one computerized anesthetic record system, which is described later, offers this form of data entry as an option. With anticipated future developments in hardware and software, voice recognition may eventually offer the easiest and most natural form of off-line data input (see Chapter 2).

On-Line Data Collection

During on-line data collection, the computer is connected directly to the data source. This means that data transfer is rapid, complete, and free from human interference. Data may be made available on-line in an analog or digital form.

Analog Data Collection

Most signals from medical equipment are presented as varying *analog voltages*—for example, an arterial pressure waveform. The signal must, therefore, be processed to a digital form that the computer can accept. This is achieved by an analog-to-digital converter (ADC) that produces binary output in proportion to the voltage received by the unit. The signal can be sampled at varying rates; sampling too slowly gives an inaccurate representation of the original signal (Fig. 21–1), whereas frequent sampling provides more accuracy (Fig. 21–2).

Complex waveforms can be analyzed to produce a set of simple sine waves of different frequencies and amplitudes (Fourier transformation). To produce an accurate representation of any waveform, sampling must occur at twice the rate of the highest frequency in the waveform (Nyquist theorem). A blood pressure wave, for example, requires a sampling rate of 50–100 samples/second; an electrocardiogram complex requires about 200–1000 samples/second.

The ADC must be calibrated or scaled according to the amplitude of the waveform. Provision must be made for a negative phase on the wave such as may occur when recording a central venous pressure wave. The maximum resolution of the waveform amplitude depends on the type of ADC used. An 8-bit ADC allows resolution of 2^8, or 256 steps, which is adequate for analysis of a blood pressure wave. For higher resolution, 16-bit converters are available and can give a resolution in excess of 64,000 steps. An ADC may require special software that interrupts the computer's main program to look for data from the converter. Thus, on-line data collection using an ADC can range from relatively simple capture of a slowly changing voltage to complex programs for collecting and analyzing rapidly varying signals.

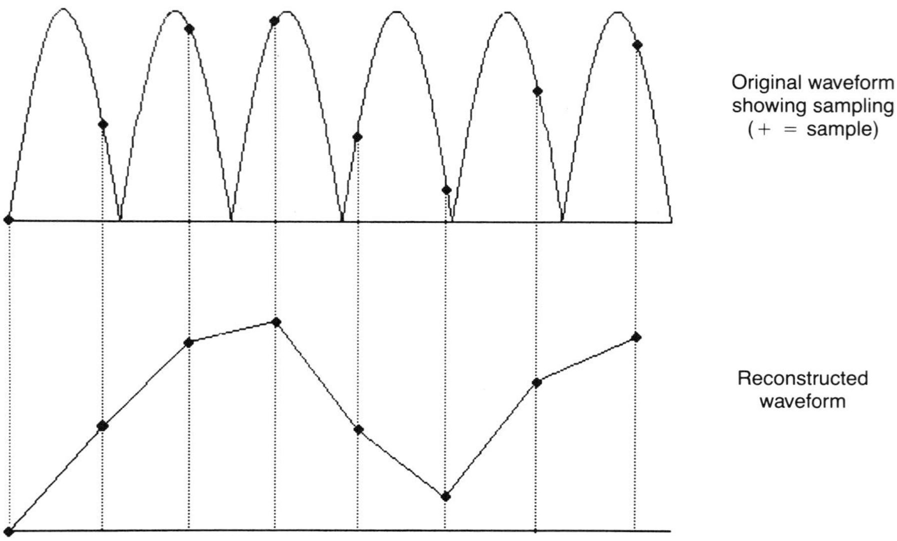

Figure 21–1. Sampling of the waveform at an incorrect rate *(top)* results in a reconstructed waveform *(bottom)* that differs markedly from the original waveform.

Digital Data Collection

An increasing number of modern patient monitors contain their own dedicated microprocessor. Preprocessed information can therefore be transferred to the computer. The computer processor load is reduced, and signal analysis programs are not required. Dedicated processors within monitoring equipment often can signal the computer when information is available for transfer.

RS 232. Special interfaces have been developed to transfer information between processors. The most common of these is known as the RS 232 interface. This consists of a multicore cable connector that allows transfer of data one bit at a time. The rate of data transfer, known as the baud rate, has to be preset and identical in both systems. Standard baud rates are 1200, 2400, 9600, and 14,400 bits/second. A baud rate of 1200 signifies transfer of about 120 characters per second. The pattern of the bits to be transferred must also be identical, because data may be sent as 5, 6, 7, or 8 bits per character. The system can also be configured to check whether data have been received correctly by the second system.

Medical Information Bus. A system known as the Medical Information Bus allows standardization of data transfer protocols, data structure, and connectors. It greatly reduces the effort required to interconnect monitoring systems and subsequently extract information from these systems. Electrical safety is extremely important if devices are connected to patients and all equipment must conform to international standards (IEC 601/1). These standards emphasize the problems of leakage current and electrical isolation when connecting computers to medical instrumentation. Isolated power supply, isolating transformers, and optical links have been used to isolate patients from computer equipment.[11]

Advantages of On-Line Collection

The advantages of on-line data collection include rapid transfer of the information into the computer. Because this transfer is totally independent of the operator, bias and

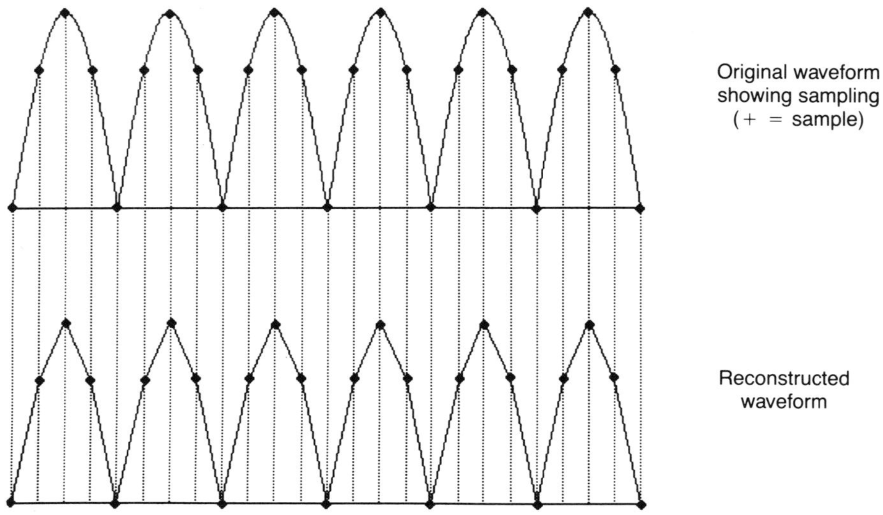

Figure 21–2. When the waveform is sampled at the correct rate, the reconstructed waveform closely resembles the original.

interpretation of the data do not occur. Information can also be obtained from several different signal sources almost simultaneously, and derived data can be calculated and displayed rapidly. However, the computer system must be able to detect and reject artifacts in the signals, and it can be relatively difficult to produce programs that perform detailed pattern recognition.[12]

If the information is supplied to the computer in digital form, preprocessed by a patient monitor, validation of data is more difficult. When accurate data are essential, such as during closed-loop control of blood pressure, the raw analog signal may have to be acquired and analyzed directly by the host computer.

OUTPUT DEVICES

The output is the result of the computer's activities as presented to the user. Several devices provide useful output for a system.

Screen Displays

Temporary display of output can be achieved with a visual display unit (cathode ray tube). The display is created as it is in a domestic television set, by the interaction of electron beams on phosphor dots on the screen, and may be either monochrome (two colors such as black and white or black and green) or multicolor. The quality of the display is improved by increasing the density of the phosphor dots. This is referred to as the *resolution* of the display, high resolution referring to higher-quality display. Most microcomputers can produce graphic displays of data, and the quality of the display depends on the number of points that the computer can address on the screen. Each point is termed a pixel, and the number of pixels determines the smoothness of curved graphs. In a monochrome system, each pixel may be on or off, whereas with a color system, each pixel can be used to display the number of colors available from the computer.

Some portable computers use a liquid crystal display (LCD) similar to those in digital watches. LCD consumes very little power, which is a major advantage in a battery-operated system. A significant disadvantage is that the angle from which the display is viewed can be critical. A small change in the viewing angle causes the display to become virtually invisible. Backlighting the display helps to overcome this problem. The newer active matrix screens, in which each pixel is controlled directly, provides a major improvement in LCD displays.

Light-emitting diodes (LEDs) arranged in a large array can also be used for display purposes. An LED is a small semiconductor device that emits light when a current is passed through it. This system has the advantage of being useable in poor lighting conditions.

The type of screen display used in any computer application depends on whether graphics will be used, what degree of resolution is required from the graphic display, and whether a color display is necessary. Power consumption, robustness, and visibility in poor ambient light may also be factors.

Printers and Plotters

Permanent copies of the computer output can be made using printers or plotting devices. Printers of different types provide different qualities of output. The most inexpensive are dot matrix printers that, as the name suggests, produce output as a series of dots in a pattern corresponding to the desired character. Daisy wheel printers are similar to electronic typewriters and contain the raised patterns of letters and characters on a wheel that spins in front of the paper. Impact printers may be excessively noisy for use in the operating environment. Alternatives to impact printers are thermal dot matrix printers, which make dot images on heat-sensitive paper, and ink jet printers, which eject a stream of ink to form each individual character.

Graphic plotters produce their output via a pen that is moved across the paper according to the computer's instructions. Plotters produce high-quality drawings and can draw on transparencies as well as on paper. However, the quality of characters produced by pen plotters is rarely totally satisfactory. Laser printers produce their output by marking the paper with a low-power laser and then passing it through a toner similar to that used by a photocopying machine. The laser-based machine produces high-quality print and graphics but are more expensive than other printers. Bubble jet printers, which are relatively quiet, produce good quality output, and are less expensive than laser printers, have improved significantly and provide a satisfactory alternative in the clinical environment.

Information can also be output in digital form for transmission to another computer. The machines may be close enough for the connections to be made directly, or a modem can be used. Modem is an abbreviation for *mod*ulator-*dem*odulator and is a device that converts electrical binary pulses into sound tones. The sounds can be transmitted by telephone and permit communication between computers almost anywhere in the world.

PROGRAMMING AND LANGUAGES

Digital computers require specific instructions in order to perform any useful function. Conventional programs organize information into data with instructions that act on the data. The step-by-step process that ensures that a given input goes through a series of simplified procedures to solve a complex problem and deliver the solution is called an algorithm. A number of algorithms are combined as a program. Programs are structured in many different ways according to the syntax of the programming language used.

LANGUAGES

Computer languages are structurally similar to human languages but with two important differences. First, they tend to be considerably more simple, with perhaps no more than several hundred ''words'' in their vocabulary. Second, the syntax rules are precise and must be obeyed rigidly, whereas in human language such rules can sometimes be disregarded without loss of meaning. Programs are known as software and are stored in the computer's RAM along with data.

Many different programming languages have been developed for different applications. For example, FORTRAN, a contraction of *for*mula *tran*slation, was developed to handle scientific and technical calculation. COBOL (*co*mmon *b*usiness-*o*riented *l*anguage) was developed for business applications such as data base management and accounting. PASCAL is a highly structured, multipurpose language but can be difficult for nonprogrammers to use. BASIC (*b*eginner's *a*ll-*s*ymbolic *i*nstruction *c*ode) is a simple language that is very similar to English and was developed to introduce people to computer programming. Modern versions of BASIC incorporate the structured approach of PASCAL but retain ease of use.

A newer generation of higher-level languages, including LISP (*lis*t *p*rocessing), have been produced that form the basis of the developing field of artificial intelligence (AI). Artificial intelligence attempts to create thought processes within a computer that are similar to those of a human. Traditional programming deals with information on two levels: the program (instructions) and the data that are acted on by the program. AI programs have an additional level containing knowledge. This results in a program of much greater power and complexity that may be able to make judgements on a situation.

At present, AI is progressing in three main fields: visual recognition, natural language recognition, and expert systems development. Of the three, only expert systems are developing at a significant rate. The aim of an expert system is to achieve a level of decision making and judgement similar to human skills in a specialized field. Problem-solving expert systems already exist in areas such as medical diagnosis and prescription. Development of an expert system involves high cost because of the considerable amount of programming time required, especially in acquiring and representing knowledge in the system. Requirements for rapid instruction execution and large memory capacity can still exceed the most advanced systems. Thus, widespread application of AI may not occur for several years.[13]

INTERACTION WITH COMPUTERS

The ease of use of a computer without detailed knowledge of the operating principles of the system is referred to as the user friendliness of the system. This can be achieved by incorporating several features into the program controlling the computer. It is extremely important to prevent the user from entering inappropriate data by checking all information as it is input to the computer. When values fall outside the expected range, the user can be queried for confirmation or re-entry. Easy correction of data must be allowed. Careful design of screen displays can assist medical and nursing staff to assimilate information quickly and accurately. The essential feature of any computer application is that it should reduce the effort of performing a task or should undertake a task that cannot be readily performed without a computer.

ANESTHETIC RECORDS

Accurate and detailed records form an integral part of the practice of anesthesia. The ever-increasing complexity of modern anesthetic techniques and equipment may leave insufficient time to record and chart cardiorespiratory variables as frequently and accurately as required.[14, 15]

Anesthetic records appeared as early as 1894. Details of the patient's physical condition and anesthetic drugs used were recorded for future reference. Since then, the anesthetic record has become more complex. However, the basic principles have remained similar to the format originally described by Cushing.

PURPOSES

The anesthetic record can provide information in three broad categories: clinical care, historical data, and continuous quality improvement.

Clinical Care

Data concerning the preoperative health of the patient and any specific risks that may be anticipated prior to administration of an anesthetic are noted. During administration of an anesthetic, records are made concurrently with patient management. Information such as administration of drugs is recorded as are cardiorespiratory responses, loss and administration of fluids, and blood products. Any unexpected events, such as an idiosyncratic reaction to a drug or an unexpected difficult intubation, are usually carefully recorded. Analysis of the electrocardiogram for dysrhythmias or ischemia is frequently performed by computer and recorded automatically (see Chapters 4 and 5). Information about the respiratory system such as respiratory rate, gas composition, and flow is determined by computers and recorded directly. Accurate intraoperative information is also immediately available to assist staff involved in postoperative care.

Many clinical research projects require a large amount of data to be collected at one time. A computer can greatly simplify this process as well as provide completely unbiased data recording. Data that are stored automatically to magnetic media are much simpler and less time-consuming to analyze.

Historical Data

Retrospective examination of anesthetic records is important in revealing potential hazards noted during previous administration of anesthetics. Early repeat use of certain anesthetic agents can be avoided. However, manual records can be lost from the patient chart, or the chart itself may be lost.

Administrative data must be extracted from which operating room utilization, staffing levels, and billing are determined. The degree of supervision of junior staff and the adequacy of their training requires documentation to ensure that adequate experience has been gained in different techniques and operations.

Review of Quality of Care (Continuous Quality Improvement)

Clinical review of anesthetic records may be undertaken for estimation of quality of care and for educational purposes, especially when unusual problems are encountered. The use of different anesthetic techniques and drugs and the frequency of complications should be documented. However, review of manual records is so tedious that it is very rarely undertaken on a large scale.

The use of an anesthetic record for medicolegal purposes requires accuracy, legibility, and completeness in recording details. In a court of law, the quality of a clinical record is taken as a reflection of the quality of the anesthetic given. Missing data and badly kept records allow conjecture by expert witnesses and reduce the chance that the anesthesiologist will be defended successfully. The basic premise is that if measurements were not recorded, they were not taken. Manually produced records can have major disadvantages in this respect, because during a crisis, the anesthesiologist is more concerned with correcting the situation than in making notes. Computerization of the anesthetic record may, therefore, offer many advantages to the practicing anesthesiologist.

COMPUTERIZED ANESTHETIC RECORDS

During anesthetic administration, the anesthesiologist spends a great deal of time examining the monitors that display information concerning the patient, determining whether the data are within an acceptable range, and, if not, deciding whether the data are accurate. The data must then be recorded on the anesthetic chart. Most of this activity is mechanical and repetitive and requires little decision-making ability.

Automatic collection of information results in greater precision of information and fewer errors from transcription. An automatic system collects data from monitors accurately and rapidly. However, data collected directly online from a monitor can contain artifacts that do not accurately reflect the patient's true status. With modern monitors, artifact rejection is very efficient, and so the need to correct data is rare. However, provision should be made to correct or annotate any spurious result.

Automated data collection is much faster than are manual methods and continues when the clinician is fully occupied with other aspects of patient care. Both the American Society of Anesthesiologists and the Association of Anaesthetists of Great Britain and Ireland recommend the recording of anesthetic data every 5 minutes. Clearly, in many situations this would be very difficult, if not impossible, without a suitable automated anesthetic record system (Fig. 21–3).

The computer record is absolutely objective and records transient fluctuations in physiologic parameters with complete accuracy. A human operator may ''smooth'' fluctuations such as a single low blood pressure reading to produce a more acceptable record.[16] Such fluctuations are very common and would appear to have little significance, but their demonstration by an automatic system may have medicolegal implications. Widespread use of automatic systems and regular demonstration of such events would reassure the legal profession of the benign nature of these transient changes. Many anesthesiologists fear that an automatic anesthetic record may require more explanation than a conventional manual record would. However, most legal experts consider that the overall cost of anesthetic litigation would be reduced by the use of automated systems.

Large quantities of data can be stored on magnetic media, resulting in a major reduction in space required for paper storage.[17] Once data have been stored in computers, recall and analysis of data are many times faster than are manual searches and calculation. Record systems should be organized in such a way that useless data do not fill valuable storage capacity. Equally important, useful information should not be missed. The problem of what data to store and what to reject has not been completely resolved. Most departments usually begin by storing excessive information but realize within 6–12 months what is actually valuable and worth storing for the long term.

DESIRABLE FEATURES

For successful complete computerization of anesthetic records, several attributes must be considered, including accurate and complete data entry from monitors, easy manual data entry, real-time record generation, adaptability, easy interfacing with existing equipment in available workspace, and use of standard anesthesia record forms.

Accurate and Complete Recording of Data

Direct transfer from patient monitors via ADC or RS 232 using suitable software achieves complete data recovery. The Medical Information Bus may assist with standardization of interfacing to medical instrumentation.

The rate of data acquisition should be considered. Frequent sampling of physiologic variables will generate a large data file. If the operation is prolonged and the patient

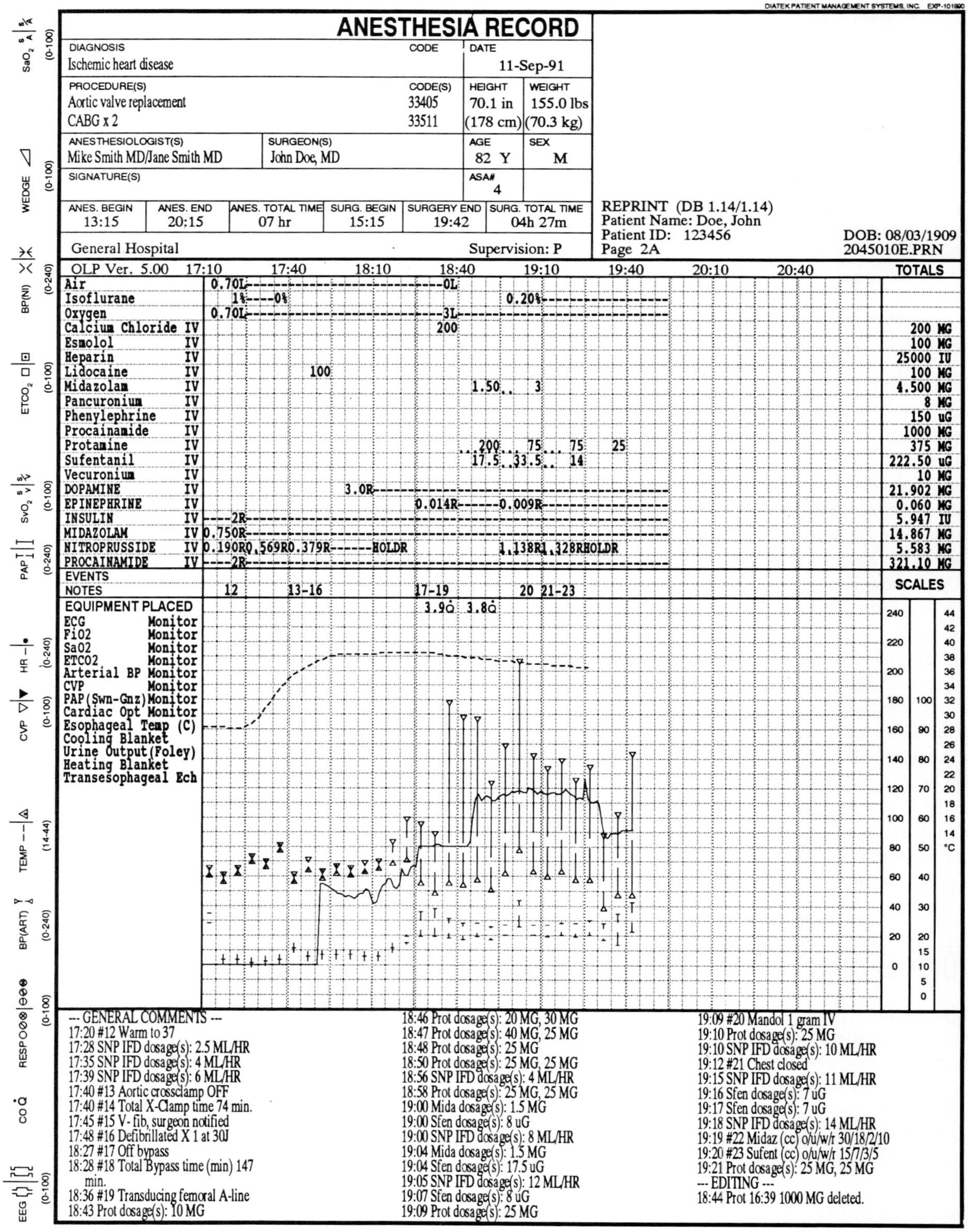

DIATEK PATIENT MANAGEMENT SYSTEMS, INC. EXP-101890

ANESTHESIA RECORD

DIAGNOSIS: Ischemic heart disease	CODE	DATE: 11-Sep-91	
PROCEDURE(S): Aortic valve replacement; CABG x 2	CODE(S): 33405; 33511	HEIGHT: 70.1 in (178 cm)	WEIGHT: 155.0 lbs (70.3 kg)
ANESTHESIOLOGIST(S): Mike Smith MD/Jane Smith MD	SURGEON(S): John Doe, MD	AGE: 82 Y	SEX: M
SIGNATURE(S)		ASA#: 4	

ANES. BEGIN	ANES. END	ANES. TOTAL TIME	SURG. BEGIN	SURGERY END	SURG. TOTAL TIME
13:15	20:15	07 hr	15:15	19:42	04h 27m

General Hospital — Supervision: P

REPRINT (DB 1.14/1.14)
Patient Name: Doe, John
Patient ID: 123456
DOB: 08/03/1909
Page 2A
2045010E.PRN

OLP Ver. 5.00 — 17:10, 17:40, 18:10, 18:40, 19:10, 19:40, 20:10, 20:40

Agent	Entries	TOTALS
Air	0.70L--------0L	
Isoflurane	1%----0% … 0.20%--------	
Oxygen	0.70L--------3L--------	
Calcium Chloride IV	200	200 MG
Esmolol IV		100 MG
Heparin IV		25000 IU
Lidocaine IV	100	100 MG
Midazolam IV	1.50.. 3	4.500 MG
Pancuronium IV		8 MG
Phenylephrine IV		150 uG
Procainamide IV		1000 MG
Protamine IV	..200... 75... 75 25	375 MG
Sufentanil IV	17.5..33.5.. 14	222.50 uG
Vecuronium IV		10 MG
DOPAMINE IV	3.0R--------	21.902 MG
EPINEPHRINE IV	0.014R-----0.009R--------	0.060 MG
INSULIN IV	---2R--------	5.947 IU
MIDAZOLAM IV	0.750R--------	14.867 MG
NITROPRUSSIDE IV	0.190R0.569R0.379R------HOLDR 1.138R1.328RHOLDR	5.583 MG
PROCAINAMIDE IV	---2R--------	321.10 MG
EVENTS / NOTES	12, 13-16, 17-19, 20, 21-23	SCALES

EQUIPMENT PLACED: 3.9Q̇ 3.8Q̇
ECG Monitor
FiO2 Monitor
SaO2 Monitor
ETCO2 Monitor
Arterial BP Monitor
CVP Monitor
PAP(Swn-Gnz)Monitor
Cardiac Opt Monitor
Esophageal Temp (C)
Cooling Blanket
Urine Output(Foley)
Heating Blanket
Transesophageal Ech

--- GENERAL COMMENTS ---
17:20 #12 Warm to 37
17:28 SNP IFD dosage(s): 2.5 ML/HR
17:35 SNP IFD dosage(s): 4 ML/HR
17:39 SNP IFD dosage(s): 6 ML/HR
17:40 #13 Aortic crossclamp OFF
17:40 #14 Total X-Clamp time 74 min.
17:45 #15 V- fib, surgeon notified
17:48 #16 Defibrillated X 1 at 30J
18:27 #17 Off bypass
18:28 #18 Total Bypass time (min) 147 min.
18:36 #19 Transducing femoral A-line
18:43 Prot dosage(s): 10 MG
18:46 Prot dosage(s): 20 MG, 30 MG
18:47 Prot dosage(s): 40 MG, 25 MG
18:48 Prot dosage(s): 25 MG
18:50 Prot dosage(s): 25 MG, 25 MG
18:56 SNP IFD dosage(s): 4 ML/HR
18:58 Prot dosage(s): 25 MG, 25 MG
19:00 Mida dosage(s): 1.5 MG
19:00 Sfen dosage(s): 8 uG
19:00 SNP IFD dosage(s): 8 ML/HR
19:04 Mida dosage(s): 1.5 MG
19:04 Sfen dosage(s): 17.5 uG
19:05 SNP IFD dosage(s): 12 ML/HR
19:07 Sfen dosage(s): 8 uG
19:09 Prot dosage(s): 25 MG
19:09 #20 Mandol 1 gram IV
19:10 Prot dosage(s): 25 MG
19:10 SNP IFD dosage(s): 10 ML/HR
19:12 #21 Chest closed
19:15 SNP IFD dosage(s): 11 ML/HR
19:16 Sfen dosage(s): 7 uG
19:17 Sfen dosage(s): 7 uG
19:18 SNP IFD dosage(s): 14 ML/HR
19:19 #22 Midaz (cc) o/u/w/r 30/18/2/10
19:20 #23 Sufent (cc) o/u/w/r 15/7/3/5
19:21 Prot dosage(s): 25 MG, 25 MG
--- EDITING ---
18:44 Prot 16:39 1000 MG deleted.

Figure 21–3. A computer-generated automated anesthesia record provides not only a legible record but also a summary with total amounts of drugs and fluids administered.

is stable, much of this information in unnecessary. Infrequent sampling, however, may miss transient events or sudden rapid deterioration of the patient's condition.

In practice, sampling at 5-minute intervals provides adequate information for a complete anesthetic record. Any changes within this time obviously can still be detected by the presence of the vigilant anesthesiologist. Data compression techniques assist and greatly reduce the volume of data stored, with only minimal loss of data resolution.

Manual Data Entry

Manual data entry should be simple and easy. Systems have been described using standard computer keyboards with single-key selection of data from menus, touch screen entry, and voice recognition. The system should ideally require no more time to enter information than is required with a manual method.

Real-Time Recording

Data should be easily available for examination during anesthesia. Physiologic data are best represented graphically as trend plots; however, provision should also be made for entry of drug and fluid data and free text information.

Adaptability and Interfacing

The system must be easily adaptable for the individual user. Individual anesthesiologists should be able to preselect their individual requirements and recall these at the beginning of a working session. Standard monitors should be interfaced easily to provide data for the record system. As previously stated, most modern monitors have standard signal or data output, so connection to a computerized system is relatively straightforward. The system should function in the available work space. Modern operating rooms are often filled with sophisticated equipment, and so space is limited. Computers used in the operating environment should therefore be as unobtrusive as possible. Some records systems are manufactured as an integral part of the anesthetic machine, obviating the need of the use of further floor space. Other systems have used portable or laptop computers for this task.

The completed anesthetic record can be produced either in the operating room using a bubble jet printer or with a centralized laser printer, depending on the local requirements. Ideally, it should be possible to store all information in a database in a form that will allow easy retrieval for reports such as the workload of the department and of each individual anesthesiologist. It is of increasing importance that data such as the use of pulse oximetry, frequency of hypotension, and critical incidents be analyzed for quality assurance.

AVAILABLE ANESTHETIC RECORD SYSTEMS

Many automated records systems of varying degrees of sophistication are commercially available. Automatic data acquisition from patient monitors is common to all systems, but off-line data entry, data display, data storage, and record production varies according to the manufacturer's perception of what is desirable in a records system.

In addition to the commercial systems, many systems have been produced by anesthesiologists and bioengineers in their own hospitals. Because these systems have been produced "in-house," they can be readily altered to fulfill local needs; new approaches can be tested, and valuable experience is gained as to the actual requirements of anesthesiologists working in the operating environment.

Three levels of computerization of anesthetic records have emerged. At the simplest level, features concerning the anesthetic, such as duration, type of operation, monitoring used, and complications, are entered onto a separate card or sheet. The sheets are then collected at a central point, and the data are entered into the computer database. The number of features can range from a few dozen to over a hundred. The frequency of occurrence of each item in the database can then be printed out at suitable intervals to form a record of work activity, operating room utilization, or junior experience. Problems with this type of record system involve data collection and entry into the computer. It can be difficult to ensure total compliance of all staff members, and it may be tedious to enter large volumes of relatively uninteresting information.

The next level includes portable computers situated on the anesthetic machine to collect relevant data at the source. In addition to purely administrative information, more clinical details of drugs and fluids can be entered. The information can then be downloaded into the database of a larger system for analysis.

Finally, the goal of an anesthetic record system is to capture all patient information at the source. For this purpose, an automated computerized system of the ARCHIVE type is necessary. These are quite expensive at present, but with recognition of the need for such systems and volume production, the cost will decrease.

BENEFITS OF ANESTHETIC RECORD SYSTEMS

Some authorities view introduction of the automated anesthetic record as inevitable, because manual records are often inaccurate, biased, incomplete, and illegible, and they divert attention from more important tasks of the anesthesiologist.[18] In support of this, a confidential enquiry into the accuracy of manual anesthetic records reported a 55% rate of occasional data omission or falsification.[19] It may be possible to reduce the observer bias, missed readings, and errors of memory that affect manual anesthetic records by using automated records systems. A comparison of handwritten and computer-generated anesthetic records showed that low values for blood pressure and heart rate and high values for end-tidal CO_2 were recorded significantly more often when data were recorded with the computerized record system than with manual recording.[20] Errors in anesthetic records are not confined to physiologic data. An assessment of the accuracy of text entries with a manually compiled anesthetic record showed that the mean proportion of omissions was 35% and that the mean proportion of incorrect entries was 3.4%.[21] The cost/benefit ratio of automated anesthetic record systems has been considered,[22] but detailed results from further studies are required to justify the purchase of systems for this reason.

INTENSIVE CARE MONITORING SYSTEMS

Anesthesiologists are frequently involved in critical care medicine. Many forms of monitoring are common to both operating room and intensive care units. It is well recognized that diagnostic accuracy increases when more relevant data are presented.[23] In the management of critically ill patients, large amounts of data are produced over short periods to detect detrimental changes as quickly as possible. To recognize significant changes, it is important that data be presented in an informative manner. Properly applied computer techniques greatly assist in the process of trend plotting (see Chapter 22).

Several workers have shown dramatic increases in the amount of time spent in direct patient care by nurses following implementation of automatic data collection by computer.[24, 25] The computerized data collection system continues to function through critical situations when medical and nursing staff are fully occupied and otherwise unable to record data. In the operating room, the endless gathering, recording, and processing of data is relegated to the ever-attentive, tireless computer, freeing the anesthesiologist to provide corrective action when required.

Many systems have been described that have had varying degrees of success. Most successful are systems based on modern microcomputers and microcomputer networks.[26, 27] The requirements of such systems are as follows: (1) the output of the system provides relevant, accurate, reliable, accessible, and familiar information at the patient's bedside; (2) the output must be appropriate to local requirements; (3) retrieval of information must be simple for all users; and (4) data entry must be simple to improve accuracy and prevent reductions in the time spent in patient care.

These systems work satisfactorily only if they are seen to benefit the patients and the staff does not oppose the system.

COMPUTERIZED ANESTHETIC ADMINISTRATION SYSTEMS

All drugs used in anesthesia have adverse effects, and the aim of any system for drug administration is to titrate drug delivery to achieve the desired clinical effect while minimizing unwanted and toxic side effects. Many of the newer drugs in anesthesia are given intravenously, and there is increasing interest in the use of computer systems to assist with their administration. When blood concentration and clinical effect are closely related in a drug, its administration can be improved by applying pharmacokinetics. Pharmacokinetics describes the relationship between the dose of a drug and the changes in blood and tissue concentrations that occur with time through dilution, elimination, and redistribution. A pharmacokinetic model using a complex series of mathematical equations can be constructed to define these changes. This mathematical model consists of a hypothetical central compartment into which the drug is delivered and from which the drug is removed by the processes of metabolism and redistribution into one or more peripheral compartments (Fig. 21–4).

Computerized infusion systems have been developed that use a pharmacokinetic model operating in real time to calculate the infusion rates necessary to achieve and maintain the theoretic target blood concentrations selected by the anesthesiologist.[28–30] The calculated infusion rates are transmitted automatically by the computer to the infusion pump so that the anesthesiologist delivers drugs by titrating the target blood concentration instead of infusion rates against the response of the patient.[31] This type of target-controlled infusion (TCI) system relieves the anesthesiologist from the need to calculate continuously the blood concentration of the drug. It allows control of intravenous drugs that is as easy as and more exact than the control possible with inhalational agents employing a vaporizer, because the drug is being delivered directly into the patient's blood, whereas the uptake of inhalational agents is subject to the variations in uptake from the lungs.[32]

These TCI systems do not measure drug concentration on-line but produce a predicted or target concentration based on population kinetics. There will, therefore, always be some variation between the target and the true concentrations achieved in the individual patient. However, it is possible to use different kinetic parameters for different patient populations.[33] In addition, the pharmacokinetic variation may be less than differences in patient pharmacody-

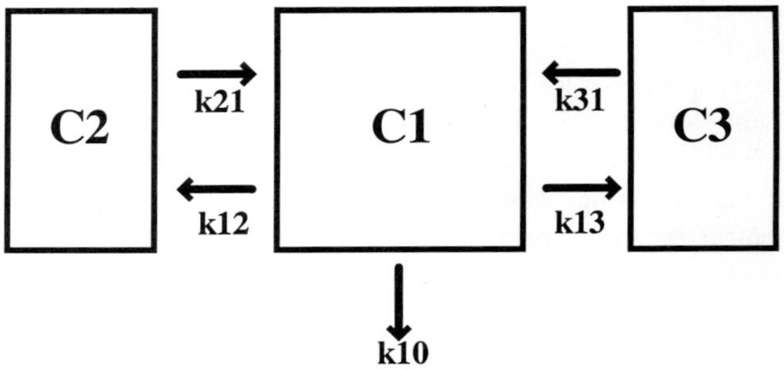

Figure 21–4. Three-compartment pharmacokinetic models. The elimination and redistribution to the peripheral compartments of drug (C2 and C3) added to the central compartment of drug (C1) is described by the rate constants. These constants are obtained from population studies and can be incorporated into a computer program.

namics. For example, there is no single blood concentration of propofol that will produce satisfactory anesthesia in all patients for all degrees of surgical stimulation.[34] TCI systems can be expected to become a routine component of anesthesia within the next few years.

CLOSED-LOOP ANESTHESIA

One additional approach to drug administration is to employ a monitor of anesthetic depth to determine the effect of the drug and use this measurement to control directly the delivery of the anesthetic. The input signal to the control system must provide an accurate index of anesthetic depth and be able to produce satisfactory anesthesia in a spontaneously breathing patient. This requires adequate cardiovascular and respiratory function, minimal or no movement during surgery, and complete avoidance of patient awareness during the procedure. In addition, the control system must be robust and reliable, and its response must be sufficiently rapid. A variety of measurement techniques have been assessed to measure the depth of anesthesia,[35] and three have been used to control the automatic delivery of anesthetic drugs.

Systolic arterial blood pressure has been used to change the inspired concentration of a volatile agent during surgery,[36] and median frequency of the electroencephalogram has been used as the input signal to control administration of methohexitone.[37] However, both of these systems were used only when satisfactory anesthesia had been established and only in patients who had received neuromuscular blocking drugs.

The auditory evoked response may be a better measure of anesthetic depth, because it results in a similar signal when used with approximately equipotent doses of different types of volatile and intravenous anesthetics and appears to respond appropriately to changing degrees of stimulation. A single parameter derived from the auditory evoked response has been used to control the administration of propofol anesthesia to patients breathing spontaneously from induction (during body surface surgery) to recovery.[38] Closed-loop control systems incorporating such modeling concepts appear promising, not only as powerful anesthetic research tools, because they should provide unbiased control of anesthetic depth, but as future tools for the administration of anesthetic drugs in a controlled manner to produce the desired clinical effect, accurately and automatically.

REFERENCES

1. Dickinson CJ: A Computer Model of Human Respiration. Lancaster, MTP, 1977.
2. Smith NT, Quinn ML, Flick J, et al: Automatic control in anesthesia: A comparison in performance between the anesthetist and the machine. Anesth Analg 1984; 63:715–722.
3. Blackburn JP: Computers and the anaesthetist. *In* Scurr C, Feldman S (eds): Scientific Foundations in Anaesthesia. London: Heinemann, 1982; 600–609.
4. Zissos A, Strunin L: A micro-computerized anaesthetic record system. Can J Anaesth 1982; 29:168–173.
5. Murchie JC, Kenny GNC: Comparison of keyboard, light pen and voice recognition as methods of data input. Int J Clin Monit Comput 1988; 5:243–246.
6. Prentice JW, Kenny GNC: Medical students' attitudes to computer assisted learning in anaesthesia. Med Educ 1986; 29:57–59.
7. Kenny GNC, Madsen S, Davis PD: Data entry by light pen. Int J Biomed Comput 1985; 17:27–30.
8. Colvin J, Kenny GNC: Automatic control of blood pressure after cardiac surgery. Anaesthesia 1989; 44:37–41.
9. Bailey JS, Wyatt R, Allwood JM: The nurse to computer interface. *In* Paul JP, Jordan MM, Ferguson-Pell MW, Andrews BJ (eds): Computing in Medicine. London: MacMillan, 1982; 289–293.
10. Smith NT, Brien RA, Pettus DC, et al: Recognition accuracy with a voice-recognition system designed for anesthesia record keeping. J Clin Monit 1990; 6:299–306.
11. Kenny GNC, Davis PD: Computer techniques in critical care medicine. *In* Ledingham IMcA, Hanning CD (eds): Recent Advances in Critical Care Medicine. Edinburgh: Churchill Livingstone, 1983; 197–209.
12. Beneken JEW, Blow JA, Meijler AP: Computerized data acquisition and display in anaesthesia. *In* Parkash O (ed): Computing in Anaesthesia and Intensive Care. Boston: Martinus Nijhoff, 1984; 25–43.
13. Zissos A, Strunin L: Computers in anaesthesia. Can J Anaesth 1985; 32:374–384.
14. Prentice JW, Kenny GNC: Microcomputer-based anaesthetic record system. Br J Anaesth 1984; 56:1433–1437.
15. Lunn JN, Mushin WW: Mortality Associated with Anaesthesia. London: Nuffield Provincial Hospitals Trust, 1982.
16. Block FE: Automated record keeping. Med Innovat Q Rev 1987; 1:1–3.
17. Hunter AR: Computing in anaesthesia and intensive care. Anaesthesia 1984; 39:487–490.
18. Hamilton WK: Will we see automated record keeping systems in common use in anesthesia during our lifetime? J Clin Monit 1990; 6:333–334.
19. Galletly DC, Rowe WL, Henderson RS: The anaesthetic record: A confidential survey on data omission or modification. Anaesth Intensive Care 1991; 19:74–78.
20. Thrush DN: Are automated anesthesia records better? J Clin Anesth 1992; 4:386–389.
21. Rowe Galletly DC, Henderson RS: Accuracy of text entries within a manually compiled anaesthetic record. Br J Anaesth 1992; 68:381–387.
22. Vickers M: Automated anaesthesia records: Economic aspects. *In* Kenny GNC (ed): Automated Anaesthetic Records. London: Bailliere Tindall, 1990; 225–235.
23. Jenkin MA, Cheezum L, Essick V, et al: Clinical patient management and the integrated health care system. Med Instrum 1968; 12:217–221.
24. Miller J, Preston TD, Dann PE, et al: Charting versus computer in a post-operative cardiothoracic intensive care unit. Nurs Times 1978; 74:1423–1425.
25. Sheppard LC: The computer in the care of the critically ill patient. Proc Inst Electron Electric Eng 1979; 67:1300–1306.
26. Phillips GD: Computer-based monitoring and data analysis in anaesthesia and intensive care. Anaesth Intensive Care 1982; 10:229–232.
27. Reid JA, Kenny GNC: Data collection in the intensive care unit. J Microcomput Applic 1984; 7:257–269.
28. Alvis JM, Reves JG, Govier AV, et al: Computer-assisted continuous infusions of fentanyl during cardiac anaesthesia: Comparison with a manual method. Anesthesiology 1985; 65:41–49.
29. Schüttler J, Kloos S, Schwilden H, Stoeckel H: Total intravenous anaesthesia with propofol and alfentanil by computer-assisted infusion. Anaesthesia 1988; 43(Suppl):2–7.
30. White M, Kenny GNC: Intravenous propofol anaesthesia using a computerised infusion system. Anaesthesia 1990; 45:204–209.
31. Taylor IN, White M, Kenny GNC: Assessment of the value and pattern of use of a target controlled propofol infusion system. Int J Clin Monit Comput 1994 (in press).
32. Crofts SL, Hutchison GL: General anaesthesia and undrained pneumothorax. The use of a computer controlled propofol infusion. Anaesthesia 1991; 46:192–194.
33. Marsh B, White M, Morton N, Kenny GNC: Pharmacokinetic model driven infusion of propofol in children. Br J Anaesth 1991; 67:41–48.

34. Glass PSA, Markham K, Ginsberg B, Hawkins ED: Propofol concentrations required for surgery. Anesthesiology 1989; 71:A273.
35. McFadzean WA, Mantzaridis H, Kenny GNC: Assessment of anaesthetic depth. Adv Hosp Technol 1992; 2:22–25.
36. Robb HM, Asbury AJ, Gray WM, Linkens DA: Towards a standardised anaesthetic state using enflurane and morphine. Br J Anaesth 1991; 66:358–364.
37. Schwilden H, Stoeckel H: Effective therapeutic infusions produced by closed-loop feedback control of methohexital administration during total intravenous anesthesia with fentanyl. Anesthesiology 1990; 73:225–229.
38. Kenny GNC, McFadzean W, Mantzaridis H: Closed-loop control of anesthesia. Anesthesiology 1992; 77:A328.

CHAPTER

22

Patient Data Management Systems

JOHN W. HOYT, M.D., FCCM, and
JEROME H. ABRAMS, M.D., F.A.C.S.

Computers have been used to manage information in the intensive care unit (ICU) for over 20 years.[1] Beginning with large mainframe systems that occupied entire rooms and moving to local area networks with bedside work stations, there have been attempts to automate the collection and presentation of patient care data in critical care. Despite our high-technology world, most ICUs continue to operate with pens, critical care flow sheets, and manually written orders and progress notes in the patient chart.

This chapter examines the need for computerized data in critical care and the obstacles to achieving that goal. It seems ironic that one can step into a grocery store in most cities in the United States and watch a checkout clerk use a bar code reader and computer system to tabulate the bill and adjust the store's inventory when it would be difficult to find more than a handful of ICUs similarly employing computers to manage information and facilitate patient care. Only isolated computer applications such as thermodilution cardiac output measurements are present in all intensive care units.

INFORMATION UTILIZATION

Although the information in a grocery store is quite different from that in an ICU, a six-step process is always applied to information to provide a quality service and to please customers. These steps are gathering, processing, presenting, analyzing, managing, and archiving.

Collinson and colleagues illustrate the importance of beginning this six-step process with accurate information.[2] These workers examine the wide variety of input devices available to the ICU and the resistance of ICU nurses and physicians to such devices. Healthcare workers are reluctant to change from old techniques because of fear of new technologies and concerns over increased workload.

INFORMATION GATHERING AND PROCESSING

In the case of the grocery store, information is gathered at the checkout counter as purchases are passed over the bar code reader. The bar code reader is an extremely accurate and rapid input device that is easily learned and that clearly saves time when compared to many ICU input devices. Information is acquired from each purchase and sent back to the computer for the second step, which is processing. The information includes price, taxes, and inventory such that the store can keep track of its cash flow and place orders so that stock is not depleted. The most accurate input device in the intensive care unit is the graphics tablet (rather than the QWERTY keyboard), cursor control keys, and mouse.[2]

In the ICU, many peripheral sensors gather information. These sensors include the bedside monitor obtaining continuous and automated information, the bedside nurse acquiring intermittent measurements and observations such as cardiac output and bedside assessment, and the physician examining and testing the patient. All of this information can be divided into subjective and objective data.

SUBJECTIVE DATA

Subjective data is nonquantitative patient information, which tends to be descriptive in nature. For example, the physical examination provides a large body of subjective data. The information is descriptive and very important, but only rarely quantitative. The examination of the eyes might lead to subjective statements that the pupils are round, equal, and reactive to light. Occasionally, an attempt is made at quantifying a physical finding such as a grade II/IV systolic murmur or 3+ pitting edema. These findings are placed in the patient chart, first in the history and physical examination and subsequently in the progress notes, when repeated examinations reveal changing information. Trending of this information is difficult because it is not systematically filed and requires the laborious reading of many handwritten daily progress notes in the usual patient chart. There is much observer variation in recording physical findings. Finally, most of the information from the physical examination is not quantified, so tables and graphs cannot be conveniently constructed for easy interpretation.

OBJECTIVE DATA

Most of the information collected in the ICU can be classified as objective data. For example, the hourly measurement of vital signs such as heart rate, blood pressure, and similar variables produces objective measurements of patient condition made at the bedside and recorded on the chart. This information is normally gathered automatically in today's busy intensive care unit or operating room by calibrated bedside monitors using various sensors, such as temperature probes or saline-filled catheters attached to strain gauges or pressure transducers. The information is continuous but is only intermittently recorded on a paper record to become part of the patient's chart. In the automated ICU or anesthesia record, the quality of these signals is very important to ensure accurate patient information.[3]

Physiologic Measurements

Another type of objective data is physiologic measurements such as thermal dilution cardiac output, arterial blood gases, and pulmonary capillary wedge pressure. This information is not always available from the bedside monitor and requires the intervention of a nurse, technician, or physician. A volume of thermal indicator must be intermittently injected to obtain cardiac output. Blood must be withdrawn from the patient and taken to the laboratory for blood gas analysis. A balloon on the tip of the pulmonary artery catheter must be inflated to occlude blood flow to measure pulmonary capillary wedge pressure. These activities lead to numeric information that must be recorded on the patient chart but can be trended for interpretation of patient status.

Information from continuously available vital signs is combined with information from intermittent physiologic measurements to perform calculations, creating more objective data.[4] Calculations for cardiac index, systemic vascular resistance, stroke work, and shunt are common cardiopulmonary evaluations in the contemporary ICU.[5] These calculations lead to a more accurate assessment of the patient.

Intake and Output Measurements

One of the most complex sets of data in the ICU is the patient's fluid input and output. On the input side, there is an enormous array of solutions in the ICU. They start with the simple dextrose and water and go to the exceedingly complex, three-in-one total parenteral nutrition solutions, including carbohydrate, amino acids, fat, vitamins, trace elements, insulin, H_2 receptor antagonist drug, and electrolytes in a 3-L bag to be delivered over 24 hours. It is important to record not only the volume of fluid administered but, particularly in the case of parenteral nutrition, such data as delivered carbohydrate and fat calories, grams of protein, and milliequivalents of electrolyte. There is, in addition, a wide variety of output fluids to record. Beyond simple urine output, there are other tubes and drains producing various kinds of fluids that must be recorded in character and amount.

Medication Records

Another significant source of objective data recorded by the nursing staff comes from medications. There are two forms of medication delivery in the ICU, intermittent and continuous. Record keeping for intermittent medications is standardized throughout any hospital to keep track of dose and interval between administration. Continuous medication delivery is more difficult to chart and tends to be more frequent in the ICU.[6] The best example is the continuous administration of a drug such as nitroprusside for decreasing blood pressure and systemic vascular resistance. This medication is given in a dose measured in micrograms/kilogram/minute, titrated to maintain a prescribed systolic or mean blood pressure. Changes in the dose may occur every few minutes in an unstable patient, and the charting of these frequent changes is essentially impossible in a manual system. As a result, the nurse usually records a dose of medication on the hour when blood pressure is recorded; other information about dosage is lost.

Laboratory Measurements

Laboratory data are collected more frequently on ICU patients than on other hospitalized patients. Usually electrolytes, hematocrit, and arterial blood gases are done one to three times daily, depending on the patient's status. Other laboratory information, such as coagulation studies and chemical profiles, are done two to three times per week in order to trend laboratory data. Some laboratory values, such as blood sugar and serum potassium, can be done every 2–4 hours for several days until an abnormality is corrected. This frequency of sampling blood for laboratory information requires a tabular presentation for ease of clinical interpretation. Computer technology with graphic presentation is uniquely capable of assisting with the interpretation of laboratory data.[7]

Miscellaneous Measurements

Finally, objective data are collected from various life support settings. When arterial blood gases are reported, they must be interpreted in the context of ventilator tidal volume, rate, oxygen concentration, and positive end-expiratory pressure if respiratory support is being used. Likewise, hemodynamic data must be interpreted in the light of the setting for the intra-aortic counterpulsation balloon if such a device is being employed. One must be able to trend these life support settings in order to make clinical judgements about patient improvement or deterioration. Unique computer applications allow quick interpretation of this information by the graphic display of blood gases next to ventilator settings.[8]

Each individual ICU information gatherer then processes the information. The monitor trends vital signs for later review, the bedside nurse transcribes this information into the appropriate boxes on the bedside flow sheet, and the physician records a progress note in the chart. At this point in the six-step process of information handling, data have been gathered and processed by a variety of ICU health care workers, and this information is now ready for presentation and analysis.

INFORMATION MANAGEMENT

PRESENTATION AND ANALYSIS

For patient care information to be valuable, it must be presented efficiently and quickly to expedite decision making and patient care.[9] In most ICUs, information is presented in multiple fashions. There is a critical care flow sheet of variable size and quality of construction. There is a bedside chart with history and physical examination notes, progress notes, and consultant opinions. Laboratory information may be on a separate laboratory clipboard. Analysis of all this information in the traditional ICU requires many stops by the clinician who is attempting to construct a medical picture of the critically ill patient and begin the process of clinical decision making.

Computerization of this medical record improves the quality and accuracy of clinical information.[10] Well-presented information permits clinicians to be more effective and to make more accurate decisions. The handling and presentation of information to improve patient care has been studied extensively.[11]

The bedside physician requires a presentation of information (e.g., chart, flow sheet, laboratory records) that permits analysis of information that leads to appropriate patient management decisions. The physician manages information by writing orders that are carried out by the various health care workers, such as a pharmacist preparing and delivering a continuous infusion drug, a respiratory therapist starting mechanical ventilation, or a nurse offering some form of treatment.

Even patient management can be assisted by the computerization of the care delivery process in the ICU. The Pulmonary Division at Latter Day Saints Hospital in Salt Lake City, Utah has developed computerized patient management protocols for the treatment of respiratory failure from adult respiratory distress syndrome.[12] Early results from this work seem to show a substantial reduction in patient mortality rate.[13]

ARCHIVING

The final step in the management of information in the ICU—one that is of growing significance to health care today—is the process of archiving. In the case of most critical care units, all of the manual records from bedside critical care flow sheets, handwritten physician orders, and progress notes are collected from various parts of the ICU, bundled, and transferred to medical records, where an International Classification of Diseases, 9th edition (ICD-9) code is applied, and the chart is sent to storage.

Any review of this information, particularly for quality assurance reasons, must be done manually. ICUs with sophisticated archival systems, based on computerized handling of information, can readily review archives to develop automated quality assurance and utilization reports.[14] The ability to automate reports that substantiate quality of patient care may be the final driving force that will push ICU computer systems into common use across the country.

The present-day manual archival system of intensive care records can again be contrasted with the grocery store, where computers store the day's activities and archive them in an automated fashion for monthly reports, annual reports, and quantified information about quality of performance. It would be a challenge indeed in almost any ICU to determine the number of patients admitted to the ICU with the ICD-9 diagnosis of congestive heart failure (428.0). Even more difficult would be the task of determining patient length of stay, mortality rate, incidence of mechanical ventilation, use of medications, and frequency of use of a pulmonary artery catheter. Whereas a grocery store could easily determine the sale of Heinz ketchup, the profit margin, and the inventory management, the ICU would have a great deal of difficulty answering questions about patients with congestive heart failure without a manual search of stacks of patient charts.

ANALYSIS OF CRITICAL CARE

Why is an ICU different than a grocery store? In the analysis of this question lies the reason why patient data management systems have not thrived in hospitals despite predictions to the contrary. Grocery stores are closed-shop businesses with a store manager, a clear mission, and an administrative structure. Business must be analyzed, profits determined, taxes paid, orders placed. If the business runs well, salaries are paid, profits are made, the community is fed, people are happy, and quality is perceived. If the business is managed poorly, it does not survive. The same cannot be said for ICUs.

The modern ICU is a high-technology environment for the monitoring and life support of patients with life-threatening illnesses. It has special utilities for emergency power, oxygen, compressed air, and vacuum to distinguish it from most other hospital beds. In addition, the ICU has bedside monitors for the automatic acquisition of electrocardiogram and heart rate, blood pressure, pulmonary artery pressure, and arterial oxygen saturation by pulse oximeter, to name a few measurements. A ratio of one nurse to two patients is needed to gather intermittent information, make assessments, and offer treatments. The ICU has special equipment such as devices for positive pressure ventilation and intra-aortic counterpulsation. The health care team believes that vigilance in the ICU will permit early detection of problems (chest pain and cardiac ischemia, cardiac arrhythmias and poor perfusion, respiratory failure and hypoxia) that can be quickly corrected before they harm the ICU patient. Most important in the information management process are appropriate interpretation of collected information and wise decisions, made in an expeditious fashion, about therapeutic plans for the ICU patient.

Unfortunately, unlike the grocery store, in most hospitals across the country,[15] the ICU does not have a physician manager who is responsible and accountable for the success of the business of monitoring and providing life support to patients with life-threatening illnesses. Many individual physicians admit patients to the ICU and utilize a variety of physician consultants to assist with patient management.[16] There is usually an ICU medical director, but recent data show that the medical director is rarely involved in the minute-to-minute management of the majority of ICU patients. Instead, care is provided through intermittent physician visits. The bedside nurse must, by phone calls to the admitting physician, manage the patient unless a crisis brings the admitting physician from the office, operating room, laboratory, or home to the ICU bedside. Thus, expeditious action commonly is prevented, potentially leading to higher mortality rates and longer stays.[17]

In the absence of a physician administrative and patient care manager of ICU services, as (in the form of a store manager) occurs in the grocery store, there is little accountability for the quality of ICU services. Records are not archived to permit an expeditious quality assessment. Techniques of or protocols for life support often depend on the wishes of individual admitting physicians. Physician management services ensure that, in this high-technology area, information management includes proper analysis, response, and archiving.

EMPHASIS ON QUALITY

One of the biggest changes in health care over the last 5 years is the consumer demand for evidence of quality. The Pennsylvania state government published a pamphlet on the results of cardiac surgery in all hospitals in the state providing open heart services. The data included total cost of surgery and patient mortality rate.[18] After the release of this information to the consumers of Pennsylvania, there was much chagrin on the part of health care providers. Hospitals with high mortality rates claimed to have the sickest patients. Hospitals with low mortality rates anointed themselves as centers of excellence in cardiac surgery and used the information as a marketing device to recruit more patients.

In fact, the information on cardiac surgery from Pennsylvania is missing some of the essential items available from a computerized patient data management system with appropriate archival records. Such a computer system could be applied to cardiac surgery patients or to general medical/surgical ICU patients. The principle is the same. Information must be gathered, processed, presented, analyzed, managed, and archived. In the case of Pennsylvania, there were only raw data on cost and death rate. There was no information on severity of illness, pre-existing illnesses, or differences in treatment protocols that might have permitted an understanding of hospital differences in cost and mortality rate.

In the ICU, quality of care has been a focus of research for the last 15 years. The Acute Physiology and Chronic Health Evaluation (APACHE) developed by William Knaus[19] originally was designed to compare care delivery in different ICUs with varying management styles.[20] It discovered that the ICU with the best system of management and highest level of staff collaboration had the lowest mortality rate. Now in its third generation, APACHE has a huge database that can be used to assess outcome or to analyze quality.

APACHE is not perfect for many reasons. However, it is a start on archiving information from critical care services needed to assess quality. Unfortunately, APACHE does not use a standardized (ICD-9) diagnosis system. Its diagnosis system is one of broad categories of organ-related illness such as respiratory or cardiac failure. APACHE uses deviation from 10 physiologic variables to determine the severity-of-illness score. There is much debate over the relevance of these ten variables, especially as they relate to situations such as postoperative cardiac surgery patients. There is no information in the system for comparing different treatment protocols. A national database, collecting information on diagnosis, treatment, outcome, and cost, is essential and can only be accomplished by computer applications to intensive care.

MANUAL INFORMATION GATHERING

By clinical example, it is possible to examine the use or misuse of information in the present-day ICU in the absence of a computerized patient data management system and critical care services as defined above.

D.L. is a 71-year-old female with coronary artery disease not amenable to percutaneous transluminal coronary angioplasty. A coronary artery bypass graft is performed, and the patient is admitted to the cardiovascular ICU. Surgery, anesthesia, and the immediate postoperative course are uneventful. The patient recovers from anesthesia and appears hemodynamically stable. The surgeon departs for home in the early evening and makes several phone calls to the bedside nurse in the late evening to evaluate patient status.

Throughout the evening, information is gathered by the bedside nurse. Blood pressure is recorded from an arterial catheter. Mixed venous oxygen saturation from a fiberoptic pulmonary artery catheter is trended on a bedside monitor. Chest tube drainage is measured and recorded on an hourly basis. Every 4 hours, the bedside nurse draws a sample of blood to fill a capillary tube and measure hematocrit. All of this information is processed to appropriate boxes on the ICU flow sheet. Once various pieces of information have been gathered from diverse sources and processed on the flow sheet, the data are ready for presentation.

Presentation of information in the ICU is key to the successful management of patients with life-threatening illnesses. The basis of valid presentation is juxtaposition of key elements. For example, in managing a patient in respiratory failure, the clinician wants to juxtapose blood gases alongside ventilator settings to interpret patient status (Fig. 22–1). In the case of cardiac failure, the clinician wants to juxtapose vital signs, hemodynamic measurements, and doses of inotropic therapy in order to assess the patient response to treatment (Fig. 22–2). The ICU physician can develop numerous clinical scenarios in which key pieces of information must be combined to allow expeditious interpretation of physiologic abnormalities and appropriate corrective action. Computers, when properly programmed for the management of information, do presentation particularly well. They can be programmed to automatically juxtapose key clinical elements.

Analysis of information in the ICU requires several key elements. First, the clinician must examine juxtaposed elements of clinical information and mentally establish patterns of physiologic function. Second, the clinician must make judgements about the patterns of physiologic function to make clinical diagnoses and initiate treatment. Computerized graphic ICU workstations are now facilitating this process.[21]

To return to the clinical example of the cardiac surgery patient: data began to accumulate after midnight that suggested postoperative difficulties. Blood pressure decreased to 85–90 mmHg. Systolic and mixed venous oxygen saturation decreased to below 40%. Chest tube drainage, previously 100 ml/hour, suddenly stopped. Hematocrit, 32% at the end of cardiopulmonary bypass, was now 21%. The patient was no longer awake. Extremities were cool, and the pulse oximeter was no longer able to determine arterial saturation.

To the experienced observer of the postoperative course of cardiac surgery patients, these data indicate postoperative mediastinal bleeding with occluded chest tubes and cardiac tamponade until proven otherwise. Data must be analyzed quickly to minimize end-organ damage from poor peripheral perfusion. Management of the patient in light of the information includes augmentation of intravascular volume, opening the chest to remove the blood, and returning to the operating room for evaluation of bleeding. This information must be archived so that the medical director of the ICU can, on an annual basis, examine the rate of postoperative bleeding and tamponade for each of the surgeons working in the hospital.

Manual gathering, processing, presentation, analyzing, managing, and archiving of data in most ICUs around the country cause delayed interpretation of physiologic abnormalities, slow correction of problems, and impossible interpretation of overall results such as morbidity, length of stay, and cost of care. The application of a computerized critical care medical information system with critical management services for the ICU can reduce the delays in diagnosis, treatment, and assessment of quality care.

RESPIRATORY

TIME	PaO_2	SaO_2	PH	$PaCO_2$	HCO_3	$P\bar{V}O_2$	$S\bar{V}O_2$	$PH\bar{V}$	$P\bar{V}CO_2$	CaO_2	$C\bar{V}O_2$	A-VDO_2	$\dot{Q}s/\dot{Q}t$	TOT Hgb	MODE	TIDAL VOLUME ORDERED/ EXHALED	RATE/ TOTAL RESP.	FIO_2	PEEP/CPAP (BASELINE)	PFR/ INSP. TIME	PEAK/DRIVE PRESSURE	INSP. PRESS. SUPPORT
00	93	97	7.39	40	24	40	73	7.36	42	20	16	4	28	15	SIMV	900/	12/20	.5	5	50	45	5
01																/	/					
02															SIMV	900/	12/20	.5	5	50	45	5
03																/	/					
04															SIMV	900/	10/25	.4	5	50	45	5
05	75	92	7.37	42	24	36	70	7.35	44	20	16	4	25	15		/	/					
06															SIMV	900/	8/28	.4	5	50	45	5
07	72	91	7.36	43	23	35	69	7.33	45	20	16	4	27	15		/	/					

Figure 22–1. An example of juxtaposition of information in the respiratory section of a critical care flow sheet. Critical care computerized medical information systems (CCCMISs) can gather all this information automatically from various sources and peripheral sensors and present it to the clinician for interpretation and decision making. The data can be displayed in a tabular form as seen here or in a graphic form for easier visual recognition of abnormalities. Unfortunately, only a handful of intensive care units around the country are capable of an automated collection and display of this data, increasing the work loads of the health care workers in nonautomated ICUs.

CARDIOVASCULAR														
												INFUSIONS		
TIME	BP S/D	HEART RATE	CVP	PA S/D	PCWP/LAP	CO (5 ± 1)	CI (3 ± .5)	SVRI (2000 ± 300)	SaO_2	$S\bar{V}O_2$	IABP	mcg/kg/ min./cc	mcg/kg/ min./cc	mcg/kg/ min./cc
00	120/80	95	6	35/19	17				95	69	1:1	10	3	
01	118/76	93	8	37/18	16				93	68	1:1	10	3	
02	132/85	105	6	33/17	15	5.0	2.5	3200	97	71	1:1	10	3	
03	114/70	90	10	39/20	19				93	65	1:1	10	3	
04	112/68	110	11	31/16	15				96	66	1:1	10	3	
05	125/85	98	13	32/16	14				95	68	1:1	10	3	
06	130/85	102	9	39/18	17				96	65	1:1	10	3	
07	132/90	95	10	40/20	19				92	66	1:1	10	3	
												DOBUTAMINE	DOPAMINE	

Figure 22–2. Juxtaposition of data is the key to accurate and expeditious decision making in the intensive care unit. This example of the cardiovascular section of a critical care flow sheet facilitates decision making in the intensive care unit. These data are from a patient with cardiovascular disease who is dependent on both intravenous inotropic therapy and intra-aortic balloon counterpulsation. The cardiac index (CI) of 2.5 L/minute/m^2 is only interpretable in the context of the life support information required to achieve that level of cardiac function. The manual gathering and manual processing of patient monitoring information gives the clinician quick access to a data set necessary for patient management.

AUTOMATED INFORMATION PROCESSING

Better processing of information is available today for ICUs. A powerful workstation is interfaced with the bedside monitor to gather and trend continuously monitored vital sign information. Nurses use the workstation to enter intermittent physiologic measurements such as cardiac output. The workstation is connected to the laboratory, so that values from blood sample analysis automatically enter the patient's computer chart. Infusion pumps at the bedside tell the workstation of doses of medication and intravenous fluid administration. Urine output and chest tube drainage can be measured and automatically entered into the bedside workstation.

Computers never tire and can be programmed to vigilantly monitor incoming data and alert the bedside health care team of impending problems. Imagine this workstation evaluating the cardiac surgery patient previously described. The computer trends the blood pressure, sees the decreasing hematocrit from the laboratory, measures the chest tube drainage, and records the decreasing mixed venous saturation. This set of abnormalities creates a package of data to alert the bedside nurse and physician quickly of impending disaster if an intervention does not correct the cardiac tamponade.

Another example is an ICU patient on continuous enteral nutrition and continuous intravenous infusion of insulin to control blood sugar. The physician writes an order to stop the enteral nutrition at midnight before a surgical procedure the next morning. The computer should be programmed to alert the bedside health care workers to follow blood glucose and consider stopping the insulin infusion, because the enteral nutrition has been discontinued.

Bedside workstations are connected to each other via a local area network with a file server to save data for later archival application. The local area network should contain essential information to help the physician make accurate decisions. Consider the example of aminoglycoside antibiotics. The ICU computer has a formula for size and interval of aminoglycoside dose and automatically examines patient data such as weight, creatinine, and aminoglycoside blood level to predict a subsequent dose correction and to limit drug toxicity.

In the processing of information, the computerized critical care medical information system has remarkable power. One of the most important components of the analysis of complex physiologic and metabolic problems is identification of the appropriate dimensionality of analysis. Clearly, in the ICU context, problems exist in many dimensions simultaneously and must be analyzed accordingly. An example of a multidimensional approach to a common ICU problem is the analysis of oxygen transport in patients being resuscitated according to oxygen transport variables. A response surface, a cusp catastrophe manifold, has been derived.[22] In this model, appropriate dimensionality is identified objectively, the influential variables controlling the system are allowed to vary simultaneously and nonlinearly, and the geometric response surface that describes the distribution of responses to resuscitation is explicitly derived. Another important feature of critical illness is its dynamic quality. The need for careful observation in the ICU is equivalent to the need for obtaining information about the time dependence of important clinical variables. Patient data management systems in the critical care unit allow dynamic systems analysis. An example of such a dynamic system is the creation of a ventricular pressure-volume loop from continuous cardiac output combined with a measurement of left ventricular pressure. A nonlinear oscillator model, the van der Pol's oscillator, has been successful in allowing, in research settings, the construction of the ventricular pressure-volume loop in nonischemic hearts.[23] In addition, dynamic analysis of electrocardiographic information, including the various intervals of the electrocardiogram signal, is useful to predict cardiac dysrhythmia.[24, 25]

An important component of computational power is the graphic representation of the computational results. The modern graphic capabilities of computers allow geometric interpretations of complicated systems. The graphic representation of the catastrophe manifold as a description of oxygen transport provides an intuitive, geometric display of the efficacy of treatment. The ability to construct graphs and other graphic aids allows the clinician to recognize patterns where only confusion or abstract formalism previously existed. The transition from stability to dysrhythmia to unstable dysrhythmia, as with atrial fibrillation, also achieves a geometric quality that is otherwise very difficult to comprehend.

The computerized critical care medical information system has many other applications to assist with the management of the ICU. A system for electronic mail (e-mail) facilitates staff communication about changes in ICU protocol. Access to read-only memory (ROM) can contain the entire ICU manual such that the bedside health care worker, unfamiliar with a particular protocol or medication or treatment, can easily review important information to reduce errors and improve quality.

All of this high-level computerized information processing and communication is unlikely to occur in the contemporary structure of most ICUs. Only when a collaborative management system for critical care that involves a nursing director and a medical director is present will there be both a demand and a process to analyze results and to determine quality.

REFERENCES

1. Peters RM: Perspectives in ICU computing. Int J Clin Monit Comput 1985; 2:101–105.
2. Collinson PO, Jones RG, Howes M, et al: Of mice and men—Data capture in the clinical environment. Int J Clin Monit Comput 1989; 6:217–222.
3. Clochesy JM, Henker RA: Selecting computer software applications in critical care. Dimensions Crit Care Nurs 1986; 5(3):171–177.
4. Edwards FH, Davies RS: The handheld computer in critical care medicine. Am Surg 1986; 52:452–455.
5. Shabot MM, Carlton PD, Sadoff S, et al: Graphical reports and displays for complex ICU data: A new, flexible and configurable method. Comput Methods Programs Biomed 1986; 22:111–116.
6. Dasta JF: Computers in critical care: Opportunities and challenges. Ann Pharmacol 1990; 24:1084–1092.
7. Hohnloser JH, Purner F: PADS (patient archiving and documentation system): A computerized patient record with educational aspects. Int J Clin Monit Comput 1992; 9:71–84.
8. Seiver A, Kohatsu S, Rowles D: Bedside computers in the surgical intensive care unit. Angiology 1987; 38:248–252.
9. Villalobos J, Manzano JL, Blazquez M, et al: Computerized system in intensive care medicine. Med Inform 1986; 11(3):269–275.
10. Clemmer TP, Gardner RM: Medical informatics in the intensive care unit: State of the art 1991. J Clin Monit Comput 1992; 8:237–250.
11. Kalli S, Ambroso C, Gregory R, et al: Inform: Conceptual modelling of intensive care information systems. Int J Clin Monit Comput 1992; 9:85–94.
12. Sittig DF, Gardner RM, Pace NL, et al: Computerized management of patient care in a complex, controlled clinical trial in the intensive care unit. Comput Methods Programs Biomed 1989; 30:77–84.
13. East TD, Morris AH, Wallace CJ, et al: A strategy for development of computerized critical care decision support systems. Int J Clin Monit Comput 1992; 8:263–269.
14. Shabot MM, Bjerke HS, LoBue M, et al: Quality assurance and utilization assessment: The major byproducts of an ICU clinical information system. Proc Annu Symp Comput Appl Med Care 1991; 554–558.
15. Groeger JS, Strosberg MA, Halpern NA, et al: Descriptive analysis of critical care units in the United States. Crit Care Med 1992; 20(6):846.
16. Hoyt JW, Leisifer DJ, Rafkin HS: Critical care units. *In* Wenzel RP (ed): Assessing Quality Health Care. Baltimore: Williams & Wilkins, 1992; 267–296.
17. Brown JJ, Sullivan G: Effect on ICU of a full-time critical care specialist. Chest 1989; 96:127–129.
18. A Consumer Guide to Coronary Artery Bypass Graft Surgery. Pennsylvania Health Care Cost Containment Council, November 19, 1992.
19. Knaus WA, Zimmerman JE, Wagner DP, et al: APACHE—Acute physiology and chronic health evaluation: A physiologically based classification system. Crit Care Med 1981; 9:591–597.
20. Knaus WA, Draper EA, Wagner DP, et al: An evaluation of outcome from intensive care in major medical centers. Ann Intern Med 1986; 104:410–418.
21. Higgins SB, Jiang K, Swindell BB, et al: A graphical ICU workstation. Proc Annu Symp Comput Appl Med Care 1991; 783–787.
22. Abrams JH, Barke RA, Cerra FB: Quantitative evaluation of clinical course in surgical ICU patients: The data conform to catastrophe theory. J Trauma 1984; 24(12):1028–1037.
23. Abrams JH, Irwin ED, Walvatne CS, et al: Use of a modified van der Pol's oscillator to construct ventricular pressure-volume relations. J Cardiothorac Vasc Anesth 1993; 7(2):195–199.
24. Goldberger AL, Bhargava V, West BJ: Nonlinear dynamics of the heartbeat. Physica 1985; 17D:207–241.
25. Winfree AT: When Time Breaks Down: The Three-Dimensional Dynamics of Electrochemical Waves and Cardiac Arrhythmias. Princeton: Princeton University Press, 1987.

SECTION SEVEN

Monitoring Anesthesia Delivery

CHAPTER

23

Monitoring the Anesthesia Machine

WILLIAM T. ROSS, JR., M.D.

THE CONTINUOUS FLOW ANESTHESIA MACHINE

Continuous flow anesthesia machines available for use in today's practice of anesthesia have evolved from experience and the thoughtful application of sound principles from several disciplines. This evolution can be traced through published reports of innovative technology spanning more than 100 years. More complete and specific information may be found in the several excellent texts,[1–3] manufacturers' publications,[4–7] and extensive literature concerning anesthesia equipment.

More important, reports describing failures of anesthesia machines and unexpected results from their operation have resulted in the modifications responsible for today's anesthesia machines. To understand the circumstances in which anesthesia equipment departs from its expected function (whether from malfunction or misuse), one needs to think of how the equipment can fail. The operation of equipment after failure of a portion of the assembled apparatus is referred to as a failure mode. Understanding likely failure modes significantly enhances the anesthesiologist's appreciation of his or her equipment.

The continuous flow anesthesia machine (Fig. 23–1) allows the anesthesiologist to accurately combine several gases (or vapors) to provide the gas mixtures used in the conduct of clinical anesthesia. The two major suppliers of anesthesia machines in the United States are Ohmeda (Madison, WI) and North American Drager (Telford, PA). Anesthesia machines, designed originally to be freestanding, mobile devices, are equipped with high-pressure vessels, typically E cylinders, each containing a few hundred liters of gas at high pressure.

GAS SUPPLY

The gases most often available on anesthetic machines are oxygen and nitrous oxide. Some machines have provisions for other compressed gases, such as air, helium, and carbon dioxide. Most hospitals in the United States now supply some or all of the gases used in anesthesia through built-in piping systems. The compressed gas cylinders on the anesthesia machines should be regarded as a reserve supply, available in the event of a failure of the hospital medical gas piping system. As such, they permit an anesthetic procedure in progress to be brought to a controlled conclusion.

Dependence on plumbing systems as the primary gas supply is so established that it is unwise to begin subsequent anesthetics with only E cylinders available. Reserve stocks of E cylinders are often maintained by hospital departments such as respiratory therapy or central supply that are not under the control of the anesthesia department. Stock levels may easily be too low to sustain continuation of a surgical schedule. Additionally, anesthesia ventilators utilize oxygen as the driving gas to produce tidal ventilation. Using these ventilators markedly increases the consumption of compressed oxygen[8] and places further demand on the supply and exchange of cylinders.

Full high-pressure cylinders containing oxygen or air are filled to pressures of approximately 2000 pounds/square inch gauge (psig) while nitrous oxide is supplied as a liquid. It has a vapor pressure of approximately 750 psig at room temperature. The amount of oxygen or air contained in a cylinder is proportional to the pressure in the cylinder. As a result, the amount of oxygen in a compressed gas cylinder may be accurately estimated when the pressure within the cylinder is known. The amount of liquid nitrous oxide (or any fluid for that matter) contained in a cylinder can be accurately estimated by knowing the weight of nitrous oxide (weight of cylinder plus nitrous oxide less the tare weight of the cylinder) contained within the cylinder.

In practice, the weighing of cylinders is awkward and is rarely performed except as a demonstration within a teaching environment. In addition, the tare weight of cylinders is typically unknown. Furthermore, during periods of nitrous

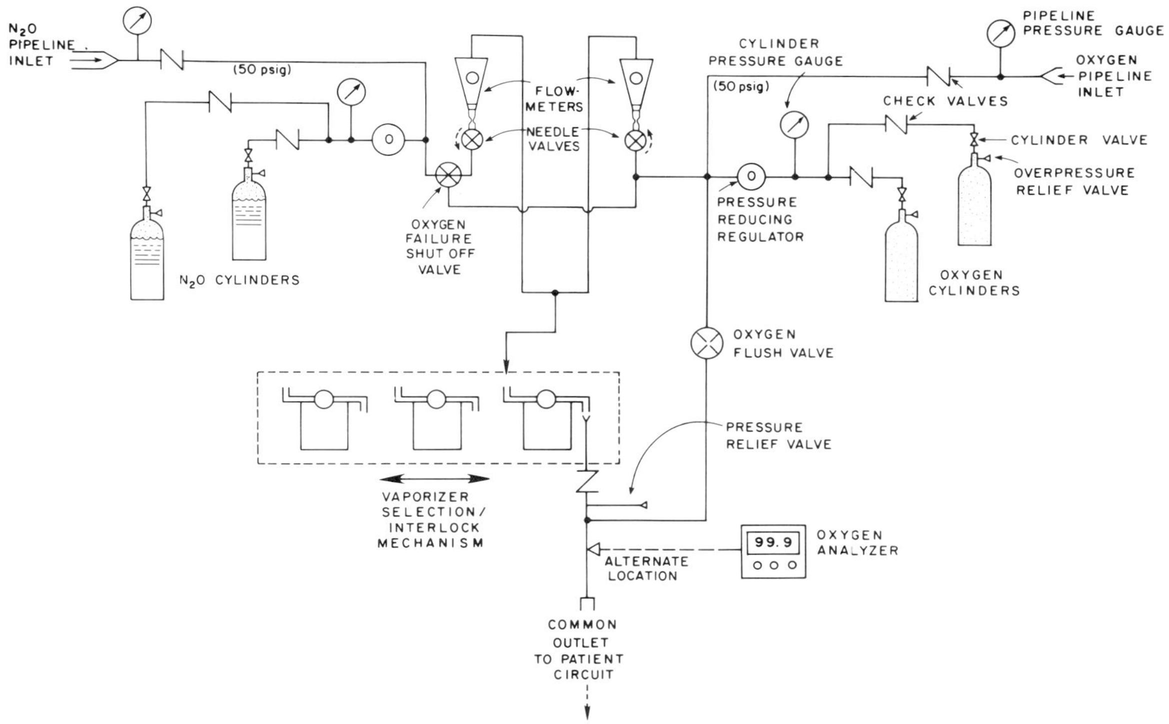

Figure 23–1. A "generic" continuous flow anesthesia machine. This diagram does not represent a specific machine but illustrates design features of various widely used machines.

oxide use, the vaporization of liquid nitrous oxide to gas sufficiently cools the cylinder and its contents to significantly reduce the vapor pressure of the liquid remaining within the cylinder. For this reason, the pressure measured in cylinders of nitrous oxide that have been subjected to significant cooling will be as much as several hundred pounds below the expected 750 psig even though they still contain liquid nitrous oxide.[9] Consequently, the amount of nitrous oxide remaining in cylinders in clinical practice is not accurately known.

Pressure and Flow Controls

The supply pipeline pressure of 50 psig is used as the intermediate or "working" pressure within the plumbing of the section of the anesthesia machine proximal to flowmeter control valves or on/off controls, such as the oxygen flush valve. The flows set by flow control valves are monitored by observing their associated flowmeters. The flow control valves used in anesthesia machines to regulate gas flow function as variable resistors and can provide, at any given setting, constant gas flow at their outlets only if presented with constant inlet pressure. Expressed mathematically, this relationship is fundamentally the same as Ohm's law for electrical circuits:

$$\text{Flow} = \frac{\text{pressure}}{\text{resistance}}$$

This association dictates that the high pressure available in high-pressure cylinders be accurately reduced to a constant working pressure. Such a requirement is met by pressure-reducing regulators adjusted to maintain a constant outlet pressure of 50 psig (or slightly less) while a variable (up to about 2000 psig), but greater, pressure is presented to the inlet.

Likewise, variations in the pressure of gas in the gas piping system result in proportional variations in the flow of that gas through a flow control valve. For example, a 10% variation in supply pressure produces a similar variation in the gas flow exiting the flow control valve in the absence of compensating adjustments of the flow control valve. Ohmeda anesthesia machines in production today are constructed with the intermediate pressure section incorporating an additional stage of regulated pressure reduction to a pressure lower than the pipeline supply pressure of 50 psig. This is done in order to achieve superior regulation of the pressure being presented to the valves controlling gas flow to the flowmeters.[5]

VAPORIZERS

Agent-specific vaporizers are used to accurately add measured concentrations of volatile anesthetics to the gas stream. These devices must be used only with the anesthetic agent for which they were designed. Anesthetic machines having more than a single vaporizer should have an interlock/exclusion mechanism to prevent more than one vaporizer from being used at a time. The interlock mechanism also serves to isolate vaporizers not selected for use from the gas stream by disconnecting both inlets and outlets of unselected vaporizers from the gas stream. This prevents vapor from an upstream vaporizer from being carried downstream and mixing with liquid anesthetic in the downstream vaporizer. Isolation of unselected vaporizers from the gas stream also serves to prevent the addition of small amounts of volatile anesthetics to the gas stream, which can result from continuing evaporation of volatile anesthetics contained within the unselected vaporizers even though the vaporizer is turned off.[10]

OXYGEN FLUSH CIRCUIT

The oxygen flush circuit permits flushing of the gas machine with a high flow of oxygen. It should be noted that the operation of the flush valve simply admits a high flow of oxygen to the outlet of the machine and neither turns off vaporizers nor provides a high flow of the anesthetic-containing gas mixture. Certain older machines had flush valves that were linked to include other functions, such as deselecting vaporizers.

Most Ohmeda anesthesia machines of recent manufacture have a check valve between the outlet of vaporizers and the junction of the oxygen flush line with the fresh gas stream (i.e., near the fresh gas outlet of the machine). This check valve prevents retrograde flow of appreciable volumes of gas back into the machine with the application of positive pressure at the machine outlet, as with positive pressure ventilation. This feature serves particularly to isolate vaporizers from the "pumping effect" of pressure fluctuations on the constancy of vaporizer output.[11] Most Drager Narkomed machines do not have an outlet check valve.[3]

FRESH GAS OUTLET

Access to the gas stream emanating from the anesthesia machine is provided at the fresh gas port. This connector provides a standardized 15-mm connecting point from which gas can be delivered to the patient breathing circuit.

RATIONALE FOR MONITORING THE ANESTHETIC MACHINE

Fundamentally, anesthetic machines fail to perform the functions for which they were designed when they provide incorrect concentrations (or proportions) of the various gases or when they deliver an incorrect absolute amount of gas. This can lead to disaster if oxygen is greatly reduced or eliminated from the gas mixture. Other serious failures can occur with less dire consequences; for example, the omission of the anesthetic agent from the gas mixture can result in failure to achieve or maintain the anesthetic state. Because gas flowing from the anesthesia machine is relied on to fill reservoir bags in anesthetic circuits and ventilators, leaks that permit the loss of gas can result in failure of ventilation when the volume of gas delivered is insufficient to adequately fill the reservoir bag or the ventilator bag.

Monitoring of the anesthesia machine as well as of the anesthetized patient can provide early recognition of problems, which is essential for their prompt correction and minimization of the likelihood of an adverse outcome.

OXYGEN DELIVERY

There is little debate that assurance of adequate delivery of oxygen to the patient breathing circuit is a crucial function of anesthetic machine monitoring. The assumption that operator vigilance prevents the occasional accidental delivery of hypoxic or anoxic breathing mixtures has been proven inaccurate.[12, 13] Extensive efforts have been made to design machines that do not permit the delivery of hypoxic gas mixtures.

One early approach was to construct machines so that the flow of oxygen could not be reduced to less than some minimum value. In this way, anoxic mixtures are prevented, although hypoxic mixtures may be accepted at some nitrous oxide flowmeter settings.

Beginning in the 1960s, anesthesia machines were equipped with fail-safe mechanisms[4, 5, 7] designed to automatically halt the delivery of gases other than oxygen in the event of failure of the oxygen supply pressure within the intermediate pressure section of the machine. Note that this system responds to oxygen supply *pressure* rather than to the *flow* of oxygen. Anesthetists must understand that with older machines, not equipped with oxygen proportion controllers, it is possible to continuously administer hypoxic gas mixtures by adjusting oxygen to low (or even to zero) flow even though the machine is equipped with a fail-safe mechanism.

The fail-safe mechanism is checked by turning on oxygen and nitrous oxide and removing the source of oxygen pressure. The flow of nitrous oxide should decline in proportion to the fall in oxygen pressure and be interrupted entirely as oxygen pressure falls below approximately 25 psig. The abruptness of cessation of nitrous oxide flow varies with the particular fail-safe device and may even vary among individual machines of the same model. Ohmeda refers to its fail-safe mechanism as a "pressure-sensor shutoff valve," whereas Drager calls it an "oxygen failure protection device" (OFPD). The operation of these devices is not tested during the checkout procedures described below. The fail-safe devices and oxygen proportion controllers on machines of recent manufacture work in tandem to make the accidental administration of hypoxic gas mixtures very unlikely.

Another design strategy has been to render machines incapable of delivering mixtures of gases containing less than 25–30% oxygen. Ohmeda and North American Drager have implemented this function by pursuing different schemes to monitor[4] or to control[4, 5] the concentration of oxygen being supplied to the patient breathing circuit. Initially, North American Drager offered pneumatic devices called oxygen ratio monitors (ORMs) that triggered an alarm when oxygen mixtures containing less than 30% oxygen were selected. More recently, Drager has offered the oxygen ratio monitor controller (ORMc), which controls the concentration of oxygen actually delivered by the anesthesia machine (by decreasing the flow of nitrous oxide) when the operator attempts to select combinations of flows of oxygen and nitrous oxide that would result in the delivery of less than 25–30% oxygen. For example, nitrous oxide is automatically adjusted downward when the operator decreases the oxygen flow such that the resulting gas mixture would contain less than 25–30% oxygen. Conversely, when nitrous oxide flow is increased such that the resulting gas mixture would contain less than 25–30% oxygen, the ORMc limits nitrous oxide flow.

The Ohmeda Modulus machine incorporates a mechanical linkage (Link 25) between the oxygen and nitrous oxide flow control valves to produce a similar result. The Link 25 proportionally increases the flow of oxygen when an attempt is made to increase the flow of nitrous oxide so that the resulting gas mixture would contain more than 70% nitrous oxide (without the compensating action of the Link 25 to maintain the oxygen concentration in the fresh gas mixture at or above 30%). The device also functions in an inverse manner so that a reduction in the flow of oxygen downward results in a proportional reduction in the flow of nitrous oxide so that the resulting concentration of oxygen in the resulting gas mixture remains at or above 30%.

OXYGEN ANALYZERS

All gas machines should be able to analyze the gas supplied to the patient for oxygen. Oxygen analyzers are durable, inexpensive, and reliable devices that specifically identify as well as quantitate oxygen in the gas stream (see Chapter 11). This may be accomplished by placing the oxygen analyzer sensor in the inspiratory limb of the patient breathing circuit or, alternatively, in the fresh gas line proximal to the breathing circuit.[14] The location of the oxygen analyzer sensor in the inspiratory limb of the patient breathing circuit is particularly advantageous when low-flow anesthetic techniques are employed with circle absorber breathing circuits, because it indicates the actual concentration of inspired oxygen. Oxygen concentration varies with time and is affected by the patient's oxygen consumption, the uptake of gases other than oxygen from the breathing circuit (e.g., nitrous oxide), and the total fresh gas flow.

On modern anesthesia machines, oxygen analysis, as just described, is used *in addition to* analysis of respiratory gases in the breathing circuit, which may include determinations of inspiratory and expiratory oxygen concentrations. Such redundancy greatly enhances safety for patients and *must not be used as an argument for eliminating basic oxygen analysis from anesthesia machines.* Furthermore, such an arrangement permits an analytic check of the oxygen supplied by a machine during machine checkout separate from any information that may be obtained from associated respiratory gas analysis devices. During anesthetic administration, a basic oxygen analyzer provides a running cross check for FIO_2 data being supplied by a respiratory gas analyzer.

PRELIMINARY TASKS IN MONITORING THE ANESTHESIA MACHINE

Monitoring the anesthetic machine includes tasks that must occur before use of the device for patient care, during anesthesia administration, and following completion of anesthesia.

PREANESTHETIC CHECK

A preanesthetic checkout of the anesthesia apparatus is a prerequisite for reliable, safe anesthesia administration. The general capabilities of the anesthesia machine to be used must be known. At a minimum, the anesthesiologist needs to know, with a high degree of certainty, whether the machine has monitors that can be turned off independently from the gas flows available on the machine and whether the machine can produce hypoxic mixtures under any circumstances, despite monitoring devices.

Although a number of anesthesia machine checkout procedures have been recommended, the United States Food and Drug Administration (FDA) published and widely disseminated an anesthesia machine checkout procedure in 1986 that was endorsed and promoted by the American Society of Anesthesiologists.[15] Several limitations of this procedure have become apparent, and the FDA Center for Devices and Radiologic Health revised the Anesthesia Apparatus Checkout procedure in 1993. Table 23–1 shows a draft of this document as of May 5, 1993.[16] This checkout procedure also is expected to find widespread acceptance.

When combined with effective preventive or progressive maintenance programs, systematically applied checkout practices should help maintain a low incidence of critical machine failures. Repeated checkouts will improve a practitioner's familiarity with the mechanics of anesthesia machines.

The introductory statement in the FDA Checkout Recommendations notes that they are valid only for anesthesia systems that conform to current standards. Presently, the applicable American Society for Testing and Materials standard is designated F 1161–88 and is entitled "Standard Specification for Minimum Performance and Safety Requirements for Components and Systems of Anesthesia Gas Machines."[17]

The FDA introductory statement further acknowledges that standards for the design and construction of anesthesia machines may change and that some machines in service antedate the current standard. It encourages modification of the checkout procedure in order to assure its utility in the face of both variations in equipment design and local variations in clinical practice with the caution that such proce-

TABLE 23–1. FDA ANESTHESIA APPARATUS CHECKOUT RECOMMENDATIONS, 1993 (DRAFT)

This checkout, or a reasonable equivalent, should be conducted before administration of anesthesia. These recommendations are only valid for an anesthesia system that conforms to current and relevant standards and includes an ascending bellows ventilator and at least the following monitors: capnograph, pulse oximeter, oxygen analyzer, respiratory volume monitor (spirometer) and breathing system pressure monitor with high and low pressure alarms. This is a guideline that users are encouraged to modify to accommodate differences in equipment design and variations in local clinical practice. Such local modifications should have appropriate peer review. Refer to the operator's manual for specific procedures and precautions.

Emergency Ventilation Equipment

*1. *Verify Backup Ventilation Equipment Is Available and Functioning*

High-Pressure System

*2. *Check Oxygen Cylinder Supply*
- a. Open O_2 cylinder and verify at least half full (about 1000 psi).
- b. Close cylinder.

*3. *Check Central Pipeline Supplies*
- a. Check that hoses are connected and pipeline gauges read about 50 psi.

Low-Pressure System

*4. *Check Initial Status of Low-Pressure System*
- a. Close flow control valves and turn vaporizers off.
- b. Check fill level and tighten vaporizers' filler caps.

*5. *Perform Leak Check of Machine Low-Pressure System*
- a. Verify that the machine master switch and flow control valves are OFF.
- b. Attach ''Suction Bulb'' to common (fresh) gas outlet.
- c. Squeeze bulb repeatedly until fully collapsed.
- d. Verify bulb stays *fully* collapsed for at least 10 seconds.
- e. Open one vaporizer at a time and repeat 'c' and 'd' as above.
- f. Remove suction bulb, and reconnect fresh gas hose.

*6. *Turn On Machine Master Switch* and all other necessary electrical equipment.

*7. *Test Flowmeters*
- a. Adjust flow of all gases through their full range, checking for smooth operation of floats and undamaged flowtubes.
- b. Attempt to create a hypoxic O_2/N_2O mixture and verify correct changes in flow and/or alarm.

Scavenging System

*8. *Adjust and Check Scavenging System*
- a. Ensure proper connections between the scavenging system and both APL (pop-off) valve and ventilator relief valve.
- b. Adjust waste gas vacuum (if possible).
- c. Fully open APL valve and occlude Y-piece.
- d. With minimum O_2 flow, allow scavenger reservoir bag to collapse completely and verify that absorber pressure gauge reads about zero.
- e. With the O_2 flush activated, allow the scavenger reservoir bag to distend fully, and then verify that absorber pressure gauge reads < 10 cmH_2O.

Breathing System

*9. *Calibrate O_2 Monitor*
- a. Ensure monitor reads 21% in room air.
- b. Verify low O_2 alarm is enabled and functioning.
- c. Reinstall sensor in circuit and flush breathing system with O_2.
- d. Verify that monitor now reads greater than 90%.

10. *Check Initial Status of Breathing System*
- a. Set selector switch to ''Bag'' mode.
- b. Check that breathing circuit is complete, undamaged and unobstructed.
- c. Verify that CO_2 absorbent is adequate.
- d. Install breathing circuit accessory equipment (e.g., humidifier, PEEP valve) to be used during the case.

11. *Perform Leak Check of the Breathing System*
- a. Set all gas flows to zero (or minimum).
- b. Close APL (pop-off) valve and occlude Y-piece.
- c. Pressurize breathing system to about 30 cmH_2O with O_2 flush.
- d. Ensure that pressure remains fixed for at least 10 seconds.
- e. Open APL (pop-off) valve and ensure that pressure decreases.

Manual and Automatic Ventilation Systems

12. *Test Ventilation Systems and Unidirectional Valves*
- a. Place a second breathing bag on Y-piece.
- b. Set appropriate ventilator parameters for next patient.
- c. Switch to automatic ventilation (Ventilator) mode.
- d. Turn ventilator ON and fill bellows and breathing bag with O_2 flush.
- e. Set O_2 flow to minimum, other gas flows to zero.
- f. Verify that during inspiration bellows delivers appropriate tidal volume and that during expiration bellows fills completely.
- g. Set fresh gas flow to about 5 L/minute.
- h. Verify that the ventilator bellows and simulated lungs fill *and empty* appropriately without sustained pressure at end expiration.
- i. *Check for proper action of unidirectional valves.*
- j. Exercise breathing circuit accessories to ensure proper function.
- k. Turn ventilator OFF and switch to manual ventilation (Bag/APL) mode.
- l. Ventilate manually and assure inflation and deflation of artificial lungs and appropriate feel of system resistance and compliance.
- m. Remove second breathing bag from Y-piece.

Monitors

13. *Check, Calibrate, and/or Set Alarm Limits of All Monitors*

Capnometer	Pulse Oximeter
Oxygen Analyzer	Respiratory Volume Monitor (Spirometer)

Pressure Monitor with High and Low Airway Pressure Alarms

Final Position

14. *Check Final Status of Machine*

a. Vaporizers off.	d. All flowmeters to zero (or minimum).
b. APL valve open.	e. Patient suction level adequate.
c. Selector switch to ''Bag.''	f. Breathing system ready to use.

*If an anesthesia provider uses the same machine in successive cases, these steps need not be repeated or may be abbreviated after the initial checkout.

dural modifications be instituted with appropriate peer review. This is clearly intended to provide flexibility in the real world; such modification will require responsible, thoughtful attention to technical detail by the anesthesiologists involved.

The testing and checkout procedures described here and in the FDA checkout procedure are abbreviated or operational test procedures. The results of such testing will suggest when further servicing of an anesthesia machine is needed. These checkout procedures cannot replace service and periodic preventive maintenance by trained service personnel. In some instances, the checkout procedures vary from the checkout procedures recommended by the equipment manufacturer. It is best to discuss such differences with the supplier or manufacturer and use the result of those discussions to establish institutional checkout procedures.

Preliminary Visual Inspection

An initial visual survey of the machine should be conducted. During a ''walk around'' inspection, the operator should verify that the apparatus has had a thorough preventive maintenance inspection within the interval established by the institution for such periodic inspections. This information should be available on an inspection sticker affixed to the machine in an obvious location. Other items to be checked during the visual inspection are the settings of controls and the absence of broken or otherwise obviously damaged machine components. Flowmeters should be observed for damage and the presence of bobbins, floats, or balls resting in the *bottom* of each flowmeter. Any sign of obvious damage to the machine should alert the anesthesiologist to the possibility of a breach of the device's integrity. For example, a damaged flowmeter shield is reason for the operator to carefully seek evidence of damage to the flowmeter itself. In addition to inspection to detect obvious gross damage, the checkout will include testing for leaks. A search for the cause of the damage should be made in order to prevent reoccurrence. Even superficial damage should be reported to enhance machine maintenance by assigned repair personnel. Signal wires, power cords, and gas and vacuum tubing should be inspected for cracks or other damage. If there is any question concerning damage to these items, they should be replaced promptly.

Initially, the pipeline-supplied gases should be connected to the machine, with all flowmeters and vaporizers turned off. However, the operator must determine that adjustable controls on the machine are set to appropriate positions before proceeding with the initial checkout. Consistent confirmation of the setting of all adjustable controls will ensure that controls have not been left in some unexpected configuration and will permit the development of personal routines, promoting efficient, thorough machine review before each anesthetic procedure.

Check of Back-Up Emergency Ventilation Equipment

Although back-up ventilation equipment is not, strictly speaking, a part of the anesthesia machine, this equipment is essential for providing safe anesthetic care. It seems prudent to include back-up equipment in the checkout. The preliminary inspection checks that back-up ventilation equipment is available and functional. The equipment should include a bag and valve apparatus to permit positive pressure ventilation and, especially for perioperative patient care, should be supplied with oxygen. Many facilities will provide oxygen from a source separate from the anesthesia machine but readily available in the operating room.

Check of High-Pressure (Cylinder) Oxygen Supply (Table 23–1, Item 2)

Cylinders mounted on the machine should be examined in their yokes for proper mounting and the presence of only one seat washer. The pressure of gas available in the cylinders mounted on the machine should be determined. If the high-pressure (cylinder) gauges indicate no pressure in the high-pressure section of the machine, the high-pressure part of the machine is depressurized; turning on a cylinder will indicate the pressure available in that cylinder.

On machines with multiple gas cylinders attached to high-pressure manifolds, an important condition routinely occurs that prevents the ready determination of gas pressure available in individual cylinders (see Fig. 23–1).

With the machine connected to the pipeline gas supply, 50–55 psig is applied to the plumbing within the machine proximal to the valves controlling the flow of gas to the flowmeters (intermediate-pressure section). In the typical machine, the pressure-reducing regulator valves have been set to deliver gas to the machine from the high-pressure cylinders at a slightly lower pressure. This feature keeps the outlet valve of the reducing regulator closed so long as the design pressure (i.e., 50–55 psig) is maintained within the internal plumbing of the intermediate-pressure section of the machine by the piped-in gases. Thus, use of gas from cylinders is minimized even if the cylinder valves remain open, as long as there is adequate pipeline pressure. In practice, however, reductions of intermediate section pressure may occur during periods of demand for high flow from the pipeline system, such as with ventilator operation or during use of flush valves.

Because the high-pressure yokes are equipped with check valves (to allow cylinders to be changed without losing high-pressure cylinder gas while remaining cylinders remain open, thus providing an uninterrupted supply of gas and preventing transfilling of high-pressure cylinders containing gas at unequal pressures), high-pressure gas will be trapped between the yoke check valve and the reducing regulator. The high pressure indicated by the cylinder gauges can be released by removing the machine from the pipeline gas supply and permitting flow from the regulator (with cylinder valves off) into the depressurized intermediate-pressure section. This latter step is not required by the FDA Checkout. The valve on each oxygen cylinder should be opened in turn while observing the cylinder pressure gauge. If more than one cylinder is present, the second cylinder's valve may also be opened to see if its pressure is greater than that of the first cylinder. If an increase in pressure is seen after opening the cylinder valve for either cylinder, the pressure indicated is the pressure in that cylinder. If no increase in pressure is observed, one cannot tell what the pressure is in that cylinder. It is acceptable to begin anesthesia if at least one oxygen cylinder contains 1000 psig.

Following the pressure check of oxygen cylinders, the respective cylinder valves should be closed. This step prevents unrecognized use of oxygen from the cylinders if the pipeline pressure drops below approximately 50 psig. Optionally, the pressure in high-pressure cylinders of other gases are checked in a similar way.

Check of Pipeline Supplies of Medical Gases (Table 23–1, Item 3)

The pipeline gas supply connections to the machine and respective pipeline pressures of 50–55 psig should be verified. Medical gas systems commonly keep the pressure of oxygen 3–5 psig greater than the pressures for nitrous oxide and compressed air. This practice ensures that inadvertent cross-connection of oxygen pipelines with either of these gases favors the flow of oxygen into nitrous oxide or air piping. Such cross-connections have resulted from plumbing errors within pipeline systems as well as from malfunction of devices connected to more than one gas in the piping system.[18]

Recommendations have been made to minimize gas leaks, particularly to prevent nitrous oxide contamination of the operating room atmosphere.[19] In response to this concern, connections between the anesthesia machine and the medical gas piping system are made with diameter-indexed safety system connectors tightened lightly, but more than finger tight, with a wrench. Quick connectors are not standardized for use in medical gas piping systems and are prone to leakage and damage while disconnected.

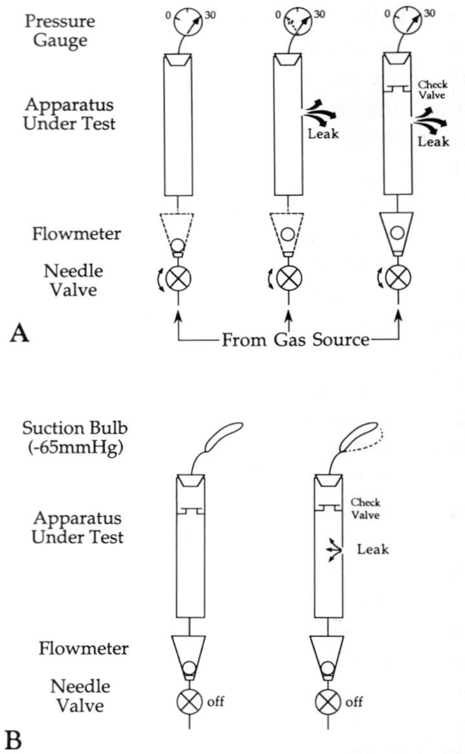

Figure 23–2. The effect of a check valve on procedures used to test a segment of tubing for leaks. (See text for discussion.)

Check of the Low-Pressure Section (Table 23–1, Items 4–7)

The low-pressure section of the anesthesia machine is that portion of the machine from the flow control valves (including the oxygen flush valve) to the fresh gas outlet. It includes flowmeters, vaporizers, and all associated plumbing. Testing of this portion of the machine is complicated by the use of unidirectional (check) valves at various locations. Check valves have been used by manufacturers in the assembly of various models of their machines. Check valves are used extensively in anesthesia machines to prevent reverse flow of gas in various portions of the machine. They are usually placed as follows:

1. In the common gas line near the fresh gas outlet to the patient breathing circuit just proximal to where the oxygen flush line joins the gas stream[20]
2. At the outlet of vaporizers to minimize the pumping effect[11] of mechanical ventilation on vaporizer output

Outlet check valves are most often present in machines manufactured by Ohmeda. The operation of check valves is typically not tested in the daily checkout of anesthesia machines but does require checking during periodic preventive maintenance.

Understanding Pneumatic Systems Containing Check Valves

The testing of pneumatic assemblies for leaks is quite straightforward, but some configurations of components can isolate one segment of an assembly from other segments. With respect to anesthesia machines, this can be particularly perplexing when a portion of the apparatus under test contains unidirectional or check valves. Figure 23–2*A* illustrates a segment of tubing connected in series with a flow control valve and a flow measuring device. The tubing can be tested for leakage most simply by placing a plug equipped with a pressure gauge in the downstream end. Flow is admitted to the tube by the flow control valve until a predetermined pressure is reached; then the flow is reduced to zero. (For testing the low-pressure section of anesthesia machines, the test pressure should be 30 cmH_2O.) If the segment of tubing is free from leaks, the pressure indicated will remain at 30 cmH_2O. On the other hand, if there is a leak, the pressure will fall promptly. In this case, the magnitude of the leak can be measured by increasing gas flow until the testing pressure of 30 cmH_2O is achieved and, by fine flow adjustments, exactly maintained. The flow indicated is the leak rate at the test pressure (e.g., 300 ml/minute at 30 cmH_2O).

When the segment of tubing under test includes a check valve downstream from the leak, the leak may be overlooked by simple pressure testing. If the segment under test is pressurized, pressure will increase on both sides of the check valve. When inlet flow ceases, the leak causes a loss of pressure in the portion of the apparatus upstream from the check valve. The fall in pressure in the upstream part of the apparatus allows the check valve to close and prevents pressure loss in the portion of the apparatus downstream from the check valve, leading to the erroneous interpretation that the entire segment of tubing being tested is free from leaks. If, as described previously, the pressure in the test segment is brought up to the test pressure using the needle valve, the leak rate can be measured by determining the flow at which pressure stops rising at the downstream end of the tubing being tested.

Figure 23–2*B* depicts another way to test a segment of tubing with an intrinsic check valve. This method permits the identification of leaks and allows go/no-go decisions to be made. Initially, all gas flow into the segment of tubing under test is turned off, and a suction bulb is attached to the downstream outlet of the tubing being tested. The bulb is squeezed repeatedly until it remains collapsed. At this point the interior of the tubing has a negative pressure of about −65 mmHg. If the plumbing being tested has no leak, the bulb will remain collapsed. If a leak is present, regardless of whether it is upstream or downstream from the check valve, ambient air will be sucked into the segment of tubing being tested and the bulb will expand. The machine will have passed the test if the bulb remains collapsed for 10 seconds or more. With typical sphygmomanometer bulbs, this represents a leak rate of approximately 120 ml/minute.

The device used for negative pressure testing for leaks can be assembled using a squeeze bulb similar to those used with sphygmomanometers but with its check valve arranged so that releasing the bulb results in negative pressure at the inlet to the bulb. The inlet to the bulb should be connected to a short piece of tubing, the other end of which is attached to a 15-mm standard tapered connector (''endotracheal tube connector'') suitable for attachment to the fresh gas outlet of the machine being checked. This test device should be tested periodically to ensure that it continues to provide a negative pressure of approximately −65 mmHg.

Check of Flowmeters (Table 23–1, Item 7)

With the machine master switch turned on, the function of the flowmeters is tested. The floats should be observed to move smoothly within the bore of each flowmeter over the full length of the flowmeter tube and should return smoothly to the base of the tube when the flow control valve is closed. Floats are designed to rotate during use. Failure to do so results in sticking or interference between the float and the tube wall, causing erroneous readings.

The oxygen proportioning system is tested by setting typical flows of oxygen and nitrous oxide, attempting to reduce the flow of oxygen to the point at which a hypoxic mixture would result and observing that there is a proportional reduction in the flow of nitrous oxide. This check should confirm that delivered oxygen concentrations are always greater than 25%.

Adjustment and Check of Scavenging System (Table 23–1, Item 8)

It is usually convenient to check and adjust the waste gas scavenging system during the early part of machine checkout. The interface between the patient breathing circuit and the conduit to the removal route should be inspected for integrity and for lack of occlusion. A common cause of partial obstruction in the scavenging system is collection of water in dependent loops of the scavenger connecting tubing. If a closed scavenging system with a reservoir bag is in use, the suction venting the scavenger must be adjusted to provide proper flow, so that the reservoir bag on the scavenging system is emptied only at the highest flows that the operator expects to use. Usually this is in the neighborhood of 10 L/minute. With the Y connection to which the patient will be connected occluded and the adjustable pressure-limiting (APL) valve open, a flow of 10 L/minute is admitted to the breathing circuit while the scavenging suction is turned off. This procedure slightly increases the pressure within the breathing circuit. Operation of the oxygen flush valve should produce a pressure increase of less than 10 cmH_2O within the breathing circuit. These steps provide a functional test of the positive pressure relief valve in a closed scavenging system and prove that the outlet of any other type of scavenging system is patent.

Similarly, with zero fresh gas flow into the patient breathing circuit, the scavenger suction on, the patient connection occluded, and the APL valve open, there should be less than 2 cmH_2O negative pressure detected in the patient breathing circuit with proper functioning of the negative pressure relief valve in the scavenging system. Other scavenging systems, such as passive systems that carry waste gases to the return vent of the nonrecirculating air conditioning system, may[7] or may not be equipped with pressure relief valves. These systems rely on patent large-bore (typically 19 mm) tubing as a conduit. Occlusion of this tubing or the direct application of suction to it must be avoided to prevent excessive positive or negative pressure from being applied to the patient breathing circuit.[21]

Check of Oxygen Analyzer (Table 23–1, Item 9)

The initial check of the oxygen analyzer should follow the manufacturer's instructions and, after a suitable warm-up interval, confirm that it reads, or can be adjusted to read, near 21% when the sensor is positioned in ambient air, well away from sources of gases that might change the ambient oxygen concentration. The sensor should be repositioned to its place on the anesthesia machine, the circuit should be flushed with a high flow of 100% oxygen, and the monitor should read 100% ± 10%. If the analyzer calibration control is adjusted while the sensor is exposed to 100% oxygen, the analyzer should be checked again to confirm a reading of 21% ± 2% in room air.

To confirm that oxygen is the only gas in the fresh gas being supplied to the patient breathing circuit, the breathing circuit should be flushed with 100% oxygen, after which a flow of 3–5 L/minute of oxygen is continued. A reading of 100% ± 10% should be noted on the oxygen analyzer, and no odor (suggesting that a vaporizer is leaking or has been left on) should be detectable by a sniff of the gas exiting the distal end of the inspiratory limb of the circuit. Concerns have been expressed regarding recommendations that anesthetists breathe from the anesthetic circuit. Alternatively, the composition of the gas being delivered from the anesthesia machine to the patient breathing circuit can be determined by using the oxygen analyzer and/or a respiratory gas analyzer. Devices for analyzing respiratory gases and their limitations are discussed in detail in Chapter 24.

Check of Breathing System Setup and of CO_2 Absorbent (Table 23–1, Item 10)

The circle absorption breathing system should be inspected to ensure that it is intact and undamaged and that all accessories for administration of the proposed anesthetic are attached. The breathing circuit should be tested with accessories connected and the ventilator/bag selector valve set to the ''BAG'' position.

If the CO_2 absorbent contains an indicator, inspection of the canister can suggest whether the absorbent has been expended. Because different indicators may be used in different formulations of absorbing compounds, the anesthesiologist must be aware of the expected color changes with the product in use.[22] The color change reflects a change in pH on the surface of the granules of absorbent; this change is most marked at the end of a period of use and may not persist overnight.

Changes of absorbent should be scheduled at regular intervals, which should be shortened as suggested by color changes observed at the *end* of periods of use. Most CO_2 absorbing circle systems are equipped with two canisters in series with the gas flow in the circle. Net flow through the canisters is from top to bottom in current machines. When the color change indicating consumption of the absorbent extends into the downstream canister of the absorber assembly, the absorbent should be changed in the upstream canister, and that canister should be placed in the downstream (lower) position in the gas stream.

Leak Testing of the Circle Absorption Breathing System (Table 23–1, Item 11)

When machines having a minimum flow of oxygen (typically in the range of 200–500 ml/minute) are tested for leaks, it will not be possible to measure leaks that are less than the minimum flow without disconnecting the machine from the pipeline gas supply. As a practical matter, leaks of 500 ml/minute or less may be accepted so long as low-flow or closed-circuit techniques are not used and sufficient total flow is available to ensure adequate ventilation of the patient. Any machine with leaks greater than 2 L/minute, including leaks in the breathing circuit, should be removed from service for repair. It is recommended that test pressures within anesthetic machines and/or breathing circuits be limited to less than 100 cmH_2O.

The procedures described below will measure the total of all leaks in gas machines (downstream from the flowmeters) having no check valves between the flowmeters and the fresh gas outlet *and* in the breathing circuit. With gas flows turned off, the Y patient connection occluded, and the APL valve closed, the breathing circuit can be pressurized to 30 cmH_2O using the oxygen flush valve. Once a pressure of 30 cmH_2O has been achieved, it should remain near 30 cmH_2O for 10 seconds. If it does not, a significant leak is present. Alternatively, machines having a continuing minimum flow of oxygen should demonstrate a continuing increase in pressure in the breathing circuit. If it appears that the pressure developed will continue to increase beyond 30 cmH_2O, it may be inferred that the anesthesia machine *and* the patient breathing circuit have no major leaks and that any leak present is less than the continuing minimum oxygen flow rate. A continuing minimum flow of oxygen of 500 ml/minute into an adult CO_2 absorbing breathing circuit will require about 10 seconds to cause a rise in pressure from 30 cmH_2O to 32 cmH_2O in the circle system. After this test, the occlusion at the Y connector is removed.

Check of Manual and Mechanical Ventilating Capability (Table 23–1, Item 12)

A second breathing bag attached to the Y connector will serve to simulate a patient's lungs. With the ventilator/bag selector valve set to the ''BAG'' position and a flow of approximately 5 L/minute established, the APL valve is adjusted to a pressure of 5–10 cmH_2O within the breathing circuit. By alternately squeezing the ''lung'' bag and the breathing bag attached to the circuit, one should demonstrate

1. Sequential inflation and deflation of the test ''lung'' without sustained positive pressure
2. Appropriate feel of breathing system resistance
3. Proper movement of the unidirectional valves in the breathing circuit

The mechanical ventilation function is checked by switching the ventilator/bag selector valve to the ''VENTILATOR'' position; a low (1 L/minute or less) flow of oxygen is set, the ventilator remains turned off, and the breathing circuit (now including the ventilator bellows) and test ''lung'' are filled using the oxygen flush valve, if necessary. The ventilator bellows (standing bellows ventilator assumed) should remain filled with less than 4 cmH_2O continuing positive pressure in the breathing circuit. The ventilator is turned on, and it is verified that the test ''lung'' inflates during the inspiratory phase of the ventilator cycle and that deflation of the ''lung'' is not restricted during the expiratory phase. It is convenient to use ventilator settings of 500 ml tidal volume with a rate of 10 breaths/minute and a fresh gas flow of 5.0 L/minute of oxygen for this ventilator checkout. The use of consistent, specific settings makes variations in results easier to identify. The breathing circuit pressure gauge and spirometer verify that pressure and flow are developed in the breathing circuit as the ventilator cycles. This portion of the checkout is completed by removing the test ''lung,'' selecting the ''BAG'' position of the ventilator/bag selector valve, opening the APL valve, reducing the oxygen flow, and setting the ventilator and the ventilation monitor to a tidal volume and rate suitable for the next patient to be anesthetized.

Check of Monitoring Equipment (Table 23–1, Item 13)

Electrical monitoring equipment for both physiologic and machine parameters is turned on and checked for proper operation as part of the checklist. Certain apparatus require a warm-up interval to assure stable operation, such as older physiologic monitors, certain oxygen analyzers, and gas analyzers. This is related either to some components reaching thermal equilibrium or to "conditioning" of electrodes. The appropriate procedures for activation and calibration of equipment are detailed in the operator's manual for each item of equipment. If the correct procedure is followed, a need for considerable calibration suggests the possibility of significant drift or erratic behavior of the monitor or its associated sensor.

INTRAOPERATIVE MONITORING OF ANESTHESIA MACHINES

Monitoring during anesthesia administration requires careful attention to the status of the patient on a continuing basis. The following discussion addresses only tasks that directly monitor the anesthesia machine; patient monitoring *per se* is addressed in Chapters 3, 4, 7–10, 12–18, and 25.

Intraoperative monitoring can be thought of as systematic verification of pressures within various portions of the machine, of proper gas flows, and of proper gas proportions, including vaporized volatile anesthetics. The operator should establish a pattern for scanning the different sources of data and should expect to check more frequently those that vary substantially over short intervals or that are judged to be particularly critical. As conditions change during the conduct of the anesthetic procedure, the order of the scan and the priority assigned to various monitoring tasks may require adjustment. For example, the initial portion of anesthetic administration demands frequent appraisal of the concentration of anesthetic agents while uptake of the anesthetic proceeds toward equilibrium, as influenced by physiologic parameters (e.g., cardiovascular responses, pattern of ventilation, absence of patient movement in response to surgical stimulation) and by measurement of the changing concentration of volatile agents in exhaled gas (e.g., mass or Raman spectroscopy, infrared absorption).

During a later phase of anesthetic maintenance, with the patient more nearly in equilibrium with the anesthetic agent, the anesthetic concentration might be monitored less frequently, and attention might be directed toward lower-priority tasks such as ensuring that the amount of liquid anesthetic in the vaporizer is adequate. Such examples illustrate the issues encountered in understanding and describing monitoring tasks during anesthesia administration (see Chapter 2). Various circumstances may dramatically affect the criteria that one might use to set priorities for establishing those parameters to be tracked most closely as well as to set tolerances. Tolerances are the limits of individual variables above or below which there must be adjustment of either the variable being monitored (e.g., volatile anesthetic concentration) or the related variables (e.g., the administration of fluids).

Monitoring a number of parameters requires ongoing assessment of the stream of continually presented data. Experienced clinicians can perform such tasks fairly well, but the presentation of increasingly large volumes of information threatens to overload them. This is demonstrated when alarms sound on operating room equipment not related to the administration of the anesthetic, and the anesthesiologist responds by searching the anesthetic machine for the source of the alarm. Manufacturers of anesthesia machines have responded to this problem by developing schemes for prioritizing the alarms and having them appear in central or common locations with instructions or other aids to help identify the proper portion of the anesthetic apparatus.

Although reports indicate that critical incidents have different origins, causes are attributed most often to human error rather than to machine failure *per se*.[2, 12, 13, 23] Understanding this, anesthetists should confirm their prior actions and continuously scan the entire clinical setting, including the anesthesia machine, for information. The anesthesiologist who is idle for very long during the conduct of anesthesia is, at least, falling behind in the gathering of information and runs the risk of missing important changes in the status of the anesthetic being conducted.

Table 23–2 provides a broad outline of parameters to be evaluated periodically during the conduct of clinical anesthesia to monitor the anesthetic machine.

PIPELINE PRESSURE MONITORING

Pipeline pressures should be monitored periodically and confirmed to remain at 50 ± 5 psig. Major fluctuations may result from high resistance in the supply lines (e.g., multiple check valves in the pipeline system) producing a large pressure drop when higher flows are called for, as when an oxygen-powered ventilator cycles or when the oxygen flush is activated. When such pressure drops are particularly large, fail-safe systems may be activated, resulting in intermittent changes in the flow of nitrous oxide or other gases. This situation indicates inadequate capacity of the oxygen pipeline system and should be corrected. It may interfere with the proper operation of oxygen-powered

TABLE 23–2. VARIABLES REQUIRING MONITORING DURING ANESTHESIA

Pipeline pressure of all gases connected to the anesthesia machine
Pressure within the high-pressure section of the anesthesia machine when the cylinder supply of gas is in use
Flowmeter indication for each gas
Concentration of oxygen within the patient breathing circuit
Pressure and flow of gas within the patient breathing circuit (i.e., ventilation)
Concentration of anesthetic agents and other gases within the patient breathing circuit
Operation of the waste gas scavenging system

equipment, particularly anesthesia ventilators, and does not permit the high flow of oxygen necessary to provide rapid oxygen flushing of the patient breathing circuit. Low pipeline pressures indicate a faulty pipeline regulator, exhaustion of the pipeline source of gas, or, rarely, substantial leaks within the pipeline system.

Close monitoring of pressure within the high-pressure portion of the anesthesia machine (i.e., within gas cylinders) during the use of the cylinder gas supplies allows the operator to estimate the amount of gas remaining on the machine. This information, together with knowledge of the flow rate being employed, can be used to calculate the expected duration of the remaining gas supply. When this procedure is carried out carefully and early, either additional cylinders can be delivered in a timely fashion or the anesthetic technique can be modified to conserve the available supply. Such estimates can be limited in several ways. The operator must recognize that the quantity of nitrous oxide remaining within the cylinders cannot be accurately estimated (see previous discussion in this chapter). If oxygen-powered equipment is used (e.g., ventilators) or the oxygen flush valve is operated, increased and unmeasured oxygen expenditure occurs.

The flow of each of the gases in the gas mixture being supplied to the anesthetized patient is usually monitored by the anesthesiologist observing the flowmeters for each gas. Although the anesthesiologist continues to be the primary monitor of gas flow, automated flow monitoring and controlling devices are becoming widespread. As described earlier, anesthesia machines presently in production and meeting the ASTM F 1161-88 standard are equipped with oxygen ratio control devices. These devices often provide the first indication that an attempt to select an incorrect proportion of oxygen has occurred. It is important for the user of an anesthesia machine to recognize that these devices rely on the critical assumption that correctly identified gases are being supplied to the apparatus. If the incorrect gas is supplied, these mechanical, pneumatic devices cannot properly report or control the proportion of oxygen actually being delivered by the anesthesia machine.[5, 14, 24] For this reason, it is particularly critical that *analytic* instruments be included on anesthesia machines to measure oxygen concentration. Knowledge of the concentration of oxygen is so fundamental to the conduct of safe anesthesia that monitors dedicated specifically to oxygen analysis are standard equipment, even though other techniques (e.g., mass spectrometry) can also identify oxygen as well as report its concentration in the gas mixture.

BREATHING CIRCUIT PRESSURE MONITORING

Monitoring pressures within the patient breathing circuit may confirm proper pressures, identify improper machine function, or indicate certain physiologic or physical problems with the patient or the endotracheal tube in the patient's airway. It has become increasingly common to have graphic display of airway pressure waveforms with respect to time during positive pressure ventilation. Sufficiently detailed information about pressures within the patient breathing circuit can be obtained from graphic displays or from careful observation of the pressure gauge in the circuit. These data allow the anesthesiologist to recognize leaks, ventilator malfunctions, disconnection of either the patient or of components of the anesthetic apparatus, changes in the physiologic condition of the patient (e.g., bronchospasm), occlusion of tubing within the anesthetic system including the endotracheal tube and scavenging system, and a closed APL valve during spontaneous ventilation.

Positive Pressure

The fact that positive pressure has been developed within the patient's airway does not assure that adequate ventilation has been achieved. Techniques to assess the adequacy of ventilation are discussed in Chapters 11, 12, 24, 25, and 27.

The location of pressure and flow measuring apparatus within the patient breathing circuit is an important determinant of the information these devices can provide. Spirometers are usually placed in the expiratory limb of the circle absorbing system. In this position, they measure the sum of the volume of gas exhaled by the patient plus the volume of fresh gas flowing through the spirometer during the interval of measurement. Pressure measuring devices are typically located downstream from the exhalation unidirectional valve (between it and the inspiratory unidirectional valve). Conditions that cause a sustained elevation of pressure within the patient's airway and in the adjacent segment of the breathing circuit, such as a positive end-expiratory pressure (PEEP) valve, will not be indicated on the pressure gauge positioned in the usual location in the patient breathing circuit. This is because the PEEP valve, positioned upstream from the expiratory unidirectional valve, in combination with a competent inspiratory unidirectional valve, isolates the segement of the breathing circuit contiguous with the patient's airway from the pressure gauge.

Negative Pressure

Negative pressures within the patient breathing circuit are abnormal and should be investigated and corrected promptly. Some causes are low total gas flow in combination with too-rapid descent of hanging bellows in certain older anesthesia ventilators, application of too great a suction to the gas scavenging system, or failure of the negative pressure relief valve of a closed scavenging system. This latter effect may result in the removal of volumes of gas from the patient breathing circuit so large that the patient cannot be ventilated properly. Ventilators utilizing hanging (ascending during inspiration) bellows may create sufficient negative airway pressure during exhalation that patients having airways with poor elastic support suffer airway closure and interference with gas exchange. This situation is managed by admitting a fresh gas flow to the breathing circuit that exceeds the maximum rate of filling of the bellows during its descent or by adjusting the ventilator to slow the rate of descent of the bellows. A major hazard of the hanging bellows arrangement is that, in the event of a disconnection of the patient or of the ventilator, the bellows continues to move in a normal fashion and is more likely to escape notice than is a standing bellows ventilator.

BREATHING CIRCUIT GAS MONITORING

The concentration of oxygen in the gas mixture being provided to the patient must be known. Flowmeter settings can be adjusted to minimize the likelihood of accidental creation of hypoxic gas mixtures. Anesthesiologists should develop the habit of increasing the flow of oxygen first when increasing total flow and of decreasing the flow of nitrous oxide first when decreasing total flow. Information concerning the oxygen concentration is available directly from an oxygen analyzer (or other analytic instrument), indirectly by calculation from flows of individual gases being employed, and from on-line analysis of gas within the patient breathing circuit.

Carbon dioxide, nitrogen, and anesthetic gases will be found in the patient breathing circuit, and analytic techniques should be applied to monitor their concentration. Analysis of the concentration of gases other than oxygen provides direct information about the progress of the patient toward equilibration with the anesthetic agents in use. This knowledge may be helpful in assessing the adequacy of ventilation or of the state of the patient's cardiac function as well as being valuable in the instructional setting for promoting a clear understanding of the uptake and distribution of anesthetic agents. Measurement of end-tidal nitrogen can assist in understanding the extent to which a patient has been denitrogenated. Intraoperative increases in exhaled nitrogen provide evidence of air embolism or of a leak in the bellows of the Drager AV-E anesthesia ventilator, which is powered by a mixture of air and oxygen. Measurement of carbon dioxide in exhaled gas provides clear evidence of the state of ventilation of the patient so long as the production of carbon dioxide remains constant (see Chapter 12).[25, 26]

Because of substantial effects of sampling site on the concentration of different gases in different portions of the anesthetic circuit, it is important to know and understand expected concentrations in the patient breathing circuit, particularly as influenced by uptake, ventilation, and fresh gas flow. End-tidal sampling of the respiratory gases of small infants may require special attention because of their small tidal volume and the pressure of leaks from uncuffed endotracheal tubes compared to the flow rate of side-stream gas analysis equipment and fresh gas flow. The details of instrumentation for the analysis and measurement of gases in the breathing circuit are discussed in Chapters 12 and 24.

Flow and pressure information from different points in the anesthesia machine and breathing circuit may be converted to electrical signals that, in turn, can be input into monitoring devices for display and recording. In anesthesia machines of recent manufacture, the monitoring of machine parameters is given high priority. Respiratory signals depicting pressure and flow within the breathing circuit are displayed in real time. The signal produced by the concentration of CO_2 in exhaled gas may be used to provide important information concerning the adequacy of ventilation, including information that can lead to the rapid diagnosis of an incorrectly placed endotracheal tube. It is clear that it is becoming increasingly difficult to describe at exactly what point monitoring of the machine ceases and physiologic monitoring of the patient begins. Indeed, one of the issues now being confronted by designers of monitoring systems for larger surgical suites is determination of monitoring priorities and display heirarchies for the integration of both physiologic monitoring of the patient and monitoring of parameters derived largely from the operation of anesthesia machines. Much of the problem relates to the need to present large amounts of monitoring information without overloading the anesthesiologist.

Gaba et al present a useful framework for understanding how anesthetic accidents evolve.[13] They describe the important elements leading to anesthetic mishaps in terms of the complexity of the interactions among equipment, the anesthesiologist, and the patient and the tightness of the coupling between the various elements of a complex system. They further described how simple incidents might interact and propagate within a complex system to develop into critical incidents or, when combined with a "substantive negative outcome," produce events that are generally recognized as accidents. Suggested strategies for recovery from such situations involve recognition and verification of a developing incident and the extent of the threat it represents, followed by the institution of life-sustaining functions and the initial application of diagnostic and corrective action, followed by specific diagnoses, treatment, and adequate follow-up to assure continued correction throughout recovery.

INNOVATIVE APPROACHES TO ANESTHETIC MACHINE DESIGN

The monitoring of functions of anesthesia machines is rapidly becoming more sophisticated, with integration of such monitoring and measurement of patient physiologic variables continuing to evolve. Integrated monitoring is designed so that turning on the machine master switch initiates monitoring of machine functions, and one cannot use the machine without the monitoring apparatus functioning—human "ingenuity" notwithstanding. For example, modern anesthesia machines have a back-up battery powering the machine monitoring functions. In the event the machine is not connected to the 120-V AC electrical service and battery power is used to power the monitoring functions, an advisory warning informs the operator of the limited power available from the battery.

Another direction apparent in the development of anesthesia machines is hardware designed so that it is not possible to administer gas mixtures containing less than 25–30% oxygen. Both American manufacturers now provide anesthesia machines that prevent the administration of less than 25–30% oxygen.

Considerable attention is now being devoted to the display of monitored information. As noted earlier, the anesthesiologist who is faced with nearly simultaneous multiple alarms can become overloaded with data, some of it appearing to conflict, to the point that effective responses to the alarms are seriously degraded. Alarms may be assigned priorities, so that the anesthesiologist can rapidly assess and plan his or her response to monitor generated messages. Schreiber and Schreiber described a scheme in which all possible alarm conditions on anesthesia machines are prioritized into a three-level classification[6]:

Warning: Requires immediate operator response
Caution: Requires prompt operator response
Advisory: Requires operator awareness that a condition exists

They provided a detailed description of the display of such prioritized alarms in the form of audible, visual, and printed or CRT-displayed messages that includes the suppression of lower-priority audible alarms until the higher-priority alarm conditions are corrected. This type of prioritized alarm indication is available on Drager and Ohmeda anesthesia machines. Alarms with prioritized indications are called for in the ASTM standard F 1161–88, in which they are designated as

Category I	High priority
Category II	Medium priority
Category III	Low priority

It may soon be the norm to display monitored variables that fall outside of predetermined limits in a central location on the anesthesia machine. Suggested courses of action might also be presented. The integration of the information resulting from the monitoring of anesthesia machine function with information resulting from physiologic monitoring of the patient will undoubtedly receive much attention.

INTEGRATED ANESTHESIA SYSTEMS

In 1978, Cooper et al reported the development of a demonstration anesthesia system that incorporated new applications of electronic control of mechanical and pneumatic functions.[27] They used electronically controlled digital valves to adjust the flow of gases and an electronically controlled injector for control of the amount of volatile anesthetic added to the gas mixture in this innovatively designed anesthesia machine. For a variety of reasons, some of which were identified in their report, as well as high costs related to product liability, development, and proof of concept costs by potential manufacturers, this design has not been incorporated into even the newest anesthesia machines. Additional sophisticated prototypes have demonstrated further refinement of computer control of "standard" anesthesia machine functions coupled with machine and respiratory monitoring.[28, 29]

Loeb et al developed the Utah Anesthesia Workstation.[28] This device is a standard anesthesia machine enhanced with computer-driven display, control, and monitoring of gas flows and pressures as well as display, control, and monitoring of ventilation. The work station control function can be operated in any of three modes. It can function as a conventional "manual" anesthesia machine, in an "electronic control" mode, or in an "autopilot" mode. In the electronic control mode, the anesthesiologist selects the *flows* for oxygen, nitrous oxide, and anesthetic vapor. In the autopilot mode, the anesthesiologist selects the *concentrations* desired, and the computer calculates and sets the flows necessary to achieve them. The work station provides elaborate monitoring of the progress of the anesthetic, displays pressures, flows, and CO_2 concentrations on a breath-by-breath basis, and detects common and uncommon problems with the anesthetics being conducted.

STANDARDS AND GUIDELINES

The continued evolution of anesthesia machines is confirmed by the ongoing development of new standards to describe their construction. The role of standards and guidelines in shaping the way anesthesia machines and related devices are used should be understood by those who use and are involved in the acquisition of these devices.

ORGANIZATIONS

A number of organizations have written standards concerning various aspects of the construction and use of anesthesia machines and of apparatus that support anesthesia practice. Standards characteristically represent the combined efforts of several groups (e.g., manufacturers, users, distributors, and regulators) concerned with a particular issue. As such, published standards are consensus documents developed by parties of differing, even competing, interests. Although standards may seem flawed from some perspectives, they are pragmatic instruments developed by knowledgeable people and are useful in the everyday world of commerce and practice.

Standards do not, by themselves, have the force of law. They may be adopted voluntarily or, in other instances, be given the force of law by reference to state or local codes or laws. For example, the National Fire Protection Association's documents are often cited by building codes. Therefore, compliance becomes mandatory before a building meets the requirements of the building code. In a general manner, whether mandated by law or not, compliance with published standards by practitioners and institutions assures good practice as agreed on by those intimately familiar with the field. In most instances, standards undergo periodic review and revision. Most institutions must plan to comply with such revisions from time to time. This can be accomplished most easily if they stay abreast of trends in the field and develop practical plans for compliance with evolving standards. The responsibility for decision making in institutional policy, risk management, and purchasing resides with informed anesthesia clinicians, administrators, risk managers, and biomedical engineers.

The American Society for Testing and Materials, the International Standards Organization, and the European Committee for Standardization are working toward standards for anesthesia work stations. This effort will involve standardized specification of most mechanical and pneumatic components presently included on anesthesia machines as well as ventilators, vaporizers, and scavenging devices. In addition to specifying the manner in which these will be monitored, the developing standards must describe schemes for integrating the information obtained into sophisticated alarm and warning systems. Detailed protocols for routing anesthesia data along with physiologic data for display, analysis, and record-keeping are yet to be determined.

Compressed Gas Association

The Compressed Gas Association is a voluntary organization of the manufacturers of compressed gases and products related to the use of compressed gases. This group has published standards describing the color coding of compressed gas cylinders, safety connecting systems (diameter-index safety system, thread-index safety system) to prevent the accidental cross-connection of gas cylinders and piping systems, the construction of cylinders for service as high-pressure gas storage, and the pin-indexed safety system to prevent the connection of improper gas cylinders to yokes intended for specific gases. Some of the Compressed Gas Association standards provide examples of very specific methodologies to be used—for example, the descriptions of safety systems for interconnection of gas vessels and piping systems outline the fittings in such detail that different manufacturers are able to produce connectors that are compatible and interchangeable.

National Fire Protection Association

The National Fire Protection Association has prepared standards that are widely applicable to building design and construction including, but not limited to, health care facilities. In the course of their work, this association has written standards dealing with electrical safety, the handling of medical gases, and medical gas piping systems that are the most widely recognized standards applied to health care facilities. Although these standards do not relate directly to anesthesia machines, understanding the underlying principles is vital to those who provide anesthesia care.

American Society of Testing and Materials

The American Society of Testing and Materials assembles knowledgeable committees to define and publish standards in order to permit the interchange of information and ideas between groups interested in a wide variety of technical disciplines. The work of the society relating to anesthesia equipment and machines has been conducted by the ASTM F-29 Committee since 1983. This committee has published the current standard for performance and safety for components and systems of anesthesia gas machines.[17]

Other Organizations

The United States Department of Transportation has developed detailed regulations governing the manufacture, marking, testing, and transportation of containers for gases and other fluids. This includes the cylinders utilized in the practice of anesthesia that contain compressed gases. The Underwriter's Laboratories have published standards that pertain to devices and components used in conjunction with anesthesia machines.

Organizations and legislation have appeared to promote the safety of medical devices and the dissemination of information concerning problems with or failure of various medical devices, including anesthesia machines. The Anesthesia Patient Safety Foundation addresses safety issues related to anesthesia, including issues that pertain directly to anesthesia machines.

The Safe Medical Devices Act of 1990 requires user facilities to report to the FDA instances in which medical devices have contributed to the serious injury, illness, or death of a patient. Ehrenwerth and Eisenkraft have summarized the important elements of this act.[3]

The Appendix lists addresses and phone numbers of organizations that write standards or guidelines applicable to anesthesia machines. Most publish a directory of available publications and provide information concerning their areas of expertise.

REFERENCES

1. Dorsch JA, Dorsch SE: Understanding Anesthesia Equipment: Construction, Care and Complications, 3rd Ed. Baltimore: William & Wilkins, 1994.
2. Petty C: The Anesthesia Machine. New York: Churchill Livingstone, 1987.
3. Ehrenwerth J, Eisenkraft JB: Anesthesia Equipment: Principles and Applications. St. Louis: Mosby, 1993.
4. Schreiber P: Safety Guidelines for Anesthesia Systems. Telford, PA: North American Drager, 1984.
5. Bowie E, Huffman LM: The Anesthesia Machine: Essentials for Understanding. Madison, WI: Ohmeda/BOC Healthcare Group, 1985.
6. Schreiber P, Schreiber J: Anesthesia System Risk Analysis and Risk Reduction. Telford, PA: North American Drager, 1987.
7. Cicman J, Himmelwright C, Skibo V, Yoder J: Operating Principles of Narkomed Anesthesia Systems. Telford, PA: North American Drager, 1993.
8. Grogono AW, Travis JT: Anesthesia ventilators. *In* Ehrenwerth J, Eisenkraft JB (eds): Anesthesia Equipment: Principles and Applications. St. Louis: Mosby, 1993; 140–171.
9. Jones PL: Some observations on nitrous oxide cylinders during emptying. Br J Anaesth 1974; 46:534–538.

10. Cook TL, Eger EI, Behl RS: Is your vaporizer off? Anesth Analg 1977; 56:793–800.
11. Keet JE, Valentine GW, Riccio JS: An arrangement to prevent pressure effect on the vernitrol vaporizer. Anesthesiology 1963; 24:734–737.
12. Cooper J, Newbower R, Long C, McPeek B: Preventable anesthesia mishaps: A study of human factors. Anesthesiology 1978; 49:399–406.
13. Gaba DM, Maxwell M, DeAnda A: Anesthetic mishaps: Breaking the chain of accident evolution. Anesthesiology 1987; 66:670–676.
14. Mazze RI: Therapeutic misadventures with oxygen delivery systems: The need for continuous in-line oxygen monitors. Anesth Analg 1972; 51:787–792.
15. Anesthesia Apparatus Checkout Recommendations. American Society of Anesthesiologists Newsletter, October, 1986; 50:5–6.
16. Anesthesia Apparatus Checkout Recommendations, 1993 (Draft May 5, 1993). Division of Technical Development, Center for Devices and Radiological Health, Food and Drug Administration, Rockville, MD.
17. American Society for Testing and Materials: Standard specification for minimum performance and safety requirements for components and systems of anesthesia gas machines. Designation: F 1161–88. Philadelphia, PA: 1989.
18. Bageant RA, Hoyt JW, Epstein RM: Error in a pipeline gas concentration: An unanticipated consequence of a defective check valve. Anesthesiology 1981; 54:166–169.
19. Whitcher C, Piziali RL: Monitoring occupational exposure to inhalational anesthetics. Anesth Analg 1977; 56:778–785.
20. Comm G, Rendell-Baker L: Back pressure check valves a hazard. Anesthesiology 1982; 56:327–328.
21. Hamilton RC, Byrne J: Another cause of gas scavenging line obstruction. Anesthesiology 1979; 51:365–366.
22. Anonymous: How to monitor Sodasorb exhaustion. Sodalines Lexington, MA: Dewey and Almy Division of WR Grace, June, 1987.
23. Epstein RM, Rackow H, Lee ASJ, Papper EM: Prevention of accidental breathing of anoxic gas mixtures during anesthesia. Anesthesiology 1962; 23:1–4.
24. Cooper JB, Newbower RS, Kitz RJ: An analysis of major errors and equipment failures in anesthesia management: Considerations for prevention and detection. Anesthesiology 1984; 60:34–42.
25. Weil MH, Bisera J, Trevino RP, Rackow EC: Cardiac output and end-tidal carbon dioxide. Crit Care Med 1985; 13:907–909.
26. Spargo PM: The use of end-tidal P_{CO_2} monitoring to detect pulmonary embolism during Swan-Ganz catheter removal. Anesthesiology 1985; 63:A293.
27. Cooper JB, Newbower RS, Moore JW, Trautman ED: A new anesthesia delivery system. Anesthesiology 1978; 49:310–318.
28. Loeb RG, Brunner JX, Westenskow DR, et al: The Utah anesthesia workstation. Anesthesiology 1989; 70:999–1007.
29. Sykes MK, Sugg BR, Hahn CEW, et al: A new microprocessor-controlled anaesthetic machine. Br J Anaesth 1989; 62:445–455.

Appendix

ORGANIZATIONS THAT HAVE DEVELOPED STANDARDS APPLICABLE TO ANESTHESIA MACHINES AND EQUIPMENT

Compressed Gas Association
1735 Jefferson Davis Highway
Suite 1004
Arlington, VA 22202-4102
(703) 412-0900

National Fire Protection Association
1 Batterymarch Park
Quincy, MA 02269
(617) 770-3000

American National Standards Institute
11 West 42nd Street
New York, NY 10036
(212) 642-4900

American Society for Testing and Materials
1916 Race Street
Philadelphia, PA 19103
(215) 299-5400

Underwriter's Laboratories, Inc.
333 Pfingsten Road
Northbrook, IL 60062
(708) 272-8800

ORGANIZATIONS REPORTING EQUIPMENT PROBLEMS AND PROMOTING SAFE ANESTHESIA PRACTICES

Anesthesia Patient Safety Foundation
520 N. Northwest Highway
Park Ridge, IL 60068
(708) 825-5586

Emergency Care Research Institute (Publisher of Health Devices Alerts)
5200 Butler Pike
Plymouth Meeting, PA 19462
(215) 825-6000

CHAPTER 24

Monitoring Anesthetic Gases

KEITH D. KNOPES, M.D., and
BERNICE R. HECKER, M.D.

With the revolution in technology, the role of the anesthesiologist now includes monitoring not only physiologic or pharmacologic variables but inspired and expired anesthetic and other respiratory gases. The routine monitoring of inspired oxygen and expired carbon dioxide is an accepted standard of anesthesiology practice. This technology is also widely used in the intensive care unit (ICU).

The application of mass spectrometry to the field of monitoring anesthetic gases allows real-time measurement of multiple inspired and expired gases, including the anesthetic vapors. Other methods of measurement include infrared and Raman scattering spectrophotometry.

In addition to monitoring patients during anesthesia, the monitoring of anesthetic gases is useful in assessing occupational exposure in the operating room. The information obtained is helpful in analyzing the risk of exposure, in detecting leaks, and in determining the sources of exposure.

INDICATIONS AND USES OF ANESTHETIC GAS MONITORING

Improved engineering designs have made mass spectrometry cost-effective through the use of time-shared sampling. With the advent of new applications of Raman scattering for gas analysis, it is possible to purchase single devices for single-patient monitoring at a reasonable cost. The availability of these respiratory gas monitors allows routine use in clinical, teaching, and research areas.

CLINICAL INDICATIONS

Routine use of mass spectrometry and Raman spectroscopy in clinical anesthesia permits continuous monitoring of all gases of interest to the practicing anesthesiologist. In addition to reporting values for the volatile anesthetic agents, these instruments simultaneously measure oxygen, carbon dioxide, nitrogen, and nitrous oxide. This technology provides a greater amount of information than do polarographic devices for monitoring oxygen or infrared spectroscopy for detecting carbon dioxide. Oxygen and carbon dioxide analyzers, however, provide an additional layer of safety when used with mass spectrometry or Raman spectral analysis. This redundancy of systems is appropriate for anesthesia monitoring.

On-line measurement of respiratory and anesthetic gases is important to both clinical care and patient safety. The continuous measurement feature points out the difference between inspired and expired gas mixtures. An astute clinician uses these differences to draw conclusions that have direct consequences on patient care. Table 24–1 lists some examples of critical events, the detection of which often prevents anesthetic misadventures.

Construction of a gas delivery system for operating rooms is a complicated engineering project. A multitude of errors may occur during installation that include, but are not limited to, using improper fittings, mislabeling, crossing pipelines, and contamination by other gases, water, and foreign matter.[1] Deaths have occurred owing to errors in installation of gas delivery systems.[2] The gas source for delivery systems may be remote from the operating rooms in order to facilitate easy delivery of the gas supply. Therefore, a hospital remodeling project may introduce dangerous modifications to the gas delivery system that are un-

TABLE 24–1. CRITICAL EVENTS DETECTED BY ANESTHETIC GAS ANALYSIS

Errors in gas delivery system
Anesthesia machine malfunction
Vaporizer malfunction
Errors in vaporizer contents
Anesthesia circuit leaks
Circuit disconnections
Esophageal intubation
Endotracheal cuff leaks
Poor mask fit
Hypoventilation
Airway obstruction
Air embolism

known to the anesthesiologist. These critical alterations have been recognized by analysis of the inspired gas mixture, before they harmed patients.[1] Obviously, a system that measures all the gases presented to the breathing circuit provides more information than does an instrument measuring any single gas and, perhaps, improves patient safety.

CLINICAL USES

Measurement of Oxygen

Continuous monitoring of oxygen by mass spectrometry or other techniques is redundant, because most anesthesia machines have polarographic monitors of the inspiratory oxygen concentration delivered to the anesthesia circuit (see Chapter 11). However, the additional inspired and expired values confirm the adequate delivery of oxygen to the patient.

Measurement of Carbon Dioxide

Simultaneous monitoring of carbon dioxide allows continuous evaluation of ventilation (see Chapter 12). The mass spectrometer uses the detection of the CO_2 waveform to trigger various alarm states. The most important alarm is the ''no breath'' or apnea state. The rapid detection of CO_2 is used routinely to confirm tracheal intubation. During maintenance of anesthesia, the detection of CO_2 confirms the integrity of the circuit. If disconnection occurs, the no breath alarm sounds as the mass spectrometer fails to detect an expiratory waveform. The quantification of the analog waveform into digital information gives the anesthesiologist further information on the adequacy of ventilation.

Astute clinicians use end-tidal CO_2 measurements for important clinical observations. An example is the detection of higher than anticipated CO_2 measurements in a child undergoing repair of total anomalous pulmonary venous return.[3] While the patient was on cardiopulmonary bypass, the end-tidal CO_2 remained mildly elevated over expected levels of less than 0.5%. This suggested the presence of a systemic-to-pulmonary shunt. Exploration of the great vessels revealed a patent ductus arteriosus. Ligation decreased the CO_2 to less than 0.2%. Careful observation and continuous gas analysis directly benefit patients.

Measurement of CO_2 identifies problems with the CO_2 absorber in a circle system. This would be seen as the presence of inspired CO_2. An alternative explanation is malfunction of the unidirectional valve on the inspiratory limb of the circuit. Therefore, the presence of increased inspired CO_2 requires direct inspection of the circle system of the anesthesia machine.

Measurement of Nitrogen

Continuous on-line measurement of nitrogen yields much useful information for the anesthesiologist. The standard of care for induction of patients with a full stomach is a rapid-sequence induction following preoxygenation (denitrogenation) of the patient. This may be accomplished by several minutes of quiet breathing of 100% oxygen via a tight-fitting face mask.[4] Alternatively, four deep breaths of 100% oxygen may be used.[5] Gas analysis monitors nitrogen washout. When the end-tidal nitrogen is less than 5% of the exhaled gases, it is safe to proceed with the rapid induction of general anesthesia.

Continuous analysis of respiratory gases is a very effective monitor of the integrity of anesthesia delivery systems. Nitrogen is washed out of the lungs in a matter of minutes. Although it may take hours for all the nitrogen to be washed out of body tissues, the end-tidal concentration is usually about 1–3% during the first few hours as the nitrogen diffuses out of the tissues and finds its way to the lungs for excretion and detection by the analyzing instrument. Therefore, a sudden increase in the percentage of nitrogen in the exhaled gas mixture is diagnostic of the introduction of air from outside the anesthesia gas delivery system. Sources of this air could be leaks in the circuit or endotracheal cuff or a venous air embolism.[6–8] In the case of venous air embolism, the increased end-tidal nitrogen precedes changes in precordial Doppler sounds.

Mass spectrometry has been used to detect disconnection of the fresh gas ''down-inflow.''[9] This disconnection occurred in an anesthesia circuit with a descending bellows type of ventilator. The combination of this ventilator with a small-diameter fresh gas inflow prevented detection of the disconnection by the low-pressure alarm. The only indication was the rapid increase in nitrogen detected by the mass spectrometer. The additional information obtained by simultaneous mass spectrometric analysis of all anesthetic gases greatly benefits the anesthesiologist in the detection and diagnosis of critical incidents.

Measurement of Anesthetic Vapors

Vaporizers. Anesthetic gas measurement is useful in the calibration and monitoring of vaporizer function. Uncalibrated vaporizers require knowledge of the vapor pressure, temperature, and gas flows to correctly calculate the concentration of anesthetic vapor delivered to the patient. Although multiple nomograms and pocket aids have been developed, errors can occur, and the inadvertent overdose of anesthetic vapor is still a real problem. Continuous anesthetic gas analysis significantly adds to patient safety by correctly reporting the delivered concentration of vapor.

Temperature-compensated and flow-calibrated vaporizers have been developed that allow the clinician to ''dial-in'' a desired percentage of vapor delivered. However, these complex devices can malfunction, and they require regular scheduled maintenance and calibration. Continuous measurement of the delivered vapor indicates when the vaporizer needs calibration. A routine check of vaporizer function is easily accomplished by connecting the sampling tube of the gas measurement instrument to the fresh gas flow outlet at the anesthesia machine by means of a T-piece and directly sampling the vaporizer output.

Analysis of anesthetic gases also detects leaks in the vaporizer system. Many newer anesthesia machines are equipped with more than one vaporizer in series. The possibility of leaking is detected when the mass spectrometer displays a signal for an ''unknown'' vapor. This display occurs when the instrument simultaneously detects two vapors. The computer analysis display also reports unknown vapor conditions when a vaporizer has been contaminated by the addition of the wrong agent.[10] For example, if enflurane has been added to a vaporizer containing halothane, both agents are presented to the sampling port simultaneously. As in the situation for a leaking vaporizer, the mass spectrometer reports the detection of an unknown vapor.

Closed-Circuit Anesthesia. Low-flow or closed-circuit anesthesia has seen episodic popularity. The benefits include better respiratory gas humidification, a clinically significant decrease in heat loss, and cost-effective anesthetic administration, because less anesthetic vapors and gases are used. However, most anesthesiologists routinely use an open circuit with higher fresh gas flows primarily because of the fear of delivering a hypoxic inspiratory gas mixture. If the oxygen added to the circle system is less than that consumed by the patient, the rebreathed gases become hypoxic. This may occur quite rapidly if nitrous oxide is included in the gas mixture. It is obvious that continuous monitoring of the anesthetic gases alerts the anesthesiologist to the need for more oxygen in the circuit.

GAS ANALYSIS IN THE ICU

The routine clinical use of respiratory gas analysis has extended from the operating room to the ICU.[11–14] Routine ICU use includes monitoring CO_2 to confirm tracheal placement of endotracheal tubes and regulating ventilation parameters to control hypoventilation and hyperventilation. Information from the measurement of respiratory gases has been used in calculating alveolar-arterial oxygen tension difference, minute volume, dead space, ventilation/perfusion ratio, and O_2 consumption (see Chapter 27). Derived variables have been used as extubation criteria. Routine ICU use depends on the time-sharing of a mass spectrometer to be cost-effective. It seems unlikely that this costly instrument and installation will be a common feature in most ICU settings, because the information most necessary in patient care can be obtained in more cost-effective ways. However, units such as a Raman spectrometer may be economically feasible for routine use in the ICU. Such an instrument on a mobile cart could be used for episodic measurements at the bedside.

TEACHING

Many teaching institutions have installed anesthesia gas analyzers to aid in the teaching of medical students and residents. Analog and trending displays are very useful in many demonstrations of normal and altered physiology during anesthesia. The concept of nitrogen washout is demonstrated on the user interface using the trend line for nitrogen. Alterations in ventilation and gas mixtures can be used to demonstrate simple principles used clinically to care for patients. The introduction of different anesthetic circuits, gas flows, and ventilation results in very different patterns of respiratory gas exchange. Attention to the change in anesthetic gas concentration with time improves student understanding of gas exchange.

The concept of uptake and distribution is a most difficult one for many students of anesthesiology. Such complex pharmacokinetic principles are difficult to understand from texts or lectures. Mass spectrometer data are used by the clinical teacher to demonstrate these concepts to the student by examination of the gas concentration-time curves. A further extension of this teaching is the pharmacodynamic results of vaporizer, gas flow, and gas mixture manipulations. Alveolar concentrations can be adjusted to a specific fraction of minimum alveolar concentration. During closed-circuit anesthesia, the calculation of metabolic oxygen requirements and their changes with depth of anesthesia give students insight into the physiologic changes caused by various anesthetic agents.

RESEARCH

In addition to the uses discussed previously, the measurement of anesthetic gases has a well-established place in clinical and basic research, but its full potential is yet to be discovered. It is very useful in establishing the steady state in studies involving the depth of anesthesia in humans and animals. Instruments have been adapted for measuring halothane metabolites[15] and examining tissue uptake of nitrous oxide.[16] This powerful technology will continue to widen our knowledge base about the pharmacokinetic, pharmacodynamic, and metabolic consequences of anesthetic vapors and gases.

MASS SPECTROMETRY

THEORY

Molecular Ion Generation

The basic purpose of the mass spectrometer is to provide measurable products of the ionization process. This results in a product that, when measured, indicates the content of the sample being measured. This process of ionization begins with the ion source (Fig. 24–1). A stream of bombarding electrons is generated by an incandescent filament. These electrons interact with a stream of vaporized sample molecules (sampled from the breathing circuit) to form ions of the parent molecules. These molecular ions may then go on to fragment, yielding the fragmentation mass spectrum.

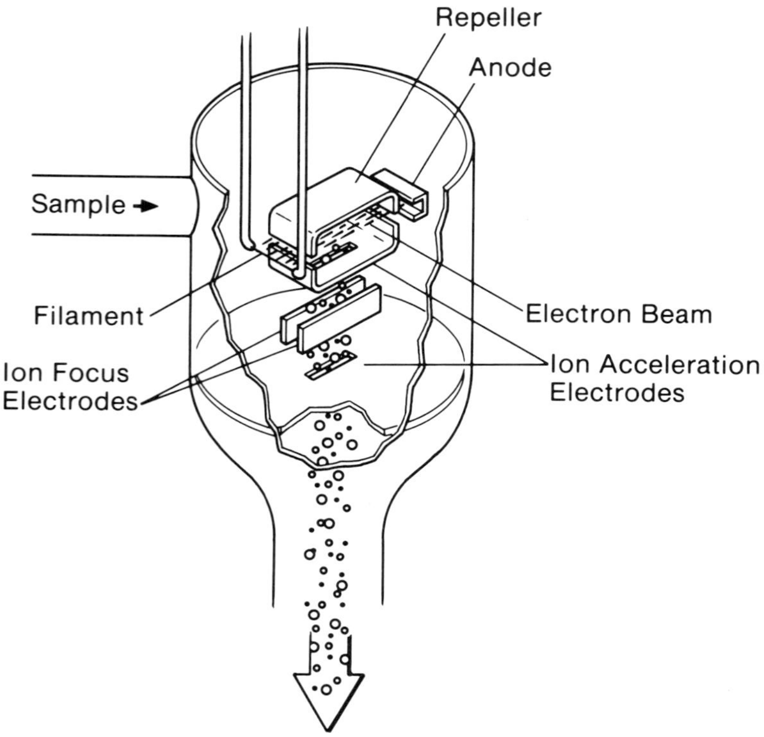

Figure 24–1. The ion source is a stream of electrons generated by an incandescent filament that interacts with the sample to form ions of the parent molecule. (From McLafferty FW: Interpretation of Mass Spectrometry. Reading, MA: WA Benjamin, 1973; 6. © University Science Books, Mill Valley, California.)

Ion Separation

Once the ions are formed, they must be separated for counting based on their mass-to-change (M/C) ratios. Common techniques of separation are magnetic deflection, time-of-flight, quadrupole lens, radio frequency, cyclotron resonance, and cycloidal focusing. The most widely applied methods of separation of the molecular ions in clinical use are the quadrupole lens and magnetic sector techniques.[17]

Quadrupole Lens. The quadrupole lens makes use of a changing magnetic field induced between two electrodes charged with a combined direct and alternating current signal.[18] The stream of molecular ions is then directed through the magnetic field, which accomplishes the ion separation based on the unique M/C ratio of each. A single detector collects and detects the ions. The results are synchronously reported, allowing the computation of the relative contribution of each ion to the mass spectrum.

Magnetic Sector. A different approach is used in a magnetic sector mass spectrometer. This method directs the stream of molecular ions through a magnetic field where the ions are deflected based on their M/C ratio. After the separation, the individual ion paths end at a series of detectors that report the raw data for analysis based on the relative amounts of each ion in the mass spectrum. An alternative design makes use of a varying magnetic field that changes the degree of ion deflection. This brings a different M/C ratio into focus on a detector slit that focuses the selected ion stream on the detector (Fig. 24–2).

Detector

Once the ions generated by the bombarding electrons in the ion source have been separated by these strategies, they are detected by collection plates. As the positive molecular ions contact the collector, a current of electrons is generated in proportion to the number of molecular ions. The resulting current is amplified and presented for analysis. Research instruments can make use of electron multiplier circuits that make possible the detection of a single ion arriving at the collector. Instruments used in clinical monitoring are not required to be so sensitive, thus making the cost of an instrument more reasonable.

Spectral Interpretation

Once the ions in the mass spectrum have been generated, separated, and detected, the instrument must provide easily interpretable results. The molecular ion, M^+, is that ion produced with the highest M/C ratio in the mass spectrum. However, detection of the molecular ion alone is insufficient to differentiate among the various gases encountered in the clinical setting, because some have the same mass number. Also, the ions generated during the fragmentation of various gases and vapors (especially halogenated hydrocarbons) cause generation of species that overlap the characteristic peaks of other components of the gas sample. Therefore, sophisticated computer programming for analysis of the mass spectrum is necessary in order to provide usable clinical data.

SAMPLING

The mass spectrometer was adapted for measurement of respiratory gases in 1952.[19] It was not until the 1960s that routine commercial use of this technology became avail-

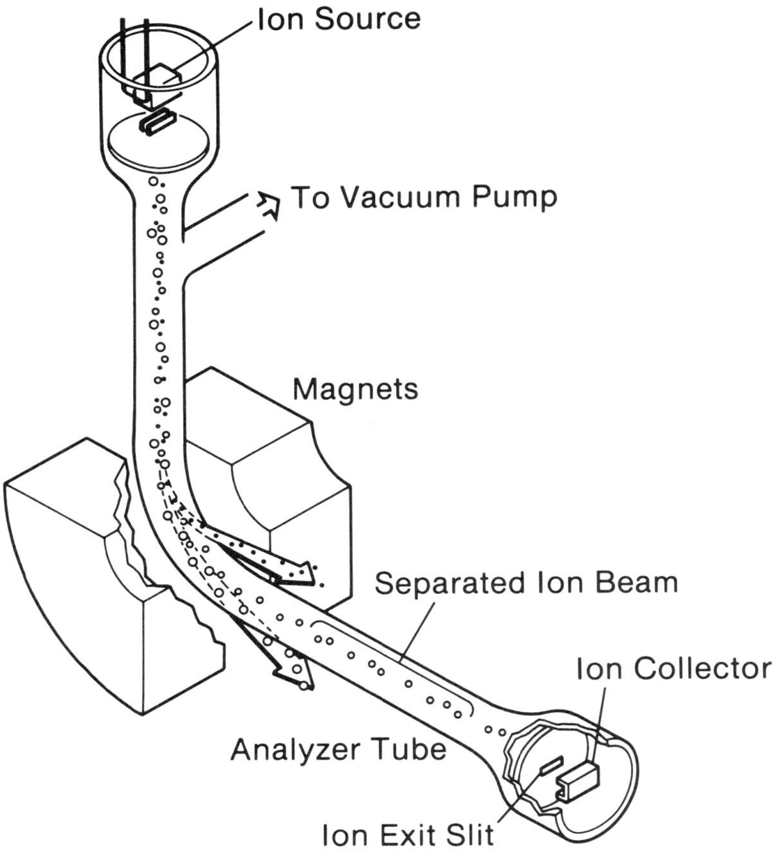

Figure 24–2. The path of ions through a varying magnetic field changes the degree of ion deflection so that ions of different mass-to-charge ratios are focused on the detector slit of the collection plates. As ions contact the collector, a current is generated in proportion to the number of molecular ions. The current is amplified and analyzed. (From McLafferty FW: Interpretation of Mass Spectrometry. Reading, MA: WA Benjamin, 1973; 7. © University Science Books, Mill Valley, California.)

able. A key feature in the adaptation of mass spectrometry to the clinical arena is the development of multipatient applications.[20] The measurement of anesthetic gases during anesthesia required multiple samplings with a small time increment between measurements. Central placement of one instrument connected to multiple sampling sites by long capillary tubing makes this possible.[21] The small diameter of the capillary tubing allows multiple breath samples to be "stored" in the tubing with very little diffusion or mixing. The mass spectrometer may then sample each tube in turn. During the sampling interval, the instrument may quickly sample several breaths from the capillary tube and provide an analog display of the concentration-time profile with digital reports of the inspired and expired end-tidal values.

The application of multiline capillary sampling systems made the clinical use of mass spectrometry economical, easy to use, and reliable. Time sharing makes the high cost of mass spectrometry practical for multipatient use. A schematic of multipatient adaptation is presented in Figure 24–3. The use of long, small-diameter catheters and a bank of solenoid sampling valves allows systematic, time-shared sampling from multiple locations. A vacuum pump pulls the sample past the inlet. The introduction of plastic catheters for sampling can lead to error introduced by the absorption of gases by the catheter. This error is considered so small as to be clinically insignificant. The use of disposable sampling apparatus eliminates the risk of infectious contamination. Sampling sites include the Y-piece of the circle system, a side port of the Rovenstine angle attached to the mask or endotracheal tube, or other portions of the anesthetic circuit.

SYSTEM MAINTENANCE

The time-shared mass spectrometer is a complex mechanical and electronic instrument that requires daily maintenance and calibration. The improvement in computer technology and its application to the user interface have made the daily care of these instruments much easier. However, meticulous care must be taken. The commercially available devices monitor themselves electronically to ensure that the values reported are within realistic parameters, or an alert condition results. Daily logs of maintenance procedures and calibration are essential to aid in trouble-shooting should a major system failure occur.

Calibration and Standardization

A daily manual calibration is recommended for most commercial instruments. This involves establishing zero references of the electronics and calibrating sensitivities. If electrical steady state is confirmed by the absence of baseline drift, gas calibration is performed. Gas calibration is accomplished using standard gas mixtures (including oxy-

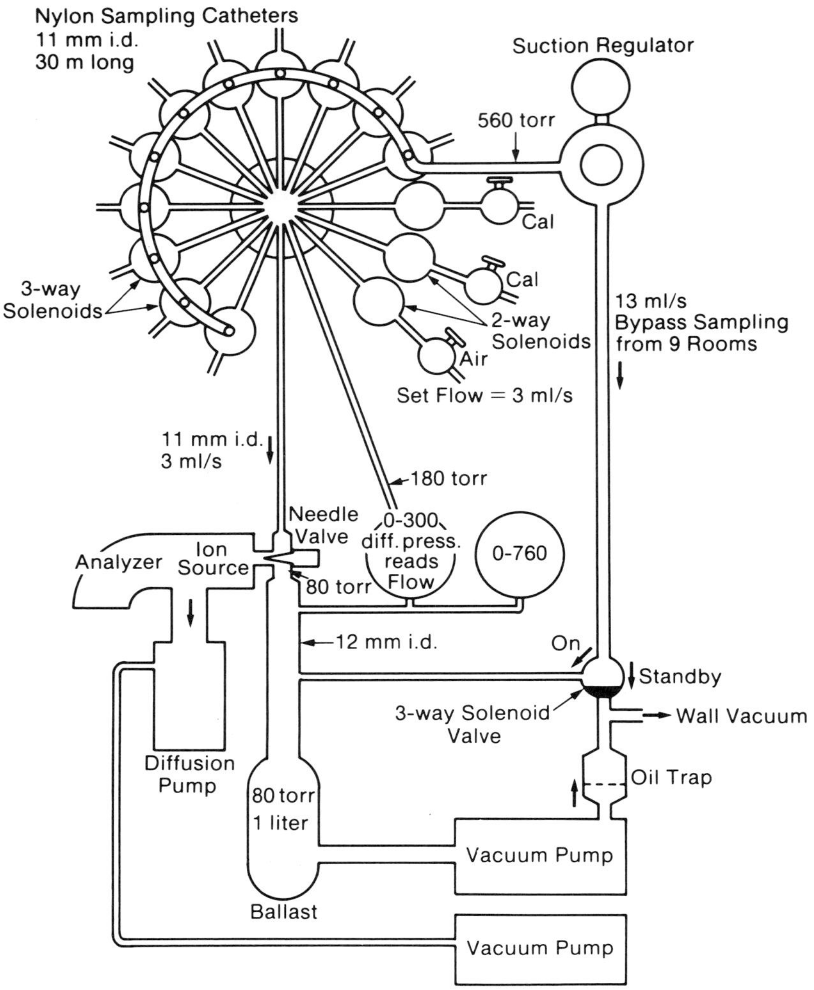

Figure 24–3. Time-shared mass spectrometer system allowing sampling from 10 rooms by way of the three-way solenoids. (From Ozanne GM, Young WG, Mazzei WJ, Severinghaus JW: Multipatient anesthetic mass spectrometry: Rapid analysis of data stored in long catheters. Anesthesiology 1981; 55:62–70.)

gen, nitrous oxide, air, carbon dioxide, and a volatile agent) supplied in cylinders. The instrument samples a known gas mixture at regular intervals during operation and adjusts its own calibration.

Reliability

Clinical mass spectrometry has resulted in a surprisingly reliable instrument, given its great complexity. The system maintains close calibration without significant technician intervention for many days. However, service is still frequent and requires a qualified technical support person to maintain the instrument daily. In addition to daily calibration, gas cylinders need regular replacement, vacuum pumps require checking and changing of oil, and the user interface stations may get damaged in daily use. The most common problems involve the sampling systems, which may become blocked owing to tubing kinks or foreign matter. Mechanical damage to other parts of the sampling or measuring portions of the instrument also occurs. The spectrometer collecting plates and filaments require regular replacement over months or years.

Sources of Error

Commercial mass spectrometers have many ways of handling sampling sources of error. One problem is the overlap in the patterns of inspiratory and expiratory gases. A spectrum overlap eraser circuit is often used to help with this problem. However, these alterations in data analysis may themselves introduce error.[18]

A significant error in measurement occurs with the introduction of unmeasured ions into the sample stream. Commercially designed clinical mass spectrometers include collection plates and ion counters for the respiratory and anesthetic gases. Very low- or high-molecular-weight species with limited fragmentation spectra are not detected by such instruments. An example of such a gas is helium.[22] Its low molecular weight prevents it from being measured. Therefore, any contribution that helium makes to the gas sample measured is not included in the calculated gas totals or percentages. Only dry gas totals are determined. Water vapor is ignored. If 50% helium were to be used in the inspired mixture, the mass spectrometer would report the totals and percentages of the remaining gas as twice their true values. This misinformation could lead the anesthesiologist to treat the incorrect information in ways injurious to the patient. For example, the end-tidal CO_2 would be reported as twice its true value. This might lead the anesthesiologist to hyperventilate the patient, with resultant metabolic alkalosis. As the use of helium (primarily for laser surgeries) and other gases is introduced into clinical practice, mass spectrometers require modification to remove these sources of error.

The sampling system, consisting of long distances of plastic tubing, may be a source of error.[18, 23] The longer the tubing system, the greater the error due to diffusion. Water vapor condenses on the walls of the tubing. This thin film of water absorbs small amounts of nitrous oxide, CO_2, and the volatile anesthetic agents, slowing their transit to the instrument. These sample tubing–induced errors are small and of no clinical significance. However, research data are influenced by even small sources of error. Thus, dedicated single-station instruments yield superior research data.

Condensate, blood, or secretions occasionally block the sampling tubing. A filter placed at the inlet of the sampling line minimizes obstruction from secretions, soda lime, or other particulate matter.

Errors in data interpretation are also common with the mass spectrometer. Many anesthesiologists assume that the end-tidal concentration is always an accurate reflection of the arterial partial pressure. However, with several conditions, this is not the case.[24] Any barrier to anesthetic gas transfer in the lung is reflected in a higher end-tidal pressure than an arterial partial pressure. Ventilation-perfusion abnormalities represent such a situation. Increased ventilation-perfusion mismatch results in less uptake into the blood. When there are large differences between inspired and end-tidal values, the error is magnified. It is important to note that ventilation-perfusion abnormalities are exaggerated by anesthesia, thus further adding to the error.

Cost/Benefit Ratio

There is no doubt that the initial capital investment (approximately \$100,000) is significant for a mass spectrometer installation. The cost per anesthetizing location decreases with the increasing number of locations serviced. However, as the number of sampling locations is increased, so are the service and maintenance costs. A stand-alone, single-station instrument costs about \$65,000. The requirement of a trained technician to perform daily service and trouble-shooting is an ongoing expense, as are parts and calibration gases. Improvements in design are moderating the cost and improving ease of use.

The addition of mass spectrometry introduces a certain redundancy to existing monitoring equipment. Most anesthesia machines are equipped with inspiratory oxygen monitors, and many hospitals have invested in capnography for each operating room. Redundancy, however, improves safety. The comparisons between operating an aircraft and administering an anesthetic have been made for many years. Redundancy in monitoring may be a safety feature common to both.

Sound clinical critical incident reporting and research have yet to be applied to mass spectrometry in the operating room. Therefore, the dollar cost/benefit ratio is only speculation at this point. There can be little doubt, however, that prevention of harm secondary to a critical incident is worth a significant number of dollars, given the litigious nature of our society today. The benefits of improved anesthetic management with the use of continuous mass spectrometry are difficult to quantify. There are no data to support decreased recovery time, monetary savings from decreased anesthetic use, or better patient outcome during routine anesthesia uncomplicated by critical events. However, these data would also be difficult to obtain. Therefore, the case for the routine use of mass spectrometry must be based on the prevention of critical events related to anesthesia.

RAMAN SCATTERING SPECTROSCOPY

Most of the commercial development of monitors of anesthetic gases followed long use of similar detection principles in the chemistry laboratory. This is certainly true for Raman scattering spectroscopy.[25]

THEORY

Raman scattering results when light strikes gas molecules. A photon of light strikes a molecule in the gas, and some of the photon's energy is converted to rotational and vibrational energy of the atoms in the molecule. The resultant loss of energy yields a re-emitted photon with a lower frequency. This characteristic frequency shift is due to a lower energy state and is measured as the Raman light scattering. The scattered light is measured at right angles to the light source as separate peaks in the spectra, resulting in easy determination of the concentration of each of the respiratory and anesthetic gases of clinical interest.

This scattered light is one millionth the intensity of the source light. Separating the Raman scattering from the source light was not feasible until laser-generated monochromic light became available. Therefore, laser beam–generated photons of a single wavelength permit easy measurement of the frequency shifts and have made Raman spectroscopy clinically useful. An argon laser source generates ultraviolet light with a wavelength of 488 nm and is well suited to operating room implementation.[26]

ADVANTAGES AND PROBLEMS

This type of analysis has some advantages. The cost of the instrument allows individual instruments at each location, providing continuous on-line data. The gases are unaltered by analysis and can be returned to the anesthesia circuit without harm to the patient. Raman scattering is unaffected by monatomic gases such as helium. The technology has the theoretic possibility of very rapid response times.[26]

The commercial success of Raman spectroscopy will depend on improvements in engineering design. The instruments currently under development have higher signal-to-noise ratios than those of mass spectrometers. Their reliability and accuracy compared with mass spectrometry has been established.[27] The laser source is an essential and costly element in the system. Therefore, the lifetime of the laser is important in the consideration of maintenance costs. Currently, argon lasers require significant power and may require annual replacement.

OTHER METHODS OF MONITORING ANESTHETIC GASES

Alternative methods, such as ultraviolet analysis and the silicone rubber absorption method for detecting and quantifying anesthetic gases, have been used for decades. Oxygen analyzers are standard equipment on many anesthesia machines. A commonly used detector is designed around a polarographic method (see Chapter 11). Infrared spectrophotometry is used in most single-station capnographs for the monitoring of CO_2 (see Chapter 12). Table 24–2 lists the commercially available instruments.

As interest intensifies for less expensive, smaller, more reliable, and easier to use instrumentation, new technologies are under development for operating room monitoring of anesthetic gases. An example is the piezoelectric quartz crystal analysis of gases.

PIEZOELECTRIC DETECTORS

Piezoelectric quartz crystals have been recognized as an alternative detector of halogenated anesthetic gases.[28] The natural resonant frequency of a quartz crystal coated by a lipophilic layer changes in proportion to the partial pressure of a halogenated anesthetic gas. The instrument supplies the electric field to the piezoelectric quartz crystal and measures the changes in the resonant frequency. Data are reported as volumes-per cent of anesthetic vapor. This method cannot distinguish among the different inhaled anesthetic vapors and must be calibrated for each agent individually by means of a dial on the instrument face.[26] Nitrous oxide and water vapor introduce error into the measurement, particularly for isoflurane.[29] If the nitrous oxide and water vapor are held constant, an electronic offset can be used to remove the error caused by them. However, the significance of the introduced error may influence clin-

TABLE 24–2. COMMERCIALLY AVAILABLE RESPIRATORY GAS INSTRUMENTS

Technology	Gas	Merits	Demerits	Company	Model	Cost Range
Mass spectrometry	ALL	System adaptability for multimonitoring and recording	Time-shared; time lag and sample delay	Marquette PPG Biomedical	Advantage System SARA System	\$140,000–\$160,000
Raman spectrometry	ALL	Freestanding; upgradable for new agents	Size	Ohmeda	Rascal II	\$17,000
Infrared absorption	CO_2 N_2O Vapors	Distinguishes agents very precisely Most models automatically identify the anesthetic agent	Sensitive to water droplets and flow rate	BCI Criticare Datascope Datex Marquette Ohmeda Nellcor PPG Biomedical Puritan-Bennett Siemens Spacelabs	9100 602-3 4100 ID Ultima MGA-IR 5250 N-2500 SARA Cap AG 254 734G 90514	\$10,000–\$12,000
Photoacoustic detection	CO_2 N_2O Vapors			Hewlett-Packard	M1025B	\$10,000–\$12,000
Magnetic-acoustic detection	O_2	Real-time FIO_2 and ETO_2 (end tidal)		Hewlett-Packard	M1025B	\$10,000–\$12,000
Galvanic cell	O_2	Stability	Cost of disposable cell	BCI Criticare Datascope Marquette Ohmeda PPG Biomedical Siemans Spacelabs	9100 602-3 4100 ID MGA-IR 5250 SARA Cap AG 734G 90514	\$10,000–\$12,000
Paramagnetic sensor	O_2	Fast response time; insensitive to ambient variables		Datex Puritan-Bennett	Ultima 254	\$10,000–\$12,000

Courtesy of Dennis J. McMahon, Chief Anesthesia Technologist, Virginia Mason Clinic.

ical data for low concentrations of the anesthetic vapors, because heated, humidified gases increase the measured concentration.[27]

Piezoelectric quartz crystal instruments can be made available at each anesthetizing location at a very low cost. Cost and the ease of use of the instrument make piezoelectric quartz crystal monitors practical for limited installations. The Engstrom multigas monitor for anesthesia is an example of this technology.

OCCUPATIONAL EXPOSURE TO ANESTHETIC GASES

ANALYSIS OF RISK

Anesthesiologists have been aware of the effects of exposure to inhaled anesthetic gases for many decades. In the early portion of this century, when open-drop ether was still in use, operating room personnel experienced headache, nausea, and inability to concentrate. The innovation of improved operating room ventilation greatly reduced these reactions. However, it has been almost 30 years since the first concerns regarding long-term effects of trace anesthetics were first appreciated.

A higher incidence of malignancies in anesthesiologists than in the general population was one of the initial clues to this problem.[30] Up to this time, trace anesthetics were thought to be inert and quickly eliminated, thus causing no harm. However, discoveries documenting the biotransformation of these agents forced a review of this mistaken concept and strengthened interest in improving scavenging techniques.[31] In 1974, *Anesthesiology* published a landmark study by Cohen and coworkers, who reported that working in the operating room resulted in a significant risk to health.[32] This and subsequent studies point to chronic exposure to trace anesthetic agents as a major health hazard, increasing the risk of spontaneous abortion,[33, 34] congenital anomalies in offspring,[35] cognitive defects,[36, 37] cancer,[28] and renal or hepatic disease.[38–40] Drug-metabolizing enzymes also are stimulated after anesthetic exposure.[41–43] Headache and nausea are also reported after chronic environmental exposure.[44] However, more recent studies have failed to confirm some of these risks (Table 24–3).[45]

TABLE 24–3. POTENTIAL* HEALTH HAZARDS RESULTING FROM OCCUPATIONAL ANESTHETIC EXPOSURE

Increased spontaneous abortion rate[33, 34]
Increased rate of congenital malformation (teratogenicity)[35]
Increased risk of hepatic disease[39, 40]
Increased risk of renal disease[40]
Impairment of motor and cognitive skills[36, 37]
Increased incidence of cancer[30]
Headache, nausea[44]
Enzyme induction[41–43]

*Although some experimental and epidemiologic evidence strongly suggests a health hazard from chronic anesthetic gas exposure, other causes have not been completely excluded.

Routine use of scavenging systems minimizes such exposure. Industry-wide standard practice now requires routine checks for sources of exposure, detection of leaks, and implementation of techniques to minimize exposure.

SOURCES OF EXPOSURE

Anesthetic gases are supplied from the wall outlet and from the anesthesia machine itself with the vaporization of volatile anesthetics. Spilling volatile anesthetics during vaporizer filling markedly increases environmental contamination. Trace contamination from the high-pressure sources and anesthesia machine flowmeters is not adequately scavenged. Removal of this source of contamination requires detection of the leak and proper machine maintenance to prevent the occurrence of leaks. A program of regular simple testing detects these leaks, allowing for their correction (see Chapter 23).[46]

The patient-anesthesia machine interface may be a significant source of operating room pollution. General anesthesia administered with a poorly fitting mask exposes every member of the operating team to large amounts of anesthetic gases. It is the duty of the anesthesiologist to use meticulous technique and provide a leak-proof mask fit (Fig. 24–4*A*). A good case may be made for the use of endotracheal intubation to protect operating room personnel from gas leaks due to poorly performed ''mask'' anesthesia (Fig. 24–4*B*). If the patient is intubated, care must be taken to ensure against cuff leaks. If positive pressure ventilation is used, a small cuff leak may allow significant amounts of gas to leak into the operating room environment. Anesthetic gas flows should be discontinued prior to intubation or patient suctioning.

The routine use of well-designed scavengers was a significant advance in improving air quality in the operating room. Scavenging systems consist of a gas-capturing assembly, a disposal assembly, and an interface to allow positive and negative pressure relief. However, the scavenger itself may not work properly if neglected in the routine evaluation of the anesthesia machine (see Chapter 23). Most modern scavenging systems have multiple connections that may be sources for leaks. A reservoir bag made of rubber is often built into the system in order to protect the patient from the vacuum source. These reservoirs are often not replaced and are degraded by the very agents they are made to scavenge. Excess circuit gases must be disposed of properly, using a nonrecirculating air conditioning system, an independent vacuum system, an adsorber, or a passive through-wall system.

The anesthesia machine is only one source of operating room pollution. Another source is the extracorporeal circuit when volatile anesthetics are used during cardiopulmonary bypass. The extracorporeal circuit must be scavenged to prevent leakage of significant halogenated vapors into the operating room.[47–49] In orthopedic surgery, the plastic cements that are mixed in the operating room just before use are known to cause headaches and nausea among operating

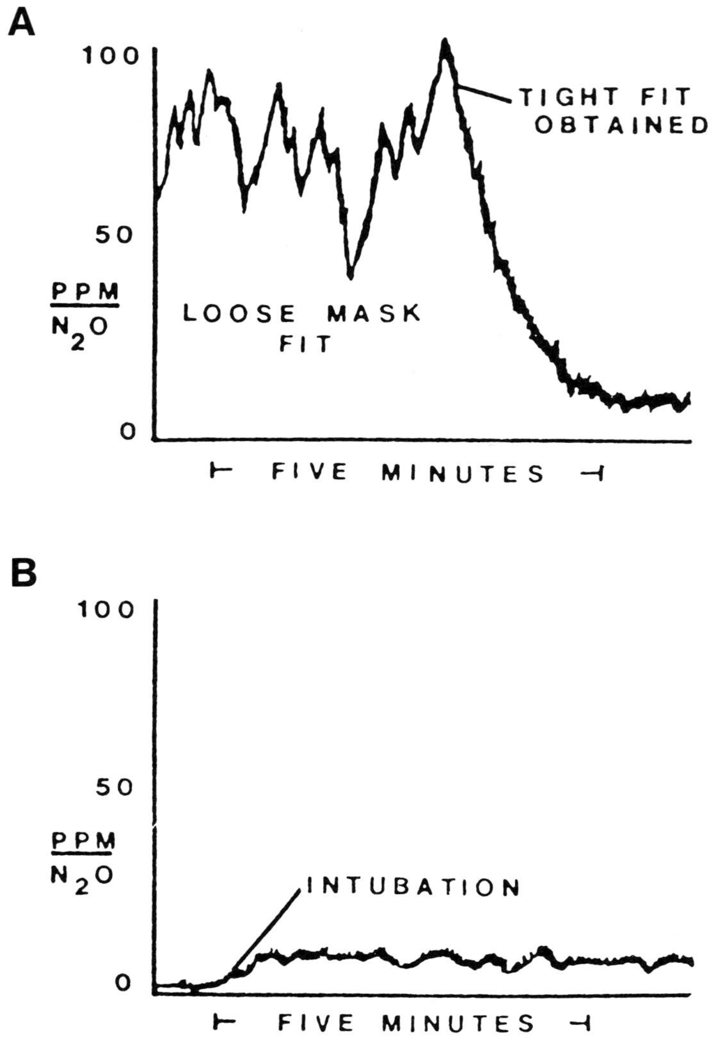

Figure 24–4. *A*, The effect of a poorly fitting mask on environmental concentrations of nitrous oxide (N_2O parts per million). With proper mask application, the nitrous oxide concentration rapidly decreases. *B*, The benefits of endotracheal intubation on the maintenance of low environmental concentrations of N_2O. (From Lecky JH [ed]: Waste anesthetic gases in operating room air: A suggested program to reduce personnel exposure. Park Ridge, IL: American Society of Anesthesiologists Ad Hoc Committee on Effects of Trace Anesthetic Agents on Health of Operating Room Personnel; 9,10. Reprinted with permission from the American Society of Anesthesiologists, ASA, 520 N. Northwest Highway, Park Ridge, Illinois 60068-2573.)

room personnel. These vapors are best handled by mixing the cement under a vacuum hood.

DETECTION OF LEAKS

The first step in detecting leaks is to establish that the operating room environment is polluted by anesthetic gases. Several methods have become accepted for monitoring exposure to anesthetic gases.[50, 51]

In the average operating room, nitrous oxide leaking at about 3 L/minute results in a concentration of 160 ppm without scavenging.[52] An infrared analyzer can be used to detect the amount of operating room pollution by nitrous oxide. An advantage to this technique is its ability to give real-time on-line data. This ability to report instantly the presence of leaks can also be used to pinpoint their sources. Samples obtained over a longer period give a better idea about the average concentration of the polluting agent.

Methods of Environmental Monitoring

Control concentrations of nitrous oxide should be measured at least every quarter year from the operating room after it has been out of use for 2 hours. Additional samples are also taken at various times during operating room use. Methods used for such sampling include continuous infrared (see Chapter 12),[50] time-weighted averaging, and ''grab'' samples.

Time-Weighted Average. The evacuated canister method of sampling is an example of time-weighted average sampling.[51] An evacuated canister fitted with a flow-controlled inlet valve continually samples the operating room air for later analysis. The canister is quite small and easily attached to a belt to sample air close to the carrier. The canister is ''opened'' in the laboratory, where a mass spectrometer determines the average amounts and species of the operating room gases collected.

''Grab'' Sampling. A leak-free inert container or syringe is used to obtain instantaneous samples of operating room air. When such samples are obtained intraoperatively, they evaluate the effectiveness of anesthetic techniques, equipment leakage, scavenger efficiency, and operating room ventilation. Grab samples can be analyzed by either infrared or chromatographic methods.

Acceptable Limits. The National Institute for Occupational Safety and Health proposes that acceptable environmental levels in operating rooms are time-weighted averages less than 25 ppm for nitrous oxide and 0.5 ppm for halogenated agents used with nitrous oxide.[53] When halogenated agents are used alone, the acceptable limit is 2 ppm.[53] When increased levels are detected, attention should be directed to modify anesthetic practice, check the anesthesia machine and gas hoses for leaks, and verify effective operation of the scavenging and ventilation systems.

REFERENCES

1. Krenis LJ, Berkowitz DA: Errors in installation of a new gas delivery system found after certification. Anesthesiology 1985; 62:677–678.
2. Feeley TW, McClelland KJ, Malhotra IV: The hazards of bulk oxygen delivery systems. Lancet 1975; 1:1416–1418.
3. Means LJ, Beckman DJ, Brown JW, King H: Detection of systemic to pulmonary shunt by end-tidal carbon dioxide concentration. Anesth Analg 1987; 66:1055–1056.
4. Heller ML, Watson TR: The role of preliminary oxygenation prior to induction with high nitrous oxide mixtures. Anesthesiology 1962; 23:219–230.
5. Gold MI, Duarte I, Muravchick S: Arterial oxygenation in conscious patients after 5 minutes and after 30 seconds of oxygen breathing. Anesth Analg 1981; 60:313–315.
6. Lanier W: Intraoperative air entrainment with Ohio[R] Modulus™ anesthesia machine. Anesthesiology 1986; 64:266–268.
7. Matjasko J, Petrozza P, Mackenzie CF: Sensitivity of end-tidal nitrogen in venous air embolism detection in dogs. Anesthesiology 1985; 65:418–423.
8. Matjasko J, Gunzelman J, Delaney J, Mackenzie CF: Sources of nitrogen in the anesthesia circuit. Anesthesiology 1986; 65:229.
9. Ghanooni S, Wilks DH, Finestone SC: A case report of an unusual disconnection. Anesth Analg 1983; 62:696–697.
10. Munshi C, Dhamee S, Bardeen-Henschel A, Dhruva S: Recognition of mixed anesthetic agents by mass-spectrometer during anesthesia. J Clin Monit 1986; 2:121–134.
11. Roberts MJ, Boustred ML, Hinds CJ: A multipatient mass spectrometer based system for the measurement of metabolic gas exchange in artificially ventilated intensive care patients. Intensive Care Med 1983; 9:339–343.
12. Rikes JB, Haberman B: Expiratory gas monitoring by mass spectrometry in a respiratory intensive care unit. Crit Care Med 1976; 4:223–229.
13. Prakash O, Meij S: Use of mass spectrometry and infrared CO_2 analyzer for bedside measurement of cardiopulmonary function during anesthesia and intensive care. Crit Care Med 1977; 5:180–184.
14. Yakulis R, Snyder JV, Powner D, et al: Mass spectrometry monitoring of respiratory variables in an intensive care unit. Respir Care 1978; 23:671–679.
15. Sharp JH, Trudell JR, Cohen EN: Volatile metabolites and decomposition products of halothane in man. Anesthesiology 1979; 50:2–8.
16. Crocker D, Koka BV, Filler RM, et al: Tissue uptake and excretion of nitrous oxide in pediatric anesthesia. Anesth Analg 1974; 53:779–785.
17. McLafferty FW: Interpretation of Mass Spectrometry. Reading, MA: WA Benjamin, 1973.
18. Salamonsen RF, Tulloh AM, Boyd T: Adaptation of the quadrupole mass spectrometer to multipatient anaesthesia gas monitoring. Anaesth Intensive Care 1986; 14:163–173.
19. Comroe JH: The functions of the lung. *In* Harvey Lecture, vol 48. New York: Academic, 1952; 110–144.
20. Ozanne GM, Young WG, Mazzei WJ, Severinghaus JW: Multipatient anesthetic mass spectrometry: Rapid analysis of data stored in long catheters. Anesthesiology 1981; 55:62–70.
21. Severinghaus JW, Ozanne GM: Multi-operating room monitoring with one mass spectrometer. Acta Anaesthesiol Scand Suppl 1978; 70:186–187.
22. Williams EL, Benson DM: Helium-induced errors in clinical mass spectrometry. Anesth Analg 1988; 67:83–85.
23. Davies NJH, Denison DM: The uses of long sampling probes in respiratory mass spectrometry. Respir Physiol 1979; 37:335–346.
24. Eger EI, Bahlman SH: Is the end-tidal anesthetic partial pressure an accurate measure of the arterial anesthetic partial pressure? Anesthesiology 1971; 35:301–303.
25. Long DA: Raman Spectroscopy. New York: McGraw-Hill, 1977.
26. VanWagenen RA: Dedicated monitoring of anesthetic and respiratory gases by Raman scattering. J Clin Monit 1986; 2:215–222.
27. Westenskow DR, Smith KW, Coleman DL, et al: Clinical evaluation of a Raman scattering multiple gas analyzer. Anesthesiology 1989; 70:350–355.
28. Hayes JK, Westenskow DR, Jordan WS: Monitoring anesthetic vapor concentrations using a piezoelectric detector: Evaluation of the Engstrom EMMA. Anesthesiology 1983; 59:435–439.
29. Linstromberg JW, Muir JJ: Cross-sensitivity in water vapor in the Engstrom EMMA. Anesth Analg 1984; 63:75–78.
30. Bruce DL, Eide KA, Linde HW, Eckenhoff JE: Causes of death among anesthesiologists: A 20 year survey. Anesthesiology 1968; 29:565–569.
31. Cascorbi HF, Blake DA, Helrich M: Differences in the biotransformation of halothane in man. Anesthesiology 1970; 32:119–123.
32. Cohen EN, Brown BW, Bruce DL, et al: Occupational disease among operating room personnel: A national study. Anesthesiology 1974; 41:321–340.
33. Mazze RI, Fujinaga M, Rice SA, et al: Reproductive and teratogenic effects of nitrous oxide, halothane, isoflurane, and enflurane in Sprague-Dawley rats. Anesthesiology 1986; 64:339–344.
34. Cohen EN, Bellville JW, Brown BW: Anesthesia, pregnancy, and miscarriage. Anesthesiology 1971; 35:343–347.
35. Askrog V, Harvald B: Teratogen effect of inhalation anesthetics. Nord Med 1970; 83:498–500.
36. Bruce DL, Bach MJ, Arbit J: Trace anesthetic effects on perceptual cognitive and motor skills. Anesthesiology 1974; 40:453–458.
37. Bruce DL, Bach MJ: Psychological studies of human performance as affected by traces of enflurane and nitrous oxide. Anesthesiology 1975; 42:194–196.
38. Spence AA, Cohen EN, Brown BW, et al: Occupational hazards for operating room-based physicians. JAMA 1977; 238:955–959.
39. Burting JE, Hennekens CH, Mayrent SL, et al: Health experiences of operating room personnel. Anesthesiology 1985; 62:325–330.
40. Cohen EN, Brown BW, Bruce DL, et al: A survey of anesthetic health hazards among dentists. J Am Dent Assoc 1975; 90:2191–2196.
41. Brown BR, Sagalyn AM: Hepatic microsomal enzyme induction by inhalation anesthetics: Mechanism in the rat. Anesthesiology 1974; 40:152–161.
42. Linde HW, Berman ML: Nonspecific stimulation of drug-metabolizing enzyme by inhalation anesthetic drugs. Anesth Analg 1971; 50:656–667.
43. Ross WT, Cordell RR: Proliferation of smooth endoplasmic reticulum and induction of microsomal drug metabolizing enzymes after ether or halothane. Anesthesiology 1978; 48:325–331.
44. Whitcher CE, Cohen EN, Trudell JR: Chronic exposure to anesthetic gases in the operating room. Anesthesiology 1971; 35:348–353.
45. Ericson HA, Källén AJB: Hospitalization for miscarriages and delivery outcome among Swedish nurses working in operating rooms 1973–1978. Anesth Analg 1985; 64:981–988.
46. Lecky JH: The mechanical aspects of anethestic pollution control. Anesth Analg 1977; 56:769–774.
47. Annis JP: Scavenging system for the Harvey blood oxygenator. Anesthesiology 1976; 45:359–360.
48. Miller JD: A device for the removal of waste anesthetic gases from the extra-corporeal oxygenator. Anesthesiology 1976; 44:181–184.
49. Muravchik S: Scavenging enflurane from extracorporeal pump oxygenators. Anesthesiology 1977; 468–470.
50. Isley AH, Crea J, Cousins MJ: Evaluation of infrared analysis used for monitoring waste anesthetic gas levels in operating theatres. Anaesth Intensive Care 1980; 8:436–440.
51. Gray WM, Burnside GW: The evacuated canister method of personal sampling. Anaesthesia 1985; 40:288–294.
52. Whitcher C, Piziali RL: Monitoring occupational exposure to inhalation anesthetics. Anesth Analg 1977; 56:778–785.
53. National Institute for Occupational Safety and Health: Criteria for a recommended standard . . . occupational exposure to waste anesthetic gases and vapors. DHEW (NIOSH) Publ No 77–140, 1977.

SECTION EIGHT

Miscellaneous Monitors

CHAPTER

25

Stethoscopy and Thermometry

CAROL L. LAKE, M.D.

STETHOSCOPY

Pathologic noises emanating from the body were noted in the seventeenth and eighteenth centuries. Initial efforts to hear these noises were by direct application of the physician's ear to the patient's chest or abdomen. Laënnec, faced with the inability to auscultate the heart of an obese patient, recalled the observation that a hollow tube amplified sounds. He placed one end of a rolled tube of paper against the patient's chest and the other in his ear, creating the first stethoscope.[1] Other landmarks in the development of stethoscopy are described in Chang's historical review[1] and in Chapter 1.

INDICATIONS

A precordial or esophageal stethoscope should be used in all anesthetic procedures, no matter how brief. Stethoscopy provides an uncomplicated, nonelectric method to qualitatively assess heart and lung function.

TYPES

Precordial

Precordial weighted stethoscopes are available in three sizes—small, medium, and large—for application with double-sided tape disks to the precordium or sternal notch (Fig. 25–1). However, a simple stethoscope made from the rubber plunger tip of an appropriate-sized, disposable syringe and fitted with a 14-gauge intravenous catheter to connect the lumen to an earpiece is an inexpensive, disposable alternative.[2] Various types of rubber or plastic tubing connect the stethoscope to monaural or standard binaural earpieces. The presence and quality of heart and lung sounds are commonly assessed using precordial stethoscopes. However, no data on the frequency response or effects of different types and lengths of tubing on the transmission of sounds exist.[3]

Esophageal

An esophageal stethoscope is an inexpensive, simple monitor of heart and lung sounds introduced into anesthesia practice more than 3 decades ago (Fig. 25–2*A*).[4] It consists of a catheter fitted with openings in the distal 2–3 cm, which are covered by a rubber cuff. Esophageal stethoscopes do not require electricity or complicated technologic interpretation. Examples of clinical situations detected with esophageal stethoscopy include dysrhythmias, ventilator disconnection or malfunction, wheezing, and quality of heart tones, including murmurs.[5] More sophisticated versions of the esophageal stethoscope incorporate thermistors (Fig. 25–2*B* and electrocardiograph (ECG) electrodes (Fig. 25–2*C*).[6] The advantages of monitoring the ECG from the esophagus are discussed in Chapter 5.[7] In addition to the risks of esophageal damage from passage of the probe, esophageal burns from leakage currents can occur when stethoscopes are connected to electrically powered ECG and temperature modules.[8]

Amplified

Small lightweight microphones attached to precordial or esophageal stethoscopes amplify the heart and breath sounds via direct, hard-wired, or telemetric devices. The output of these battery-operated devices can be monitored through earphones.

Doppler

Doppler probes of 2.4 MHz transmit and reflect ultrasound from the heart of both infants and adults. The optimal location for cardiac monitoring is the third or fourth intercostal space to the right of the sternum. However, the probe should be placed where sound transmission is best, particularly in response to rapid injection of fluid through a central venous catheter. Precordial Doppler probes are usu-

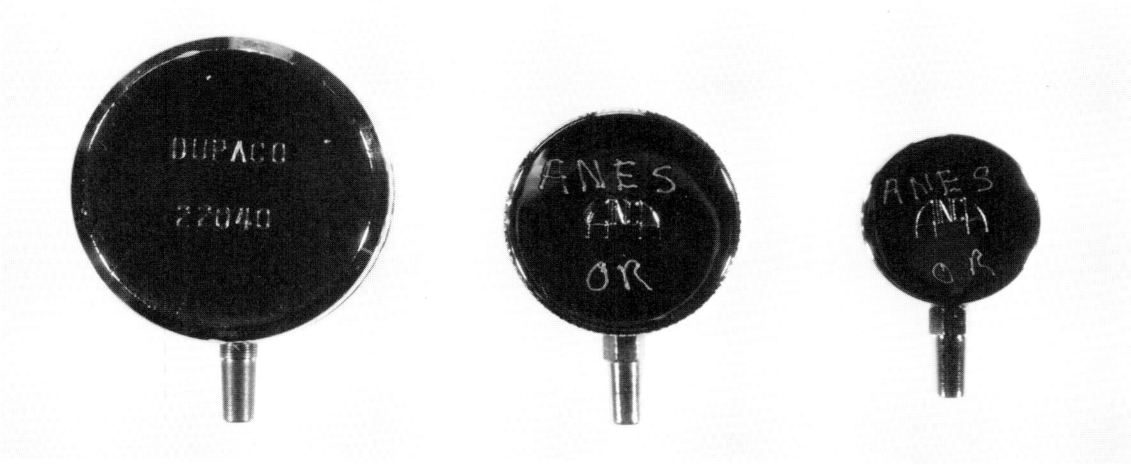

Figure 25–1. Weighted precordial bell-type stethoscopes for use in adults, children, and infants. They can also be placed over the trachea at the sternal notch for better transmission of breath sounds. A double-sided adhesive disk secures the stethoscope to the skin.

ally used for detection of venous air embolism rather than for routine cardiac monitoring. Unlike the normal cardiac sounds, air embolism causes a characteristic high-pitched scratching noise.[9] An unfortunate disadvantage of Doppler technology is interference by electrocautery.

COMPLICATIONS

Loss of an esophageal stethoscope into the stomach coincident to placement of a nasogastric tube and a second esophageal stethoscope has been reported.[10] Stethoscopes may fracture with retention of fragments in the gastrointestinal tract. Misidentification of the esophagus containing a stethoscope for the trachea or the internal jugular vein containing a ventriculojugular shunt catheter has been reported in children.[11] Misplacement of stethoscopes into the trachea instead of the esophagus causes significant gas leakage around the endotracheal tube cuff, which may preclude adequate ventilation.[12] Loss of the cuff of the esophageal stethoscope can occur, especially with repeated use. Inadvertent fixation of the stethoscope during surgical repairs around the nasopharynx or esophagus can be avoided by using a precordial device or by verifying mobility of the stethoscope during surgical procedures in the area. Esophageal stethoscopes are flammable at clinically used oxygen and nitrous oxide concentrations if a source of ignition is nearby.[13]

THERMOMETRY

PHYSIOLOGY OF THERMOREGULATION

Heat Gain

Body heat is primarily produced by metabolism in the liver and skeletal muscles. Basal heat production ranges from 65 to 85 kcal/hour. Heat is produced by voluntary muscle activity (exercise), involuntary muscle activity (shivering), and nonshivering thermiogenesis (NST). During moderate work or exercise, heat production increases to 300 kcal/hour. With maximum work, heat production increases to 600 kcal/hour or more. Heat generated from muscular contraction is transferred to blood flowing through the muscle bed. The temperature of the body core as well as blood exiting from the liver or lower extremities increases during exercise.

NST, an oxygen-consuming, heat-producing mechanism stimulated by the sympathetic nervous system, is the major mechanism for heat production in infants. It results from byproducts of glucose metabolism, fatty acid metabolism, and gluconeogenesis. In infants, fatty acids are liberated from triglycerides because of lipase release (stimulated by norepinephrine) in brown fat and oxidized in muscle, white fat, brain, and liver or re-esterified or oxidized in brown fat. Brown fat, accounting for 2–6% of body weight, is located between the scapulae, around kidneys, adrenals, vertebrae, neck blood vessels, and mediastinum, and in the axillae. It causes the infant's neck and interscapular skin to be warmer than other body parts during cold exposure. Microscopically, brown fat contains numerous mitochondria, densely packed with cristae and respiratory chain components.[14] NST is more energy-efficient than shivering thermiogenesis, which is, nevertheless, fully developed in infants. It is unaffected by neuromuscular blockade[15] but is blocked by sympathectomy, ganglionic blockade, and beta-adrenergic blockade.

Heat Loss

Physiologic Mechanisms

Convection, conduction, and radiation from the skin surface and lungs normally dissipate the heat produced and protect the body from thermal damage. The thermoregula-

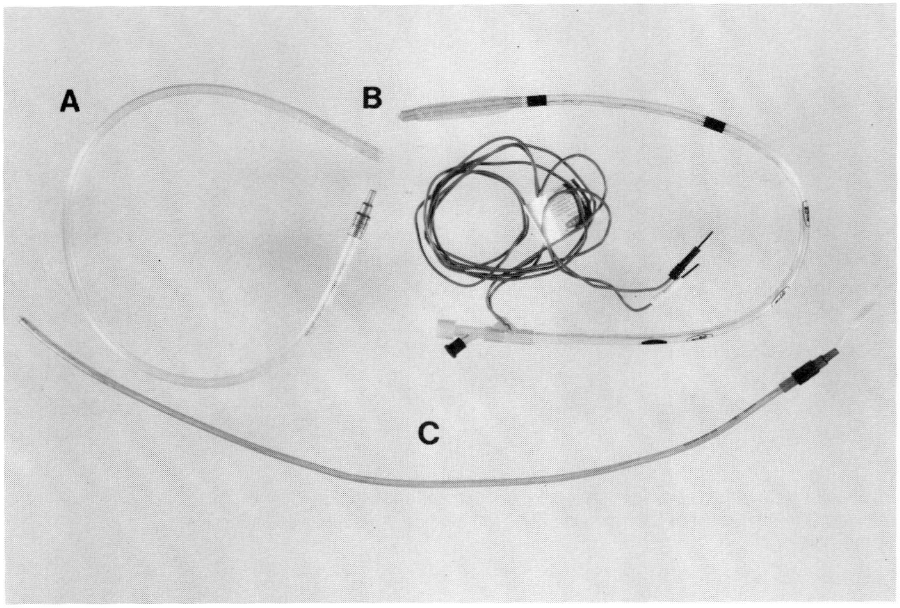

Figure 25–2. Esophageal stethoscopes of various types. *A* is an adult stethoscope. Stethoscope *B* is modified with two electrodes for monitoring the electrocardiogram. Stethoscope *C* has an integral thermistor for monitoring esophageal temperature.

tory center is located in the anterior and posterior hypothalamus, the anterior temperature-sensitive area known as the Aronsohn-Sachs center and the posterior, temperature-insensitive area known as the Krehl-Isenschmidt center.[16] The hypothalamic temperature changes as heated blood from muscle flows into the area. The posterior hypothalamus receives sensory input of temperature changes, and the anterior hypothalamus adjusts the mechanisms controlling heat loss and production. An increase in hypothalamic temperature induces systemic dilatation of skin vessels and secretion of sweat to offset the increase, a process known as the Benzinger reflex.[17] Cold impulses arriving in the posterior hypothalamus induce shivering to initiate heat production. However, in the presence of normal or increased body temperature, the anterior hypothalamus overrides the posterior center, preventing heat production. Because hypothalamic temperature is integral to thermal equilibrium, its temperature should probably be regarded as the ''core temperature.''

In addition to the central thermoreceptors, peripheral thermoreceptors are found in the skin. From these receptors, cold impulses (activated at skin temperatures of < 40°C and maximal at 30–35°C) travel through the A delta nerve fibers, whereas warm impulses are carried by the C fibers (activated at 30–35°C and maximal at 40–45°C).[18]

Alterations in the core temperature away from its set point initiates changes in heat production or heat loss. To maintain a balance between heat production and heat loss, the autonomic nervous system varies the blood supply to the body surface, causing shivering or sweating.[19] If the environmental temperature is cool, a thermal gradient between the body surface and the environment allows rapid dissipation. If environmental temperature is increased to body surface temperature or greater, heat is lost only by vaporization of sweat. Maximal rates of sweat vaporization are limited by atmospheric humidity, air movement, and rate of sweating. At conditions of increased humidity, heat loss through sweat vaporization is limited, and body temperature increases. Practically, the amount of heat loss through sweating is about 650 kcal/hour.[20]

In addition to sweating, cardiovascular changes occur in

TABLE 25–1. PHYSIOLOGIC CONSEQUENCES OF TEMPERATURE ALTERATIONS

Increased Temperature
Increased respiratory work
Increased cardiac work
Increased oxygen demand
Hypovolemia
Acidosis (respiratory and metabolic)
Decreased Temperature
Patient discomfort
Increased oxygen demand (shivering)
Decreased drug disposition
Decreased myocardial contractility and compliance
Impaired coronary autoregulation (coronary perfusion dependent on diastolic pressure)[120, 121]
Decreased total myocardial oxygen consumption (oxygen consumption/beat same or increased)[120]
Cardiac dysrhythmias (atrial and ventricular, ventricular fibrillation around 28°C, asystole with profound hypothermia), J point elevation on ECG, conduction disturbances (increased P-R interval, A-V block, widening of the QRS complex), bradycardia, and Osborne wave (secondary wave following S wave)
Peripheral vasoconstriction (increased systemic vascular resistance, decreased microcirculatory flow, increased hematocrit)
Decreased cerebral blood flow and $CMRO_2$
Central nervous system depression, delirium, and coma (EEG slowing between 30 and 35°C, decreased EEG amplitude below 30°C, isoelectricity of increasing duration below 22°C)
Decreased oxygen availability (oxyhemoglobin dissociation curve shifted to left)
Sympathetic stimulation
Hyperglycemia
Thrombocytopenia and impaired platelet thromboxane synthesis
Decreased anesthetic requirements and delayed anesthetic emergence

humans exposed to hot environments (Table 25–1). These changes include increased cardiac output, tachycardia, decreased hepatic and splanchnic blood flow, decreased systemic vascular resistance, and reduced effective arterial volume. In adequately conditioned and heat-acclimatized humans, maximum cardiac output increases, peak heart rate decreases, stroke volume increases, and sweat composition and volume change to limit volume and sodium loss. However, these compensatory mechanisms are overwhelmed by prolonged exposure to high environmental temperatures. Sweating ceases, cardiac output and stroke volume decrease, and cutaneous blood flow is reduced while core temperature increases. The end result is heat stroke, which is characterized by rectal temperature greater than 41.1°C, delirium, and coma.[20] Even physically conditioned and heat-acclimatized individuals may suffer heat stroke during extreme exertion.

Nonphysiologic Mechanisms

Infants have considerable difficulty maintaining their core temperature in the face of changing ambient temperatures. They have a small body mass acting as a heat generator, but a large surface area for heat loss (ratio of surface to mass = 3:1). Heat loss is also increased in infants because of their lack of subcutaneous tissue and decreased motor tone.

Thermoregulation increases oxygen consumption in infants in proportion to the ambient–to–skin surface temperature gradient.[21] Thus, the thermoregulatory range of infants is significantly limited compared with that of adults. Minimum ambient temperature for thermoregulation is 22°C in an infant compared with 0°C in an adult. Minimum oxygen consumption in infants occurs at environmental temperatures of 32–34°C, the neutral thermal state, in which there is less than a 2-degree gradient between environmental and abdominal skin temperature.[22] Thus, the usual recommendations are to maintain operating room temperature at 27°C for premature infants, at 26°C for infants up to 6 months of age, and at 25°C for infants from 6 months to 24 months of age.[23] However, most operating room personnel are most comfortable with relative humidities of less than 50%, temperatures of 18°C, and an air exchange rate of 25 times/hour or greater.[24]

In humans, heat loss occurs in two phases: (1) transfer of heat from body core to skin surface (internal temperature gradient) and (2) heat dissipation (the external temperature gradient). Heat loss is determined by the skin and environmental temperatures, the thermal transfer coefficient, and surface area. Tissue thickness, body size, and blood flow determine thermal transfer coefficients. Heat transfer from the core to the surface of the body creates an internal temperature gradient. Vasoconstriction decreases cutaneous blood flow and increases tissue insulation, attempting to increase the internal temperature gradient and reduce conductive and convective heat loss.

Heat loss across the external temperature gradient is affected by evaporation, convection, conduction, and radiation. Evaporative heat losses through the skin and respiratory systems depend on minute ventilation, air flow velocity, and relative humidity (specifically the difference between vapor pressures in the environment and on the skin surface). The transfer of heat to the air currents (convection) is influenced by air velocity, specific heat of the flowing gas, surface area, and ambient temperature. Because of high air turnover rates in operating rooms, convection causes about 25% of body heat loss.[23, 25] Trapping a layer of air between the skin and the environment reduces heat loss by convection.

Heat loss by conduction depends on a temperature gradient between contacting surfaces and is affected by surface area and the thermal conductivity of the surface. Wetting increases conduction by 25–30 times.[23] The transfer of heat between two objects in the form of electromagnetic energy is radiant heat loss. It is independent of environmental temperature but dependent on the radiating surface area and proportional to the temperature difference between skin and surrounding environment.[15, 25] Radiation is the largest source of heat loss (65%) for the human body.[23]

INDICATIONS FOR TEMPERATURE MEASUREMENT

The measurement of body temperature by some route is a standard of care during all anesthetic procedures. The risk of both malignant hyperthermia and accidental hypothermia necessitate continuous observation of temperature. A specific indication for temperature monitoring is induced hypothermia, either by surface or by perfusion (extracorporeal circulation) cooling.

Measurements of skin, core, and mean body temperature are typically made or calculated in the perioperative period. Accurate assessments of skin temperature require measurements at four or more sites.[26] Mean body temperature in neutral or warm environments is calculated as

$$T_{body} = (0.66 \times T_{core}) + (0.34 \times T_{skin})$$

where T_{core} is core temperature, T_{body} is mean body temperature, and T_{skin} is mean skin temperature.[27] Total body heat (TBH) is determined as

$$\text{TBH} = \text{mean temperature} \times \text{weight (kg)} \times \text{specific heat}$$

where the specific heat of the human body is 3.475 $kJ°C^{-1}$.[28]

METHODS

Body temperature was first measured by John Hunter in 1776 using a mercury-in-glass thermometer under the tongue. Glass thermometers are still used clinically but are usually impractical perioperatively in semiconscious patients.

Thermistors, Thermocouples

A thermistor or thermally sensitive resistor includes semiconductive elements (heavy metal oxides such as manganese, iron, zinc, cobalt, nickel) in which electrical resistance varies with temperature. Electrodes are attached to a bead of the metal oxide, which is sealed into a small measuring tip. Large changes in resistance correspond to changes in temperature, allowing a rapid response time. Thermistors are usually accurate to ± 5°C over a range from −80 to +150°C, but narrower ranges improve linearity.[29]

In a thermocouple, voltage is produced by the electromotive force (Seebeck effect) between two dissimilar metals (usually copper and constantan, a mixture of copper and nickel), which depends on the temperature difference between two junctions maintained at different temperatures, a standard thermoneutral or "cold" junction and the probe end of the thermocouple. One of the junctions is maintained as the "reference" junction; the other becomes the "measuring" junction, located within the probe. The electromotive force generated is proportional to the temperature difference between the two junctions.[29] Thermocouples have several advantages, including small size and reproducibility. A problem with thermocouples involving the reference junction is the Peltier effect, in which a current passed around the thermocouple circuit creates cold at one junction and heat at the other, so that the reference junction does not remain thermoneutral.

Liquid-Crystal Devices

Adhesive liquid-crystal temperature detectors measure skin temperature over ranges of 92–104°F and 34–40°C (Fig. 25–3). Skin temperature on the forehead is usually close to oral temperature but demonstrates considerable individual variation. Although temperatures measured with liquid crystal thermometry correlate well with forehead skin temperature, their correlation with temperatures monitored at other sites is poor (r = 0.54 to esophageal or tympanic probes).[30] Vaughan and colleagues reported that, compared with tympanic membrane thermometry, liquid-crystal strips failed to accurately track temperature trends in postanesthetic patients.[31] Their data suggest that temperature in the body shell is an unreliable indicator of core temperature.[31] Skin thermistors are also unreliable indicators of malignant hyperthermia, because peripheral vasoconstriction is an initial feature of the syndrome.

Despite their inaccuracy, the convenience of liquid-crystal thermometers makes them useful for continuous temperature monitoring in operating rooms and postanesthesia care units and during the sympathetic blockade of peripheral nerve blocks. For perioperative use, the sensors are applied to the forehead, whereas during sympathetic blocks, they are applied to the involved extremity. Advantages include safety (completely noninvasive) and low cost. Disadvantages include difficulties with adhesion secondary to skin secretions, susceptibility to external thermal influences such as radiant heat lamps or air currents, allergic reactions to adhesive backing, and inaccuracy and imprecision.[30–32]

Infrared Thermometry

Another method of clinical thermometry is an infrared tympanic probe, which determines temperature by measuring the infrared radiation given off by an object. It consists of an otoscope-like probe covered by a disposable speculum, which is introduced into the external auditory canal like an otoscope. The sensor in the probe gathers emitted infrared radiation for about 1 second and then transfers that information to an analog-to-digital converter and microprocessor. A liquid crystal displays the resultant temperature on a base module. Accuracy of this technology has been documented with *in vitro* water baths as well as *in vivo*. Clinical trials demonstrate a correlation coefficient of the infrared tympanic probe with pulmonary artery thermistor of 0.98[33] and with esophageal temperature.[18] Aural canal and tympanic thermometry accurately assess hypothalamic temperature.[18] Advantages of this technology include the speed of determination, reduced potential for cross-contamination, and the absence of need for direct contact and temperature equilibrium of the device with the measuring surface.

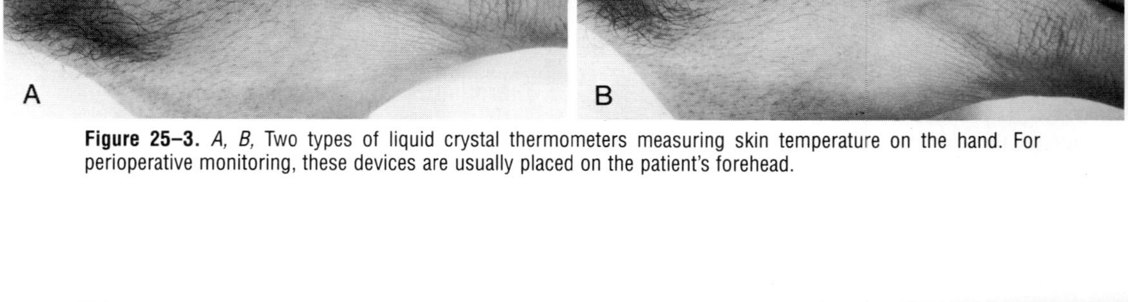

Figure 25–3. *A, B,* Two types of liquid crystal thermometers measuring skin temperature on the hand. For perioperative monitoring, these devices are usually placed on the patient's forehead.

SITES

Sites used for measurement of body temperature include the skin, nasopharynx, esophagus, bladder, rectum, axilla, and tympanic membrane. Central sites for temperature monitoring include the esophagus, nasopharynx, tympanic membrane, and pulmonary artery. Intermediate sites are the bladder and rectum. The skin is the most common peripheral site.

The choice of sites depends on the purpose of the measurements. Usually, either specific organ temperature or core (total body) temperature is needed. Temperatures measured in the tympanic membrane or nasopharynx estimate brain temperature. Esophageal temperature approximates myocardial temperature. Cork and coworkers report the greatest precision (correlation between tympanic membrane and other sites) and accuracy (accuracy defined by difference from the tympanic membrane temperature) for temperature measurements in the urinary bladder, nasopharynx, and esophagus.[34] Axilla, great toe, and forehead temperatures are less accurate than those obtained at the other sites.[34]

Tympanic Membrane

The efficacy and convenience of tympanic thermometry was documented more than 2 decades ago. Measurement of tympanic membrane temperature as an index of brain temperature is particularly prudent, because thermal homeostasis depends on anterior hypothalamic temperature.[35] At the tympanic membrane, the thermoelectric sensor is in the vicinity of the internal carotid artery, the major cerebral blood supply.[36] The tympanic membrane and surrounding structures are supplied by branches of the external carotid artery, including the internal maxillary and posterior auricular arteries. Tympanic temperatures parallel temperatures measured from an ideally placed esophageal thermistor, except that tympanic temperatures are lower by about 0.2°C.[36] The tympanic membrane may be the optimum site during profound hypothermic circulatory arrest.[37]

An otoscopic examination to document patency of the auditory canal should precede tympanic or external auditory canal thermometry. The presence of cerumen may render measurements inaccurate.

Nasopharyngeal

Nasopharyngeal temperatures estimate brain temperature, particularly when the thermistor is carefully positioned behind the soft palate. However, air leakage around tracheal tube cuffs affects nasopharyngeal probe accuracy.[38] Another disadvantage is the possibility of epistaxis or adenoidal bleeding in children.

Esophageal

Esophageal temperatures are affected by ventilation (particularly when the thermistor is placed at the mid or upper esophagus),[38] thoracotomy, or rapid infusion of cold fluids and blood, which cools the heart and great vessels. Variations of 1–6°C have been reported, depending on the location of the tip of the probe within the esophagus,[36, 38, 39] varying with tracheal intubation, tracheal extubation, and intrathoracic manipulation. Kaufman noted that coolest portion of the esophagus was where both heart and breath sounds were best heard, and the warmest point was 12–16 cm past the position of best cardiorespiratory sounds.[39] Compared with the lower esophagus, temperature at the tracheal bifurcation is about 1°C lower and at the atrium about 0.5°C lower.[40] The ideal location for the thermistor is about 45 cm from the nostril so that its tip is between the heart and descending thoracic aorta and below the pulmonary veins.[41] However, this suggestion assumes that the distance between the teeth and the heart is similar in all individuals. Accurate positioning of the probe in relation to the heart is achieved by auscultation through an integral esophageal stethoscope (Fig. 25–2*C*). Whitby and Dunkin noted that temperatures in the lower esophagus approximated cerebral temperatures in the absence of rapid infusions of cold fluids or an open thorax.[38]

Contraindications to esophageal temperature measurements are bronchoscopy, esophagoscopy, laryngoscopy, certain facial or oral surgical procedures, and patients with esophageal pathology (varices, Zenker's diverticulum). However, Ritter and coworkers inserted esophageal stethoscopes in patients with varices undergoing hepatic transplantation without any incidents of bleeding.[42] Normal esophageal temperature are from 36.9 to 37.7°C.[29]

Bladder

Urinary catheters with thermistor tips have been available for more than a decade, providing a safe, continuous, and convenient method for temperature measurement.[43] Both urine volume and bladder temperature are simultaneously measured. Bladder temperature is usually 0.2°C higher than rectal temperature, 0.7°C greater than esophageal temperature, and 3.5°C more than skin temperature (thumb).[44] During extracorporeal cooling and rewarming, temperature in the urinary bladder changes more rapidly than does rectal temperature.[45] Lilly noted excellent correlation between urinary bladder and esophageal, rectal, and pulmonary artery temperatures; the strongest correlation occurred with pulmonary artery temperatures during extracorporeal rewarming.[43] Nevertheless, the advantages of bladder temperature monitoring may be outweighed by the risks of bladder catheterization if a urinary catheter is not otherwise indicated.

Rectum

The rectum is distant from the central nervous system and the heart and, therefore, has little thermal significance. Several sources of inaccuracy of rectal temperatures are the presence of heat-producing bacteria in the rectum, insulation by feces, and cold blood returning from the legs.[46] Temperatures measured in the rectum often differ substantially from those measured in other areas. For this reason, rectal temperatures should be considered erroneous if they differ from other points. However, rectal temperatures may be useful indicators of the temperature of poorly perfused tissues (Fig. 25–4).[29] Rectal thermometry is relatively contraindicated during surgical procedures in the lower pelvis or during organ transplantation because of the infection risk in an immunocompromised patient. The risk of rectal perforation should always be considered during placement of probes, particularly in infants and children. Normal rectal temperatures are 36.9–37.7°C.[29]

Skin

Skin temperature is lower than core temperature, and the skin-to-core gradient decreases during general anesthesia.[47] Factors altering thermal conduction, convection, and radiation affect skin temperature, so that the measured temperature is a balance between metabolic heat production and cutaneous loss. The forehead and axilla are common skin sites to monitor temperature. Axillary temperature normally ranges from 35.3 to 36.7°C.[29] However, measurement is affected by pressure on the probe and by sweat production.

Other Sites

During cardiopulmonary bypass, temperatures of the venous blood returning to the extracorporeal circuit and arterial blood leaving the circuit are routinely measured. Muscle temperatures can be measured with a 25-gauge needle thermistor. Because a special probe is required, muscle temperatures are infrequently measured. However, muscle temperatures are quite responsive to blood flow. During extracorporeal cooling and rewarming, muscle remains warmer during hypothermia and cooler after rewarming.

Temperature can be measured in the pulmonary artery through the thermistor used for thermodilution cardiac output determinations. However, temperatures from this site are affected by ventilation, use of topical pericardial hypothermia, and cold cardioplegia solutions. In the absence of topical hypothermia and cardioplegia, pulmonary artery temperatures indicate core temperature. After discontinuation of cardiopulmonary bypass, pulmonary artery temperatures tend to be lower than temperatures at nasopharyngeal, rectal, and other sites.[48]

In the perioperative period, temperature on the great toe of cardiac surgical patients has been advocated as an indicator of peripheral perfusion because of the dependence of its temperature on cutaneous blood flow. This temperature also correlates well with cardiac output.[49] However, this temperature does not indicate skin temperature.[50]

COMPLICATIONS OF THERMOMETRY

Tympanic membrane temperature probes have a reported complication rate of less than 3%, with the primary complication being bleeding from the external auditory canal.[51] Other complications from the tympanic site include tympanic membrane perforation.[52] As described earlier, burns are possible when temperature probes are electrically operated and leakage currents are present.[8]

ALTERATIONS IN TEMPERATURE IN PERIOPERATIVE PERIOD

Induced Hypothermia

Hypothermia has been used in both neurosurgery and cardiac surgery to decrease the metabolic rate and allow

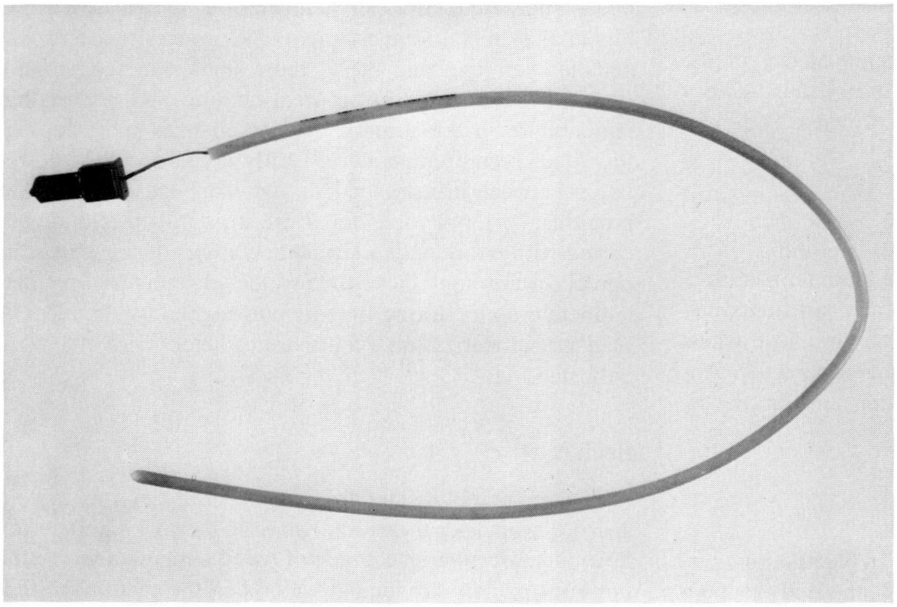

Figure 25–4. A disposable rectal temperature thermistor.

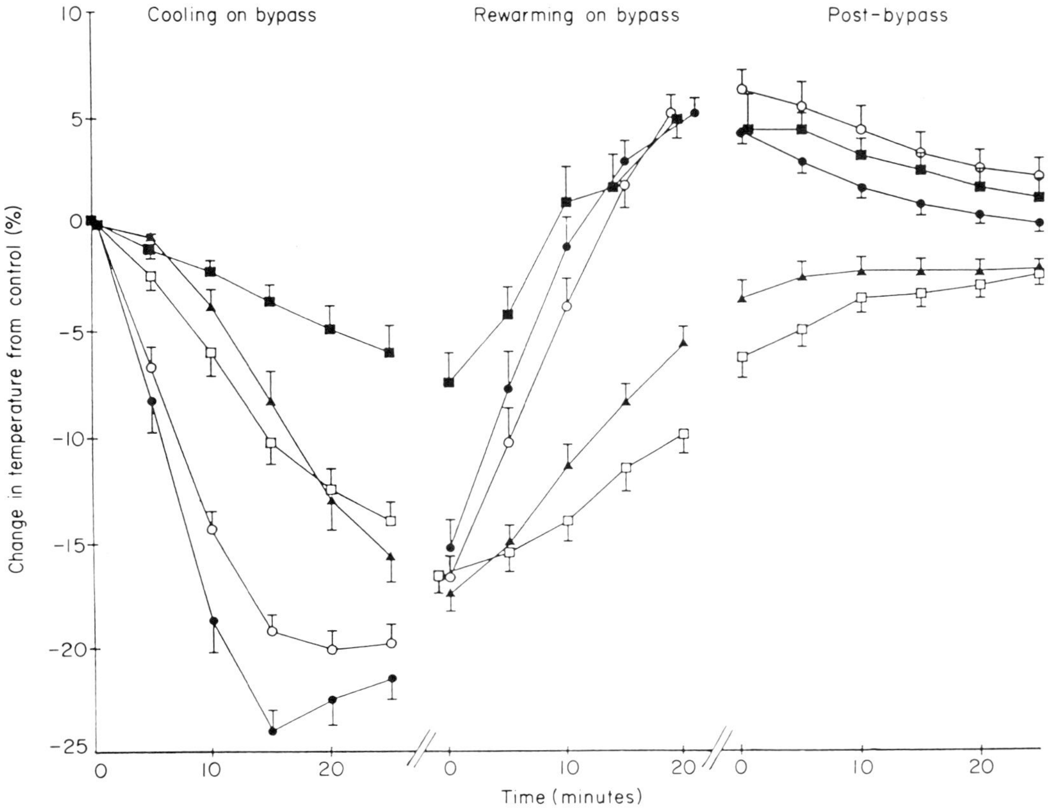

Figure 25–5. Changes in temperature as a percentage of control temperature during extracorporeal cooling and rewarming. Cooling and rewarming occurred most rapidly in the esophagus. Rewarming also occurred more rapidly in the nasopharynx *(open circles)* than in the bladder *(solid triangles)*, rectum *(open squares)*, or skin *(solid squares)*. Bladder temperature decreased more slowly during cooling and increased more slowly during rewarming than esophageal temperature did *(solid circles)*. Bladder temperatures remained below nasopharyngeal, esophageal, and skin temperatures after bypass. (From Bone ME, Feneck RO: Bladder temperatures as an estimate of body temperature during cardiopulmonary bypass. Anaesthesia 1988; 43:181–185, with permission of author and publisher.)

complex intracranial and intracardiac repairs. However, it is infrequently used in neurosurgery because of the prolonged time required for surface cooling and rewarming of the requisite anticoagulation if extracorporeal techniques are used. Some degree of hypothermia is used in most centers during cardiopulmonary bypass in both adult and pediatric patients. Profound hypothermia to esophageal temperatures of 10–12°C is used in children with congenital cardiac lesions or occasionally in adults with lesions of the aortic arch. Hypothermia with circulatory arrest provides ideal surgical conditions, decreases the duration of cardiopulmonary bypass, and prevents myocardial rewarming from washout of cardioplegia solutions by noncoronary collateral circulation.

Cold induces intense stimulation of thermoregulatory mechanisms, including sympathetic stimulation, vasoconstriction, shivering, and specific responses in the cardiorespiratory, central nervous, renal, hepatic, and endocrine systems. Anesthesia blunts both the sympathetic and shivering responses to hypothermia.

During surgery, hypothermia is induced by either surface or core cooling. Core cooling with an extracorporeal circuit causes significant differences in the temperature measured at various sites (Fig. 25–5). The rate of decrease in temperature is greatest in the esophagus and least in the rectum.[44] During perfusion cooling, bladder temperature is similar to rectal temperature but differs significantly from nasopharyngeal, esophageal, and skin temperatures.[44] During hypothermia, renal oxygen consumption decreases more rapidly than oxygen consumption in other organs, decreasing renal blood flow.

During perfusion rewarming, esophageal and nasopharyngeal temperatures demonstrated the greatest rate of rise, with increases in bladder and rectal temperatures occurring more slowly (Fig. 25–5).[44] Lilly and colleagues noted that urinary bladder temperature consistently increased faster than rectal temperature and correlated well with pulmonary artery temperature during extracorporeal rewarming.[43] Changes in esophageal and nasopharyngeal temperatures reflect blood flow from the extracorporeal circuit to the vital organs. Temperatures measured from these sites tend to overshoot the control values during rewarming.[44]

After perfusion hypothermia and rewarming, core temperature often decreases (''afterdrop'') after cessation of extracorporeal circulation. Afterdrop is defined as the difference between the nasopharyngeal temperature at the termination of bypass and the lowest nasopharyngeal temperature reached after bypass.[48] Ramsay and coworkers noted that the urinary bladder temperature at termination of bypass most closely indicated the amount of afterdrop and was minimized by a bladder temperature greater than 36.2°C.[48] The subsequent period of rewarming occurring 2–4 hours following extracorporeal cooling is accompanied by marked increases in oxygen consumption, carbon dioxide production, and shivering.[53, 54] Patients who do not exhibit shivering consume less oxygen during this period.[53]

Accidental Hypothermia

Hypothermia is defined as a reduction of core temperature to less than 35–36°C. In hospital settings, hypothermia commonly occurs in neonates exposed to cold environmental conditions or in adults anesthetized in cold operating rooms or transfused with unwarmed blood and fluids.[55, 56] Core temperature usually decreases during the early minutes of anesthesia because of uncovering of the patient, use of wet and cold preparation solutions, and losses due to the anesthetic administration system. Alterations in temperature at various measuring sites are shown in Figure 25–6.

Patients at risk for intraoperative hypothermia include the elderly[57] and patients with major burns, paraplegia, quadriplegia, cachexia, trauma, hypothyroidism, adrenal insufficiency, diabetes, uremia, epilepsy, and cirrhosis. During anesthesia, temperature decreases about 1.1°C/hour at age 80 years versus only 0.3°C/hour at age 20 years.[58] Burned patients are unable to limit passage of water vapor through the skin, and their peripheral thermoregulatory mechanisms are impaired. Cachectic patients may have lost both muscle mass responsible for heat production and insulating fat. Paraplegia and quadriplegia disrupt the thermosensory pathways as well as the motor pathways responsible for shivering, impairing both autonomic and behavioral thermoregulation. Exposure of large surfaces of the abdominal or thoracic cavities increases intraoperative heat loss (Table 25–2).[56, 59, 60] Neonates are particularly prone to hypothermia because of their large ratio of body surface area to heat-producing mass, decreased capacity to increase metabolic rate, limited energy stores, lack of insulating fat, and decreased shivering. Elderly patients are more prone to hypothermia in the perioperative period than are younger individuals.[61, 62] Aged humans are likely to become hypothermic because of immobility, impaired sensation, decreased shivering response, loss of muscle mass, reduced threshold for thermoregulatory vasoconstriction in response to cold (particularly during anesthesia),[63] and inability to maintain their core-to-surface temperature gradient. About

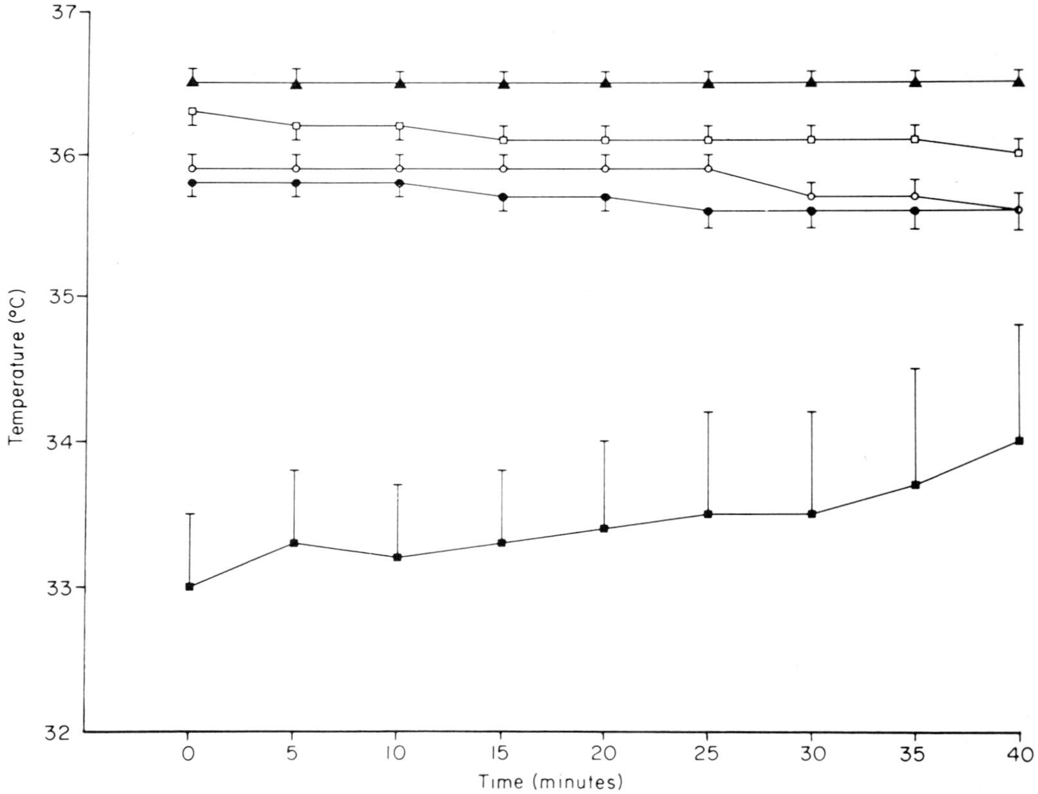

Figure 25–6. During the prebypass period, skin temperature *(solid squares)* is lower than internal body temperatures measured in the esophagus *(solid circles)*, nasopharynx *(open circles)*, rectum *(open squares)*, and bladder *(solid triangles)*. (From Bone ME, Feneck RO: Bladder temperature as an estimate of body temperature during cardiopulmonary bypass. Anaesthesia 1988; 43:181–185, with permission of author and publisher.)

60% of adult patients have hypothermia on arrival in postanesthetic care units.[57]

The human body loses heat by radiation, conduction, convection, and evaporation, as well as through the respiratory tract. Decreases in environmental temperature are first sensed by cutaneous cold-sensitive thermoreceptors. Warm-sensitive receptors in the anterior hypothalamus are stimulated by temperatures greater than 44°C, whereas cold-sensitive receptors are inactive until the environmental temperature is less than 24°C.[25]

Anesthetic Effects on Thermoregulation

General Anesthetic Effects on Thermoregulation. Body temperature is reduced to a greater degree during general than during regional anesthesia.[62] During general anesthesia, three phases of heat loss occur. Initially, hypothermia results from redistribution of heat from the central core to the peripheral shell of the body. This initial hypothermia can be minimized by preinduction, skin-surface warming with an electric blanket for 90 minutes in adult patients (Fig. 25–7).[64] A small amount of heat loss also occurs during surgical skin preparation, particularly with cold, alcohol-based solutions. Thermal losses during surgical preparation can be minimized by radiant warming, water-based solutions, and skin-drying after washing.[65]

Heat loss to the environment continues to exceed metabolic heat production during the second phase, reaching a plateau at 34–35.5°C in several hours.[66] Normally, thermoregulatory mechanisms respond quickly, causing vasoconstriction to decrease heat loss when decreases in temperature of < 0.4°C occur.[67] This thermoregulatory threshold is the central temperature at which significant peripheral vasoconstriction occurs.[68] However, anesthetized humans have altered thermoregulatory responses (determined by skin-surface temperature gradients between forearm and fingertip temperature and venous occlusion volume plethysmography)[69] during the third phase of hypothermia during anesthesia with halothane, isoflurane, or fentanyl and respond only to changes of 2.5–4°C.[70–72] Thus, peripheral thermoregulatory vasoconstriction occurs at a threshold temperature about 2.5°C below normal thermoregulatory levels during general anesthesia in both infants and adults.[73, 74] Thermoregulatory vasoconstriction, primarily in the extremities, reduces heat loss and the rate of core cooling in the third phase by 25%.[75, 76] However, during isoflurane anesthesia, vasoconstriction induced by thermoregulatory mechanisms decreases heat loss about 25%.[76]

Effects of Regional Anesthesia on Thermoregulation. Peripheral thermal receptors, particularly the warm-sensitive receptors, are blocked by regional anesthesia.[25] Patients receiving regional anesthesia rewarm less readily in the postoperative period because of continued vasodilation and muscle flaccidity.[57] During peridural anesthesia, administration of cold intravenous fluids, alterations in metabolic heat production, and environmental heat loss are insufficient to explain the 1–2°C decrease in central temperature. Instead, it is due to redistribution of body heat.[77] Suppression of vasoconstriction by epidural anesthesia increases heat loss to a small extent, and compensatory shivering thermiogenesis occurs.

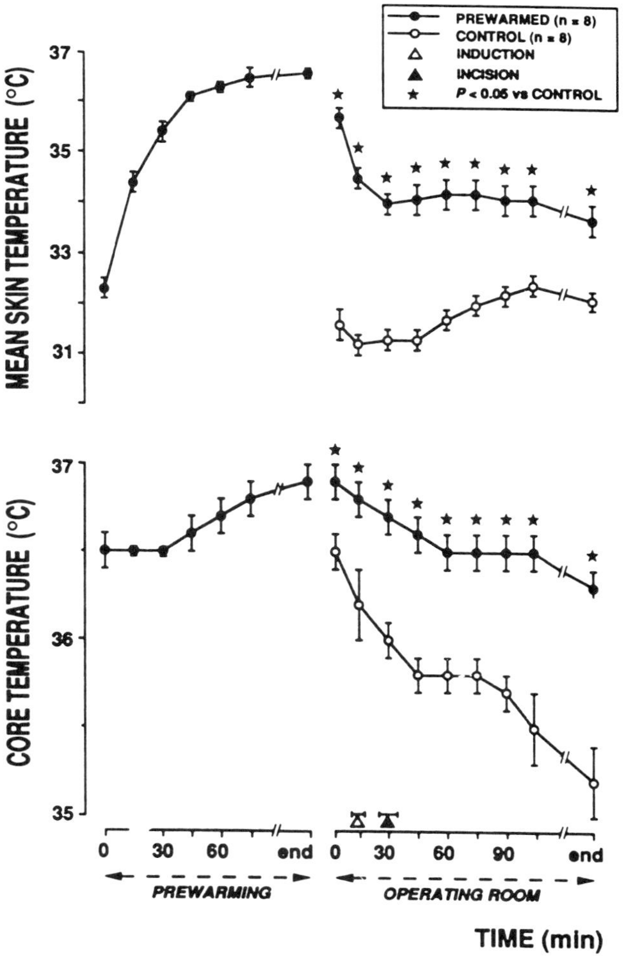

Figure 25–7. Prewarming of the skin of adult patients prior to surgical procedures minimizes the hypothermia that develops after induction of anesthesia. When prewarming is combined with intraoperative surface warming with an electric blanket, near normothermia is maintained, and postoperative shivering is prevented. (From Just B, et al: Prevention of intraoperative hypothermia by preoperative skin-surface warming. Anesthesiology 1993; 79:214–218, with permission of author and publisher.)

Effects of Hypothermia on Organ Systems

Total body metabolism decreases about 7–8% per degree Celsius as temperature decreases. Thus, metabolic rate is about 50% of normal at 28°C. Despite the decrease in metabolic rate, aerobic metabolism continues at low temperatures provided that adequate oxygen is delivered (see Table 25–1).

Heart and Circulatory Effects. In response to sympathetic activation during cooling, heart rate, stroke volume, and peripheral vascular tone increase, and shivering occurs. Shivering, the involuntary rhythmic contraction of muscle, is mediated through hypothalamic pathways. It ceases at temperatures below 27°C. During shivering, oxygen consumption and calorigenesis are increased,[53] but convective and radiant heat losses are also increased by the increased muscular activity.[56] Ralley and coworkers noted significant reductions in mixed venous oxygen tension even when cardiac output increased in shivering patients after cardiac surgery.[53] This finding indicates an imbalance between whole-body oxygen supply and demand, mandating that shivering patients always receive supplemental oxygen. A greater incidence of myocardial ischemia has been reported in hypothermic patients with peripheral vascular disease on the first postoperative day.[78]

As hypothermia develops, fluid shifts from the vascular space, increasing the hematocrit. Despite the shift of blood to the central compartment, cardiac output decreases beginning at 32°C. By 30°C, cardiac output is reduced 30–40%.[25] Hypovolemia and increased blood viscosity may further reduce cardiac output. Systemic vascular resistance increases with hyperviscosity. Microcirculatory flow is reduced.

Central Nervous System Effects. The effects of hypothermia on the central nervous system include depression of membrane conduction and neurochemical processes. As hypothermia progresses, alterations in the electroencephalogram (EEG) occur. The EEG remains normal to temperatures of 35°C. Between 30 and 35°C, the predominant rhythm slows. At temperatures of 32°C, responses to stimuli are slowed, ataxia is present, and there is slight clumsiness. The amplitude of the EEG decreases below 32°C. Below 32°C, delirium, followed by stupor and coma, occurs. Pupillary dilatation is seen below 30°C. Slower EEG rhythms predominate between 24 and 29°C. Periods of isoelectricity of ever-lengthening duration develop below temperatures of 22°C.[79] Anesthetic requirements decrease, so that minimum alveolar concentration decreases about 7% per degree Celsius.[80]

However, aerobic brain metabolism continues at low temperatures although the cerebral metabolic rate for oxygen ($CMRo_2$) slows concomitantly with temperature reduction. Cerebral blood flow also decreases with hypothermia (about 7% per degree Celsius)[56] because of decreased cardiac output, increased cerebrovascular resistance, and greater viscosity. At electrocerebral silence, there is no further reduction in $CMRo_2$. The preservative effects of hypothermia on the brain are greater than those predicted by decreased $CMRo_2$ alone. The "no reflow" phenomenon after ischemia is prevented by hypothermia.

Respiratory Effects. Respiratory rate initially increases as hypothermia ensues. Between 30 and 34°C, the respiratory response to carbon dioxide decreases (CO_2 response curve shifts to the right). Because carbon dioxide production decreases with hypothermia, respiratory alkalosis is often present. Dead space may increase owing to bronchodilation as temperature decreases if spontaneous respiration continues.

Hypoxic pulmonary vasoconstriction is reduced during hypothermia.[81] Ventilatory response to hypoxia may also be reduced, although it has been incompletely studied.[82] However, respiratory drive does not cease until 24°C.[56] Resistance in the pulmonary circulation increases with hypothermia. There is little change in lung compliance. Hypothermic patients should be fully rewarmed prior to extubation because of these effects on the respiratory system.

The oxyhemoglobin dissociation curve shifts to the left, diminishing release of oxygen at the tissue level. The affinity of oxygen for hemoglobin increases about 6% per degree Celsius. The question of assessment of acid-base disturbances during hypothermia is a controversial one addressed in detail in Chapter 27.

Hepatic and Renal Effects. Renal blood flow and oxygen consumption are reduced by hypothermia. Glomerular filtration rate decreases progressively during cooling. Because both renal blood flow and glomerular filtration rate decrease, filtration fraction is unchanged. Because tubular function requires active enzymatic processes, tubular function is decreased, reducing the concentrating effects of the renal tubules. Antidiuretic hormone release is suppressed, because cold-induced vasoconstriction is interpreted by the kidney as volume overload, resulting in diuresis of urine produced by glomerular filtration. Hemoconcentration also results from capillary sequestration of fluid.

Hepatic enzymatic and excretory processes are reduced with hypothermia. Blood flow to the liver is reduced, but blood shifts from the periphery to the splanchnic circulation. Drug metabolism is reduced. The liver is also a site for sequestration of platelets during hypothermia. Coagulopathy during hypothermia results from thrombocytopenia, decreased activity of clotting cascade, and slight decrease in platelet function.

Endocrine Effects. Because peripheral utilization of glucose and release of insulin decrease during hypothermia, blood glucose increases.[83] Parenteral insulin has little effect, but the hyperglycemia reverts to normal or near normal with rewarming. The stress response described previously causes release of adrenal cortical and medullary hormones (epinephrine and norepinephrine).[84, 85] In response to cold, the hypothalamus releases thyrotropin-releasing hormone, stimulating secretion of thyroxine and triiodothyronine to increase metabolic rate.

Profound hypothermia is compatible with life for brief periods because of the decreased metabolic rate and oxygen demand. However, prolonged hypothermia is not tolerated and usually causes death because of cardiac electrical conduction disturbances. Rewarming in therapeutic applications of hypothermia is usually with extracorporeal circulation at a gradient of no more than 10°C. In accidental hypothermia, surface methods are usually employed, coupled with supportive treatment of associated cardiac, respiratory, and coagulation problems.

Methods to Prevent or Minimize Perioperative Hypothermia

Postoperative hypothermia delays drug clearance, enhances peripheral vasoconstriction, and causes shivering. Shivering may occur because the patient is actually cold or because of a discrepancy between the actual core temperature (normal) and the thermostat set point (elevated), which activates heat generation.[86] For these reasons, both prevention and treatment are mandatory. Modalities to prevent or treat the mild to moderate hypothermia seen in the perioperative period include covering the patient with impervious insulation material, increasing the environmental temperature, using warmed respiratory gases and intravenous fluids, using forced air convection blankets, and using pharmacologic agents to reduce shivering (clonidine, ketanserin, meperidine, dexmedetomidine, chlorpromazine, droperidol, and nondepolarizing neuromuscular blockers).[87] The mechanism of improvement with clonidine is central thermoregulatory impairment, which decreases the thermoregulatory threshold for shivering and peripheral vasoconstriction.[88]

Environmental Warming. Warmer operating rooms (greater than 21°C) minimize decreases in temperature in adults as compared with unwarmed rooms.[89–91] The "critical ambient temperature" appears to be 21°C or 70°F for stability of patient temperature between 36 and 37.5°C.[90, 91] Room temperatures of 24–26°C are necessary to prevent any heat loss.[23] However, for a naked adult patient to maintain temperature without significant energy use requires ambient temperatures of 27–33°C.[23] The room temperatures must also be modified for patients with large ratios of surface area to body mass, those receiving large volumes of unwarmed intravenous fluids, those undergoing body cavity surgery, and those in a deeply anesthetized state.[90] However, Roizen and colleagues noted no difference in temperature in the postanesthetic period between patients undergoing surgical preparation and draping in a cold room and those in a warm operating room.[92] Temperatures at the beginning of surgery were lower in patients in the cold room.[92]

Patient Covering. Because radiation and convection account for as much as 80% of heat loss perioperatively, covering the patient as much as possible is beneficial. Covering the scalp prevents the 50% radiation of heat from the head. Warmed blankets reduce heat loss more than unwarmed blankets, but the effect is transient.[93] Sessler and coworkers noted that reflective paper drapes and unheated paper/plastic quiltlike blankets (blankets of forced-air convection devices) prevented heat loss better than did cloth, plastic, or paper drapes.[94] Body heat is conserved when increasing amounts of the patient's body surface area are covered with reflective materials.[94, 95] However, Radford and Thurlow were unable to prevent intraoperative hypothermia with reflective blankets.[96]

Forced Air Convection Blankets. The application of forced-air warming devices to adults, children, and infants over body surfaces uninvolved in the surgical procedure prevents intraoperative hypothermia more effectively than do circulating water mattresses.[97] The efficacy of these devices is maintained when approximately 25% of body surface area is available for warming in adults. In fact, these devices are so effective that continuous monitoring of the patient's core temperature is essential to prevent hyperthermia. Despite initial concerns to the contrary, Zink and Iaizzo failed to demonstrate increased airborne bacterial wound contamination during intraoperative forced-air convective warming.[98] Finally, some investigators suggest that a specific brand of forced-air warmer may be more efficient than other similar devices.[99]

Radiant Heating. Murphy and coworkers demonstrated that radiant heat lamps stopped postanesthetic shivering (in animals) even without rewarming the core temperature.[100] Sharkey and colleagues showed that radiant heat lamps, but not warm blankets, terminated postanesthetic shivering within 10 minutes of application.[101] Other methods of radiant heat include frequently changed warm blankets or an active warming blanket. Operations in infants can be performed in specially modified radiant warmers to minimize heat loss. However, as shown by Sessler and Moayeri, radiant warming is less effective than forced-air convection or circulating-water blankets.[102]

Thermal Mattresses. Thermal mattresses that circulate thermostatically controlled water minimize heat loss by increasing the conduction of heat from the environment to the patient. A layer of cotton sheet is placed over the mattress to prevent direct pressure of the fluid cells on poorly perfused skin. The level of the reservoir fluid should be noted before activating the unit. During operation, the temperature of the circulating fluid must be noted to prevent excessive temperatures and patient burns.

Although thermal mattresses are efficacious in infants,[103] they fail to maintain body temperature in adults.[89, 91, 104] This finding probably is due to the lack of a highly perfused surface area in contact with the blanket.[104] Combination of a thermal mattress (38–40°C) and a heated humidifier preserved body heat better than either method alone (Fig. 25–8).[104]

Fluid and Blood Warming. Warming of room-temperature intravenous fluids (1000 ml) to body temperature requires about 15 calories. In the anesthetized patient who is unable to increase caloric production, body temperature decreases.[23, 105] Body temperature decreases about 0.5°C after administration of 1 L of 4°C blood over 15 minutes.[23, 56] The efficacy of various blood warmers in delivering blood at temperatures above 32°C at rates of 150 ml/minute was reviewed by Russell.[55] Active heating of fluid in the delivery tubing (Hotline, Level 1 Technologies, Marshfield, MA) more effectively maintains the temperature of the delivered fluid at flow rates up to 3000 ml/hour than do dry-wall warmers.[61] At higher flow rates (3000–6000 ml/hour), the delivery temperature of the active heating device was similar to that of dry-wall devices.[61]

Humidifiers. Heated humidifiers are an excellent way to prevent and treat heat loss in the perioperative period.[104, 106–108] They prevent patients from warming and humidifying cold, dry gases from the anesthetic circuit and, compared with use of unhumidified gases, maintain temperature.[104, 109, 110] Preheating of the humidifier prior to use increases its effectiveness.[25] Airway temperature should always be measured

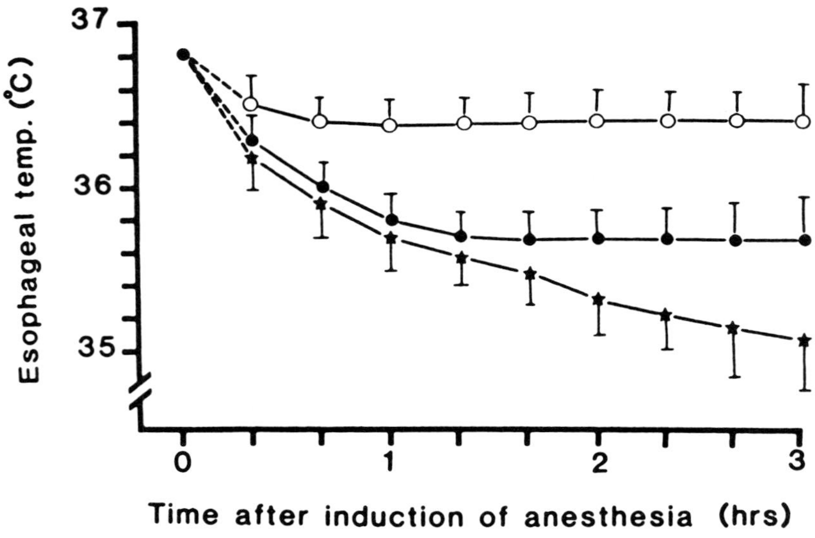

Figure 25–8. Combination of warming mattress and heated humidifier during abdominal aortic surgery *(open circles)* maintains esophageal temperature better than humidifier alone *(closed circles)* or no active warming *(stars)*. (From Tollofsrud SG, et al: Peroperative hypothermia. Acta Anaesthesiol Scand 1984; 28:511–515, with permission of author and publisher.)

and maintained at 38°C or less when humidifiers are used in order to prevent airway burns or tracheobronchial edema.[22, 108]

A study of outpatients noted that warmed humidified gases during anesthesia resulted in warmer patients arriving in the postanesthetic unit who had shorter postoperative stays.[111] Ralley and coworkers noted the inability of heated humidified gases to prevent decreases in temperature after discontinuation of hypothermic cardiopulmonary bypass.[112] However, humidified gases minimize damage to the cilia of the respiratory mucosal cells.

Even passive, unheated humidifiers (heat and moisture exchangers, artificial "noses") maintain body temperature better than is the case without humidification. However, they fail to provide benefits similar to heated devices.[113] They do limit the intraoperative temperature decrease by about 1°C.[114]

Other Methods. Vasodilator therapy with nitroprusside during extracorporeal rewarming of cardiac surgical patients speeds rewarming, restores core temperatures after cardiopulmonary bypass, and prevents postbypass cooling.[115]

Malignant Hyperthermia

Malignant hyperthermia (MH) is an uncommon syndrome triggered by stress or certain anesthetic agents that causes uncontrolled calcium flux in skeletal muscle, resulting in increased temperature, muscle rigidity, and respiratory and metabolic acidosis.[116] The defect involves an abnormal sensitivity of the calcium channel in the sarcoplasmic reticulum to calcium. Abnormally increased calcium ion in the cellular cytoplasm explains the heat production, muscle rigor, and glycogenolysis associated with the syndrome (Table 25–2).[117]

Etiology

In susceptible humans, hyperthermia is triggered by various anesthetic agents but can also occur in nonanesthetic settings. Anesthetic agents that trigger MH include succinylcholine, halothane, enflurane, desflurane, and isoflurane. MH is inherited as an autosomal dominant trait with variable penetrance, and a mutation in the ryanodine receptor gene may be responsible, as indicated by genetic linkage and biochemical investigations.[117] An increased incidence has been noted in idiopathic scoliosis, Duchenne muscular dystrophy, strabismus, ptosis, central core disease, and other musculoskeletal diseases. Susceptibility is suggested by family history, presence of increased creatine kinase, and skeletal muscle contracture to caffeine, as well as by molecular genetic linkage studies. Frequency is variable, ranging from 1 in 14,000 to 1 in 190,000 anesthetic procedures.[116]

Symptoms

Symptoms of MH include spasm of the masseter muscles with difficulty in opening the mouth for intubation, general muscular rigidity, tachycardia with dysrhythmias, increased carbon dioxide production, tachypnea, peripheral cyanosis, and hyperthermia. Laboratory studies reveal severe meta-

TABLE 25–2. CAUSES OF INTRAOPERATIVE TEMPERATURE ALTERATIONS

Increased Temperature
Malignant hyperthermia, thyrotoxicosis, pheochromocytoma
Infections (endotoxins)
Drugs
Chemical reactions (hardening of plaster casts, methylmethacrylate cement)
Excessive environmental warming (heating lamps, heated humidifiers, blankets, heavy surgical drapes)
Decreased Temperature
Exposure to cold operating room environment
Intravenous, intraperitoneal, intrathoracic administration of cold fluids
Skin preparation with cold solutions
Vasodilatation secondary to spinal, epidural, or other regional anesthesia
Hypothyroidism (myxedema)
Trauma or burn patients unable to compensate for heat loss
Deliberate hypothermia (surface or extracorporeal cooling)

bolic acidosis with pH less than 7.0, hypercarbia, decreased mixed venous Po_2, and hyperkalemia. Arterial oxygenation is usually adequate. Hyperphosphatemia, hemoconcentration, hyperglycemia, acute renal failure resulting from acute tubular necrosis caused by excessive myoglobin release from muscle, disseminated intravascular coagulation, and central nervous system dysfunction resulting from brain temperatures exceeding the lethal upper limit of 42–43°C occur in later stages.[118]

Therapy

Therapy consists of general supportive treatment including hyperventilation with oxygen, intravenous fluids, discontinuation of triggering agents, control of metabolic acidosis with bicarbonate, control of hyperkalemia with dextrose-insulin infusions, and control of dysrhythmias with procainamide or other agents. Attempts should be made to cool the patient with external methods, gastric or peritoneal lavage, lavage of an open body cavity, or administration of iced intravenous fluids. Monitoring during the episode should include intra-arterial and central venous catheters, a urinary bladder catheter, ECG, and, if possible, a muscle temperature probe. Otherwise, temperature can be measured in the esophagus or other common sites. The definitive therapy is dantrolene, given in initial doses of 2.5 mg/kg body weight, with additional increments every 5–10 minutes if no reduction of temperature, acidosis, tachycardia, or muscle rigidity occurs to a total dose of 10 mg/kg. Therapy with dantrolene should commence even while supportive measures are being applied, because it must be given while muscle perfusion is adequate. Dantrolene alters calcium release but does not affect its uptake. It also causes muscle weakness and hepatic dysfunction.

The choices for anesthesia in MH-susceptible patients include local anesthetics given in regional techniques such as epidural or subarachnoid block of thiopental, nitrous oxide, narcotics, benzodiazepines, ketamine, propofol, and nondepolarizing neuromuscular blocking drugs (with the possible exception of curare). An anesthesia machine with clean tubing, new soda lime, and empty vaporizers, whose fresh gas flow has been analyzed for absence of volatile anesthetics, is satisfactory for administration of anesthesia to an MH-susceptible patient. Pretreatment with oral dantrolene to a dose of 4–7 mg/kg body weight during the 24 hours prior to surgery effectively prevents MH.[119]

REFERENCES

1. Chang L: Development and use of the stethoscope in diagnosing cardiac disease. Am J Cardiol 1987; 60:1378–1382.
2. Dunteman E, Hirshberg GE: A simple alternative precordial stethoscope. Anesthesiology 1993; 78:1188–1189.
3. Webster TA: Now that we have pulse oximeters and capnographs, we don't need precordial and esophageal stethoscopes. J Clin Monit 1987; 3:191–192.
4. Smith C: An endo-esophageal stethoscope. Anesthesiology 1954; 15:566.
5. Petty C: We do need precordial and esophageal stethoscopes. J Clin Monit 1987; 3:192–193.
6. Baker AB, McLeod C: Oesophageal multipurpose monitoring probe. Anaesthesia 1983; 38:892–897.
7. Kates RA, Zaidan JR, Kaplan JA: Esophageal lead for intraoperative electrocardiographic monitoring. Anesth Analg 1982; 61:781–785.
8. Parker EO: Electrosurgical burn at the site of an esophageal temperature probe. Anesthesiology 1984; 61:93–95.
9. Maroon JC, Albin MS: Air embolism diagnosed by Doppler ultrasound. Anesth Analg 1974; 53:399–402.
10. Kugler J, Stirt JA, Finholt D, Sussman MD: The one that got away: Misplaced esophageal stethoscope. Anesthesiology 1985; 62:643–645.
11. Schwartz AJ, Downes JJ: Hazards of a simple monitoring device, the esophageal stethoscope. Anesthesiology 1977; 47:64–65.
12. Goto H, Hackman LT, Arakawa K: Tracheal insertion of an esophageal stethoscope. Anesth Analg 1977; 56:584–585.
13. Simpson JI, Wolf GL: Flammability of esophageal stethoscopes, nasogastric tubes, feeding tubes, and nasopharyngeal airways in oxygen- and nitrous oxide-enriched atmospheres. Anesth Analg 1988; 67:1093–1095.
14. Himms-Hagen J: Cellular thermiogenesis. Annu Rev Physiol 1976; 38:315–351.
15. Davis PJ: Thermoregulation of the newborn. *In* Cook DR, Marcy JH (eds): Neonatal Anesthesia. Pasadena: Appleton Davies, 1988; 63–70.
16. Hall GM: Body temperature and anaesthesia. Br J Anaesth 1978; 50:39–44.
17. Benzinger TH: On physical heat regulation and the sense of temperature in man. Proc Natl Acad Sci USA 1959; 45:645–659.
18. Imrie MM, Hall GM: Body temperature and anaesthesia. Br J Anaesth 1990; 64:346–354.
19. Atkins E, Bodel P: Fever. N Engl J Med 1972; 286:27–34.
20. Knochel JP: Environmental heat illness. Arch Intern Med 1974; 133:841–864.
21. Adamson K Jr, Gandy G, James L: The influence of thermal factors upon oxygen consumption of the newborn infant. J Pediatr 1965; 66:495–508.
22. Heiser MS, Downes JJ: Temperature regulation in the pediatric patient. Semin Anesth 1984; 3:37–42.
23. Lilly RB: Inadvertent hypothermia. Refresher Courses in Anesthesiology 1986; 15:93–107.
24. Wyon DP, Lidwell OM, Williams REO: Thermal comfort during surgical operations. J Hyg Camb 1968; 66:229–248.
25. Morley-Forster PK: Unintentional hypothermia in the operating room. Can Anaesth Soc J 1986; 33:516–527.
26. Ramanathan NL: A new weighting system for mean surface temperature of the human body. J Appl Physiol 1964; 19:531–533.
27. Colin J, Timbal J, Houdas Y, et al: Computation of mean body temperature from rectal and mean skin temperatures. J Appl Physiol 1971; 31:484–489.
28. Burton AC: The average temperature of the tissues of the body. J Nutr 1935; 9:264–267.
29. Holdcroft A: Body Temperature Control in Anaesthesia, Surgery, and Intensive Care. London: Balliere Tindall, 1980.
30. Lacoumenta S, Hall GM: Liquid crystal thermometry during anaesthesia. Anaesthesia 1984; 39:54–56.
31. Vaughan MS, Cork RC, Vaughan RW: Inaccuracy of liquid crystal thermometry to identify core temperature trends in postoperative adults. Anesth Analg 1982; 61:284–287.
32. Lees DE, Schuette W, Bull J, et al: An evaluation of liquid-crystal thermometry as a screening device for intraoperative hyperthermia. Anesth Analg 1978; 57:669–674.
33. Shinozaki T, Deane R, Perkins FM: Infrared tympanic thermometer: Evaluation of a new clinical thermometer. Crit Care Med 1988; 16:148–150.
34. Cork RC, Vaughan RW, Humphrey LS: Precision and accuracy of intraoperative temperature monitoring. Anesth Analg 1983; 62:211–214.
35. Benzinger TH: Clinical temperature. New physiological basis. JAMA 1969; 209:1200–1206.
36. Benzinger M: Tympanic thermometry in surgery and anesthesia. JAMA 1969; 209:1207–1211.
37. Hickey PR, Andersen NP: Deep hypothermia circulatory arrest: A review of pathophysiology and clinical experience as a basis for anesthetic management. J Cardiothorac Anesth 1987; 1:137–155.
38. Whitby JD, Dunkin LJ: Cerebral, oesophageal, and nasopharyngeal temperatures. Br J Anaesth 1971; 43:673–676.

39. Kaufman RD: Relationship between esophageal temperature gradient and heart and lung sounds heard by esophageal stethoscope. Anesth Analg 1987; 66:1046–1048.
40. Severinghaus JW: Temperature gradients during hypothermia. Ann N Y Acad Sci 1962; 80:515–521.
41. Piironen P: Effects of exposures to extremely hot environments on temperatures of the tympanic membrane, the oesophagus, and the rectum of men. Technical Documentary Report No. AMRL-TDR-63-85, Wright-Patterson Air Force Base, Ohio, 6570th Aerospace Medical Research Laboratory, 1963.
42. Ritter DM, Rettke SR, Hughes RW, et al: Placement of nasogastric tubes and esophageal stethoscopes in patients with documented esophageal varices. Anesth Analg 1988; 67:280–282.
43. Lilly JK, Boland JP, Zekan S: Urinary bladder temperature monitoring: A new index of body core temperature. Crit Care Med 1980; 8:742–744.
44. Bone ME, Feneck RO: Bladder temperature as an estimate of body temperature during cardiopulmonary bypass. Anaesthesia 1988; 43:181–185.
45. Moorthy SS, Winn BA, Jallard MS, et al: Monitoring urinary bladder temperature. Heart Lung 1985; 14:90–93.
46. Stupfel M, Severinghaus JW: Internal body temperature gradients during anesthesia and hypothermia and effect of vagotomy. J Appl Physiol 1956; 9:380–386.
47. Bissonnette B, Sessler DI, LaFlamme P: Intraoperative temperature monitoring sites in infants and children and the effect of inspired gas warming on esophageal temperature. Anesth Analg 1989; 69:192–196.
48. Ramsay JG, Ralley FE, Whalley DG, et al: Site of temperature monitoring and prediction of afterdrop after open heart surgery. Can Anaesth Soc J 1985; 32:607–612.
49. Joly HR, Weil MH: Temperature of the great toe as an indicator of the severity of shock. Circulation 1969; 39:131–138.
50. Matthews HR, Meade JB, Evans CC: Peripheral vasoconstriction after open-heart surgery. Thorax 1974; 29:343–348.
51. Webb GE: Comparison of esophageal and tympanic temperature monitoring during cardiopulmonary bypass. Anesth Analg 1973; 52:729–733.
52. Wallace CT, Marks WE, Adkins WY, Mahafey JE: Perforation of the tympanic membrane, a complication of tympanic thermometry during anesthesia. Anesthesiology 1974; 41:290–291.
53. Ralley FE, Wynands JE, Ramsay JG, et al: The effects of shivering on oxygen consumption and carbon dioxide production in patients rewarming from hypothermic cardiopulmonary bypass. Can J Anaesth 1988; 35:332–337.
54. Sladen RN: Temperature and ventilation after hypothermic cardiopulmonary bypass. Anesth Analg 1985; 64:816–820.
55. Russell WJ: A review of blood warmers for massive transfusion. Anesth Intensive Care 1974; 2:109–130.
56. Roe CF: Temperature regulation in anaesthesia. *In* Hardy JD, et al (eds): Physiological and Behavioral Temperature Regulation. Springfield, IL: Charles C Thomas, 1970; 727–740.
57. Vaughan MS, Vaughan RW, Cork RC: Postoperative hypothermia in adults: Relationship of age, anesthesia, and shivering to rewarming. Anesth Analg 1981; 60:746–751.
58. Fox RH, Woodward PM, Exton-Smith AN, et al: Body temperatures in the elderly: A national study of physiological social and environmental conditions. Br Med J 1973; 1:200–206.
59. Newman BJ: Control of accidental hypothermia: Occurrence and prevention of accidental hypothermia during vascular surgery. Anaesthesia 1971; 26:177–187.
60. Dyde LA, Lunn HF: Heat loss during thoracotomy. Thorax 1970; 25:355–358.
61. Presson RG, Bezruczko AP, Hillier SC, McNiece WL: Evaluation of a new fluid warmer effective at low to moderate flow rates. Anesthesiology 1993; 78:974–980.
62. Frank SM, Beattie C, Christopherson S, et al: Epidural versus general anesthesia, amnient operating room temperature, and patient age as predictors. Anesthesiology 1992; 77:252–257.
63. Kurz A, Plattner O, Sessler DI, et al: The threshold for thermoregulatory vasoconstriction during nitrous oxide/isoflurane anesthesia is lower in elderly than in young patients. Anesthesiology 1993; 79:465–469.
64. Just B, Trevien V, Delva E, Lienhart A: Prevention of intraoperative hypothermia by preoperative skin-surface warming. Anesthesiology 1993; 79:214–218.
65. Sessler DI, Sessler AM, Hudson S, Moayeri A: Heat loss during surgical skin preparation. Anesthesiology 1993; 78:1055–1064.
66. Sessler DI, Hynson J, McGuire J, et al: Thermoregulatory vasoconstriction during isoflurane anesthesia minimally decreases heat loss. Anesthesiology 1992; 76:670–675.
67. Sessler DI, Moayeri A, Stoen R, et al: Thermoregulatory vasoconstriction decreases cutaneous heat loss. Anesthesiology 1990; 73:656–660.
68. Sessler DI, Olofsson CI, Rubinstein EH: The thermoregulatory threshold in humans during nitrous oxide-fentanyl anesthesia. Anesthesiology 1988; 69:357–364.
69. Rubinstein EH, Sessler DI: Skin-surface temperature gradients correlate with fingertip blood flow in humans. Anesthesiology 1990; 73:541–545.
70. Sessler D, Olofsson C, Rubinstein E, et al: The thermoregulatory threshold in humans during halothane anesthesia. Anesthesiology 1988; 68:836–842.
71. Stoen R, Sessler D: The thermoregulatory threshold is inversely proportional to isoflurane concentration. Anesthesiology 1990; 72:822–827.
72. Hitt BA, Mazze RI, Cook TL, et al: Thermoregulatory defect in rats during anesthesia. Anesth Analg 1977; 56:9–15.
73. Sessler DI, Olofsson CI, Rubinstein EH, Beebe JJ: The thermoregulatory threshold in humans during isoflurane anesthesia. Anesthesiology 1988; 68:836–842.
74. Bissonnette B, Sessler DI: The thermoregulatory threshold in infants and children anesthetized with isoflurane and caudal anesthesia. Anesthesiology 1990; 73:1114–1119.
75. Belani K, Sessler DI, Sessler AM, et al: Leg heat content continues to decrease during the core temperature plateau in humans anesthetized with isoflurane. Anesthesiology 1993; 78:856–863.
76. Sessler DI, McGuire J, Hynson J, et al: Thermoregulatory vasoconstriction during isoflurane anesthesia minimally decreases cutaneous heat loss. Anesthesiology 1992; 76:670–675.
77. Hynson JM, Sessler DI, Glosten B, McGuire J: Thermal balance and tremor patterns during epidural anesthesia. Anesthesiology 1991; 74:680–690.
78. Frank SM, Beattie C, Christopherson R, et al: Unintentional hypothermia is associated with postoperative myocardial ischemia. Anesthesiology 1993; 78:468–476.
79. Hicks RG, Poole JL: EEG changes with hypothermia and cardiopulmonary bypass in children. J Thorac Cardiovasc Surg 1979; 78:823–830.
80. Vitez T, White PF, Eger EI: Effect of hypothermia on halothane MAC and isoflurane MAC in the rat. Anesthesiology 1974; 41:80–81.
81. Benumof JL, Wahrenbrock EA: Dependency of hypoxic pulmonary vasoconstriction on temperature. J Appl Physiol 1977; 42:56–58.
82. Regan MJ, Eger EI: Ventilatory responses to hypercapnia and hypoxia at normothermia and moderate hypothermia during constant-depth halothane anesthesia. Anesthesiology 1966; 27:624–633.
83. Benzing G, Frances PD, Kaplan S, et al: Glucose and insulin changes in infants and children undergoing hypothermic open heart surgery. Am J Cardiol 1983; 52:133–136.
84. Wood M, Shand DG, Wood AJJ: The sympathetic response to profound hypothermia and circulatory arrest in infants. Can Anaesth Soc J 1980; 27:125–131.
85. Turley K, Roizen M, Vlahakes GJ, et al: Catecholamine response to deep hypothermia and total circulatory arrest in the infant lamb. Circulation 1980; 62(Suppl):175–179.
86. Flacke JW, Flacke WE: Inadvertent hypothermia: Frequent, insidious, and often serious. Semin Anesth 1983; 2:183–196.
87. Joris J, Banache M, Bonnet F, et al: Clonidine and ketanserin both are effective treatment for postanesthetic shivering. Anesthesiology 1993; 79:532–539.
88. Delaunay L, Bonnet F, Liu N, et al: Clonidine comparably decreases the thermoregulatory thresholds for vasoconstriction and shivering in humans. Anesthesiology 1993; 79:470–474.
89. Lewis DG, Mackenzie A: Cooling during major vascular surgery. Br J Anaesth 1972; 44:859–864.
90. Morris RH: Influence of ambient temperature on patient temperature during intra-abdominal surgery. Ann Surg 1971; 173:230–233.
91. Morris RH, Wilkey BR: The effect of ambient temperature on patients monitored during surgery, not involving body cavities. Anesthesiology 1970; 32:102–107.
92. Roizen MF, Sohn YJ, L'Hommedieu CS, et al: Operating room

temperature prior to surgical draping: Effect on patient temperature in recovery room. Anesth Analg 1980; 59:852–855.
93. Sessler DI, Shroeder M: Heat loss in humans covered with cotton hospital blankets. Anesth Analg 1993; 77:67–72.
94. Sessler DI, McGuire J, Sessler AM: Perioperative thermal insulation. Anesthesiology 1991; 74:875–879.
95. Bourke D, Wurm H, Rosenberge M, Russell S: Intraoperative heat conservation using a reflective blanket. Anesthesiology 1984; 60:151–154.
96. Radford P, Thurlow AC: Metallised plastic sheeting in the prevention of hypothermia during neurosurgery. Br J Anaesth 1979; 51:237–239.
97. Kurz A, Kurz M, Pieschl G, et al: Forced-air warming maintained intraoperative normothermia better than circulating-water mattresses. Anesth Analg 1993; 77:89–95.
98. Zink RS, Iaizzo PA: Convective warming therapy does not increase the risk of wound contamination in the operating room. Anesth Analg 1993; 76:50–53.
99. Giesbrecht GG, Ducharme MB, McGuire JP: Comparison of three forced-air patient warming systems. Anesthesiology 1994; 80:671–679.
100. Murphy MT, Lipton JM, Loughran MB, Gieseke AH: Postanesthetic shivering in primates: Inhibition by peripheral heating and by taurine. Anesthesiology 1985; 63:161–165.
101. Sharkey A, Lipton JM, Murphy MT, Giesecke AH: Inhibition of postanesthetic shivering with radiant heat. Anesthesiology 1987; 66:249–252.
102. Sessler DI, Moayeri A: Skin-surface warming: Heat flux and central temperature. Anesthesiology 1990; 73:218–224.
103. Goudsouzian NG, Morris RH, Ryan JF: The effects of warming blanket on maintenance of body temperature in anesthetized infants and children. Anesthesiology 1973; 39:351–353.
104. Tollofsrud SC, Gundersen Y, Anderson R: Peroperative hypothermia. Acta Anaesthesiol Scand 1984; 28:511–515.
105. Boyan CP, Howland WS: Blood temperature: A critical factor in massive transfusion. Anesthesiology 1961; 22:559–563.
106. Stone DR, Downs JB, Paul WL, Perkins HM: Adult body temperature and heated humidification of anesthetic gases during general anesthesia. Anesth Analg 1981; 60:736–741.
107. Pflug AE, Aasheim GM, Foster C, Marten RW: Prevention of postanesthesia shivering. Can Anaesth Soc J 1978; 25:43–49.
108. Tausk HC, Miller R, Roberts RB: Maintenance of body temperature by heated humidification. Anesth Analg 1976; 55:719–723.
109. Shanks CA: Humidification and loss of body heat during anaesthesia. II. Effects in surgical patients. Br J Anaesth 1974; 46:863–865.
110. Bissonnette B, Sessler DI, LaFlamme P: Passive and active inspired gas humidification. Anesthesiology 1989; 71:350–354.
111. Conahan TJ, Williams GD, Apfelbaum JL, Lecky JH: Airway heating reduces recovery time (cost) in outpatients. Anesthesiology 1987; 67:128–130.
112. Ralley FE, Ramsay JG, Wynands JE, et al: Effect of heated humidified gases on temperature drop after cardiopulmonary bypass. Anesth Analg 1984; 63:1106–1110.
113. Goldberg ME, Jan R, Gregg CE, et al: The heat and moisture exchanger does not preserve body temperature or reduce recovery time in outpatients undergoing surgery and anesthesia. Anesthesiology 1988; 68:122–123.
114. Haslam KR, Nielsen CH: Do passive heat and moisture exchangers keep the patient warm? Anesthesiology 1986; 64:379–381.
115. Noback CR, Tinker JH: Hypothermia after cardiopulmonary bypass: Amelioration by nitroprusside-induced vasodilation during rewarming. Anesthesiology 1980; 53:277–280.
116. Strazis KP, Fox AW: Malignant hyperthermia: A review of published cases. Anesth Analg 1993; 77:297–304.
117. MacLennan DH, Philips MS: Malignant hyperthermia. Science 1992; 256:789–794.
118. Gronert GA: Malignant hyperthermia. Anesthesiology 1980; 53:395–423.
119. Gronert GA, Milde JH, Theye RA: Dantrolene in porcine malignant hyperthermia. Anesthesiology 1976; 44:488–495.
120. Buckberg GD, Brazier JR, Nelson RL, et al: Studies of the effects of hypothermia on regional myocardial blood flow and metabolism during cardiopulmonary bypass. The adequately perfused beating, fibrillating and arrested heart. J Thorac Cardiovasc Surg 1977; 73:87–94.
121. McConnell DH, Brazier JR, Cooper N, et al: Studies of the effects of hypothermia on regional myocardial blood flow and metabolism during cardiopulmonary bypass. J Thorac Cardiovasc Surg 1977; 73:95–101.

CHAPTER

26

Monitoring Hemostasis

ROGER A. MOORE, M.D.

During every invasive surgical procedure, the hemostatic control mechanisms of the body are stimulated. For most operations, the intricate balances among the vascular, the coagulation factor, and the platelet control mechanisms are sufficient to ensure adequate intraoperative hemostasis; however, inherited conditions or acquired derangements in one or more of the hemostatic control mechanisms can lead to intraoperative situations requiring the intervention of the anesthesiologist. A primary problem in these situations is the need for rapid and accurate diagnosis so that direct and specific therapeutic interventions can be initiated. The "shotgun approach" to blood component therapy (concomitant administration of plasma, platelets, and erythrocytes) is no longer acceptable.[1] In addition to the older tests such as platelet count, prothrombin time, and partial thromboplastin time, a variety of devices are now available for use by the clinician for the intraoperative management of hemostasis.

The initial step in the evaluation of hemostasis is establishing the actual blood loss through measurement and estimation. Blood in operative suction containers, if not contaminated with irrigating solutions, is directly measured. The amount of blood on sponges, surgical drapes, surgeons' gowns, and the operating room floor is more difficult to determine. Usually, an estimate is made by visual inspection. As for sponges, the cumbersome measurement of hemoglobin concentration in the effluent of washed sponges can be performed. An estimate based on the difference between the wet and dry weights of sponges (assuming 1 ml of blood weighs 1 gm) is more commonly used. If measured and estimated blood loss is over the expected level for a specific surgical procedure, a hemostatic *derangement* should be considered.

The first medical devices brought into the operating room for the evaluation of hemostasis answered the need for monitoring anticoagulation during the extracorporeal circulatory techniques of open heart surgery. Complete inhibition of the coagulation system with heparin is an absolute requirement during extracorporeal circulation. More recently, the development of transplant surgical techniques has led to other medical instrumentation that allows more accurate diagnosis and management of the severe coagulation derangements that occur. At present, there is no "perfect" medical device or test for the intraoperative evaluation of coagulation. Each device or test has certain advantages and limitations. To adequately understand these devices, one should thoroughly understand the basic principles governing hemostatic control mechanisms.

MECHANISMS OF HEMOSTASIS

VASCULAR INTEGRITY

The first line of defense in hemostasis is maintenance of vascular integrity. However, the elderly patient, the debilitated patient, or the patient receiving certain pharmacologic agents (e.g., steroids) may have compromised vascular defenses, increasing the bleeding tendency. The patient with compromised vascular defenses may be brought to the anesthesiologist's attention preoperatively by the presence of a prolonged bleeding time (increased bleeding time might also be due to platelet dysfunction).

Once a blood vessel is incised, unless hemostatic control mechanisms intervene, the intravascular fluids pour from the vessel. The driving force for the blood loss is the difference between the pressure inside the vessel and the pressure outside. Vascular mechanisms that come into play for the control of bleeding can be divided into immediate effects and delayed effects.[1]

Immediate Effect

An immediate effect is constriction of the vessel wall at the site of injury, thereby reducing blood flow to the severed vessel. The importance of simple vasoconstriction for stemming blood loss should not be underestimated. According to Poiseuille's law, any reduction in the radius of the bleeding vessel is translated into an exponential decrease in blood loss from the vessel.[5]

$$F = \frac{(P_1 - P_2) \times \pi \times r^4}{8 \times \lambda \times L}$$

where F = blood flow, $P_1 - P_2$ = pressure difference over length of vessel, r = the vessel radius, λ = the coefficient of viscosity, and L = the length of the vessel. Therefore, by constricting the bleeding vessel, blood loss can be reduced significantly. The primary mechanism for inducing this vascular constriction is the release of a cyclo-oxygenase product of arachidonic acid metabolism called thromboxane A_2 (Fig. 26–1). Thromboxane A_2 is released from granules within activated platelets and serves as both a potent vasoconstrictor and an inducer for platelet aggregation.[2, 3]

Delayed Effects

A delayed vascular mechanism for limiting blood loss is an increase in extravascular tissue pressure resulting from the extravasation of blood into the surrounding tissues as well as the leakage of edema fluid into these tissues. The increase in extravascular tissue pressure from the extravasated blood and edema fluid balances the intravascular pressure, thereby nullifying the primary determinant promoting bleeding and the pressure differential. The increased extravascular tissue pressure serves the same physiologic function as pressure bandages applied directly to a bleeding site or the use of positive end-expiratory pressure for intrathoracic bleeding.[6]

If a large vessel is severed, preventing normal hemostatic mechanisms from controlling the bleeding, the continued blood loss eventually leads to contraction of the intravascular volume and a resultant decrease in blood pressure. The decrease in blood pressure, in combination with a reflex redistribution of blood flow away from the periphery and to the vital organs by the central nervous system, serves as an extremely effective end-stage hemostatic control mechanism. The value of this mechanism for limiting blood loss is well known intraoperatively, when techniques using anesthetic agents[7] or other pharmacologic hypotensive agents[8] produce deliberate hypotension and effectively reduce intraoperative blood loss.

COAGULATION FACTORS

One of the first events leading to hemostasis is formation of a hemostatic plug through activation of the coagulation cascade. The coagulation cascade allows a small stimulus for coagulation to be amplified by a series of sequential enzymatic steps, leading to the formation of a fibrin clot at the bleeding site. This enzymatic amplification of coagulation stimuli can occur through two pathways: the intrinsic pathway and the extrinsic pathway (Fig. 26–2). The end

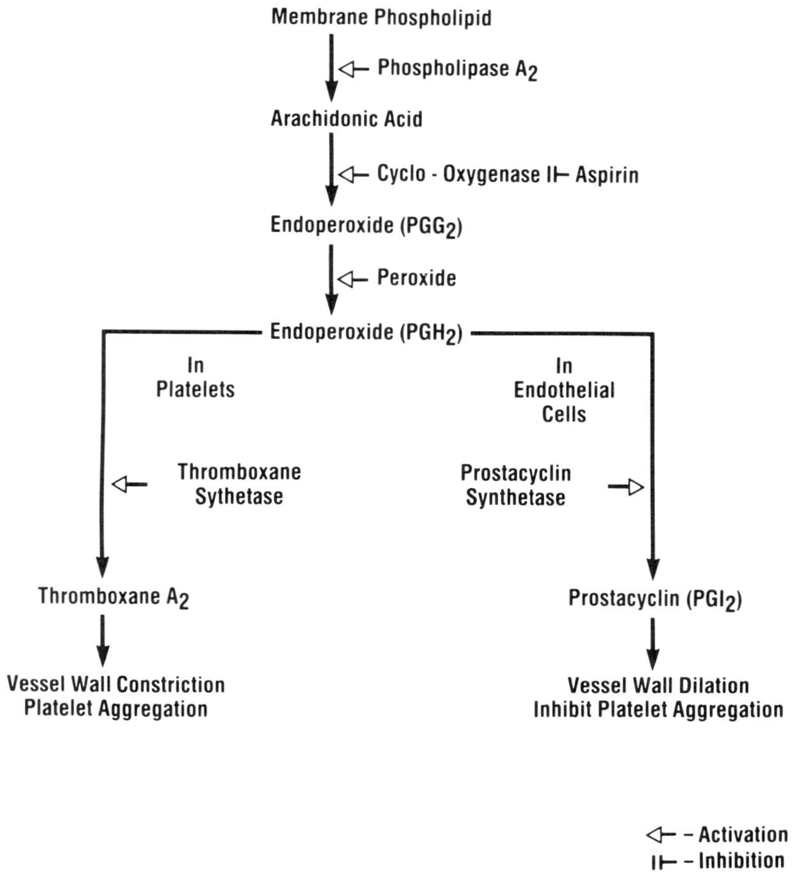

Figure 26–1. The metabolism of arachidonic acid by the cyclo-oxygenase pathway leads to the production of thromboxane A_2 in platelets and prostacyclin in vascular endothelial cells. These two products of arachidonic acid metabolism have opposite effects on vascular wall reactivity and platelet activity. The cyclo-oxygenase metabolism of arachidonic acid can be inhibited with aspirin.

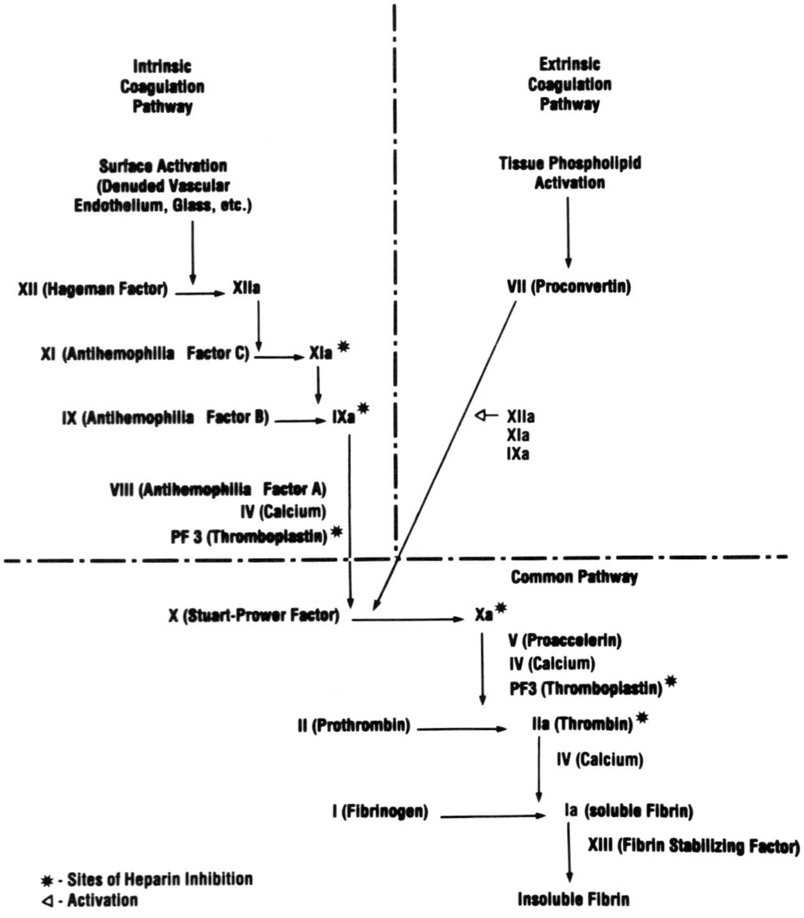

Figure 26–2. The coagulation cascade allows a small stimulus for clot formation to be amplified, resulting in the formation of a fibrin clot. The coagulation cascade is made up of three pathways—the intrinsic pathway, the extrinsic pathway, and the final common pathway. Heparin's effect is exerted primarily on the activated serum proteases (XIa, IXa, Xa, IIa) and thromboplastin (platelet factor 3).

result of activation of either pathway is the conversion of fibrinogen to fibrin, but each pathway is initiated by different stimuli. Upon contact with foreign surfaces, including such diverse substances as collagen, glass, and denuded vascular endothelium, the intrinsic pathway is activated with conversion of inactive factor XII to active factor XIIa. This is followed by sequential activation of factor XI and factor IX, with factor IX combining with factor VIII, calcium, and platelet factor 3. This latter conglomerate leads to the conversion of inactive factor X to its activated form (Xa), which is the first step in the final common pathway.

As an alternative method for activation of the final common pathway, the extrinsic coagulation pathway can be induced through the activation of factor VII by contact with tissue phospholipid. Tissue phospholipid is commonly released by damaged tissue as well as during platelet activation. The end result of activation of the extrinsic pathway is the same as for activation of the intrinsic pathway—stimulation of the final common pathway and formation of a fibrin clot. In this discussion, the activities of the intrinsic and extrinsic pathway are rigidly separated, but in reality, crossovers between these pathways can occur, with activated factor VIII producing direct activation of intrinsic pathway factors.[4]

The final common pathway consists of conversion by activated factor X (Xa) of prothrombin (II) to thrombin (IIa), which induces the conversion of fibrinogen (I) to fibrin (Ia). The initial clot that results from activation of the final common pathway is helpful in providing hemostasis, but this clot is relatively unstable and friable. Through the action of factor XIIIa, increased cross-linkage between the fibrin strands is stimulated, thereby converting the unstable clot into a solid, insoluble plug, providing better hemostatic control.

Although the coagulation cascade's ability to amplify a small stimulus for clot formation through a series of enzymatic steps is a major advantage, its complexity can be a primary weakness. Interruption of any of the enzymatic steps, through congenital abnormalities, pharmacologic interventions, or acquired conditions, results in abnormal clot formation. For the most part, a relative deficiency in the serum level of a coagulation factor does not play a major role in reducing hemostasis, because normal clot formation only requires between 10% and 50% of the normal amount of each factor.[9, 10] A decrease in a coagulation factor below the required level, however, can compromise overall clot formation. As the ability to identify which coagulation factor is deficient in a bleeding patient improves, therapeutic factor replacements can be tailored to the specific deficiency. At present, a number of coagulation factors are available through recombinant techniques.[11] These recombinant factors have the advantage over plasma-derived factors of being rapidly reconstitutable, disease-free, hypoallergenic, and effective as a replacement therapy.

However, even though a direct cause-effect relationship between the level of coagulation factor and the adequacy of clot formation is presumed, this relationship does not always exist. For example, in classic factor VIII–deficient hemophilia, the bleeding tendency is usually inversely related to the serum level of factor VIII.[10] However, some patients with extremely low factor VIII levels undergo surgery without hemostatic difficulty, whereas others with seemingly adequate factor VIII levels develop major hemostatic problems. Despite the growing knowledge of the coagulation system, whether or not an individual patient with an individual factor deficiency will have intraoperative bleeding problems is not easily predicted. Fortunately, commonly used anesthetic agents do not directly affect most coagulation-promoting or -inhibiting systems.[12]

PLATELETS

As important to the hemostatic process as the coagulation cascade is platelet activation. Normally, platelets circulate through the blood vessels in an inactive smooth-surfaced form. When an inactive platelet comes into contact with a damaged blood vessel, the platelet immediately changes from its smooth-surfaced form to a spiny-surfaced form (Fig. 26–3). This change to the spiny-surfaced form increases the platelet's adhesiveness and leads to primary aggregation.[13] The platelet's shape change is thought to be due to the release of adenosine diphosphate from the injured vessel's wall.

The primary aggregation induced by adenosine diphosphate is potentially reversible; if no further stimulation for platelet activation occurs, the primary platelet aggregate dissipates, with reversion of the platelets to their inactive smooth-surfaced form. However, if the stimulus for aggregation persists and reaches a threshold level, a release reaction occurs, and the platelets discharge cytoplasmic granules containing a variety of substances, including adenosine diphosphate, serotonin, platelet factor 4, platelet factor 3, and catechols. The increased level of platelet activation leads to irreversible or secondary aggregation.

The secondary platelet aggregate acts as a base for the formation of a hemostatic plug, and during secondary aggregation, platelets release platelet factor 3. Platelet factor

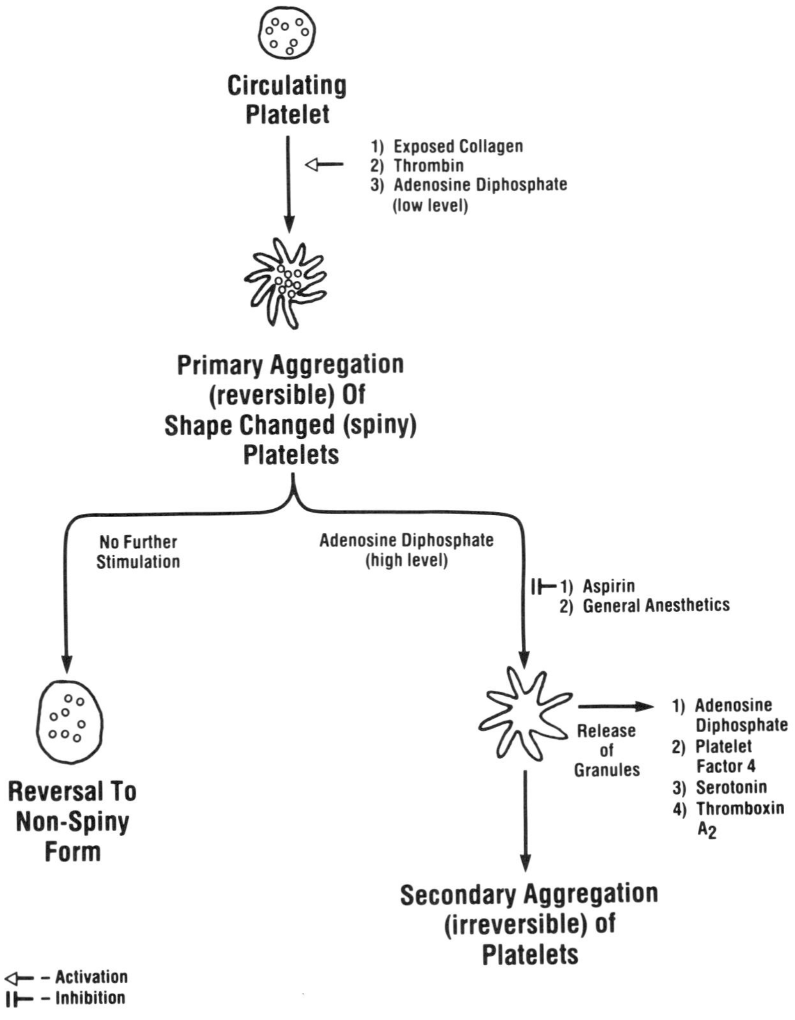

Figure 26–3. Smooth-surfaced circulating platelets can be stimulated to undergo a shape change to a spiny form by exposure to collagen, thrombin, and low levels of adenosine diphosphate. Spiny platelets can undergo primary aggregation, which is completely reversible in the absence of further stimulation. However, in the presence of continued adenosine diphosphate stimulation, platelet granule release occurs, leading to irreversible secondary aggregation.

3 is a cofactor with IXa, VIII, and ionized calcium to form a complex that activates the final common pathway in the coagulation cascade.[13] Platelet factor 3 may also initiate the extrinsic coagulation pathway. Therefore, platelets not only are involved in producing the initial hemostatic plug but also act as major modifiers and modulators of the coagulation cascade.[14] In addition, during secondary aggregation, thromboxane A_2 is released from the platelets, leading to constriction of the vessel wall and further stimulation of platelet aggregation.[2, 3] Although the role of thromboxane A_2 in maintenance of hemostasis is obviously advantageous in peripheral vessels, its release in coronary vessels may play a central role in initiating unstable angina episodes[13] as well as coronary thrombosis.[15] Thromboxane A_2 synthesis inhibitors, such as low-dose acetylsalicylic acid, are suggested prophylactic measures for prevention of myocardial infarctions in patients with coronary artery disease.[16–18]

Functional platelet counts of greater than 100,000/μl are necessary in order to have normal template bleeding times.[19] Below functional platelet counts of 50,000–75,000/μl, intraoperative hemostasis may be inadequate. The major point is that functional platelets are the primary determinant of platelet adequacy, and absolute platelet counts are not adequate indicators of circulating platelet function. Platelets are usually counted using phase-contrast microscopy. A variety of clinical conditions adversely affect platelet function, including such diverse conditions as von Willebrand's disease and uremia, as well as a number of commonly used pharmacologic agents.

Conversely, hyperactive platelet function can be found in a variety of clinical situations, including idiopathic thrombocytopenic purpura and post-chemotherapeutic bone marrow recovery. Qualitative tests of platelet function, not quantitative tests of platelet number, should be used to make clinical decisions regarding the need for platelet infusion. The Ivy bleeding time (whole blood) has been used to indicate both platelet and vascular competency, but the results of this test do not correlate consistently with the potential for increased intraoperative bleeding.[20, 21] One reason for the inconsistency with the Ivy bleeding time is that the test procedure must be followed rigorously and exactly. When performed rigorously, this test has been successfully used as a preoperative predictor of patients who will develop excessive bleeding after coronary artery bypass grafting.[22]

During performance of a bleeding time, venous pressure is maintained at 40 mmHg using a sphygmomanometer cuff. Standard incisions of 9 mm in length and 1 mm in depth are made on the volar surface of the forearm. Every 30 seconds, the bleeding edges are blotted with filter paper until bleeding ceases. The normal bleeding time is 4.5 ± 1.5 minutes. The Ivy bleeding time is relatively insensitive as an indicator of hemostasis. Bleeding times return to normal in 2 days after aspirin ingestion, whereas more sensitive platelet function tests are adversely affected for 6 days or more.[21]

The question of adequate platelet function is even more confusing. For instance, during cardiopulmonary bypass, a complex constellation of platelet defects occurs, including alpha granule release, impairment of aggregation, and the continued circulation of as much as 58% of platelets with impaired function. If only platelet number were evaluated in the postbypass period, a significant underestimation of platelet function would result.[23, 24] Unlike coagulation factors, platelet function is adversely affected by a variety of preoperative and intraoperative conditions.[13, 25] For example, a variety of premedications adversely affects platelet function.[13, 25] Hypothermia produces a reversible inhibition of platelet activity,[26] which makes maintenance of postbypass body temperature a primary therapeutic intervention for patients with hemostatic derangements.

Finally, the choice of anesthetic agent may have a major effect on intraoperative platelet function. Although all investigators do not agree,[27, 28] the general consensus from both *in vitro* and *in vivo* studies is that all of the commonly used inhalation anesthetic agents cause a dose-dependent inhibition of platelet function.[29–32] Preservation of platelet function during cardiopulmonary bypass has been accomplished using reversible pharmacologic interventions that inhibit platelet activation. Some suggested interventions include trimethaphan,[33] nitroprusside,[34] nitroglycerine,[35] and aprotinin.[36] In addition, thrombolytic therapy, which is being used increasingly in patients with acute myocardial infarctions, produces a complex interaction affecting platelet integrity that is not easily anticipated.[37]

MECHANISMS OF ANTICOAGULATION

The body's mechanisms of hemostasis are intricately related through positive and negative feedback systems. The mechanisms for formation and lysis of thrombus, for aggregation and inactivation of platelets, for activation and inhibition of plasminogen, and for dilation and constriction of vessels are all in delicate balance.

PROTEIN C SYSTEM

As important to hemostasis as the clot-promoting systems are the activities of the balancing systems of clot inhibition and lysis. The role of the protein C system in inhibition of clot formation has been elucidated (Fig. 26–4). Protein C is a naturally occurring vitamin K–dependent anticoagulant that contains the protein residue gamma-carboxyglutamic acid, as do the other vitamin K–dependent factors (II, VII, IX, X).[38, 39] The inactive, zymogen form of protein C is converted to its active, enzymatic form (Ca) through enzymatic cleavage by thrombin. The activated protein C then functions as a potent anticoagulant through inactivation of coagulation factors V and VIII. Thrombin is normally only a mild activator of protein C, but when thrombin combines with a capillary endothelial receptor (thrombomodulin), the protein C conversion to an active state increases some 20,000 times.[40] In addition, the com-

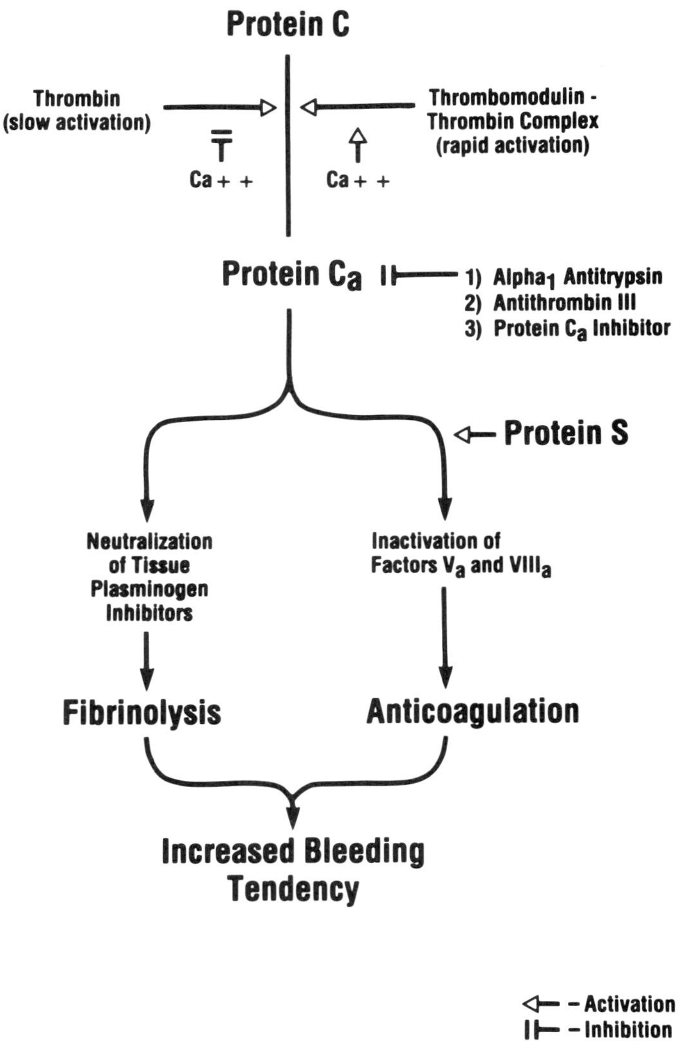

Figure 26–4. The protein C system is actively involved in promoting fibrinolysis and anticoagulation. In the presence of calcium chloride, thrombin, and an endothelial cell wall molecule (thrombomodulin), protein C is rapidly converted to its enzymatically active form, C_a. Protein C_a neutralizes tissue plasminogen inhibitors, thereby promoting fibrinolysis. In addition, with the help of protein S, protein C_a inactivates factors V and VII, leading to an increased anticoagulant state.

bination of thrombin with thrombomodulin removes thrombin from the circulation, thereby reducing the amount of fibrinogen converted to fibrin. Protein C also has an effect on the fibrinolytic pathway. Activated protein C neutralizes tissue plasminogen inhibitors, with the direct result being increased fibrinolysis.

The activity of the protein C system is made even more complex by the presence of an additional vitamin K–dependent plasma protein called protein S.[38] The purpose of protein S is the modulation of protein C's conversion to its active form. Therefore, a genetic or an acquired deficiency of either protein C or protein S could lead to a hyperthrombotic state.[38, 41] Also, the presence of normal levels of protein C, but of an abnormal type, may be responsible for hyperthrombotic states.[42, 43] Derangements in the protein C system during extracorporeal circulation have been linked to increased bleeding tendencies in patients following open heart surgery.[45] Also, infusions of activated protein C have been suggested as a possible alternative to heparin as an anticoagulant[40] as well as for the treatment of acute disseminated intravascular coagulation (DIC).[44] An inherited heterozygous deficiency of protein C occurs with a prevalence rate of 1 in 300. Many investigators feel that patients with a deficiency of protein C are at increased risk for venous thromboembolic disease[46–48]; others do not.[49]

Not only does the vessel wall contain thrombomodulin for modulation of the protein C system, but the vascular endothelial tissue also contains prostacyclin.[50] Unlike the platelet cyclo-oxygenase product of arachidonic acid (thromboxane A_2), prostacyclin acts as a potent vasodilator and inhibitor of platelet aggregation. Therefore, through the thromboxane A_2 and the prostacyclin systems, nature has set up another mechanism to balance normal hemostasis against overwhelming thrombosis. Obviously, imbalances in either system from acquired or pharmacologic disruptions can lead to hemostatic problems.

FIBRINOLYSIS

The primary system preventing clot formation from causing overwhelming thrombosis is the fibrinolytic system. Induction of the fibrinolytic system occurs early in the initiation of clot formation (Fig. 26–5). The first step in the coagulation cascade on exposure of blood to vascular collagen is the conversion of factor XII to its active state, XIIa. Factor XIIa then initiates the coagulation cascade through the intrinsic pathway. However, factor XIIa has another important function—conversion of plasminogen to the nonspecific serine protease, plasmin.[51] Therefore, as soon as clot formation is stimulated, clot lysis is induced. Plasmin formation is also stimulated by a number of other tissue plasminogen activators.

Both plasmin and plasminogen have high chemical affinities for the fibrin molecule. As clot formation progresses, these factors are actively incorporated into the growing clot. The active plasmin molecule immediately begins enzymatically cleaving fibrin strands in the clot, leading to its dissolution and the release of fibrin split products. Only in the area of greatest stimulation for clot formation (at the wall of the severed vessel) can the clot-promoting systems overcome the clot-dissolving systems. The fibrin split products released during fibrin breakdown also act as substitute fibrin monomers during the polymerization of fibrin. Because fibrin split products are inadequate substitutes for fibrin monomers, the result is the formation of friable, abnormal, easily destroyed clots. Finally, plasmin also destroys other coagulation factors, including factors V and VIII and fibrinogen.[51, 52]

One can understand why an imbalance in the fibrinolytic system could lead to major derangements in the hemostatic process. Excessive plasmin production might rapidly lead to a fibrinolytic state in which all clot is dissolved and further clot formation is impaired. The body's mechanism for preventing this situation is an additional plasma glycoprotein called alpha$_2$ antiplasmin, which rapidly inactivates serum plasmin.[4, 51] A congenital deficiency of alpha$_2$ antiplasmin can lead to a fibrinolytic state, which may be reversible with a fibrinolytic inhibitor such as tranexamic acid.[53] In spite of alpha$_2$ antiplasmin's presence, overstimulation of the fibrinolytic system can lead to clinical bleeding, whereas overinhibition increases the risk of widespread thromboses.

Thrombolysis

Manipulation of the fibrinolytic system via pharmacologic agents has gained increased application as a method for destroying unwanted systemic thrombus.[54, 55] Both urokinase and streptokinase are fibrinolytic agents that function like plasmin. Their primary clinical application has been to

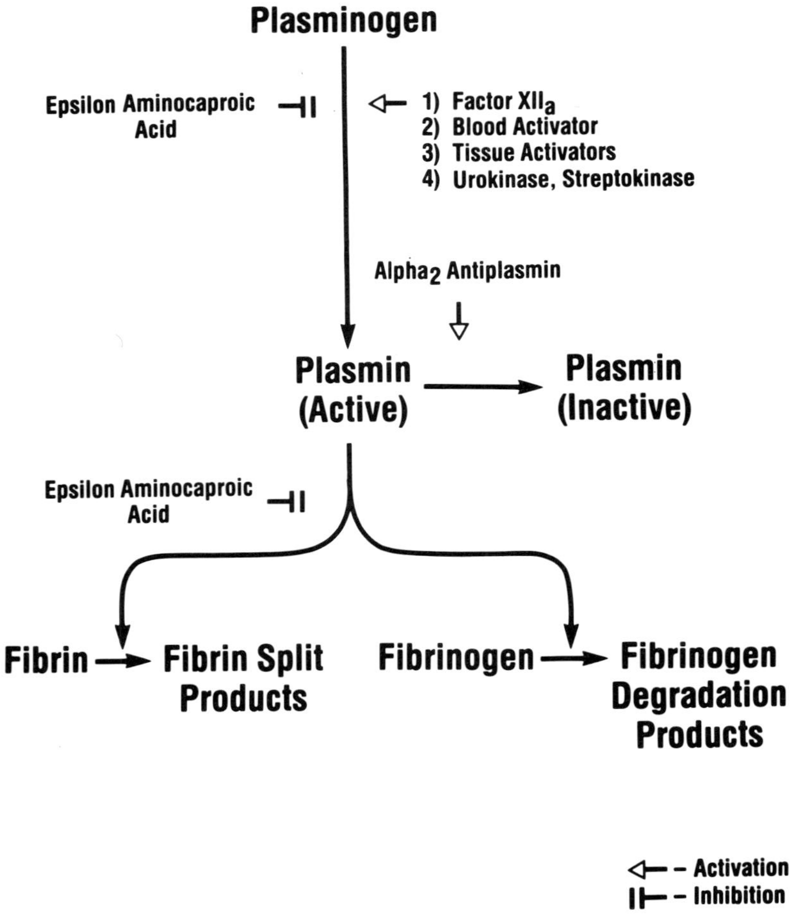

Figure 26–5. The fibrinolytic system acts as the primary balance to clot-promoting systems in the body. Inactive plasminogen is converted to plasmin by a variety of factors, including factor XIIa (the first step in clot formation through the intrinsic pathway). Plasmin actively destroys fibrin and fibrinogen, leading to clot dissolution. Epsilon aminocaproic acid acts through inhibition of plasmin formation as well as direct inhibition of active plasmin. Overwhelming fibrinolysis is prevented by alpha$_2$ antiplasmin's destruction of active plasmin.

dissolve coronary thrombi during and after myocardial infarction.[56, 57] These agents effectively improve regional myocardial blood flow and left ventricular function during a myocardial infarction.[52, 60, 61] The primary disadvantage associated with these agents is severe generalized fibrinolysis,[62] leading to significant bleeding complications[60] and prolonged derangements of coagulation (2 days or more). Emergency surgery in patients receiving thrombolytic therapy can result in complex and difficult coagulation problems.[63]

A direct tissue plasminogen activator is also available[57] that can be substituted for the other kinases and may be preferable to them.[58, 59] Tissue plasminogen activator destroys clot by direct conversion of plasminogen to plasmin. Therefore, the body's natural defenses can destroy the resultant plasmin, leading to a short half-life for the drug (5–8 minutes) and the absence of prolonged derangements in hemostatic control.[51]

PHARMACOLOGY AND COAGULATION

ANTICOAGULANTS

Heparin

The initial intraoperative introduction of coagulation-monitoring devices was specifically aimed at evaluating the adequacy of anticoagulation during extracorporeal circulation. The variability of heparin's dose response–dose effect relationship negated the use of a predetermined dosage for providing an accurate level of anticoagulation and led to intraoperative coagulation-monitoring devices, which allow reliable, accurate, and reproducible assessment of the patient's state of anticoagulation.[64] Heparin is a mucopolysaccharide discovered by McLean in 1916.[65] The molecular weight of heparin varies between 15,000 and 18,000 daltons, depending on the number of saccharide units in the chemical structure. The relatively large size of this molecule prevents it from crossing the blood-placental barrier and, for the most part, keeps it within the intravascular space.

Low-molecular-weight heparin produced by digestion of the larger heparin molecule can also be used clinically. The main advantage of low-molecular-weight heparin is its minimum effect on platelets.[66] However, potential disadvantages include weaker anticoagulant effect, longer half-life, and inability to easily reverse its anticoagulation with protamine. Its usefulness during open heart surgery is limited.

Structure-Activity Relationship

For the most part, only 25–30% of the heparin molecule is responsible for over 95% of the anticoagulant activity.[67] The portion of the heparin molecule most involved in producing anticoagulation is a specific tetrasaccharide sequence: L-iduronic acid, N-acetylated D-glucosamine-6 sulfate, D-glucuronic acid, and N-sulfated D-glucosamine-6 sulfate.[68] Part of the difficulty in predicting heparin's action in any individual patient is related to the varying amounts of specific tetrasaccharide in each heparin molecule. The amount of this tetrasaccharide can vary greatly, depending on the mammalian source from which the heparin is extracted,[68] the organ system from which it is obtained,[69] and the pharmaceutic extraction process used for its refinement. In addition, different lots of heparin obtained from the same organ system and the same mammalian species can have widely variable anticoagulant activities based on a milligrams-per-milliliter sample. For these reasons, the pharmaceutic companies report heparin in units per milliliter rather than in milligrams per milliliter.

Also, a threefold variability can exist between patient responses to a specific anticoagulant bolus dose of heparin.[64, 70] Individual variations in intravascular volume, age, sex,[71] and serum antithrombin III levels,[69, 72] as well as previous exposure to heparin therapy,[73] all contribute to the variability in individual patient responses to a specific dose of heparin. It is this variability that negates the use of heparin-dosing protocols as successful and acceptable mechanisms for providing reliable anticoagulation.[64]

Another variable is the half-life of heparin, which can vary as much as fourfold among individuals.[64] Normally, the half-life of heparin is determined by first-order kinetics and is approximately 1.5 hours.[70, 72] However, because heparin inactivation occurs by reticuloendothelial system uptake,[74] differences in the activation and integrity of the reticuloendothelial system among patients also cause variability in the serum half-life for the drug.

Finally, individuals with antiheparin antibodies and increased levels of platelet factor 4 (an antiheparin) have reduced efficacy from a dose of heparin.[76, 77] In fact, an infusion of recombinant platelet factor 4 has been suggested as an improved alternative for reversal of heparin in patients following cardiovascular surgery.[75] Use of platelet factor 4 instead of protamine for heparin reversal would avoid potentially catastrophic protamine reactions.[78–82]

Antithrombin III

If a bolus of heparin is placed in a test tube of clotted blood, the clot is not affected. Therefore, heparin's action occurs prior to clot formation. Heparin is not in and of itself an anticoagulant. Heparin produces anticoagulation through its interaction with the serum protein antithrombin III. Antithrombin III inactivates serine proteases in the coagulation cascade (activated coagulation factors XIa, IXa, Xa, and IIa).[66, 76, 83] By itself, antithrombin III is a fairly weak enzyme; but, in combination with heparin, a configurational change occurs in its structure, allowing a 200–10,000-fold increase in activity.[68]

As might be expected, individuals with low levels of antithrombin III are more difficult to anticoagulate with heparin than are individuals with normal levels of antithrombin III.[72] Approximately 1 in 2000 individuals has depressed antithrombin III levels due to an inherited heterozygous defect. Patients homozygous for antithrombin III deficiency usually die prior to birth or in the early newborn period owing to overwhelming thromboses. In addition, a variety of clinical conditions, including liver disease, pregnancy, and debilitating illness, depress serum levels of antithrombin III.[84] The antithrombin III not only affects the coagulation cascade but neutralizes plasmin in the fibrinolytic system.[84] Antithrombin III deficiency may be responsible for as many as 2% of clinical cases of venous thrombosis.[84]

Dose

Owing to heparin's lack of effect on factor VII, low-dose heparin therapy primarily affects the intrinsic pathway with prolongation of the partial thromboplastin time (PTT) and maintenance of a relatively normal prothrombin time (PT). At higher doses, heparin's effect on factors in the final common pathway also leads to prolongation of the PT.

Coumarin

Coumarin, which inhibits the formation of vitamin K–dependent factors (II, VII, IX, and XII), primarily affects the extrinsic pathway in low doses with prolongation of the PT and little effect on the PTT.[9] As coumarin doses are increased, the PTT is also prolonged, owing to common final pathway effects.

Platelet Inhibitors

Prostacyclin

Prostacyclin is a cyclo-oxygenase product of arachidonic acid metabolism found naturally in vascular endothelial walls (see Fig. 26–1). The chemical name for prostacyclin, (5Z)-9-deoxy-6,9α-expoxy-Δ^5-$PGF_{1\alpha}$, has the shorthand designation of PGI_2. The primary physiologic effects of PGI_2 are vascular dilatation and inhibition of platelet aggregation. Prostacyclin's effect on platelet aggregation is thought to occur through direct stimulation of platelet adenylate cyclase, leading to increased platelet adenosine monophosphate (cAMP). The increased cAMP inhibits Ca^{2+} mobilization, thereby preventing the calcium-dependent, platelet-dense granule release that causes platelet aggregation.[85] Interestingly, unlike most prostaglandins, PGI_2 is not destroyed during passage through the lungs, and most of the PGI_2 activity is generated by lung tissue.

The future importance of PGI_2 in medical therapy is its potential use as a heparin substitute or at least as a preserver of platelets. During extracorporeal circulation[86, 87] and hemodialysis,[88] platelet activation and consumption can occur in spite of adequate anticoagulation. Unlike heparin, PGI_2 has an *in vitro* half-life of only a few minutes, inhibits platelets without affecting the coagulation cascade, and, when it is metabolized, allows the platelets to return to full active function. The primary problem associated with the clinical use of PGI_2 is vasodilatation, leading to systemic hypotension. PGI_2 has been used as a safe and effective substitute for heparin during hemodialysis, both clinically[88] and experimentally.[89]

Unlike its use during hemodialysis, use of PGI_2 as a sole substitute for heparin during extracorporeal circulation is not recommended. Although PGI_2 would preserve platelets during extracorporeal circulation, surface activation of other coagulation components could lead to a tragic thrombotic episode. The primary value of PGI_2 during extracorporeal circulation is as an adjunct to anticoagulation with heparin, in order to preserve platelet function after bypass. In spite of adequate anticoagulation, extracorporeal circulation leads to a significant release of platelet-dense granules causing platelet aggregation and consumption.[87, 90] An infusion of PGI_2 during bypass prevents dense granule release and preserves platelet function.[87]

Iloprost

During cardiac surgery, a prostacyclin analog called iloprost (ZK36374) has been effectively used.[90–92] Iloprost has a half-life of 15–30 minutes, is 10 times more potent than PGI_2, and allows a complete return of platelet function once it is metabolized. In addition, iloprost causes less hypotension than PGI_2 does. Though iloprost can preserve postbypass platelet activity in the routine open heart surgical patient,[90] its primary clinical value has been the preservation of platelets in patients with heparin-induced thrombocytopenia.[91, 92] Heparin-induced thrombocytopenia is a relatively rare complication of heparin therapy. One to five days after initiation of heparin therapy, a sudden, severe drop in the platelet count and the occurrence of thrombotic episodes herald the onset of heparin-induced thrombocytopenia.[93, 94] If one of these patients receives a bolus of heparin prior to bypass, a sudden thrombotic episode secondary to massive platelet aggregation and the appearance of severe postbypass bleeding owing to the loss of platelets might occur. An iloprost infusion started prior to giving the bolus of heparin effectively prevents the thrombocytopenic response and allows preservation of the patient's platelets throughout the bypass period.[91, 92]

Ancrod

Another anticoagulant substitute that has been suggested to replace heparin is ancrod, which is an anticoagulant derived from the venom of the Malayan pit viper.[95] Ancrod functions as an anticoagulant by selectively producing defibrinogenation through the digestion of the arginine-glycine link in fibrinogen's alpha chain. The result is an aggregate of fibrinogen monomers that can sustain only end-to-end linkages.[99] The inability to cross-link between the monomers ensures a friable and unstable conglomerate. Ancrod has been found to be as effective as heparin for anticoagulation during open heart surgery,[96] hemodialysis,[97] and thrombotic conditions.[98] In one study, 20 patients requiring open heart surgery were effectively and successfully anticoagulated for bypass with an infusion of ancrod.[96] The target fibrinogen level for adequate anticoagulation with ancrod is 0.40–0.80 g/L. However, because fibrinogen may be important in wound healing, use of ancrod might delay postoperative wound closure.[100]

Aspirin

Aspirin, or acetylsalicylic acid, was first introduced into clinical practice in 1899. Aspirin is an effective prophylactic agent for preventing myocardial infarction.[17, 18] The beneficial effect of aspirin in atherosclerotic heart disease seems to be primarily mediated through its platelet-inhibitory action. Aspirin irreversibly inhibits the platelets' ability to release adenosine diphosphate,[16, 20, 101] which prevents secondary aggregation. The aspirin-induced inhibition of adenosine diphosphate lasts for the life of the platelet. Therefore, a patient taking aspirin might have a normal platelet count but effectively have no platelet function. A second role of aspirin in preventing myocardial infarction is the inhibition of thromboxane A_2 synthesis. Thromboxane A_2, by causing coronary constriction, may induce ischemic episodes that can be prevented by prophylactic pretreatment with aspirin.[16, 17]

For similar reasons, aspirin is used following coronary artery bypass surgery to improve postoperative graft patency.[102, 103] In spite of aspirin's beneficial effect for patients with ischemic heart disease, its preoperative use in patients without heart disease who are undergoing major surgical procedures may increase their risk for intraoperative hemorrhage.[104] For 5–7 days following a single dose of aspirin, normal platelet function may be compromised, but not all investigators have found that the resultant prolongation of the bleeding time necessarily leads to increased perioperative bleeding.[20] Because aspirin does cross the placental barrier, and maternal ingestion of aspirin does induce neonatal hemostatic derangements, use of aspirin during pregnancy should be discouraged.[105]

COAGULANTS

Epsilon Aminocaproic Acid

Epsilon aminocaproic acid is a synthetic lysine analog that effectively inhibits the fibrinolytic system. It occupies the lysine binding sites on plasminogen and plasmin, preventing the esteric binding of these molecules with the lysine residues on fibrinogen and fibrin. At serum levels of 13 mg/dl, epsilon aminocaproic acid combines with both plasminogen activator and plasminogen, thereby preventing the formation of active plasmin. At higher serum levels of 130 mg/dl, epsilon aminocaproic acid directly inhibits already-formed plasmin. The drug is rapidly excreted by the kidneys, and approximately 80% of an intravenous dose is cleared within 3 hours. Owing to the small size of the molecule, epsilon aminocaproic acid penetrates the entire extravascular space, which slows complete elimination of the drug (total elimination can take 12–36 hours).[106]

Clinical Indications

The primary clinical indications for the use of epsilon aminocaproic acid include alpha$_2$ antiplasmin deficiency, fibrinolytic drug overdoses, and excessive plasminogen activation. Increased accumulation of serum plasmin in the body leads to a state in which adequate clot formation would be impossible. The mechanism for preventing this state is a serum protein called alpha$_2$ antiplasmin. However, in patients with an inherited or acquired deficiency of alpha$_2$ antiplasmin, plasmin levels may be 10 times normal. For these patients, epsilon aminocaproic acid effectively reduces the hyperfibrinolytic state and stabilizes the coagulation equilibrium.[107] Alternatively, tranexamic acid can be used in this situation.[53]

Another major use of epsilon aminocaproic acid is the reversal of hyperfibrinolytic states produced by fibrinolytic drugs. Increasingly, fibrinolytic drugs are being used during acute myocardial infarctions as a method for re-establishing coronary perfusion.[53–55, 108–110] If a patient receives an overdose of an antifibrinolytic drug or requires emergency coronary artery bypass graft surgery,[63] the hyperfibrinolytic state can be controlled with the use of epsilon aminocaproic acid. However, use of shorter-acting tissue-type plasminogen activators in patients with evolving myocardial infarctions decreases the need for pharmacologic intervention to reverse the fibrinolytic state.[111]

More controversial is the use of epsilon aminocaproic acid at times of increased plasminogen activation. Patients with cyanotic congenital heart disease are in an increased fibrinolytic state,[112–114] possibly owing to peripheral stasis and hypoxia leading to low-level activation of coagulation and fibrinolysis. Use of epsilon aminocaproic acid in the patient with cyanotic heart disease effectively corrects the hemostatic defect[112] and reduces perioperative bleeding during open heart surgery.[114] Prophylactic use of epsilon aminocaproic acid has been advocated for reducing bleeding during all cardiopulmonary bypass operations, because an increased fibrinolytic state is frequently found following sternotomy and cardiopulmonary bypass.[115–118] An argument against the routine use of fibrinolytic inhibitors in the postbypass period is that the fibrinolysis is usually self-limited, lasting only 1–2 hours. Finally, use of epsilon aminocaproic acid in patients with disseminated intravascular coagulation impedes the body's natural defense for recanalization of thrombosed vessels.[119–121]

Another clinical use for epsilon aminocaproic acid is in patients with subarachnoid hemorrhage[122]; however, cerebral thrombosis is a known complication of this intervention.[123] Epsilon aminocaproic acid is also used to control the severe fibrinolytic state occurring during liver transplant surgery.[124, 125] Unfortunately, no current medical instrument can rapidly and accurately direct the use of epsilon aminocaproic acid for balancing the fibrinolytic system. However, concentrations of fibrinogen and its degradation products can be measured, as described later.

Tranexamic Acid

Tranexamic acid is an analog of epsilon aminocaproic acid but with significantly greater potency. Like epsilon aminocaproic acid, it is water-soluble and is rapidly distributed throughout the extravascular fluid volume.[126] Like epsilon aminocaproic acid in postcardiopulmonary bypass studies, tranexamic acid effectively inhibits fibrinolysis and reduces postoperative blood loss.[127, 128] And like epsilon aminocaproic acid, tranexamic acid may predispose patients to thrombosis.[129]

Aprotinin

Aprotinin is a soluble polypeptide with a molecular weight of 6512 daltons that has been used to enhance hemostasis during open heart surgical procedures.[130, 131] Several studies indicate impressive reductions in postoperative blood loss of between 30 and 80% with the use of aprotinin.[130–132] The mechanism for aprotinin's observed hemostatic qualities has not been fully elucidated but is thought to be primarily through inhibition of the contact phase of coagulation,[132] with secondary reduction of fibrinolysis and preservation of platelet function. On contact with surfaces, the kallikrein system amplifies the conversion of factor XII to factor XIIa. Aprotinin's primary effect may be to inhibit kallikrein, slowing the conversion of factor XII to factor XIIa[132] and prolonging celite-activated clotting times and activated partial thromboplastin times. Additionally, high levels of aprotinin (100–400 KIU/ml) inhibit the second phase of platelet aggregation,[133] which accounts for the reduced thromboxane levels observed in patients receiving aprotinin during cardiopulmonary bypass.[134] Finally, aprotinin acts as a potent inhibitor of plasmin and, therefore, has the expected antifibrinolytic activity.[133]

Although there are concerns of renal damage due to aprotinin's high affinity for renal tissue, clinical studies have failed to associate renal dysfunction with aprotinin.[130, 133] Also, some patients previously exposed to aprotinin have shown hemodynamically significant allergic responses on repeat exposure.[130, 135] Aprotinin is undergoing active investigation for use in open heart surgical procedures.

Desmopressin Acetate

Desmopressin acetate (1-deamino-8-D-arginine vasopressin) is a synthetic vasopressin analog that differs from vasopressin in its reduced vasoactive responsiveness. Clinically, this drug improves the hemostatic state of patients with mild hemophilia, von Willebrand's disease, and anemia. Although the exact mechanism for desmopressin acetate's action is unclear, it appears to promote hemostasis through the release of von Willebrand factor and coagulation factor VIII:C from endothelial cells.[136, 137]

Clinical trials of desmopressin acetate have provided mixed results. Following open heart surgical procedures, some investigators have found significant decreases in blood loss,[136, 150] but others have not.[138–142] Because of these conflicting results, a final determination of desmopressin acetate's value in hemostatic control is not available. It may be that specific subgroups of patients will benefit from desmopressin acetate, such as those taking aspirin,[143] those undergoing complex operative procedures,[144] or those with identified reductions in coagulation.[145] It has been argued that the observed increase in von Willebrand factor during desmopressin acetate infusions concurrent with a surgical procedure is simply the stress response to surgery.[146, 147]

Desmopressin also causes significant adverse hemodynamic responses. Significant and occasionally severe reductions in blood pressure have been noted in association with desmopressin acetate infusions.[138, 140–142, 148] The hypotension seems to be primarily produced by a non–histamine-mediated relaxation of vascular smooth muscle.[149]

TECHNIQUES FOR INTRAOPERATIVE EVALUATION OF COAGULATION

Numerous instruments have been developed for the intraoperative evaluation of hemostasis. Characteristics that might increase a specific instrument's value include accuracy and the usefulness of information provided, simplicity of use, reproducibility of results, compactness, quietness, quick availability of results, minimum operator's time or attention demand, use of stable long-lasting reagents, and cost-effectiveness in both price and maintenance.[151]

HEPARIN LEVEL DEVICES

Anticoagulation with heparin occurs in two stages. First, following a bolus dose of heparin, heparin is distributed throughout the intravascular space, producing a specific serum level. Second, the serum heparin interacts with antithrombin III to produce anticoagulation. The division of anticoagulation with heparin into these two stages is artificial, but medical instrumentation for evaluation of heparin has been developed in accord with these stages. Devices aimed at the evaluation of heparin level include the automated protamine titration system and the fluorometric substrate analysis system. Heparin effect is evaluated by automated, activated clotting time systems.

Protamine Titration

Protamine sulfate is a low-molecular-weight protein extracted from the sperm of salmon and other fish. The strongly basic nature of protamine allows it to combine with the strongly acidic heparin to form a stable salt, thereby reversing the anticoagulant activity of heparin. The development of both manual and automated protamine titration tests is based on two primary characteristics of protamine sulfate. First, 1 mg of protamine sulfate completely neutralizes 100 U of heparin activity.[152] Second, protamine sulfate in excess acts as an anticoagulant and delays clot formation *in vitro.*

The earliest use of protamine titration for evaluation of anticoagulation was the placement of a series of test tubes in a 37°C heated block. Increasing concentrations of protamine sulfate were sequentially placed into the test tubes. By adding a specific volume of blood containing the unknown amount of heparin into each of the test tubes and observing which of the test tubes clotted first, the heparin level in the unknown blood sample could be estimated closely. Test tubes containing excess protamine or excess heparin would be delayed in clot formation, whereas the test tube containing an amount of protamine most closely approximating the level of heparin in the unknown sample would undergo clot formation first. Unfortunately, in spite of the usefulness of this method, the anesthesiologist had to spend a lot of time adding the samples of protamine and blood and constantly tipping the test tube to assess clot formation. Automation of this technique was a logical step.

Automated Protamine Titration

HemoTec, Inc. (Englewood, CO) has been the leader in the development of an automated system for protamine titration. HemoTec first produced the Hepcon/System A-10 for performing protamine titrations during open heart surgical procedures. This system uses a disposable cartridge containing four assay chambers with increasing amounts of protamine in each chamber. A series of cartridges can be purchased containing different ranges of protamine levels. The choice of cartridge must be based on the anesthesiologist's expectation of the existing heparin level. After aliquots of heparinized blood are placed in each of the cartridge's assay chambers, the cartridge is placed within the analyzer, and air is bubbled up through each of the chambers. The top of each assay chamber contains a silicon-coated fiber mesh that debubbles blood rising to the chamber's top while capturing any fibrin and clot. As more clot accumulates in the silicon mesh, the cartridge's blood level slowly falls until a photosensitive cell registers increased light transmission (the endpoint for clot formation) (Fig. 26–6). Using the amount of heparin within the assay chamber, the calculated blood volume of the patient using height and weight nomograms, and the extracorporeal circuit priming volume, the Hepcon/System A-10 internally calculates the expected total amount of heparin within the patient.[153]

The HemoTec, Inc., Hepcon/System B-10 was the next machine designed for the evaluation of heparin level after extracorporeal circulation (Fig. 26–7). In addition to protamine titration, this system performs activated clotting time (ACT) and determines heparin dose-response curve. Protamine titration with the Hepcon/System B-10 is performed by placing 0.8 ml of blood containing an unknown heparin level into four assay chambers that contain increasing amounts of protamine in a premade cartridge (Fig. 26–8). Each assay chamber has a small "flag" mechanism attached to a plunger that fits inside the chamber. When a protamine titration is performed, the plunger is raised automatically and allowed to drop inside the chamber, causing the reagents and blood to mix. The plunger's drop rate slows as fibrin formation occurs; this decrease in drop rate is detected by a photo-optical system, which is indicated on the machine's face. In addition to protamine titration, this machine also has cartridges allowing the performance of ACTs, heparin dose responses (to determine a patient's sensitivity to heparin), partial thromboplastin times, and prothrombin times.

HemoTec, Inc.'s newest addition is the Hemostasis Monitoring System (Hepcon/HMS), which performs protamine titrations, heparin dose responses, and ACTs (Fig. 26–9). These tests detect the plunger drop rate in each assay cham-

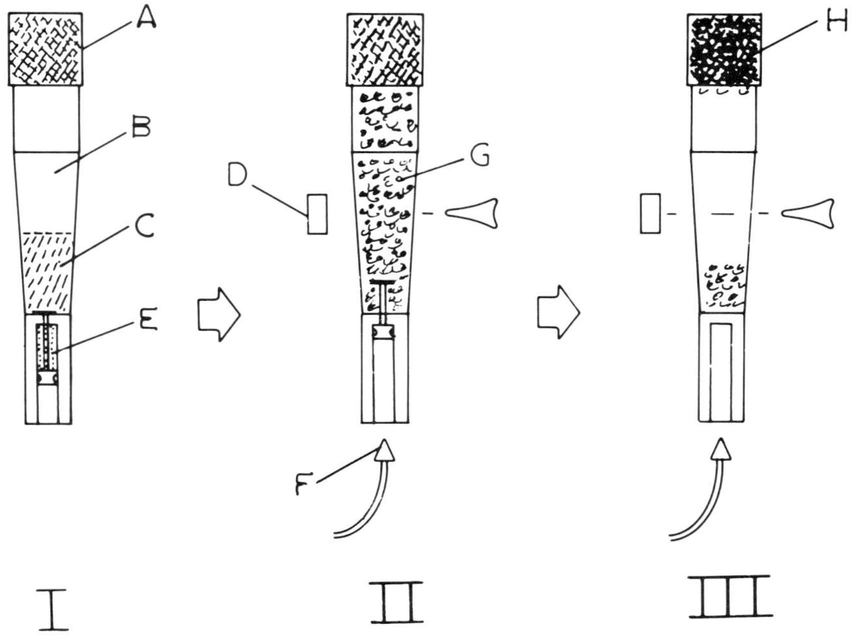

Figure 26–6. Cartridges for the Hepcon/System A-10 are made up of four assay chambers for the evaluation of automated protamine titrations. *I*, A single assay chamber in the cartridge consists of foam mesh (A) located above a reaction chamber (B), into which the sample of blood is placed (C). Reagents including protamine are located in the reagent chamber (E). *II*, To run a protamine titration, the cartridge is placed within the Hepcon system detector module and air (F) is bubbled through the bottom of the chamber, causing the protamine and blood (G) to mix. An optical detection system (D) evaluates light transmission through the chamber. *III*, The foam mesh (H) captures clotted blood, and non-clotted blood is defoamed and returned to the reaction chamber. As clot capture increases, a change in optical transmission signals which of the four assay chambers has undergone clot formation first. On the basis of this information, the amount of heparin in the unknown sample of blood can be estimated. (From Baugh R: Detection of whole blood coagulation. Am Clin Prod Rev 1984; 3:2.)

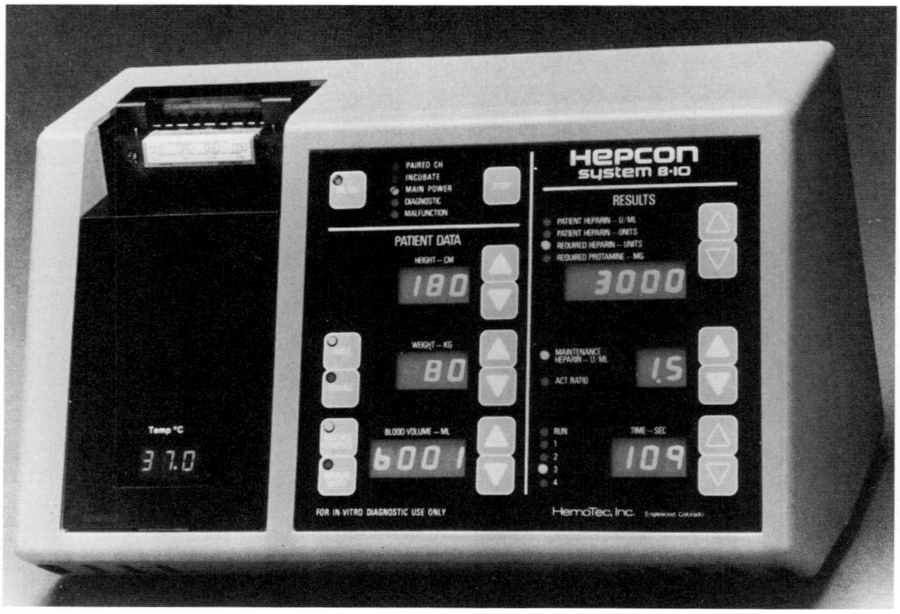

Figure 26–7. The Hepcon/System B-10. The primary purpose of this machine is to perform automated protamine titrations after open heart surgical procedures. When a protamine titration is performed, the amount of heparin within the patient, as well as the amount of protamine necessary for reversal, is computed according to the test result and the patient's height and weight, which are entered prior to running the test. Activated clotting times, heparin dose-response curves, prothrombin times, and partial thromboplastin times can also be obtained. (Courtesy of HemoTec, Inc., Englewood, CO.)

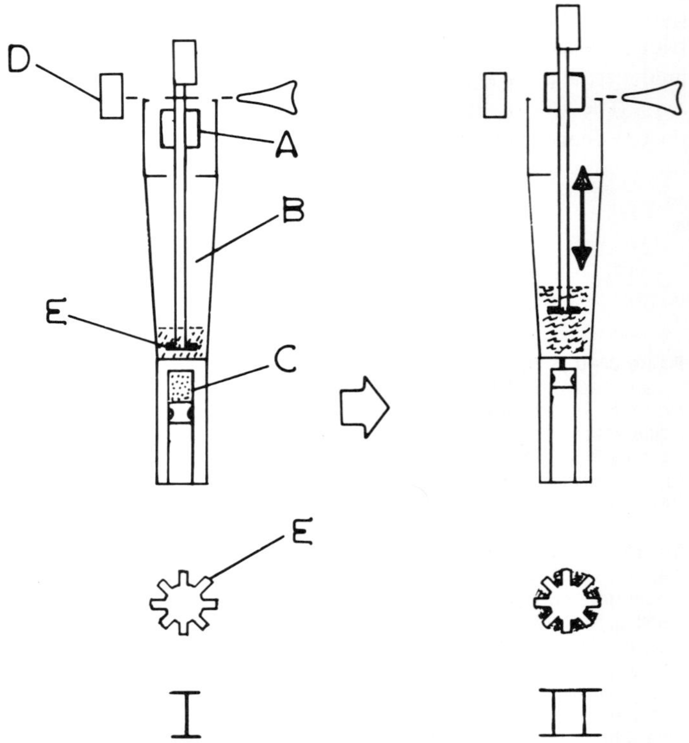

Figure 26–8. The Hepcon/System B-10 utilizes a four-chamber cartridge for evaluating protamine titration. A schematic representation of one of the plunger assay chambers is shown. *I,* An assay chamber is made up of (A) a small flange on the plunger shaft used by the optical system (D) to measure the drop rate of the plunger. In addition, there is a flange disk (E) at the bottom of the plunger shaft. The assay chamber is made up of a reaction chamber (B) containing the blood sample and a reagent chamber (C) containing the protamine. *II,* When a protamine titration is performed, protamine and blood are mixed by the plunger being elevated and dropped. Clot detection occurs when the drop rate of the plunger is slowed to a rate predetermined to indicate clot formation. (From Baugh R: Detection of whole blood coagulation. Am Clin Prod Rev 1984; 3:3.)

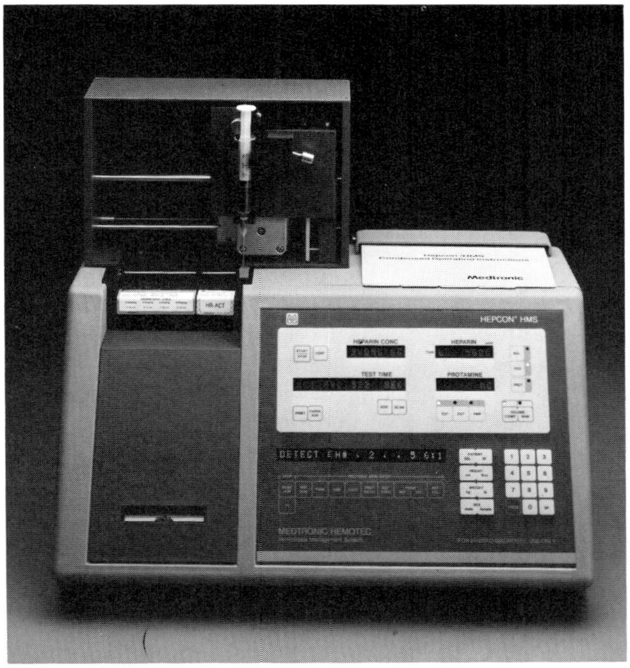

Figure 26–9. The Hepcon Hemostasis Monitoring System (HMS). This machine performs protamine titrations, heparin dose responses, and activated clotting times. (Courtesy of HemoTec, Inc., Englewood, CO.)

ber of the cartridge, as in the Hepcon/System B-10. A cartridge for performance of a heparin dose-response curve prior to heparinization allows evaluation of a patient's response to a heparin dose.[154] Patients with antithrombin III deficiencies[155–157] and patients at risk for heparin resistance because of antiheparin antibodies, preoperative intra-aortic balloon pump use, preoperative heparin infusion,[158] or use of intravenous nitroglycerin[159] can be identified preoperatively. Early heparin dose-response cartridges were unacceptably inaccurate[160] but have since been improved.

Advantages of each of the protamine titration systems include simplicity of use, rapidity of results, reliability of information, and ease of intraoperative use.[161–163] A disadvantage is the cost of the machines, both in initial capital outlay and in individual cartridge use. Even with refrigeration, reagents within the cartridges are outdated in only 60 days, requiring the constant replacement of unused cartridges.

Protamine Dose Assay. A device called a Hemochron (described later) can determine the protamine dosage required to neutralize heparin after cardiopulmonary bypass. Special tubes containing 0, 10, 30, and 40 μg of protamine as well as 12 mg of diatomaceous earth are used to conduct a modified protamine titration. On a special graph that plots protamine concentration against ACT, a plot is made of the patient's control ACT (ACT prior to heparinization), ACT when the patient is being evaluated ("status ACT"), and the ACT in one of the special tubes (tube chosen according to expected heparin concentration in the patient). Based on the graph produced, a relatively accurate determination of the amount of protamine needed for complete heparin reversal can be calculated. An additional correction factor based on the potency of the protamine should also be applied (e.g., the correction factor is 1 if 100 U of heparin are neutralized by 1 mg of protamine). Weak protamines require a greater protamine dose and require a correction factor greater than 1.

After the administration of protamine, the ACT is repeated using a control tube (no protamine) and a tube containing 10 μg protamine. If both tubes demonstrate control ACTs, no additional protamine is necessary. If the ACT is prolonged in both tubes, a coagulopathy or protamine excess may be present. If the tube containing protamine demonstrates an ACT shorter than the control tube ACT, additional protamine is necessary and can be calculated from the graph described.

Fluorometric Substrate Analysis

Another medical device available for the intraoperative determination of heparin level is the fluorometric substrate analysis test, or Protopath system (Dade Division of the American Hospital Supply Corp., Miami, FL).[164] This device allows accurate intraoperative evaluation of heparin level, but performance of the test requires separation of plasma from the red blood cell fraction. A second instrument called the STATSEP plasma separator (Instrumentation Laboratories, Lexington, MA) allows rapid plasma separation such that both plasma separation and performance of the heparin level analysis can be accomplished in 5 minutes.[165]

Performance of a Protopath system evaluation depends on the chemical interaction of heparin, antithrombin III, and thrombin (Fig. 26–10). A sample of plasma with an unknown heparin level is mixed with a diluted pool of normal plasma containing antithrombin III to eliminate test inaccuracies due to individual variations in antithrombin III levels. A known standard aliquot of thrombin also is added to this mixture, thereby resulting in the formation of antithrombin III–heparin-thrombin complexes, plus excess thrombin remaining in solution. The amount of excess thrombin is inversely proportional to the amount of heparin in the unknown plasma sample. A thrombin-sensitive fibrinogen analog (D-phenylalanine-proline-arginine-5-amidoisophthalic acid, dimethyl ester, diacetate, or D-Phe-Pro-Arg-AIE) is added to this solution.[166] The excess thrombin remaining in solution enzymatically cleaves the fibrinogen analog and in doing so releases the fluorophore, AIE. Fluorometric analysis of the resulting fluorescence using the Protopath instrument allows a determination of the heparin level. The heparin level is inversely related to the excess thrombin remaining in solution and, therefore, inversely proportional to the amount of fluorescence. A comparison of fluorescence level with standardized curves allows determination of the heparin level with an accuracy of 0.02–0.05 U/ml.[167]

An advantage of the Protopath technique is that it provides an accurate determination of heparin level unaffected by the presence of intermediate procoagulant, fibrinogen,

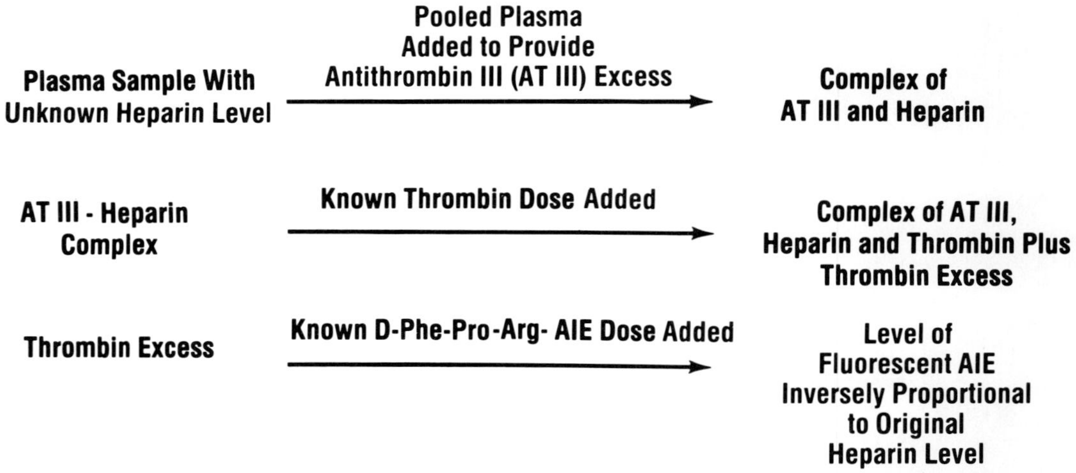

Figure 26–10. The fluorometric substrate analysis of heparin level, or Protopath technique, evaluates heparin level through a sequence of chemical interactions. The end result is the release of a fluorescent molecule in an amount inversely proportional to the original heparin level. Use of calibrated nomograms allows the heparin level to be identified accurately.

antithrombin III,[165] or hypothermia.[168] The disadvantages of the Protopath technique include the need to develop standardized curves for each set of fluorometric kits, each type of heparin, and each lot of heparin.[167] In addition, at least daily calibrations of the equipment are necessary in order to ensure continued accuracy. Finally, the meticulous aliquoting of chemical, as well as the need for strict attention to incubation times and other assay parameters, distracts the anesthesiologist from direct patient care functions. Although the Protopath technique has been successfully used intraoperatively for the evaluation of residual heparinization,[165, 168] the primary objection to its routine use during open heart surgery is the same as for any heparin level test.

In spite of its disadvantages for evaluating heparinization, the Protopath assay may be extremely important for the evaluation of intraoperative hemostasis in the future. Through the use of different fluorometric kits, this system can also evaluate other components of coagulation, including plasminogen level[169] and antithrombin III level.[170] As more complete evaluations of intraoperative coagulation become necessary, the versatility and specificity of this system may increase its clinical role in the intraoperative evaluation of total hemostasis.

Usefulness of Intraoperative Heparin Level Devices

A proposed advantage for protamine titration devices is the ability to continuously and accurately assess heparin levels during cardiopulmonary bypass. However, whether heparin level tests provide the information needed to make decisions during open heart surgery is unclear. During open heart surgery, the patient's coagulation status must be assessed (1) prior to heparin administration, (2) after heparin administration but before initiation of cardiopulmonary bypass, (3) after heparin administration during hypothermic cardiopulmonary bypass, and (4) immediately before and after reversal of heparin with protamine.

Prior to administration of heparin, protamine titration tests normally provide little information except for the occasional patient in whom either circulating natural heparin-like anticoagulants exist[9] or residual heparin from preoperative therapy is still present. Generally speaking, the protamine titration assay is of little value in assessing overall coagulation. In addition, the use of protamine titration tests for determining adequacy of anticoagulation prior to the initiation of cardiopulmonary bypass can be exceedingly dangerous.[161] In normal patients, serum levels of heparin of 4 U/ml are adequate for anticoagulation. However, the great variability in patient responses to heparin, especially patients with acquired or congenital antithrombin III deficiencies, can lead to intraoperative tragedies if the decision to initiate cardiopulmonary bypass is based only on the serum heparin level.[84] Antithrombin III–deficient patients may have serum heparin levels three or four times greater than the normal patient and still not have adequate inhibition of the coagulation cascade. In addition, a combination of patient variability and test variability leads to an overall inherent inaccuracy in protamine titration tests of 26% or more.[161, 162]

Following heparin administration and during hypothermic cardiopulmonary bypass, heparin level tests such as protamine titration and fluorometric substrate analysis provide more accurate information on heparin levels than do heparin effect–type tests. Normally, the initiation of cardiopulmonary bypass decreases serum heparin from 3–4 U/ml of blood to 1.5–2 U/ml. However, the anesthesiologist should not be concerned with the heparin *level* during hypothermia and hemodilution, but with the anticoagulant effect. As long as fibrin formation is inhibited, the actual heparin level is unimportant.

The major clinical value of an automated protamine titration analysis or fluorometric substrate analysis during open heart surgical procedures is to determine doses of protamine to reverse heparin and to decide if inadequate heparin reversal is the cause of excessive postoperative bleeding.[151] In addition, protamine titration assays can assist in diagnosing postoperative bleeding secondary to heparin rebound.[163]

HEPARIN EFFECT DEVICES

Rational conduct of open heart surgical procedures requires anticoagulation evaluation based on heparin effect rather than on heparin level. In light of heparin's effect on multiple serine proteases in the coagulation cascade, it is not surprising that a variety of heparin effect tests have been proposed and utilized for determination of adequate anticoagulation. Some of these tests include the whole blood clotting time,[157, 171] activated PTT,[166, 171–173] thrombin time,[174] and ACT.[157, 171–173] For the purpose of intraoperative management of anticoagulation, the ACT is the gold standard against which all other heparin effect tests are evaluated. Although the whole blood clotting time provides essentially the same information as the ACT, the excessive time required to get the information makes the whole blood clotting time of little practical value for procedures requiring extracorporeal circulation. An ACT of 187 seconds corresponds to a whole blood clotting time of 30 minutes or more.[151]

The activated PTT has been advocated as a possible alternative to the ACT for evaluation of heparin anticoagulation. However, interpretation of the results of activated PTTs is more difficult, because the reported results have a nonlinear relationship with changing heparin blood levels.[171, 173] The nonlinearity of the activated PTT to serum heparin level is particularly striking at the higher levels of heparin necessary for cardiopulmonary bypass. Another disadvantage of the activated PTT is its lack of sensitivity compared with the ACT in the presence of low heparin levels.[175]

The thrombin time has also been presented as a possible alternative to the ACT for assessment of adequate heparinization. The thrombin time can be performed relatively easily, quantitatively, reproducibly, and comparatively rapidly (6–12 minutes).[174] The disadvantages of the thrombin time are a requirement for calibrated equipment and the need for more active involvement by the individual running the test.

Activated Clotting Time

Hattersley[176] was the first to describe a method for obtaining consistent reproducible clotting times much faster than with whole blood clotting time by accelerating the clotting process with diatomite. This ACT was faster and more reliable than the Lee-White (whole blood) clotting time, and although it was temperature-sensitive (the sample had to be kept at 37°C), the results were not adversely affected by such variables as differing amounts of diatomaceous earth (4–46 mg), diameters of test tubes used for performing the test (10–20 mm), or volumes of blood used for the test procedure (1–3 ml).[176] Owing to the speed and reliability of the test result, the ACT rapidly gained clinical acceptance, but it was cumbersome to perform in the operating room, because it required the operator to constantly tilt a test tube and assess clot formation.

Automation of the ACT was clinically introduced in 1974 in the form of the Hemochron system (International Technidyne Corp., Edison, NJ). Although the automated test results took 10–15 seconds longer than manual methods, the delay was consistent at all levels of anticoagulation and provided excellent correlations with handheld methodology.[177]

The Hemochron automated activated clotting system utilizes a disposable test tube containing diatomaceous earth and a bar magnet (Fig. 26–11). The fresh whole blood sample to be tested is immediately placed in the test tube, and the tube is inserted into the Hemochron machine while the coagulation timer is set to 0 seconds (Fig. 26–12). The Hemochron machine heats the blood sample to 37°C while slowly rotating the test tube. As the test tube turns, the bar magnet retains its position at the bottom of the tube. As clot formation begins, fibrin strands bind the bar magnet, preventing it from maintaining its position at the bottom of the tube. As the magnet is displaced, a magnet sensor circuit is broken, resulting in stoppage of the timer. This automated system of ACT fulfills nearly all the criteria for an intraoperative device that evaluates heparinization.[84]

The addition of a variety of test tubes has expanded the value of this machine for intraoperative hemostatic monitoring. Besides the ACT tubes, tubes are available for the performance of a protamine dose assay, activated PTT, PT, thrombin time, and heparinase activated clotting time. The heparinase test tube contains the enzyme heparinase, which instantly destroys any heparin in the sample of blood.[178] This test is useful when a patient arrives in the operating room already on a heparin drip, and a baseline activated clotting time is desired.

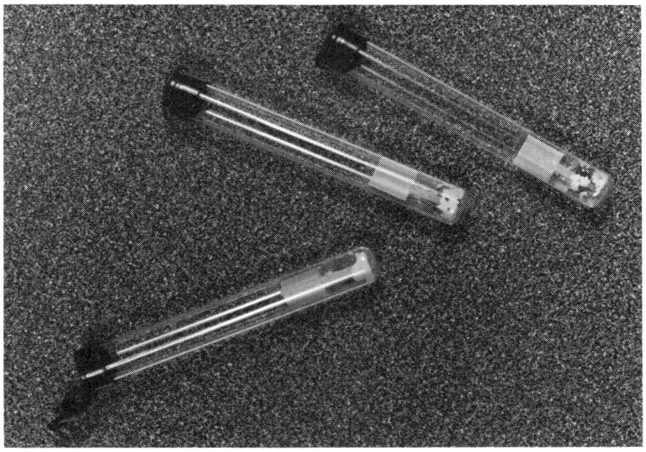

Figure 26–11. The Hemochron activated clotting time system utilizes a test tube containing diatomite for activation of the intrinsic coagulation pathway. A bar magnet at the bottom of the test tube moves freely as the tube is rotated in the analyzer. When fibrin strands prevent the magnet's free movement, a sensor in the machine is activated, indicating clot formation. (Courtesy of International Technidyne Corp.)

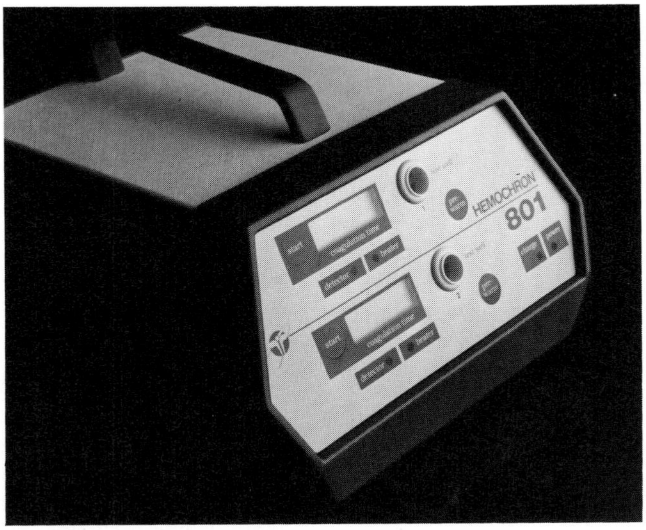

Figure 26–12. The Hemochron 801 performs an activated clotting time using a test tube containing diatomite and a bar magnet into which a sample of blood is placed. Using different test tubes, the Hemochron 801 also can perform protamine dose responses, activated partial thromboplastin times, prothrombin times, thrombin times, and heparinized activated clotting times. (Courtesy of International Technidyne Corp.)

HemoTec, Inc. has also developed a machine for the evaluation of ACTs. The HemoTec ACT system uses a disposable cartridge with a noncelite coagulation activator, into which an aliquot of blood is placed. The mechanism for assessing clot formation is similar to the automated protamine titration Hepcon/System B-10 and Hepcon/HMS. A small plunger is raised and dropped inside an assay cartridge, allowing the whole blood and activator to be mixed. Fibrin accumulation on the plunger and in the blood slows the drop rate to a point predetermined to indicate clot formation. The simplicity of use and reliability of the information obtained with the HemoTec ACT are similar to those of the Hemochron ACT. If aprotinin is used for hemostatic purposes, the noncelite activator used in the HemoTec cartridges is not affected by the aprotinin, which allows a more accurate evaluation of the ACT.[179]

The primary advantage of the ACT over other heparin effect tests is the constant linear relationship between a plot of the ACT and the milligram-per-kilogram heparin dose for any individual patient. In 1975, Bull and coworkers[173] studied this linear dose-response relationship in the context of anticoagulation for open heart surgery and suggested that a dose-response plot be made for each individual during the heparinization process. The slope of the dose-response plot is different for each patient and depends on such diverse factors as the patient's volume of distribution, antithrombin III level, platelet factor 4 level, and other variables. However, once the plot is formed, it can be used as a guide for providing additional heparin for that patient[73] and for directing reversal of heparin with protamine after extracorporeal circulation.[180] The plot is produced by charting a baseline ACT (preheparin) followed by a plot of a repeat ACT once the patient is provided a specific milligram-per-kilogram dose of heparin (Fig. 26–13). A line is extended from the baseline point to the heparinized ACT point; the slope of this plot is specific for the patient receiving heparin. It is recommended that the baseline ACT be obtained following surgical incision, because surgery induces a thromboplastic response with an accelerated ACT.[181] If the baseline is established *prior* to surgery, a "normal" ACT obtained later, following protamine reversal, might be falsely accepted as indicating adequate protamine neutralization.

A normal baseline ACT is in the range of 110–130 seconds, using automated methods. A low baseline ACT should alert the anesthesiologist to the presence of a hypercoagulable state,[182, 183] leading to possible heparin resistance.[184, 185] Initial studies indicated that an ACT between 300 and 600 seconds was usually acceptable for initiation of extracorporeal bypass.[173] In their original paper, Bull and colleagues[64] suggested an optimal clotting time of 480 seconds, although adequate anticoagulation was achieved when the ACT was over 300 seconds. As a result of this publication, heparin protocols based on timed heparin doses were abandoned, and ACTs of over 300 seconds became the criteria for initiation and maintenance of cardiopulmonary bypass.

In 1978, Young and coworkers[186] investigated fibrin monomer production (an indication of ongoing coagulation) at varying ACTs. They found that an ACT of less than 400 seconds was not adequate, and their study led to the recommendation that ACTs be kept over 400 seconds. At present, the level of ACT most optimal for performance of cardiopulmonary bypass remains controversial. In one study,[187] ACTs were allowed to fall below 300 seconds during cardiopulmonary bypass without an observed increase in postoperative bleeding. However, until a definitive study is performed to exactly define the safest level for an ACT, maintenance of an ACT over 400 seconds is reasonable during cardiopulmonary bypass.

Manufacturers of heparin level medical devices have criticized the use of ACTs as inaccurate and unreliable indicators of heparin level during hypothermia[188, 189] and hemodilution.[173, 189] At face value, this criticism is correct. However, it must be emphasized that during hypothermic cardiopulmonary bypass, the objective is to provide an adequate level of anticoagulation, not a stable heparin level. The ACT during both hypothermia and hemodilution continues to serve as an accurate indicator of the overall coagulation state. In addition, Cohen[190] has shown that the ACT–heparin dose plot continues to be linear under hypothermic conditions for ACTs below 500 seconds. Therefore, during hypothermia, ACTs greater than 500 seconds indicate the presence of more than adequate anticoagulation. However, in the postbypass period, ACTs can be prolonged during infusions of fresh frozen plasma, most likely because of the resultant increase of plasma antithrombin III in the fresh frozen plasma.[191]

One area in which heparin level tests may have an advantage over the ACT is determining the adequacy of prota-

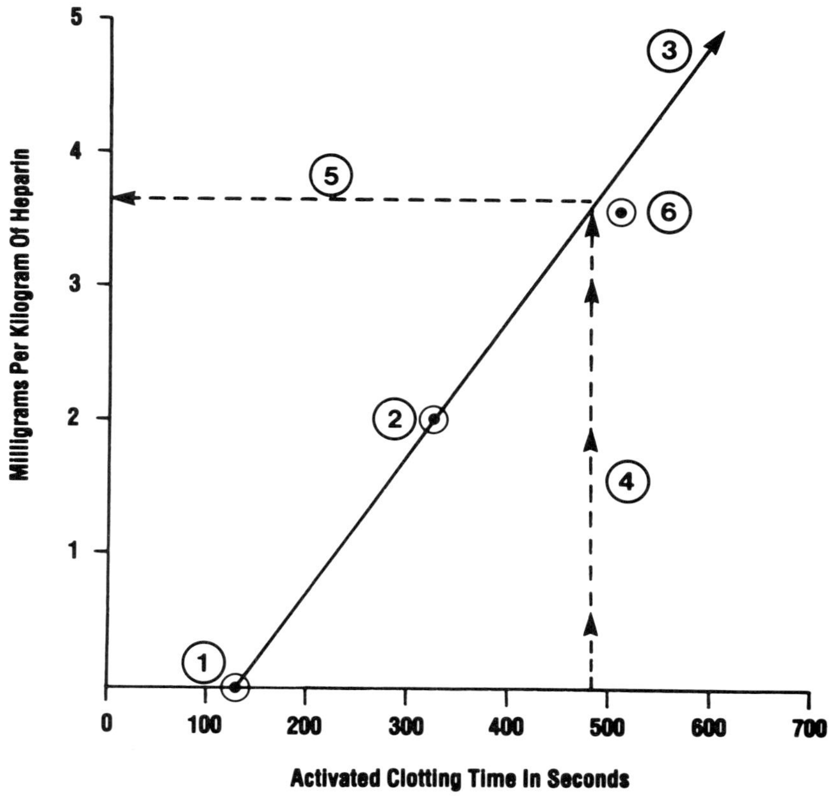

Figure 26–13. A linear relationship exists for each patient between the measured activated clotting time and the milligrams-per-kilogram dose of heparin. This relationship allows the prediction of additional heparin doses during anticoagulation and the amount of protamine necessary for heparin reversal. Generation of a heparin dose-activated clotting time plot is performed by (1) plotting the baseline activated clotting time on a graph of the activated clotting time versus milligrams-per-kilogram dose of heparin, (2) plotting a second activated clotting time performed after giving the patient a milligrams-per-kilogram dose of heparin, and (3) connecting a line between the two plotted points. (4) If a greater level of anticoagulation is desired, a line can be extended from the desired activated clotting time until it intersects the plot line (in the example shown, an activated clotting time of 480 is desired). (5) By extending a second line (perpendicular to the ordinate) from the point of intersection, the additional milligrams-per-kilogram dose of heparin can be determined. (6) A repeat activated clotting time should be performed once the additional heparin is given to ensure that the original activated clotting time–milligrams-per-kilogram-heparin dose plot was accurate.

mine reversal. Although a heparin dose–activated clotting time plot can be used to determine the protamine reversal dose, difficulty occurs when the ACT does not return to baseline following the administration of protamine. In this situation, if a protamine titration device is not available, the typical clinical approach is to administer an additional dose of protamine and repeat the ACT. If the ACT at that point returns to baseline, the cause for the elevated ACT is excess heparin. On the other hand, if the ACT remains elevated or increases, derangements in the coagulation system should be suspected.

In spite of the ACT's value in evaluating heparinization, its use as an indicator of other hemostatic derangements is poor. The ACT is relatively insensitive for the detection of residual heparin compared to activated partial thromboplastin time.[192, 193] Because normal clot formation depends on only 20–50% of each component of the coagulation system, the ACT does not indicate anything about relative deficiencies of specific coagulation factors. In addition, a total absence of factor VII would go unrecognized, because diatomaceous earth stimulates only the intrinsic pathway.

The ACT is also an inadequate indicator of platelet function. Normal ACTs can be observed even in the presence of severe thrombocytopenia, although there is evidence that prostacyclin inhibition of platelet function does prolong ACT.[194] Finally, the ACT only provides information on coagulation up to the time of fibrin formation. Coagulation events occurring after fibrin formation, such as clot retraction, cross-linkage (factor XIII), and fibrinolysis, are not evaluated. In spite of the inadequacies of the automated ACT, this test continues to be the most valuable intraoperative medical device for ensuring adequate anticoagulation and avoidance of catastrophic thrombotic episodes during cardiac surgery.[195]

PARTIAL THROMBOPLASTIN AND PROTHROMBIN TIME ANALYZERS

Although the results are not usually immediately available, intraoperative determinations of PT, PTT, and fibrinogen are helpful in the management of patients receiving massive transfusions, undergoing hepatic transplantations, exhibiting disseminated intravascular coagulation, and receiving thrombolytic therapy.

The PTT measures coagulation in the intrinsic system and final common pathway, and heparin effect is easily demonstrated with this test. The test is performed by centrifuging citrated blood and placing the plasma in tubes containing calcium and partial thromboplastin reagent. After incubation for 30 seconds, the tube is tilted until clotting occurs (normally in 73–84 seconds). A ''partial'' thromboplastin cannot compensate for deficiencies of factors VIII, IX, X, XI, and XII, resulting in prolonged clotting times. Activation with kaolin or diatomaceous earth can shorten the PTT.

A ''complete'' thromboplastin is used in determining the PT. The one-stage method for evaluating PT is used to determine defects in the extrinsic system. With this method, the plasma obtained from centrifugation of citrated blood is added to calcium and thromboplastin. The resultant time to clot formation is the PT. Reference values for PTs are in the range of 11–15 seconds, or the value may be given as a percentage of a control value obtained in a ''normal'' patient.

Fibrinogen is converted to fibrin, which is measured using a standard biochemical protein assay. Normal values are in the range of 170–370 mg/dl. The presence of fibrinolysis (spontaneous lysis of clot normally occurs over 24–48 hours), caused by either endogenous or exogenous thrombolytic agents, thereby producing either primary or secondary fibrinolysis, can be determined using the euglobulin lysis test (ELT). The ELT is significantly shortened when fibrinolytic activity is present. Also, latex agglutination tests can be used, which detect the fibrinogen degradation product fragments D and E.

The Ciba Corning Biotrack 512 coagulation system (Fig. 26–14), a handheld machine, was devised for the rapid performance of PTs and activated PTTs on small amounts of blood. A drop of blood placed on a disposable test cartridge travels through a microcapillary channel containing dry reagents within the lumen. As clotting occurs, the blood's movement through the capillary channel stops, and a reading based on the time to clot formation is digitally provided. Results from the Biotrack 512 correlate well with laboratory-performed PTTs.[196, 197] However, determinations of PT performed by the Biotrack 512, compared with laboratory evaluations, serve only as approximations.[197] Whether this machine has an intraoperative role has yet to be determined. However, the Biotrack 512 has competition from both the Hemochron and HemoTec instruments, which also have PT and PTT capabilities.

VISCOKINETIC DEVICES

Medical instrumentation for evaluating anticoagulation has been stimulated by the development of extracorporeal circulation and other surgical interventions. Advances in transplant surgery, particularly liver transplantation, emphasize the need for intraoperative evaluation of the rapidly changing coagulation states of these patients.[124] Heparin-monitoring devices are of little value for these patients, so other coagulation-monitoring devices are being used. The Thromboelastograph (Haemoscope Corp., Morton Grove, IL) and the Sonoclot Coagulation Analyzer (Sienco, Inc., Morrison, CO) evaluate viscokinetic changes in blood during the clotting process in order to indicate abnormalities in coagulation.

Thromboelastograph

Although its appearance in the operating room is relatively recent, thromboelastography was developed during World War II[198] and was used clinically in the 1960s for managing anticoagulation with subcutaneous heparin.[199] More recently, it has been used as an intraoperative indicator of the rapidly changing coagulation state during liver transplant surgery,[124, 200] as an indicator of postcardiopulmonary bypass coagulopathies,[204, 205] and for the evaluation of coagulation during massive blood loss.[206]

The operating principle of the Thromboelastograph is the evaluation of changes in blood viscosity as it undergoes coagulation. The core of the machine is a cylindric stainless steel cup into which a blood sample is placed (Fig. 26–15). A piston is suspended in the cup from a wire so that torque placed on the wire is electrically amplified through a recorder-printer. The cup is heated to 37°C and undergoes horizontal, oscillatory rotations of 4°45′ at 9-second intervals.[207] When the blood is in its liquid state, the cup's rotation is not transmitted to the piston, and the recorder-printer indicates no deviation. As coagulation begins to occur, the increase in viscosity of the blood, as well as the deposition of fibrin strands between the cup and the piston leads to incremental increases in piston deviation, increased torque on the suspension wire, and recording of the changing viscokinetic pattern of blood.[207]

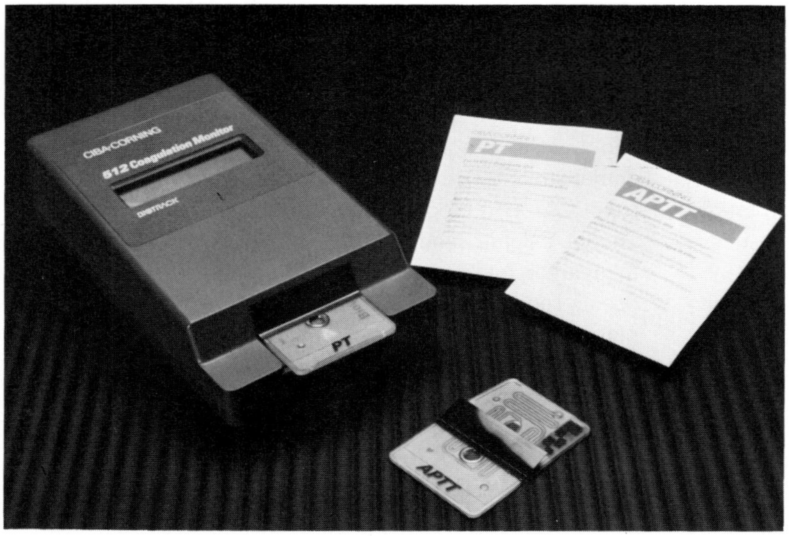

Figure 26–14. The Ciba Corning Biotrack 512 Coagulation System, a hand-held machine devised for the rapid performance of prothrombin times and activated partial thromboplastin times. (Courtesy of Ciba Corning Co.)

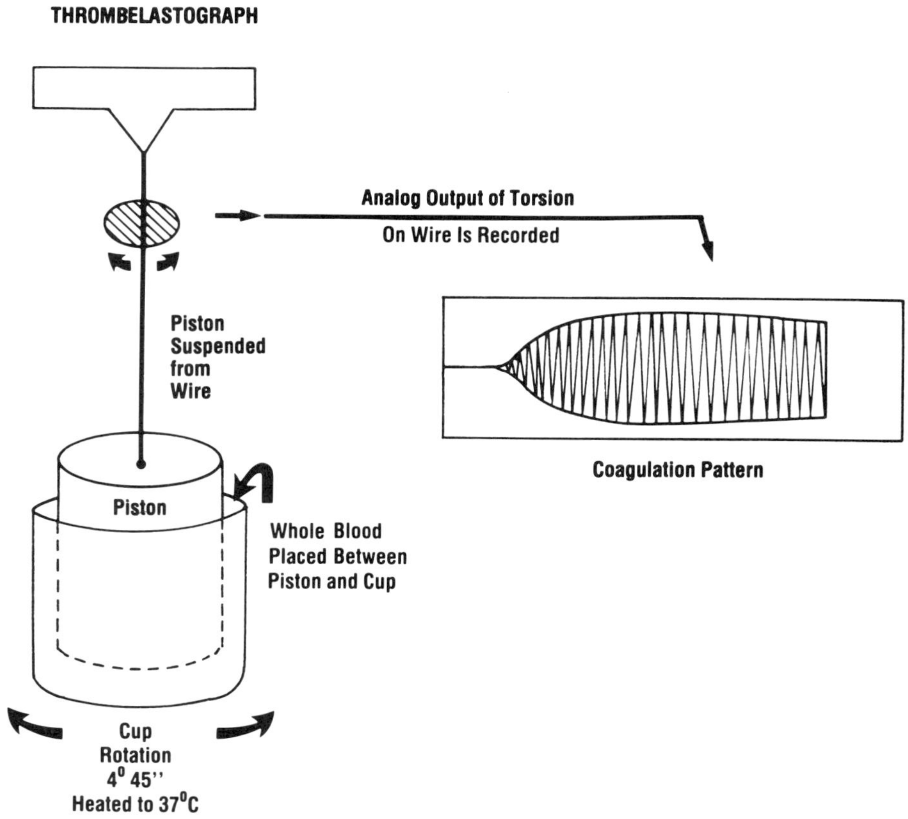

Figure 26–15. The Thromboelastograph evaluates the viscokinetic changes occuring in blood as it undergoes clot formation. This evaluation is performed by suspending a piston on a wire inside a rotating cup. As coagulation occurs, the rotation of the cup is transmitted to the piston. The resulting change is recorded as an analog output of the torsion on the suspension wire.

A representative example of the Thromboelastograph pattern generated during normal coagulation is shown in Figure 26–16. The R time (reaction time) corresponds to the time between the taking of the sample of blood and the occurrence of the first oscillatory movements. In a patient with normal coagulation, this is usually between 6 and 8 minutes. The k time is the period between onset of clot formation and a point at which the oscillatory amplitude is 20 mm. The combination of R and k times gives a value called the coagulation time, which is normally between 10 and 12 minutes. The angle generated by the slope of the line drawn between the time oscillatory movement first begins and the clot formation rate is designated the alpha angle, which is normally greater than 50°. The maximum amplitude (MA) is the point of greatest oscillatory deviation and is normally between 50 and 70 mm. Finally, the amplitude of oscillation 60 minutes after the MA is called the A_{60}. A whole blood clot lysis index indicating the rate of fibrinolysis can be calculated by dividing the A_{60} by the product of the MA and 100. Normally, this value is greater than 85% and decreases in the presence of active fibrinolysis.[124] Another indicator of fibrinolysis is the time following the MA for clot dissolution to occur, and this is called the F time, which is usually greater than 300 minutes. All of these values are for nonactivated samples. Parameters of coagulation may be obtained more rapidly with the use of coagulation activators.

The advantage of thromboelastography compared with

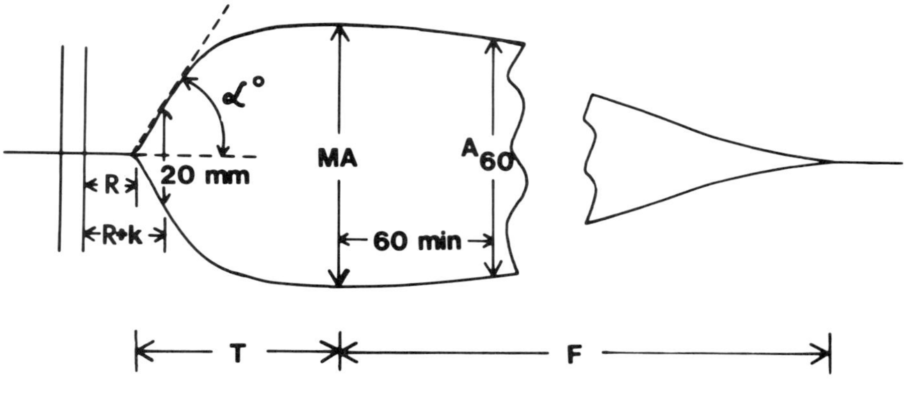

Figure 26–16. The Thromboelastograph generates individual coagulation patterns that are specific for a variety of clotting disorders. The characteristics of a normal coagulation pattern are represented schematically (R = reaction time, R + k = coagulation time, alpha slope = clot formation rate, MA = maximum amplitude, A_{60} = amplitude 60 minutes after MA, T = whole blood clotting time, F = whole blood lysis time). (Reprinted with permission from the International Anesthesia Research Society from Intraoperative changes in blood coagulation and thromboelastographic monitoring in liver transplantation by Kang YG, Martin DJ, Marquez J, et al., Anesthesia and Analgesia, 1985; 64:891.)

heparin-monitoring instruments is that more information is obtained concerning clot integrity, including rate of formation, strength, and long-term stability.[208] In addition, indirect evidence is obtained concerning coagulation factor levels, platelet integrity, and the occurrence of fibrinolysis. Clinical decision making for liver transplant patients based on thromboelastography has been successful in directing epsilon aminocaproic acid therapy and reducing both blood and coagulation factor transfusion.[124, 125, 200] The Thromboelastograph R time has been found to correlate positively with the activated PTT, and the MA correlates with both the functional platelet count and the fibrinogen level. In addition, the whole blood lysis time (F) is positively correlated with the ELT.[124]

Aside from liver transplant surgery, the Thromboelastograph has been used to monitor both the hypercoagulable and the fibrinolytic states after thrombotic episodes[199] and during the postpartum period.[209] Use of the Thromboelastograph for assessment of heparinization prior to open heart surgery is questionable, but it has been used to assess postbypass coagulopathies.[204, 205] Preoperative evaluation of cardiac surgical patients to determine increased risk for excessive blood loss has not been successful,[201] nor has intraoperative thromboelastographic evaluation for predicting postoperative bleeding.[202] Also of concern is the lack of relationship between postbypass D-dimer levels (an indication of fibrinolysis) and the presence of fibrinolysis revealed on thromboelastography. These results may indicate that thromboelastography is a more sensitive tool for evaluating fibrinolysis.[203] Future uses of the Thromboelastograph may well include monitoring plasminogen activator therapy for patients with acute myocardial infarction[62, 210] and for patients in fibrinolytic states during emergency myocardial revascularization.[63]

Sonoclot

The Sonoclot system evaluates the viscokinetic changes occurring during clot formation and provides information similar to that obtained with the Thromboelastograph. The Sonoclot system was developed in response to perceived disadvantages of the early Thromboelastograph system, including nonportability, lack of ruggedness, complexity of use, and lack of computerization.[211]

The Sonoclot analyzer records the changing mechanical impedance of clotting blood against a vibrating, oscillating probe. The probe has an oscillatory amplitude less than 1 μm and an oscillatory frequency of less than 200 Hz, and the sample of blood is warmed to 37°C (Fig. 26–17).[212] As the blood undergoes coagulation, a record of the changing mechanical impedance is converted to an analog output and recorded on a chart.[213] The resultant pattern, or "signature," resembles one half of the Thromboelastograph pattern (Fig. 26–18). The T_1 time, or onset of clot formation time (normal 80–130 seconds in the activated cuvette), corresponds to the Thromboelastograph R time. The Sonoclot rate of coagulation slope (normal 15–30 U/minute) corresponds to the Thromboelastograph alpha slope. One difference in the Sonoclot signature is the presence of an inflection or hump on the upward slope indicating a peak and the occurrence of a downward slope (normal greater than 2 U/minute) indicating clot retraction. Both the Thromboelastograph and the Sonoclot require the recognition of character-

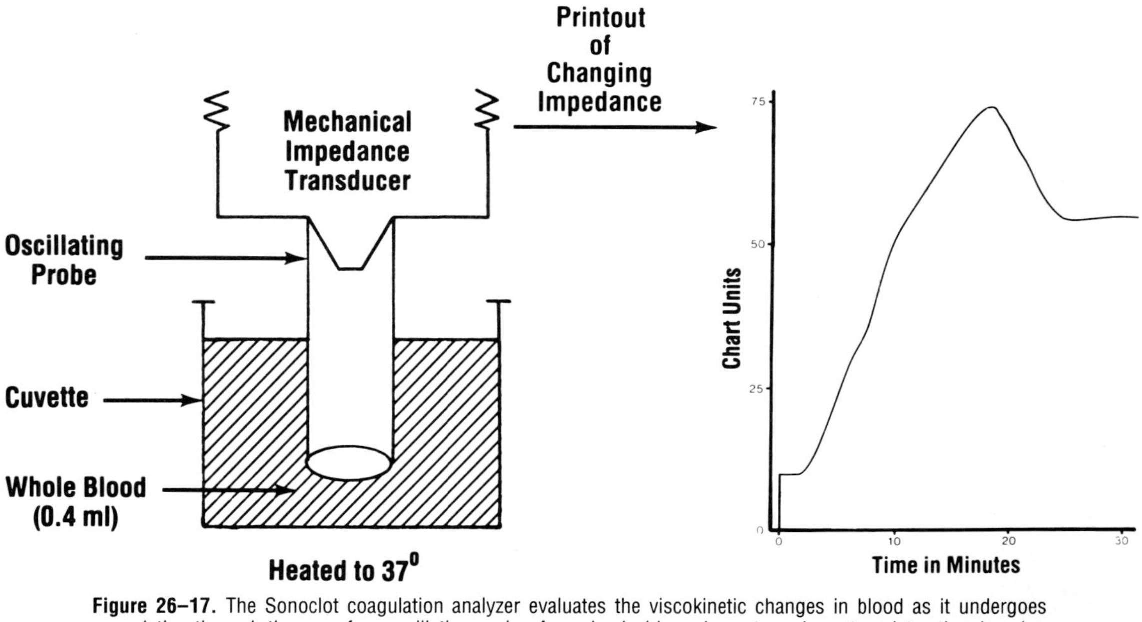

Figure 26–17. The Sonoclot coagulation analyzer evaluates the viscokinetic changes in blood as it undergoes coagulation through the use of an oscillating probe. A mechanical impedance transducer translates the changing impedance into a pattern (signature) of the blood as it undergoes clot formation.

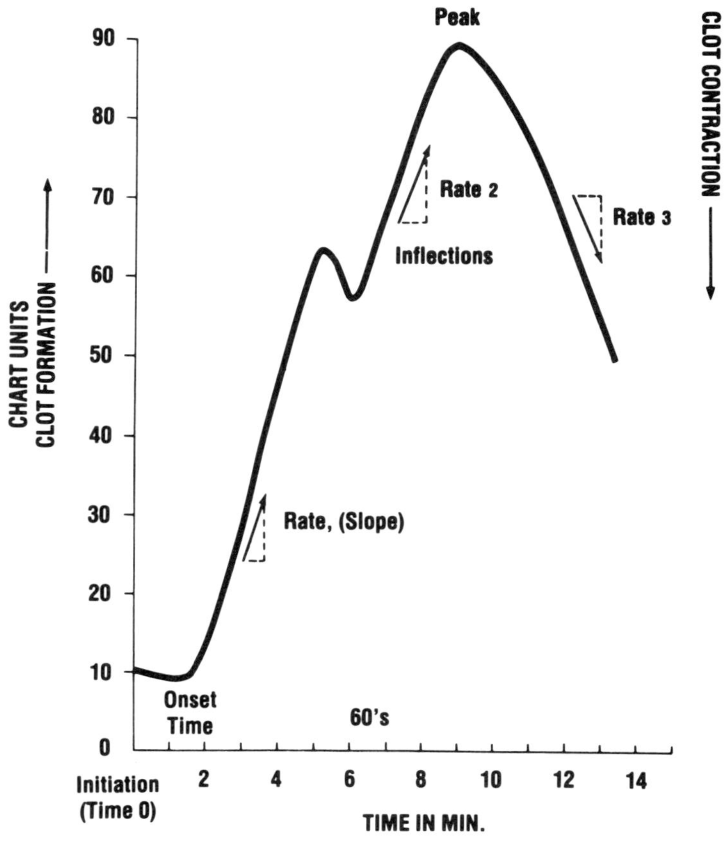

Figure 26–18. The Sonoclot signature is generated by the changing impedance on a vibrating probe placed in blood as it undergoes coagulation. The *initiation time* corresponds to the time the probe is immersed in the blood sample. The *onset time* indicates the intial formation of fibrin. *Upsloping rates* correspond to the rate of fibrin formation and platelet activation. The inflection seen on the upslope is a function of both platelet aggregation and contraction of the first fibrin strands. The *peak* corresponds to completion of fibrin formation, and the *downsloping rate* is produced by platelet-induced contraction of the fibrin clot. (Modified from Sienco, Inc., product literature.)

istic clotting patterns in order to identify coagulation disorders.

The Sonoclot analyzer has been proposed as an effective instrument for the qualitative evaluation of platelet function.[213] In the presence of either thrombocytopenia or dysfunctional platelets, changes in the Sonoclot signature include a lag in the coagulation onset time, a decrease in slope (rate), loss of the upward slope inflection (thought to correspond to initial platelet-induced contraction of fibrin strands), and dampening of both the primary peak and the resultant downslope (from platelet-mediated clot contraction). As with the Thromboelastograph, the Sonoclot pattern does not indicate the exact cause of a coagulation abnormality. Delays in onset time, depression of the upward slope, and dampening of the inflection occur with decreased levels of factors II, V, VIII, IX, X, and XI.[213] These changes also occur in the presence of heparin.

Clinically, the Sonoclot analyzer has been used for predicting patients at increased risk for thromboembolic episodes following surgery[214] and for evaluating coagulation during hypothermic cardiopulmonary bypass.[215] However, despite the length of time this instrument has been available, there are few studies indicating its value in evaluating and managing hemostatic derangements. As a way of increasing the versatility, specificity, and usefulness of the Sonoclot, additional cuvettes to evaluate activated clotting time, heparin level, and other coagulation parameters are being developed.

SPECIAL CONCERNS IN COAGULATION MONITORING

MASSIVE BLOOD LOSS—LIVER TRANSPLANT SURGERY

Advances in the development of devices for the intraoperative evaluation of coagulation have been a direct result of the need to monitor the severe coagulation derangements occurring during liver transplant surgery.[124, 125, 200] The combination of a need for massive blood component therapy during these operative procedures and the recommendations concerning curtailment and caution in blood component use[1, 216] emphasizes the need for accurate assessment of coagulation. Most of the interest in avoidance of homologous blood product transfusion has arisen from the fear of acquired immunodeficiency syndrome (AIDS) virus,[217, 218] despite the rarity of AIDS virus in donor blood with the new screening techniques.[1] However, recipients of blood provided by an AIDS virus–positive donor have a 70% or greater risk of becoming seropositive for this disease.[219]

The patient undergoing liver transplantation is of particular interest for coagulation monitoring owing to the wide range of coagulation derangements occurring during the perioperative period. These patients often have pre-existing coagulation defects due to the inadequate generation of liver-dependent coagulation factors and deficiencies in platelet activity from both endogenous abnormalities and preoperative medications. During the operative procedure, major changes in fibrinolysis, platelet activity, and coagulation factor levels occur. Overstimulation of the fibrinolytic system can become a major problem owing to increases in serum tissue plasminogen activator levels during dissection and removal of the diseased liver.

Aside from the coagulation problems directly associated with the diseased liver, a major problem during liver transplantation is massive blood loss.[124] Previous studies have defined massive blood loss as the loss of one, up to one and one-half, times a patient's blood volume.[220, 221] However, during the course of liver transplantation, the patient's estimated blood volume may be replaced 12 or more times. Problems associated with massive transfusion encompass a variety of metabolic abnormalities, including increased serum potassium, free hemoglobin, and pH[200, 222, 223] and decreased 2,3-diphosphoglycerate and ionized calcium. Platelets and coagulation factors decrease during massive transfusion. Platelet counts decrease more slowly than expected, owing to maintenance of platelet levels through release of splenic and bone marrow reserves.[221] However, in some patients, a single estimated blood volume exchange decreases platelet count well below 50,000/μl.[224] Depletions of the labile clotting factors, particularly factors V and VIII, also occur during massive transfusion.[220]

AUTOLOGOUS BLOOD USE AND INTRAOPERATIVE SALVAGE

Autotransfusion

In conjunction with the recommendations for decreased use of homologous red blood cell and component therapy,[216] preoperative collection of autologous blood and intraoperative salvage of blood from the surgical field is extensively utilized. The collection of autologous blood preoperatively, as a method of supplying blood for surgery when major blood loss is expected, is not new.[225, 227] Normal, healthy volunteers with phlebotomies of 3–5 U of blood/week for as many as 23 weeks can maintain a stable hemoglobin by using intravenous iron dextran supplementation to increase erythropoiesis.[228] In nonhealthy patients, preoperative phlebotomy of up to 4 U of blood (1 U every 48 hours) during the 10 days prior to a scheduled surgical procedure has been performed with resultant hematocrits of over 30% when iron dextran is provided.[229] Use of autologous blood not only avoids the risks associated with homologous blood transfusion but also has the advantage of being richer in 2,3-diphosphoglycerate, platelets, and labile clotting factors.[230] The fresher the blood, the greater the amount of available clotting factors V and VIII. One method of autologous blood use is removal of blood immediately prior to the surgical procedure using hemodilution techniques.[225, 226, 230, 231] By reinfusing the freshly taken blood during the surgical procedure, total blood loss can be decreased 25–95%.[225, 226, 230]

Intraoperative salvage of blood lost during the surgical procedure decreases homologous blood transfusion. Intraoperative blood salvage dates back to the late 1800s,[218] but it was not until the Vietnam War that a device was developed specifically for the rapid intraoperative autotransfusion of lost blood (Bentley Laboratories, Inc., Santa Ana, CA). The Bentley autotransfusion machine consisted of a roller-head pump attached to tubing leading from the surgical field. Blood was aspirated from the surgical field into a reservoir, where it was defoamed and filtered prior to reinfusion back to the patient.[218, 232, 233] Disadvantages of this system included the requirement for anticoagulation of either the scavenged blood or the patient and the risk of inadvertent infusion of large air emboli during blood reinfusion.

Thus, the Bentley system was abandoned and superseded by devices for rapid red blood cell washing and reinfusion of scavenged blood,[233] including commercially available devices from Haemonetics Corp. (Braintree, MA) and Electromedics (Englewood, CO). Reinfusion can be accomplished in as little as 3 minutes. The washing process removes non–red blood cell debris suctioned from the surgical field, activated clotting factors, free hemoglobin, pharmaceutic agents including heparin, and normal clotting factors. Unfortunately, bacteria, cancer cells,[218] and microfibrillar collagen hemostat[234] are not removed with the washing cycles. Although the scavenging systems return red blood cells, the reinfused blood is depleted of platelets and coagulation factors. Therefore, increased use of these devices necessitates improved intraoperative coagulation-monitoring devices to evaluate whether coagulation component infusions are required.

FUTURE DEVELOPMENTS

The need for specific, reliable, and rapid intraoperative evaluation of all components leading to hemostasis continues to increase. Future development of medical instrumentation for the evaluation of intraoperative hemostasis will most likely occur along two lines.

First, present medical instrumentation will be refined and expanded to allow more specific and accurate evaluations of particular components of the hemostatic system. This is already happening in the expansion of both the Hemochron and HemoTec ACT machines and the Sonoclot viscokinetic analyzer. Special cuvettes or cartridges will allow the evaluation of specific components of the coagulation system as well as of other factors involved in the hemostatic process.

Second, the expansion of monoclonal antibody research will most likely lead to the development of simple immunobiologic assays that can rapidly, specifically, and accurately evaluate derangements in coagulation. As the cost of monoclonal antibody production decreases and the intraoperative need for such specific evaluation increases, such assays should become more available. Organon Teknika Corporation introduced a quantitative Micro-ELISA Test for prothrombin fragment 1.2. The test uses a murine monoclonal antibody specific for the 1.2 fragment of prothrombin, which is released during activation of prothrombin to thrombin. Though this test cannot be used intraoperatively because of the need for exact aliquoting and long incubation periods, it does point to future intraoperative tests that might provide rapid and exact information concerning specific portions of the hemostatic process. In spite of expected advances in the intraoperative evaluation of hemostasis, maintaining the intricate balance of the various hemostatic factors will remain a challenge.

Acknowledgment

The author thanks Mariela Velasquez for her excellent help in the preparation of this chapter.

REFERENCES

1. McCullough J: The nation's changing blood supply system. JAMA 1993; 269:2239–2245.
2. Oates JA, FitzGerald GA, Branch RA, et al: Clinical implications of prostaglandin and thromboxane A_2 formation. N Engl J Med 1988; 319:689–761.
3. Oates JA, FitzGerald GA, Branch RA, et al: Clinical implications of prostaglandin and thromboxane A_2 formation. N Engl J Med 1988; 319:761–767.
4. Ellison N: What the anesthesiologist should know about coagulation. International Anesthesia Research Society Review Course Lectures. Cleveland: International Anesthesia Research Society, 1986; 127–132.
5. Arterial blood pressure. *In* Goudsonzian N, Karamanian A (eds): Physiology for the Anesthesiologist, 2nd Ed. Norwalk, CT: Appleton-Century-Crofts, 1984; 55–85.
6. Hoffman WS, Tomasello DN, Mac Vaugh H: Control of postcardiotomy bleeding with PEEP. Ann Thorac Surg 1982; 34:71–73.
7. Thompson GE, Miller RD, Stevens WC, Murray WR: Hypotensive anesthesia for total hip arthroplasty: A study of blood loss and organ function (brain, heart, liver, and kidney). Anesthesiology 1978; 48:91–96.
8. Lawson NW, Thompson DS, Nelson CL, et al: Sodium nitroprusside-induced hypotension for supine total hip replacement. Anesth Analg 1976; 55:654–662.
9. Ellison N: Diagnosis and management of bleeding disorders. Anesthesiology 1977; 47:171–180.
10. Rizza CR: Coagulation factor therapy. Clin Hematol 1976; 5:113–133.
11. White GC, McMillan CW, Kingdon HS, et al: Use of recombinant antihemophilic factor in the treatment of two patients with classic hemophilia. N Engl J Med 1989; 320:166–170.
12. Richard LC, Buller HR, Bovill J, Ten Cate JW: Influence of anesthesia on coagulation and fibrinolytic proteins. Br J Anaesth 1983; 55:869–872.
13. Barrier MJ, Ellison N: Platelet function. Anesthesiology 1977; 46:202–211.
14. Mustard JF: Anesthetics and platelets [Editorial]. Anesthesiology 1971; 34:401–402.
15. Davies MJ, Thomas A: Thrombosis and acute coronary-artery lesions in sudden cardiac ischemic death. N Engl J Med 1984; 310:1137–1140.
16. Weksler BB, Pett SB, Alonso D, et al: Differential inhibition by aspirin of vascular and platelet prostaglandin synthesis in atherosclerotic patients. N Engl J Med 1983; 308:800–805.
17. Cairns JA, Gent M, Singer J, et al: Aspirin, sulfinpyrazone, or both in unstable angina. N Engl J Med 1985; 313:1369–1375.
18. Preliminary report: Findings from the aspirin component of the ongoing physicians' health study. N Engl J Med 1988; 318:262–264.
19. Harker LA, Slichter SJ: The bleeding time as a screening test for evaluation of platelet function. N Engl J Med 1972; 287:155–159.
20. Amrein PC, Ellman L, Harris WH: Aspirin-induced prolongation of bleeding time and perioperative blood loss. JAMA 1981; 245:1825–1828.
21. Hindman BJ, Koka BV: Usefulness of the post-aspirin bleeding time. Anesthesiology 1986; 64:368–370.
22. Ferraris VA, Gildengorin V: Predictors of excessive blood use after coronary artery bypass grafting. J Thorac Cardiovasc Surg 1989; 98:492–497.
23. Rinder CS, Mathew JP, Rinder HM, et al: Modulation of platelet surface adhesion receptors during cardiopulmonary bypass. Anesthesiology 1991; 75:563–570.
24. Rinder CS, Bohnert J, Rinder HM, et al: Platelet activation and aggregation during cardiopulmonary bypass. Anesthesiology 1991; 75:388–393.
25. Hicks GL, Jensen LA, Norsen LH, et al: Platelet inhibitors and hydroxyethyl starch: Safe and cost-effective interventions in coronary artery surgery. Ann Thorac Surg 1985; 39:422–425.
26. Valeri R, Cassidy G, Khuri S, et al: Hypothermia-induced reversible platelet dysfunction. Ann Surg 1987; 205:175–181.
27. Litchtenfeld KM, Schiffer CA, Helrich M: Platelet aggregation during and after general anesthesia and surgery. Anesth Analg 1979; 59:293–296.
28. Gotta AW, Gould P, Sullivan CA, et al: The effect of enflurane and fentanyl anaesthesia on human platelet aggregation *in vivo*. Can Anaesth Soc J 1980; 27:319–321.
29. Dalsgaard-Nielsen J, Risbo A, Simmelkjaer P, Gormsen J: Impaired platelet aggregation and increased bleeding time during general anesthesia with halothane. Br J Anaesth 1981; 53:1039–1041.
30. Walter F, Vulliemoz Y, Verosky M, Triner L: Effects of halothane on the cyclic 3′,5′-adenosine monophosphate enzyme system in human platelets. Anesth Analg 1980; 59:856–861.
31. Fauss BG, Meadows JC, Bruni CY, Qureshi GD: The *in vitro* and *in vivo* effects of isoflurane and nitrous oxide on platelet aggregation. Anesth Analg 1986; 65:1170–1174.
32. Ueda I: The effects of volatile general anesthetics on adenosine diphosphate induced platelet aggregation. Anesthesiology 1971; 34:405–408.
33. Hines R: Preservation of platelet function during trimethaphan infusion. Anesthesiology 1990; 72:834–837.
34. Hines R, Barash PG: Infusion of sodium nitroprusside induces platelet dysfunction *in vivo*. Anesthesiology 1989; 70:611–615.
35. Graybar G, Lobar D, Jones J: Comparison of nitroprusside and nitroglycerine in perioperative blood loss with open heart surgery. Crit Care Med 1980; 240–242.
36. Lavee J, Savion N, Smolinsky A, et al: Platelet protection by aprotinin in cardiopulmonary bypass: Electron microscopic study. Ann Thorac Surg 1992; 53:477–481.
37. Coller BS: Platelets and thrombolytic therapy. N Engl J Med 1990; 322:33–41.
38. Kazmier FJ: Thromboembolism, coumarin necrosis, and protein C. Mayo Clin Proc 1985; 60:673–674.
39. Rick ME: Protein C and protein S. JAMA 1990; 263:701–703.
40. Clouse LH, Comp PC: The regulation of hemostasis: The protein C system. N Engl J Med 1986; 314:1298–1304.
41. Peters C, Casella JF, Marlar RA, et al: Homozygous protein C deficiency: Observations on the nature of the molecular abnormality and the effectiveness of warfarin therapy. Pediatrics 1988; 81:272–276.
42. Matsuda M, Sugo T, Sakata Y, et al: A thrombotic state due to an abnormal protein C. N Engl J Med 1988; 19:1265–1268.
43. Bomzer CA, Bertina RM, Briet E, et al: Protein C deficiency and the risk of venous thrombosis [Letter]. N Engl J Med 1988; 318:930–932.
44. Gerson WT, Dickerman TD, Bovill EG, Golden E: Severe acquired protein C deficiency in purpura fulminans associated with disseminated intravascular coagulation: Treatment with protein C concentrate. Pediatrics 1993; 91:418–422.
45. Knobl PN, Zilla P, Fasol R, et al: The protein C system in patients undergoing cardiopulmonary bypass. J Thorac Cardiovasc Surg 1987; 94:600–605.
46. Griffin JH, Evatt B, Zimmerman TS, et al: Deficiency of protein C in congenital thrombotic disease. J Clin Invest 1981; 68:1370–1373.
47. Broekmans AW, van der Linden IK, VeltKamp JJ, Bertina RM: Prevalence of isolated protein C deficiency in patients with venous thrombotic disease and in the population [Abstract]. Thromb Haemost 1983; 50:350.
48. Pabinger-Fasching I, Bertina RM, Lechner K, et al: Protein C deficiency in two Austrian families. Thromb Haemost 1983; 50:810–813.

49. Miletich J, Sherman L, Broze G Jr: Absence of thrombosis in subjects with heterozygous protein C deficiency. N Engl J Med 1987; 317:991–996.
50. Fitzgerald DJ, Roy L, Catella F, FitzGerald GA: Platelet activation in unstable coronary disease. N Engl J Med 1986; 315:983–998.
51. Jaffe AS, Sobel BE: Thrombolysis with tissue-type plasminogen activator in acute myocardial infarction. JAMA 1986; 255:237–239.
52. Laffel GL, Braunwald E: Thrombolytic therapy: A new strategy for the treatment of acute myocardial infarction. N Engl J Med 1984; 311:710–717.
53. Aoki N, Sakata Y, Matsuda M, et al: Fibrinolytic states in a patient with congenital deficiency of α_2-plasmin inhibitor. Blood 1980; 55:483–488.
54. Marder VJ, Sherry S: Thrombolytic therapy: Current status (first of two parts). N Engl J Med 1988; 318:1512–1520.
55. Marder VJ, Sherry S: Thrombolytic therapy: Current status (part two). N Engl J Med 1988; 318:1585–1594.
56. Mentzer RL, BS, Budzynski AZ, Sherry S: High-dose, brief-duration intravenous infusion of streptokinase in acute myocardial infarction: Description of effects in the circulation. Am J Cardiol 1986; 57:1220–1226.
57. White HD, Rivers JT, Maslowski AH, et al: Effect of intravenous streptokinase as compared with that of tissue plasminogen activator on left ventricular function after first myocardial infarction. N Engl J Med 1989; 320:817–824.
58. Loscalzo J, Braunwald E: Tissue plasminogen activator. N Engl J Med 1988; 319:925–931.
59. Haber E, Quertermous T, Matsueda GR, et al: Innovative approaches to plasminogen activator therapy. Science 1989; 243:51–56.
60. ISAM Study Group: A prospective trial of intravenous streptokinase in acute myocardial infarction (I.S.A.M.). N Engl J Med 1986; 314:1465–1471.
61. Kennedy JW, Ritchie JL, Davis KB, et al: The western Washington randomized trial of intracoronary streptokinase in acute myocardial infarction. A 12-month follow-up report. N Engl J Med 1985; 312:1073–1078.
62. Cowley MJ, Hastillo A, Vetrovec GW, et al: Fibrinolytic effects of intracoronary streptokinase administration in patients with acute myocardial infarction and coronary insufficiency. Circulation 1983; 67:1031–1038.
63. Goldberg M, Colonna-Romano P, Babins NA: Emergency coronary artery bypass surgery following intracoronary streptokinase. Anesthesiology 1984; 61:601–604.
64. Bull BS, Korpman RA, Huse WM, Briggs BD: Heparin therapy during extracorporeal circulation. Problems inherent in existing heparin protocols. J Thorac Cardiovasc Surg 1975; 69:674–684.
65. McLean J: The thromboplastic action of cephalin. Am J Physiol 1916; 16:250–257.
66. Salzman EW: Low-molecular-weight heparin. Is small beautiful? N Engl J Med 1986; 315:957–959.
67. Lam LH, Silbert JE, Rosenberg RD: The separation of active and inactive forms of heparin. Biochem Biophys Res Commun 1976; 69:570–577.
68. Rosenberg RD, Lam L: Correlation between structure and function of heparin (mucopolysaccharide/anticoagulant function). Proc Natl Acad Sci U S A 1979; 76:1218–1222.
69. Novak E, Sekhar NC, Dunham NW, Coleman LL: A comparative study of the effect of lung and gut heparins on platelet aggregation and protamine neutralization in man. Clin Med 1972; July:22–27.
70. Estes JW, Poulin PF: Pharmacokinetics of heparin. Thromb Diath Haemorrh 1974; 33:26–37.
71. Jick H, Slone D, Borda IT, Shapiro S: Efficacy and toxicity of heparin in relation to age and sex. N Engl J Med 1968; 279:284–286.
72. Blauhut B, Nacek S, Kramar H, et al: Activity of antithrombin III and effect of heparin on coagulation in shock. Thromb Res 1980; 19:775–782.
73. Cloyd GM, D'Ambra MN, Akins CW: Diminished anticoagulant response to heparin in patients undergoing coronary artery bypass grafting. J Thorac Cardiovasc Surg 1987; 94:535–538.
74. Perry MO, Horton J: Kinetics of heparin administration. Arch Surg 1976; 111:403–409.
75. Cook JJ, Niewiarowski S, Yan Z, et al: Platelet factor 4 efficiently reverses heparin anticoagulation in the rat without adverse effects of heparin-protamine complexes. Circulation 1992; 85:1102–1109.
76. Anderson EF: Heparin resistance prior to cardiopulmonary bypass. Anesthesiology 1986; 64:504–507.
77. Palmer NR, Rick ME, Rick PD, et al: Circulating heparin sulfate anticoagulant in a patient with a fatal bleeding disorder. N Engl J Med 1984; 310:1696–1699.
78. Morel DR, Zapol WM, Thomas SJ, et al: C5a and thromboxane generation associated with pulmonary vaso- and broncho-constriction during protamine reversal of heparin. Anesthesiology 1987; 66:597–604.
79. Colman RW: Humoral mediators of catastrophic reactions associated with protamine neutralization. Anesthesiology 1987; 66:595–596.
80. Ullman DA, Bloom BS, Danker PR, et al: Protamine-induced hypotension in a two-year-old child. J Cardiothorac Vasc Anesth 1988; 2:497–499.
81. Weiss ME, Nyhan D, Peng Z, et al: Association of protamine IgE and IgG antibodies with life-threatening reactions to intravenous protamine. N Engl J Med 1989; 320:886–892.
82. Horrow JC: Protamine allergy. J Cardiothorac Vasc Anesth 1988; 2:225–242.
83. Ellison N: Heparin: New information on an old drug [Editorial]. J Cardiothorac Anesth 1987; 1:377–378.
84. Rosenberg RD: Actions and interactions of antithrombin and heparin. N Engl J Med 1975: 292:146–151.
85. Gorman RR: Modulation of human platelet function by prostacyclin and thromboxane A_2. Fed Proc 1979; 38:83–88.
86. Coppe D, Wonders T, Snider M, Salzman EW: Preservation of platelet number and function during extracorporeal membrane oxygenation by regional infusion of prostacyclin. *In* Vane JR, Bergstrom S (eds): Prostacyclin. New York: Raven, 1979; 371–383.
87. Malpass TW, Hanson SR, Savage B, et al: Prevention of acquired transient defect in platelet plug formation by infused prostacyclin. Blood 1981; 57:736–740.
88. Zusman RM, Rubin RH, Cato AE, et al: Hemodialysis using prostacyclin instead of heparin as the sole antithrombotic agent. N Engl J Med 1981; 304:934–939.
89. Woods HF, Ash G, Weston MJ, et al: Prostacyclin can replace heparin in hemodialysis in dogs. Lancet 1978; 2:1075–1077.
90. Kappa JR, Horn MK III, Fisher CA, et al: Efficacy of iloprost (ZK36374) versus aspirin in preventing heparin-induced platelet activation during cardiac operations. J Thorac Cardiovasc Surg 1987; 94:405–413.
91. Ellison N, Kappa JR, Fisher CA, Addonizio VP Jr: Extracorporeal circulation in a patient with heparin-induced thrombocytopenia. Anesthesiology 1985; 63:336–337.
92. Kappa JR, Ellison N, Fisher CA, Addonizio VP: The use of iloprost (ZK36374) to permit cardiopulmonary bypass in 2 patients with heparin-induced thrombocytopenia [Abstract]. Anesthesiology 1985; 63:A32.
93. Smith JP, Walls JT, Muscato MS, et al: Extracorporeal circulation in a patient with heparin-induced thrombocytopenia. Anesthesiology 1985; 62:363–365.
94. Bell WR, Tomasulo PA, Alving BM, Duffy TP: Thrombocytopenia occurring during the administration of heparin. Ann Intern Med 1976; 85:155–160.
95. Reid HA, Chan KE, Thean PC: Prolonged coagulation defect (defibrinogenation syndrome) in Malayan viper bite. Lancet 1963; 1:621–626.
96. Zulys VJ, Teasdale SJ, Michel ER, et al: Ancrod (Arvin) as an alternative to heparin anticoagulation for cardiopulmonary bypass. Anesthesiology 1989; 71:870–877.
97. Hall RJC, Young C, Sutton GC, et al: Anticoagulation by ancrod for haemodialysis. Br Med J 1970; 4:591–593.
98. Lowe GDO, Morrice JJ, Fulton A, et al: Subcutaneous ancrod after operation for fractured hip. A dose ranging and feasibility study. Thromb Haemost 1978; 40:134–143.
99. Ewart MR, Hatton MWC, Basford JM, et al: The proteolytic action of Arvin on human fibrinogen. Biochem J 1970; 603–609.
100. Sharp AA: Clinical use of arvin. Thromb Diath Haemorrh Suppl 1971; 45:69.
101. Weiss HJ, Aledort LM, Kochwa S: The effect of salicylates on the hemostatic properties of platelets in man. J Clin Invest 1968; 47:2169–2180.
102. Chesebro JH, Clements IP, Fuster V, et al: A platelet-inhibitor-drug trial in coronary-artery bypass operations. Benefit of perioperative dipyridamole and aspirin therapy on early postoperative vein-graft patency. N Engl J Med 1982; 307:73–78.

103. Chesebro JH, Fuster V, Elveback LR, et al: Effect of dipyridamole and aspirin on late vein-graft patency after coronary bypass operation. N Engl J Med 1984; 310:209–214.
104. Rubin RN: Aspirin and postsurgery bleeding. Ann Intern Med 1978; 89:1006.
105. Stuart MJ, Gross SJ, Elrad H, Graeber JE: Effects of acetylsalicyclic-acid ingestion on maternal and neonatal hemostasis. N Engl J Med 1982; 307:909–912.
106. McNicol GP, Fletcher AP, Alkaersig N, Sherry S: The absorption, distribution, and excretion of epsilon-aminocaproic acid following oral or intravenous administration to man. J Lab Clin Med 1962; 59:15–24.
107. Aoki N, Sakata Y, Matsuda M, Tateno K: Fibrinolytic states in a patient with congenital deficiency of alpha$_2$-plasmin inhibitor. Blood 1980; 55:483–488.
108. Kennedy JW, Ritchie JL, Davis KB, Fritz JK: Western Washington randomized trial of intracoronary streptokinase in acute myocardial infarction. N Engl J Med 1983; 309:1477–1482.
109. Markis JE, Malagold M, Parker JA, et al: Myocardial salvage after intracoronary thrombolysis with streptokinase in acute myocardial infarction. Assessment by intracoronary thallium-201. N Engl J Med 1981; 305:777–782.
110. Khaja F, Walton JA, Brymer JF, et al: Intracoronary fibrinolytic therapy in acute myocardial infarction. Report of a prospective randomized trial. N Engl J Med 1983; 308:1306–1318.
111. Van der werf F, Ludbrook PA, Bergmann SR, et al: Coronary thrombolysis with tissue-type plasminogen activator in patients with evolving myocardial infarction. N Engl J Med 1984; 310:609–614.
112. Gralnick HR: Aminocaproic acid in preoperative correction of hemostatic defect in cyanotic congenital heart disease. Lancet 1970; 2:1204–1205.
113. Brodsky I, Gill DN, Lusch CJ: Fibrinolysis in congenital heart disease. Preoperative treatment with aminocaproic acid. Am J Clin Pathol 1969; 51:51–57.
114. McClure PD, Izak J: The use of epsilon-aminocaproic acid to reduce bleeding during cardiac bypass in children with congenital heart disease. Anesthesiology 1974; 40:604–608.
115. Midell AI, Hallman GL, Bloodwell RD, et al: Epsilon-aminocaproic acid for bleeding after cardiopulmonary bypass. Ann Thorac Surg 1971; 11:577–582.
116. Lambert CJ, Marengo-Rowe AJ, Leveson JE, et al: The treatment of post-perfusion bleeding using aminocaproic acid, cryoprecipitate, fresh-frozen plasma, and protamine sulfate. Ann Thorac Surg 1979; 28:440–441.
117. Sterns LP, Lillehei CW: Effect of epsilon aminocaproic acid upon blood loss following open-heart surgery: An analysis of 340 patients. Can J Surg 1967; 10:304–307.
118. DelRossi AJ, Cernaianu AC, Botros S, et al: Prophylactic treatment of postperfusion bleeding using EACA. Chest 1989; 96:27–30.
119. Naeye RL: Thrombotic state after a hemorrhagic diathesis, a possible complication of therapy with epsilon-aminocaproic acid. Blood 1962; 19:694–701.
120. Charytan C, Purtilo D: Glomerular capillary thrombosis and acute renal failure after epsilon aminocaproic acid therapy. N Engl J Med 1969; 280:1102–1104.
121. Gibbon JH, Camishion RC: Problems with hemostasis with extracorporeal apparatus. Ann N Y Acad Sci 1964; 115:195–198.
122. Adams HP, Nibbelink DW, Torner JC, Sahs AL: Antifibrinolytic therapy in patients with aneurysmal subarachnoid hemorrhage. A report of the cooperative aneurysm study. Arch Neurol 1981; 38:25–29.
123. Hoffman EP, Koo AH: Cerebral thrombosis associated with amicar therapy. Radiology 1979; 131:687–689.
124. Kang YG, Martin DJ, Marquez J, et al: Intraoperative changes in blood coagulation and thromboelastographic monitoring in liver transplantation. Anesth Analg 1985; 64:888–896.
125. Kang YG, Navalgund A, Russell M, Starzl TE: Antifibrinolytic therapy during liver transplantation. Anesthesiology 1985; 63:A92.
126. Spiess BD: The contribution of fibrinolysis to postbypass bleeding. J Cardiothorac Vasc Anesth 1991; 5:13–17.
127. Horrow J, Hlavacek J, Strong MD, et al: Prophylactic tranexamic acid decreases bleeding after cardiac operations. J Thorac Cardiovasc Surg 1990; 99:70–74.
128. Horrow J, Van Riper DF, Parmet J, et al: Tranexamic acid, not demopressin or both, decreases bleeding after opern heart surgery. Anesthesiology 1990; 73:A63.
129. Davies D, Howell DA: Tranexamic acid and arterial thrombosis. Lancet 1977; 1:49.
130. Dietrich W, Barankay A, Hähnel CH, et al: High-dose aprotinin in cardiac surgery: Three years' experience in 1,784 patients. J Cardiothorac Vasc Anesth 1992; 6:324–327.
131. Vedrinne C, Girard C, Jegaden O, et al: Reduction in blood loss and blood use after cardiopulmonary bypass with high-dose aprotinin versus autologous fresh whole blood transfusion. J Cardiothorac Vasc Anesth 1992; 6:319–323.
132. Dietrich W, Spannagl M, Jochum M, et al: Influence of high-dose aprotinin treatment on blood loss and coagularion patterns in patients undergoing myocardial revascularization. Anesthesiology 1990; 73:1119–1126.
133. Royston D: High-dose aprotinin therapy: A review of the first five years' experience. J Cardiothorac Vasc Anesth 1992; 6:76–100.
134. Nagaoka H, Innami R, Murayama F, et al: Effects of aprotinin on prostaglandin metabolism and platelet function in open heart surgery. J Cardiovasc Surg 1991; 32:31–37.
135. Böhrer H, Bach A, Fleischer F, et al: Adverse haemodynamic effects of high-dose aprotinin in a pediatric cardiac surgical patient. Anaesthesia 1990; 45:853–854.
136. Salzman EW, Weinstein MJ, Weintraub RM, et al: Treatment with desmopressin acetate to reduce blood loss after cardiac surgery. A double-blind randomized trial. N Engl J Med 1986; 314:1402–1406.
137. Mannucci PM: Desmopressin (DDAVP) for treatment of disorders of hemostasis. Prog Hemost Thromb 1986; 8:19–43.
138. Reich DL, Hammerschlag BC, Rand JH, et al: Desmospressin acetate is a mild vasodilator that does not reduce blood loss in uncomplicated cardiac surgical procedures. J Cardiothorac Vasc Anesth 1991; 5:142–145.
139. Ansell J, Klassen V, Lew R, et al: Does desmopressin acetate prophylaxis reduce blood loss after valvular heart operations? A randomized, double-blind study. J Thorac Cardiovasc Surg 1992; 104:117–123.
140. Salmenperä M, Kuitunen A, Hynynen M, et al: Hemodynamic responses to desmopressin acetate after CABG: A double-blind trial. J Cardiothorac Vasc Anesth 1991; 5:146–149.
141. Hackmann T, Gascoyne RD, Naiman SC, et al: A trial of desmopressin (1-desamino-8-D-arginine vasopressin) to reduce loss in uncomplicated cardiac surgery. J Cardiothorac Vasc Anesth 1989; 321:1437–1443.
142. Frankville DD, Harper GB, Lake CL, et al: Hemodynamic consequences of desmopressin administration after cardiopulmonary bypass. Anesthesiology 1991; 74:988–996.
143. Lethagen S, Rugarn P: The effect of DDAVP and placebo on platelet function and prolonged bleeding time induced by oral acetylsalicylic acid intake on volunteers. Thromb Haemost 1992; 67:185–186.
144. Salzman EW: Desmopressin and surgical hemostasis. N Engl J Med 1990; 322:1085.
145. Mongan PD, Hosking MP: The role of desmopressin acetate in patients undergoing coronary artery bypass surgery. Anesthesiology 1992; 77:38–46.
146. Guay J, Reinberg C, Poitras B, et al: A trial of desmopressin to reduce blood loss in patients undergoing spinal fusion for idiopathic scoliosis. Anesth Analg 1992; 75:405–410.
147. Rickles FR, Hoyer LW, Rick ME, et al: The effects of epinephrine infusion in patients with von Willebrand's disease. J Clin Invest 1976; 57:1618–1625.
148. Israels SJ, Kobrinsky NL: Serious reaction to desmopressin in a child with cyanotic heart disease. N Engl J Med 1989; 320:1563–1564.
149. Jahr JS, Marquez J, Cottington E, et al: Hemodynamic performance and histamine levels after desmopressin acetate administration following cardiopulmonary bypass in adult patients. J Cardiothorac Vasc Anesth 1991; 5:139–141.
150. Czer L, Bateman T, Gran R, et al: Prospective trial of DDAVP in treatment of severe platelet dysfunction and hemorrhage after cardiopulmonary bypass. Circulation 1985; 72(Suppl 3):130.
151. Jobes DR, Schwartz AJ, Ellison N, et al: Monitoring heparin anticoagulation and its neutralization. Ann Thorac Surg 1981; 31:161–166.
152. Chargaff E, Olson KB: Studies on the chemistry of blood coagulation. Studies on the action of heparin and other anticoagulants. The influence of protamine on the anticoagulant effect in vivo. J Biol Chem 1937; 122:153–167.
153. Hill AG, Lefrak EA: Monitoring heparin and protamine therapy during cardiopulmonary bypass procedures. Pro Am Sect 1978; 6:10–13.

154. Hill AG, Groom RC, Marino JA, et al: More precise heparin and protamine management during cardiopulmonary bypass. Proc Am Acad Cardiovasc Perf 1990; 11:12–16.
155. Esposito RA, Culliford AT, et al: Heparin resistance during cardiopulmonary bypass. J Thorac Cardiovasc Surg 1983; 85:346–353.
156. Anderson EF: Heparin resistance prior to cardiopulmonary bypass. Anesthesiology 1986; 64:504–507.
157. Mabry CD, Read RC, et al: Identification of heparin resistance during cardiac and vascular surgery. Arch Surg 1979; 114:129–134.
158. Marciniak E, Gockerman JP: Heparin-induced decrease in circulating antithrombin—III. Lancet 1977; 581–584.
159. Habbab MA, Haft JI: Heparin resistance induced by intravenous nitroglycerin. Arch Intern Med 1987; 147:857–860.
160. Gravlee GP, Brauer SD, Roy RC, et al: Predicting the pharmacodynamics of heparin: A clinical evaluation of the Hepcon System 4. J Cardiothorac Vasc Anesth 1987; 1:379–387.
161. Bull MH, Huse WM, Bull BS: Evaluation of tests used to monitor heparin therapy during extracorporeal circulation. Anesthesiology 1975; 43:346–353.
162. Gravlee GP, Brauer SD, Roy RC, et al: Predicting the pharmacodynamics of heparin: A clinical evaluation of the Hepcon System 4. J Cardiothorac Vasc Anesth 1987; 1:379–387.
163. Pifarre R, Babka R, Sullivan HJ, et al: Management of postoperative heparin rebound following cardiopulmonary bypass. J Thorac Cardiovasc Surg 1981; 81:378–381.
164. Mitchell GA, Gargiulo RJ, Huseby RM, et al: Assay for plasma heparin using a synthetic peptide substrate for thrombin. Thromb Res 1978; 13:47–52.
165. Umlas J, Taff RH, Gauvin G, Swierk P: Anticoagulant monitoring and neutralization during open heart surgery—A rapid method for measuring heparin and calculating safe reduced protamine doses. Anesth Analg 1983; 62:1095–1099.
166. Choo IHF, Didisheim P, Doerge ML, et al: Evaluation of a heparin assay method using a fluorogenic synthetic peptide substrate for thrombin. Thromb Res 1982; 25:115–123.
167. Anido G, Freeman DJ: Heparin assay and protamine titration. Am J Clin Pathol 1981; 76:410–415.
168. Hughes DR, Faust RJ, Didisheim P, Tinker JH: Heparin monitoring during cardiopulmonary bypass in man: Use of fluorogenic heparin assay to validate activated clotting time. Anesth Analg 1982; 61:189–190.
169. Pochron SP, Mitchell GA, Albareda I, et al: A fluorescent substrate assay for plasminogen. Thromb Res 1978; 13:733–739.
170. Mitchell GA, Hudson PM, Huseby RM, et al: Fluorescent substrate assay for antithrombin III. Thromb Res 1977; 12:219–225.
171. Schriever HG, Epstein SE, Mintz MD: Statistical correlation and heparin sensitivity of activated partial thromboplastin time, whole blood coagulation time, and automated coagulation time. Am J Clin Pathol 1973; 60:323–329.
172. Dauchot PJ, Berzina-Moettus L, Rabinovitch A, Ankeney JL: Activated coagulation and activated partial thromboplastin times in assessment and reversal of heparin-induced anticoagulation for cardiopulmonary bypass. Anesth Analg 1983; 62:710–719.
173. Bull BS, Huse WM, Brauer FS, Korpman RA: Heparin therapy during extracorporeal circulation. II. The use of a dose-response curve to individualize heparin and protamine dosage. J Thorac Cardiovasc Surg 1975; 69:685–689.
174. Cohen JA, Frederickson EL, Kaplan JA: Plasma heparin activity and antagonism during cardiopulmonary bypass with hypothermia. Anesth Analg 1977; 56:564–570.
175. Donahoo KM, Taylor CA, Baugh RF, Soloway HB: A promising new multifunction instrument for monitoring heparin therapy. Adv Ther 1985; 2:150–159.
176. Hattersley PG: Activated coagulation time of whole blood. JAMA 1966; 196:436–440.
177. Hill JD, Dontigny L, de Leval M, Mielke C: A simple method of heparin management during prolonged extracorporeal circulation. Ann Thorac Surg 1974; 17:129–134.
178. Baugh RF, Deemar KA, Zimmermann JJ: Heparinase in the activated clotting time assay: Monitoring heparin-independent alterations in coagulation function. Anesth Analg 1992; 74:201–205.
179. Wang JS, Lin CY, Hung WT, et al: Monitoring of heparin-induced anticoagulation with Kaolin-activated clotting time in cardiac surgical patients treated with aprotinin. Anesthesiology 1992; 77:1080–1084.
180. Esposito RA, Culliford AT, Colvin SB, et al: The role of the activated clotting time in heparin administration and neutralization for cardiopulmonary bypass. J Thorac Cardiovasc Surg 1983; 85:174–185.
181. Gravlee GP, Whitaker CL, Mark LJ, et al: Baseline activated coagulation time should be measured after surgical incision. Anesth Analg 1990; 71:549–553.
182. Weinberg S, Phillips L, Twersky R, et al: Hypercoagulability in a patient with a brain tumor. Anesthesiology 1984; 61:200–202.
183. Fyman PN, Gotta A, Casthely PA, et al: Factor IX–induced hypercoagulable state. Anesthesiology 1985; 62:515–516.
184. Hanowell ST, Kim YUD, Rattan V, MacNamara TE: Increased heparin requirement with hypereosinophilic syndrome. Anesthesiology 1981; 55:450–452.
185. Esposito RA, Culliford AT, Colvin SB, et al: Heparin resistance during cardiopulmonary bypass. The role of heparin pretreatment. J Thorac Cardiovasc Surg 1983; 85:346–353.
186. Young JA, Kisker CT, Doty DB: Adequate anticoagulation during cardiopulmonary bypass determined by activated clotting time and the appearance of fibrin monomer. Ann Thorac Surg 1978; 26:231–240.
187. Metz S, Keats AS: Low activated coagulation time during cardiopulmonary bypass does not increase postoperative bleeding. Ann Thorac Surg 1990; 49:440–444.
188. Culliford AT, Gitel SN, Starr N, et al: Lack of correlation between activated clotting time and plasma heparin during cardiopulmonary bypass. Ann Surg 1981; 193:105–111.
189. Thomas SJ, Gitel SN, Starr NJ, et al: Activated clotting time and heparin levels during hypothermic cardiopulmonary bypass. Anesthesiology 1980; 53:S115.
190. Cohen JA: Activated coagulation time method for control of heparin is reliable during cardiopulmonary bypass. Anesthesiology 1984; 60:121–124.
191. Barnette RE, Shupak RC, Pontius J, et al: In vitro effect of fresh frozen plasma on the activated coagulation time in patients undergoing cardiopulmonary bypass. Anesth Analg 1988; 67:57–60.
192. Hooper TL, Conroy J, McArdle B, et al: The use of the hemochron in assessment of heparin reversal after cardiopulmonary bypass. Perfusion 1988; 3:295–300.
193. O'Neill AI, McAllister C, Corke CF, et al: A comparison of five devices for the bedside monitoring of heparin therapy. Anaesth Intensive Care 1991; 19:592–601.
194. Moorehead MT, Westengard JC, Bull BS: Platelet involvement in the activated coagulation time of heparinized blood. Anesth Analg 1984; 63:394–398.
195. Kind DO, Kane PB: Blood clot formation during multiple cardiopulmonary bypass procedures necessitated by massive hemorrhage. Anesth Analg 1978; 57:273–276.
196. Ansell J, Tiarks C, Hirsh J, et al: Measurement of the activated partial thromboplastin time from a capillary (fingerstick) sample of whole blood. J Clin Pathol 1991; 95:222–227.
197. Nuttall GA, Oliver W, Beynen FM, et al: Intraoperative measurement of APTT and PT by portable laser photometer. Anesth Analg 1991; 72:S201.
198. Franz RC, Coetzee WJC: The thromboelastographic diagnosis of hemostatic defects. Surg Annu 1981; 13:75–107.
199. Eliot RS, von Kaulla KN, Blount SG: Thromboelastographic studies with a twenty-four-hour schedule for subcutaneous heparin. Circulation 1961; 24:1206–1214.
200. Kang Y, Borland LM, Picone J, et al: Intraoperative coagulation changes in children undergoing liver transplantation. Anesthesiology 1989; 71:44–47.
201. Dorman BH, Spinale FG, Bailey MK, et al: Identification of patients at risk for excessive blood loss during coronary artery bypass surgery: Thromboelastograph versus coagulation screen. Anesth Analg 1993; 76:694–700.
202. Wang JS, Lin CY, Hung WT, et al: Thromboelastogram fails to predict postoperative hemorrhage in cardiac patients. Ann Thorac Surg 1992; 53:435–439.
203. Whitten CW, Allison PM, Latson TW, et al: Thrombelastographic fibrinolysis does not correlate with levels of D-Dimers after cardiopulmonary bypass. Anesthesiology 1991; 75:A432.
204. Spiess BD, Tuman KJ, McCarthy RJ, et al: Thromboelastography as an indicator of post-cardiopulmonary bypass coagulopathies. J Clin Monit 1987; 3:25–30.
205. Tuman KJ, Spiess BD, Schoen RE, Ivankovich AD: Use of thromboelastography in the management of von Willebrand's disease dur-

ing cardiopulmonary bypass. J Cardiothorac Anesth 1987; 1:321–324.
206. Tuman KJ, Spiess BD, McCarthy RJ, Ivankovich AD: Effects of progressive blood loss on coagulation as measured by thrombelastography. Anesth Analg 1987; 66:856–863.
207. von Kaulla KN: Continuous automatic recording of fibrin formation and fibrinolysis: A valuable tool of coagulation research. J Lab Clin Med 1957; 49:304–312.
208. Zuckerman L, Cohen E, Vagher JP, et al: Comparison of thrombelastography with common coagulation tests. Thromb Haemost 1981; 46:752–756.
209. Kang YG, Abouleish E: Thrombelastography in obstetrics. Anesthesiology 1981; 55:A304.
210. Koren G, Weiss AT, Hansin Y, et al: Prevention of myocardial damage in acute myocardial ischemia by early treatment with intravenous streptokinase. N Engl J Med 1985; 313:1384–1389.
211. von Kaulla KN, Ostendorf P, von Kaulla E: The impedance machine: A new bedside coagulation recording device. J Med 1975; 6:73–87.
212. Chandler WL, Schmer G: Evaluation of a new dynamic viscometer for measuring the viscosity of whole blood and plasma. Clin Chem 1986; 32:505–507.
213. Saleem A, Blifield C, Saleh SA, et al: Viscoelastic measurement of clot formation: A new test of platelet function. Ann Clin Lab Sci 1983; 13:115–124.
214. Kurica K, Holmes J, Peck S, et al: Hypercoagulation and predictability of thromboembolic phenomena in total hip and total knee surgery. Thromb Haemost 1981; 46:17.
215. Goto H, Nonami R, Hamasaki Y, et al: Effect of hypothermia on coagulation. Anesthesiology 1985; 63:A107.
216. Committee on Blood and Blood Products: Questions and Answers about Transfusion Practices. Park Ridge, IL: American Society of Anesthesiologists, 1992; 1–44.
217. Miller RD, Bove JR: Acquired immunodeficiency syndrome (AIDS) and the blood products. Anesthesiology 1983; 58:493–494.
218. Council on Scientific Affairs: Autologous blood transfusions. JAMA 1986; 256:2378–2380.
219. Menitove JE: Status of recipients of blood from donors subsequently found to have antibody to HIV. N Engl J Med 1986; 315:1095–1096.
220. Zauder HL: Massive transfusion. Int Anesth Clin 1982; 20:157–170.
221. Miller RD, Robbins TO, Tong MJ, Barton SL: Coagulation defects associated with massive blood transfusions. Ann Surg 1971; 174:794–801.
222. Abbott TR: Changes in serum calcium fractions and citrate concentrations during massive blood transfusions and cardiopulmonary bypass. Br J Anaesth 1983; 55:753–759.
223. Kahn RC, Jascott D, Carlon GC, et al: Massive blood replacement: Correlation of ionized calcium, citrate, and hydrogen ion concentration. Anesth Analg 1979; 58:274–278.
224. Coté CJ, Liu LM, Szyfelbein SK, et al: Changes in serial platelet counts following massive blood transfusion in pediatric patients. Anesthesiology 1985; 62:197–201.
225. Hallowell P, Bland JHL, Buckley MJ, Lowenstein E: Transfusion of fresh autologous blood in open-heart surgery. J Thorac Cardiovasc Surg 1972; 64:941–948.
226. Ochsner JL, Mills NL, Leonard GL, Lawson N: Fresh autologous blood transfusions with extracorporeal circulation. Ann Surg 1973; 177:811–817.
227. Barbier-Bohm G, Desmonts JM, Couderc E, et al: Comparative effects of induced hypotension and normovolemic hemodilution on blood loss in total hip arthroplasty. Br J Anaesth 1980; 52:1039–1043.
228. Hamstra RD, Block MH: Erythropoiesis in response to blood loss in man. J Appl Physiol 1969; 27:503–507.
229. Newman MM, Hamstra R, Block M: Use of banked autologous blood in elective surgery. JAMA 1971; 218:861–863.
230. Kramer AH, Hertzer NR, Beven EG: Intraoperative hemodilution during elective vascular reconstruction. Surg Gynecol Obstet 1979; 149:831–836.
231. Jobes DR, Gallagher J: Acute normovolemic hemodilution. Int Anesth Clin 1982; 20:77–95.
232. Stehling LC, Zauder HL, Rogers W: Intraoperative autotransfusion. Anesthesiology 1975; 43:337–345.
233. Rosenblatt R, Dennis P, Draper LD: A new method for massive fluid resuscitation in the trauma patient. Anesth Analg 1983; 62:613–616.
234. Robicsek F, Duncan GD, Born GVR, et al: Inherent dangers of simultaneous application of microfibrillar collagen hemostat and blood-saving devices. J Thorac Cardiovasc Surg 1986; 92:766–770.

CHAPTER

27

Arterial Blood Gas Analysis

CHARLES G. DURBIN, JR., M.D., FCCM

Since the discovery of oxygen in the air, humans have been fascinated by the function of this gas in biologic systems. The prevailing view that the universe was made up of the four primary elements—earth, water, air, and fire—was gradually replaced in the nineteenth century by the more general theories of chemistry. The existence of oxygen and carbon dioxide in the blood was discovered in the early 1800s, but it was not until the middle of the twentieth century that the full significance of these discoveries was apparent.

The utility of chemical measurements has depended in large part on the equipment used to make the measurements. The clinical use of blood gases and acid-base information has depended on the reliability of available methods of measurement. The blood gas and acid-base data discussed in this chapter are shaped by the equipment and technology that are used to obtain the values of these variables. It is essential that the capabilities and limitations of the equipment be kept foremost in mind when using the measured data for clinical applications and decisions. The limitations of methods and techniques are discussed in this chapter.

HISTORY

Credit for discovering the elemental gas, oxygen, is given to Priestley, who in 1774 collected the gas over water in a closed vessel. He also discovered that it was produced by green plants and was necessary to sustain animal life or a candle flame. Davy proved that both oxygen and carbon dioxide were present in blood by using vacuum extraction techniques. A device used for this type of analysis is illustrated in Figure 27–1. It was constructed and used by Zuntz in the 1880s and was remarkably accurate. Even today, the industry standard for blood gas analysis depends on such a technique. The time required to perform the measurement as well as the amount of blood required makes this technique impractical for frequent use in patients. Modern methods of analysis depend on selectively permeable membranes and the electrochemical activity of the gases present.

Clark, in 1953, covered a platinum oxygen electrode with cellophane and created a way of accurately and rapidly measuring oxygen partial pressure (Po_2) in blood. The Clark electrode remains the basis of the electrochemical measurement of Po_2 today.

Modern measurement devices, such as the one shown in Figure 27–2, combine analysis of oxygen, carbon dioxide (CO_2), and blood pH in a rapid and accurate manner. This device (produced by Ciba Corning Diagnostics) includes automatic measurement of sodium, potassium, and calcium levels as well as blood gas analysis, as seen in Figure 27–3. Maintenance is streamlined, and calibration checks are automatic. Most modern equipment provides data that have an accuracy of ± 2–3% of the actual variables.

INDICATIONS FOR Po_2 MONITORING

Arterial Po_2 (Pao_2) is usually measured intermittently. The goal of this technique of monitoring is to direct changes in inspired oxygen (FIo_2) or ventilatory support. It is also a way to follow the progression of pulmonary disease or to identify the need for acute intervention, such as with acute development of bronchospasm. The clinical assessment of decreased oxygen is very poor, because cyanosis is frequently undetected at dangerously low levels of oxygen in the arterial blood. Continuous measurement of arterial oxygen saturation (pulse oximetry—see Chapter 11) allows estimation of the Pao_2 for continuous monitoring of patients at risk of hypoxia.

Continuous indwelling arterial blood gas sensors have been introduced.[1] These are fine-wire optode devices that can be placed through a 20-gauge arterial catheter and provide continuous monitoring of Pao_2, Pco_2, and pH.[2,3] These devices have been placed into clinical trials. They appear to be stable, accurate, and tolerant of the abuses of the clinical environment for at least several days.[4] These devices are bulky and expensive, and their value and reliability are yet to be determined. Being continuous, they provide ongoing information that alerts the clinician to potential problems. When used in some patients, these devices may

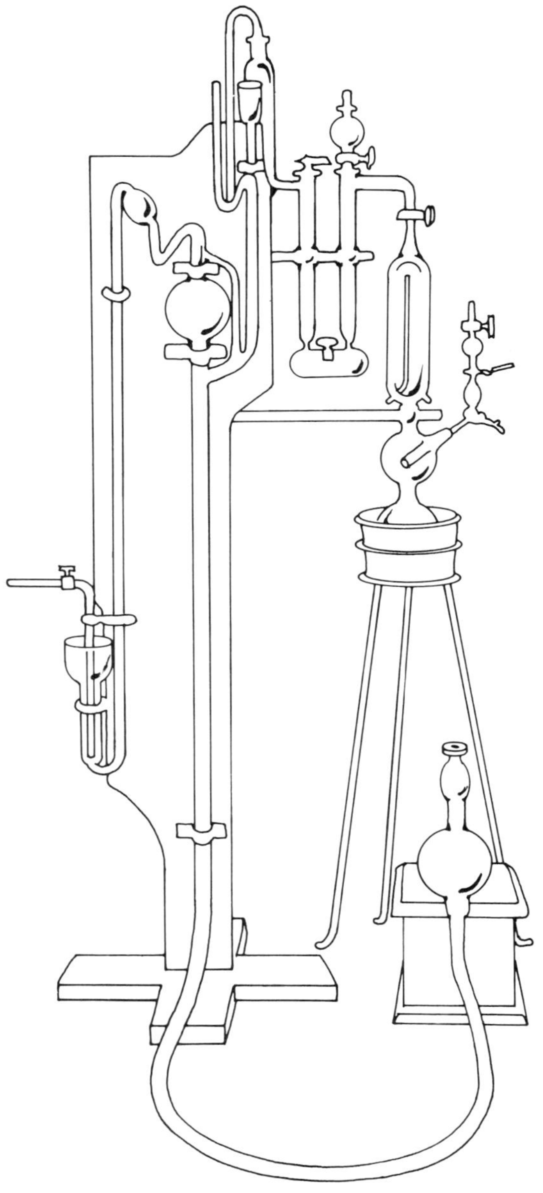

Figure 27–1. A vacuum extraction device for measuring gases dissolved in blood. It was designed and built by Nathan Zuntz, of Bonn, Germany, in the 1880s. (Modified from Astrup P, Severinghaus JW: The History of Blood Gases, Acids and Bases. Copenhagen: Munksgaard, 1986; 164.)

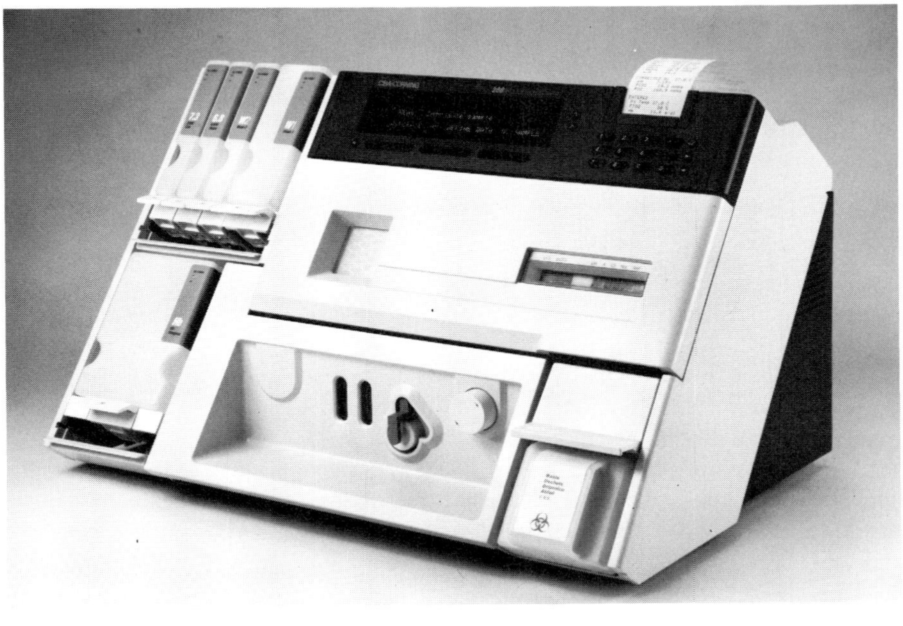

Figure 27–2. The 288 Blood Gas System, produced by Ciba Corning Diagnostics, rapidly analyzes a blood sample for blood gas partial pressures. It is microprocessor-driven, automatically calibrated, and very accurate.

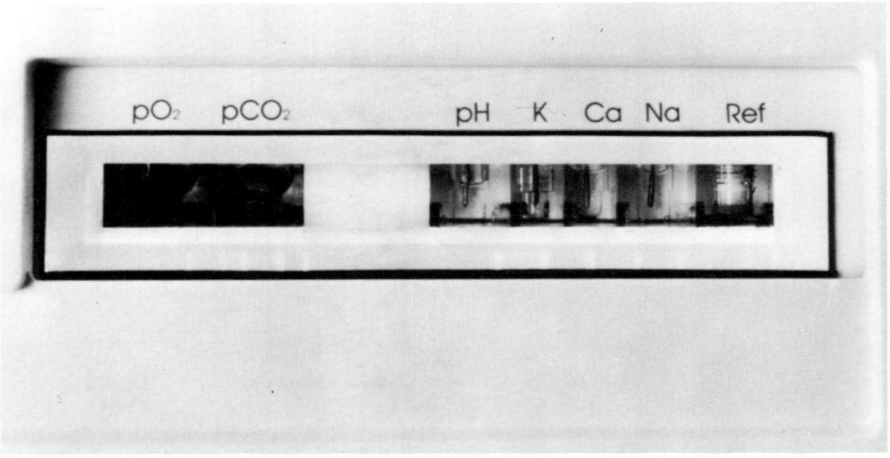

Figure 27–3. Close-up of the electrode bank of the automatic analyzer shown in Figure 27–2 shows that analysis of calcium, sodium, and potassium concentration also is available.

be cost-effective, reducing the need for other forms of blood gas sampling and shortening length of hospital stay.[5]

Transcutaneous sensors can also provide continuous information regarding oxygenation (see Chapter 11). These devices heat the skin to increase local blood flow and measure an ''arterialized'' value. The measurements are affected by the volume status and blood pressure of the patient as well as by the oxygen content of the blood.[6] This may be important information, but the cause of a deterioration in oxygenation is not specifically related to arterial oxygenation (Fig. 27–4). Sensors have also been adapted to measure conjunctival Po_2.[7, 8] These are useful in anesthetized patients for short periods, but they are of little use in awake subjects for continuous monitoring.[9]

ARTERIAL BLOOD GAS SAMPLING

SAMPLE COLLECTION

Samples for intermittent blood gas measurement are collected by direct arterial puncture with a small-gauge, sterile needle or from an indwelling arterial catheter. Indications for insertion, techniques for placement, and complications from arterial catheters are discussed in Chapter 7. Direct arterial puncture is usually carried out after infiltrating the skin with a small amount of local anesthetic (without a vasoconstrictor). A small metal needle that has been flushed with a solution containing 0.5–2 mg of heparin/L is inserted into a palpable artery after use of sterilizing skin preparation. A butterfly needle or a hypodermic needle attached to a small (1–3 ml) syringe is used, and pulsatile flow is confirmed. After an adequate sample is withdrawn (0.2–1.5 ml, depending on the specific analyzer), the needle is removed, and manual pressure is applied over the puncture site for 1–2 minutes. The site should be examined after this compression and again in several minutes for the development of a hematoma. Infection from a single arterial puncture is rare; pain from hematoma formation is common. Spasm, clot, and ischemia may occur and must be treated in order to prevent permanent disability. This direct sampling technique is contraindicated in patients who are anticoagulated. An indwelling arterial catheter may be of less risk under this circumstance. Raynaud's disease and other vasospastic conditions are relative contraindications to repeated direct arterial punctures.

When a blood sample is obtained from an arterial catheter, care must be taken to avoid contamination of the sample with the flushing solution. Three times the dead space amount of fluid must be withdrawn and discarded to produce an uncontaminated sample. A simple way to do this is to note the volume that is withdrawn until blood just appears in the aspirating syringe; this is approximately 80% of the dead space volume. Removing four times this volume guarantees an adequate sample.[10]

SAMPLE HANDLING

The syringe should be capped and sealed and immediately processed in a blood gas machine. If there is to be a delay before performing the analysis (longer than 20–30 minutes), the sample should be placed on ice in order to reduce the metabolic activity of the white blood cells, which will alter the values. When a patient has leukemia or another cause of an elevated white blood cell count, this metabolic change in the sample may be quite significant.[11] The effects of dilution with heparin flush are indicated in Table 27–1. The primary abnormality induced by this type of contamination is in the $Paco_2$ measurement. Because the CO_2 content is directly proportional to the Pco_2 of the blood and very little CO_2 is present in the heparin solution, the $Paco_2$ is markedly reduced in the contaminated sample. The calculated bicarbonate concentration is similarly affected. Commercially prepared heparin-coated syringes in both glass and plastic obviate the problem of contamination by the heparin solution.

The use of glass syringes for blood gas sampling has been debated, because plastic is semipermeable to O_2 and CO_2. The rate of change in these values is very slow and not clinically important if samples are analyzed in a reasonably short time (less than 2 hours).

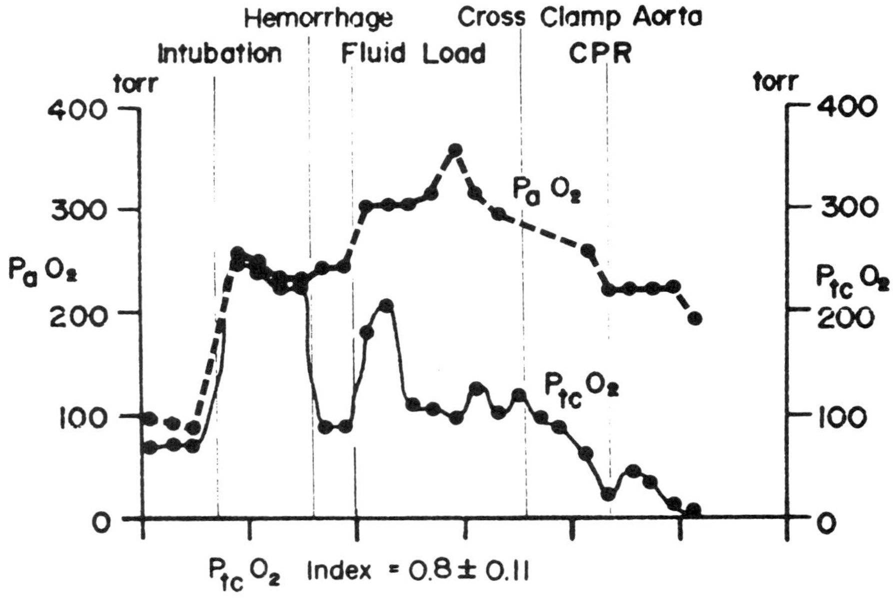

Figure 27–4. Various clinical events can cause changes in the transcutaneous oxygen saturation ($P_{tc}O_2$). In this example, both $Ptco_2$ and arterial oxygen partial pressure (Pao_2) are being monitored. The difference between arterial and transcutaneous values reflects the change in cutaneous perfusion occurring with changes in volume status and cardiac output. (From Tremper KJ, Shoemaker WC: Transcutaneous oxygen monitoring of critically ill adults, with and without low flow shock. Crit Care Med 1981; 9(10):706–709, © by The Williams & Wilkins Company, 1981.)

VARIABILITY OF OXYGEN MEASUREMENTS

When basing an intervention on a measurement of Pao_2, it is important to keep in mind the variability of this value as determined from the analyzer. If laboratory or commercially prepared standards are used for quality control, the variability of Po_2 on repeated measurements on the same machine is very small, 1–4 mmHg standard deviation at clinical levels of Pao_2. This variability depends on the composition of the standard and its temperature. Warm fluorocarbon solutions demonstrate the least variation; cool aqueous solutions demonstrate the most.[12] Failure to meet these accuracy levels should initiate machine repair. Variation between different analyzers is much greater, however. As much as 10–15 mmHg of difference in Pao_2 around a "true" Pao_2 of 60 mmHg may occur between different analyzers.[12]

Variability in Pao_2 also results from patient factors. With continuous monitoring, often the Pao_2 varies quite widely in response to clinical interventions. Occasionally, large changes are seen without discernible causes. Repeated, intermittent arterial blood gases in clinically stable patients often show marked variation.[13] When a Pao_2 value is interpreted, this large variability must be borne in mind. Interpretation must be based on developing trends rather than on the absolute value.

TABLE 27–1. EFFECT OF HEPARIN SOLUTION ON BLOOD GAS VALUES

Blood Heparin	100% 0%	50% 50%	0% 100%
With Normal Blood Gases*			
Pco_2 (mmHg)	44.9	18.8	3.2
Po_2 (mmHg)	143.5	152.5	171.4
pH	7.41	7.44	6.11
HCO_3^- (mEq/L)	28.2	12.7	0.1
With Low Oxygen and Bicarbonate*			
Pco_2 (mmHg)	16.2	7.2	0.1
Po_2 (mmHg)	45.1	48.1	171.4
pH	7.25	7.25	6.11
HCO_3^- (mEq/L)	16.2	7.2	0.1

*Top section illustrates the effect on a relatively normal sample; the bottom section shows the effect on a hypoxic sample with metabolic acidosis. The major effects of dilution are on the Pco_2 measurement and bicarbonate calculation.

INDEXES OF OXYGENATION

Various calculated expressions are used to describe the severity of oxygenation deficit. Some of these are listed in Table 27–2. The ease of determination, accuracy, and the influence of extrapulmonary factors vary among these measures.

ALVEOLAR-ARTERIAL OXYGEN PARTIAL PRESSURE DIFFERENCE (A-a GRADIENT)

The expected Pao_2 varies with the inspired fraction of oxygen. The relationship between the ideal alveolar concentration of oxygen and the inspired oxygen fraction is shown in the alveolar air equation:

$$PAO_2 = FIO_2(Pb - 47) - Paco_2/R$$

where PAO_2 = the ideal alveolar partial pressure of oxygen, FIO_2 = the inspired oxygen fraction, Pb = the barometric pressure in mmHg, 47 = the vapor pressure of water in mmHg at 37°C, $Paco_2$ = the partial pressure of carbon dioxide in the blood, and R = the respiratory quotient (the volume of CO_2 produced for each volume of oxygen consumed). The term $Paco_2/R$ is a measure of the oxygen that is being removed by the blood flowing through the lungs in relation to the amount of oxygen being brought into the lungs by ventilation. The difference between this ideal

TABLE 27–2. CLINICAL PARAMETERS OF OXYGENATION

	Factors Influencing Value		
Index Parameter	*FIO_2*	*Cardiac Output*	*Oxygen Consumption*
A-a gradient	√	√	√
Oxygenation ratio	0	√	√
A-a ratio	0	√	√
Venous admixture	0	0	0

value for oxygen and the actual measured value is called the alveolar-arterial oxygen difference, or the A-a gradient for oxygen (A-aPO_2).

Calculating and following the A-a gradient is a clinical tool to monitor deficits in oxygenation. Changes in this number are produced by several mechanisms. A-aPO_2 depends on the inspired oxygen fraction (as indicated in the previous equation). A "normal" gradient is about 5–10 mmHg on room air, but it increases to 50–70 mmHg on an FIO_2 of 1.0. Other causes of an increased gradient include abnormal cardiac function with a decreased cardiac output, lung disease with increased resistance to diffusion of oxygen, ventilation-perfusion mismatching, or intrapulmonary or intracardiac shunting. Decreased A-aPO_2 is seen with increased cardiac output, systemic sepsis, left-to-right intracardiac shunts, and failure to utilize oxygen in the tissues as occurs in cyanide or carbon monoxide poisoning.

Calculation of A-aPO_2 is useful when changing the FIO_2 of a patient on mechanical ventilation. For example, PaO_2 of 246 mmHg is obtained from an intubated, ventilated patient. The FIO_2 is 1.0. The A-aPO_2 is calculated

$$PAO_2 = 1.0(760 - 47) - 40/0.8$$

assuming the barometric pressure is 760 mmHg, the $PaCO_2$ is normal (40 mmHg), and the respiratory quotient is 0.8.

$$PAO_2 = 663$$
$$A\text{-}aPO_2 = 663 - 246 = 417$$

To change the FIO_2 to produce a PaO_2 of 100 mmHg, the same equation is solved for FIO_2:

$$PAO_2 - PaO_2 = 417$$
$$\text{Setting } PaO_2 = 100$$
$$PAO_2 = 517$$
$$517 = FIO_2\,(760 - 47) - 40/0.8$$
$$FIO_2 = (517 + 40/0.8)/(760 - 47) = 0.80$$

The assumptions made in this calculation are that equilibration took place before the first blood sample was obtained and that no change occurred in A-aPO_2. As implied previously, the A-aPO_2 changes with changes in FIO_2. Because, in this example, the new FIO_2 was lower than the previous setting, the gradient would also be lower, thus providing a margin of safety.

OXYGENATION RATIO

A method to eliminate the effects of changes in A-aPO_2 caused by changes in FIO_2 is to divide the PaO_2 by the FIO_2. This number is referred to as the oxygenation ratio. To use this parameter in the example shown previously:

$$PaO_2/FIO_2 = 246/1.0 = 246$$

to obtain a $PaO_2 = 100$, then

$$100/FIO_2 = 246$$
$$FIO_2 = 100/246 = 0.41$$

This result differs significantly from the previous method (a lower new FIO_2 was obtained) and reflects the fact that the A-aPO_2 decreases as FIO_2 is reduced.

ARTERIAL-ALVEOLAR OXYGEN RATIO

Another index of gas exchange is the ratio of arterial to alveolar O_2 (a/APO_2).[14] This index, like the oxygenation ratio above, is less affected by FIO_2, more constant than A-aPO_2, and most constant above alveolar oxygen values of 200 mmHg.[15] Normal a/APO_2 values range from 0.7–0.8. It offers no advantage in comparison to the oxygenation ratio. Factors such as cardiac output and oxygen consumption affect this and the other monitors discussed above. Lung pathology is not specifically quantitated.

VENOUS ADMIXTURE (SHUNT FRACTION)

The best estimate of oxygenation defect is provided by venous admixture or intrapulmonary shunt calculation. The formula for this is:

$$\dot{Q}s/\dot{Q}t = (CaO_2 - Cc O_2)/(C\bar{v}O_2 - Cc O_2)$$

where CaO_2 = arterial content of oxygen, $C\bar{v}O_2$ = mixed venous content of oxygen, and CcO_2 = estimated pulmonary capillary content of oxygen. This takes into account the effects of changes in cardiac output (reflected in $C\bar{v}O_2$) and oxygen consumption. It is a helpful reflection of pulmonary pathology. The determination of the factors in the shunt equation is described later.

MONITORING OF OXYHEMOGLOBIN

OXYHEMOGLOBIN DISSOCIATION CURVE

The discussion up to this point has been about the partial pressure of oxygen in the blood. The total amount of oxygen dissolved in blood is quite small, however, and would be quickly exhausted if it were not for the large amount of hemoglobin present in red blood cells. Hemoglobin reversibly binds large quantities of oxygen and acts as a reservoir for this essential gas. The physiochemical basis of this process is the tertiary structure of hemoglobin and its ferrous core.

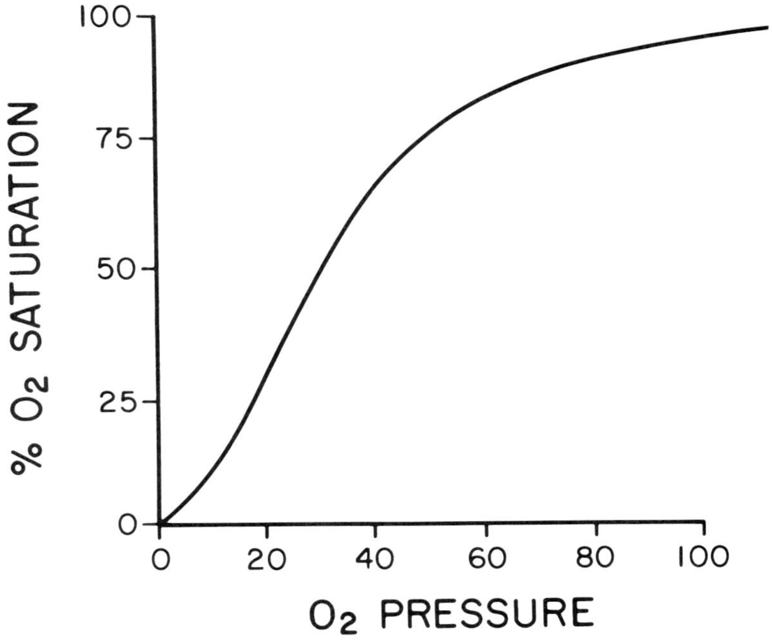

Figure 27–5. The relationship between the Po_2 and the percentage saturation of hemoglobin. The position of this curve is affected by many factors, which are explained in the text. The sigmoid shape of the curve is due to facilitated binding of successive oxygen molecules.

Hemoglobin consists of four heme subunit proteins clustered around a ferrous ion. There are four binding sites in each molecule of hemoglobin (one on each heme subunit). As the first O_2 molecule is bound, the other chains rotate, and the binding of the next O_2 molecule is easier (more easily bound). This configurational change occurs with the addition of each successive O_2 molecule, until all four binding sites are occupied.[16, 17] This allosteric cooperation accounts for the shape of the oxyhemoglobin dissociation curve (Fig. 27–5).

The relationship between oxygen saturation and Po_2 is important to remember in clinical practice. A simple rule of thumb is that at a Po_2 of 40 mmHg, hemoglobin is about 70% saturated; at 60 mmHg, it is about 90% saturated. The "40, 50, 60; 70, 80, 90 rule" is illustrated in the following easy-to-recall form:

Po_2	40	50	60
% Saturation	70	80	90

In 1904, Bohr discovered the sigmoid shape of the oxyhemoglobin dissociation curve of whole blood. He also described the effect of carbon dioxide tension on the position of this curve. A leftward shift of the curve, facilitating uptake of O_2, occurs when CO_2 is released in the lungs. This is known as the Bohr effect.

Measurement

Hemoglobin saturation is easily measured by determining the light absorbance in the visual and infrared spectral range in a co-oximeter. Oxygenated blood absorbs light in a different pattern than that of deoxygenated blood. The absorbance spectra for these species are illustrated in Figure 27–6. By comparing the absorbance at several wave lengths, the percentage of saturated hemoglobin can be calculated. Current co-oximeters use at least four different wave lengths and calculate carboxyhemoglobin and methemoglobin percentages as well as the percentage of oxygen saturation of normal hemoglobin.

Alterations in Oxyhemoglobin Dissociation

Various conditions such as those listed in Table 27–3 affect the position of the oxyhemoglobin dissociation curve. Major factors shifting the curve to the right (reducing hemoglobin affinity for oxygen) are acidosis (respiratory or metabolic), fever, and increased 2,3-diphosphoglycerate (2,3-DPG). Minor factors include increased hemoglobin concentration, exogenous cortisol, hyperaldosteronism, and hyperthyroidism. Factors that shift the curve to the left

TABLE 27–3. FACTORS AFFECTING HEMOGLOBIN-OXYGEN AFFINITY

Causes of Increased Oxygen Affinity
Hypothermia
Respiratory alkalosis
Metabolic alkalosis
Decreased 2,3-diphosphoglycerate (2,3-DPG)
Decreased serum phosphate
Anemia
Hypothyroidism
Factors That Decrease Oxygen Affinity
Fever
Respiratory acidosis
Metabolic acidosis
Increased 2,3-DPG
Steroid administration
Hyperaldosteronism
Hyperthyroidism
Polycythemia

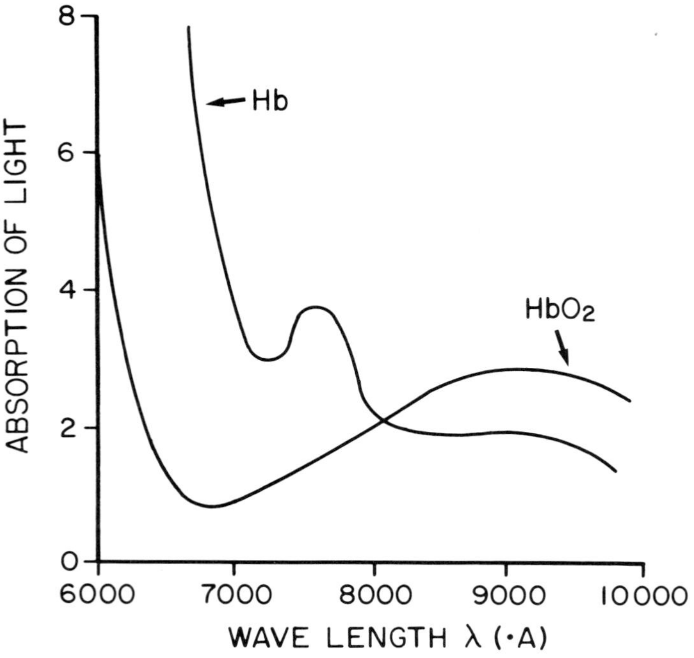

Figure 27–6. Absorption of light of oxygenated and deoxygenated hemoglobin. Comparing the absorption at several wavelengths allows calculation of the percentage saturation.

(producing more avid binding of oxygen) are cold, alkalosis, reduced 2,3-DPG, anemia, hypothyroidism, carboxyhemoglobin, and methemoglobin.[18] Genetic hemoglobin variants have various effects on the curve. The clinical significance of these changes in hemoglobin oxygen affinity has not been established.[19]

P_{50}

A useful way to describe the shift in the oxyhemoglobin dissociation curve quantitatively is to calculate or determine experimentally the Po_2 at which the blood sample is 50% saturated. This is called the P_{50} value. A normal value for this number is about 27 mmHg. If the P_{50} is greater than this normal value, the curve is shifted to the right. If it is less, the curve is shifted to the left. The magnitude of the shift is indicated by the degree of deviation from this normal value.

OXYGEN CONTENT

The oxyhemoglobin dissociation curve is useful in that it allows determination of the amount of oxygen carried by hemoglobin, and hemoglobin is the major reservoir of oxygen. The actual amount of molecular oxygen dissolved in blood or plasma is directly related to the partial pressure of oxygen and is quite small in relation to the amount bound to hemoglobin. The following equation describes the amount of oxygen in arterial blood:

$$Cao_2 = (\text{Hbg} \times 1.36 \times Sao_2) + 0.0031 \times Pao_2$$

$$\text{Content} = \text{Bound} + \text{Dissolved}$$

where CaO_2 = the oxygen content in liters of oxygen/100 ml of whole blood, Hbg = the hemoglobin content in gm/100 ml of blood, 1.36 = the milliliters of oxygen in a fully saturated gram of hemoglobin, Sao_2 = arterial saturation, and 0.0031 = the amount of oxygen dissolved in plasma per mmHg of oxygen partial pressure.

OXYGEN TRANSPORT

The amount of oxygen that is available to the body often is described using the concept of oxygen transport.

$$\text{Oxygen transport} = Cao_2 \times CO \times 10$$

where CO = cardiac output. More appropriately called oxygen availability, this product estimates the total available arterial oxygen (in ml) per minute. When oxygen transport is inadequate, this concept allows a rational therapeutic approach by addressing each of the components of the delivery system independently.

Although this oxygen transport parameter is useful conceptually, there are several problems in using it clinically. Because hemoglobin is almost fully saturated if Pao_2 is greater than 60 mmHg, tissues can only use more oxygen if they can increase flow (cardiac output) or increase extraction (resulting in a lower venous saturation). When flow or cardiac output is limited, extraction is increased. The tissues are able to extract only some of the available oxygen, and this fraction varies among different tissues. The heart is efficient at removing the available oxygen and removes as much as 90% of the oxygen delivered (coronary sinus [venous] hemoglobin saturation may fall as low as 5%).[20] Other organs may become hypoxic at much higher venous oxygen contents, such as the brain, which begins to fail at a Pvo_2 of about 30 mmHg (cerebral venous blood falls to about 50% saturated).

A-V OXYGEN DIFFERENCE

Comparing the oxygen content of the venous blood with the amount available in the arterial blood gives a measure of the utilization of oxygen. $C(a\text{-}v)O_2$, or the arteriovenous oxygen content difference, is easily calculated if a mixed venous blood sample can be obtained (usually from a pulmonary artery or central venous catheter). $C(a\text{-}v)O_2$ is usually 5–6 vol%, but it may increase to 8–10 vol% in stress states (increased total body oxygen extraction). A problem with this parameter, as well as with the oxygen availability parameter described previously, is that the entire body is averaged in the calculations. Critical regional differences in supply and demand matching are not reflected in these overall indexes. Monitoring of tissue oxygenation is discussed in Chapter 11. Mixed venous PO_2 ($P\bar{v}O_2$) gives some indication of total body oxygen supply and demand balance.

OXYGEN UTILIZATION COEFFICIENT

A measure of the efficiency of extraction of oxygen is the ratio of oxygen consumption divided by oxygen transport (UC). This estimate of the ratio of supply to demand can be approximated by subtracting $S\bar{v}O_2$ from 1.

$$UC = 1 - S\bar{v}O_2$$

This assumes an arterial saturation of greater than 92%. Usually UC falls between 0.2 and 0.3; when it reaches 0.5 (meaning that half of the delivered oxygen is used), tissue hypoxia often occurs.

ARTERIAL OXYGENATION

HYPOXIA

Physiologic Effects

Oxygen is essential to all tissues for energy generation through oxidative phosphorylation in the Krebs cycle. Anaerobic metabolism is much less efficient and not satisfactory for most organs for long periods. Oxygen is transported by the blood (bound to hemoglobin and freely dissolved) and must diffuse to the mitochondria from the capillaries. There are almost no tissue stores of oxygen in the body. Oxygen must be continually delivered in order to maintain organ function and prevent cellular death. The driving force for oxygen delivery from blood to tissues is diffusion down a partial pressure gradient. The partial pressure of oxygen in the mitochondrion is probably less than 2 mmHg.[21] Oxygen extraction from blood by the (normal) brain seems to fail when venous blood reaches 20 mmHg. This may occur at a PaO_2 of 25–35 mmHg depending on the hemoglobin type, concentration, and blood flow. Other organs may tolerate lower venous (and arterial) oxygen partial pressures.

Complete interruption of oxygen delivery, anoxia, results in rapid disruption of organ function and, if it persists for more than a short period, organ death. Anoxia tolerance varies from organ to organ. Irreversible brain injury occurs after only 3–5 minutes of anoxia. The heart may resume normal function after several hours without oxygen.

When PaO_2 is monitored in the clinical arena, two conditions need to be avoided, hypoxia and hyperoxia. Although the definition of hypoxia varies from organ to organ, a PaO_2 of 55 mmHg or less or a saturation of 88% is usually considered to be hypoxia.[22] At this point on the oxyhemoglobin dissociation curve, there is still a large quantity of bound oxygen (90% of capacity). The use of high inspired concentrations of oxygen to achieve this desired level of PaO_2 may be associated with development of pulmonary oxygen toxicity.[23] Abnormalities of gas exchange and pathologic anatomic changes in lung structure occur. In extreme cases, the adult respiratory distress syndrome follows high inspired oxygen concentrations.[24]

Causes

Hypoventilation

The simplest cause of low PaO_2 is hypoventilation on room air. It can be seen from the alveolar gas equation described earlier in this chapter that a high $PaCO_2$ (hypoventilation) results in a low PaO_2 when the FIO_2 is low, even with normal pulmonary function. The effect of increasing $PaCO_2$ is shown in Table 27–4. By simply increasing the FIO_2, this cause of hypoxia can be overcome. For example, the PaO_2 of a patient with a $PaCO_2$ of 80 mmHg would only be 44 mmHg on room air; this would improve dramatically to 108 mmHg by increasing the FIO_2 slightly to 0.30. Hypoventilation is often seen as a consequence of general anesthesia, especially when narcotics are employed. The practice of administering an increased FIO_2 to patients recovering from anesthesia is based on this consideration.[25]

Decreased Inspired Oxygen

A second cause of low PaO_2 that can be entirely explained by the alveolar gas equation is the effect of decreased FIO_2, such as occurs at high altitude. Table 27–5 illustrates the effect on PaO_2 of increased height above sea level. Once again, this cause of hypoxia can be overcome by increasing the inspired oxygen fraction. This is the rea-

TABLE 27–4. EFFECT OF HYPERCARBIA ON PaO_2

$PaCO_2$ Room Air (mmHg)	PaO_2 Room Air (mmHg)	PaO_2 30% FIO_2 (mmHg)
40	92	156
50	80	144
60	68	132
70	56	120
80	44	108
90	32	96
100	20	84

The predicted PaO_2 due to a rise in $PaCO_2$ on room air (21% FIO_2) and on 30%. A normal, unchanging alveolar-to-arterial gradient is assumed in performing the calculations.

TABLE 27–5. EFFECT OF INCREASED ALTITUDE AND DECREASED FIO_2 ON PO_2

Altitude (Feet)	Barometric Pressure	Alveolar Po_2	Arterial Po_2
0	760	149	99[1]
2000	707	138	88[1]
4000	656	127	77[1]
6000	609	118	68[1]
8000	564	108	58[1]
10000	523	100	50[1]
12000	483	91	41[1]
14000	446	83	41[2]
16000	412	76	34[2]
18000	379	69	27[2]
20000	349	63	21[2]
30000	226	37	0[2]

The fall in barometric pressure is shown as altitude increases. The alveolar partial pressure and estimated arterial partial pressure of oxygen are illustrated. The (A-a) Po_2 is assumed to be 0, the $Paco_2$ is assumed to be 40 mmHg[2] or 25 mmHg[2], and the respiratory quotient is assumed to be 0.8.

son that mountain climbers and pilots employ oxygen masks at high altitudes.

Diffusion Defects

The idea of a mechanical intrapulmonary diffusion defect (thickened alveolar membranes) for oxygen has been suggested. Because oxygen is more limited by diffusion than CO_2 and several other gases are, an increase in the thickness of the alveolar-capillary membrane could theoretically decrease Pao_2 by preventing adequate O_2 passage in the lung. A pulmonary function test, the carbon monoxide diffusion capacity, was purported to correlate with an increase in the thickness of this membrane (see Chapter 12). This led to the concept of alveolar-capillary block, which was used to explain the hypoxia seen in a wide variety of pulmonary diseases.

The clinical significance of this pathophysiologic mechanism has been questioned. In Figure 27–7, it can be seen that during transit through the pulmonary circulation, the average red cell is fully saturated in less than 0.25 seconds, one third the time spent in contact with the gas exchange membrane. Even in patients whose diseases cause massive thickening of this membrane (interstitial fibrosis, alveolar proteinosis), oxygenation is complete during the normal red cell transit time. It is only during periods of reduced transit time (such as with increased cardiac output from exercise or fever) that desaturation occurs. This cause of arterial hypoxia can be easily overcome by slight increases in the FIO_2. The use of portable, low-flow oxygen delivery devices has markedly improved the lifestyle of patients suffering from diseases causing this form of oxygenation failure.

Ventilation-Perfusion Mismatching

The most important cause of oxygenation failure is ventilation-to-perfusion mismatching ($\dot{V}/\dot{Q}$ mismatching). One extreme example of this problem is "shunt," in which there is perfusion of areas that have no ventilation. Unlike the causes of hypoxia discussed in the preceding paragraphs, this cause of hypoxia is not overcome by simply increasing the FIO_2. To separate the effects of $\dot{V}/\dot{Q}$ mismatching from true shunt, 100% O_2 may be administered; any residual oxygenation deficit is due to true shunt rather than to $\dot{V}/\dot{Q}$ mismatching. The curves in Figure 27–8 illustrate the relationship of FIO_2 to PaO_2 with various degrees of intrapulmonary shunt (extrapulmonary venous-to-systemic shunts behave analogously). Thirty percent inspired oxygen fails to correct the hypoxia caused by a shunt greater than 15%.

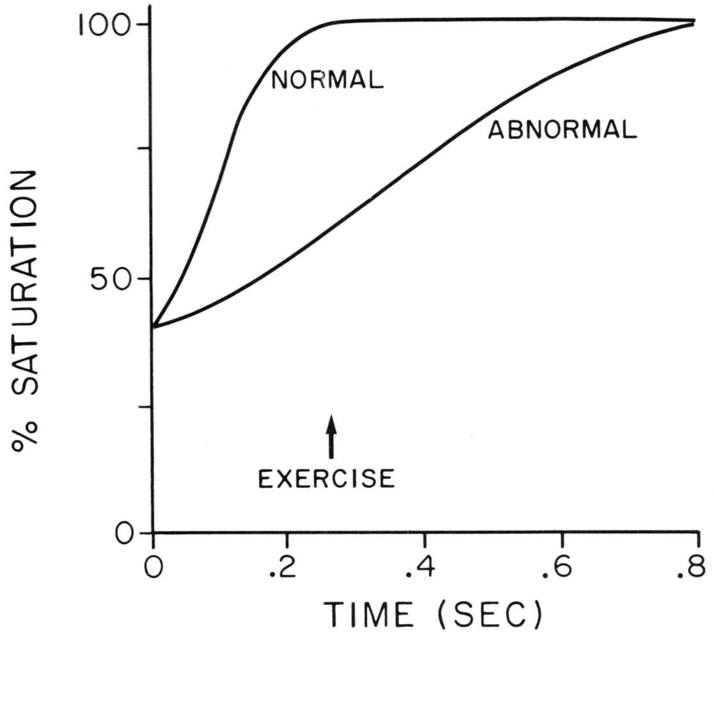

Figure 27–7. The time spent by a red cell in transit through the pulmonary bed. Full saturation with oxygen is obtained in about one third of this time. Even in extremely abnormal alveoli with thickened walls, saturation is complete during the normal passage. Exercise shortens transit time and may cause desaturation in the extremely diseased lung by this mechanism. See the text for details.

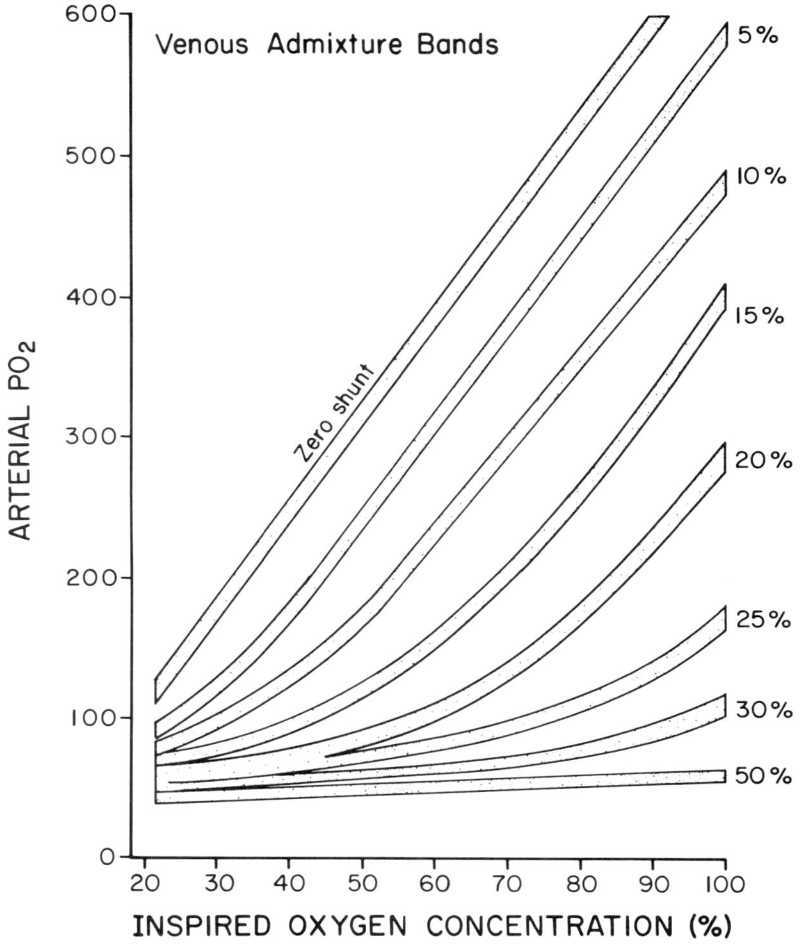

Figure 27–8. Bands showing the range of Pa_{O_2} expected with various amounts of venous admixture or shunt. Knowing the Pa_{O_2} and the inspired oxygen allows a guess at the percentage of shunt present. (Modified from Nunn JF: Applied Respiratory Physiology. London: Butterworth, 1987; 371.)

Therapeutic Approaches to Hypoxia

Diseases that lead to $\dot{V}/\dot{Q}$ mismatching and shunt include cardiogenic pulmonary edema, adult respiratory distress syndrome, pneumonia, pulmonary embolism, volume overload, inhalation burn injury, respiratory distress syndrome of the newborn, use of antineoplastic agents, and other diverse conditions. The therapeutic goal is treatment of the primary problem; however, maintenance of an acceptable Pa_{O_2} is essential for recovery. The main therapies used to increase Pa_{O_2} are increased FI_{O_2} and raised airway pressure. The goal in treatment of this class of disease is to maintain oxygenation on a nontoxic FI_{O_2}. Pulmonary oxygen toxicity occurs in less than 24 hours at an FI_{O_2} of 100%.[26] FI_{O_2} levels of 40–60% are probably acceptable at sea level indefinitely.

Positive end-expiratory pressure (PEEP) is a useful and popular method of raising airway pressure. PEEP decreases shunt and increases lung volume (functional residual capacity).[27] The effectiveness of this form of therapy is increased if the lung pathology is uniformly distributed throughout both lungs. Because cardiac output may decrease with the application of PEEP, the actual Pa_{O_2} may decrease owing to a lower $P\bar{v}_{O_2}$, despite improvement in lung function and reduction of intrapulmonary shunt.

Table 27–6 lists several methods that have been suggested in order to decide on the "best" PEEP level. On one extreme is the group headed by Kirby and coworkers, who believe that PEEP is therapeutic and should be used to maximum effect regardless of the cardiovascular or barotraumatic effects.[28] The other side of the debate is illustrated by Petty and Fowler, who suggest that PEEP is toxic and should be employed only if high levels of FI_{O_2} are ineffec-

TABLE 27–6. METHODS PROPOSED TO DETERMINE THE IDEAL LEVEL OF PEEP

Pa_{O_2} is acceptable
Static lung compliance is maximum*
Intrapulmonary shunt is 15% or less†
PEEP is lowest, and FI_{O_2} is up to 80%‡
FI_{O_2} is less than or equal to 40%
Smallest end-tidal to arterial carbon dioxide gradient§

*Suter PM, Fairley HB, Isenberg MC: Optimum end expiratory pressure in patients with acute pulmonary failure. N Engl J Med 1975; 292:284–289.

†Gallagher J, Civetta JM: Goal-directed therapy of acute respiratory failure. Anesth Analg 1980; 59:831–834.

‡Petty TL, Fowler AA: Another look at ARDS. Chest 1982; 82:98–104.

§Murray IP, Modell JH, Gallagher TJ, Banner MJ: Titration of PEEP by the arterial minus end-tidal carbon dioxide gradient. Chest 1984; 85:100–104.

tive in preventing severe hypoxia (Petty and Fowler's work was done at an altitude over 5000 feet, and an FIO_2 of 100% is equivalent to an FIO_2 of only 78% at sea level).[29] Most clinicians make early use of some low level of end-expiratory pressure (10–12 cmH_2O) in patients at risk for developing hypoxic lung disease, and it appears that the incidence of the syndrome of adult respiratory distress is waning, or its severity is decreasing.

Because the side effects of positive pressure ventilation and PEEP are significant and always impact the cardiovascular system,[30] monitoring of cardiac function is usually indicated when these modalities are employed. This is often assisted by use of a flow-directed pulmonary artery catheter, which may be used to optimize cardiac filling, cardiac output, and shunt fraction ($\dot{Q}s/\dot{Q}t$). The insertion techniques, use, and complications of this device are described in Chapter 8. Calculation of $\dot{Q}s/\dot{Q}t$ is performed with the following equation:

$$\dot{Q}s/\dot{Q}t = (CaO_2 - CcO_2)/(C\bar{v}O_2 - CcO_2)$$

where CaO_2 is calculated from arterial saturation and measured hemoglobin, and $C\bar{v}O_2$ is calculated from a mixed venous sample obtained from the distal port of the pulmonary artery catheter. Care must be taken to aspirate this sample slowly (usually over 20–30 seconds) in order to avoid arterializing the blood. CcO_2 is estimated from the following equation:

$$CcO_2 = 1.36 \times Hbg \times 100\% + 0.0031 \times PAO_2$$

This calculation is performed assuming that pulmonary capillary blood is fully oxygen-saturated and that there is no alveolar-pulmonary capillary gradient for oxygen. These assumptions are not correct, but the errors introduced are small and inconsequential for clinical management decisions.

The usefulness of the shunt calculation is that it removes the effect of changes in cardiac output from the intrapulmonary effects of airway pressure therapy. Although there is no *a priori* reason to believe that shunt is the pathologic problem in adult respiratory distress syndrome, clinicians who monitor and treat changes in shunt fraction report the lowest mortality in this condition.[31, 32] The use of PEEP to improve pulmonary compliance makes physiologic sense. However, mechanical difficulties in measuring pulmonary compliance and conflicting results by various investigators have made it a less useful parameter to optimize PEEP. All authors agree that PEEP should be used to avoid high concentrations of inspired oxygen.

The cardiac effects of PEEP (and positive airway pressure) include reduced venous return, increased right ventricular afterload,[33] decreased left ventricular afterload, and leftward shift of the intraventricular septum.[34] Possible effects of PEEP are reduced cardiac compliance[35] and reduced contractility.[36] Some authors have actually shown an increase in contractility with elevated airway pressure.[37] Because airway pressure may be reflected in vascular pressures, the absolute values of filling pressure are altered when increased airway pressures are employed. As much as half of the PEEP may be reflected in the ventricular filling pressure and should be subtracted from the measured value.[38] Cardiac status should be assessed by observing the changes in filling pressures and cardiac output occurring after volume challenges and not on the actual values determined during monitoring.

The effects of changes in the level of PEEP on the cardiovascular system are rapid, occurring in less than a minute. The effects on arterial blood gases are more gradual, requiring at least 10–15 minutes to reach a new steady state. The same is true for FIO_2, although evidence suggests that a shorter equilibration period may be acceptable to assess the results of a change in FIO_2.[39]

HYPEROXIA

Hyperoxia (PaO_2 greater than 75 mmHg) in the premature infant is associated with the development of blindness due to retrolental fibroplasia. The exact cause of this problem is not known, although oxygen may be one of several factors responsible.[40] Hyperoxia (at greater than 1.5 atm as seen in divers or in patients in hyperbaric chambers) stimulates the central nervous system and causes seizures.

Hyperoxia has several short-term therapeutic uses (Table 27–7). Administration of 100% oxygen is therapeutic in carbon monoxide poisoning. Hyperbaric oxygen may also be employed in this circumstance (if a hyperbaric chamber is readily available). Systemic or venous air embolism is an indication for high FIO_2 in order to reduce the size of the bubble. Denitrogenation of the blood creates a pressure gradient for nitrogen to leave the bubble. Tension pneumocephalus[41] or pneumothorax may be improved by a high PaO_2, but direct removal of the trapped air is the normal therapeutic approach. In prolonged or difficult obstetric delivery, fetal metabolic status may be improved when maternal PaO_2 is elevated above 200 mmHg. When a fluorocarbon blood substitute is used to replace red cells, 100% oxygen must be used to raise the amount of dissolved oxygen to acceptable levels (at least 5 vol%).[42] Administration of high FIO_2 is practiced in patients with chest pain presumed to be due to myocardial infarction or ischemia in order to prevent hypoxia from early pulmonary edema and to improve cardiac oxygenation. Hyperoxia has been shown to improve cerebral function in patients after cerebral artery

TABLE 27–7. THERAPEUTIC USES OF INCREASED FIO_2

Carbon monoxide poisoning
Venous air embolism
Arterial air (or other gas) embolism
Fetal distress (maternal hyperoxia)
Acute myocardial ischemia
Cerebral ischemia
Pneumothorax
Pneumocephalus
Fluorocarbon blood substitute
Anaerobic infections

occlusion, but the risks from oxygen toxicity have not made this a standard practice for long-term (greater than 24 hours) treatment.[43]

CARBON DIOXIDE AND pH

Investigations into pH and CO_2 measurements originated with concerns over fermentation processes in the 1800s. Pasteur demonstrated that control of acidity was essential for proper brewing and creation of wine from grapes. Nernst developed the theory of electrochemical activity, which led Oswald to the development of the hydrogen electrode capable of measuring pH. The equipment was refined and used on blood by Hasselbalch, Belcher, Astrup, and others. Gasometric techniques developed by Van Slyke enabled researchers and clinicians to determine the P_{CO_2} accurately. Today, the measurement of P_{CO_2}, pH, and P_{O_2} is combined in a single machine capable of analyzing as little as 50–100 μl of blood.

TRANSPORT OF CARBON DIOXIDE

The end products of cellular respiration are carbon dioxide and water. The human body produces about 12,000 mEq of acid in the form of CO_2 every 24 hours. This tremendous load is excreted by the lungs in the form of volatile acid (CO_2), and body pH is tightly maintained. A smaller amount of fixed acid is excreted by the kidneys. This amounts to about 1 mEq/kg of body mass each day. These two systems are responsible for the control of body acid-base balance and maintenance of optimal pH for metabolic function of individual organs and the whole body.

In order for ventilation to be efficient in acid removal, metabolic CO_2 must be transported to the lungs. CO_2 is relatively insoluble in blood and is predominantly carried as bicarbonate, which is produced by reaction with water as shown in the following chemical equation:

TABLE 27–8. FORMS AND AMOUNT OF CO_2 CARRIED IN WHOLE VENOUS BLOOD

Dissolved CO_2	1.27	mmol/L
Carbonic acid (undissociated)	0.0012	mmol/L
Bicarbonate ion	10.3	mmol/L
Carbamino compounds (hemoglobin)	1.7	mmol/L
Total	23.3	mmol/L

O_2 saturation is 70%, hemoglobin is 12–14 gm/100 ml.

$$CO_2 + H_2O \rightleftharpoons H_2CO_3 \rightleftharpoons H^+ + HCO_3^-$$

In order for this system of CO_2 transport to work, the normally slow conversion of CO_2 to bicarbonate is facilitated by the enzyme carbonic anhydrase, located primarily in red blood cells. Hemoglobin and other proteins serve as carriers for some of the CO_2 produced. The relative amounts of CO_2 carried in each of these forms are indicated in Table 27–8.

Hemoglobin acts as a buffer when oxygen is released at the tissue level. This allows some of the H^+ produced from carbonic acid to be neutralized by hemoglobin. This is referred to as the Haldane effect. As illustrated in Figure 27–9, when a solution of oxygenated free hemoglobin at pH 7.3 is deoxygenated, the solution pH increases to 7.5. As oxygen is released at the tissues, the buffering effect of hemoglobin allows less pH change than would otherwise occur with the production of carbonic acid. This makes hemoglobin a most important buffer.

Most of the important parts of the CO_2 transport system occur inside red cells. Major ion and chemical shifts are indicated in Figure 27–10. To maintain electrical neutrality inside the red cell, chloride ion is exchanged for bicarbonate. This is termed the chloride shift (or Hamberger effect). Potassium ion is excreted from the cell as well. The

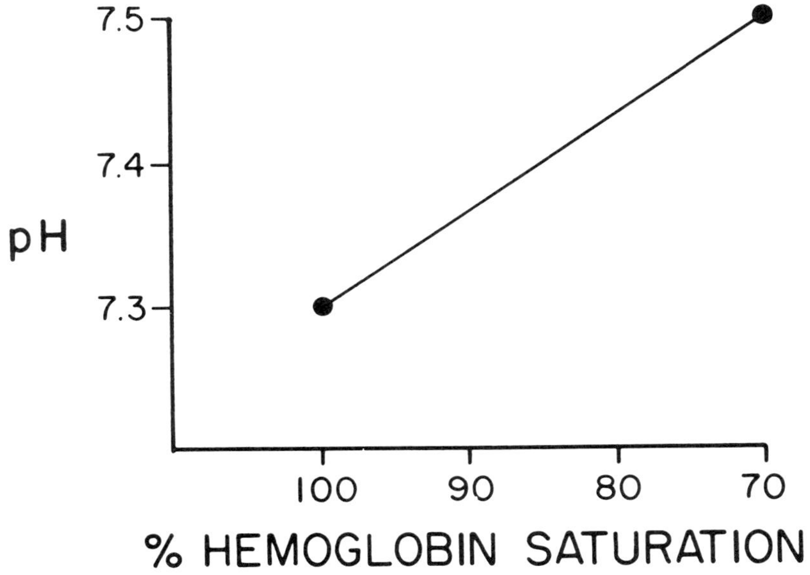

Figure 27–9. The effect of desaturating a solution of hemoglobin. The pH increases as the oxygen saturation decreases. This is referred to as the Haldane effect.

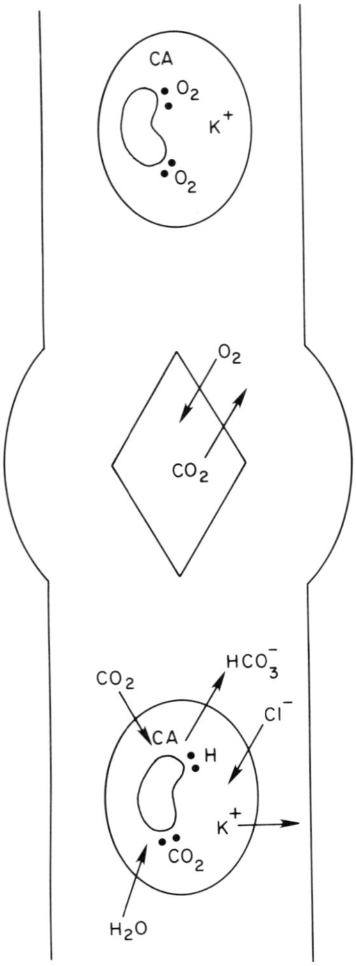

ARTERIAL

	Blood	Red Cells
pCO_2 (torr)	40	42
pO_2 (torr)	100	100
pH	7.40	7.14
HCO_3^- (meq/L)	24	10
K^+ (meq/L)	4.0	140
Cl^- (meq/L)	105	5
Hematocrit	40	

CAPILLARY BED

VENOUS

	Blood	Red Cells
pCO_2 (Torr)	46	50
PO_2 (Torr)	40	40
pH	7.36	7.04
HCO_3^- (meq/L)	28	14
K^+ (meq/L)	4.5	137
CL^- (meq/L)	103	7
Hematocrit	43	

Figure 27–10. The transition of blood from arterial to venous. (CA = carbonic anhydrase.) The chemical composition and blood gas changes are illustrated. An important change is the increase in levels of hematocrit and potassium. Other details are explained in the text.

total number of particles in the red cell increases because of these events, and water passively enters the cell along an osmotic gradient. The red cell swells, resulting in a venous hematocrit level that is slightly greater than the arterial (6–10%) change. Venous potassium levels are similarly elevated. These differences should be kept in mind when analyzing blood drawn from arterial catheters and comparing the results with normal venous values.

Buffer systems consist of a weak acid or base and its salt. These systems change in pH by increasing or decreasing the amount of their dissociated form when a stronger acid or base is added to the system. The general behavior of such buffers is illustrated for a theoretic buffer system in Figure 27–11. As acid or base is added to the system, the pH tends to remain unchanged. A buffer system is most resistant to changes in pH and is most efficient at buffering around its pK. The pK is the pH at which the weak acid or base is half dissociated.

The general chemical dissociation formula for a weak base is shown in the following equation:

$$BOH \rightleftharpoons OH^- + B^+$$

where BOH = a weak base, OH^- = the hydrogen ion acceptor, and B^+ = a cation available to form a salt. When a strong acid is combined with a weak base, the following equation describes the buffer system formed:

$$\text{strong base} + \text{weak base} \rightleftharpoons \text{weak acid} + \text{neutral salt}$$

pH is defined as the negative logarithm of the hydrogen ion concentration of an aqueous solution. K = the ionization constant for an acid or a base. K can be defined in the following way for a weak acid:

$$K[HA] = [H^+] \times [A^-]$$

where [HA] = the concentration of the unionized acid, $[H^+]$ = the concentration of the hydrogen ion, and $[A^-]$ = the concentration of the salt-forming radical (or base). Rearranging this equation yields

$$[H^+] = K[HA] / [A^-]$$

Taking the negative logarithm of both sides yields

$$-\text{Log}\,[H^+] = pH = -\text{LogK} + \text{Log}\,\{[A^-] / [HA]\}$$

By convention, pK is the negative logarithm of K. pH can be defined in terms of any of its buffer pairs, as suggested by the following general formula:

$$pH = pK + \text{Log}\,\{[\text{base}] / [\text{acid}]\}$$

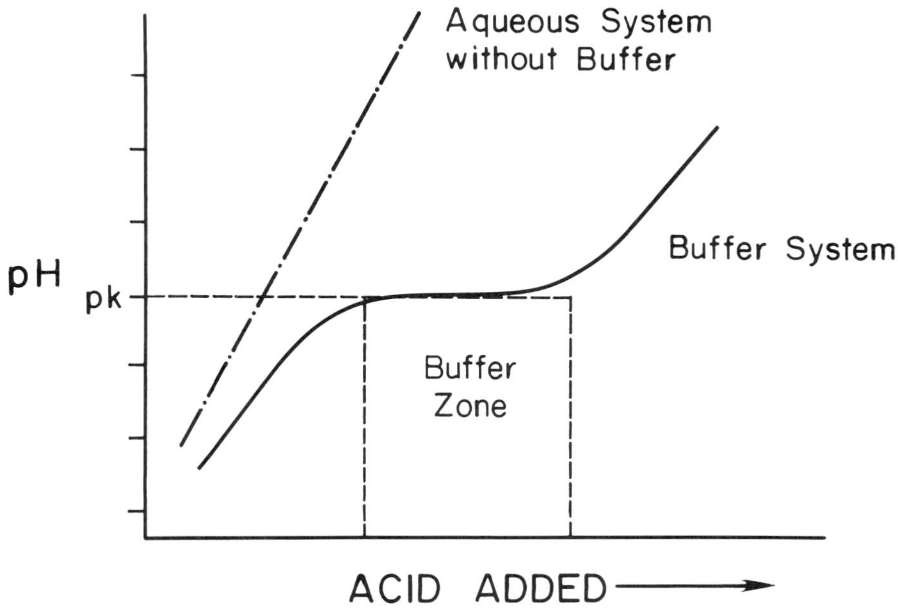

Figure 27–11. The performance of a "typical" buffer system. A buffer system is most resistant to change near its pK. The effect on pH of an aqueous system without buffer is contrasted in the dotted line.

Because bicarbonate is present in the blood in large quantities, the use of carbonic acid in this equation yields the following description of blood pH:

$$pH = pK + Log\{[HCO_3^-]/[H_2CO_3]\}$$

The pK for this reaction is 3.5, far from the usual blood pH.[44] By expressing this equation in terms of CO_2 (because there is approximately 600 times more CO_2 than H_2CO_3 in blood), the apparent pK becomes 6.1, and the classic Henderson-Hasselbalch form of the equation is

$$pH = 6.1 + Log\{[HCO_3^-]/(s \times PCO_2)\}$$

where s = the solubility constant for CO_2. Even at this pK, this buffer system would not be a very satisfactory one to maintain a physiologic pH of 7.40. However, because the CO_2 can be continually removed from the system, the pH can be easily regulated. This is called an open system.

The importance of ventilation in the maintenance of acid-base balance is demonstrated during apnea, when the blood pH rapidly falls to very low levels in several minutes. This is illustrated in Figure 27–12. To change the pH by an equivalent amount using renal compensatory mechanisms takes several days.

Use of the term pH is somewhat confusing in clinical practice because it represents logarithmic changes in hydrogen ion concentrations. As seen in Figure 27–13, the hydro-

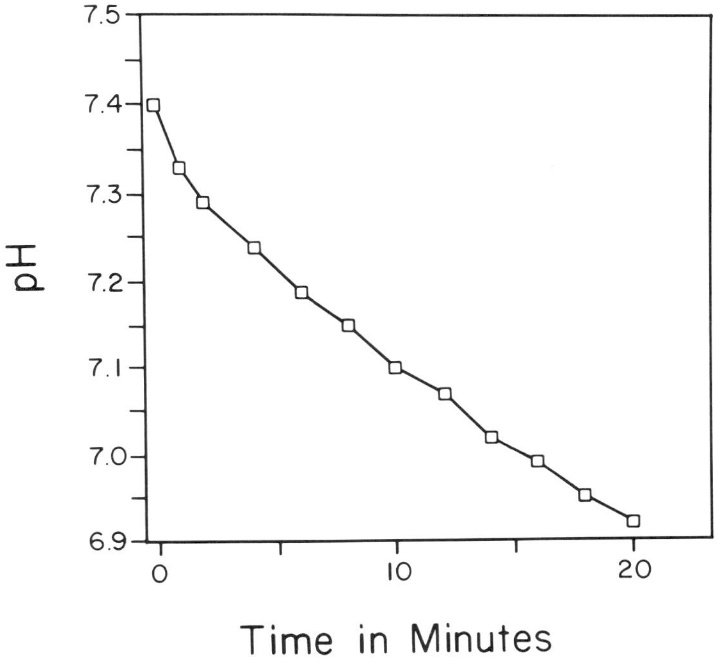

Figure 27–12. pH changes over time during apnea. The importance of the respiratory system to acid-base balance is discussed in the text.

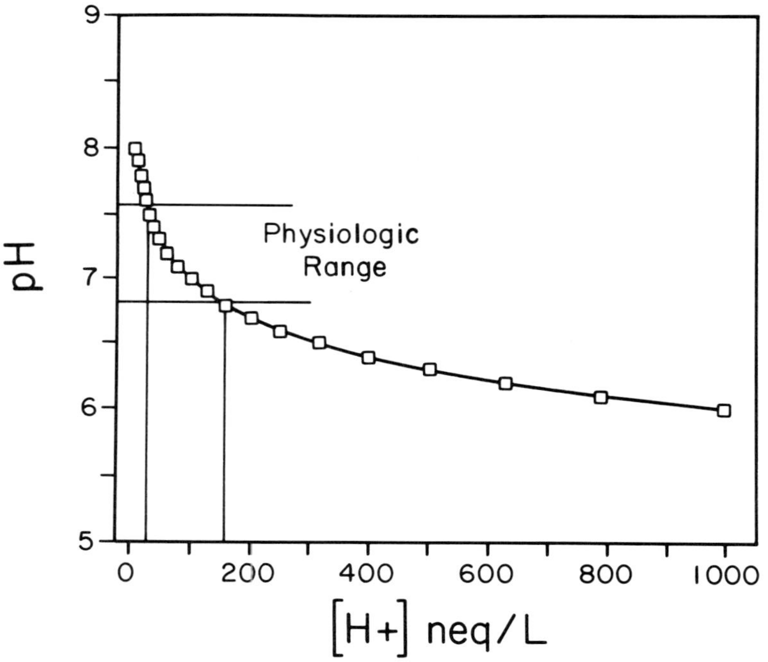

Figure 27–13. The relationship between pH and actual hydrogen ion concentration. The normal range is quite wide.

gen ion concentration changes by a factor of 10 between pH of 7.00 and 8.00. At a normal pH of 7.40, the hydrogen ion concentration is about 40 nEq/L. When we consider how tightly controlled most body chemicals are (such as potassium or sodium), it is surprising to see that hydrogen ion is normally allowed to vary between 32 and 45 nEq/L (pH 7.35–7.45).

CLINICAL ACID-BASE MANAGEMENT

Respiratory disorders are defined from the value of the $Paco_2$. If the $Paco_2$ is greater than 45 mmHg, respiratory acidosis is present. This is often called hypoventilation; however, this word carries the connotation of a patient who is breathing slowly and shallowly. Patients may, in fact, be hyperventilating in a clinical sense (breathing rapidly or deeply with an elevated minute ventilation). To avoid confusion, increased $Paco_2$ is called ''respiratory acidosis'' or ''hypercapnia'' throughout the remainder of this chapter. Respiratory alkalosis is defined as a $Paco_2$ less than 35 mmHg. This is not referred to as ''hyperventilation'' but as ''hypocapnia'' or ''respiratory alkalosis.'' In referring to the various components of acid-base balance derangement, processes are identified with the suffix ''-osis'' regardless of the blood pH. The pH of the blood is referred to as ''-emia.'' For example, a patient with a low pH due to metabolic acidosis may have partial respiratory compensation (pH < 7.35 and $Paco_2 < 35$); this would be described as acidemic (low blood pH) from metabolic acidosis (the metabolic process) with respiratory alkalosis or hypocapnia (the respiratory process).

The major problem in dealing with the interpretation of acid-base information is separation of the metabolic and respiratory components. There are six primary disorders: metabolic alkalosis and acidosis, and acute and chronic respiratory alkalosis and acidosis. For every primary disorder, there is a partial or complete compensatory response in the other system. When a disorder is treated, it is essential to identify the initiating (primary) disturbance, because this may require therapy. Treatment must not be applied to the compensatory reaction.

Many systems of analysis have been developed to deal with the problem of identifying the primary disorder and secondary response. Several of these approaches are described later in this chapter. None of the systems is totally effective or always produces the correct answer. Whenever there is more than a single primary disorder, no system is capable of sorting out the components and directing therapy. The clinical status of the patient and her or his response to attempted correction of a disturbance provide the information needed to correctly proceed in diagnosis and treatment.

When blood gas results are reported from an automated analyzer, the Pco_2 and the pH are measured with electrodes having an accuracy of 2–3%. The values for bicarbonate, standard bicarbonate, or base excess are calculated from nomograms based on the Henderson-Hasselbalch equation or other nomograms based on the behavior of blood or plasma in a test tube *(in vitro)*. These derived parameters were devised in attempts to separate the metabolic or fixed component (renal) from the respiratory component ($Paco_2$) of the acid-base status. Table 27–9 lists the normal values for some of these proposed parameters. Some of these indexes attempt to remove the respiratory component of the disorder. This is done by equilibrating the sample with a gas mixture having a $Paco_2$ of 40 mmHg and a Po_2 of 100

TABLE 27–9. METABOLIC INDEXES OF ACID-BASE BALANCE

Parameter	Range of Normal (mEq/L)
Plasma bicarbonate	22–26
Total CO_2	23–27
CO_2 combining power	21–27
Standard bicarbonate	21–25
Whole buffer base	45–50
Base excess	−3 to +3

mmHg under standard conditions at normal body temperature (37°C).

Total CO_2 includes bicarbonate and dissolved CO_2. It is based on extraction techniques and is not very different from plasma bicarbonate (dissolved CO_2 is only 1/20 the amount of bicarbonate).[45] No correction is made for the respiratory system contribution in either of these indexes.

CO_2 combining power was suggested as a way to account for the respiratory contribution to the disorder. Plasma is equilibrated with gas having a P_{CO_2} of 40 mmHg. The total CO_2 (and bicarbonate) is determined and should approximate the ''corrected'' metabolic contribution to acid-base balance. Theoretic problems with this calculated variable are that it is based only on the plasma component of blood (as indicated previously, hemoglobin plays a significant buffering role clinically), and it is an *in vitro* correction factor.

Standard bicarbonate, proposed by Astrup, is the bicarbonate of whole blood equilibrated under standard conditions of P_{CO_2} and temperature and includes the *in vitro* buffering contribution of hemoglobin.[46]

Whole buffer base includes the addition of the ''unmeasured'' buffers (amino acid protein components) to plasma bicarbonate. It does not account for the contribution from changes in hemoglobin oxygenation, which may buffer pH at the tissue level. Whole buffer base is normally 45–50 mEq/L. It is not calculated under standard conditions.

Base excess is the amount of acid (or base) needed to return a sample of whole blood to normal pH under standard conditions of P_{CO_2}, P_{O_2}, and temperature.[47] It is also an *in vitro* method for estimating the body's metabolic attempt to correct for abnormalities in acid-base status. The normal value for base excess is 0.

All these methods describe *in vitro* techniques to define the metabolic components of an acid-base disorder. Deviations from normal values are proposed to indicate a metabolic derangement. A problem of interpretation of these parameters is that compensation does occur, and ''normal'' values are not necessarily appropriate.[48]

TEMPERATURE CORRECTION OF ARTERIAL BLOOD GASES

Solubility of carbon dioxide and oxygen in blood depends on blood temperature. Blood gas analyzers are maintained at 37°C. Whether to correct the values obtained from patients with abnormal body temperatures to 37°C has been debated for many years. Temperature-correction formulas have been derived by cooling or heating anaerobically maintained blood (or plasma) samples and measuring blood gases in analyzers maintained at the same temperature as the sample. Reference or ''normal'' values are those obtained from samples having normal blood gas values at 37°C; the mathematical formulas ''correct'' them to this normal range.[49] Deviations in calculated values are assumed to indicate an abnormality.

Clinical and experimental data suggest that temperature-correcting blood gases may be inappropriate. Study of poikilothermic animals indicates that if their blood is obtained at several different temperatures and analyzed in a machine at 37°C, the values obtained are identical to the ''normal'' values obtained and analyzed at 37°C. In humans in cold environments, blood obtained from cold distal arteries has the same values as blood obtained from warm central arteries when both are analyzed at 37°C. If the values were temperature-corrected, the cold sample would be alkalotic (lower Pa_{CO_2}) and have a lower Pa_{O_2}.

The effects of temperature change on enzyme system activities parallel changes in hydrogen ion activity. To maintain neutrality, that is, the same relative activity of $[H^+]$ and $[OH^-]$, the solution must become slightly alkalotic as temperature decreases. The increased solubility of CO_2 accomplishes this change. A ''normal'' value should be obtained when the sample is warmed. No artificial *in vitro* correction is necessary or appropriate.[50] These concepts are well discussed by Rahn and colleagues.[51]

Clinical evidence also refutes temperature correction of blood gases. Profoundly hypothermic animals given sodium bicarbonate to normalize temperature-corrected blood gases invariably develop profound alkalemia and suffer myocardial damage on rewarming.[52] Hypothermic patients given little or no bicarbonate have normal acid-base balance when returned to normothermia.[53]

Temperature correction of Pa_{O_2} is usually performed, because O_2 solubility is also affected by temperature. Because metabolic activity is altered by temperature, the need for oxygen delivery should parallel its solubility. Temperature-correcting the Pa_{O_2} reduces the measured Pa_{O_2} value and may artifactually indicate the need for increased FI_{O_2}. However, the risks of administration of extra oxygen for a short period (increasing the FI_{O_2}) are minimal, and the extra margin of safety is justified.

DISORDERS OF ACID-BASE EQUILIBRIUM

The use of ''significance bands'' as described by Arbus and associates[54] helps identify the primary disorder and the expected compensatory response range. As seen in Figure 27–14, the six primary disorders can be identified in graphic form.[55] These disorders are acute respiratory alkalosis, chronic respiratory alkalosis, metabolic alkalosis,

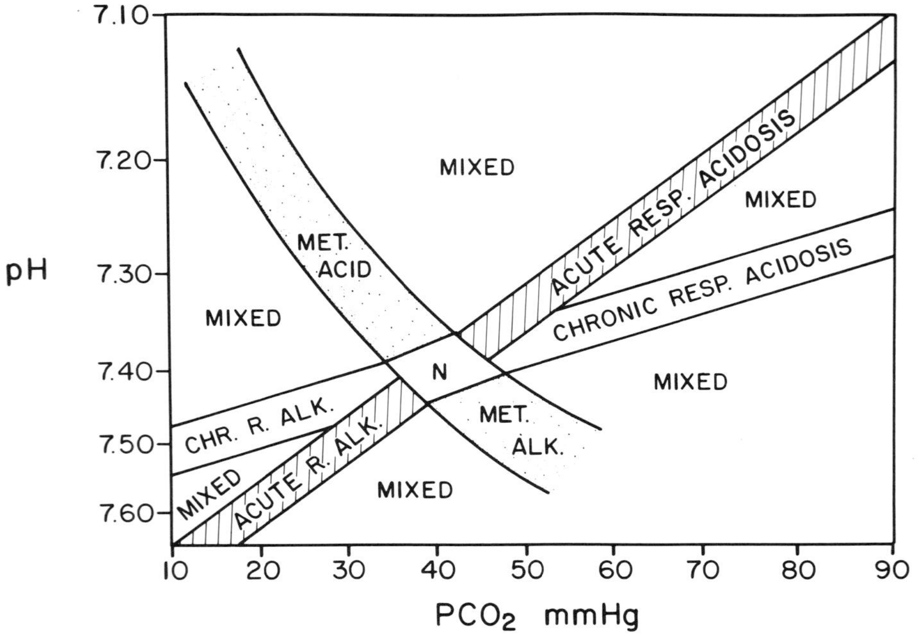

Figure 27–14. Significance bands describing the expected range of compensation for the primary disorders. See text for details. (Reprinted [modified] with permission from the International Anesthesia Research Society from Acid-base disorders: Application of total body carbon dioxide titration in anesthesia, by Levesque PR, Anesthesia and Analgesia, 1975; 54:307.)

acute respiratory acidosis, chronic respiratory acidosis, and metabolic acidosis.

To use the graphic method to identify the types of derangements present, plot the pH against the Pa_{CO_2}. The intersection identifies the type of problem. For example, a pH of 7.54 with a Pa_{CO_2} of 25 indicates "acute respiratory alkalosis" with appropriate metabolic compensation. The areas marked "mixed" identify situations in which more than one primary disorder is present or the degree of compensation is inappropriate or incomplete. No system separates the components when more than a single primary disorder is present. The clinical situation must be known in order to appropriately diagnose the problem. Further information can be obtained by making interventions and repeating the measurements. Only primary derangements should be treated, and then only if certain limits are exceeded and symptoms are present.

The data used to design the "significance bands" in Figure 27–14 were obtained by observing groups of patients with only one primary disorder and recording their range of compensation. These data have been collected and summarized.[56] Table 27–10 summarizes the *in vivo* compensation that occurs in response to a primary disorder. To utilize this information, simply use the correction factor to predict the compensated value. Any deviation from this expected value indicates a second (or third) primary disorder, which may require independent assessment and treatment.

ARTERIAL VERSUS VENOUS ACID-BASE BALANCE

Because there is very little difference between arterial and venous P_{CO_2}, usually only 4–5 mmHg, a venous sample can be used to evaluate acid-base status. Bicarbonate is calculated from the pH and is also only slightly lower in venous samples. Malignant hyperthermia may be confirmed in the operating room by a venous blood sample, because this hypermetabolic state is characterized by early develop-

TABLE 27–10. COMPENSATORY RESPONSES TO THE SIX PRIMARY DISORDERS

Primary Disorder	Compensatory Response (Expected)	Magnitude of Response (Predicted)
Respiratory alkalosis (acute)	Decreased bicarbonate	$[HCO_3^-]$ decreases 2 mEq/L for each 10-mmHg decrease in Pa_{CO_2}
Respiratory alkalosis (chronic)	Decreased bicarbonate	$[HCO_3^-]$ decreases 5 mEq/L for each 10-mmHg decrease in Pa_{CO_2}
Metabolic alkalosis	Increased Pa_{CO_2}	$Pa_{CO_2} = 0.9 \times [HCO_3^-] + 9$
		$Pa_{CO_2} = 0.9 \times [HCO_3^-] + 15.6$
		Pa_{CO_2} = base excess + 40.6
Respiratory acidosis (acute)	Increased bicarbonate	$[HCO_3^-]$ increases 1 mEq/L for each 10-mmHg increase in Pa_{CO_2}
Respiratory acidosis (chronic)	Increased bicarbonate	$[HCO_3^-]$ increases 3.5 mEq/L for each 10-mmHg increase in Pa_{CO_2}
Metabolic acidosis	Decreased Pa_{CO_2}	$Pa_{CO_2} = 1.5 \times [HCO_3^-] + 8$
		$Pa_{CO_2} = 1.8 \times (\text{base excess} - 24) + 8$
		Pa_{CO_2} = Last two digits of the pH

The direction of the expected response is indicated as well as several rules of thumb for determining the magnitude of the compensatory response.

ment of a mixed metabolic and respiratory acidosis.[57] Venous acid-base balance is an excellent monitor for this syndrome. In the case of a patient with cardiorespiratory arrest when external chest compressions are being performed, a large discrepancy between arterial and venous blood gases may exist.[58] The venous PCO_2 may reflect the adequacy (or inadequacy) of the artificial circulation and tissue acid-base status. The end-tidal PCO_2 may be a useful monitor of tissue acidosis, because it reflects venous and tissue PCO_2 in this circumstance.[59, 60]

ACUTE RESPIRATORY ALKALOSIS

$PaCO_2$ decreases when alveolar ventilation exceeds carbon dioxide production (Table 27–11). This results in a rise in pH. An immediate change in total CO_2 and base excess follows the change in $PaCO_2$. This amounts to a decrease of 2 mEq/L of bicarbonate (1.8 base excess units) for each 10-mmHg change in $PaCO_2$. This immediate compensation is not due to renal mechanisms; it is most likely due to local tissue factors. After several hours, renal retention of acid begins. This fall in the metabolic component (bicarbonate fall) continues, and the disorder becomes chronic with more complete compensation.

As seen in Table 27–11, many of the causes of hypocapnia have no specific therapy. Respiratory alkalosis reduces cerebral blood flow and may improve intracranial compliance in patients with brain injury or tumor. No treatment would be appropriate, because this is a normal protective response. Anxiety can often be treated with anxiolytic agents or reassuring discussions with the patient. Hypoxia (PaO_2 less than 55 mmHg) affects the peripheral chemoreceptors (aortic and carotid bodies) and increases minute ventilation. Other disorders may be treated, but therapy is not appropriate for the hypocapnia *per se*.

TABLE 27–11. CAUSES OF RESPIRATORY ALKALOSIS

Hypoxemia
Decreased pulmonary compliance
Pulmonary edema
Adult respiratory distress syndrome
Pulmonary fibrosis
Infection
Septic syndrome
Pneumonia
Fever
Bronchospasm (early)
Pulmonary embolism
Drugs
Doxapram hydrochloride
Theophylline
Progesterone
Salicylates
Pregnancy
Central nervous system disorders
Cirrhosis
Excessive mechanical ventilation
Anxiety
Psychogenesis

Some of these conditions may require primary treatment; however, low $PaCO_2$ is usually never itself treated.

TABLE 27–12. CAUSES OF METABOLIC ALKALOSIS

Diuretic use
Nasogastric suction
Vomiting
Diarrhea (containing chloride)
Antacid administration
Transfusions (citrate)
Drugs
Carbenicillin
Penicillin
Hypokalemia
Hypercalcemia
Primary hyperaldosteronism

CHRONIC RESPIRATORY ALKALOSIS

When hypocapnia persists for several hours or longer, renal mechanisms are activated, and further compensation occurs. Renal compensation occurs naturally in inhabitants of high altitudes. Some patients can completely compensate for respiratory alkalosis and obtain a normal pH. This is unusual with other disorders. For every 10-mmHg fall in $PaCO_2$, there is up to a 5-mEq/L decrease in bicarbonate (4 base excess units), as seen in Table 27–10.[61] It may take several weeks to normalize pH in this circumstance.

METABOLIC ALKALOSIS

Because metabolic disorders develop slowly, and respiratory compensation occurs immediately, there is no chronic or acute distinction. Despite this fact, the respiratory response elicited may be quite variable. No definite reasons for this variability have been identified. A normal or low $PaCO_2$ suggests a coexisting respiratory alkalosis. Several formulas have been proposed to predict the respiratory compensation seen in metabolic alkalosis. The $PaCO_2$ was equal to $0.9 \times$ [bicarbonate] + 12 (range, 9–16) in a group of patients in whom alkalosis was induced by a variety of methods.[62] Other authors have found less of a compensatory respiratory acidosis, as indicated in Table 27–10.[63]

There are many causes of this common abnormality of acid-base balance. Some are listed in Table 27–12. Diuretic use with hypokalemia and hypochloremia is a frequent cause. Acid and chloride loss from the gastrointestinal tract, antacid administration, certain antibiotics, and some endocrine abnormalities are also implicated. Some causes are treatable by replacement of chloride and potassium. There are several significant, undesired side effects of metabolic alkalosis. These include increased total body oxygen consumption, myocardial depression, increased frequency of cardiac arrhythmias, desensitized respiratory center, and hypoxia on room air (see causes of low PaO_2, discussed previously).

ACUTE RESPIRATORY ACIDOSIS

Disorders that decrease the efficiency of pulmonary carbon dioxide excretion may increase $PaCO_2$. Acute changes in the metabolic component result in pH being returned toward normal. Normal people with acute elevation in Pa_{CO_2} show an approximately 1-mEq/L increase in bicarbonate for each 10-mmHg increase in Pa_{CO_2} (about 0.8 base excess units) owing to tissue and hemoglobin buffers.[64] Renal regulation takes much longer but is far more complete.

The causes of acute respiratory acidosis include drug effects on the respiratory center or neuromuscular transmission and upper or lower airway obstruction. Narcotics and sedatives, general anesthetics, bronchospasm, upper airway occlusion, and rebreathing of exhaled CO_2 are causes of acute CO_2 retention (Table 27–13).

The physiologic effects of acute hypercapnia are usually fairly benign. If hypoxia is avoided, hypercapnia increases heart rate and blood pressure through sympathetic stimulation. It shifts the hemoglobin saturation curve to the right. Dysrhythmias and enhanced cardiac contractility result. Serum potassium increases. If the Pa_{CO_2} increases above 80–90 mmHg, anesthesia or CO_2 narcosis usually results. In patients with head injury or brain tumors, increased cerebral blood flow may cause increased intracranial pressure and herniation of brain tissue.

Treatment of acute hypercapnia is directed at relief of the underlying cause rather than at the pH change. Occasionally, it is necessary to correct the pH with exogenous base. The use of bicarbonate is controversial in that more CO_2 is produced, and the pH may remain unchanged. Also, because the CO_2 can freely diffuse into cells, the intercellular pH may actually fall further. Nonbicarbonate buffers such as tris(hydroxymethyl)aminomethane (THAM) have been suggested for this use.[65, 66] Carbicarb (a mixture of sodium carbonate and sodium bicarbonate) has been recently tested and found not to increase Pa_{CO_2} as much as sodium bicarbonate does.[67]

TABLE 27–13. CAUSES OF RESPIRATORY ACIDOSIS

Chronic obstructive pulmonary disease
Acute bronchospasm
Primary alveolar hypoventilation syndrome
Ondine's curse
Pickwickian syndrome
High-level spinal cord injury
Myasthenia gravis
Multiple sclerosis
Muscular dystrophies
Bulbar polio
Guillain-Barré syndrome
Narcotic drug effects
Neuromuscular-blocking drugs
Airway obstruction
General anesthetics
Mechanical ventilation
Rebreathing
Intentional
Equipment failure

CHRONIC RESPIRATORY ACIDOSIS

When an elevated Pa_{CO_2} persists for longer than 6–10 hours, the metabolic response is more complete. Hypercapnia causing acidemia stimulates retention of bicarbonate. Compensation does not return blood pH to normal if Pa_{CO_2} is greater than 55 mmHg. An increase of 3.5 mEq/L of bicarbonate (3 base excess units) for every 10-mmHg rise in Pa_{CO_2} is seen in response to this primary disorder.[68] CO_2 retention is a result of ventilation-perfusion mismatch in chronic lung disease. End-stage restrictive lung disease (such as kyphoscoliosis) may also result in hypercapnia.[69] Ondine's curse and the pickwickian syndrome are conditions in which the central nervous system center controlling respiratory drive becomes less sensitive to changes in pH, with a resultant elevation in Pa_{CO_2}. As a consequence of this abnormality, pulmonary hypertension and right heart failure frequently follow prolonged elevations of Pa_{CO_2}. Hypoxia on room air (described previously) also occurs as a consequence of elevated Pa_{CO_2}.

The treatment of the elevated CO_2 should be directed at the underlying cause. Ventilatory muscle weakness, fatigue,[70] and malnourishment[71] contribute to elevated CO_2 in chronic pulmonary disease. Diaphragm rest and nutritional improvement can favorably affect gas exchange. Conditioning exercises may also improve muscle strength and endurance.[72] High glucose loads during parenteral feeding can increase CO_2 production by stimulating fat synthesis and may worsen respiratory failure.[73] Drugs that have been used to reduce Pa_{CO_2} include estrogens, caffeine, aminophylline, and doxapram hydrochloride.[74] Surgical procedures to correct airway obstruction and obesity have been successful in treating the pickwickian syndrome. Positive pressure ventilation reverses the CO_2 retention, but this may mean indefinite commitment to artificial ventilation. The use of noninvasive ventilation, especially at night during sleep, may improve function and prolong life in terminal patients with very high Pa_{CO_2} levels.[75]

METABOLIC ACIDOSIS

When acid products decrease the serum bicarbonate, the respiratory center and peripheral chemoreceptors are stimulated, and ventilation increases. This response is proportional to the degree of change in bicarbonate and may be delayed 12–24 hours. This delay is due to the slow transfer of bicarbonate across the blood-brain barrier. Central nervous system pH changes due to changing blood bicarbonate concentrations occur after blood pH changes. When the brain is involved in the process causing metabolic acidosis, this delay is absent. The expected Pa_{CO_2} in compensation for a decreased bicarbonate is about $1.5 \times [\text{bicarbonate}] + 8$.[76] Another rule of thumb is that the Pa_{CO_2} should be equal to the first two decimal point digits of the pH (e.g., a pH of 7.25 should have a Pa_{CO_2} of about 25) (see Table 27–10).

The causes of metabolic acidosis are listed in Table 27–14. These are divided into two groups: those with acid accumulation, called high anion gap, and those with bicar-

TABLE 27–14. CAUSES OF METABOLIC ACIDOSIS

Normal Anion Gap	Elevated Anion Gap
Renal tubular acidosis	Renal failure
Diarrhea	Ketoacidosis
Carbonic anhydrase inhibitors	Starvation
Ureteral diversions	Ethanol ingestion
Hyperalimentation	Methanol ingestion
Renal failure (early)	Ethylene glycol ingestion
Acid indigestion	Salicylates
Hyperchloremia	Lactic acidosis
	Nephrotic syndrome
	Seizures
	Circulatory failure
	Cyanide poisoning
	Carbon monoxide poisoning

bonate loss, called normal anion gap. The anion gap is calculated as the serum sodium minus the sum of the chloride and bicarbonate. This accounts for unmeasured anions, such as proteins, phosphate, sulfate, and others. The anion gap is usually 10–12 mEq/L. An increase in the anion gap means an accumulation of unmeasured acid products such as lactic acid.

The underlying cause of the acidosis should be treated, if possible. The following formula is useful to calculate the required amount of bicarbonate if correction of a deficit is deemed desirable, usually a blood pH less than 7.15:

Bicarbonate dose (mEq) = base excess $\times$ 0.2 $\times$ weight (kg)
or

Bicarbonate dose (mEq) = (24 − [HCO_3^-]) $\times$ 0.2 $\times$ weight (kg)

These approximations allow about half the deficit in plasma to be corrected. The effect of treatment on acid-base parameters should be closely monitored. Data suggest that aggressive correction of the deficit in metabolic acidosis may be associated with paradoxical central nervous system depression and respiratory arrest.[77] The levels and balance of potassium, phosphate, and magnesium should also be considered in these disorders and during therapy. Complications often result from other electrolyte imbalances.

COMBINED ACID-BASE DISORDERS

The disorders described in the preceding sections were single primary disorders with the appropriate, expected compensatory responses. More than one primary disorder may be present. This is indicated when the expected response to the first disorder is not seen. For a detailed description of these combined disorders, which are beyond the scope of this chapter, the reader should consult the excellent review by Narins and Emmett.[56]

OTHER MONITORS

The discussion of acid-base monitoring and clinical implications is based on the fact that the total body's contribution to metabolic activity is averaged in the blood. This sample only approximates what is happening in each separate tissue. Monitors of tissue pH, PCO_2, K^+, and PO_2 are being developed in laboratories and have been used in animals and some humans. Tissue probes are closer to the intracellular environment, where the abnormalities originate and have their most significant effects. Other technologies, such as magnetic resonance imaging, accurately identify intracellular metabolic derangements and may lead to the development of monitoring at the cellular level.

REFERENCES

1. Peterson JI, Fitzgerald RV, Buckhold DK: Fiberoptic probe for measurement of oxygen partial pressure. Anal Chem 1984; 56:62–67.
2. Zimmerman JL, Dellinger RP: Initial evaluation of a new intra-arterial blood gas system in humans. Crit Care Med 1993; 21:495–500.
3. Eberhart RC: Indwelling blood compatible chemical sensors. Surg Clin North Am 1985; 65:1025–1040.
4. Shapiro BA, Mahutte CK, Crane RD, Gilmore IJ: Clinical performance of a blood gas monitor: A prospective, multicenter trial. Crit Care Med 1993; 21:487–494.
5. Shapiro BA: *In Vivo* monitoring of arterial blood gases and pH. Respir Care 1992; 37:1087–1095.
6. Severinghaus JW: Transcutaneous blood gas analysis. Respir Care 1982; 27:152–159.
7. Podolsy S, Wertheimer J, Harding S: The relationship of conjunctival and arterial blood gases oxygen measurements. Resuscitation 1989; 18:31–36.
8. Brown M, Vender JS: Noninvasive oxygen monitoring. Crit Care Clin 1988; 4:493–509.
9. Shufflebarger C, Jehle D, Cottington E, Martin M: Transconjunctival oxygen monitoring as a predictor of hypoxemia during helicopter transport. Am J Emerg Med 1986; 4:501–503.
10. Bourke DL: Errors in intraoperative hematocrit determination. Anesthesiology 1976; 45:357–359.
11. Fox MJ, Brody JS, Weintraub LR, et al: Leukocyte larceny: A cause of spurious hypoxemia. Am J Med 1979; 67:742–746.
12. Ong ST, David D, Snow M, Hanson JE: Effect of variations in room temperature on measured values of blood gas quality-control materials. Clin Chem 1983; 29:502–505.
13. Thorson SH, Marini JJ, Pierson DJ, Hudson LD: Variability of arterial blood gas values in stable patients in the ICU. Chest 1983; 84:14–18.
14. Gilbert R, Keighley JF: The arterial-alveolar oxygen tension ratio. An index of gas exchange applicable to varying inspired oxygen concentrations. Am Rev Respir Dis 1974; 109:142–145.
15. Gilbert R, Auchincloss JH, Kuppinger M, Thomas MV: Stability of the arterial/alveolar oxygen partial pressure ratio. Crit Care Med 1979; 7:267–272.
16. Perutz NF: Stereochemistry of cooperative effects in hemoglobin. Nature 1970; 228:726–739.
17. Perutz NF: Hemoglobin structure and respiratory transport. Sci Am 1978; 239:92–125.
18. Shappell SD, Lenfant CJM: Adaptive, genetic, and iatrogenic alterations of the oxyhemoglobin-dissociation curve. Anesthesiology 1972; 37:127–139.
19. Schumacker PT, Long GR, Wood LDH: Tissue oxygen extraction during hypovolemia: Role of hemoglobin P_{50}. J Appl Physiol 1987; 62:1801–1807.
20. Rubio R, Berne RM: Regulation of coronary blood flow. Prog Cardiovasc Dis 1975; 43:105–122.
21. Nunn JF: Applied Respiratory Physiology. London: Butterworth, 1987; 241–473.
22. Block AJ, Cherniac RM, Christopher KL, et al: Problems in prescribing and supplying oxygen for medicare patients. Am Rev Respir Dis 1986; 134:340–341.
23. Durbin, CG Jr: Pulmonary oxygen toxicity. Respir Care 1993; 39:1–12.
24. Deneke SM, Fanburg BL: Normobaric oxygen toxicity of the lung. N Engl J Med 1980; 303:76–86.
25. Marshall BE, Wyche MQ: Hypoxemia during and after anesthesia. Anesthesiology 1972; 37:178–209.

26. Davis WB, Rennard SI, Bitterman PB, Crystal RG: Pulmonary oxygen toxicity: Early reversible changes in human alveolar structures induced by hyperoxia. N Engl J Med 1983; 309:878–883.
27. Roes DM, Downes JB, Heenan TJ: Temporal responses of functional residual capacity and oxygen tension to changes in positive end-expiratory pressure. Crit Care Med 1981; 9:79–82.
28. Kirby RR, Downs JB, Civetta JM, et al: High level end expiratory pressure (PEEP) in acute respiratory failure. Chest 1975; 67:156–163.
29. Petty TL, Fowler AA: Another look at ARDS. Chest 1982; 82:98–104.
30. Dofinsky PM, Whitcomb ME: The effect of PEEP on cardiac output. Chest 1983; 84:210–216.
31. Gallagher J, Civetta JM: Goal-directed therapy of acute respiratory failure. Anesth Analg 1980; 59:831–834.
32. Miller RS, Nelson LD, DiRusso SM, et al: High-level positive end-expiratory pressure management in trauma-associated adult respiratory distress syndrome. J Trauma 1992; 33:284–290.
33. Luce JM: The cardiovascular effects of mechanical ventilation and positive end-expiratory pressure. JAMA 1984; 252:807–811.
34. Jardin F, Farcot JC, Boisante L, et al: Influence of positive end-expiratory pressure on left ventricular performance. N Engl J Med 1981; 304:387–392.
35. Haynes JB, Carson SD, Whitney WP, et al: Positive end-expiratory pressure shifts left ventricular pressure-area curves. J Appl Physiol 1980; 48:670–676.
36. Prewitt RM, Wood LDH: The effect of positive end-expiratory pressure on ventricular function in dogs. Am J Physiol 1979; 236:H534–544.
37. Buda AJ, Pinsky MR, Ingels NB, et al: Effects of intrathoracic pressure on left ventricular performance. N Engl J Med 1979; 301:453–459.
38. Chapin JC, Downs JB, Douglas ME, et al: Lung expansion, airway pressure transmission, and positive end-expiratory pressure. Arch Surg 1979; 114:1193–1197.
39. Mathews PJ: The validity of Pa_{O_2} values 3, 6, and 9 minutes after an FI_{O_2} change in mechanically ventilated heart-surgery patients. Respir Care 1987; 32:1029–1034.
40. Lucey JF, Dangman B: A reexamination of the role of oxygen in retrolental fibroplasia. Pediatrics 1984; 73:82–96.
41. Kitahata LM, Katz JD: Tension pneumocephalus after posterior fossa craniotomy: A complication of the sitting position. Anesthesiology 1976; 44:448–450.
42. Faithfull NS: Fluorocarbons: Current status and future applications. Anaesthesia 1987; 42:234–242.
43. Kapp JR: Neurological response to hyperbaric oxygen—A criterion for cerebral revascularization. Surg Neurol 1981; 15:43–46.
44. Roughton JWF: Transport of oxygen and carbon dioxide. *In* Fenn WO, Rahn H (eds): Handbook of Physiology, Section 3, Respiration, Vol 1. Washington, DC: American Physiological Society, 1964; 800.
45. Van Slyke DD, Cullen GE: Studies of acidosis. 1. Bicarbonate concentration of blood plasma: Its significance and its determination as measure of acidosis. J Biol Chem 1917; 30:289–346.
46. Astrup P: New approach to acid-base metabolism. Clin Chem 1961; 7:1–15.
47. Astrup P, Jorgensen K, Siggaard Andersen O, Engle K: Acid-base metabolism: A new approach. Lancet 1960; 1:1035–1039.
48. Schwartz WB, Relman AS: A critique of the parameters used in the evaluation of acid-base disorders. N Engl J Med 1963; 268:1382–1388.
49. Andritsch RF, Muravchick S, Gold MI: Temperature correction of arterial bloodgas parameters: A comparative review of methodology. Anesthesiology 1981; 55:311–316.
50. Ream AK, Reitz BA, Silverberg G: Temperature correction of Pa_{CO_2} and pH in estimating acid-base: An example of the emperor's new clothes? Anesthesiology 1982; 56:41–44.
51. Rahn H, Reeves RB, Howell BJ: Hydrogen ion regulation, temperature, and evolution. Am Rev Respir Dis 1975; 112:162–165.
52. Becker H, Vinten-Johansen J, Buckberg GD, et al: Myocardial damage caused by keeping pH 7.40 during deep systemic hypothermia. J Thorac Cardiovasc Surg 1981; 82:810–820.
53. Blayo MC, LeCompte Y, Pocidalo JJ: Control of acid-base status during hypothermia in man. Respir Physiol 1980; 42:287–298.
54. Arbus CS, Hebert LA, Levesque PR, et al: Characterization and clinical application of the "significance band" for acute respiratory alkalosis. N Engl J Med 1969; 280:117–123.
55. Levesque PR: Acid-base disorders: Application of total body carbon dioxide titration in anesthesia. Anesth Analg 1975; 54:299–307.
56. Narins RG, Emmett M: Simple and mixed acid-base disorders: A practical approach. Medicine 1980; 59:161–187.
57. Durbin CG: Malignant hyperthermia syndrome: Identification and management. *In* Berry FA (ed): Anesthetic Management of Difficult and Routine Pediatric Patients. New York: Churchill Livingstone, 1986; 414–415.
58. Grundier W, Weit MH, Rackow EC, et al: Selective acidosis in venous blood during human cardiopulmonary resuscitation: A preliminary report. Crit Care Med 1985; 13:886–887.
59. Garnett AR, Ornato JP, Gonzalez ER, Johnson EB: End-tidal carbon dioxide monitoring during cardiopulmonary resuscitation. JAMA 1987; 257:512–515.
60. Adrogué HJ, Rashad MN, Gorin AB, et al: Assessing acid-base status in circulatory failure. Differences between arterial and central venous blood. N Engl J Med 1989; 320:1312–1316.
61. Lahiri S, Milledge JS: Acid-base in Sherpa altitude residents and lowlanders at 4880 M. Respir Physiol 1967; 2:323–334.
62. Fulop M: Hypercapnia in metabolic alkalosis. N Y State J Med 1976; 76:19–22.
63. Goldring RM, Cannon PJ, Heinemann HO, Fishman AP: Respiratory adjustment to chronic metabolic alkalosis in man. J Clin Invest 1968; 47:188–202.
64. Brackett NC, Cohn JJ, Schwartz WB: Carbon dioxide titration curve of normal man: Effect of increasing degrees of acute hypercapnia on acid-base equilibrium. N Engl J Med 1965; 272:6–12.
65. Minuck M, Sharma GP: Comparison of THAM and sodium bicarbonate in resuscitation of the heart after ventricular fibrillation in dogs. Anesth Analg 1977; 56:38–45.
66. Manfredi F, Sieker HO, Spoto AP, Saitzman HA: Severe carbon dioxide intoxication: Treatment with organic buffer (trishydroxymethyl aminomethane). JAMA 1960; 173:999–1003.
67. Gazmuri RJ, von Planta M, Weil MH, Rackow EC: Cardiac effects of carbon dioxide–consuming and carbon dioxide–generating buffers during cardiopulmonary resuscitation. J Am Coll Cardiol 1990; 15:482–490.
68. Brackett NC, Wingo CF, Muren O, Solano JT: Acid-base response to chronic hypercapnia in man. N Engl J Med 1969; 280:124–130.
69. West JB: Causes of carbon dioxide retention in lung disease. N Engl J Med 1971; 284:1232–1236.
70. Arora NS, Rochester DF: Respiratory muscle strength and maximal voluntary ventilation in undernourished patients. Am Rev Respir Dis 1982; 126:5–8.
71. Hunter MAB, Cary MA, Larsh HW: The nutritional status of patients with chronic obstructive pulmonary disease. Am Rev Respir Dis 1981; 124:376–381.
72. Sonnes LJ, Davis JA: Increased exercise performance in patients with severe COPD following inspiratory resistive training. Chest 1982; 82:436–439.
73. Covelli HD, Black JW, Olsen MS, Beekman JF: Respiratory failure precipitated by high carbohydrate loads. Ann Intern Med 1981; 95:579–581.
74. Aubier M, De Troyer A, Sampson M, et al: Aminophylline improves diaphragm contractility. N Engl J Med 1981; 305:249–277.
75. Hill NS: Noninvasive ventilation. Does it work, for whom, and how? Am Rev Respir Dis 1993; 147:1050–1055.
76. Albert MS, Dell RB, Winters RW: Quantitative displacement acid-base equilibrium in metabolic acidosis. Ann Intern Med 1967; 66:312–322.
77. Morris LR, Murphy MB, Kitabchi AE: Bicarbonate therapy in severe diabetic ketoacidosis. Ann Intern Med 1986; 105:836–840.

CHAPTER

28

Perioperative Biochemical Monitors

WILLIAM P. ARNOLD III, M.D.

The anesthesiologist depends on many biochemical analyses to gather information not available from either physical examination or other monitors. In recent years, reliance on intraoperative laboratory data has become routine, especially in more extensive surgical procedures. Although the relevance of laboratory data is usually well understood by the clinician, the nuts and bolts of the assays that produce these data are less clear. This chapter reviews the basis of biochemical tests commonly used during the perioperative period while highlighting the role of the acute or "stat" clinical laboratory. Emphasis is placed on the details of the assay rather than on the myriad of clinical implications discussed in general textbooks of anesthesiology. Included are reasons for inaccuracies, errors in sample handling by persons obtaining blood for analyses (e.g., effects of anticoagulants, sample volume), the importance of understanding the various methods employed by the clinical chemist, and the effects of different assay methods on interpretation of results (e.g., serum sodium and pseudohyponatremia). For a detailed discussion of the gamut of determinations performed by the clinical chemist, the reader is encouraged to consult a comprehensive textbook of clinical chemistry.[1]

THE ACUTE LABORATORY

Our ability to provide intensive perioperative care has been significantly advanced by improvements in the methods employed by clinical chemistry laboratories and especially by the creation of satellite facilities, called acute or stat laboratories, located close to acute care areas.

An acute laboratory, dedicated only to those assays required for the perioperative management of critically ill patients and those undergoing extensive surgical procedures, is an essential part of many hospitals. Although these laboratories may be physically separated from the main clinical laboratory, they usually remain under the administrative and operational control of the clinical chemist.[2] This is extremely important, because full-time personnel are more aware of the need for quality control and maintenance of analytic equipment than are those to whom the laboratory is only a means to an end.[3, 4]

The proximity of the laboratory to the ward or operating room permits a positive, ongoing interaction between the clinician and the clinical chemist. A close relationship between the disciplines is important, because it encourages discussion of a variety of factors that may affect results. These include such things as the time that a sample is obtained, the effects of various anticoagulants, the patient's condition, and the source of the sample (whether it is central or peripheral venous, arterial, or capillary).[4] It also instills a sense of active participation on the part of the clinical chemist that would otherwise be absent because of the remoteness of the main laboratory.[5]

ASSAY METHODS IN THE ACUTE LABORATORY

FLAME PHOTOMETRY

Flame photometry is still used by some clinical laboratories to determine the concentrations of various ions in body fluids, including sodium, potassium, and lithium. Certain ions, when heated, emit colors. The wavelength of the color produced by a given ion is characteristic of that ion—for example, 589 and 766 nm (yellow and red-violet) for sodium and potassium, respectively.

In practice, a salt-containing solution is injected into a flame. After the water in the sample has been evaporated, the molecules of the salt are dissociated into an atomic vapor. A small number of the atoms are subsequently excited by the heat, resulting in the displacement of electrons into higher orbitals. Almost immediately, these atoms return to their ground state and in doing so release light of a specific wavelength, which is used to identify that ion. The intensity of the color is directly proportional to the concentration of the ion in question. It is measured by a phototube, the output of which is displayed as a concentration. Sodium and potassium may be measured simultaneously with this method. Lithium is usually added to the sample as an internal standard to compensate for variables that otherwise might result in quantitative inaccuracies. A separate phototube is used for each ion. Standard solutions of the ions in question must be used to calibrate the instrument, because it is impossible to calculate independently the light intensity emitted by a given concentration of sodium or potassium.[6]

Flame photometry used to be an important method in the acute laboratory, but it has been displaced by newer methods. One of the main objections to the technique was the need to have explosive gas (propane) in the laboratory to provide a source for the flame.[1]

ION-SELECTIVE ELECTRODES

The ion-selective electrode (ISE) is the mainstay for assaying electrolytes in the modern acute laboratory. Although it is not important for the clinician to understand all of the nuances of these devices, a basic understanding of their operation aids in interpretation of results and in understanding the occasional differences between results determined with ISEs and results from other methods used in central clinical chemistry laboratories.

ISEs are basically batteries that develop a voltage or potential between two electrodes in contact with the sample. The potential is proportional to the concentration of a specific ion being assayed (Fig. 28–1). The potential is mathematically related to the concentration by the Nernst equation:

$$E = E_0 + \frac{RT}{nF} \ln(fC)$$

where: E = electrical potential
E_0 = constant potential
R = universal gas constant
T = temperature
n = charge of the ion being measured
F = Faraday's constant (96,500 coulombs)
C = concentration of the ion being measured
f = activity coefficient of ion being measured

Because ISEs respond to a difference in potential, they are referred to as *potentiometric* sensors. Some measuring devices respond to current instead of voltage and are thus *amperometric* sensors. An example of the latter is the Clark oxygen electrode, a modification of which is used in some glucose analyzers.[1]

All ISEs are composed of a reference electrode and a measuring electrode, each of which may be thought of as a half-cell.[1] The voltage between the two electrodes is displayed as the activity of ion being assayed. The reference electrode is usually composed of either a silver wire covered with a coating of silver chloride or mercury in contact with calomel (Hg_2Cl_2). The electrode is immersed in an internal filling solution of KCl or other constituents of known concentration that, in turn, via a liquid-liquid junction, forms a salt bridge with the solution being measured. The measuring electrode is a metallic conductor that is immersed in an internal solution containing a known concentration of the ion being measured. This solution is separated from the sample in question by a membrane that is selectively responsive to the ion. A potential develops across the membrane as the result of an exchange of ions in the outer layers of the membrane. The potential difference between the measuring and reference electrodes is proportional to the concentration of the ion being assayed. This difference is detected by a sensitive voltmeter, converted to the appropriate units, and displayed as a concentration.

Some ISEs require that the sample be diluted prior to assay (indirect potentiometry), whereas others detect ions

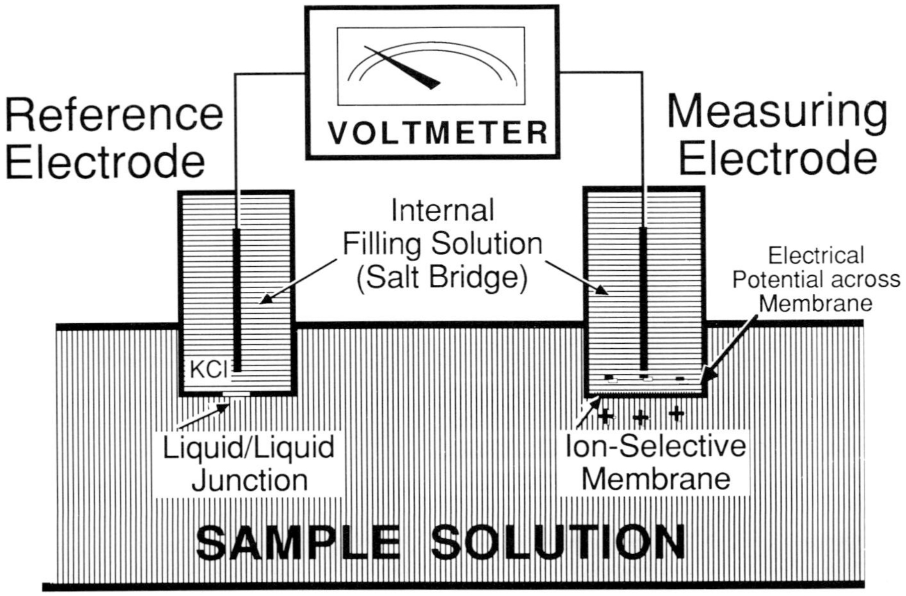

Figure 28–1. Diagram of an ion-selective electrode. (See text for details.)

in undiluted samples (direct potentiometry). Results from diluted samples are reported in units of "concentration" of an ion, whereas those from undiluted samples are reported as "activities" of that ion.[1] Although this distinction may seem arcane, it becomes important when interpreting results (see Activity versus Concentration).

The prototype of the ISE is the pH electrode. It consists of a calomel reference electrode and a measuring electrode containing a solution of 0.1 N hydrogen chloride (HCl) that is separated from the sample by a thin membrane made of glass composed of oxides of sodium, silicon, and calcium. This glass membrane is selective for hydrogen ions. When the electrode is placed into a sample, a potential develops across the membrane. Hydrogen ions in the sample cause the oxides on the outer surface of the glass to become charged. Similarly, the HCl in contact with the inner surface of the membrane induces a charge in the oxides on that surface. An electrical potential develops across the glass membrane that is proportional to the number of hydrogen ions in the sample. The potential that develops between the reference and measuring electrodes is converted to pH units. All other ISEs work by essentially the same principle.[1]

ISEs have been developed to measure Na^+, K^+, Ca^{2+}, F^-, Cl^-, and others. All are potentiometric sensors. The keys to the function of these various electrodes are the membranes that make each electrode selective for only the ion being measured. Like the pH electrode, the membrane in the sodium electrode is made of glass. The glass is composed of a mixture of oxides of silicon, sodium, and aluminum that is selective for sodium.

The membrane in widespread use for determining potassium consists of a collodion sheet impregnated with valinomycin, a cyclic antibiotic that is a highly selective binder of potassium ions.[7] The selectivity results in part from the conformation of the valinomycin molecule, the central cavity of which is about the size of the potassium ion. Glass electrodes have been developed to measure potassium, but they have proved to be less selective for the ion.[7]

A membrane composed of a liquid ion exchanger was developed in 1967 for the detection of ionized (or free) calcium.[8] The membrane contains the calcium salt of a disubstituted phosphoric acid. When the electrode and its reference half-cell come into contact with a sample, an electrical potential proportional to the concentration of ionized calcium in the sample develops across the membrane. Ionized calcium may be measured in serum, plasma, or whole blood. When whole blood is assayed, erythrocytes may alter the liquid junction potential of the reference electrode, resulting in artifactual increases in calcium activities (and sodium and potassium, to a lesser extent). This problem has been eliminated by substituting sodium formate for potassium chloride in the salt bridge of the electrode.[9]

In practice, these membranes are not absolutely selective. Sodium electrodes in common use are a thousand times more selective for sodium than for potassium. Potassium electrodes have about ten thousand times more affinity for potassium than for sodium.[6] The calcium electrode is capable of measuring free calcium in solutions containing a 1000-fold greater concentration of sodium or potassium ions.[9] Thus, at clinical concentrations of these ions, interference is unlikely. Clinically important details regarding interference with the output of electrodes will be discussed in the sections dealing with specific ions.

ACTIVITY VERSUS CONCENTRATION

Most assay methods, including flame photometry and indirect potentiometry, determine the "concentration" of the total amount of ion in plasma or serum. In contrast, direct potentiometry measures only the concentration of the free unbound ion in plasma water, a value more accurately termed "activity". Activity refers to the amount of ion that is physiologically active rather than to the total amount of ion (see Osmolality). It must be stressed that activities are determined in plasma water rather than in the entire plasma volume. This is an important distinction when considering the significance of reported values, because physiologic control mechanisms regulate the concentrations of ions in the water phase rather than in the entire plasma volume.[10] Even though ISEs respond to activity rather than to concentration, results are usually reported in units of concentration. Activity is related to concentration by the following formula:

$$A = \gamma c$$

where A = activity, γ = the activity coefficient, and c = the concentration of the ion.[11]

The difference between activity and concentration becomes important in certain diseases, such as hyperlipidemia and hyperproteinemia. In these diseases, lipids or proteins displace water from the portion of the plasma that they occupy and will similarly displace all material dissolved in the water phase. Thus, the volume occupied by ions is significantly smaller than the total volume of the plasma. An example of this phenomenon is the pseudohyponatremia associated with hyperlipidemia. It is an artifactual occurrence solely dependent on the method used to measure sodium. Assays requiring dilution of the sample, such as flame photometry and indirect potentiometry, are inaccurate when used to assay sodium in lipemic serum, because the differences between activity and concentration diminish if the sample is diluted prior to assay.[10, 12] With lipemic serum, either of these methods produces results that may be as much as 15–25 mmol/L lower than the physiologically correct value as determined by direct potentiometry, which does not involve dilution of the sample.[12] Values determined by indirect potentiometry in hyperlipemic plasma may also be incorrect.[12] Perfluorocarbon emulsions, used experimentally as blood substitutes, also displace water in plasma. As expected, these compounds have a similar effect on laboratory values.[13]

SAMPLE HANDLING

Laboratory results sometimes are changed significantly by improper methods of sample collection and transportation. Details that may seem insignificant have the potential to alter results enough to modify clinical decisions. The specific factors that are relevant to individual analytes will be discussed in the sections on these compounds. This section covers some of the general aspects of sample handling that affect results but that may be overlooked, especially during the intensive management of critically ill patients.[1, 3]

SAMPLE COLLECTION

Variability

Arterial or venous blood samples obtained in the operating room or intensive care unit are usually anticoagulated with heparin and sent to the acute laboratory in a syringe immediately after collection. Results from these specimens may not be identical to those determined in a central laboratory on samples sent from the ward. A variety of things may unknowingly cause differences between routine and stat samples, leading to confusion or misinterpretation. Some of the more common factors affecting the routine samples are discussed in the following sections.

Position

Changes in body position alter the concentrations of many blood constituents. It is widely recommended that patients be seated or supine for at least 15 minutes prior to phlebotomy. The increase in hydrostatic pressure from standing causes significant shifts of the filterable components of blood into cells, resulting in hemoconcentration and a decrease in plasma volume from 12% in healthy individuals to as much as 30% in those who are ill.[14] Standing increases serum potassium, calcium, total protein, albumin, and some enzyme activities when compared to the supine position.[15] The Scandinavian Committee on Reference Values suggests that persons at bed rest and ambulatory individuals who have been seated for 15 minutes represent different reference populations[16] (see Reference Values versus Normal Values). Thus, patient position during phlebotomy for preoperative laboratory values affects the reported results.

Venipuncture

The technique of venipuncture used by the phlebotomist may alter test values. Tourniquets cause venous stasis, resulting in increased protein concentration, concomitantly increased protein-bound constituents, release of certain intracellular chemicals, and decreased pH as lactate accumulates.[1] If the fist is pumped during phlebotomy, increases in plasma potassium of more than 1 mmol/L have been observed,[17] and further increases in lactate are likely. The decrease in pH increases the concentration of ionized calcium.[18] Some authors, however, have reported that a tourniquet decreases[15] or has no effect on the concentration of serum potassium.[19]

Vacuum Tubes

Both vacuum tubes that aspirate blood through a needle and vigorous manual aspiration may artificially increase the plasma concentration of intracellular constituents by causing hemolysis.[1, 20] An erroneous increase in potassium concentration is the most common result of hemolysis seen in the acute laboratory (see Potassium). The activities of many enzymes, including lactate dehydrogenase, aspartate aminotransferase, acid phosphatase, creatine kinase, and alanine aminotransferase, are fallaciously increased if hemolysis is present.[20] In contrast, hemolysis has no effect on observed concentrations of albumin, total protein, calcium, chloride, creatinine, glucose, sodium, urea, and many other constituents.[21]

Tube Filling Order. The order in which tubes are filled should be indicated, because it may affect certain constituents. The notable effect is on potassium, the concentration of which is slightly higher (0.1 mmol/L) in the initial few milliliters of blood removed during phlebotomy.[20]

Tube Composition. Glass tubes made of soda lime release trace elements, such as magnesium and calcium, into the sample and may spuriously increase the observed values. Tubes composed of borosilicate do not have this effect.[1]

Anticoagulant

Commercially prepared tubes containing known quantities of specific anticoagulants are commonly used if whole blood or plasma is required for testing. The anticoagulant in the tube is indicated by the color of the stopper (Table 28–1).[1] By convention, tubes with either red or yellow tops contain no anticoagulant and are thus used to collect serum after the blood has been allowed to clot. The values for certain analytes, including calcium, glucose, inorganic phosphorus, potassium, and total protein, vary considerably between serum and plasma. Occasionally, the differences are great enough to influence clinical decisions (see also Potassium). Therefore, it is important to consider which anticoagulant has been used when interpreting results.[22]

Heparin is the most common anticoagulant in specimens

TABLE 28–1. CODING OF STOPPER COLOR

Color	Additive	Use
Gray	Oxalate, fluoride and iodoacetate	To inhibit glycolysis in plasma or whole blood
Yellow	None	Interior of tube sterile
Green	Heparin	Plasma or whole blood
Red	None	Serum
Blue	Citrate	Plasma or whole blood
Lavender	EDTA	Plasma or whole blood

Modified from Young DS, Bermes EW Jr: Specimen collection and processing: Sources of biological variation. *In* Tietz NW (ed): Textbook of Clinical Chemistry. Philadelphia: WB Saunders, 1986; 482.

assayed in the acute laboratory. It is an acidic heterogeneous polymer of D-glucuronic acid and D-glucosamine containing sulfuric acid ester groups. Heparin readily forms salts and is commonly supplied as the sodium salt, although preparations containing lithium or other cations are also available. Heparin is prepared commercially from bovine lung and porcine intestinal mucosa. It functions immediately by neutralizing several activated clotting factors.[23]

Final concentrations of heparin needed to anticoagulate samples of blood are said to be 1 U of heparin/ml of sample,[23] 2 U/ml,[1] and 20 U/ml.[1] The dead space volume of a 3-ml disposable syringe is about 60 μl.[24] Commercially prepared heparin is usually supplied in a concentration of 1000 U/ml. If a 3-ml syringe, the dead space of which contains heparin, is filled completely with blood, the concentration of heparin in the blood will be approximately 15 U of heparin/ml of blood. For most assays, this concentration should have minimal effect on laboratory results. However, heparin may alter certain values if more than the recommended amount is added to the sample. For example, 10–50 U of sodium heparin/ml of blood increases the observed value for sodium by 0.5–2 mmol/L.[1, 25] In contrast to these small changes, heparin significantly decreases the observed values for ionized calcium (see Calcium).

Although anticoagulants other than heparin are not normally used for perioperative chemical analyses, they are frequently used for routine analyses (Table 28–1). If an improper anticoagulant is used, results may be significantly altered. Fluoride, a preservative for glucose, is a potent inhibitor of many enzymes. Ethylenediaminetetra-acetic acid (EDTA) interferes with methods used to determine chloride. Both citrate and EDTA, used in coagulation and hematologic studies, decrease calcium activities by chelation. Oxalates also bind calcium. Iodoacetate inhibits creatine kinase.[1, 3]

Sampling from Catheters and Tubing

Most samples are obtained intraoperatively from indwelling catheters. For results of these assays to be correct, the samples must be drawn properly. A volume nearly that of the tubing must be withdrawn from an arterial catheter before blood-tinged fluid appears, and accurate results can be assured only after withdrawing six times the volume of the tubing.[26] Similar recommendations hold true for samples drawn from central venous catheters.[27] Dilutions of the sample by the flush solution in the line will alter results significantly and must be avoided.

Risk of Infection

Any biologic sample may contain pathogens responsible for occupationally acquired diseases. Human immunodeficiency virus type 1 (HIV-1), the etiologic agent in acquired immunodeficiency syndrome (AIDS), is a frequent topic of discussion, debate, and controversy among many specialties, including anesthesiology.[28–31] The several types of hepatitis are far more common occupationally incurred illnesses and are also of concern.

HIV-1 may be transmitted by parenteral inoculation, with likelihood of transmission usually being related to the volume of the inoculum. Although transfusion of blood containing HIV-1 carries a high risk, a small inoculum, such as that from a needle stick (the volume of which is less than 2 μl)[32] is associated with a low incidence of transmission of the virus. However, at least one case may have resulted from merely compressing a puncture site following an unsuccessful attempt to cannulate a radial artery.[33] The minimum dose required to infect humans is unknown. The reported incidence of HIV-1 infection in health care workers having a history of percutaneous contact with the virus is 0.3% per exposure (95% Cl 0.13 to 0.70%).[34] The most common preventable exposures are from needle sticks during attempts to recap needles and from improperly discarded objects. Nearly 10% of the exposures occur in laboratories.[35]

The overall incidence of AIDS in health care workers is nearly identical to that in the general population. In both groups, the disease is common only in those individuals who have exhibited high-risk behavior.[36] In contrast to AIDS, the likelihood of health care workers developing hepatitis from contact with infected patients or specimens is much higher. The incidence of seropositivity following parenteral inoculation with hepatitis B ranges from 19% to 27%. The risk of infection strongly correlates with the extent of blood contact and the frequency of needle accidents.[37]

Because every patient may be infected with communicable pathogens, not all of which can be identified preoperatively, the Centers for Disease Control have recommended that all patients be treated as if they are infective.[36] Similarly, all laboratory specimens should be considered infective. Gloves should be worn while obtaining and processing samples. Needles should be handled with extreme caution and should not be recapped. Containers should be sturdy and covered in order to prevent leakage during transport. Blood that is discarded following analysis should be either incinerated or poured into a sanitary sewer. Warning labels are not needed if all specimens are treated with the same precautions. The Occupational Safety and Health Administration (OSHA) has made employers responsible for developing enforcible plans for exposure control.[38]

Transportation of Samples

Transportation may adversely affect laboratory results. Factors such as cellular metabolism[39] and pH changes[18] may occur during delays in forwarding samples. It is critically important that certain specimens be kept on ice, especially if there are delays between collection and analysis. Pneumatic transport systems may subject samples to harmful vibration and forces of acceleration if they are rapidly propelled. Cells may rupture during transport and release intracellular contents, especially if specimen containers are inadequately cushioned or are only partially filled with blood. Although most tube systems can transport samples safely, such systems should be evaluated before they are used for this purpose.[40] Messengers need to be aware of the critical importance of their role in providing rapid, safe transport of hand-carried samples.

SPECIFIC ANALYTES

The following sections discuss specific analytes (the sample being analyzed) commonly measured in the acute laboratory, with emphasis on factors that may affect results. Although each section contains brief discussions of the physiologic role of each analyte, the reader should refer to other texts for more extensive discussions of these functions.

GLUCOSE

Specimen Collection

Both arterial and venous blood may be obtained in the perioperative period, but for many analytes, including glucose, the results from these two sources are not strictly comparable. Arterial and capillary blood may contain significantly higher concentrations of glucose than does venous blood.[41, 42] There is little difference between arterial and venous values in fasting patients. However, during infusion of solutions containing glucose, arterial values may be as much as 70 mg/dl greater than venous values in samples drawn simultaneously.[43]

Precautions must be taken to prevent glycolysis by the cellular components of blood after a sample has been obtained. In the absence of a metabolic inhibitor, blood with normal hematologic values undergoes a decrease in glucose concentration of about 10 mg/dl (0.56 mmol/L) of blood per hour when stored at 25°C.[1] Erythrocytes at 37°C will metabolize glucose at a rate of up to 18 mg/dl (1 mmol/L) of blood per hour,[44] whereas leukocytes metabolize about half this amount over the same period.[45] Leukocytosis may decrease the concentration of glucose as much as 65 mg/dl over 1–2 hours if no glycolytic agent has been added to the sample.[46] The most effective antiglycolytic agents are fluoride and iodoacetate (gray-colored stopper). Samples that are analyzed immediately after having been drawn need not contain these agents. The clinician must be aware, however, that results may be affected significantly if processing is delayed.[39]

Methods of Analysis

Glucose is usually measured in plasma or serum rather than in whole blood. It is also measured in urine as a screening test for diabetes and also to guide perioperative glucose control in diabetic patients. Values for glucose in whole blood are about 10% lower than in plasma. The explanation is as follows, and is similar to that for pseudohyponatremia (see Activity versus Concentration). Glucose is limited to the water phase of blood. Its concentration in the aqueous phases of both red cells and plasma is identical.[47] However, erythrocytes contain 20% less water than an equivalent volume of plasma. Thus, there is less glucose per unit volume of red cells, because the portion of the red cell that is nonaqueous excludes glucose. Consequently, a given volume of blood contains less glucose than does the same volume of plasma.

Immobilized enzymes are used as reagents in the assay of glucose. The enzyme glucose oxidase is immobilized or bonded to an adsorbent such as cellulose or agarose. It then participates in, but is not consumed by, the following chemical reaction:

$$\text{glucose} + O_2 \xrightarrow{\text{glucose oxidase}} \text{gluconic acid} + H_2O_2$$

The change in oxygen concentration with respect to time as measured with a Clark oxygen electrode reflects the glucose concentration in the sample. Because the Clark oxygen electrode is used to detect the disappearance of oxygen, some mention of its operation is warranted before discussing the use of immobilized enzymes in the assay for glucose.

The Clark method for detecting oxygen is an amperometric, or current-measuring, assay. In amperometric assays, a constant voltage is applied to two electrodes in an electrochemical cell. The analyte, which must be capable of being oxidized or reduced, is brought into contact with the cell. It is ionized by the voltage, and a current proportional to the analyte's concentration flows through the cell. The current is measured and displayed as the concentration of the analyte in question. The Clark electrode works by this principle. It consists of a platinum cathode maintained at a potential of -0.65 V and a silver–silver chloride anode in phosphate buffer containing potassium chloride. The electrode is separated from the solution being tested by a membrane permeable to oxygen. Oxygen diffuses across the membrane and is reduced at the cathode, and current proportional to the amount of oxygen in the sample flows through the electrode.[48]

A multitude of time-consuming, complex methods have been developed for assaying glucose.[6] Rapid methods such as the amperometric glucose oxidase method are used in acute laboratories. The glucose analyzer contains a membrane to which glucose oxidase has been bound (Fig. 28–2). The catalytic ability of the enzyme is not altered by the membrane. The enzyme may be used for multiple assays and is stable for months.[49] As with all assays involving enzymes, temperature and other reaction conditions must be painstakingly controlled.

To perform the assay, the operator injects a precisely measured sample into the analyzer. It is assumed that all of the glucose in the sample is oxidized to gluconic acid. The P_{O_2} in the reaction mixture is continuously measured by a Clark oxygen electrode as the reaction proceeds. The

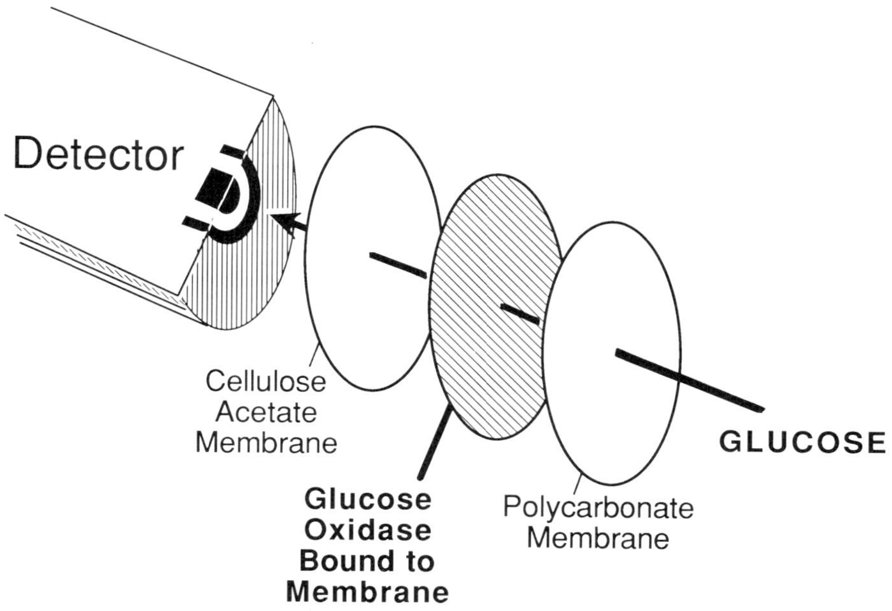

Figure 28–2. Diagram of a glucose analyzer that employs immobilized enzyme. Glucose oxidase is bound to the membrane in the center. Depending on the specific analyzer, the amperometric detector, shown on the left, measures either the decrease in oxygen or the increase in hydrogen peroxide produced during the conversion of glucose to gluconic acid. A similar method may be used to assay lactate, by substituting lactate oxidase for glucose oxidase, and measuring hydrogen peroxide. (Modified from Clark LC Jr, Noyes LK, Grooms TA, Moore MS: Rapid micromeasurement of lactate in whole blood. Crit Care Med 12[5]:461–464, © by Williams & Wilkins, 1984.)

amount of oxygen consumed during the reaction, which is proportional to the concentration of glucose in the sample, is recorded by an electronic circuit. Results are displayed as the concentration of glucose in the sample and are available within 20 seconds.[50] Similar amperometric methods for glucose have been developed to measure the appearance of hydrogen peroxide rather than the disappearance of oxygen.[51]

The glucose oxidase method is also used for urinary or blood glucose determinations. Reagents are impregnated into filter paper, making a convenient paper strip for urine testing. Values for glucose determined in capillary blood obtained by cutaneous puncture accurately reflect those from a clinical laboratory.[52]

Reference Ranges

To some extent, reference ranges for glucose depend on the assay method. They also are influenced by the techniques of the individual laboratory. For the glucose oxidase-oxygen rate method, the range is 65–110 mg/dl.[6] Normally, glucose is absent in the urine until the plasma levels exceed 150–300 mg/dl. This variability results from variation in the rate of delivery of glucose to the proximal tubule and tubular reabsorption efficiency. See Presentation of Results for a discussion of the differences between reference ranges and normal values.

Sources of Inaccuracy

Results of glucose assays are affected by the source of the sample (arterial or venous) and the duration between collection and analysis if inhibitors of glycolysis have not been added to the sample. Results may also be influenced by drugs that a patient is taking preoperatively. Acetylsalicylic acid and indomethacin increase, caffeine has a variable effect on, and ibuprofen has no effect on apparent values for glucose when assayed by a variety of methods.[53] Ascorbic acid at high therapeutic levels decreases glucose slightly.[54] None of these changes are major. In contrast, acetaminophen, which has become a drug of abuse, significantly interferes with the amperometric-H_2O_2 method of glucose analysis when large amounts of the drug are ingested. Thus, glucose values are falsely elevated after ingestion of large quantities of acetaminophen.[55]

Physiologic Role

Glucose is an essential source of energy. It is the primary substrate for the phosphorylation of adenosine to adenosine triphosphate. It is converted to glycogen for storage in the liver and may also be converted to fat. It may be formed from sources other than carbohydrates by gluconeogenesis. Its concentration in blood is regulated by insulin, which enhances the transfer of glucose into cells, and by several other hormones, including glucagon, epinephrine, and cortisol, which increase its concentration. Glucose is an absolute requirement for proper function of the central nervous system, which cannot store glucose.[1]

LACTATE

Specimen Collection

Lactate concentrations were measured during anesthesia well before the development of rapid measurement techniques.[56] The significance of isolated lactate analyses in anesthetized patients was questioned decades ago, but the ratio of lactate to pyruvate (L/P ratio) was felt to be a marker of oxygenation in these patients, and thus of some importance.[57] Later work demonstrated that the L/P ratio is not always an accurate indicator of oxygenation at the cellular level.[58] Although changes in lactate concentration occur in the anesthetized patient, the perioperative utility of the information is still somewhat unclear, especially if examined without regard to other physiologic and biochemical data.[59]

Method of Analysis

An analyzer has been developed that measures lactate in less than 1 minute in either whole blood or plasma.[60] The method is identical in principle to the amperometric-H_2O_2 technique for glucose. Immobilized lactic oxidase catalyzes the following reaction:

$$\text{lactate} + O_2 \xrightarrow{\text{lactic oxidase}} \text{pyruvate} + H_2O_2$$

Hydrogen peroxide is detected amperometrically. The rapidity of the method makes it suitable for both acute and research laboratories.

Reference Ranges

Normal arterial blood lactate concentrations are 9.7–16.3 mg/100 ml at rest. Lactate concentrations increase with physical exercise.

The clinical significance of these measurements in the physiologic role perioperative period continues to be investigated. Plasma lactate levels have been measured in conjunction with other tests during hepatic transplantation. In one report, lactate increased at a rate of 2.6 mmol/L/hour prior to hepatectomy in 12 recipients. Lactate increased less rapidly during the anhepatic phase but increased acutely and then decreased when the allograft was perfused after vascular anastomosis. The magnitude of the decrease in plasma lactate concentrations after reperfusion may predict subsequent hepatic function.[61]

OSMOMETRY

Biologic fluids contain dissolved particles of widely differing sizes, ranging from ions such as hydrogen, sodium, and chloride to proteins. Semipermeable membranes permit some small particles to cross while inhibiting the passage of others. The particles are distributed across cell membranes in part by osmosis, a measurable phenomenon. Because water freely crosses biologic membranes, there is osmotic equilibrium throughout the body.

Osmometry is the measurement of the concentration of solute particles in a solvent such as water, without regard to the identity of the particles. It is based on the measurement of any one of four related physical properties, also known as colligative properties, that are common to all solutions containing particles. These properties are osmotic pressure, boiling point, vapor pressure, and freezing point. Changes in these variables are related to the collective concentrations of all of the particles in solution. The first two increase and the latter two decrease as the solute concentration is increased.

Osmosis refers to the flow of water across a semipermeable membrane. The direction in which water travels is governed by the difference in concentrations of the solutions on the two sides of the membrane. Generally, the flow of water is toward the side containing the greater number of solute particles. That is, water flows down its concentration gradient. An example of osmosis is the swelling and lysis of red cells when placed in distilled water.

Osmotic pressure is strictly defined as the hydrostatic pressure required to prevent changes in volume when solutions containing solutes of differing concentrations are separated by a semipermeable membrane. The contribution of small molecules is determined by measuring the osmolality of a solution. The effect of large molecules is assessed by measuring colloid osmotic pressure.[1, 6]

OSMOLALITY

The molarity of a solution is the number of moles of a compound per liter of water. Molality is the number of moles per kilogram of water. Concentrations are usually reported in moles per liter—that is, with respect to the *volume* of water rather than to its mass. In contrast, molality is applied to osmometry because the calculations are simpler with respect to mass than to volume.

Osmolality is the number of moles of particles per kilogram of water. It is directly related to the molal concentration of all of the solutes in a liquid. If a solution contains only noncharged particles, the numeric values for molality and osmolality are identical. Solutions of salts composed of monovalent ions, such as sodium chloride, yield two moles of particles/mole of salt (assuming complete dissociation), making the osmolality twice the molality. Calcium chloride dissociates into three particles, so its osmolality is three times its molality. Actually, most salts are not completely dissociated in solution. For example, sodium chloride is only about 93% dissociated in physiologic solutions, making its actual osmolality only 1.86 times its molality. The true osmolality is equal to the molal "activity" of the compound, which reflects the biologically effective concentration of the ions in solution (see Activity versus Concentration).[6]

Specimen Collection

Osmolality may be measured in either serum or plasma. If plasma is analyzed, heparin is the appropriate anticoagulant, because others increase the observed osmolality.[62]

Method of Analysis

Osmolality is determined by measuring any of the four colligative properties of solutions. In practice, only decreases in freezing point and vapor pressure are used routinely. Freezing point depression is most commonly used because of its ease and relative simplicity. The change in freezing point is directly related to the number of particles in a solution. This principle is used ''therapeutically'' by road maintenance engineers to melt ice and snow by increasing the osmolality of the precipitate and thus decreasing its freezing point. Each mole of particles added to pure water lowers the freezing point of the solution by 1.858°C. The freezing point of a solution containing 285 mOsm/L is thus −0.53°C.

By definition, the freezing point of liquid is the temperature at which the liquid and crystalline phases of a substance are in equilibrium. It is this temperature that is determined by a freezing point osmometer (Fig. 28–3). In practice, a small sample, typically 25–250 μl, is injected into the osmometer. The sample is first supercooled to −5°C to −7°C, a temperature well below its freezing point. Crystallization is then induced by vigorous stirring. As freezing proceeds, the heat of fusion released by the developing ice crystals warms the sample. After rapid freezing has stopped, an equilibrium temperature is attained between crystals and liquid. This plateau temperature is measured with a thermistor and is reported as the osmolal concentration of the sample.[1, 6]

Sources of Inaccuracy

Changes in vapor pressure also reflect the osmolality of a solution. The vapor pressure, or dew point, of an aqueous solution at 25°C is decreased by 0.3 mmHg/mole of particles. The vapor pressure osmometer measures the dew point temperature of a sample and converts the observed decrease into milliosmoles per liter. The volume sampled is less than 10 μl, making the technique useful in pediatrics.[1, 6] Drawbacks of the method include the inability to detect volatile solutes that contribute to the osmolality of plasma, such as ethanol and other compounds of interest in acute poisoning.[63] It also gives erroneously high readings with lipemic sera.[64]

Reference Range

The normal osmolality of blood is 300 mOsm/kg with a range of 278–305 mOsm/kg. Urinary osmolality varies from 40 to 1350 mOsm/kg.

Physiologic Role

Serum osmolality alone does not permit an accurate assessment of the state of hydration. Evaluation of osmolality is important primarily to determine major deviations in serum water content and to screen for exogenous substances such as alcohol.[65] To do either, the observed and calculated osmolalities must be compared. The primary solutes contributing to the osmolality of serum are sodium, glucose, and blood urea nitrogen (BUN). Several empirical equations, each utilizing the observed values for these analytes, have been proposed for use in calculating serum osmolality.[65–67] One of these follows:

$$\text{Calculated osmolality} = 2 \times \text{sodium} + \text{glucose}/18 + \text{BUN}/2.8$$

where sodium is in mEq/L, and glucose and BUN are in mg/dl.[65] Differences between observed and calculated values, referred to as the osmolal gap, result primarily from decreased serum water content, as in hyperlipidemia and hyperproteinemia, or in the presence of low-molecular-weight substances such as ethanol, mannitol, and toxins. An osmolal gap of greater than 10 mOsm/kg suggests that one or more of these compounds is present.[65] Glycine may also contribute to the osmolal gap during transurethral resection of the prostate. Urine osmolality of greater than 600 mOsm/L demonstrates that the kidney is able to concentrate urine. Lower values are nondiagnostic.[6]

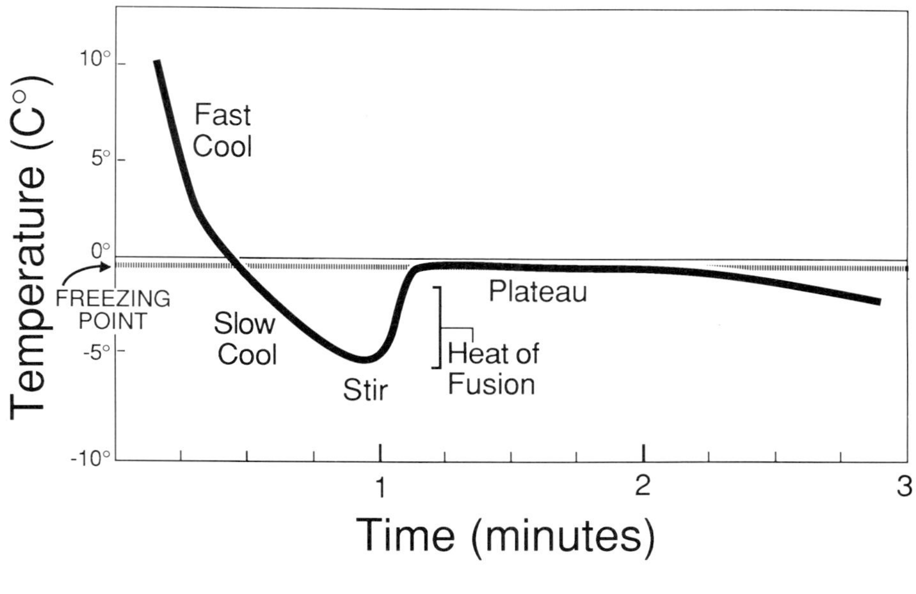

Figure 28–3. Temperature changes in a freezing point osmometer. (See text for details.)

COLLOID OSMOTIC PRESSURE

Specimen Collection

Colloid osmotic pressure (COP, or oncotic pressure) is osmotic pressure produced by large molecules in solution. In plasma, it is generated primarily by albumin and to a lesser extent by globulins. Owing to their large molecular weights (30,000 daltons and more), proteins have small molal concentrations in plasma. These macromolecules contribute less than 2 mOsm/kg of water to the osmolality of plasma as determined by freezing point depression.

Methods of Analysis

COP may be calculated if the concentrations of plasma proteins are known, although the calculated values are inaccurate in patients receiving intravenous colloid solutions and in critically ill patients.[30, 31]

COP is measured with a colloid osmometer. This device consists of a chamber divided into two compartments by a membrane permeable to molecules smaller than 30,000 daltons. The membrane separates the sample from physiologic saline, which is in contact with a pressure transducer. When serum or plasma from either arterial or central venous blood is injected into the osmometer, saline crosses the membrane by osmosis and enters the sample. After equilibrium has been reached, the pressure in the saline compartment will have decreased by a value equal to the COP of the sample.[68] This value is presented on a digital display in millimeters of mercury.

Reference Range

COP in normal human plasma averages about 25 mmHg. It decreases with age and bed rest, and is lower in females.

Sources of Inaccuracy

Peripheral venous blood should not be used for analysis, because stasis induced by a tourniquet will drive intravascular water into tissues and artifactually increase the COP in the sample.[68] Dextran will increase COP significantly in plasma, because it develops pressure that is several times greater than that of equimolar solutions of proteins.[1]

Physiologic Role

COP, in combination with pulmonary capillary wedge pressure, is felt by some to be clinically important in the diagnosis and treatment of pulmonary edema caused by left ventricular failure[66] (see Chapter 8). The gradient between COP and wedge pressure is normally about 10 mmHg. In patients with pulmonary edema, it is significantly lower.[69] Other authors question the clinical utility of the measurement, especially in patients with chronic hypoproteinemia.[70]

SODIUM

Specimen Collection

Sodium may be determined in whole blood, serum, or plasma. Hemolysis, unless severe, has little effect on determined values for sodium because its concentration in red cells is only 10% of its plasma concentration. Sodium values are minimally affected by venous stasis, time of sampling, postural changes, prolonged bed rest, eating, and exercise. Values will be increased by 1–20 mmol/L if sodium heparin is used to anticoagulate the sample.[3, 25]

Method of Analysis

Sodium is most commonly determined with an ISE. Flame photometry may also be used, but the risk of explosion makes this method less attractive.[1]

Reference Range

The reference range for serum sodium is 136–146 mmol/L. It is applicable from infancy through old age.[1]

Sources of Inaccuracy

Spuriously low values for sodium result when the analyte is assayed by flame photometry or indirect potentiometry in sera from patients with hyperlipidemia or hyperproteinemia[12] (see Activity versus Concentration).

Physiologic Role

Sodium is the major cation in extracellular water. Dietary intake and renal excretion of sodium are equal in the absence of pathology. Because sodium salts make up more than 90% of the solutes in plasma, they are responsible for most of its osmolality. The volume of the extracellular fluid is directly related to the quantity of sodium in the fluid. It is closely regulated by renal mechanisms involving the renin-angiotensin-aldosterone system and other hormones.[71]

Plasma sodium concentrations in the perioperative period are measured routinely. Some authors, however, believe that plasma sodium measurements are unhelpful except to diagnose such things as primary aldosteronism and to determine causes of the alteration in neurologic state seen with acute water overload. The decrease in sodium commonly seen postoperatively usually results from water overload rather than from lack of sodium, especially because the stress of surgery causes secretion of antidiuretic hormone. At times, the results are misinterpreted. For example, unless results are evaluated in conjunction with serum osmolality, the differentiation of postoperative fluid overload from sodium loss cannot be made with certainty.[72]

POTASSIUM

Specimen Collection

Because the intracellular concentration of potassium is nearly 40 times greater than its plasma concentration, and its concentration in red blood cells is 25 times greater than in plasma, great care must be exercised during phlebotomy and subsequent analysis to avoid contaminating the sample with potassium of cellular origin (see Sources of Inaccuracy). Preferably, an anticoagulant should be added when the sample is obtained.[3, 73]

Method of Analysis

In the acute laboratory, potassium is usually assayed with an ISE. This method is rapid and accurate and avoids the dangers imposed by flame photometers (see Assay Methods).

Reference Range

The reference range for potassium is 3.5–5.0 mmol/L.

Sources of Inaccuracy

Determined concentrations for potassium vary greatly between serum and plasma. Although samples referred to the acute laboratory are usually anticoagulated, the routine samples assayed in a central laboratory frequently are not. This may result in confusion if results from different laboratories are compared. The average concentration in serum is 0.4 mmol/L higher than in plasma, but the range is quite wide: −0.6 to +1.4 mmol/L.[22, 51, 73] Similar differences have been observed between venous serum and arterial plasma (Fig. 28–4), the latter values being comparable to those in venous plasma.[74] These differences result from the release of potassium from platelets during clotting. Although there is a positive correlation between higher platelet counts and increases in serum versus plasma potassium in the same patient, there is such great variability between patients that prediction of the quantitative effect of thrombocytosis on potassium is impossible.[75] Potassium may also be released from white blood cells during the process of clotting, although this source is only important with extreme leukocytosis.[76]

Potassium values are increased by hemolysis because of the great disparity between its intracellular and extracellular concentrations. A hemoglobin concentration of at least 20 mg/dl is required for visual recognition of hemolysis.[1] Plasma potassium increases linearly with increases in free hemoglobin (Fig. 28–5). Eighty mg/dl of free hemoglobin, a concentration easily detected by inspection, increases potassium concentrations by only 1.04 times when assayed by either flame photometry or ISE. In contrast, 660 mg/dl produces a 1.4-fold increase.[21] Thus, although hemolysis causes significant increases in the observed concentrations of potassium, the visual threshold for detecting free hemoglobin in serum or plasma corresponds to only a slight increase in potassium.

If an anticoagulated sample of blood is not analyzed rapidly, the plasma should be removed from the cellular components, because glucose metabolism by the cells has been shown to affect the concentration of potassium. Potassium in plasma is very stable after the cells have been removed.[3]

Physiologic Roles

Potassium, whose concentration in cells approximates 150 mmol/L, is the predominant intracellular cation. About

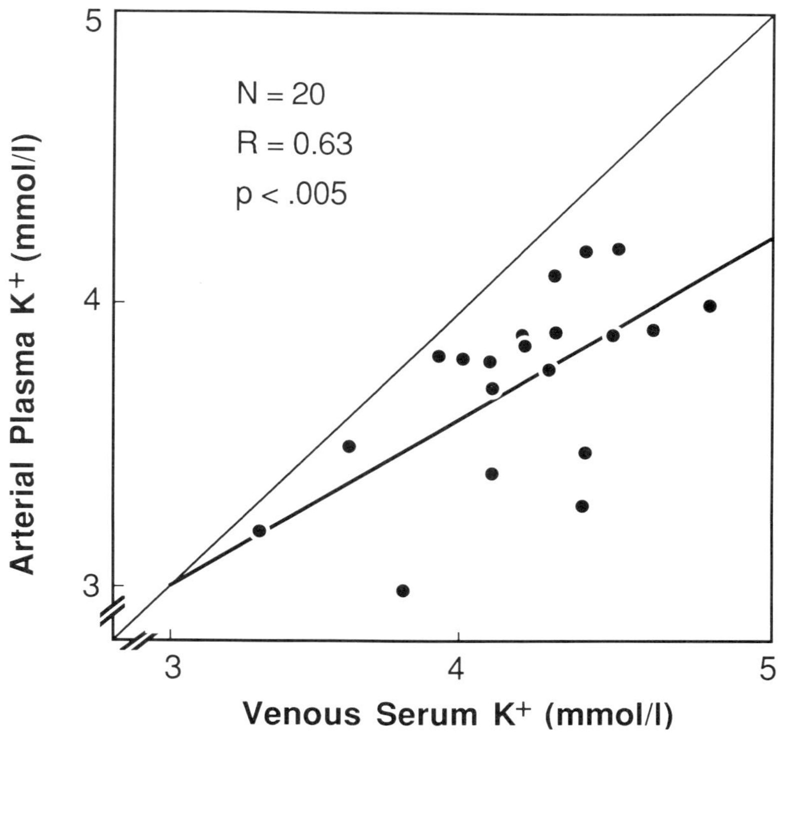

Figure 28–4. Arterial plasma versus venous serum potassium. The dotted line running from the lower left corner to the upper right corner represents the line of identity. All venous values are below the line. (Modified from Ward CF, Arkin DB, Benumof J, Saidman LJ: Arterial versus venous potassium: Clinical implications. Crit Care Med 6[5]:335–336, © by Williams & Wilkins, 1978.)

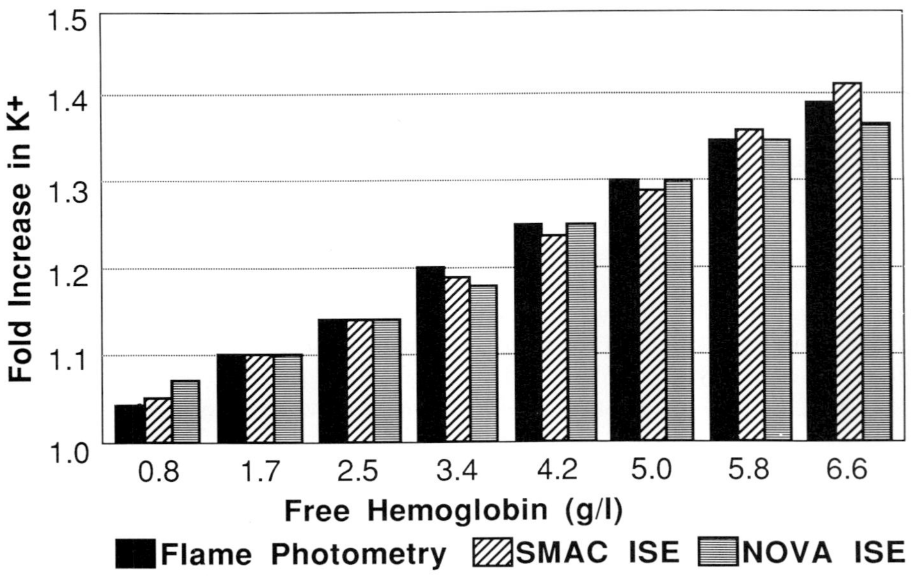

Figure 28–5. Effect of hemolysis on potassium. Free hemoglobin was obtained by freeze-fracturing red cells from the sample prior to assay. Results were determined on the sample by flame photometry and indirect and direct potentiometry (SMAC [Technicon] and NOVA I [Nova] ion-selective electrodes, respectively). Significant increases do not occur below the visual threshold for hemolysis. (Data from Sonntag O: Haemolysis as an interference factor in clinical chemistry. J Clin Chem Clin Biochem 1986; 24:127–139.)

98% of the roughly 3500 mmol of potassium found in the hypothetic 70-kg person is intracellular. In contrast, its concentration in extracellular fluid ranges from 3.5 to 5 mmol/L in healthy individuals. Maintenance of the appropriate ratio of intracellular to extracellular potassium is essential to the proper functioning of the cardiovascular and neuromuscular systems. Alterations in the delicate internal harmony may be caused by such things as metabolic acidosis and hypertonicity of body fluids (including infusion of hypertonic solutions), both of which cause hyperkalemia; catecholamines, which have a biphasic effect; and insulin, which decreases plasma potassium.[77] A major external influence on potassium homeostasis is diuretic use. In a study of over 2000 nonrandomly selected ambulatory patients older than 65 years, 40% of women and 30% of men were on at least one diuretic drug. Serum potassium concentrations were most influenced by thiazides and averaged 0.44 mmol/L lower than those of age-matched controls.[78]

CHLORIDE

Specimen Collection

Concentrations of chloride are commonly measured in serum, urine, and cerebrospinal fluid. However, chloride concentrations provide the least useful information of the four measured electrolytes. Samples should be separated from cellular constituents to prevent shifts in ionic equilibrium secondary to metabolism and pH alterations. Under aerobic conditions, loss of carbon dioxide changes the distribution of chloride between plasma and cells. However, chloride is stable for prolonged periods in plasma, serum, and other acellular fluids stored at or below room temperature.

Method of Analysis

Chloride in serum or cerebrospinal fluid is measured in an ISE, either by quantitative displacement of thiocyanate by chloride from mercuric thiocyanate with subsequent formation of a red ferric thiocyanate complex or with a semiautomated coulometric-amperometric technique. The mercuric/ferric thiocyanate method is most frequently used and is quite accurate and precise. Ion selective electrodes are being increasingly used and are also precise and accurate.

Reference Range

The normal serum chloride is 98–110 mmol/L. In the cerebrospinal fluid, the concentration is 120–132 mmol/L. Because urinary chloride varies with diet, the average chloride excretion ranges from 110–250 mmol/day. Chloride does not vary with either age or gender.

Sources of Inaccuracy

With the ferric/thiocyanate method, the chemical reaction is very temperature-sensitive, and temperature must be carefully controlled to ensure accuracy. All of the analysis methods for chloride will demonstrate positive interference from other halides.

Physiologic Role

Decreased serum chloride concentrations are present in patients with metabolic acidosis (uncontrolled diabetes), Addisonian crisis, prolonged vomiting (pyloric stenosis, nasogastric suction, or high intestinal obstruction), salt-losing nephritis, and metabolic alkalosis (increased bicarbonate causes reciprocal decreases in chloride). Chloride concentrations increase in respiratory alkalosis, renal tubular acidosis, and dehydration.

CALCIUM

Specimen Collection

One must be cautious when obtaining whole blood for calcium assay. Although heparin is the only suitable anticoagulant, it binds free calcium and produces major decreases in the reported values for ionized calcium (Fig. 28–6). The decrease is directly related to the concentration of heparin in the sample, and is reported to range from 0.002[11] to 0.01 mmol/L[79] for each unit of heparin per milliliter of sample. Some recommend that the heparin concentration should be less than 10 U/ml of blood.[24] These data suggest that if less than 2 ml of blood is added to heparin contained in the dead space of a 3-ml disposable syringe, the observed value will be significantly less than the actual calcium activity.

The observed value for ionized calcium is inversely related to the pH of the specimen. As pH increases, protein binding of free calcium also increases, thus decreasing the ionized fraction of calcium. If the sample is exposed to air or transported in a tube only partially filled with blood, its pH increases as CO_2 is lost, and reported values are artifactually low. To avoid these changes, samples should be collected anaerobically, as they are for the determination of blood gases.[1, 18, 80] Perioperative samples for analysis of ionized calcium are usually obtained from indwelling catheters, which avoids the problems induced by stasis from the use of a tourniquet (see Venipuncture).

Method of Analysis

Historically, ionized calcium was first assayed in biologic and clinical fluids in 1934 by exposing hearts from "healthy, full-blooded frogs of medium size" to the sample in question.[81] The resulting amplitude of contraction of the heart, as recorded on a smoked kymograph drum, was a function of the concentration of ionized calcium in the specimen. Unknown values were quantified by comparing the resulting contractions with those produced by reference solutions.[81]

Several instruments incorporating ISEs are now available for assaying ionized calcium. The technology has been progressively refined since the development of the first calcium electrode in 1967[8] but is still evolving as experience with the technique accumulates. For example, although whole blood rather than plasma or serum is preferred for assay,[82] erythrocytes may falsely increase the observed value for ionized calcium by up to 11%. This results from a positive voltage created by red cells at the junction between the sample and the reference electrode (see Fig. 28–1). This has been eliminated by altering the electrolyte solution in the reference electrode.[9] Values determined with instruments from different manufacturers may differ by as much as 8%, in part because of differences in electrode design. However, the reproducibility of the individual instruments is excellent.[83]

Reference Range

Reference intervals for ionized calcium in the absence of disease are 1.05–1.30 mmol/L or 4.2–5.2 mg/dl.[11] Even though clinical research on ionized calcium was first reported as long ago as 1935,[84] appropriate reference ranges for the analyte are still being disputed. In question is exactly what is being measured, the *activity* or the *concentration* of ionized calcium (see Activity versus Concentration).[85] The activity of calcium ion in the plasma of healthy individuals is about 0.38 mmol/L. Most analyzers divide the observed activity by an activity coefficient of 0.304 to give a substance concentration of about 1.25 mmol/L or 5.0 mg/dl.[85] However, certain disease states alter this activity coefficient. It is lower with severe hypernatremia and higher with hyperlipemia or hyperproteinemia, making the true substance concentration higher or lower, respectively.[85]

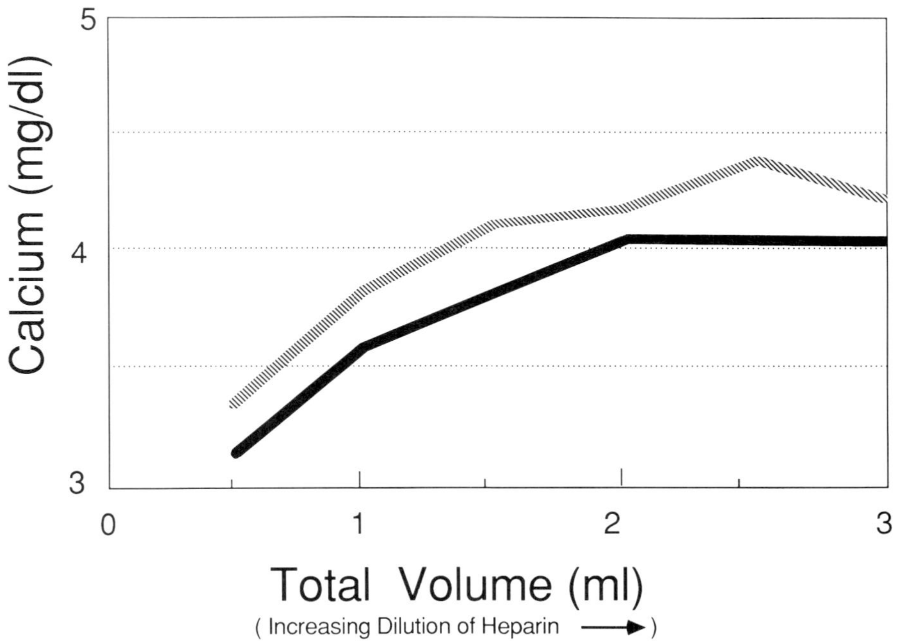

Figure 28–6. Effect of heparin on ionized calcium. Aliquots of arterial blood ranging from 0.5 to 3 ml were drawn into syringes, the dead spaces of which contained heparin (1000 units/ml of heparin). All samples were analyzed for ionized calcium with a NOVA ion-selective analyzer. The data shown are from two patients. (Protocol approved by committee.)

Sources of Inaccuracy

Inaccuracies in the reported values for ionized calcium may be caused by errors in sample collection, by transportation, by delays between collection and analysis, and by the method used for assay. Already discussed are such things as the amount of heparin in the sample, the effects of increases in pH resulting from loss of CO_2, and certain technical features. Temperature-dependent increases in ionized calcium occur with storage of heparinized whole blood. At 4°C, 20°C, and 37°C, the increases are 0.02, 0.04, and 0.08 mmol/L, respectively, over 4 hours. These changes are due to glycolysis and lactic acid formation.[18] If the concentrations of electrolytes in the specimen differ significantly from their reference ranges, the observed value for ionized calcium will be affected. At sodium concentrations of 112 and 168 mmol/L, ionized calcium will be respectively 4% less than and 4% greater than its value when the sodium concentration is normal. In contrast, potassium has no effect on the assay.[11] These effects vary in magnitude with analyses from different manufacturers.[86]

Physiologic Role

Calcium, the fifth most abundant element (and the most abundant mineral element) in the human body, is incredibly important to both anatomic structure and physiologic function. More than 99% of the 1–2 kg of calcium in the adult is in bone. The remainder is found in cells, blood, and extracellular fluid. Extraskeletal calcium is involved in a myriad of regulatory and metabolic functions. Some of these include the release of central and peripheral neurotransmitters, contraction of cardiac and skeletal muscle, secretion of hormones (including insulin, adrenocorticotropic hormone, corticosteroids, prolactin, leuteinizing hormone, oxytocin, and vasopressin), and a vital role in blood coagulation. Calcium is the major inorganic second messenger for the regulation of cellular function.

Circulating calcium accounts for less than 1% of total body calcium. It exists in three states: protein-bound (45%), ionized (45%), and complexed to small anions including citrate, phosphate, and bicarbonate (10%). The ionized or free calcium is the only fraction of physiologic importance and is responsible for calcium's regulatory effects.[1, 87] The cardiovascular effects of ionized calcium have been detailed by Drop.[88]

PROTEINS

Hematocrit

Specimen Collection

Hematocrit is determined in whole blood drawn into an anticoagulant that does not affect the size of erythrocytes.

Method of Analysis

The blood sample is centrifuged in a tube of uniform bore. After centrifugation, the hematocrit percentage is determined as the height of the red cell column in millimeters divided by the total height of the column in millimeters times 100.

Reference Range

The reference range for hematocrit in males is 41–53%, whereas in females it is 36–46% of the packed red cell volume.

Sources of Inaccuracy

A single determination is usually accurate for routine work. However, hematocrits determined in capillary tubes are often performed in duplicate. Errors arise if the sample is not centrifuged for adequate rates and times to assure complete packing of the cells. About 5% of the packed cell volume is actually trapped plasma. The hematocrit is usually more accurate than either erythrocyte count or hemoglobin.

Physiologic Role

The concentration of erythrocytes and their content of oxygen-carrying hemoglobin is one of the factors affecting tissue oxygen delivery. However, in many clinical conditions, the actual hematocrit is most useful as an indicator of whether to administer blood or crystalloid to a given patient (i.e., is the patient anemic?) rather than as a tool for timing blood administration. Acute hemorrhage causes concomitant loss of plasma and erythrocytes, so that hematocrit may remain normal although total erythrocyte mass is severely decreased. Similar problems occur with acute shifts of fluids between intravascular and extravascular space in shock or acute cardiac failure.

Myoglobin

Myoglobin is an oxygen-binding protein found in skeletal and cardiac muscle.

Specimen Collection

Myoglobin is analyzed in either serum or urine. Nonlipemic, nonhemolyzed serum is preferred. Urine samples should be collected without preservative. If either serum or urine cannot be analyzed within 24 hours, serum specimens should be frozen, and urine specimens should be refrigerated at 2–8°C.

Method of Analysis

Although many methods are available to analyze serum or urine myoglobin, most are lacking in sensitivity, difficult to control qualitatively, or unavailable in acute laboratories. The most commonly used are the latex agglutination or radioimmunoassay methods. Latex agglutination is easy to perform because latex beads coated with antibody to myoglobin readily agglutinate in the presence of myoglobin. A visual reading of the extent of agglutination provides qualitative evidence of the presence of myoglobin.[6]

The radioimmunoassay method is more sensitive and detects concentrations as low as 15 ng/ml.[6] It can also be performed with shortened incubation times as a stat procedure, with results available in 1 hour.

Reference Range

Normally, very low levels of myoglobin are found in serum: 20–60 ng/ml in females and 20–70 ng/ml in males. Myoglobin concentrations increase with age, so children have lower myoglobin concentrations than adults do. Myoglobin also varies with race, with black men having higher levels than caucasians do.

Sources of Inaccuracy

Myoglobin concentrations exhibit circadian variation, with the highest levels occurring in the morning and the lowest occurring between 6 and 11 P.M.[89]

Physiologic Role

Myoglobin must be differentiated from hemoglobin in the urine, because both cause positive tests for protein and occult blood. The two substances can be differentiated by electrophoresis, ultrafiltration, gel filtration, absorption spectra, or solubility. In addition, red cells will be absent on microscopic examination of the urine when myoglobinemia is present.

Increases in serum myoglobin occur after myocardial infarction, shock, crush injuries, vigorous exercise, or other skeletal muscle trauma. Myoglobin concentrations can be used as early indicators of myocardial infarction and of reinfarction, because they decrease more rapidly than creatine kinase does.[6] Evaluation of muscle damage in muscular dystrophy or myopathies and after malignant hyperthermia or administration of succinylcholine is facilitated by myoglobin assay. The released myoglobin is excreted in the urine, causing it to become cola- or coffee-colored. Copious amounts of myoglobin in the urine may occlude renal tubules, impairing renal function.

PSEUDOCHOLINESTERASE AND DIBUCAINE NUMBER

The enzyme pseudocholinesterase (PCE) is interesting to anesthesiologists because it biotransforms succinylcholine. About 1 in 1500–2500 patients has an atypical variant of pseudocholinesterase that is incapable of metabolizing succinylcholine, although it retains the ability to metabolize other substrates. Thus, PCE's ability to inactivate succinylcholine is not predictable with methods commonly used to assay its activity but may be determined by assaying the enzyme with and without dibucaine and comparing the respective activities. Because of its lack of substrate specificity, PCE has been given a variety of names, including cholinesterase, nonspecific cholinesterase, and butyrylcholinesterase.[90]

SPECIMEN COLLECTION

PCE activity may be assayed in either serum or plasma. Conventionally, it is determined in serum removed from a red-topped tube after clot retraction has occurred. Heparin is a suitable anticoagulant if the activity of the enzyme is desired in plasma, although the differences in PCE activity between serum and plasma are usually not clinically significant. Five milliliters of blood is plenty of serum for assay. Many methods use less than 100 μl of sample, but the excess becomes important if the assay needs to be repeated. The enzyme is extremely stable in serum and may be stored in a refrigerator for weeks with little change in activity. Samples used for quality control may be frozen and stored for months to years, although repeated freezing and thawing will decrease the activity.

METHOD OF ANALYSIS

PCE is an enzyme capable of biotransforming a host of substrates. For this reason, many methods using many different substrates has been developed. Substrates that are frequently used to assay the enzyme include benzoylcholine, butyrylthiocholine, and propionylthiocholine. Benzoylcholine requires the use of a recording ultraviolet spectrophotometer, and it is more cumbersome than the latter two, which are colorimetric methods that can be performed easily by automated analyzers.

By assaying PCE in the absence and presence of a given concentration of dibucaine, the ability of the enzyme to metabolize succinylcholine may be predicted (Table 28–2). The extent of the inhibition of PCE activity by dibucaine is reported as the dibucaine number (DN), as shown in the following formula:

$$\text{Dibucaine number} = \left\{1 - \left(\frac{\text{Activity with dibucaine}}{\text{Activity without dibucaine}}\right)\right\} \times 100$$

Classically, benzoylcholine was used as the substrate in this determination. A dibucaine concentration of 1×10^{-5} M inhibited the normal enzyme by about 80%, whereas the abnormal enzyme, which is incapable of biotransforming succinylcholine, was inhibited by only about 25%.[91] A 10-fold greater concentration of dibucaine produces the same differential inhibition of normal versus atypical PCE if butyrylcholinesterase is used as the substrate. The advantage of the latter method is that it has been modified for use on

TABLE 28–2. DIBUCAINE NUMBERS

Patient	PCHE Activity (Reference Range: 7–17 IU)	Plasma Cholinesterase + Dibucaine	Dibucaine Number	Duration of Succinylcholine
A	10	2	80	5 minutes
B	4	1	75	15 minutes
C	4	3	25	3 hours

an automated analyzer, yielding results within 30 minutes of sample collection.[92]

REFERENCE RANGE

The lack of substrate specificity of PCE has resulted in the development of many assays for the enzyme, each of which has its own reference range. Thus, a given activity must be compared to the reference range for the specific method used to determine that activity.

In contrast, the reference ranges for DNs are independent of the method of assay. For DNs, values for the normal, heterozygous, and atypical variants are 75 or greater, 40–70, and 30 or less, respectively.

SOURCES OF INACCURACY

At very low activities of PCE, DNs may be unreliable if the activity determined in the presence of dibucaine is less than the lower linear limit of the assay. In this case, the apparent extent of inhibition of activity of genetically normal enzyme by dibucaine may be less than the actual inhibition, leading to the incorrect interpretation that the enzyme is other than genetically normal. This is usually of academic rather than clinical interest, because the duration of action of succinylcholine is frequently prolonged regardless of its phenotype if the enzyme activity is extremely low.

PHYSIOLOGIC ROLE

PCE is important in the elimination of succinylcholine. The ability of genetically normal PCE to metabolize succinylcholine is so great that the duration of action of the drug is usually not significantly prolonged in patients with activities far below the lower end of the reference range, as long as the enzyme is genetically normal. In contrast, the activity of genetically atypical enzyme may fall within the reference range of the assay and yet be completely incapable of metabolizing succinylcholine. Thus, enzyme activity alone can not be used to predict the duration of action of succinylcholine unless the drug itself is used as the substrate in the assay. Although this method has been used as a research tool, it is too cumbersome for use in the clinical laboratory.

The DN can be used to predict the duration of action of succinylcholine, whereas reference to PCE activity alone may be misleading, as shown in Table 28–3. Patients A and B have genetically normal enzyme, whereas patient C has the dibucaine-resistant variant. Patient B has decreased PCE activity.

Atypical enzymes other than the dibucaine-resistant variant have been identified using other inhibitors of the enzyme, such as fluoride, chloride, formaldehyde, and urea. Of these, the most well evaluated compound is fluoride. The fluoride-resistant variant has an incidence of about 1 in 155,000.[93] The incidence of the other variants is less well documented.

TABLE 28–3. URINALYSIS

Test	Reference Range of Normal Urine Findings
pH	4.6–8.0
Specific gravity	1.015–1.025
Glucose	Negative on dipstick (<0.5 gm/24 hours)
Sodium	130–260 mEq/24 hours
Potassium	25–100 mEq/24 hours
Protein	Negative on dipstick (40–150 mg/24 hours)
Osmolality	38–1400 mOsm/kg
Urine sediment	3–5 WBC/HPF
	Occasional RBC
	Occasional mucus
	Occasional bacteria

The role of PCE, other than its ability to metabolize succinylcholine and other ester-containing drugs such as tetracaine and 2-chloroprocaine, is still in question. It may be involved in the metabolism of certain steroids and fatty acids.

RENAL FUNCTION

Tests of renal function, including BUN, creatinine, and urinalysis, are performed preoperatively as well as perioperatively. Preoperative assessments of renal function permit alterations in intraoperative management to enhance perfusion and glomerular filtration. In the postoperative period, determinations of quality and quantity of urine are diagnostic in the differentiation of prerenal, renal, or postrenal azotemia.

BLOOD UREA NITROGEN

Urea is the major end-product of nitrogen metabolism, so production depends on dietary intake. In the kidney, urea is excreted and partially reabsorbed. During dehydration, more urea is reabsorbed, resulting in increased BUN.

Specimen Collection

The urease/glutamate dehydrogenase assay described below requires serum or heparinized plasma. Because fluoride will inhibit urease, fluoride-preserved serum cannot be used. Serum and urine samples should be kept at 4–8°C to avoid bacterial degradation of urea.

Method of Analysis

The most commonly used method of BUN measurement is a coupled enzymatic spectrophotometric assay. In the assay, urease catalyzes the formation of ammonia from urea. The amount of ammonia formed is detected in a nicotinamide-adenine dinucleotide/reduced form of nicotinamide-adenine dinucleotide (NAD/NADH) indicator reaction involving glutamate dehydrogenase that is monitored at 340 nm.

Reference Range

Serum concentrations vary with diet, age, and analytic method. Reference ranges for adults using the urease/glutamate dehydrogenase method are 50–170 mg/L or 1.8–6.1 mmol/L. Higher values are found in males and in the elderly.

Sources of Inaccuracy

Both endogenous enzymes and exogenous ammonia may affect results. If the sample is diluted prior to assay, no significant interference from bilirubin, lipemia, hemoglobin, or other nitrogenous substances occurs.[6]

Physiologic Role

Urea is the endpoint of protein catabolism in the liver. Because BUN varies with dietary intake, state of hydration, renal function, and hepatic function, the metabolic situation must always be considered in evaluating BUN. However, because BUN is filtered at the glomerulus and passively reabsorbed in the proximal tubules, it does provide a semiquantitative assessment of renal function.

CREATININE

Creatinine is more reliable than BUN as a measure of glomerular filtration rate. If creatinine production is constant, plasma creatinine is inversely related to the glomerular filtration rate.

Specimen Collection

Creatinine is measured in plasma, serum, or urine. Except for the ammonium salt of heparin, the anticoagulants heparin and fluoride do not interfere in enzymatic methods.[6] With the Jaffé reaction, specimens are stable for 7 days at refrigerated temperatures, but enzymatic methods require immediate separation of serum from erythrocytes.

Method of Analysis

Creatinine is determined using the Jaffé reaction, in which creatinine reacts with sodium picrate to form a red Janovsky complex whose absorbance is measured spectrophotometrically at 510–520 nm. Enzymatic methods that hydrolyze creatinine to creatine before its spectrophometric measurement with creatine kinase are used in automated analyses.

Reference Range

Serum creatinine depends on rate of production and rate of excretion. The reference range is 0.6–1.3 mg/dl. Muscular individuals may have concentrations as high as 1.6 mg/dl.

Sources of Inaccuracy

Fuller's earth is used to adsorb the creatinine and isolate it from potential interferents. Substances known to interfere in the Jaffé reaction include uric acid, protein, pyruvate, acetoacetate, glucose, aminohippurate, ascorbic acid, and cephalosporin antibiotics.[6]

Physiologic Role

Because creatinine in blood is derived from muscle creatine, the principle source of creatinine is muscle metabolism. Normally, there is fairly constant turnover of 1–2% of muscle creatine, depending on the individual's age, gender, and size. Renal excretion by filtration removes creatinine from the serum, making serum creatine a good indicator of glomerular filtration.

Because the reference range is large, owing to considerable individual variation, glomerular filtration can be severely impaired before creatinine concentrations exceed the reference range. Plasma creatinine may not increase significantly for hours to days after complete cessation of glomerular filtration, because the level rarely increases more than 1.5 mg/dl/day. The clearance of creatinine, a better indicator of glomerular filtration than either BUN or creatinine, can be measured using either 2- or 24-hour samples of urine with the following equation:

Creatinine clearance (ml/minute) =
urine creatinine × urine volume/plasma creatinine

Creatinine clearance is corrected by surface area by multiplying by 1.73/body surface area. Reference ranges are 90–120 ml/minute when corrected for surface area.

URINE

Sample Collection

Urine output is determined perioperatively by collection of urine in a graduated vessel connected to an indwelling urethral catheter. Most patients requiring continuous evaluation of urinary output will require indwelling catheters despite the risk of urinary tract infection. Voided specimens are used for preoperative evaluation of renal function. Fresh specimens can be examined at any time for glucose and specific gravity and microscopically for casts, erythrocytes, leukocytes, and microorganisms.

Obstruction of the lower urinary tract or external urinary drainage system should always be corrected prior to assuming that decreased urine output is from renal causes. Likewise, extracellular fluid volume and hemodynamic function must be adequate before prerenal causes are excluded.

Methods of Analysis

Various tests are performed on urine. Specific gravity is measured, even though it only roughly correlates with urine osmolarity. A calibrated hydrometer specific for urine specific gravity determinations is used. The hydrometer is allowed to float freely in the specimen, and the scale on the stem is read at the lowest line of the meniscus. Correction factors should be applied to the hydrometer number for temperature, glucose, and protein as follows:

Add or subtract 0.001 to the reading for each 3°C that the temperature is above or below the calibration temperature of the hydrometer.
Subtract 0.003 for each 1 gm/dl of protein present.
Subtract 0.004 for each 1 g/dl of glucose.[1]

Glucose is determined as indicated previously. Urine protein is determined by the benzethonium chloride turbidimetric method.

Microscopic analysis of the urine is usually performed in a qualitative, rather than quantitative, fashion. A drop of centrifuged urine sediment suspended in a known volume of urine is examined under a microscope, and the number of the various elements per high power field (HPF) is reported. Supravital staining of the sediment further facilitates identification of specific elements. Casts are cylindrical bodies formed in the distal and collecting tubules from erythrocytes (red cell casts), epithelial cells, or cells and cellular debris with protein (hyaline casts). These casts indicate the presence of glomerular or tubular disease.

Because the rate of urinary sodium excretion depends on intake, the fractional excretion of sodium is a more useful indicator of renal function. Fractional excretion of sodium is calculated by dividing the urinary/plasma sodium concentration ratio by the urinary/plasma creatinine concentration ratio. Values below 1% indicate prerenal dysfunction, whereas values over 2–3% indicate compromised tubular function.

Reference Range

The reference ranges for urine protein, sugar, electrolytes, specific gravity, pH, and other substances are given in Table 28–4. Microscopic examination of the urine should reveal few erythrocytes or leukocytes and no casts in healthy humans. Pus cells indicate urinary tract infection. Erythrocytes and red cell casts indicate glomerulonephritis. Epithelial casts or hyaline casts are present in patients with nephrotic syndrome or chronic renal insufficiency.

Sources of Inaccuracy

Measurement of specific gravity using a urinometer will be erroneous if the urinometer is not allowed to float freely in the urine specimen or if correction factors for temperature are not applied. Gross proteinuria or glucosuria also affect specific gravity determinations, as indicated previously.

Physiologic Changes

Glomerular filtration and tubular reabsorption rates determine urine output. In the perioperative period, urine output should be 0.5–1 ml/kg/hour. Complete bladder emptying must be assured by insertion of an indwelling catheter together with suprapubic compression, positional changes, and flushing of the catheter with saline or air to avoid intraluminal obstruction.

Proteinuria occurs because of increased glomerular permeability, defective tubular reabsorption, abnormal secretion of protein into the urinary tract, and abnormal proteins causing protein overload because of increased plasma proteins. Benign types of proteinuria include those caused by exercise, pyrexia, or posture. Proteinuria due to defective glomerular permeability indicates the presence of serious conditions such as primary renal disease, diabetes, or immune complex disorders.

Acute renal failure is defined as a rapid progressive decrease of renal function associated with azotemia and oliguria. Oliguria lasts about 7–10 days, with ranges from a few hours to several weeks. Even after urine volume begins to increase, BUN may continue to increase.

However, in certain phases of renal failure in some patients, urine output is increased. Polyuric renal failure is present when urine output exceeds 2.5 L/day; nonoliguric renal failure is present when the output is 0.4–2.5 L/day. Urine volume increases after administration of mannitol in prerenal azotemia but not in acute tubular necrosis or renal failure. The differentiation of etiology of renal failure is facilitated by results of plasma and urine tests.

TABLE 28–4. RENAL FAILURE: PLASMA AND URINE TESTS

Test	Acute Renal Failure	Acute Tubular Necrosis	Prerenal Azotemia
Blood urea nitrogen (mg/dl)	>20 mg%	>20 mg%	>20 mg%
Serum creatinine (mg/dl)	>1.5 mg%	>1.5 mg%	>1.5 mg%
Urine/plasma creatinine	<20:1	<10:1	>40:1
Urine osmolality (mOsm)	<350	<350	>500
Urine/plasma osmolality	<1.1:1	<1.2:1	>1.5:1
Urine specific gravity	1.010	1.010–1.015	>1.015
Urine sodium (mEq/L)	>40	>25	<10–20
Fractional excretion of sodium	>1	>1	<1
Urine sediment	Granular and tubular casts, tubular cells	Tubular cell casts	Hyaline casts or normal sediment

PRESENTATION OF RESULTS

REFERENCE VALUES VERSUS "NORMAL" VALUES

To interpret laboratory values, we frequently compare an observed value with published values that may loosely be called "normal". If the value in question falls between the upper and lower values, we assume that the result is "within normal limits" without, perhaps, considering what normal means. In the strict sense of the word, "normal" assumes that the results are those of a healthy population, and that the distribution of values is gaussian, with the normal range falling within two standard deviations of the mean. In most cases, the normal distribution for a specific assay is rarely this ideal.[94]

Instead, clinical laboratories report results as reference ranges or values. The concept of reference values, recommended by the International Federation of Clinical Chemistry, circumvents the difficulties caused by the use of the term normal.[1] Reference values are reported for specific populations with selection criteria based on such things as age, gender, race, physical condition, and socioeconomic factors. Some values may also be influenced by a variety of factors, including the time of day that the sample is collected and body posture at the time of collection.

The observed value for a specific patient must be interpreted with respect to the reference range appropriate for that patient. The result is "usual" if it falls within the reference range, or "low" or "high" if it is outside the range. For detailed discussions of reference values, the interested reader should consult a standard textbook of clinical chemistry.

UNITS OF MEASURE

The majority of the world has adopted the use of Système International (SI) units for reporting laboratory data. These units are intended to improve communication between the clinician and the clinical chemist and to clarify the interpretation of laboratory data. Attempts to convert to the SI in the United States and some European countries has met with great reluctance. It has been encouraged by the American National Metric Council, the American Medical Association, and the American Board of Pathology, among other organizations, but has been opposed by the American College of Clinical Pathologists and the College of American Pathologists.[95–97] Although the system seems cumbersome, many feel it will make the integration of laboratory values with patient care more scientific. Table 28–5 compares conventional units with SI units for some analytes.

Concentrations of analytes and drugs reported in SI units are expressed as moles of compound rather than as units of mass. Although the change from milligram to millimole for univalent ions presents no problem (because the numeric values are identical), values for other compounds such as glucose, which is reported as 5.5 mmol/L rather than as 100 mg/dl, may lead to confusion.

There is a scientific reason for making the transition. Substances interact physiologically according to the relative numbers of molecules rather than the masses of the individual molecules. Conventionally, Ca^{2+} is reported in milligrams per deciliter rather than in moles or millimoles per liter. The latter value, when added to the molar concentrations of other cations, provides a more precise quantification of the ionic balance of plasma. By reporting all measured cations and anions in these units, one may be able to accurately quantitate such things as the concentrations of the normally unmeasured compounds responsible for the anion gap.[98]

There are equally convincing arguments against the conversion. Many feel that the system leads to confusion that could contribute to errors in patient care. Some of the hospitals that spearheaded the conversion to SI later found that they could no longer exchange data with outside laboratories.[97] Although some journals now use only SI units, few American physicians use these units when caring for patients. Thus, these physicians are forced to read in one system and practice in another. For these and other reasons, *The New England Journal of Medicine* chose to revert to conventional units and to report SI units parenthetically for its European readers.[99] Other grounds for resistance range from economic (the cost of developing and printing new forms may be prohibitive for smaller hospitals)[97] to the feelings of some that the SI is un-American.[100] Thus, adoption of SI in the United States remains controversial.

TABLE 28–5. CONVENTIONAL AND SYSTÈME INTERNATIONAL UNITS

	Conventional		Conversion Factors		Système International	
Analyte	*Reference Ranges*	*Units*	*Conventional to SI*	*SI to Conventional*	*Reference Ranges*	*Units*
Calcium, ionized	4.2–5.2	mg/dl	0.25	4	1.05–1.30	mmol/L
Chloride	100–109	mEq/dl	1	1	100–109	mmol/L
Glucose	70–110	mg/dl	0.055	18	3.8–6.1	mmol/L
Magnesium	1.8–3.0	mg/dl	0.41	2.43	0.8–1.2	mmol/L
Potassium	3.5–5.0	mEq/L	1	1	3.5–5.0	mmol/L
Sodium	135–147	mEq/L	1	1	135–147	mmol/L
Urea nitrogen	12–20	mg/dl	0.356	2.81	3.0–6.5	mmol/L
Osmolality	280–300	mOsm/kg	1	1	280–300	mmol/L

Data from Lundberg GD, et al: Now read this: The SI units are here. JAMA 1986; 255:2329–2339.

THE FUTURE

Rapid analysis of biochemical substances in the perioperative period has become a reality. On the horizon are implantable electrodes capable of continually analyzing pH, oxygen, carbon dioxide, sodium, potassium, calcium, glucose, hormones, enzymes, and even drugs.[102] Although miniaturized sensors for a variety of analytes have been developed over the past two decades, none has yet become important clinically. Problems still to be overcome include drift, interference, inadequate structural integrity, and slow response times. To date, incorporation of an implantable reference electrode near the sensor remains an unsolved technical challenge in the development of intravascular ISEs. Development of suitable membranes and encapsulants for long-term electrodes also poses a significant technical challenge. Miniaturization of colorimetric assays using implantable fiberoptic bundles is another technique currently under development.[102] Another major hurdle is the problem of the biocompatability of materials used in implantable sensors. Development of this technology, currently in its early stages, is essential to the future of continuous biochemical analysis in the perioperative period.[103]

Whether this technology will become commonplace is presently open to speculation. Should it happen, it will provide even more on-line data than are currently available. But will it lead to improved management of patients, or provide yet another distraction from the direct patient contact that is essential to patient monitoring?

REFERENCES

1. Tietz NW (ed): Textbook of Clinical Chemistry. Philadelphia: WB Saunders, 1986; 1–1919.
2. Berger RL, Rutenberg AM, Hechtman HB, Egdahl RH: The intensive-care laboratory. Surgery 1973; 73:159–160.
3. Sonnenwirth AC, Jarett L (eds): Gradwohl's Clinical Laboratory Methods and Diagnosis, 8th Ed. St. Louis: CV Mosby, 1980; 149–209.
4. Willatts SM, Myerson K: Electrolyte measurement by clinicians. Intensive Care Med 1987; 13:411–415.
5. Evans SE, Buckley BM: Biochemists nearer the patient? Br Med J 1983; 287:1399–1400.
6. Kaplan LA, Pesce AJ (eds): Clinical Chemistry: Theory, Analysis, and Correlation. St. Louis: CV Mosby, 1984; 51–73, 232–239, 917–921, 1032–1043, 1075–1078.
7. Pioda LAR, Simon W: Determination of potassium ion concentration in serum using a highly selective liquid-membrane electrode. Clin Chim Acta 1970; 29:289–293.
8. Ross JW: Calcium-selective electrode with liquid ion exchanger. Science 1967; 156:1378–1379.
9. Siggaard-Andersen O, Fogh-Andersen N, Thode J: Elimination of the erythrocyte effect on the liquid junction potential in potentiometric measurements on whole blood using mixed salt bridge solutions. Scand J Clin Lab Invest 1983;(Suppl): 165:43–46.
10. Worth HGJ: Plasma sodium concentration: Bearer of false prophecies? Br Med J 1983; 287:567–568.
11. Ladenson JH, Bowers GN Jr: Free calcium in serum. I. Determination with the ion-specific electrode, and factors affecting the results. Clin Chem 1973; 19:565–574.
12. Ladenson JH, Apple FS, Koch DD: Misleading hyponatremia due to hyperlipidemia: A method-dependent error. Ann Intern Med 1981; 95:707–708.
13. Mullins RE, Hutton PS, Conn RB: Effects of Fluosol-DA (artificial blood) on clinical chemistry tests and instruments. Am J Clin Pathol 1983; 80:478–483.
14. Fawcett JK, Wynn V: Effects of posture on plasma volume and some blood constituents. J Clin Pathol 1960; 13:304–310.
15. Statland BE, Bokelund H, Winkel P: Factors contributing to intra-individual variation of serum constituents: 4. Effects of posture and tourniquet application on variation of serum constituents in healthy subjects. Clin Chem 1974; 20:1513–1519.
16. Felding P, Tryding N, Hyltoft Petersen P, Horder M: Effects of posture on concentrations of blood constituents in healthy adults: Practical application of blood specimen collection procedures recommended by the Scandinavian Committee on Reference Values. Scand J Clin Lab Invest 1980; 40:615–621.
17. Romano AT, Young GW Jr: Mild forearm exercise during venipuncture, and its effect on potassium determinations. Clin Chem 1977; 23:303–304.
18. Thode J, Fogh-Andersen N, Aas F, Siggaard-Andersen O: Sampling and storage of blood for determination of ionized calcium. Scand J Clin Lab Invest 1985; 45:131–138.
19. Hill AB, Nahrwold ML, Noonan D, Northrop P: A comparison of methods of blood withdrawal and sample preparation for potassium measurements. Anesthesiology 1980; 53:60–63.
20. Leppänen E, Gräsbeck R: The effect of the order of filling tubes after venipuncture on serum potassium, total protein, and aspartate and alanine aminotransferases. Scand J Clin Lab Invest 1986; 46:189–191.
21. Sonntag O: Haemolysis as an interference factor in clinical chemistry. J Clin Chem Clin Biochem 1986; 24:127–139.
22. Ladenson JH, Tsai L-M B, Michael JM, et al: Serum versus heparinized plasma for eighteen common chemistry tests: Is serum the appropriate specimen? Am J Clin Pathol 1974; 62:545–552.
23. O'Reilly RA: Anticoagulant, antithrombotic, and thrombolytic drugs. *In* Gilman AG, Goodman LS, Rall TW, Murad F (eds): Goodman and Gilman's The Pharmacological Basis of Therapeutics, 7th Ed. New York: Macmillan, 1985; 1338–1359.
24. Heining MPD, Jordan WS: Heparinization of samples for plasma ionized calcium measurement. Crit Care Med 1988; 16:67–68.
25. Shek CC, Swaminathan R: Errors due to heparin in the estimation of plasma sodium and potassium concentrations. Intensive Care Med 1985; 11:309–311.
26. Bourke DL: Errors in intraoperative hematocrit determination. Anesthesiology 1976; 45:357–359.
27. Jackson EF: The reliability of blood tests drawn from intravenous lines. Ohio Med 1972; 68:32–35.
28. Kunkel SE, Warner MA: Human T-cell lymphotropic virus type III (HTLV-III) infection: How it can affect you, your patients, and your anesthesia practice. Anesthesiology 1987; 66:195–207.
29. Bazaral M: Preoperative testing for human immunodeficiency virus infection. Anesthesiology 1987; 67:278.
30. Berry AJ: Prevention of blood-borne infections in anesthesia personnel. Anesthesiology 1988; 68:164.
31. Arden J: Managing patients with AIDS—Update. Anesthesiology 1988; 68:164–165.
32. Napoli VM, McGowan JE: How much blood is in a needle stick? J Infect Dis 1987; 155:828.
33. Centers for Disease Control: Update: Human immunodeficiency virus infections in health-care workers exposed to blood of infected patients. MMWR 1987; 36:285–289.
34. Henderson DK, Fahey BJ, Willy M, et al: Risk for occupational transmission of human immunodeficiency virus type 1 (HIV-1) associated with clinical exposures. Ann Intern Med 1990; 113:740–746.
35. McCray E: Occupational risk of the acquired immunodeficiency syndrome among health care workers. N Engl J Med 1986; 314:1127–1132.
36. Centers for Disease Control: Recommendations for prevention of HIV transmission in health-care settings. MMWR 1987; 36(Suppl 2):3–18.
37. Hadler SC, Doto IL, Maynard JE, et al: Occupational risk of hepatitis B infection in hospital workers. Infect Control 1985; 6:24–31.
38. Department of Labor, Occupational Health and Safety Administration: Occupational exposure to bloodborne pathogens. Fed Reg 1991; 56(235):64004–64182.
39. Weissman M, Klein B: Evaluation of glucose determinations in untreated samples. Clin Chem 1958: 4:420–422.

40. Steige H, Jones JD: Evaluation of pneumatic-tube system for delivery of blood specimens. Clin Chem 1971; 17:1160–1164.
41. Gibbs EL, Lennox WG, Nims LF, Gibbs FA: Arterial and cerebral venous blood: Arterial-venous differences in man. J Biol Chem 1942; 144:325–332.
42. Larsson-Cohn U: Differences between capillary and venous blood glucose during oral glucose tolerance tests. Scand J Clin Lab Invest 1976; 36:805–808.
43. Duffy T, Phillips N, Pelligrin F: Review of glucose tolerance—A problem in methodology. Am J Med Sci 1973; 265:117–133.
44. Phillips GB, Mendershausen PB: Glucose consumption by red cells of diabetic patients and normal subjects. Effect of ethanol. Clin Chim Acta 1975; 61:175–182.
45. Stjernholm RL, Manak RC: Carbohydrate metabolism in leukocytes. XIV. Regulation of pentose cycle activity and glycogen metabolism during phagocytosis. J Reticuloendothel Soc 1970; 8:550–560.
46. Schwartz MK: Interferences in diagnostic biochemical procedures. Adv Clin Chem 1973; 16:1–45.
47. Holtkamp HC, Verhoef NJ, Leijnse B: The difference between the glucose concentrations in plasma and whole blood. Clin Chim Acta 1975; 59:41–49.
48. Clark LC Jr, Clark EW: A personalized history of the Clark oxygen electrode. *In* Tremper KK, Barker SJ (eds): Advances in Oxygen Monitoring. Int Anesthesiol Clin 1987; 25(3):1–29.
49. Kunz HJ, Stasny M: Immobilized glucose oxidase used to measure glucose in serum. Clin Chem 1974; 20:1018–1022.
50. Kadish AH, Litle RL, Sternberg JC: A new and rapid method for the determination of glucose by measurement of rate of oxygen consumption. Clin Chem 1968; 14:116–131.
51. Chua KS, Tan IK: Plasma glucose measurement with the Yellow Springs glucose analyzer. Clin Chem 1978; 24:150–152.
52. Dacus J, Schultz K, Averill A, Sibai B: Comparison of capillary Accu-Chek blood glucose values to laboratory values. Am J Perinatol 1992; 6:334–336.
53. Jelić-Ivanović Z, Majkić-Singh N, Spasić P, et al: Interference by analgesic and antirheumatic drugs in 25 common laboratory assays. J Clin Chem Clin Biochem 1985; 23:287–292.
54. Wright LA, Foster MG: Effect of some commonly prescribed drugs on certain chemistry tests. Clin Biochem 1980; 6:249–252.
55. Farrance I, Aldons J: Paracetamol interference with YSI glucose analyzer. Clin Chem 1981; 27:782–783.
56. Ronzoni E, Koechig I, Eaton EP: Ether anesthesia. III. Role of lactic acid in the acidosis of ether anesthesia. J Biol Chem 1924; 61:465–492.
57. Greene NM: Lactate, pyruvate and excess lactate production in anesthetized man. Anesthesiology 1961; 22:404–412.
58. Cohen RD, Simpson R: Lactate metabolism. Anesthesiology 1975; 43:661–673.
59. Waxman K, Nolan LS, Shoemaker WC: Sequential perioperative lactate determination: Physiological and clinical implications. Crit Care Med 1982; 10:96–99.
60. Clark LC Jr, Noyes LK, Grooms TA, Moore MS: Rapid micromeasurement of lactate in whole blood. Crit Care Med 1984; 12:461–464.
61. Fath JJ, Ascher NL, Konstantinides BS, et al: Metabolism during hepatic transplantation: Indicators of allograft function. Surgery 1984; 96:664–673.
62. Smith JC Jr, Lewis S, Holbrook J, et al: Effect of heparin and citrate on measured concentrations of various analytes in plasma. Clin Chem 1987; 33:814–816.
63. Epstein FB: Osmolality. Emerg Med Clin North Am 1986; 4:253–261.
64. Mercier DE, Feld RD, Witte DL: Comparison of dewpoint and freezing point osmometry. Am J Med Technol 1978; 44:1066–1069.
65. Gennari FJ: Serum osmolality: Uses and limitations. N Engl J Med 1984; 310:102–105.
66. Dowart WV, Chalmers L: Comparison of methods for calculating serum osmolality from chemical concentrations, and the prognostic value of such calculations. Clin Chem 1975; 21:190–194.
67. Bhagat CI, Garcia-Webb P, Fletcher E, Beilby JP: Calculated vs measured plasma osmolalities revisited. Clin Chem 1984; 30:1703–1705.
68. Morissette MP: Colloid osmotic pressure: Its measurement and clinical value. Can Med Assoc J 1977; 116:897–900.
69. Luz PL, Shubin H, Weil MH, et al: Pulmonary edema related to changes in colloid osmotic and pulmonary artery wedge pressure in patients after acute myocardial infarction. Circulation 1975; 51:350–357.
70. Duncan A, Young DS: Measurements of serum colloid osmotic pressure are of limited usefulness. Clin Chem 1982; 28:141–145.
71. Fernandez P, Cox M: Basic concepts of renal physiology. *In* Priebe H-J (ed): The Kidney in Anesthesia. Int Anesthesiol Clin 1984; 22(1):1–33.
72. Morgan DB: Why plasma electrolytes? Ann Clin Biochem 1981; 18:275–280.
73. Lum G, Gambino SR: A comparison of serum versus heparinized plasma for routine chemistry tests. Am J Clin Pathol 1974; 61:108–113.
74. Ward CF, Arkin DB, Benumof J, Saidman LJ: Arterial versus venous potassium: Clinical implications. Crit Care Med 1978; 6:335–336.
75. Hartmann RC, Auditore JV, Jackson DP: Studies on thrombocytosis. I. Hyperkalemia due to release of potassium from platelets during coagulation. J Clin Invest 1958; 37:699–707.
76. Bronson WR, Devita VT, Carbone PP, Cotlove E: Pseudohyperkalemia due to release of potassium from white blood cells during clotting. N Engl J Med 1966; 274:369–375.
77. Cox M: Potassium homeostasis. Med Clin North Am 1981; 65:363–384.
78. Stewart RB, Hale WE, Marks RG: Diuretic use in an ambulatory elderly population. Am J Hosp Pharm 1983; 40:409–413.
79. Biswas CK, Ramos JM, Kerr DNS: Heparin effect on ionised calcium concentration. Clin Chim Acta 1981; 116:343–347.
80. Boink AB, Buckley BM, Christiansen TF, et al: International Federation of Clinical Chemistry (IFCC) scientific division IFCC recommendation. Recommendation on sampling, transport and storage for the determination of the concentration of ionized calcium in whole blood. Ann Biol Clin (Paris) 1991; 49:434–438.
81. McLean FC, Hastings AB: A biological method for the estimation of calcium ion concentration. J Biol Chem 1934; 107:337–350.
82. Wandrup J, Kancir C: The concentration of free calcium ions in whole blood. Scand J Clin Lab Invest 1983; 43(Suppl 165):47–48.
83. Brauman J, Delvigne CH, DeConinck I, Willems D: Factors affecting the determination of ionized calcium in blood. Scand J Clin Lab Invest 1983; 43(Suppl 165):27–31.
84. McLean FC, Hastings AB: Clinical estimation and significance of calcium-ion concentrations in the blood. Am J Med Sci 1935; 189:601–613.
85. Siggaard-Andersen O, Thode J, Fogh-Andersen N: What is "ionized calcium"? Scand J Clin Lab Invest 1983; 43(Suppl 165):11–16.
86. Grima JM, Brand MJD: Activity and interference effects in measurement of ionized calcium with ion-selective electrodes. Clin Chem 1977; 23:2048–2054.
87. Bringhurst FR, Potts JT Jr: Calcium and phosphate turnover, and metabolic actions. *In* DeGroot LJ, Cahill GF Jr, Odell WD, et al (eds): Endocrinology, vol 2. New York: Grune & Stratton, 1979; 551–585.
88. Drop LJ: Ionized calcium, the heart, and hemodynamic function. Anesth Analg 1985; 64:43–51.
89. Bombardieri T, Clericu A, Riente L, et al: Circadian variations of serum myoglobin levels in normal subjects and patients with polymyositis. Arthritis Rheum 1982; 25:1419–1424.
90. Brown SS, Kalow W, Pilz W, et al: The plasma cholinesterases: A new perspective. *In* Latner AL, Schwartz MK (eds): Advances in Clinical Chemistry, vol 22. New York: Academic Press, 1981; 1–123.
91. Kalow W, Genest K: A method for the detection of atypical forms of human serum cholinesterase. Determination of dibucaine numbers. Can J Biochem 1957; 35:339–346.
92. Arnold WP: A rapid, semi-automated method for determining dibucaine numbers. Anesthesiology 1981; 55:676–679.
93. Whittaker M: Plasma cholinesterase variants and the anesthetist. Anaesthesia 1980; 35:174–197.
94. Jones JD: Factors that affect clinical laboratory values. J Occup Med 1980; 22:316–320.
95. Lundberg GD, Iverson C, Radulescu G: Now read this: The SI units are here. JAMA 1986; 255:2329–2339.
96. Council on scientific affairs: SI units for clinical laboratory data. JAMA 1985; 253:2553–2554.
97. Christie RW, Marallo T: Experiences with conversion to système international units. N Engl J Med 1990; 323:1075–1077.
98. Young DS: Standardized reporting of laboratory data: The desirability of using SI units. N Engl J Med 1974; 290:368–373.

99. Campion EW: A retreat from SI units. N Engl J Med 1992; 327:49.
100. Powsner ER: SI quantities and units for American medicine. JAMA 1984; 252:1737–1741.
101. Michenfelder JD: Who's afraid of Blaise Pascal? Anesthesiology 1982; 56:245–246.
102. Kazacos M, Skalsky M, Skyllas-Kazacos M: A review of developments in implantable selective chemical sensors. Life Support Syst 1985; 3:189–205.
103. Galletti PM, and members of the Consensus Development Panel: Consensus conference: Clinical applications of biomaterials. JAMA 1983; 249:1050–1054.

Index

Note: Page numbers in *italics* indicate figures; those followed by t indicate tables.